AF248863

EXPERTddx™

ULTRASOUND

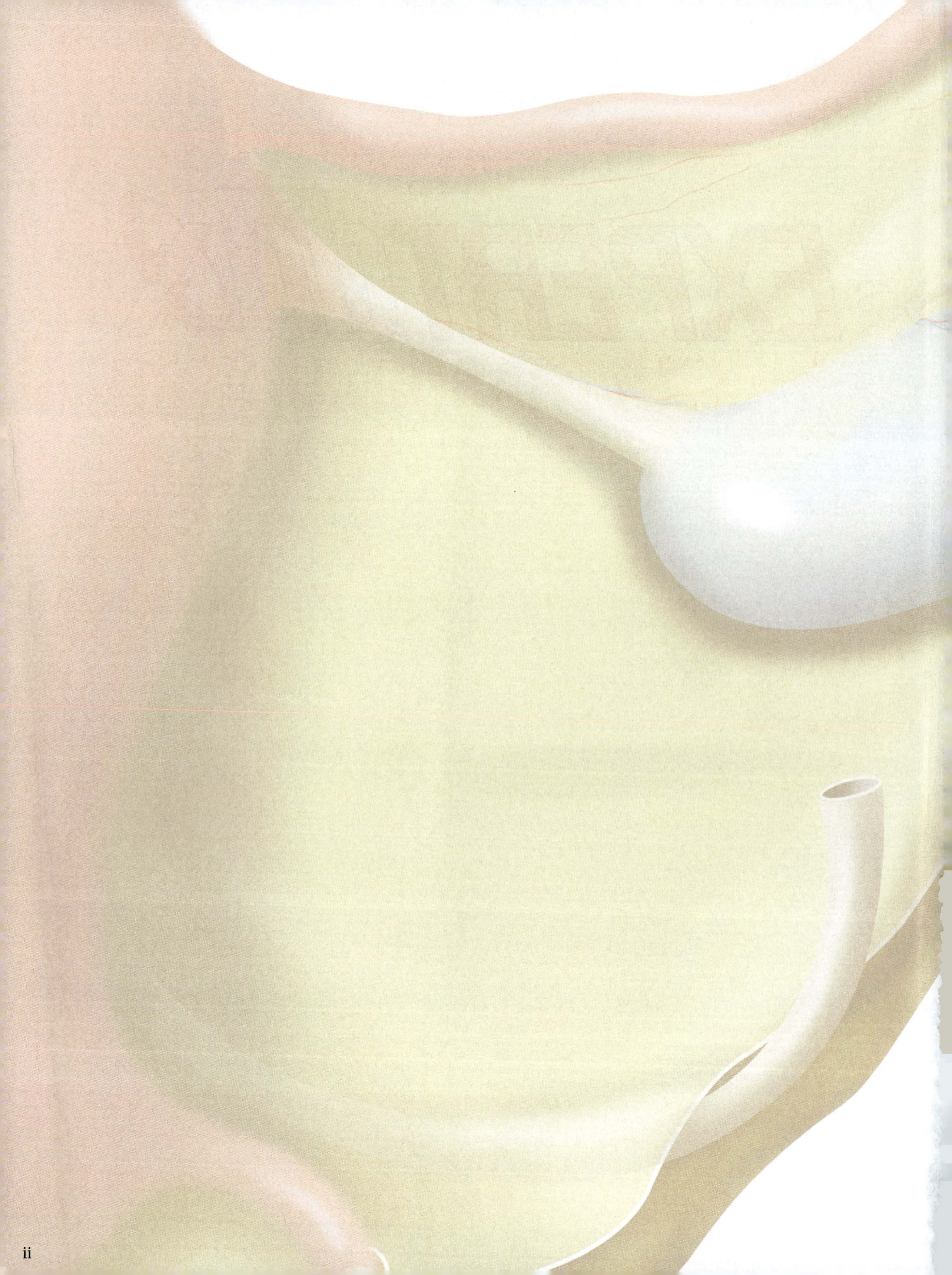

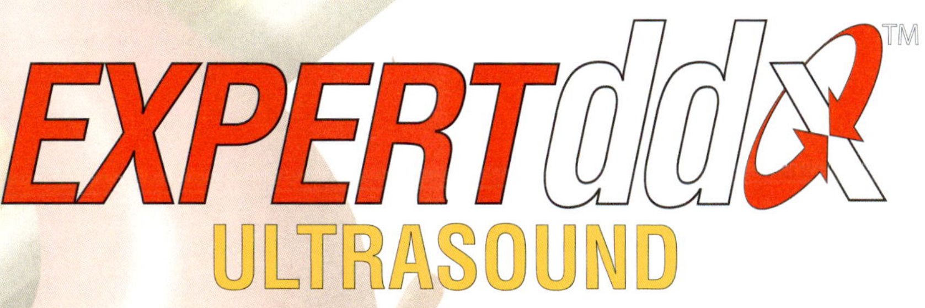

Anil T. Ahuja, MD, FRCR
Professor
Department of Diagnostic Radiology & Organ Imaging
The Chinese University of Hong Kong
Hong Kong, China

James F. Griffith, MBBCh, FRCR
Professor
Department of Diagnostic Radiology & Organ Imaging
The Chinese University of Hong Kong
Hong Kong, China

Gregory E. Antonio, MD, FRANZCR
Honorary Professor
Department of Diagnostic Radiology & Organ Imaging
The Chinese University of Hong Kong
Hong Kong, China

K.T. Wong, MBChB, FRCR
Honorary Clinical Associate Professor
Department of Diagnostic Radiology & Organ Imaging
The Chinese University of Hong Kong
Hong Kong, China

Yolanda Y.P. Lee, MBChB, FRCR
Honorary Clinical Assistant Professor
Department of Diagnostic Radiology & Organ Imaging
The Chinese University of Hong Kong
Hong Kong, China

Winnie C.W. Chu, MBChB, FRCR
Professor
Department of Diagnostic Radiology & Organ Imaging
The Chinese University of Hong Kong
Hong Kong, China

Deborah Levine, MD
Associate Radiologist-in-Chief of Academic Affairs
Co-Chief of Ultrasound
Director of Ob/Gyn Ultrasound
Beth Israel Deaconess Medical Center

Professor of Radiology
Harvard Medical School
Boston, Massachusetts

Stella S.Y. Ho, PhD, RDMS
Adjunct Associate Professor
Department of Diagnostic Radiology & Organ Imaging
The Chinese University of Hong Kong
Hong Kong, China

Bhawan K. Paunipagar, MD, DNB
Clinical Tutor
Department of Diagnostic Radiology & Organ Imaging
The Chinese University of Hong Kong
Hong Kong, China

Simon S.M. Ho, MBBS, FRCR
Honorary Assistant Professor
Department of Diagnostic Radiology & Organ Imaging
The Chinese University of Hong Kong
Hong Kong, China

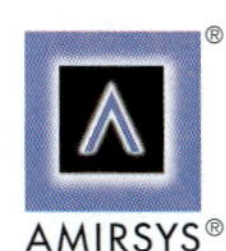

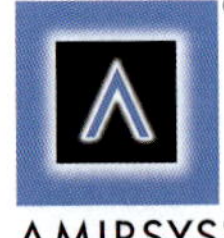

AMIRSYS®

Names you know. Content you trust.®

First Edition

Composition by Amirsys, Inc., Salt Lake City, Utah

Printed in Canada by Friesens, Altona, Manitoba, Canada

ISBN: 978-1-931884-14-3

Notice and Disclaimer

Library of Congress Cataloging-in-Publication Data

Expertddx. Ultrasound / [edited by] Anil T. Ahuja. -- 1st ed.
   p. ; cm.
   Includes index.
   ISBN 978-1-931884-14-3
   1. Diagnostic ultrasonic imaging--Atlases. 2. Diagnosis, Differential--Atlases. I. Ahuja, Anil T. II. Title: Ultrasound.
   [DNLM: 1. Ultrasonography--Handbooks. 2. Diagnosis, Differential--Handbooks. WN 39 E96 2009]
   RC78.7.U4E97 2009
   616.07'543--dc22
                    2009019984

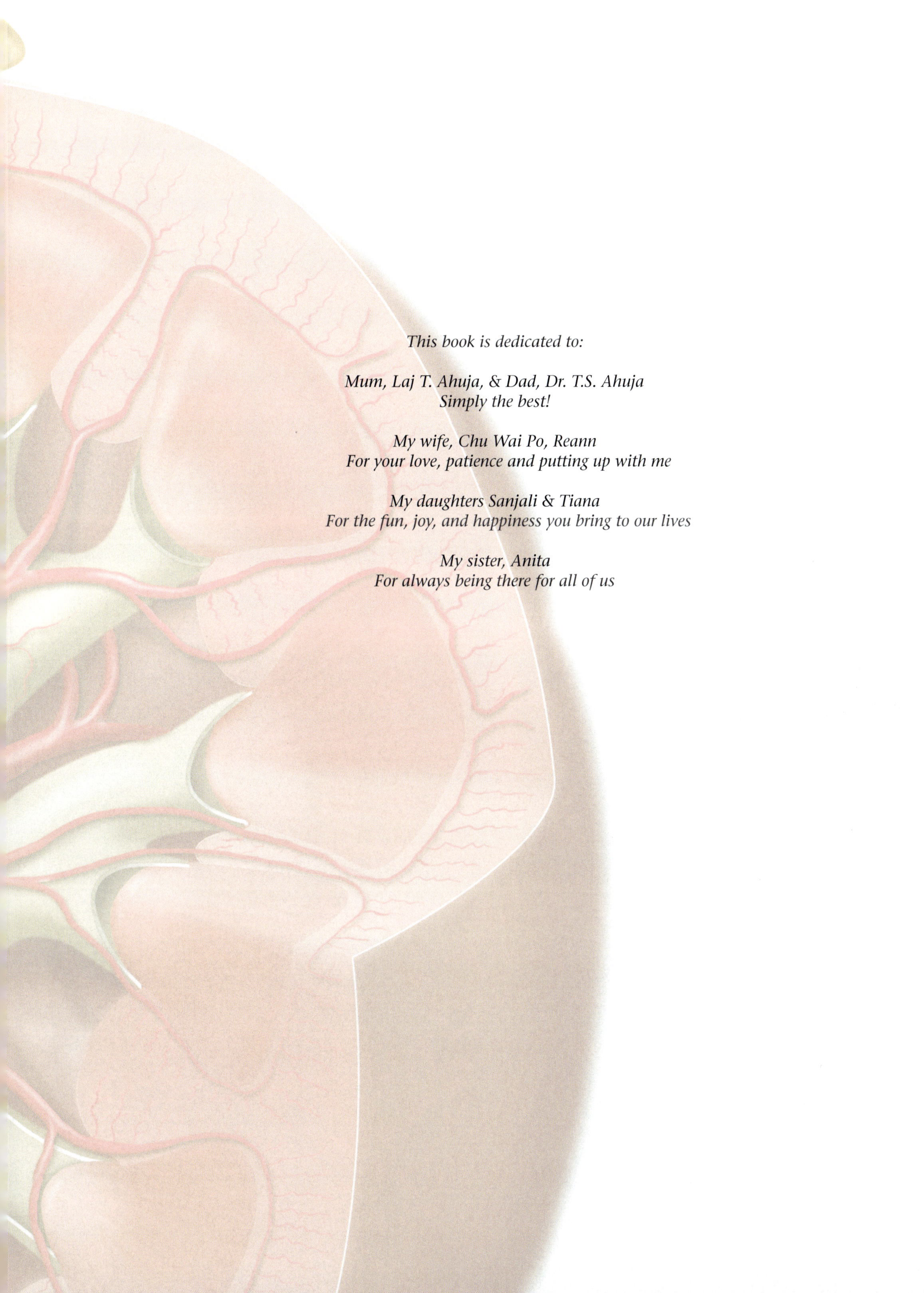

This book is dedicated to:

Mum, Laj T. Ahuja, & Dad, Dr. T.S. Ahuja
Simply the best!

My wife, Chu Wai Po, Reann
For your love, patience and putting up with me

My daughters Sanjali & Tiana
For the fun, joy, and happiness you bring to our lives

My sister, Anita
For always being there for all of us

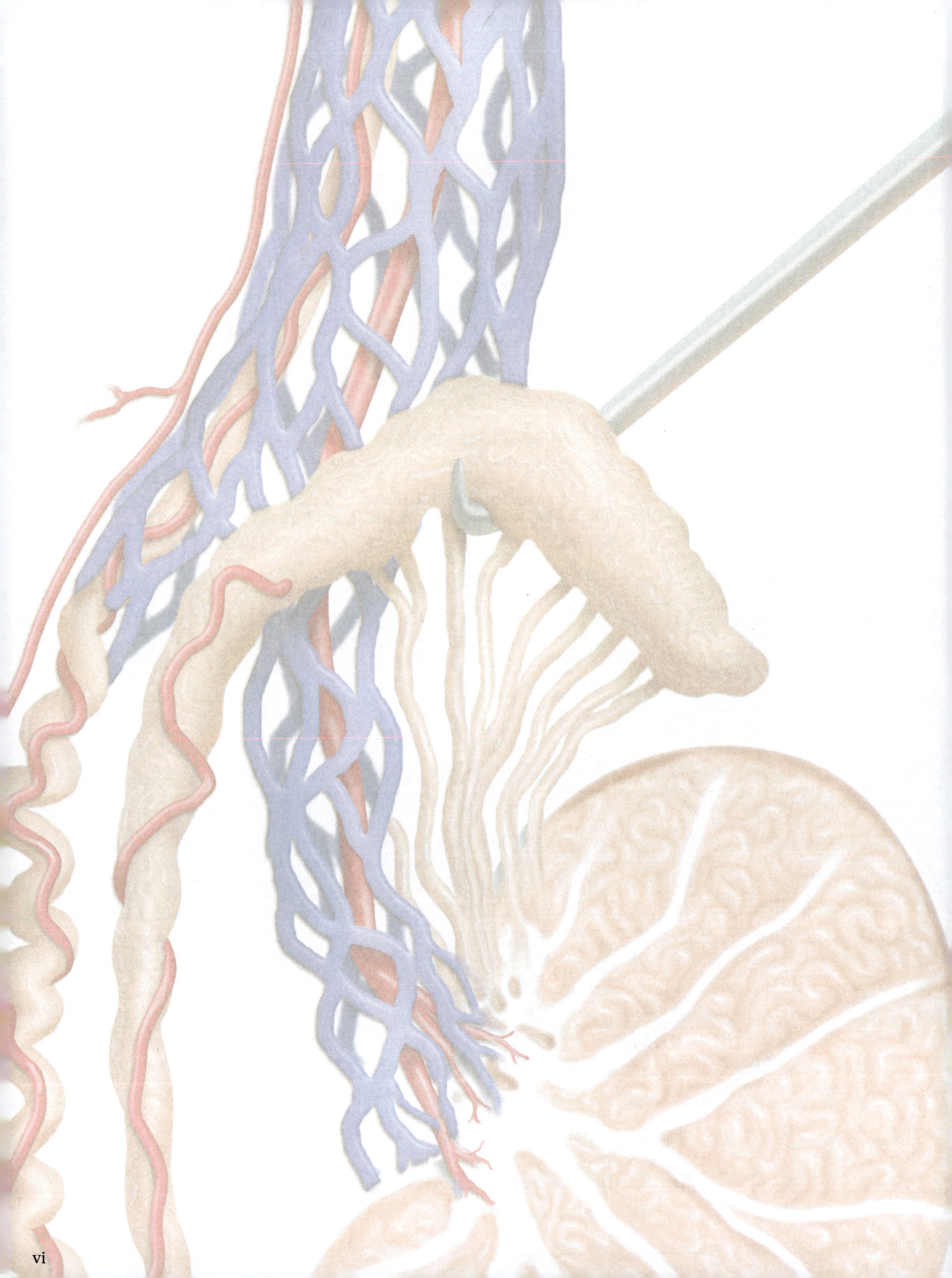

CONTRIBUTING AUTHORS

Chander Lulla, MD, DMRD
Consultant Sonologist
RIA Clinic
Mumbai, India

Vivian Y.F. Leung, PhD, RDMS
Adjunct Associate Professor
Department of Diagnostic Radiology & Organ Imaging
The Chinese University of Hong Kong
Hong Kong, China

Eric K.H. Liu, PhD, RDMS
Adjunct Assistant Professor
Department of Diagnostic Radiology & Organ Imaging
The Chinese University of Hong Kong
Hong Kong, China

Nicole Roy, MD
Associate Professor of Breast and Body Imaging
University of Utah School of Medicine
Salt Lake City, Utah

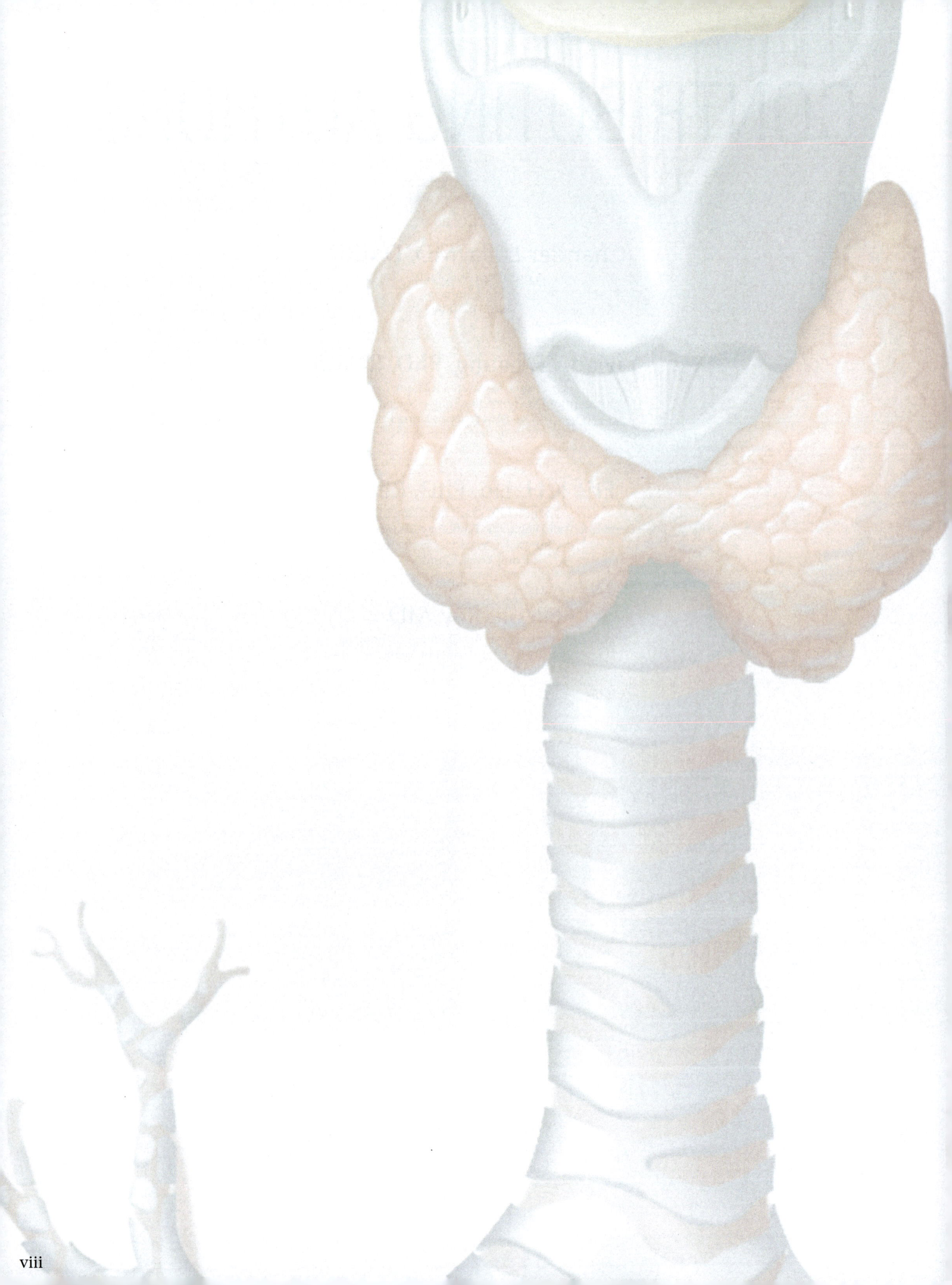

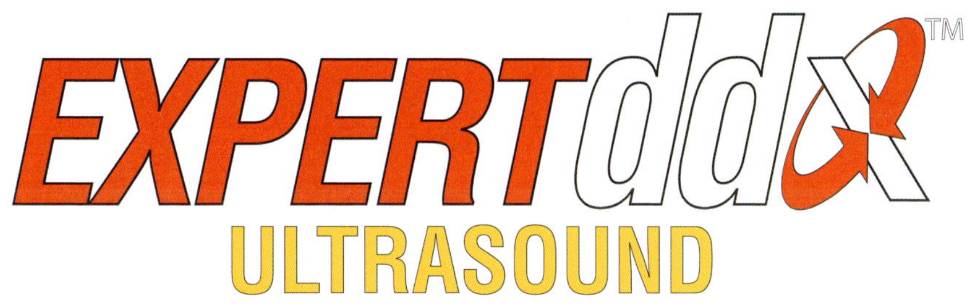

Once the appropriate technical protocols have been delineated, the best quality images obtained, and the cases queued up on PACS, the diagnostic responsibility reaches the radiology reading room. The radiologist must do more than simply "lay words on" but reach a real conclusion. If we cannot reach a definitive diagnosis, we must offer a reasonable differential diagnosis. A list that's too long is useless; a list that's too short may be misleading. To be useful, a differential must be more than a rote recitation from some dusty book or a mnemonic from a lecture way back when. Instead, we must take into account key imaging findings and relevant clinical information.

With these considerations in mind, we at Amirsys designed our Expert Differential Diagnoses series—EXPERTddx for short. Leading experts in every subspecialty of radiology identified the top differential diagnoses in their respective fields, encompassing specific anatomic locations, generic imaging findings, modality-specific findings, and clinically based indications. Our experts gathered multiple images, both typical and variant, for each EXPERTddx. Each features at least eight beautiful images that illustrate the possible diagnoses, accompanied by captions that highlight the pertinent imaging findings. Hundreds more are available in the eBook feature that accompanies every book. In classic Amirsys fashion, each EXPERTddx includes bulleted text that distills the available information to the essentials. You'll find helpful clues for diagnoses, ranked by prevalence as Common, Less Common, and Rare but Important.

Our EXPERTddx series is designed to help radiologists reach reliable—indeed, expert—conclusions. Whether you are a practicing radiologist or a resident/fellow in training, we think the EXPERTddx series will quickly become your practical "go-to" reference.

Anne G. Osborn, MD
Executive Vice President and Editor-in-Chief, Amirsys, Inc.

Paula J. Woodward, MD
Executive Vice President and Medical Director, Amirsys, Inc.

H. Ric Harnsberger, MD
CEO, Amirsys, Inc.

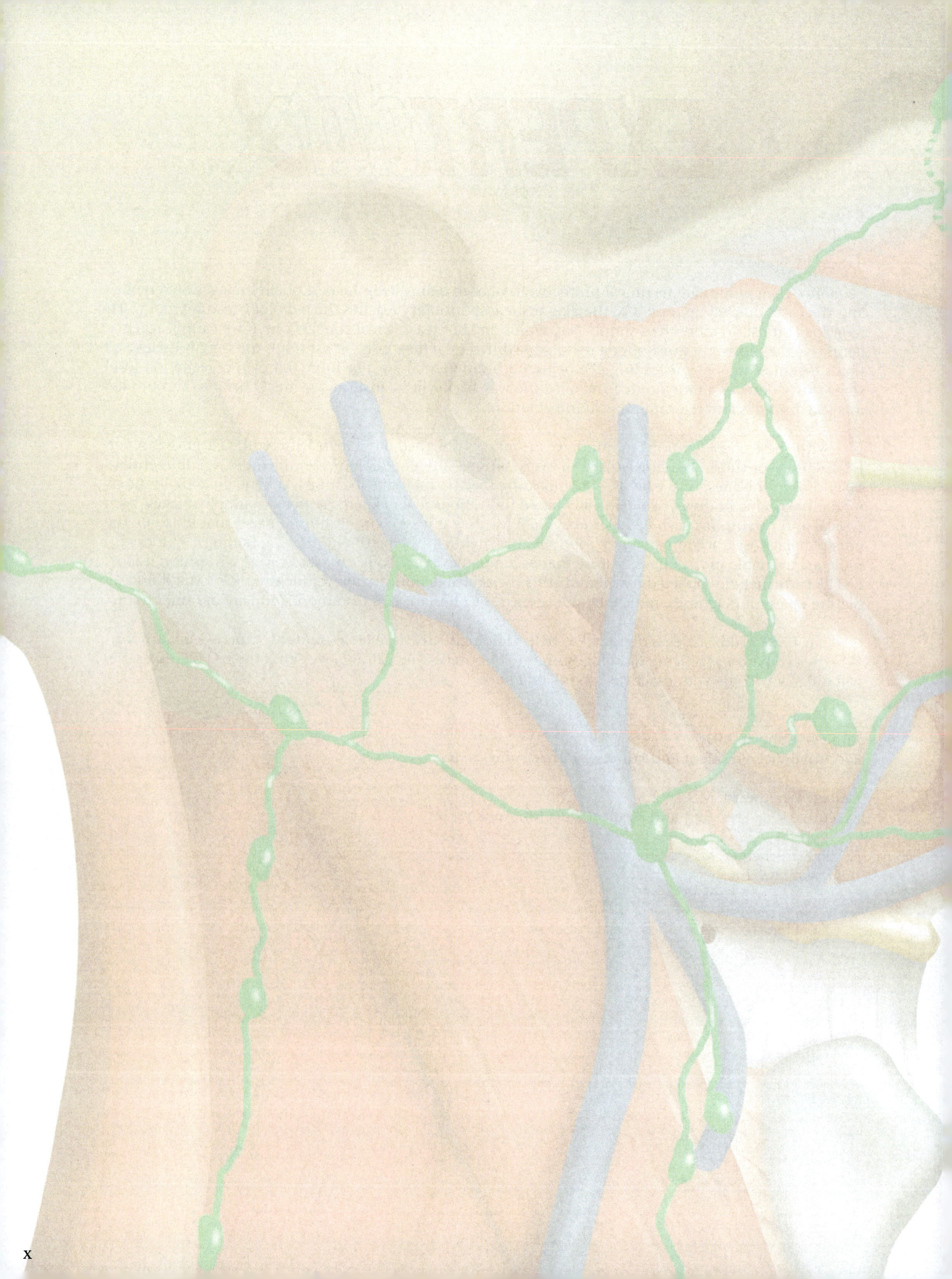

PREFACE

Despite the advances of teleradiology, in most cases ultrasound diagnosis is made on real-time examination. Because of its real-time nature, ultrasound demands a high level of skill and meticulous attention to detail.

EXPERTddx: Ultrasound is the third Amirsys book designed specifically for the practicing sonologist. Our first book, *Diagnostic Imaging: Ultrasound*, discussed the sonographic appearances of conditions commonly encountered in clinical practice. The second, *Diagnostic and Surgical Imaging Anatomy: Ultrasound*, covered key anatomy that should be familiar to any sonologist.

In *EXPERTddx: Ultrasound*, we focus on the building blocks of ultrasound diagnosis. The book looks at the discrete sonographic characteristics of a mass or lesion. Is it hypoechoic, calcified, vascular, or solid? The presence and arrangement of these discrete sonographic features enables the characterization of involved tissues, making it possible to arrive at a sonographic diagnosis/differential diagnosis. Relating this sonographic diagnosis to the clinical presentation then provides the most likely final diagnosis.

It is important to realize that a diagnosis is rarely based on one sonographic characteristic alone. Typically, any lesion shows a plethora of sonographic features, each of which provides a clue to the nature of the tissue being examined. For example, a liver mass may be hypoechoic, noncalcified, vascular, and solid all at the same time. This combination of features leads us to a differential diagnosis that includes hepatocellular carcinoma. The presence of cirrhosis, ascites, weight loss, and elevated alpha-fetoprotein narrows the possible diagnosis to hepatocellular carcinoma.

When you read *EXPERTddx: Ultrasound*, please consider each feature as a starting point in a chain of thought. Very soon you will put these features and thoughts together to rapidly arrive at a definitive diagnosis.

Although dedicated to ultrasound, this book also includes images from other modalities. This is to emphasize that ultrasound is not a standalone modality. Information gained by ultrasound can frequently complement or be supported by information obtained from other imaging modalities. Please note that this book does not discuss obstetric ultrasound, as the topic has been covered in a separate book in the same series.

I am grateful to Drs. Ric Harnsberger, Anne Osborn, and Paula Woodward for giving me the opportunity to work on this project and patiently guiding me along the process. I remain humbled by their continuing patience and faith. The production team at Amirsys has been great and contributed significantly toward the completion of this book.

Finally, a book such as this would not have been possible without the contribution of all members of the department. Once again, I have been fortunate to work with a wonderful group of colleagues interested in ultrasound. Despite their significant clinical and academic duties, they have worked hard on this project and contributed their cases, knowledge, and time. I remain forever grateful.

The journey has been hard work but also good fun. The effort has been more than compensated by the privilege of working with friends and learning from them. I hope this book will help you in your daily clinical practice.

Anil T. Ahuja, MD, FRCR
Professor
Department of Diagnostic Radiology & Organ Imaging
The Chinese University of Hong Kong

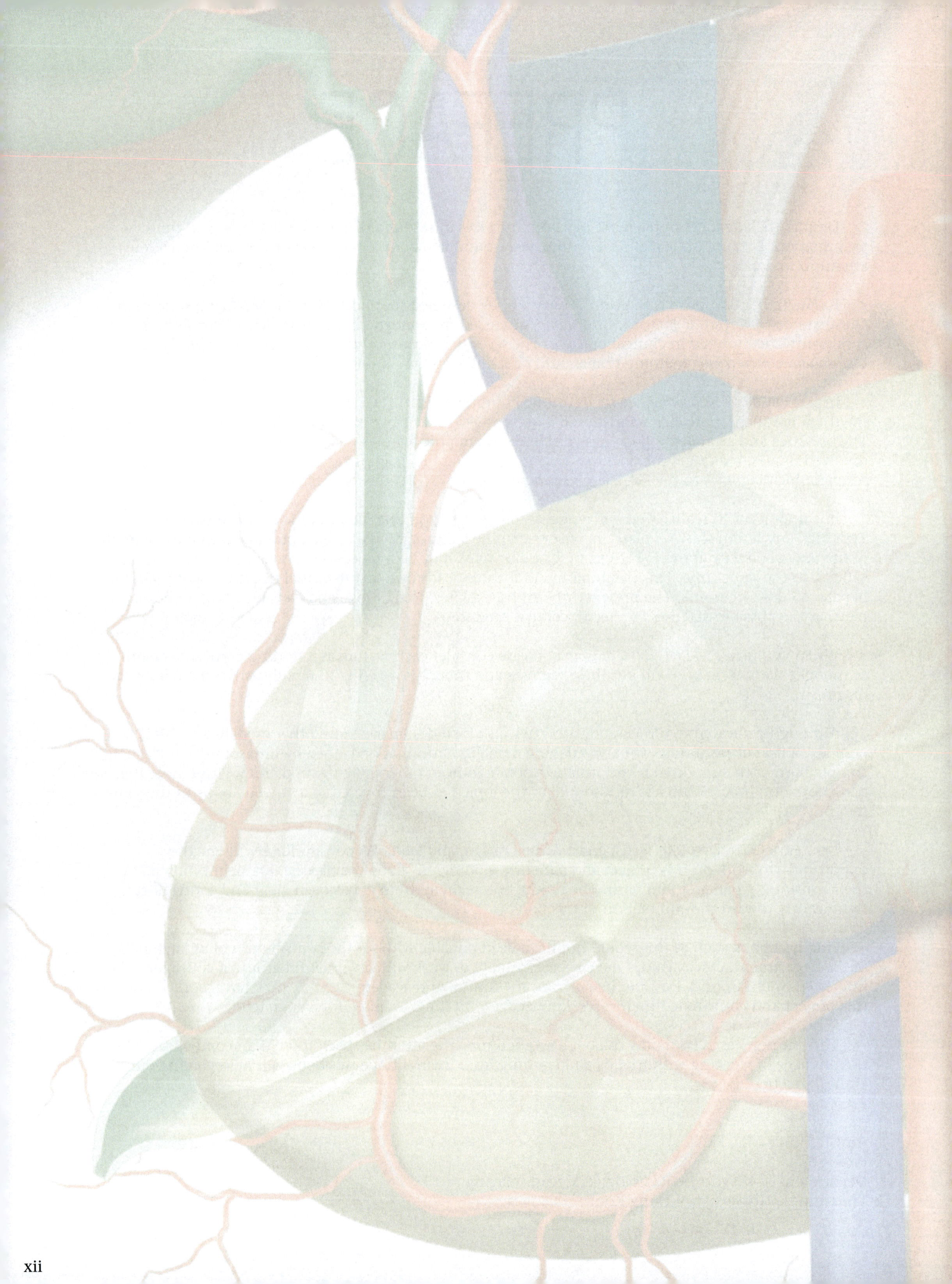

ACKNOWLEDGMENTS

Text Editing

Kellie J. Heap

Arthur G. Gelsinger, MA

Katherine Riser

Image Editing

Jeffrey J. Marmorstone

Terence Y.W. Lam

Kevin K.W. Leung

Abby Y.T. Tong

Medical Text Editing

Paula J. Woodward, MD

Marc Tubay, MD

Art Direction and Design

Lane R. Bennion, MS

Richard Coombs, MS

Contributors

Alex H.C. Chan

James S.W. Cheung

Carmen Cho, MBChB

Ann King, FRCR

William K.M. Kong

Aniruddha Kulkarni, MD

Pramod Lonikar, MBBS, DMRD

Tom W.K. Lee

Asif Momin, MD, DNB

Darshana Rasalkar, MBBS, FRCR

Sanjay Vaid

Cina Tong, MBChB

Ki Wang, FRCR

Simon C.H. Yu, FRCR

Associate Editor

Ashley R. Renlund, MA

Production Lead

Melissa A. Hoopes

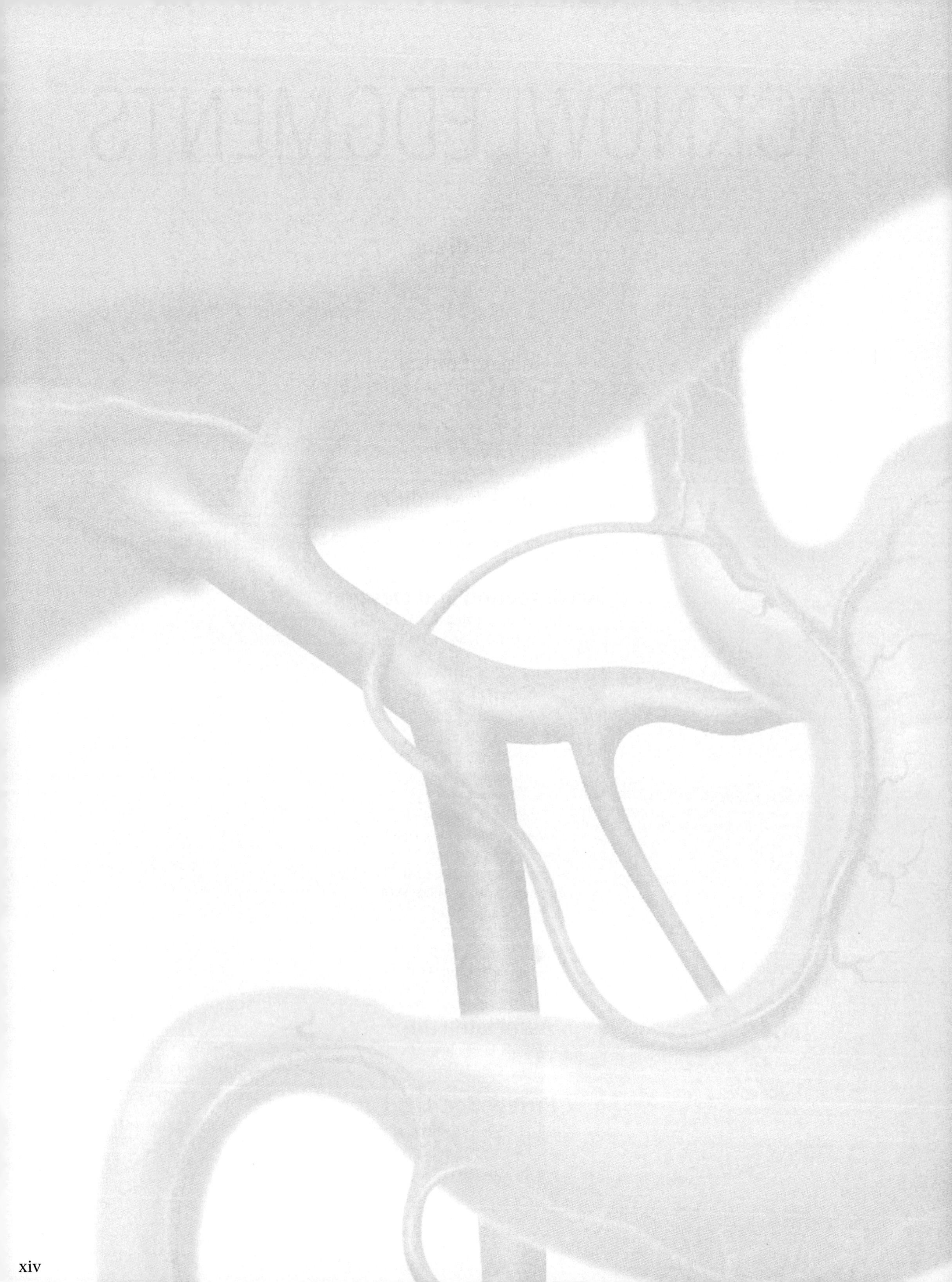

SECTIONS

Head and Neck

Thyroid/Parathyroid

Liver

Biliary System

Pancreas

Spleen

Adrenal Gland

Kidney

Abdominal Wall/Peritoneal Cavity

Bladder

Prostate

Scrotum

Female Pelvis

Vascular

Musculoskeletal

Breast

TABLE OF CONTENTS

SECTION 10
Bladder

SECTION 11
Prostate

SECTION 12
Scrotum

SECTION 13
Female Pelvis

SECTION 14
Vascular

Arteries

Veins

SECTION 15
Musculoskeletal

SECTION 16
Breast

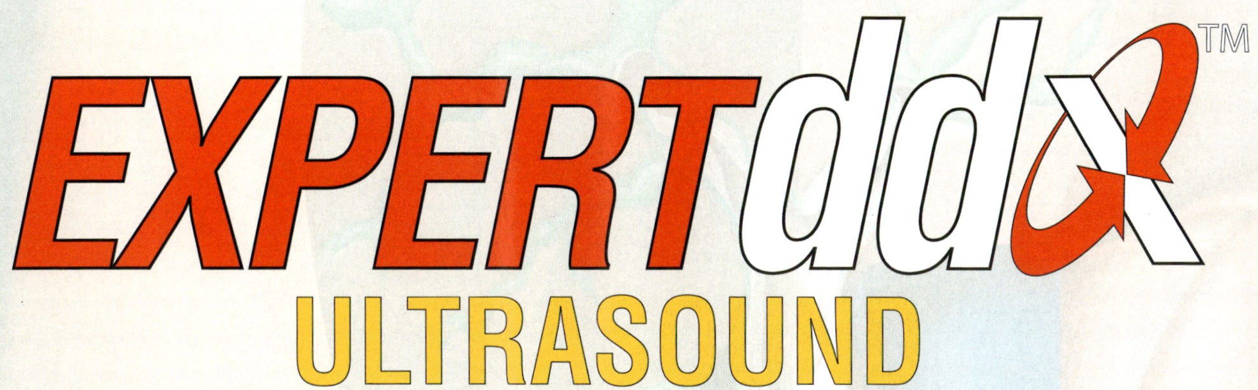

EXPERT ddx™
ULTRASOUND

SECTION 1
Head and Neck

MIDLINE NECK MASS

DIFFERENTIAL DIAGNOSIS

Common
- Lymph Nodes
- Thyroid Mass
- Pyramidal Lobe (Mimic)
- Thyroglossal Duct Cyst
- Ranula

Less Common
- Dermoid/Epidermoid
- Laryngocele
- Lateral Pharyngeal Diverticulum
- Hypopharyngeal Tumor
- Postoperative
  - Para-Stomal Recurrence
  - Colonic Interposition
  - Jejunal Pull-Up

Rare but Important
- Ectopic Thyroid

ESSENTIAL INFORMATION

Key Differential Diagnosis Issues
- During routine US of head & neck, central compartment is often overlooked
  - Establish scanning protocol that routinely includes central compartment
  - Shadowing from hyoid, laryngeal cartilage, and tracheal ring may obscure visualization of lesions in midline
    - Pay meticulous attention to detail and technique at this site to avoid mistakes
- Most abnormalities at this location are site specific and have typical US features

Helpful Clues for Common Diagnoses
- **Lymph Nodes**
  - Normal lymph nodes in central compartment generally small and obscured by tracheal ring shadowing
  - Malignant nodes in this compartment receive drainage from specific sites and give clue to origin of primary tumor (thyroid, larynx)
    - Large, round, hyper- to hypoechoic, loss of normal echogenic hilum, peripheral vascularity
  - Hypertrophied nodes in post-radiation patients (particularly with nasopharyngeal carcinoma) or those with autoimmune thyroid disease
    - Lymph nodes are benign looking with normal hilar architecture and vascularity
- **Thyroid Mass**
  - Thyroid is major organ in central neck
  - Midline thyroid nodules are common
- **Pyramidal Lobe (Mimic)**
  - 10-30% of patients have "3rd" lobe: Pyramidal lobe
    - Should be recognized as anatomic variant
  - Isolated island of tissue with fine bright echopattern of thyroid gland, superior to thyroid lobes/isthmus
  - Secondary to ascent from isthmus or adjacent part of either lobe (more often left lobe)
- **Thyroglossal Duct Cyst**
  - Occur anywhere along thyroglossal duct: Infrahyoid (75%) > hyoid (20%) > suprahyoid (15%)
    - Suprahyoid thyroglossal duct cyst (TDC) at base of tongue or posterior floor of mouth
    - At hyoid level: Anterior/ventral to hyoid
    - Infrahyoid: Embedded in strap muscles; often paramedian
  - Noninfected, nonhemorrhagic: Anechoic, thin walls, posterior enhancement, "pseudosolid" or with fluid-fluid level
  - Infected, hemorrhagic: Thick irregular walls, debris, vascularity in walls and septa
  - Thick wall or soft tissue may represent functioning thyroid tissue, infection, or malignant change (thyroid carcinoma in 1-4%)
    - Guided fine-needle aspiration and cytology (FNAC) for any TDC with solid component confirms diagnosis
  - Evaluate thyroid bed for presence or absence of normal thyroid tissue
- **Ranula**
  - Retention cyst in sublingual space, epithelial lining
  - Thin walled, anechoic, posterior enhancement
  - Thick wall with internal debris/fluid level if infected or hemorrhagic

Helpful Clues for Less Common Diagnoses
- **Dermoid/Epidermoid**
  - Dermoid: Round, well-defined, with internal echoes ± posterior enhancement

- May be heterogeneous ± fluid-fluid level; "pseudosolid" with fat content and osseo-dental structures
- Look for any soft tissue growth as 5% develop squamous cell carcinoma
  ○ Epidermoid: Well defined and homogeneously echogenic due to fat content, posterior enhancement
  ○ Define location for both: Supra-mylohyoid (sublingual) vs. infra-mylohyoid (submandibular)
    - Determines intraoral vs. external operative approach
- **Laryngocele**
  ○ 26% external, 40% mixed: Completely or partially protruded through thyrohyoid membrane
  ○ Seen as mobile echogenic lines (air) in characteristic location, exacerbated on blowing, ± fluid, debris-thickened walls
  ○ Rule out laryngeal ventricle obstruction by tumor in patients with no relevant clinical history (trumpet players, glass blowers)
- **Lateral Pharyngeal Diverticulum**
  ○ Seen as mobile echogenic lines (gas) or fluid-filled space
  ○ Empties on compression
- **Hypopharyngeal Tumor**
  ○ Pyriform fossae are inferolateral to hyoid
  ○ Solid, hypoechoic tumor filling fossa may be seen on US
- **Postoperative**
  ○ **Para-Stomal Recurrence**
    - Hypoechoic, soft tissue mass ± vascularity at surgical site
    - Evaluate nodal status, confirm recurrent tumor by FNAC
  ○ **Colonic Interposition, Jejunal Pull-Up**
    - Need to know patient history to avoid misdiagnosis of mass
    - Look for "gut signature"

Helpful Clues for Rare Diagnoses
- **Ectopic Thyroid**
  ○ Anywhere along course of thyroglossal duct
  ○ Only functioning thyroid tissue in 70-80% of cases
    - Check thyroid bed for presence of any thyroid tissue
  ○ Multinodular goiter changes may occur; 3% malignant change to papillary carcinoma

Alternative Differential Approaches
- Evaluate lesions by their specific/common location in neck, from cranial to caudal
- Lymph nodes occur at any level in midline/paramidline (often obscured by shadowing from bone, cartilage)
- Floor of mouth/suprahyoid neck
  ○ Ranula, TDC, dermoid, epidermoid, ectopic thyroid
- Infrahyoid neck
  ○ TDC, ectopic thyroid, thyroid masses, hypopharyngeal diverticula/tumor, laryngocele, para-stomal recurrence, postoperative change

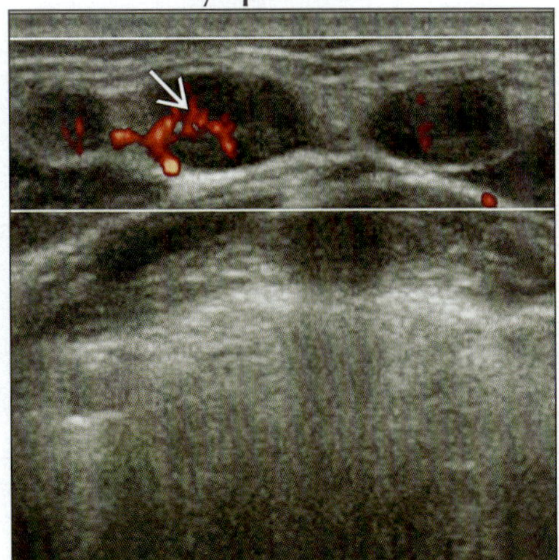

Lymph Nodes

Transverse power Doppler ultrasound shows hypertrophied midline submental neck lymph nodes in a patient with previous radiation therapy. Note central vascularity ➡ and absence of peripheral vascularity.

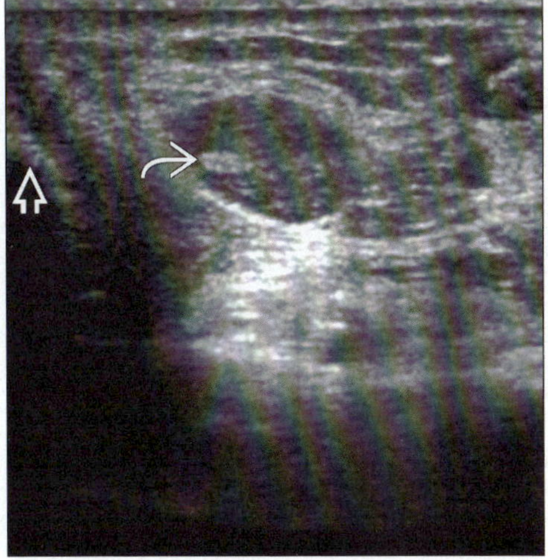

Lymph Nodes

Transverse ultrasound shows a hypertrophied node in the suprasternal region with preserved hilar architecture ➡. Note the trachea ➡.

MIDLINE NECK MASS

Lymph Nodes

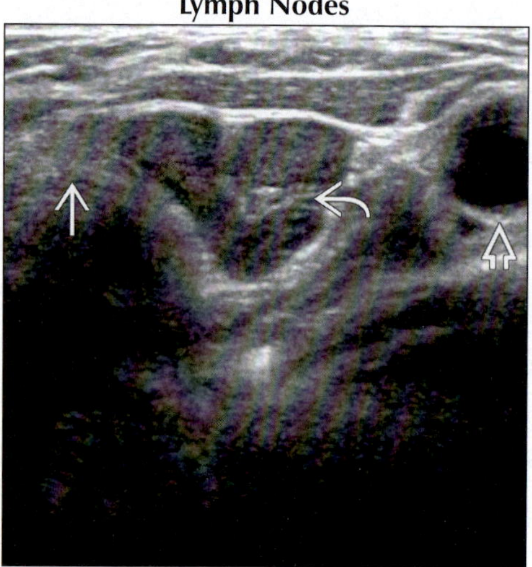

Lymph Nodes

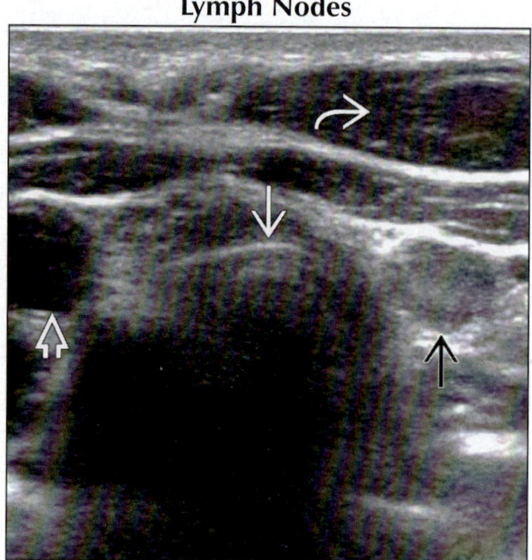

(Left) Transverse ultrasound shows a well-defined, hypoechoic, hypertrophic node in the left paratracheal location in a patient with previous radiation therapy. Note normal hilar architecture ⮕ (trachea ⮕, left CCA ⮕). (Right) Transverse ultrasound shows an enlarged node ⮕ in the left paratracheal region. Note this node is hyperechoic compared to the adjacent muscle ⮕, suggesting a metastatic node from papillary thyroid carcinoma (trachea ⮕, right CCA ⮕).

Pyramidal Lobe (Mimic)

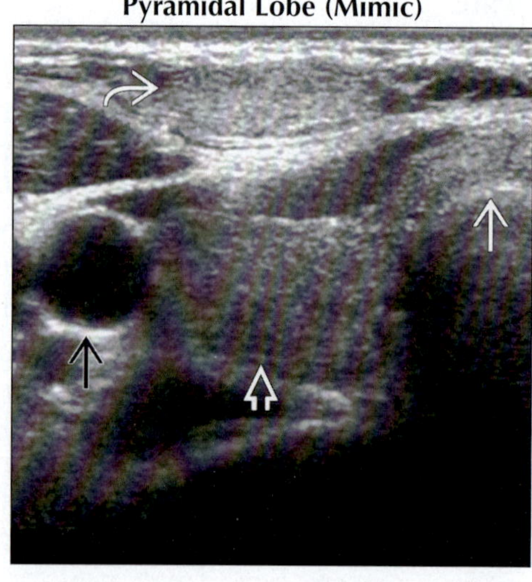

Pyramidal Lobe (Mimic)

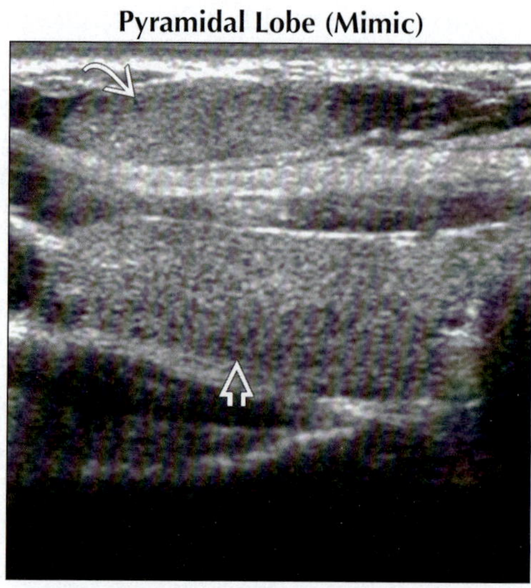

(Left) Transverse ultrasound shows an island of soft tissue ⮕ with similar echogenicity to the normal thyroid gland ⮕. Note its anterior location, just off midline (CCA ⮕, trachea ⮕). The appearance is consistent with a pyramidal lobe. (Right) Longitudinal ultrasound in the same patient shows the island of thyroid tissue ⮕ and its relation to the thyroid gland ⮕. Although pyramidal lobes are more typical on the left, in this patient, the lobe was on the right.

Thyroglossal Duct Cyst

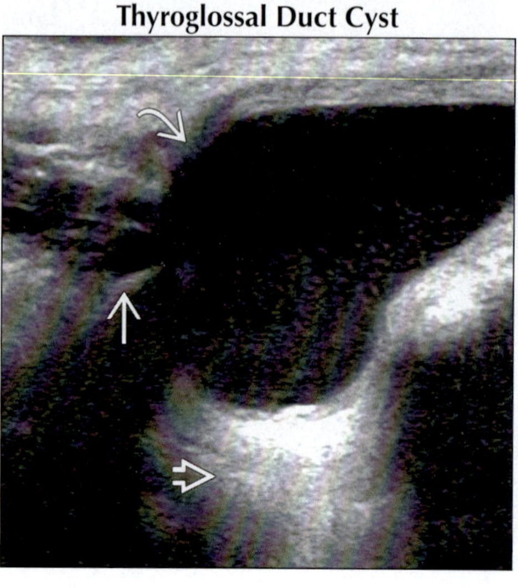

Thyroglossal Duct Cyst

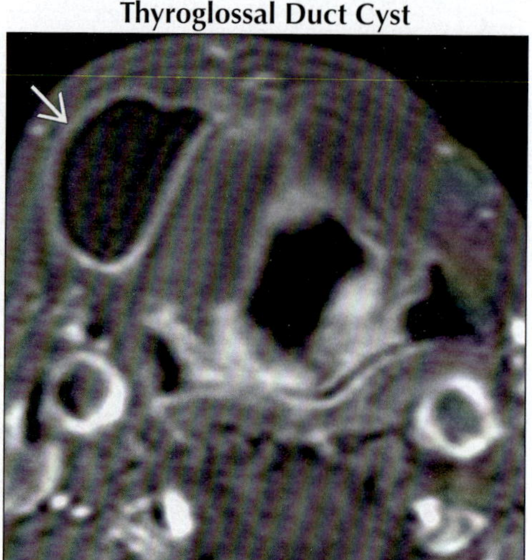

(Left) Longitudinal ultrasound shows an uncomplicated infrahyoid TDC ⮕. Note the thin wall, fluid content with small amount of debris, and posterior acoustic enhancement ⮕. The cyst's relation to the hyoid ⮕ is clearly seen. (Right) Axial T1WI+C MR with fat suppression shows enhancement of the wall ⮕ of a TDC, which is thin and regular. The internal content is hypointense and of fluid signal. No solid component is seen.

MIDLINE NECK MASS

Thyroglossal Duct Cyst

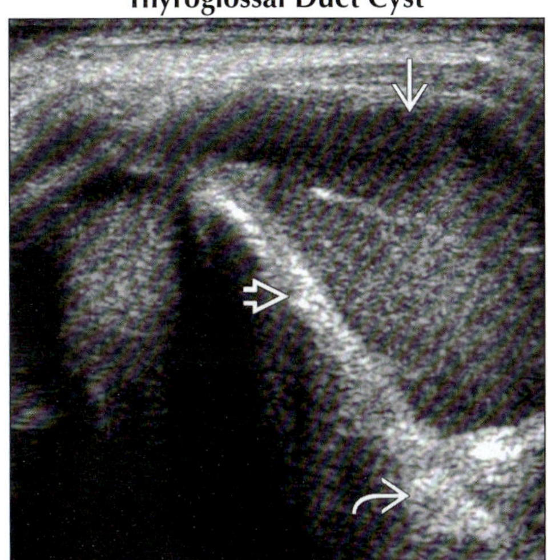

Thyroglossal Duct Cyst

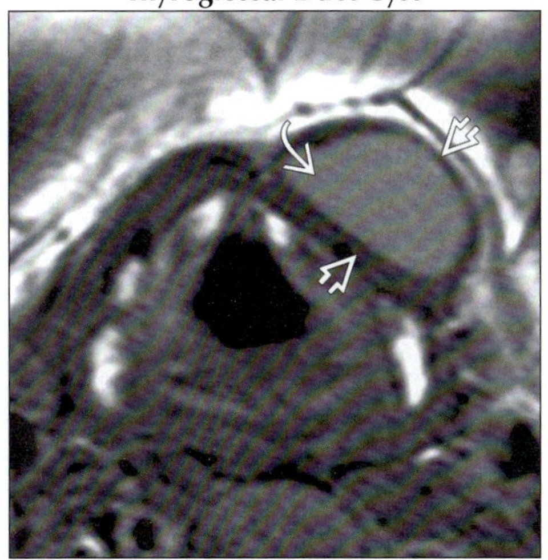

(Left) Transverse ultrasound shows an infrahyoid TDC ➡ with uniformly dispersed internal debris giving it a "pseudosolid" appearance (thyroid cartilage ⧨). Note that the posterior acoustic enhancement ➡ provides a clue to the mass's cystic nature. (Right) Transverse T1WI MR in the same patient shows hyperintense ➡ signal in the TDC ⧨ due to proteinaceous content. One would normally expect a hypointense signal in a cystic mass.

Thyroglossal Duct Cyst

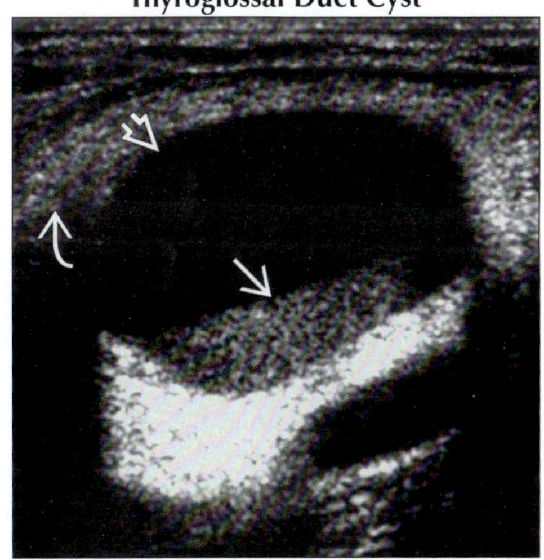

Thyroglossal Duct Cyst

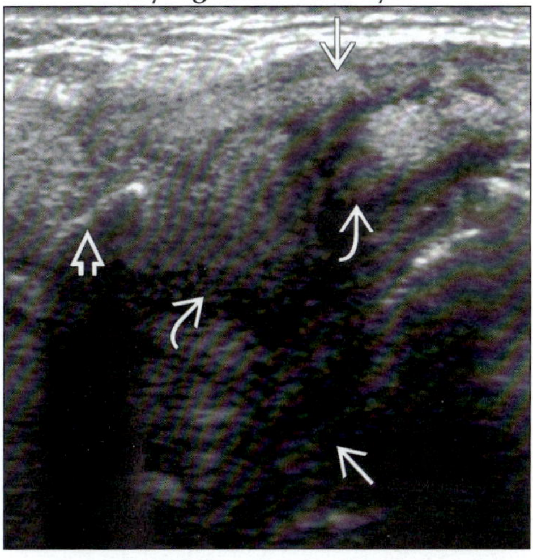

(Left) Longitudinal ultrasound shows an infrahyoid TDC ⧨ with a fluid-fluid level ➡ suggestive of a previous hemorrhage or infection (hyoid ➡). (Right) Longitudinal ultrasound shows an infrahyoid TDC ⧨ with irregular solid soft tissue ➡, suspicious of malignant change and confirmed on FNAC (hyoid bone ⧨). In patients with solid tissue, an FNAC is indicated to rule out any malignant change. This is readily done under US guidance.

Dermoid/Epidermoid

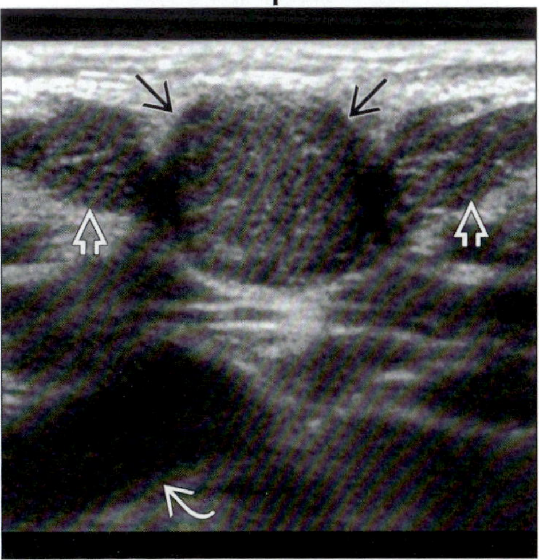

Dermoid/Epidermoid

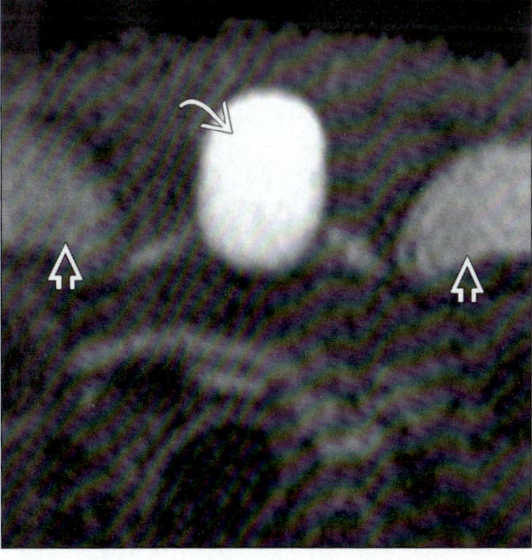

(Left) Transverse ultrasound shows a suprasternal dermoid ➡. Note its round shape, well-defined border, and echogenic internal content. The posterior acoustic enhancement is not obvious. Note the sternal head of the sternomastoid muscles ⧨ and the innominate artery ➡. (Right) Correlative axial T2WI MR with fat suppression shows the dermoid cyst with homogeneous bright fluid signal ➡. Note the medial end of the clavicles ⧨.

1

MIDLINE NECK MASS

(Left) Transverse ultrasound shows an epidermoid ⮕ at the floor of the mouth. Note the uniform, echogenic, homogeneous echopattern of the epidermoid cyst. Also present are the sublingual glands ⮕. (Right) Axial T2WI MR with fat suppression in the same patient shows the homogeneous fluid signal ⮕ typically seen in an epidermoid. On this MR, TDC is included in the differential, but the US appearance is more suggestive of an epidermoid.

Dermoid/Epidermoid

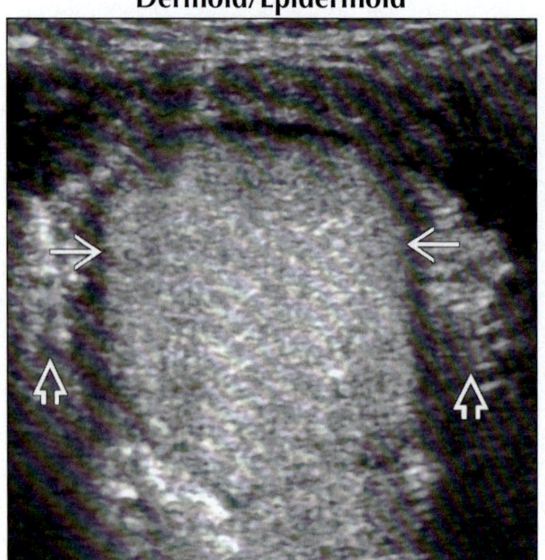

Dermoid/Epidermoid

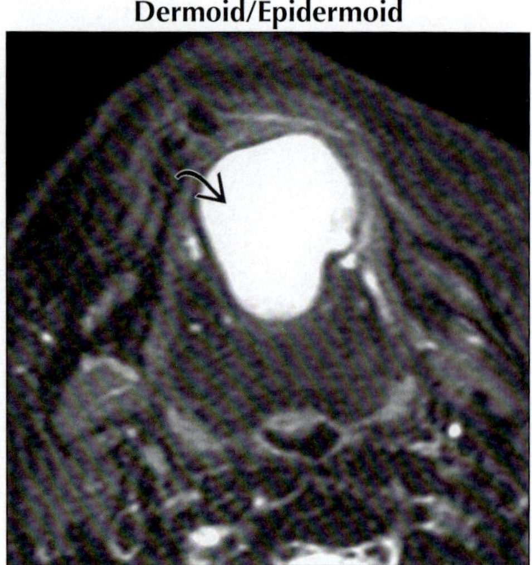

(Left) Transverse ultrasound of the right paramedian region of the neck shows a curvilinear echogenic interface ⮕ and "dirty" posterior acoustic shadowing ⮕, consistent with a laryngocele. Note the thyroid cartilage ⮕. (Right) Transverse ultrasound through the thyrohyoid membrane shows an irregular soft tissue laryngeal mass ⮕ and an associated laryngocele ⮕, seen as echogenic foci representing air. Note the left thyroid cartilage ⮕.

Laryngocele

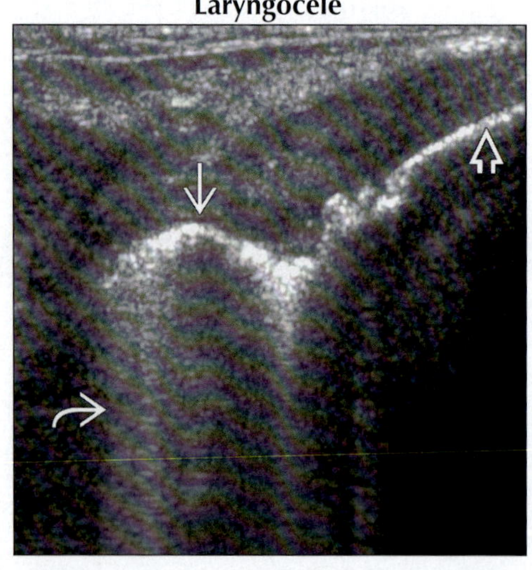

Laryngocele

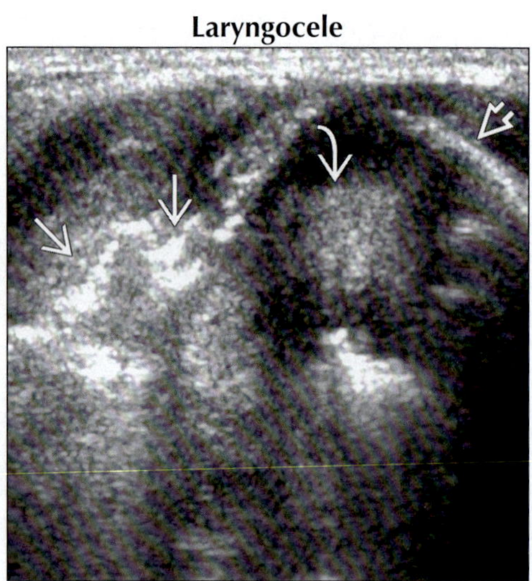

(Left) Axial CECT in the same patient shows the air-filled laryngocele ⮕ and soft tissue mass in right vocal cord ⮕. Note arytenoid ⮕ and left thyroid cartilage ⮕. CT better evaluates laryngocele and any associated abnormality. (Right) Transverse ultrasound shows an irregular, solid, hypoechoic, soft tissue mass ⮕ near the stoma ⮕, suspicious of a para-stomal recurrence. The soft tissue was vascular on Doppler, & US-guided FNAC confirmed tumor recurrence.

Laryngocele

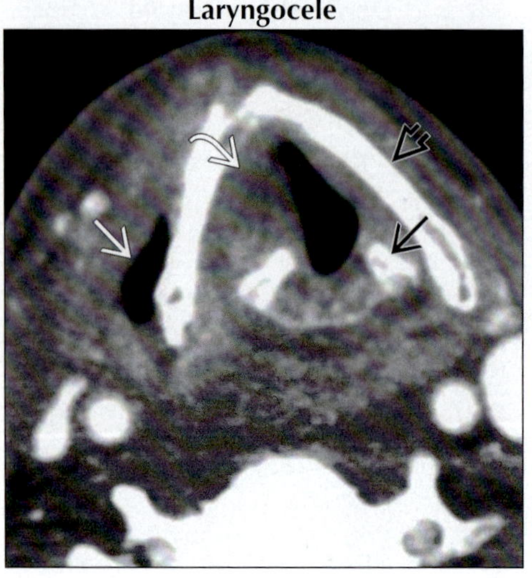

Para-Stomal Recurrence

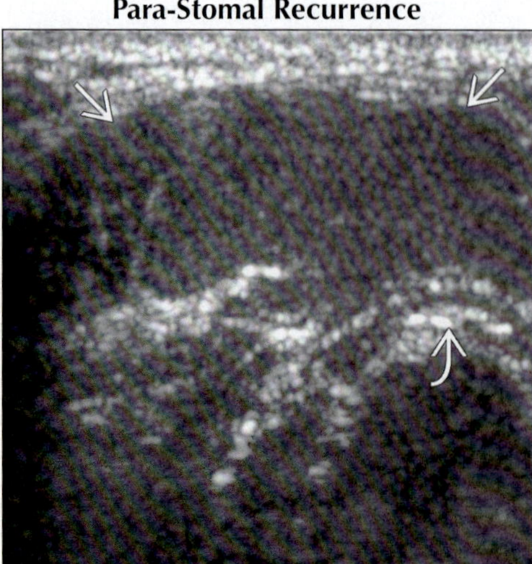

MIDLINE NECK MASS

Colonic Interposition

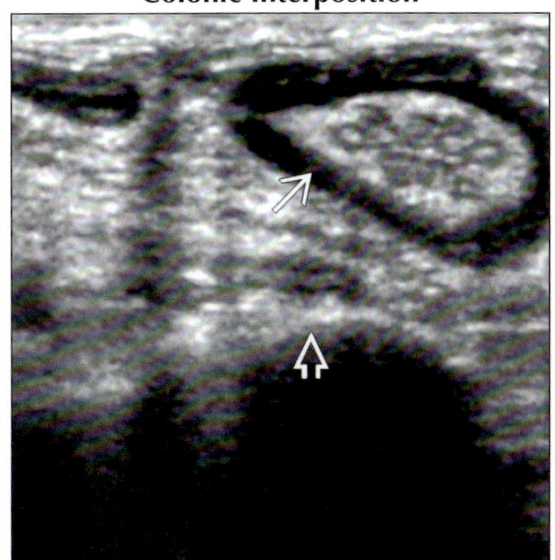

Colonic Interposition

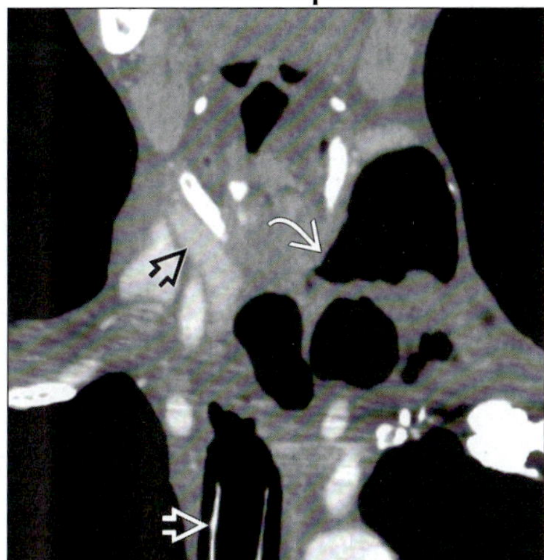

(Left) Transverse ultrasound at the midline of the neck shows a "mass" ⇨ with a "bowel" signature, a colonic pull-up in this patient. Note the vertebral body ⇨. It is helpful to be familiar with a patient's surgical history to avoid mistaking this for an abnormality. *(Right)* Coronal reformatted CECT of the same patient shows the loops of the colon ⇨ (gas-filled) in the left para-median region. Note the tracheostomy tube ⇨ and right lobe of the thyroid gland ⇨.

Jejunal Pull-Up

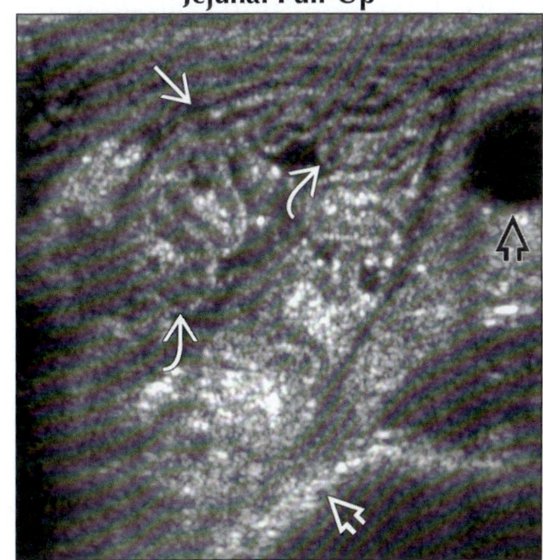

Ectopic Thyroid

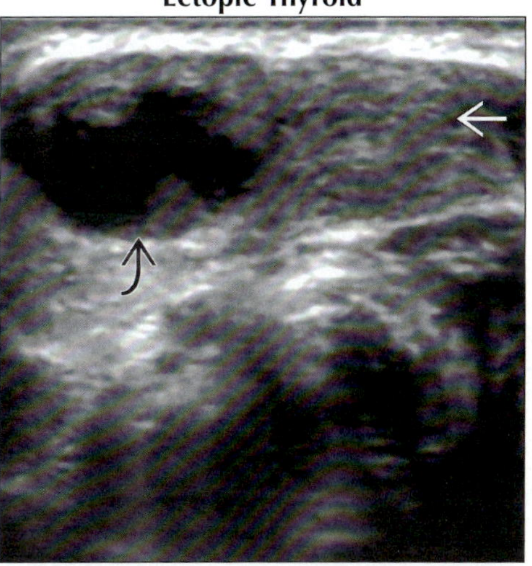

(Left) Transverse ultrasound shows a jejunal pull-up ⇨ in the neck. Note the typical mucosal folds ⇨, left CCA ⇨, & vertebral body ⇨. In such patients, mesentry with nodes may also be seen. *(Right)* Longitudinal ultrasound shows an ectopic thyroid ⇨ with a heterogeneous, thick-walled, cystic nodule ⇨. These represent changes of a multinodular goiter in an ectopic thyroid, similar to a normally located thyroid.

Ectopic Thyroid

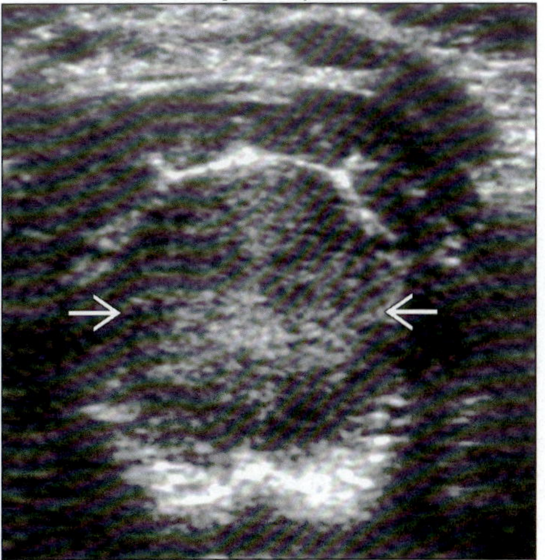

Ectopic Thyroid

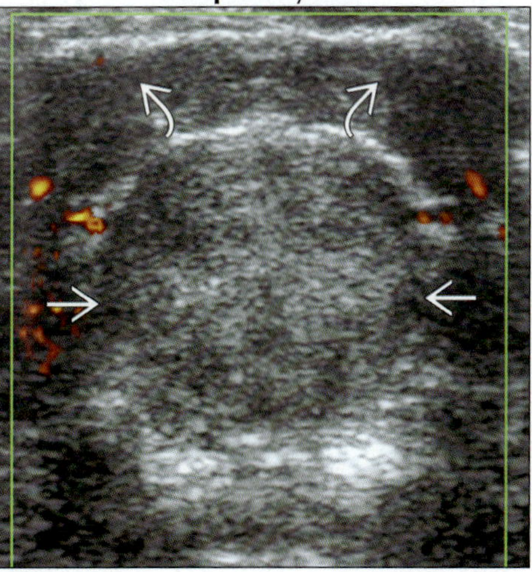

(Left) Transverse ultrasound at the floor of the mouth shows a well-defined solid "mass" ⇨ with a uniform, fine, bright, parenchymal echopattern, similar to a thyroid gland. *(Right)* Transverse power Doppler ultrasound in the same patient shows minimal flow within this mass ⇨. Note the mylohyoid muscles ⇨. This was a confirmed ectopic thyroid.

CYSTIC NECK MASS

DIFFERENTIAL DIAGNOSIS

Common
- Neck Abscess
- Metastatic Lymph Node
  - Squamous Cell Carcinoma
  - Papillary Carcinoma of Thyroid

Less Common
- Venous Vascular Malformation (VVM)
- Lymphangioma
- Acute Suppurative Thyroiditis
- Simple Ranula (SR)
- Diving Ranula (DR)

Rare but Important
- Dermoid
- Epidermoid
- 2nd Branchial Cleft Cyst (2nd BCC)
- 1st Branchial Cleft Cyst (1st BCC)
- Thymic Cyst

ESSENTIAL INFORMATION

Key Differential Diagnosis Issues
- Cystic masses in head & neck are site specific; therefore, location of mass is clue to diagnosis
  - Asymptomatic adult male
    - Solitary metastatic node from H&N SCCa is much more common than 2nd BCC, even at known site of 2nd BCC
  - Asymptomatic adult female
    - Consider possibility of metastatic node from papillary thyroid cancer
  - Guided fine-needle aspiration and cytology (FNAC) is crucial to diagnosis
- If abscess is detected on US/CT & MR may be indicated to evaluate
  - Exact anatomical location, extent, and mediastinal involvement if any
  - Relation of abscess to carotid artery and risk of carotid blow-out

Helpful Clues for Common Diagnoses
- **Neck Abscess**
  - Clinical features of acute infection in majority of cases
  - Thick-walled, irregular outlines with hypoechoic/necrotic center, ± echogenic foci with "comet tail" artifacts representing gas, ± enlarged nodes
  - Doppler: Hypervascular walls, avascular center, hypervascularity in adjacent inflammatory tissues
  - US-guided aspiration of liquefied contents helps to identify infective organism
- **Metastatic Lymph Node**
  - **Squamous Cell Carcinoma**
    - Round, heterogeneously hypoechoic, loss of hilar architecture (69-95%), cystic or coagulation necrosis
    - Doppler: Abnormal, chaotic, peripheral vascularity
  - **Papillary Carcinoma of Thyroid**
    - Round or ovoid with large cystic areas
    - Solid components contains punctate calcification and internal vascularity
    - Primary carcinoma is often in ipsilateral thyroid lobe, and its appearance is similar to metastatic node

Helpful Clues for Less Common Diagnoses
- **Venous Vascular Malformation (VVM)**
  - Often multiple with multicompartmental involvement
  - Thin walled, multiseptated with serpiginous cystic spaces, ± phleboliths (characteristic)
  - Variable hypoechoic stromal component
    - May mimic muscle or intermuscular fat on ultrasound
  - Slow venous flow
    - May be seen only on grayscale; too slow to be seen on color Doppler
  - High probe pressure may compress and obscure abnormality
  - MR is indicated to detect multiplicity, extent of abnormality
    - May extend into mediastinum
- **Lymphangioma**
  - Cystic hygroma > cavernous lymphangioma or capillary lymphangioma
  - Thin-walled, multiloculated, anechoic, cystic mass
  - Commonly in posterior triangle; septated with multicompartmental involvement
  - Thick walled and debris if complicated by infection or hemorrhage
  - No grayscale flow movement (as in VVM), no vascularity within septae or debris
  - MR may be indicated to evaluate anatomical extent in neck and mediastinal/axillary involvement

1

- US helps to guide sclerotherapy and follow-up after treatment
- **Acute Suppurative Thyroiditis**
  - Seen in children
  - Left lobe (95%) > > right lobe (5%)
  - Perithyroidal ± intrathyroidal abscess, typically around upper pole of left lobe
  - Barium study after acute episode to identify underlying pyriform fossa fistula
- **Simple Ranula (SR)**
  - Thin-walled, unilocular, anechoic, retention cyst confined to sublingual space
- **Diving Ranula (DR)**
  - Simple ranula (+ epithelial lining) ruptures into submandibular space forming pseudocyst (no epithelial lining)
  - Uni-/multilocular internal debris & thick walls

Helpful Clues for Rare Diagnoses

- **Dermoid**
  - Commonly midline, well defined, anechoic, with posterior acoustic enhancement
  - May appear pseudosolid or heterogeneous with fat content and osseodental structures
- **Epidermoid**
  - Less common than dermoid cyst
  - Often well defined, homogeneous, echogenic, representing fat content
- **2nd Branchial Cleft Cyst (2nd BCC)**
  - 95% of all branchial anomalies

- Typically posterior to submandibular gland, along anteromedial border of sternocleidomastoid muscle
  - Superficial to common carotid artery (CCA) and internal jugular vein
- US may demonstrate associated track or fistula & characteristic extension of cyst between internal carotid artery (ICA) and external carotid artery (ECA)
- Typically well defined, anechoic, thin walls, posterior acoustic enhancement, or "pseudosolid" (avascular)
- May be become infected or hemorrhagic
  - Complex cyst with thick irregular walls, septa, debris, ± vascularity
  - FNAC or excisional biopsy essential to differentiate from metastatic node
- **1st Branchial Cleft Cyst (1st BCC)**
  - 8% of all branchial anomalies
  - In/around parotid gland, external auditory canal (EAC), and angle of mandible
  - Typically seen in middle-aged woman with recurrent parotid abscesses
  - Anechoic, thin walls, posterior acoustic enhancement, or "pseudosolid"
  - MR to exclude deep sinus tract through EAC to temporal bone
- **Thymic Cyst**
  - Uncommon; occur anywhere from angle of mandible to superior mediastinum along carotid sheath
  - Well-defined anechoic cyst, commonly below level of thyroid, left > > right
  - Aspiration yields clear "watery" fluid

Neck Abscess

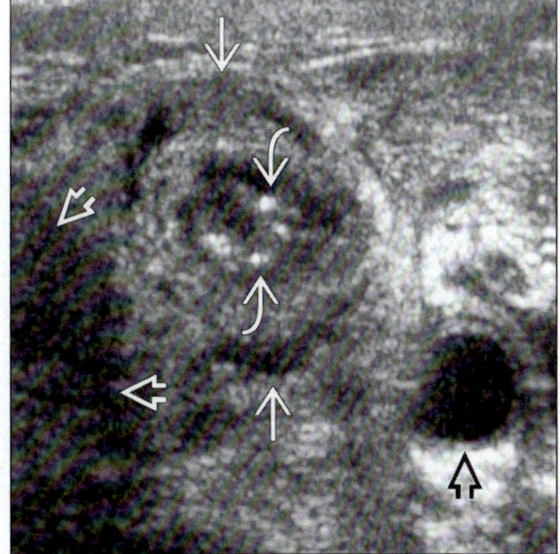

Transverse ultrasound shows an ill-defined heterogeneous abscess ➡ with internal necrosis, echogenic foci representing gas ➡, and marked surrounding edema ➡. Note relation to the CCA ➡.

Neck Abscess

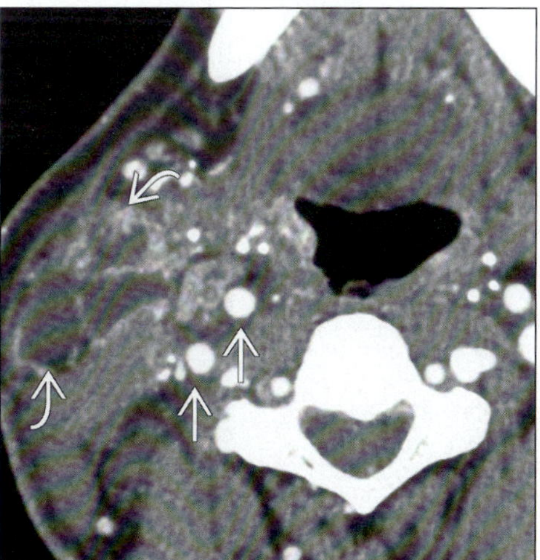

Axial CECT in the same patient shows a multiloculated rim-enhancing abscess ➡ in the right upper cervical region. Its anatomical extent and relation to major vessels ➡ are well seen on CT.

CYSTIC NECK MASS

(Left) Transverse ultrasound shows an ovoid lymph node ➡ with a large cystic area and an eccentric solid mural nodule ➡ in a metastatic lymph node from thyroid papillary carcinoma. (Right) T2WI MR with fat suppression in the same patient shows the fluid content as a hyperintense signal ➡, and the solid component is demonstrated as a hypointense nodule ⇨.

Metastatic Lymph Node

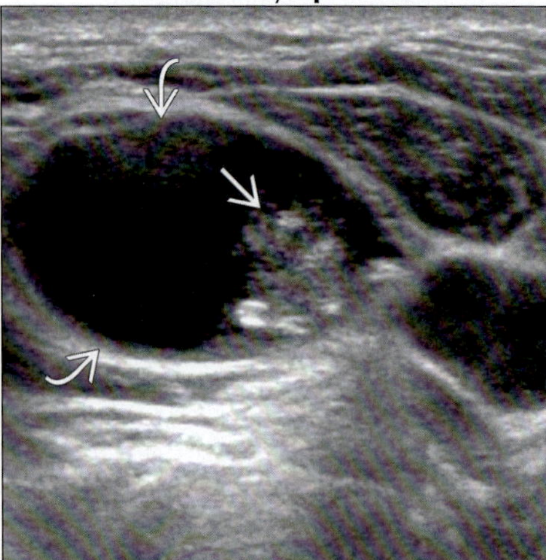

Metastatic Lymph Node

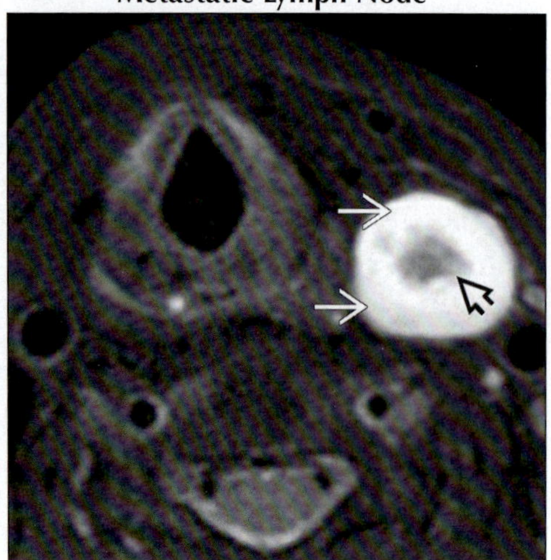

(Left) Transverse ultrasound of the left upper cervical region shows a cystic mass ➡ with thin septae ➡ and internal serpiginous vascular spaces ⇨. Note the echogenic focus ➡ with dense posterior acoustic shadowing ➡, representing a phlebolith; these features are characteristic of a VVM. (Right) Transverse power Doppler ultrasound of the VVM shows vascularity within serpiginous cystic spaces ➡. Often slow flow is better seen on grayscale US than Doppler US.

Venous Vascular Malformation (VVM)

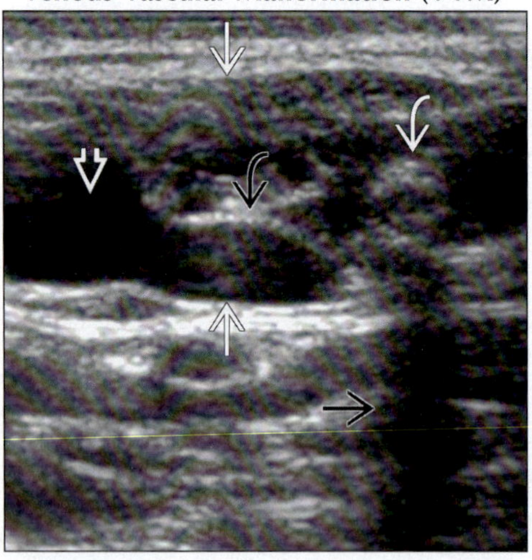

Venous Vascular Malformation (VVM)

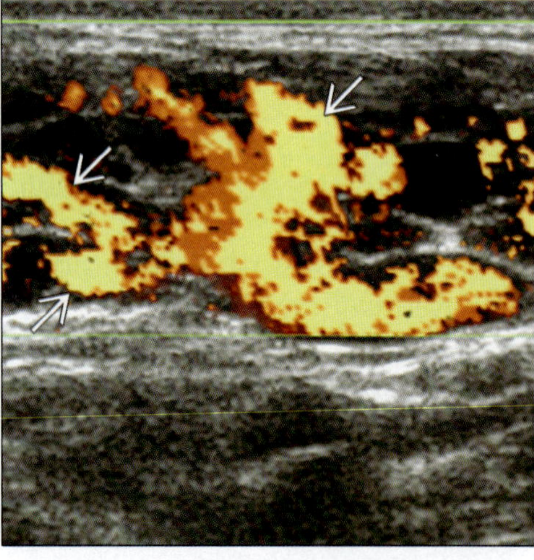

(Left) Axial T2WI MR with fat suppression of the VVM ➡ in the same patient shows the slow flow vascular space as fluid signal. The hypointense foci represent phleboliths ➡. (Right) Transverse ultrasound of the posterior triangle shows a thin-walled, septated ➡, multiloculated cystic mass ➡. Note that the cystic spaces are compartmentalized rather than serpiginous, and no phleboliths are present (vs. VVM). These are typical US features of a lymphangioma.

Venous Vascular Malformation (VVM)

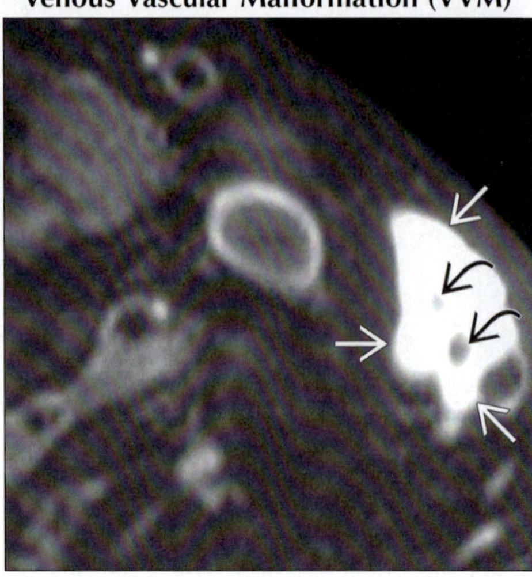

Lymphangioma

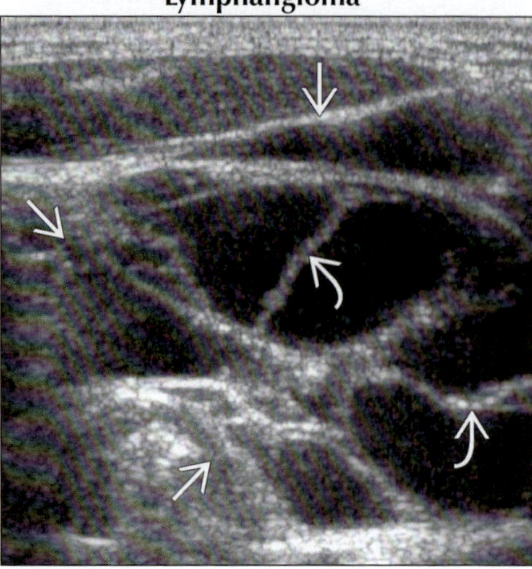

CYSTIC NECK MASS

Lymphangioma

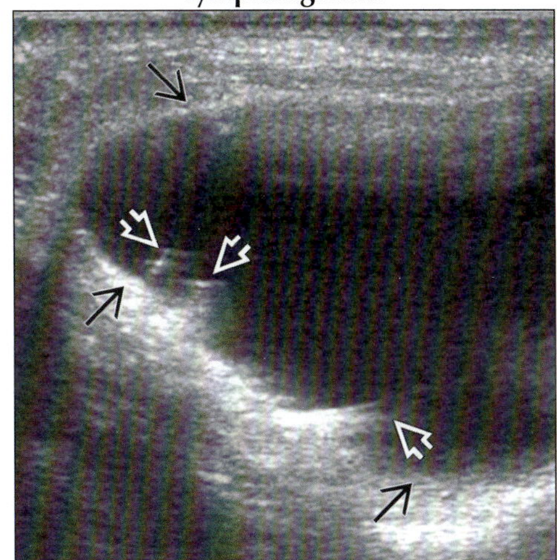

Lymphangioma

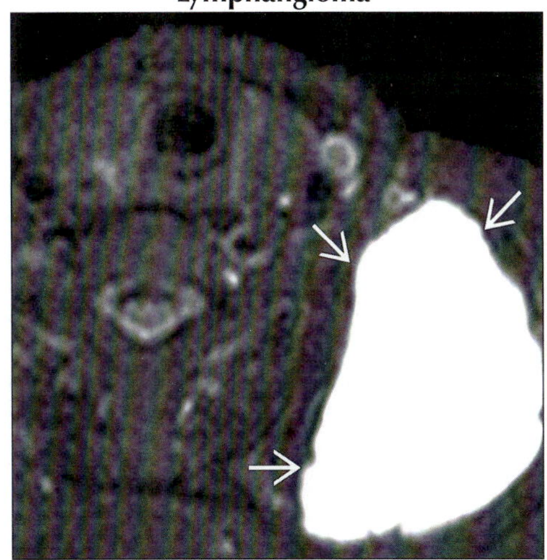

(Left) Transverse ultrasound of the left lower posterior triangle shows a well-defined, thin-walled, cystic mass ⮕ with thin internal septae ⮖ and fine debris, demonstrating a typical US appearance of a cystic hygroma. (Right) T2WI MR with fat suppression in the same patient shows a homogeneous fluid signal within the lobulated mass ⮕. MR and CECT are superior to US in evaluating anatomic extent of the abnormality.

Acute Suppurative Thyroiditis

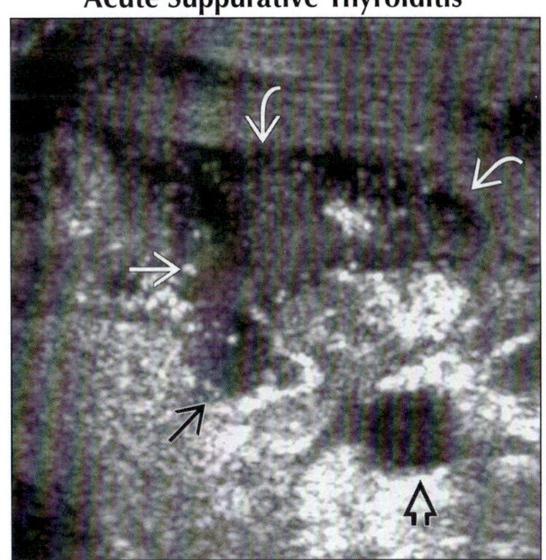

Acute Suppurative Thyroiditis

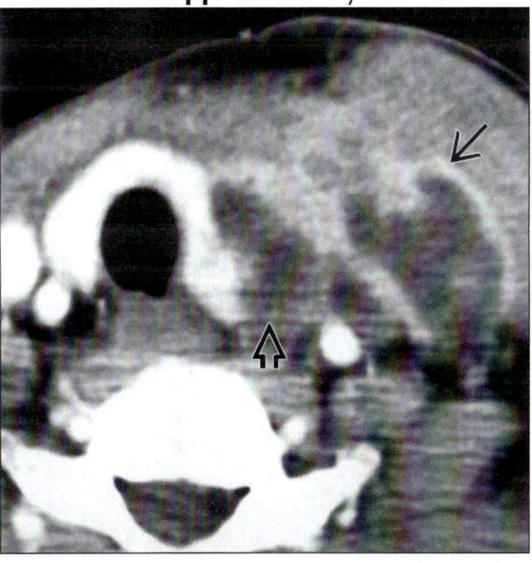

(Left) Transverse ultrasound of the left lobe of a thyroid gland shows a perithyroidal abscess ⮕ with intrathyroidal extension ⮕, consistent with acute suppurative thyroiditis. Note echogenic gas ⮕ in the abscess (CCA ⮖). (Right) Axial CECT of the neck in the same patient shows the rim-enhancing perithyroid abscess ⮕ with extension into the left lobe of thyroid ⮖. The anatomic extent is better delineated on CT than on US.

Diving Ranula (DR)

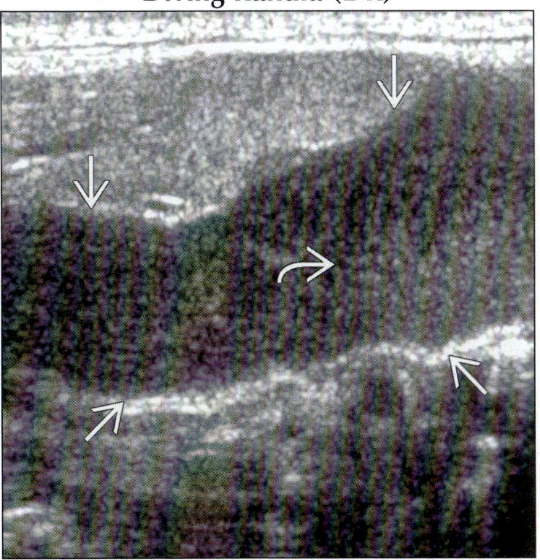

Diving Ranula (DR)

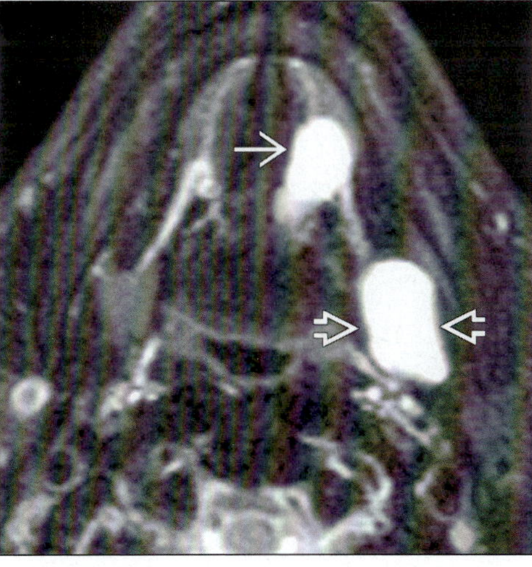

(Left) Transverse ultrasound shows a thin-walled cystic abnormality in the left posterior submandibular region ⮕, with dispersed internal debris ⮕. It was shown to communicate with the sublingual space and is consistent with a diving ranula. (Right) Axial T2WI MR with fat suppression in the same patient shows involvement of ipsilateral sublingual ⮕ and submandibular ⮖ spaces. A diving ranula is a pseudocyst with no epithelial lining.

CYSTIC NECK MASS

Simple Ranula (SR)

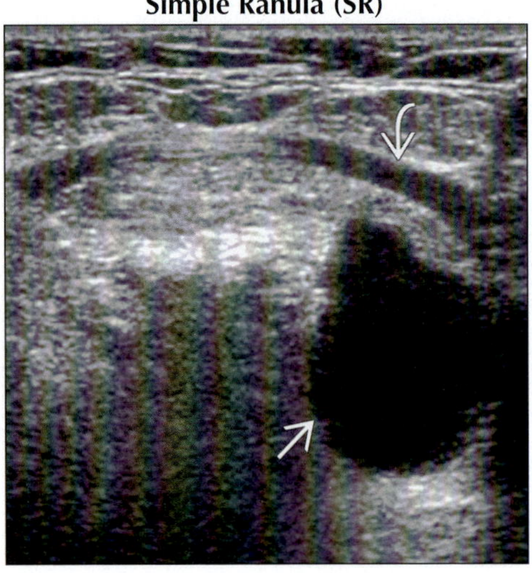

Dermoid

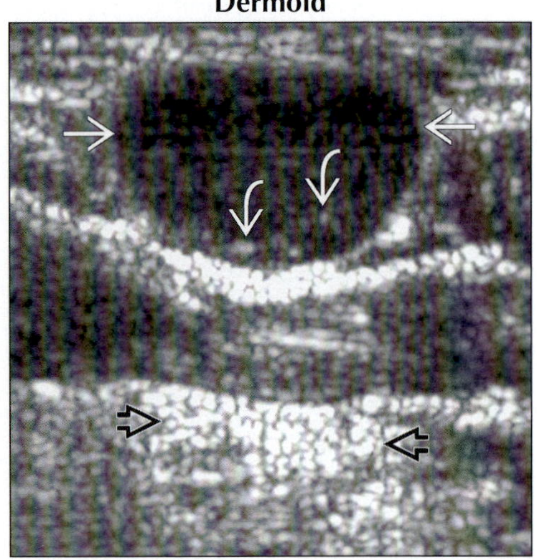

(Left) Transverse ultrasound of the submental region shows a thin-walled, unilocular, anechoic mass ➡ confined to the left sublingual space, consistent with a simple ranula. Note its relation to mylohyoid muscle ➤. Simple ranula is a retention cyst with an epithelial lining. *(Right)* Transverse ultrasound of the lower neck shows a midline dermoid cyst ➡. It is thin walled with internal debris ➤ and posterior acoustic enhancement ➤.

Dermoid

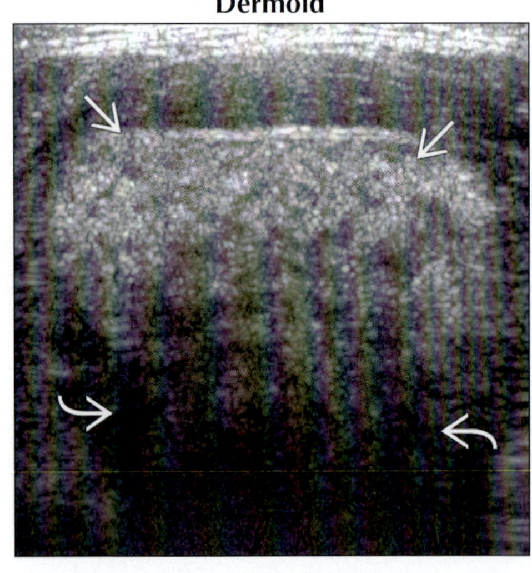

Dermoid

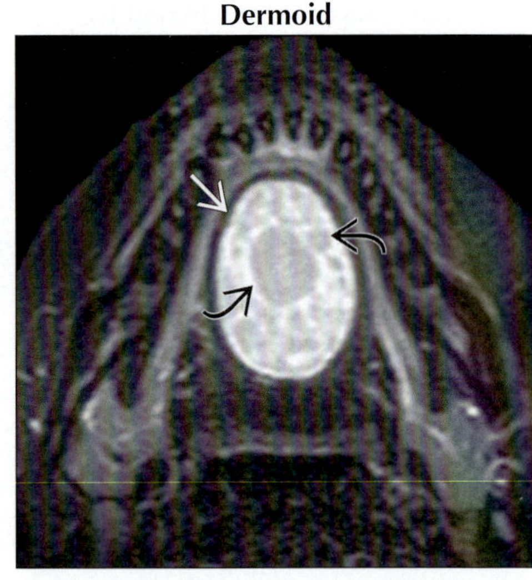

(Left) Transverse ultrasound of the submental region shows a well-defined heterogeneously echogenic mass ➡ in the floor of the mouth. Note that fat in the lesion attenuates the sound beam posteriorly ➤, making delineation of the entire mass difficult. *(Right)* Axial T2WI MR with fat suppression of the submental region in the same patient shows a midline dermoid cyst with a "sack of marbles" appearance ➡. The "marbles" ➤ represent fat globules in the dermoid cyst.

2nd Branchial Cleft Cyst (2nd BCC)

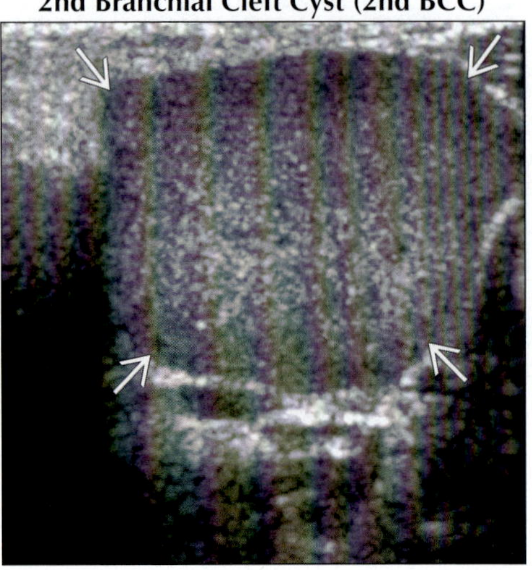

2nd Branchial Cleft Cyst (2nd BCC)

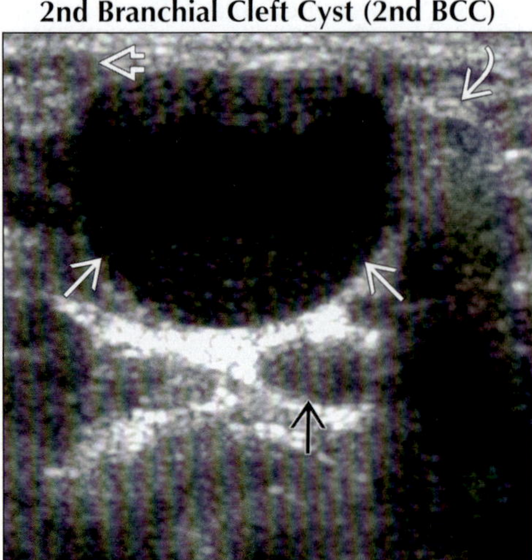

(Left) Transverse US of the left upper neck shows a 2nd BCC with a "pseudosolid" appearance ➡. Note the uniform fine internal echo pattern that mimics a solid mass (due to epithelial cells, cholesterol, mucus debris). *(Right)* Transverse US shows a typical appearance of a 2nd BCC ➡. It is thin walled, anechoic, unilocular with internal debris and posterior acoustic enhancement. (CCA ➤, sternocleidomastoid ➤, and submandibular gland ➤.)

CYSTIC NECK MASS

2nd Branchial Cleft Cyst (2nd BCC)

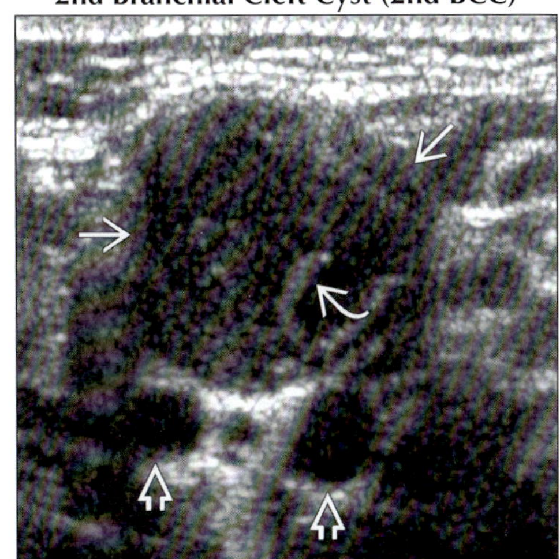

2nd Branchial Cleft Cyst (2nd BCC)

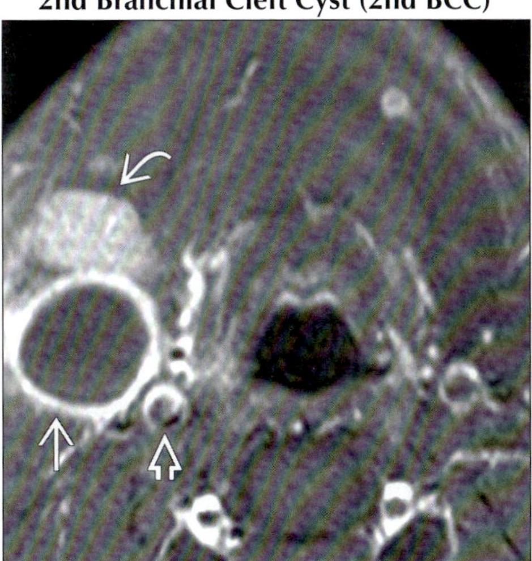

(Left) Transverse ultrasound of the left upper cervical region shows a complicated 2nd BCC ➡. Note its thick wall, internal septae ➡, and echogenic debris. (ICA/ECA ➡.) With such an appearance, always exclude a metastatic node by biopsy. (Right) Gadolinium-enhanced axial T1WI MR shows enhancement of the wall of a 2nd BCC ➡. Note the hypointense center and its relationship to the submandibular gland ➡ and CCA ➡.

1st Branchial Cleft Cyst (1st BCC)

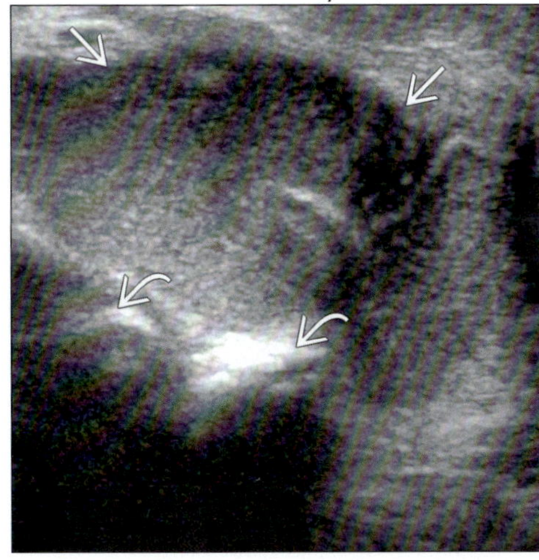

1st Branchial Cleft Cyst (1st BCC)

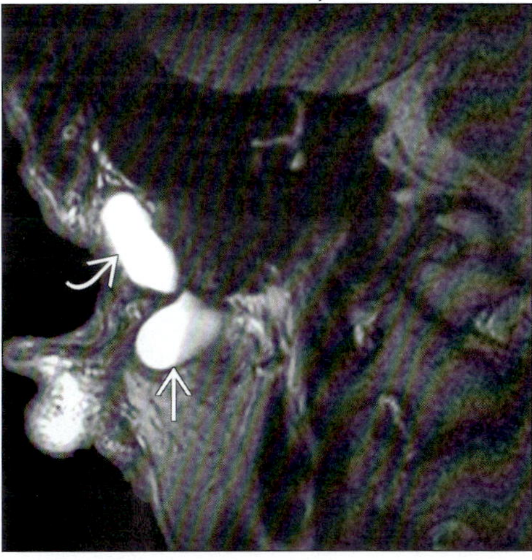

(Left) Longitudinal ultrasound of the right parotid region shows a 1st BCC ➡ with uniform homogeneous internal echoes in a "pseudosolid" pattern. Movement of debris and posterior acoustic enhancement provide clues to its cystic nature. Other congenital cysts may appear similar. Mastoid process ➡. (Right) Coronal T2WI the right parotid region in the same patient shows the deep extent of the 1st BCC ➡, reaching to the external auditory canal region ➡.

Thymic Cyst

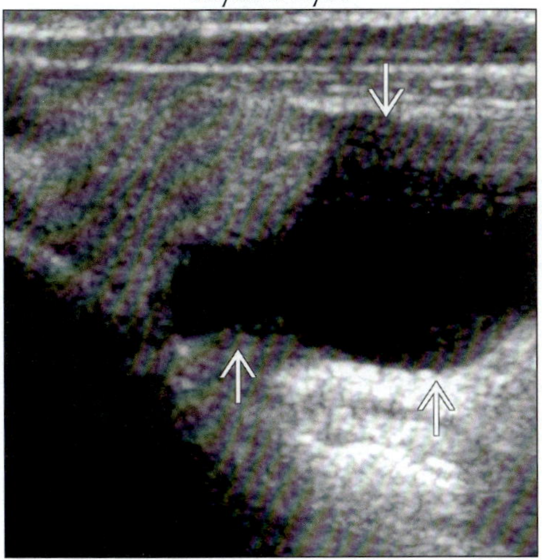

Thymic Cyst

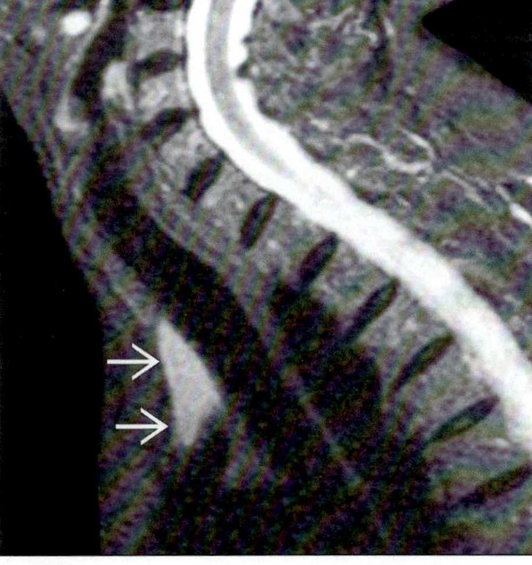

(Left) Longitudinal ultrasound of the suprasternal region shows an irregular midline unilocular cyst ➡, representing a thymic cyst, which is more common on the left. Aspiration of such a cyst yields clear "watery" fluid. These are usually discovered as incidental lesions. (Right) Sagittal T2WI MR with fat suppression of the midline suprasternal region in the same patient shows homogeneous fluid signal within the thymic cyst ➡.

NON-NODAL SOLID NECK MASS

DIFFERENTIAL DIAGNOSIS

Common
- Nerve Sheath Tumor
- Lipoma
  - Madelung Disease

Less Common
- Carotid Body Paraganglioma

Rare but Important
- Ectopic Thyroid

ESSENTIAL INFORMATION

Key Differential Diagnosis Issues
- Most common solid masses in neck are normal/abnormal lymph nodes
  - Look for clues that mass represents lymph nodes
    - Along lymph node chains, hilar architecture, vascularity, multiplicity, bilaterality
  - Clinical history helpful: Known head & neck or infraclavicular tumor, infection/inflammation signs, ↑ white cell count, fever
- Once non-nodal nature of mass is established, evaluate mass based on its location and specific characteristics
  - Nerve sheath tumors (NST) occur at known location of nerve: Vagus, brachial plexus, sympathetic chain
  - Location of carotid body paraganglioma (CBP) is specific and very good clue to diagnosis
- MR/CT may be indicated for further evaluation
  - In patients with CBP, rule out glomus jugulare & vagale as US cannot evaluate these accurately

Helpful Clues for Common Diagnoses
- **Nerve Sheath Tumor**
  - Commonly arise from vagus nerve, brachial plexus, or small cutaneous nerve
  - Transverse scan to identify tumor; longitudinal scan to evaluate continuity/nerve thickening and vascularity
  - Identification of tapering end/continuation with nerve is often tedious & requires meticulous technique
    - Use light pressure on long axis scan to prevent slipping of tumor off scan plane
  - Grayscale features
    - Well circumscribed, fusiform/oval-shaped ± tapering end(s), hypoechoic
    - Often show posterior enhancement (despite being solid), "pseudocystic"
    - ± sharply defined focal intratumoral cystic areas
    - ± mass effect on adjacent vessels (carotid arteries may be draped over surface of tumor)
    - Continuity with nerve/thickening of adjacent nerve is diagnostic
  - Color Doppler
    - Prominent intratumoral vascularity; better evaluated on longitudinal scan
    - Use light transducer pressure to avoid compression of intratumoral vessels
  - FNAC is usually not necessary if continuation with thickened nerve is seen
  - NSTs often have specific MR features to help confirm diagnosis
  - If US and MR findings are both equivocal, FNAC may be considered
    - Note: Aspiration may trigger excruciating pain (considered diagnostic by some)
- **Lipoma**
  - Posterior cervical space, submandibular space most common
  - Intermuscular > intramuscular, may be trans-spatial
  - Grayscale features
    - Well-defined, soft, compressible mass
    - Typically hypoechoic in neck (isoechoic to muscles); echogenic type of lipoma/angiolipoma is more commonly seen in trunk and limbs
    - Multiple, thin, echogenic lines oriented parallel to transducer/skin in both transverse and longitudinal planes
    - Characteristic feather-like appearance (compare with striation of muscles seen only in longitudinal plane)
  - Color Doppler
    - Absence/paucity of vascularity
  - Liposarcoma should be suspected if soft tissue stranding present ± vascularity ± necrosis ± calcification

NON-NODAL SOLID NECK MASS

- MR indicated to evaluate full extent; subsequent US-guided FNAC or excision for pathological diagnosis
  - **Madelung Disease**
    - Benign symmetrical lipomatosis
    - Diffuse lobulated lipomas in cervical and shoulder regions bilaterally
    - As fat is unencapsulated, US not able to define degree of involvement
    - CT and MR better define distribution of fat, compression of vital structures, and examination of deeper structures

Helpful Clues for Less Common Diagnoses
- **Carotid Body Paraganglioma**
  - Solid vascular tumor at carotid bifurcation is 1st clue to diagnosis
  - Always evaluate contralateral side as tumor may be bilateral
  - Grayscale features
    - Round/oval hypoechoic mass straddling carotid bifurcation
    - Typically blurred outlines despite its superficial location (probably due to dispersion of sound by multidirectional high velocity flow within tumor)
    - Homogeneous parenchymal echopattern, ± serpiginous vessels within
    - Heterogeneous parenchymal echopattern in larger tumors due to necrosis or hemorrhage within
  - Color/power Doppler
    - Profuse intratumoral vascularity

- Deeper components may appear avascular as they are not well interrogated with Doppler
- External and internal carotid arteries are splayed (by large enough tumors) & often encased without any narrowing
- Use gentle transducer pressure to avoid compressing intratumoral vessels

Helpful Clues for Rare Diagnoses
- **Ectopic Thyroid**
  - May occur anywhere along tract of thyroglossal duct
  - Represents functioning thyroid tissue in only 70-80%
  - Malignancy in 3%, typically papillary carcinoma
  - Ultrasound features
    - Midline dorsum of tongue near foramen cecum (majority) > thyroglossal duct > trachea
    - Well-defined solid mass with fine echogenic parenchymal pattern and vascularity (resembling thyroid tissue)
    - ± empty thyroid bed
    - ± changes of multinodular goiter
    - Exclude presence of papillary carcinoma (solid, hypoechoic, ill-defined, vascular tumor ± punctate calcification, cystic necrosis, associated lymph nodes)
  - Scintigraphy to confirm diagnosis and detect functioning tissue at any other location in neck

Nerve Sheath Tumor

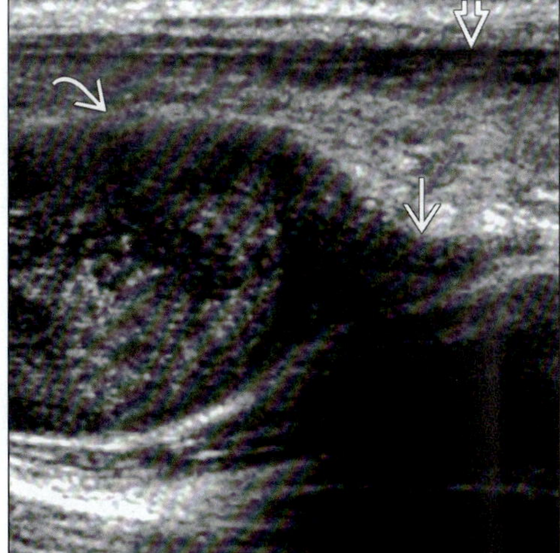

Longitudinal US shows a hypoechoic heterogeneous mass ➡ deep to the sternocleidomastoid muscle ⊟. Note its tapering end ➡, which is continuous with a thickened nerve, characteristic of a NST.

Nerve Sheath Tumor

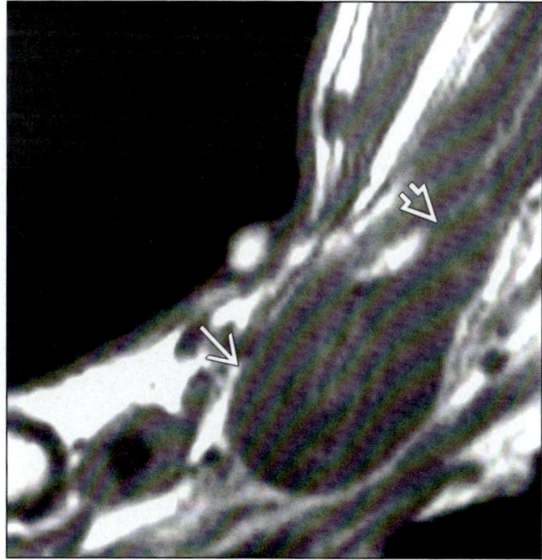

Coronal T1WI MR in the same patient shows a brachial plexus nerve sheath tumor ➡. Note its continuation with the thickened trunk ⊟ of the brachial plexus.

NON-NODAL SOLID NECK MASS

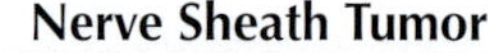

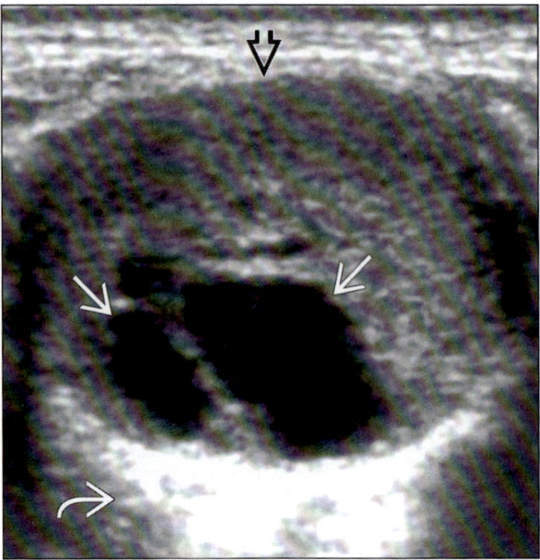

Nerve Sheath Tumor

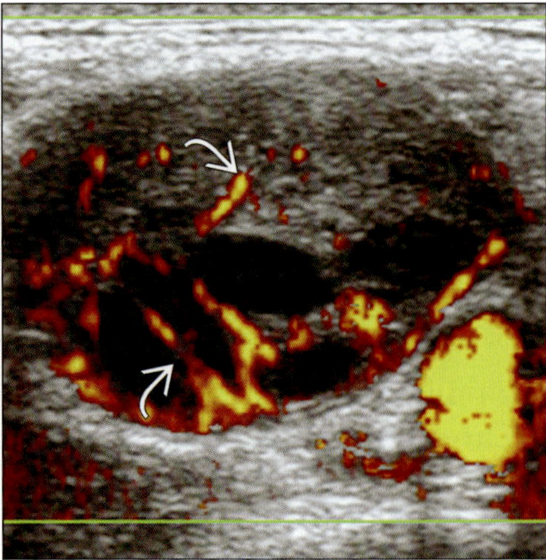

Nerve Sheath Tumor

(Left) Transverse ultrasound of a NST ⊃ shows discrete internal cystic areas ➔ and posterior acoustic enhancement ➔. The intratumoral cystic areas represent mucoid accumulation, necrosis, and hemorrhage. *(Right)* Transverse power Doppler ultrasound in the same patient shows profuse intratumoral vascularity ➔ in the NST. Use gentle transducer pressure to avoid compressing the vessels.

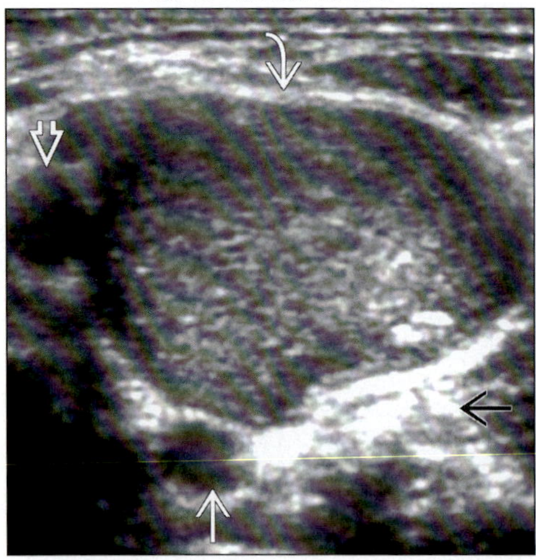

Nerve Sheath Tumor

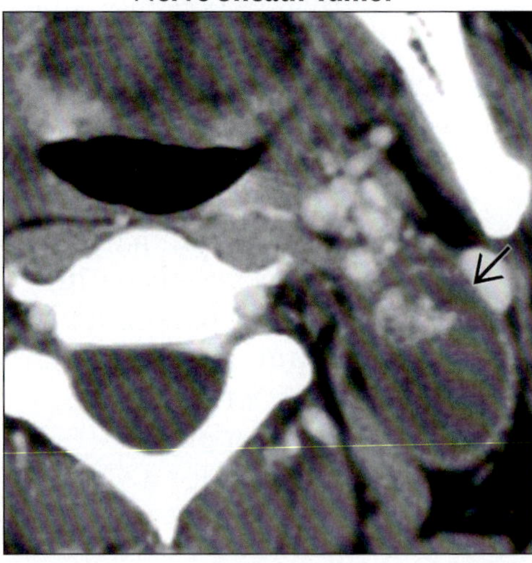

Nerve Sheath Tumor

(Left) Transverse ultrasound shows a solid NST ➔ with posterior acoustic enhancement ➔, despite its solid nature. This "pseudocystic" appearance is characteristic of a NST. The external ➔ and internal ⊃ carotid are splayed by the mass but are not encased (as opposed to carotid body paraganglioma). *(Right)* Axial CECT in the same patient shows the well-defined appearance, location, and relationship of a NST ➔ to the adjacent major vessels.

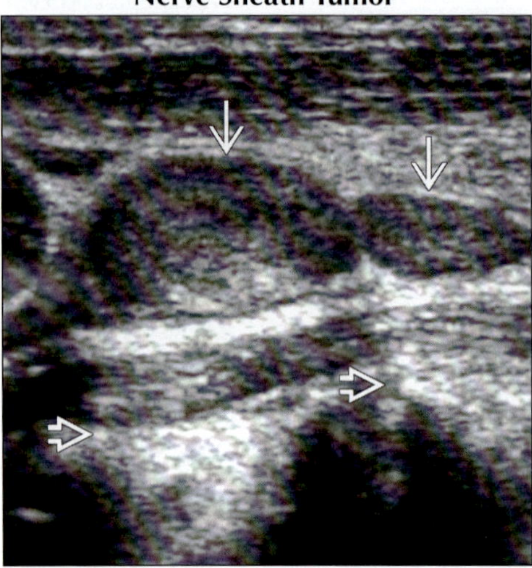

Nerve Sheath Tumor

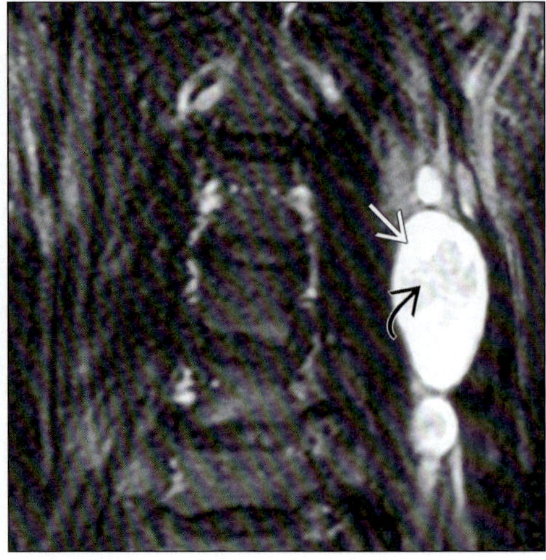

Nerve Sheath Tumor

(Left) Longitudinal ultrasound shows ovoid, well-defined, hypoechoic NSTs ➔ arranged in a chain along the vagus nerve with typical posterior acoustic enhancement ➔. *(Right)* Correlative T2WI MR with fat suppression shows multiple NSTs. Note the "target" sign with a hypo- to isointense center ➔ and hyperintense periphery ➔. US readily establishes the diagnosis, while CECT and MR better demonstrate other associated small NSTs.

1

NON-NODAL SOLID NECK MASS

Lipoma

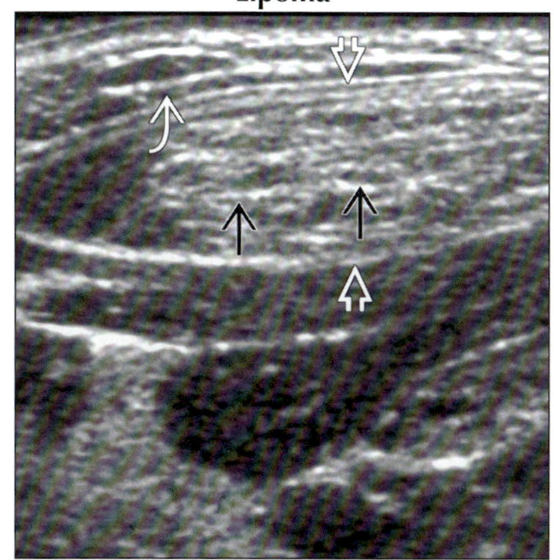

Lipoma

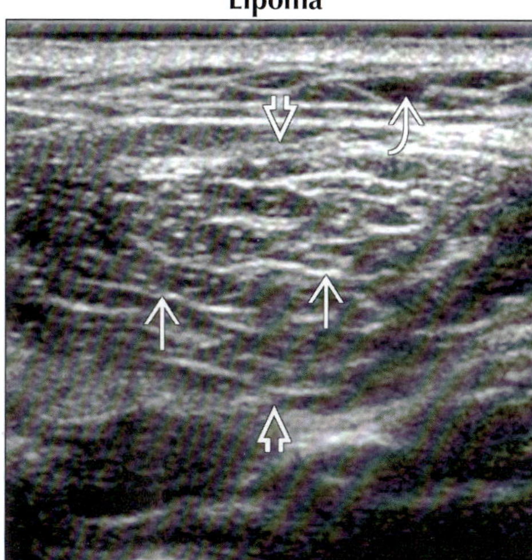

(Left) Longitudinal ultrasound shows a lipoma. Note the long horizontal echogenic stripes producing a feather-like appearance and its similarity to the adjacent muscle. *(Right)* Rotating the transducer shows that the long horizontal stripes are preserved in the transverse plane of the lipoma but not in the overlying muscle. Note similar echogenicity of the lipoma and muscles.

Madelung Disease

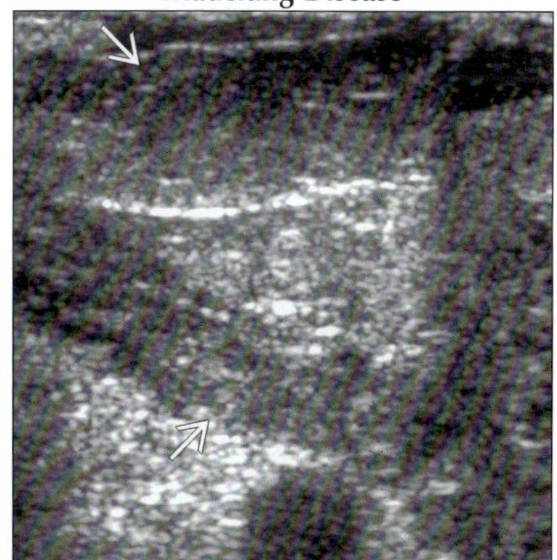

Madelung Disease

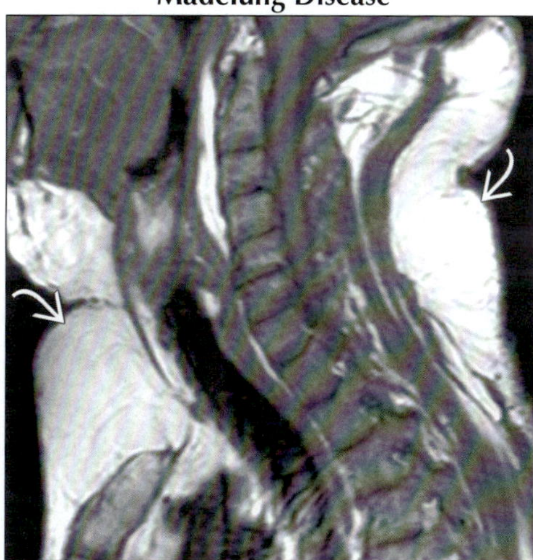

(Left) Transverse ultrasound shows a large, soft, compressible, hypoechoic mass in the subcutaneous layer of the neck with extensive involvement, consistent with Madelung disease. *(Right)* Sagittal T1WI MR in the same patient shows extensive lipomatosis in the neck. Although US readily establishes the diagnosis, CT or MR better evaluates the extent of involvement and presence of any associated tumor, which may be masked by lipomatosis.

Carotid Body Paraganglioma

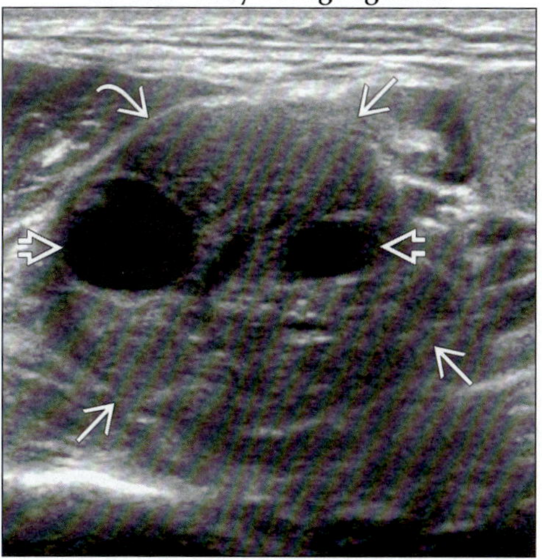

Carotid Body Paraganglioma

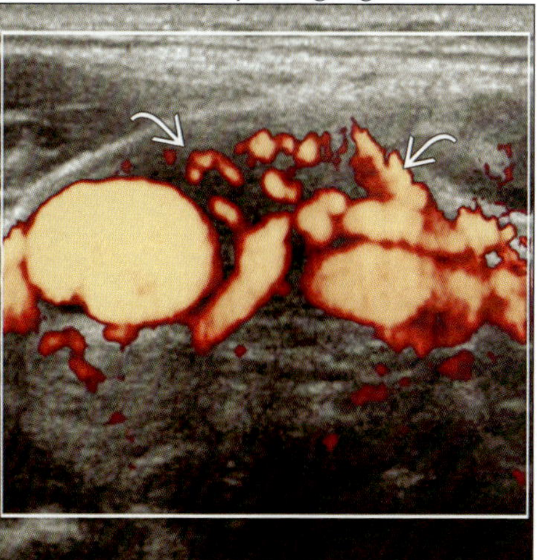

(Left) Transverse ultrasound shows a typical appearance of a CBP with a fine, heterogeneous parenchymal pattern splaying and encasing the carotid arteries without stenosis. Note that the border is typically indistinct on ultrasound despite the sharply marginated nature of the tumor. *(Right)* Transverse power Doppler ultrasound shows typical profuse intratumoral vascularity. The vascularity in the posterior aspect of the tumor is artifactually suppressed.

(Left) Transverse ultrasound shows a large CBP. Note the prominent tortuous internal vessels ⇗ and the splayed and encased arteries ⇒.
(Right) Transverse power Doppler ultrasound in the same patient shows profuse vascularity ⇒ in the tumor and splayed but patent carotid arteries ⇒. Ultrasound readily identifies a contralateral tumor but cannot evaluate glomus jugulare and vagale. CECT or MR is therefore indicated.

Carotid Body Paraganglioma

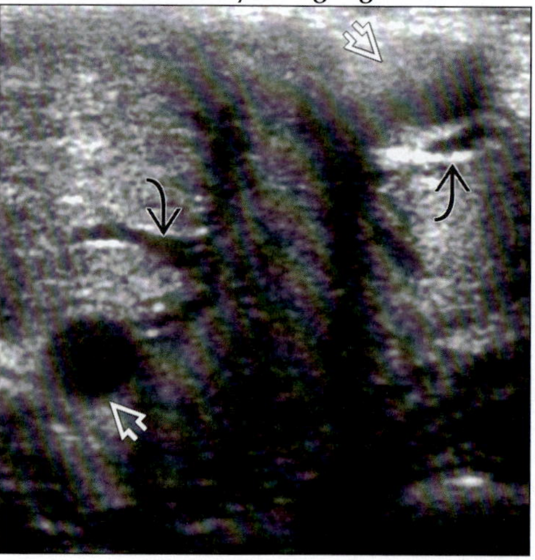

Carotid Body Paraganglioma

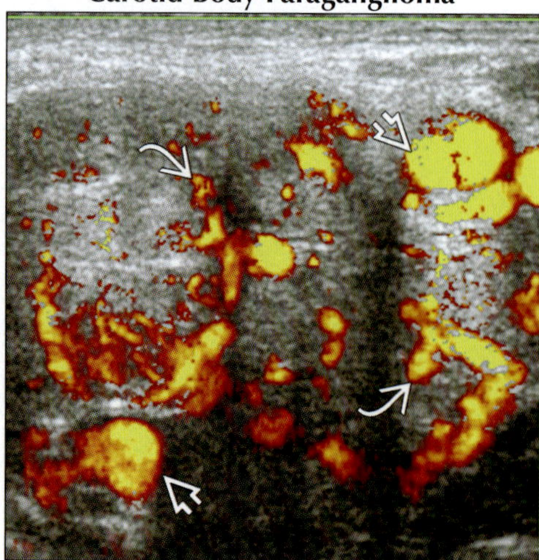

(Left) Axial T1WI MR with fat suppression shows a right CBP. Scattered signal void foci ⇒, which represent small high flow vessels, are the "pepper" in the typical "salt & pepper" appearance of CBP. Splayed carotid arteries ⇒ are also seen.
(Right) Axial T2WI MR with fat suppression shows bilateral carotid body tumors ⇒. Note the bilateral carotid artery ⇒ encasement. MRA provides a vascular road map for preoperative embolization.

Carotid Body Paraganglioma

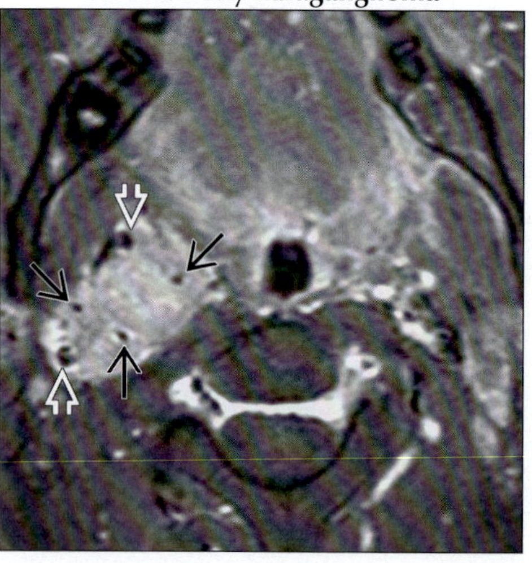

Carotid Body Paraganglioma

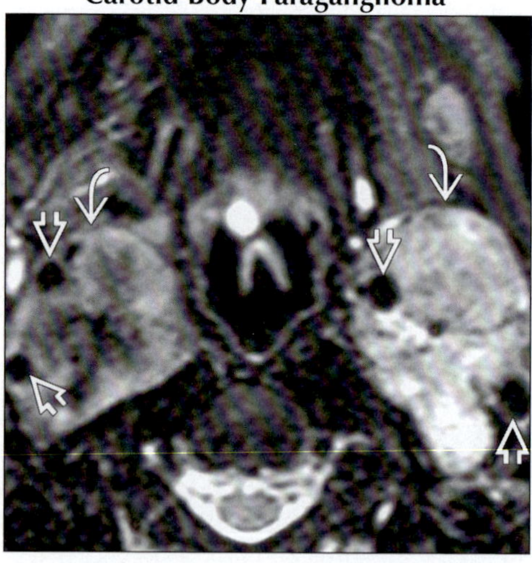

(Left) Axial NECT shows a well-defined, homogeneously hypodense mass ⇒ in the left upper cervical region. *(Right)* Axial CECT shows avid contrast enhancement ⇒ of the mass, close to that of the adjacent vessels. The carotid arteries ⇒ are splayed and partially encased. The features are typical of a carotid body paraganglioma. The coverage on CT/MR should extend from temporal bones to the lower neck.

Carotid Body Paraganglioma

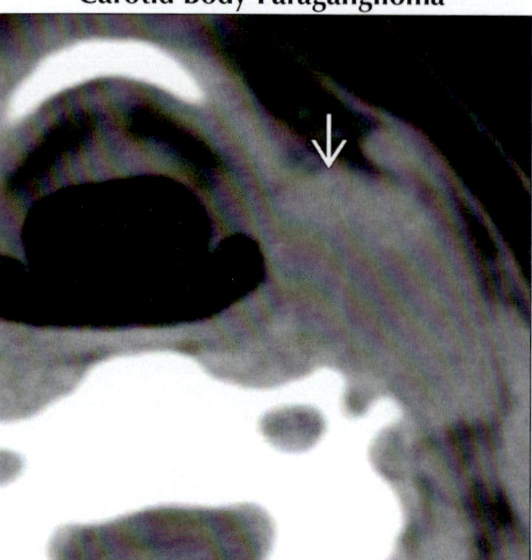

Carotid Body Paraganglioma

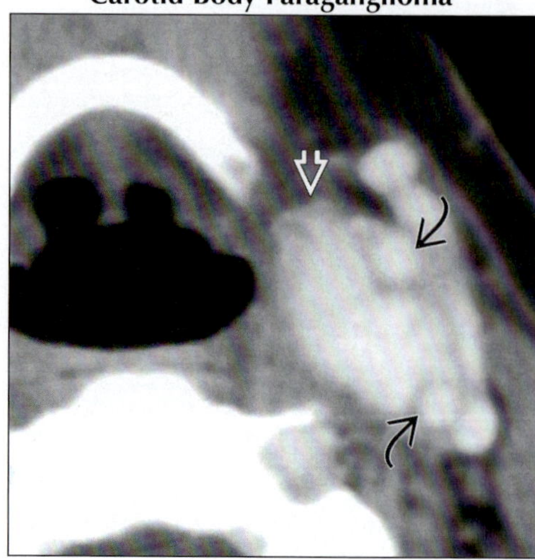

NON-NODAL SOLID NECK MASS

Ectopic Thyroid

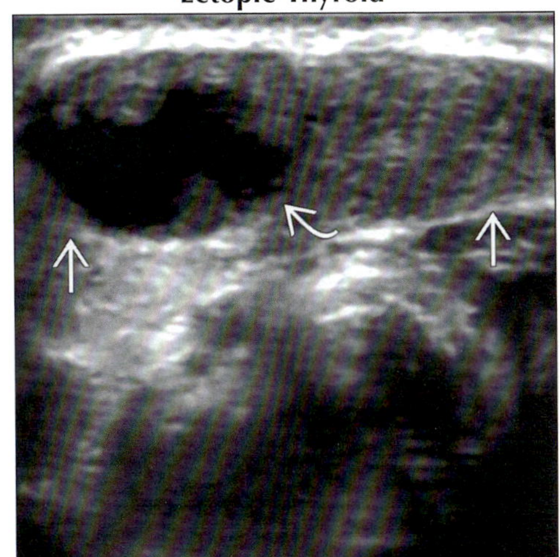

Ectopic Thyroid

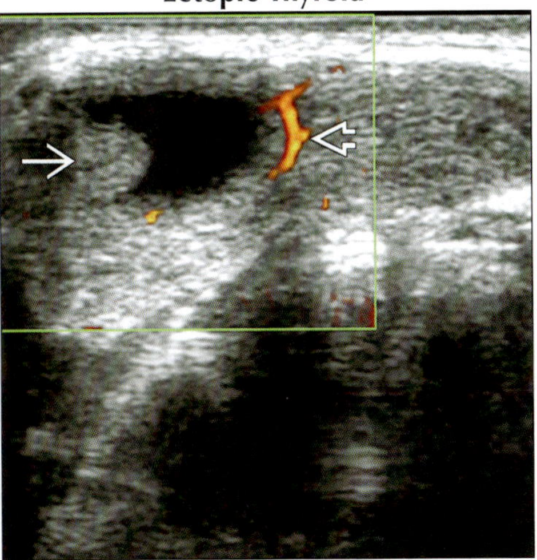

(Left) Longitudinal ultrasound shows ectopic thyroid tissue ➡ in the midline suprahyoid neck. A well-defined nodule with internal cystic change is represented within, consistent with a degenerative thyroid nodule ➡. *(Right)* Longitudinal power Doppler ultrasound in the same patient shows scant vascularity ➡ in ectopic thyroid tissue. No punctate calcification or abnormal vascularity is seen in the solid portion ➡ to suggest a papillary carcinoma.

Ectopic Thyroid

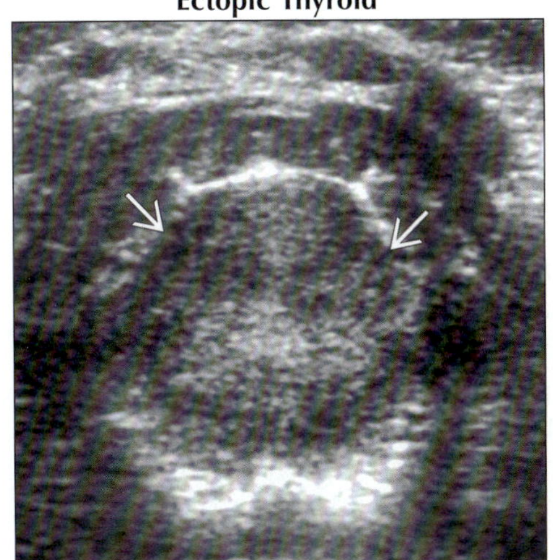

Ectopic Thyroid

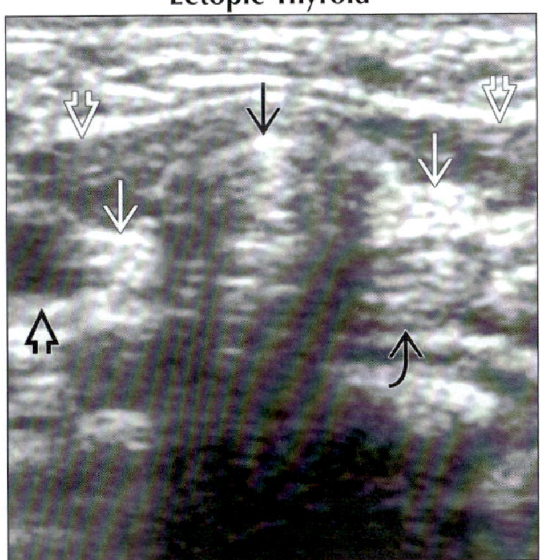

(Left) Transverse ultrasound at the floor of the mouth in the same patient shows an ectopic thyroid gland ➡ at the tongue base. Note the well-defined border and fine homogeneous parenchymal pattern. The parenchymal echopattern is reminiscent of thyroid tissue. *(Right)* Transverse ultrasound in the same patient shows an empty thyroid bed. Note the trachea ➡, esophagus ➡, paratracheal fat ➡, strap muscles ➡, and right CCA ➡.

Ectopic Thyroid

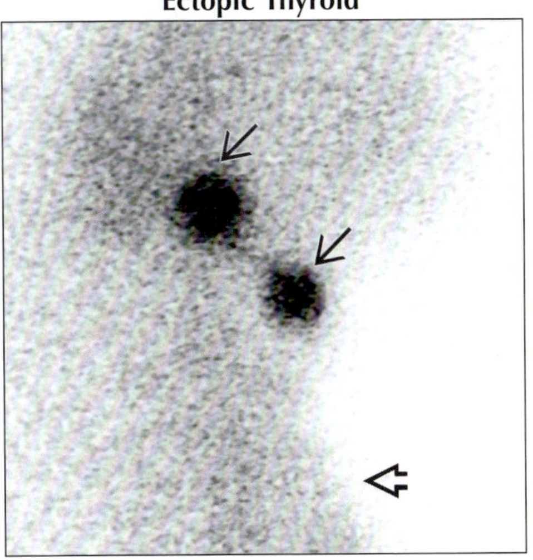

Ectopic Thyroid

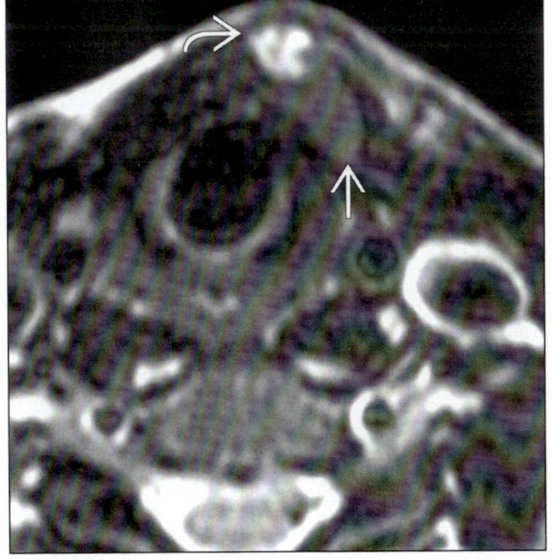

(Left) Thyroid scintigraphy in the same patient shows 2 areas of functioning ectopic thyroid tissue ➡ at the tongue base and in the suprahyoid neck. No thyroid activity is evident in the thyroid bed ➡. *(Right)* Axial T2WI MR with fat suppression in the same patient shows small ectopic thyroid tissue ➡ in the suprahyoid neck containing the degenerative nodule ➡ within.

SOLID NECK LYMPH NODE

DIFFERENTIAL DIAGNOSIS

Common
- Reactive Lymph Node
- Metastatic Lymph Node
- Lymphoma

Less Common
- Calcified Lymph Node
- Tuberculous Infection
- Autoimmune Disease
  - Systemic Lupus Erythematosus (SLE)
  - Rheumatoid Arthritis (RA)

Rare but Important
- Kikuchi Disease
- Kimura Disease
- Rosai-Dorfman Syndrome

ESSENTIAL INFORMATION

Key Differential Diagnosis Issues
- No single sonographic criterion is absolute for malignancy or benignity of lymph nodes
- Size is not reliable predictor of malignancy
  - Serial change in size on follow-up examination is more relevant
  - US able to identify small nodes, which ↑ its sensitivity but ↓ specificity
    - Addition of guided fine-needle aspiration and cytology (FNAC) ↑ specificity
- Findings suggestive of nodal abnormality
  - Round shape, absent hilus, intranodal necrosis, intranodal punctate calcification, reticulation, and disorganized intranodal vascularity

Helpful Clues for Common Diagnoses
- **Reactive Lymph Node**
  - Commonly seen in children, smokers, and patients with allergic rhinitis & recent upper respiratory tract infection
  - Common sites: Submandibular, posterior triangle > internal jugular chain > supraclavicular fossa & intraparotid region
  - Distribution often bilateral & symmetrical
  - Elliptical, homogeneously hypoechoic with normal echogenic hilar architecture
  - Vascularity is central, i.e., from hilus, branching to cortex with tapering ends
    - Dual hila sometimes seen
    - No peripheral vascularity
  - No intranodal necrosis or calcification

- **Metastatic Lymph Node**
  - Location is ipsilateral to primary tumor & in known draining sites of primary tumor
    - Always evaluate for contralateral lymphadenopathy as this may alter staging & management
  - Round, ± eccentric enlargement (eccentric cortical hypertrophy)
    - Most are hypoechoic (except metastatic nodes from papillary carcinoma, iso-/hyperechoic to muscle)
    - Intranodal necrosis: Cystic (hypoechoic) or coagulation necrosis (echogenic, mimicking hilus but not continuous with surrounding fat)
    - Necrotic nodes common in metastases from head and neck SCCa, papillary thyroid carcinoma
  - Calcification: Punctate in papillary carcinoma; coarse, dense shadowing in post-treatment nodes
  - Margins are well defined in malignant nodes, ill defined in inflammatory nodes due to periadenitis (also in post-radiation nodes)
    - If all features of malignancy but ill-defined margins, suggests extracapsular spread (poorer prognosis)
  - Nodal matting & soft tissue edema may be seen in post-treatment nodes
  - Disorganized intranodal vascularity
    - Absent hilar flow to peripheral vascularity (not originating from hilum), displaced vessels, focal avascular areas
- **Lymphoma**
  - Enlarged round node, ± multiple, hilar architecture often preserved
  - Diffuse cortical hypertrophy with reticulated pattern (seen with newer high-frequency transducers)
  - Acoustic enhancement behind solid nodes ("pseudocystic" pattern)
    - Intranodal necrosis is uncommon
  - ± surrounding tissue edema
  - Marked intranodal vascularity: Exaggerated hilar and peripheral vessels
  - Biopsy confirms diagnosis

Helpful Clues for Less Common Diagnoses
- **Calcified Lymph Node**
  - Small foci of calcification: TB, papillary carcinoma

- ○ Coarse calcification: Old TB infection, post-treatment nodes, metastasis from medullary thyroid carcinoma
- **Tuberculous Infection**
  - ○ Sonographic features very similar to malignant lymph nodes except
    - More oval than round
    - Necrosis & matting are seen earlier, i.e., in smaller nodes, and are common features
    - Surrounding edema more prominent
    - Coarse shadowing from calcification may be present (different from punctate calcifications seen in metastatic papillary carcinoma)
    - Necrotic content may discharge to form cold abscess with characteristic "collar stud" appearance
  - ○ Necrosis may be focal, ill defined, & difficult to see
    - Absent or displaced vascularity (at site of necrosis) is supportive evidence
  - ○ Appearances closely mimic metastatic nodes ± superimposed infection or pyogenic nodes
    - FNAC establishes definitive diagnosis
- **Autoimmune Disease**
  - ○ Prominent lymph nodes common in patients with autoimmune disease
    - RA and connective tissue diseases such as Sjögren syndrome, SLE, dermatomyositis
  - ○ Variable sonographic appearance of nodes
    - Reactive in majority of cases

- Cortical hypertrophy, profuse hilar vascularity seen with more active disease
- ↑ risk of lymphoma in RA, Sjögren syndrome, ± SLE and dermatomyositis

Helpful Clues for Rare Diagnoses
- **Kikuchi Disease**
  - ○ Typically young Asian female (20-30 years)
  - ○ Nodes commonly in posterior triangle
  - ○ Oval, hypoechoic, normal hilar architecture ± cortical necrosis
  - ○ ± surrounded by echogenic rim
  - ○ Profuse hilar vascularity + displaced/absent in necrotic areas
- **Kimura Disease**
  - ○ Typically in young Asian male (20-30 years)
  - ○ Nodes within parotid and in vicinity of salivary glands
  - ○ Round, well defined, homogeneous, hypoechoic, ± normal echogenic hilus, ± intranodal necrosis
  - ○ Associated soft tissue masses, salivary & subcutaneous in head & neck (in proximity of salivary glands)
- **Rosai-Dorfman Syndrome**
  - ○ Typically 10- to 20-year-old blacks with massive lymphadenopathy
  - ○ Grayscale and power Doppler features mimic malignant nodes
    - Round, absent hilus, peripheral/mixed vascularity
  - ○ Diagnosis relies on histology

Reactive Lymph Node

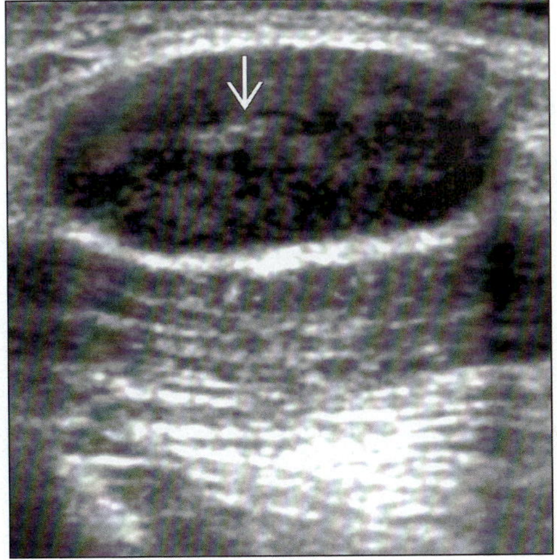

Transverse ultrasound shows a well-defined, oval, hypoechoic lymph node with normal echogenic hilum ➔.

Reactive Lymph Node

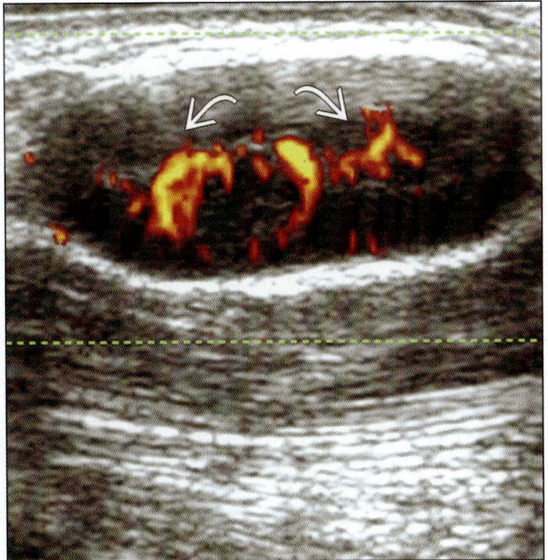

Transverse power Doppler ultrasound in the same patient shows the vessels branching out from the central hilum ➔. These are features of reactive lymph nodes.

SOLID NECK LYMPH NODE

(Left) Transverse ultrasound shows multiple metastatic lymph nodes ➯ in the internal jugular chain. They are round, heterogeneous, & hypoechoic with loss of hilar architecture. Cystic necrosis ➡ is seen in 1. (CCA ➭.) These appearances are commonly seen in nodal metastases from head and neck SCCa. *(Right)* Longitudinal power Doppler ultrasound in the same patient shows disorganized intranodal vascularity with mixed hilar ➡ and peripheral vessels ➦.

Metastatic Lymph Node

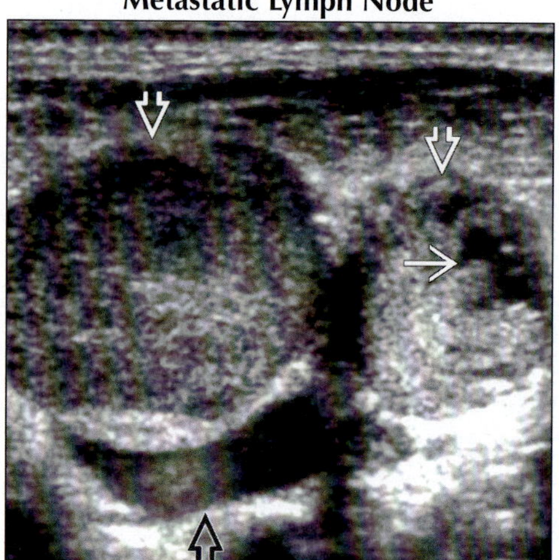

Metastatic Lymph Node

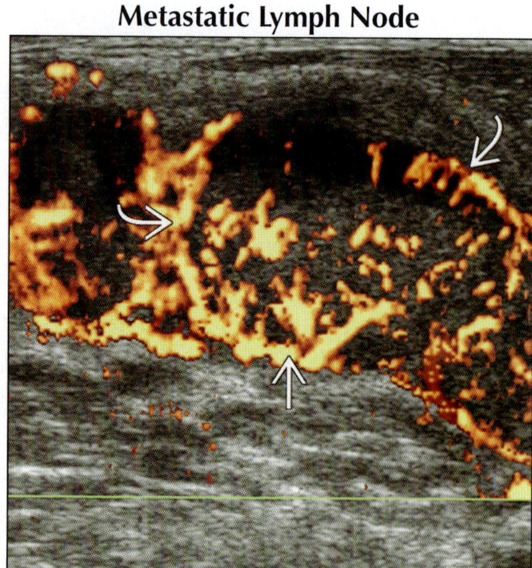

(Left) Transverse ultrasound shows eccentric cortical hypertrophy ➡ in a metastatic lymph node. The echogenic hilus ➶ is preserved. Note the nonhypertrophied part ➡ of the node. FNAC should be directed toward the hypertrophied area. *(Right)* Transverse ultrasound shows a cluster of metastatic LNs ➯ from a H&N SCCa. They are round, well defined, & heterogeneously hypoechoic with marked intranodal necrosis ➡. One appears almost completely cystic.

Metastatic Lymph Node

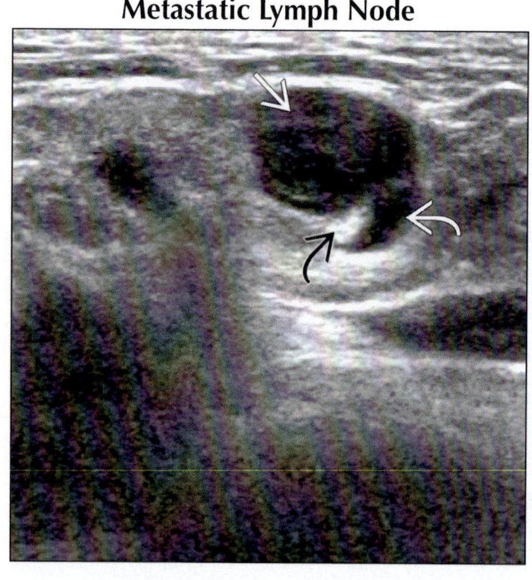

Metastatic Lymph Node

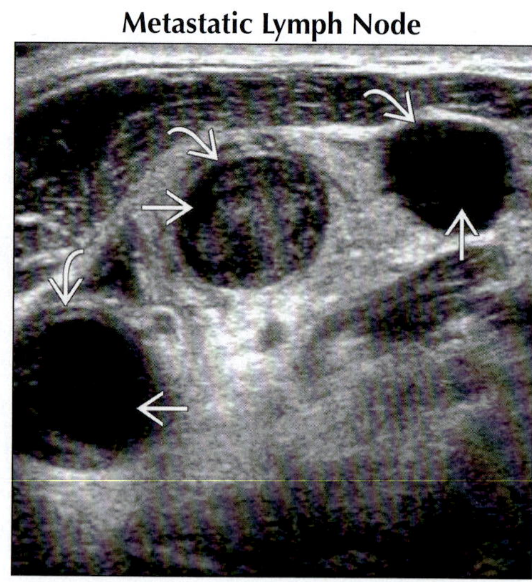

(Left) Transverse US shows round, hypoechoic, heterogeneous, metastatic lymph nodes ➯ with loss of hilar architecture and intranodal eccentric cystic necrosis ➡. Note the sternocleidomastoid muscle ➶. *(Right)* Longitudinal US shows a metastatic LN ➡ with a heterogeneous echopattern. The focal echogenic area represents coagulative necrosis ➡. Note it is not continuous with the perinodal soft tissues (vs. hilus). (CCA ➯, compressed IJV ➦.)

Metastatic Lymph Node

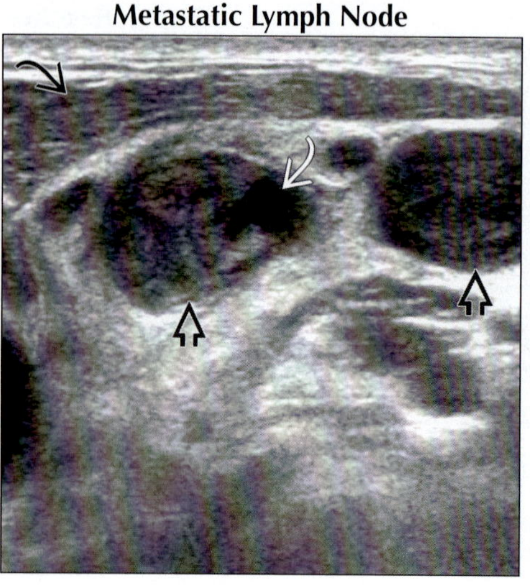

Metastatic Lymph Node

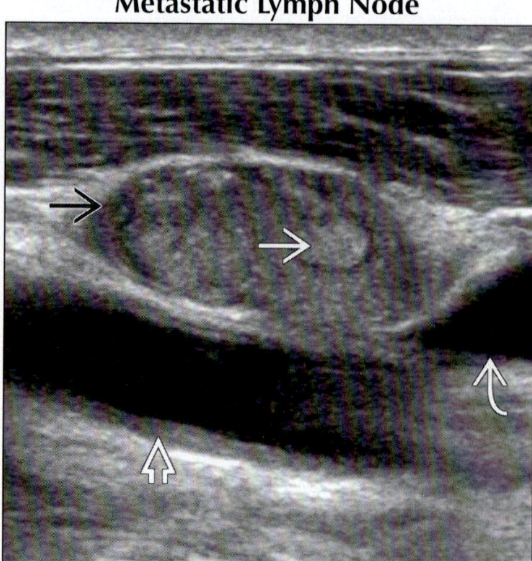

1

SOLID NECK LYMPH NODE

Metastatic Lymph Node

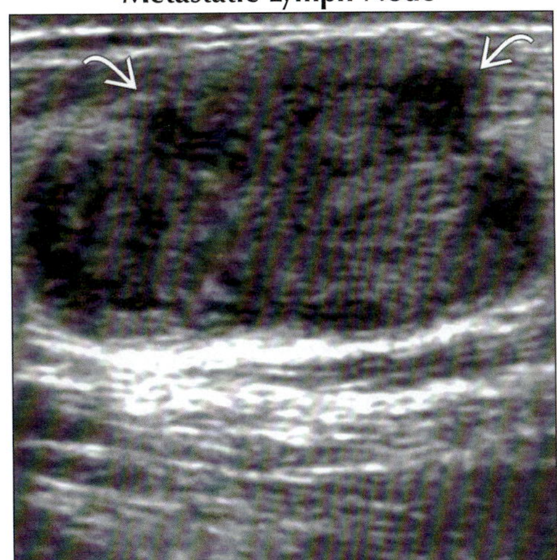

Metastatic Lymph Node

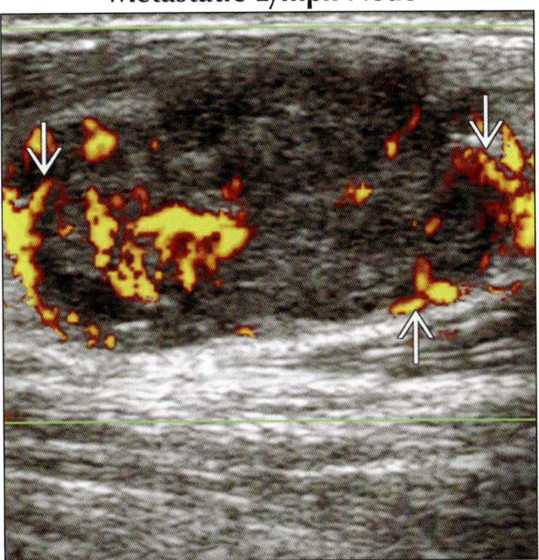

(Left) Longitudinal ultrasound shows a metastatic, heterogeneously hypoechoic lymph node with loss of hilar architecture. The superficial border is ill defined & infiltrative, consistent with extracapsular spread ➡. (Right) Longitudinal power Doppler ultrasound in the same patient shows disorganized peripheral vascularity ➡. The presence of extracapsular spread confers a poor prognosis and should be carefully looked for in metastatic nodes.

Metastatic Lymph Node

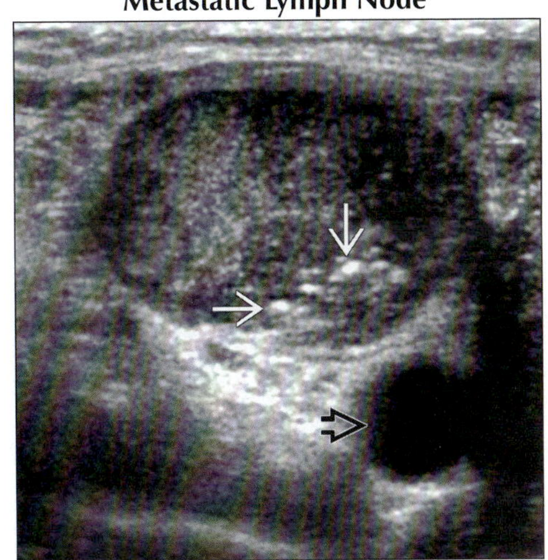

Metastatic Lymph Node

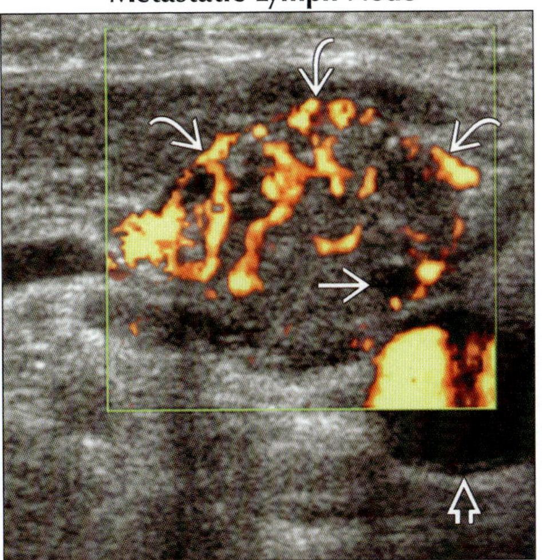

(Left) Transverse US shows a heterogeneously hypoechoic node with multiple punctate calcifications ➡, characteristic for a metastatic node from primary papillary carcinoma of the thyroid. (CCA ➡.) (Right) Transverse power Doppler ultrasound in the same patient shows profuse, disorganized, peripheral, nodal vascularity ➡. No normal hilar vascularity is seen. Note a tiny area of cystic change ➡, frequently seen in such nodes. (CCA ➡.)

Lymphoma

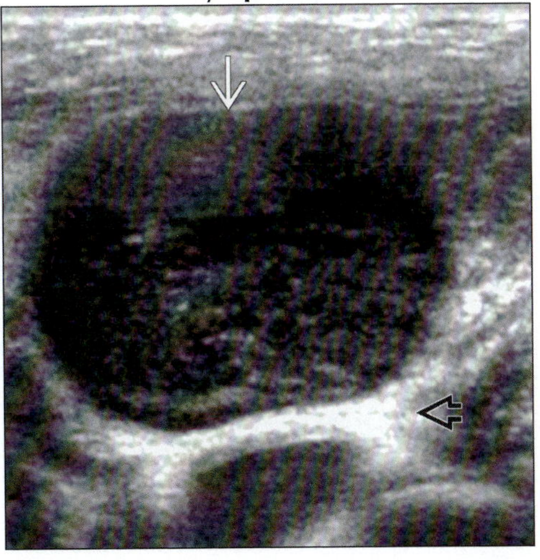

Lymphoma

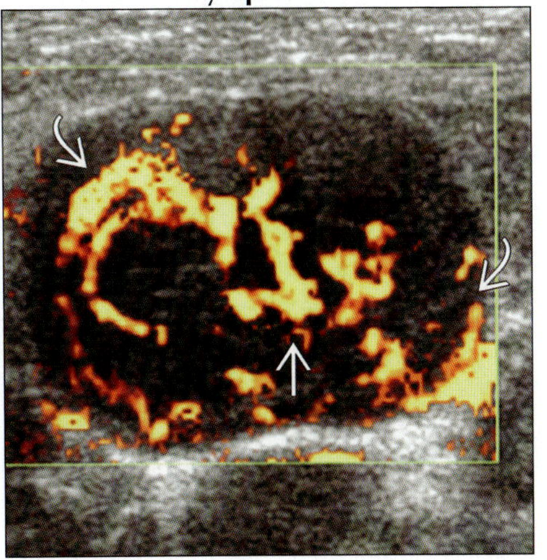

(Left) Transverse US along the internal jugular chain shows a round, solid, hypoechoic LN ➡. An interlaced network with round hypoechoic areas creates the "reticulated" pattern seen in lymphomatous LNs. Posterior acoustic enhancement ➡ is also noted. (Right) Transverse power Doppler ultrasound in the same patient shows exaggerated hilar ➡ and peripheral ➡ vascularity, a common appearance of lymphomatous nodes.

SOLID NECK LYMPH NODE

(Left) *Longitudinal ultrasound shows a chain of densely calcified lymph nodes ➡ in a patient with a previous TB infection. Also note the posterior acoustic shadowing ➡. (Right) Longitudinal ultrasound shows a LN with dense calcification ➡ and posterior shadowing ➡ in a post-treatment patient in clinical remission. The shape, cortex ➡, and echogenic hilum ➡ are otherwise preserved. Such nodes may be hypo-/avascular on Doppler.*

Calcified Lymph Node

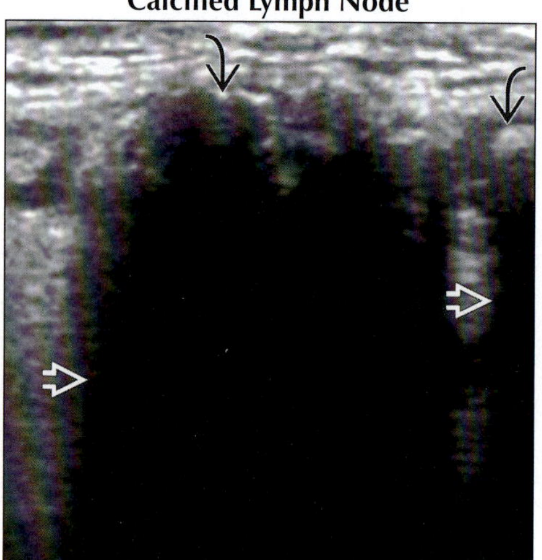

Calcified Lymph Node

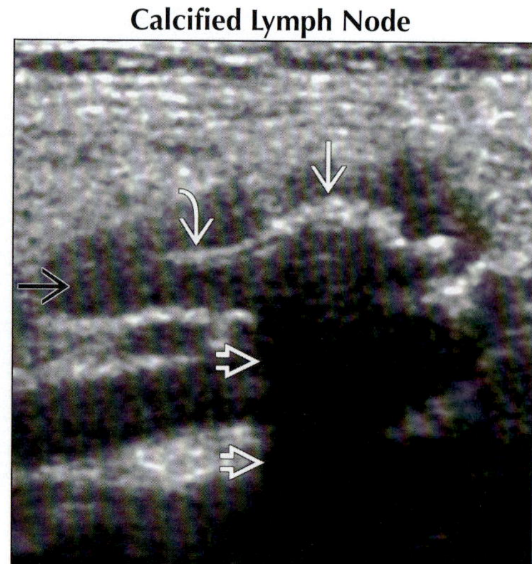

(Left) *Transverse ultrasound shows a cluster of necrotic, hypoechoic, matted lymph nodes ➡ in the upper neck posterior to the ICA ➡ & ECA ➡. A sinus tract ➡ is seen discharging from 1 of the LNs ➡. Note marked surrounding edema ➡. (Right) Longitudinal power Doppler ultrasound shows multiple, hypoechoic, matted nodes ➡ with hilar vascularity ➡ and a focal avascular area ➡ at the site of early necrosis in 1 node. The findings are consistent with TB.*

Tuberculous Infection

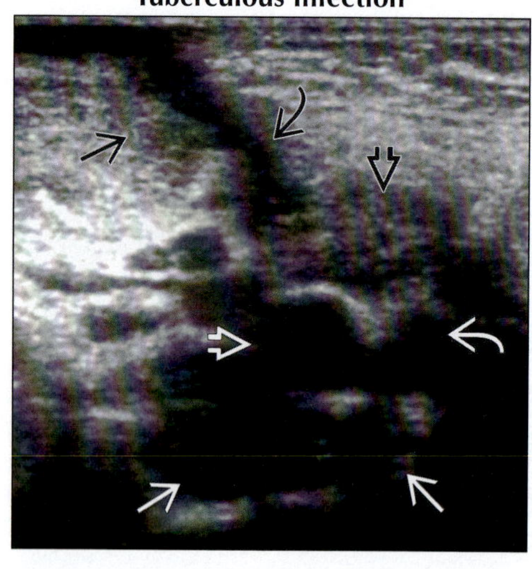

Tuberculous Infection

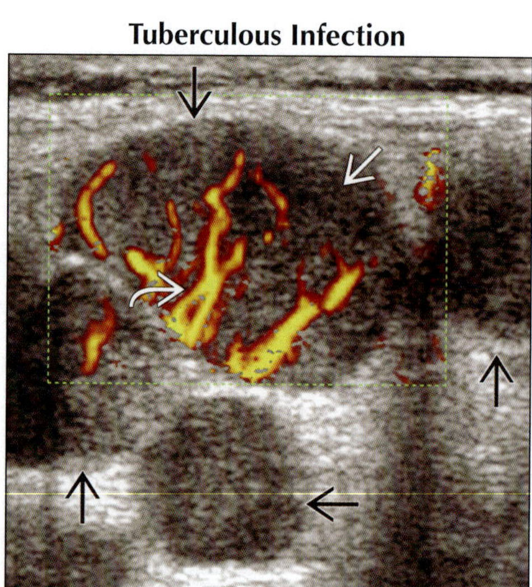

(Left) *Longitudinal power Doppler ultrasound of a patient with SLE shows a prominent LN ➡ that is elliptical and hypoechoic with benign type (hilar) vascularity ➡. This may represent a reactive or inflammatory node in the given clinical setting. (Right) Longitudinal ultrasound shows a chain of prominent LNs ➡ in the posterior triangle with preserved hilar architecture ➡. FNAC revealed Kikuchi disease, which is usually seen in young women.*

Systemic Lupus Erythematosus (SLE)

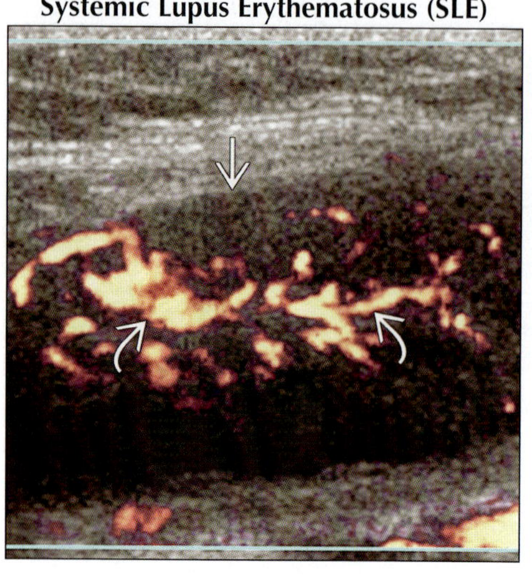

Kikuchi Disease

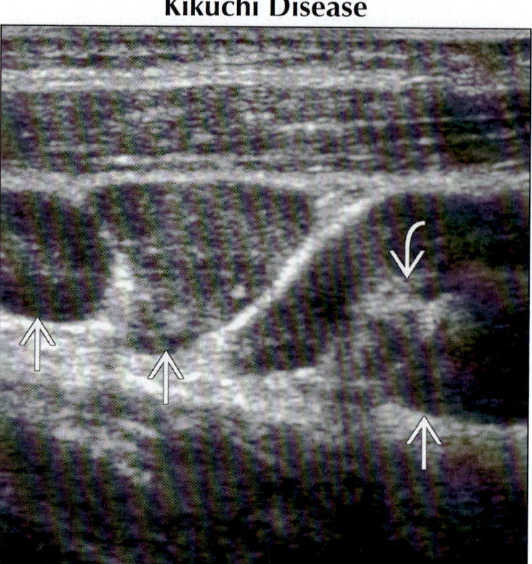

SOLID NECK LYMPH NODE

Kikuchi Disease

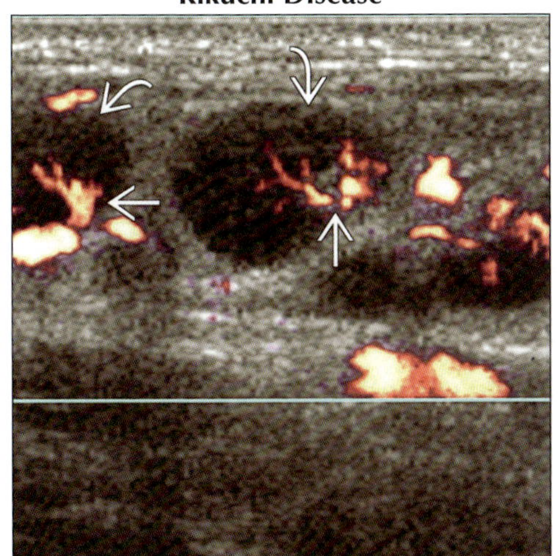

Kimura Disease

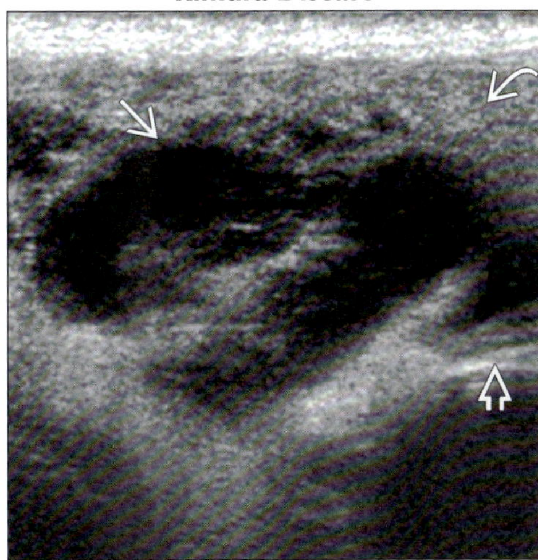

(Left) Longitudinal power Doppler ultrasound shows a benign vascular pattern in LNs ➡, which have a typical radiating hilar vascularity ➡. *(Right)* Transverse US shows an irregular, hypoechoic, soft tissue mass ➡ in the parotid gland ➡. Note the mandible ➡. Other common findings in Kimura disease include abnormal intraparotid nodes and other nodes in the vicinity of enlarged salivary glands are also common findings. Kimura disease is commonly seen in young Asian males.

Kimura Disease

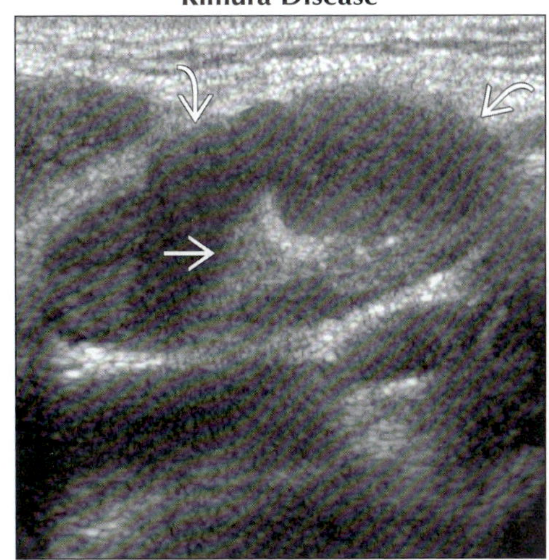

Kimura Disease

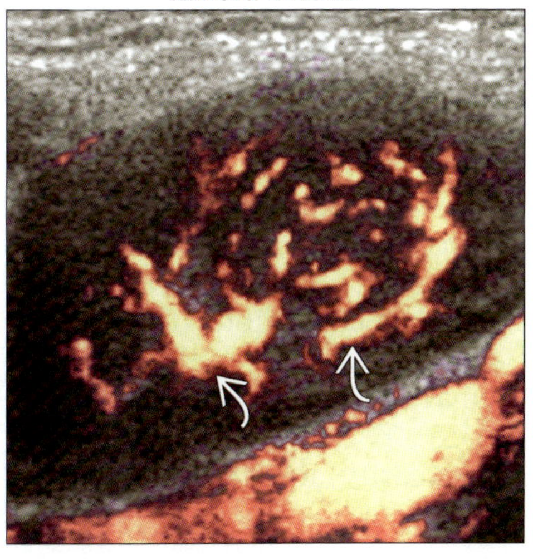

(Left) Longitudinal ultrasound in the same patient shows an enlarged, solid, hypoechoic node ➡ in the posterior triangle. The cortex is diffusely hypertrophied, but the echogenic hilar architecture ➡ is preserved. *(Right)* Longitudinal power Doppler ultrasound in the same patient shows profuse hilar vascularity ➡. Together with the intraparotid soft tissue mass, the features are suggestive of Kimura disease.

Rosai-Dorfman Syndrome

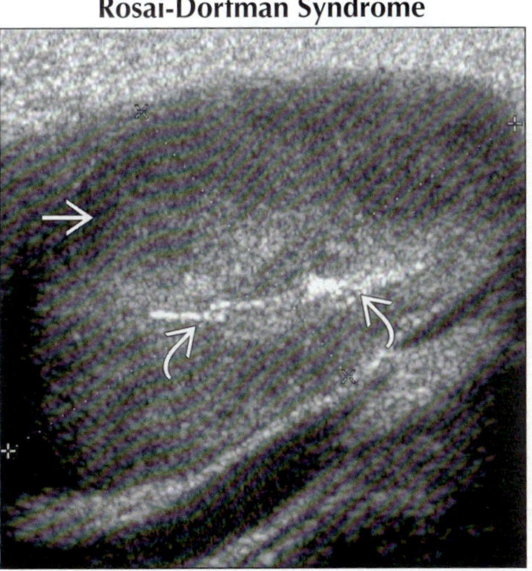

Rosai-Dorfman Syndrome

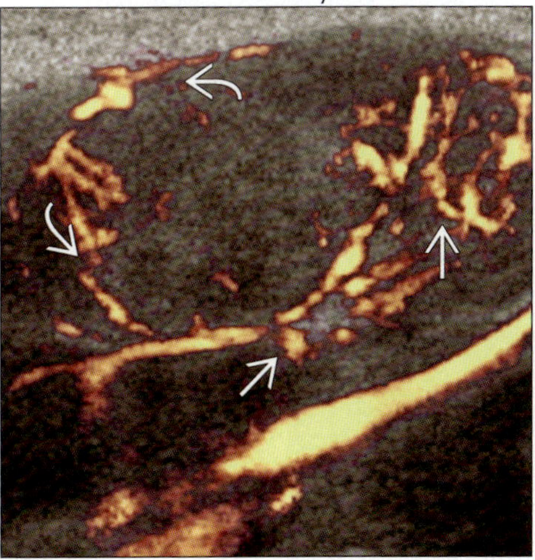

(Left) Longitudinal US shows a markedly enlarged LN in an African adolescent. Note the node's solid, hypoechoic echopattern ➡. The echogenic hilum ➡ is preserved. *(Right)* Longitudinal power Doppler ultrasound in the same patient shows both central ➡ and peripheral ➡ vascularity. The ultrasound findings and clinical setting suggest Rosai-Dorfman syndrome, but metastatic LNs must be excluded. The biopsy confirmed the diagnosis.

1

DIFFERENTIAL DIAGNOSIS

Common
- Metastatic Lymph Node, Squamous Cell Carcinoma (SCCa)
- Tuberculous Lymphadenitis

Less Common
- Metastatic Lymph Node, Papillary Thyroid Carcinoma

ESSENTIAL INFORMATION

Key Differential Diagnosis Issues
- Punctate calcification within solid component of necrotic lymph node is characteristic of metastasis from papillary carcinoma of thyroid

Helpful Clues for Common Diagnoses
- **Metastatic Lymph Node, Squamous Cell Carcinoma (SCCa)**
  - Primary: Head and neck SCCa, esophagus, lung, distant or unknown primary
    - Primary head and neck SCCa, follows expected nodal drainage of tumor
  - Round, heterogeneous, hypoechoic, loss of normal hilar architecture reported in 69-95% of involved nodes
  - Cystic necrosis is common; can be small to entirely cystic
  - Coagulative necrosis seen as echogenic foci/areas
  - Doppler: Disorganized vascularity, absent vascularity in necrotic areas

- **Tuberculous Lymphadenitis**
  - Common in young adults and new immigrants to endemic area
  - Posterior triangle ± discharging sinus ± low-grade fever
  - Heterogeneous hypoechoic lymph nodes, ovoid > rounded
  - Early necrosis seen as small cortical hypoechoic area with displaced vascularity
  - Larger necrotic nodes tend to mat together and have associated soft tissue edema (scrofula)
  - Discharge of contents of necrotic node form large subcutaneous abscess, "collar stud" abscess
  - Following fine-needle aspiration and cytology (FNAC), send specimen for culture, PCR to establish diagnosis

Helpful Clues for Less Common Diagnoses
- **Metastatic Lymph Node, Papillary Thyroid Carcinoma**
  - Round or ovoid with large cystic areas
  - Solid component contains punctate calcification and internal vascularity
  - Primary carcinoma in ipsilateral thyroid lobe may be occult
  - Lymph nodes in expected drainage areas
    - Anterior compartment and along internal jugular vein
  - Exclude contralateral neck node metastasis in tumors close to midline
  - FNAC should be directed toward solid area with calcifications

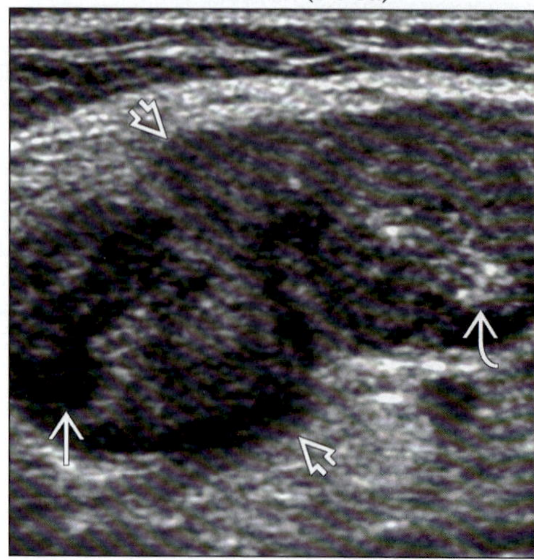

Metastatic Lymph Node, Squamous Cell Carcinoma (SCCa)

Transverse ultrasound shows round, heterogeneously hypoechoic neck nodes with cystic ➡ and coagulative ➡ necrosis. The ill-defined border ➡ is suggestive of extracapsular spread.

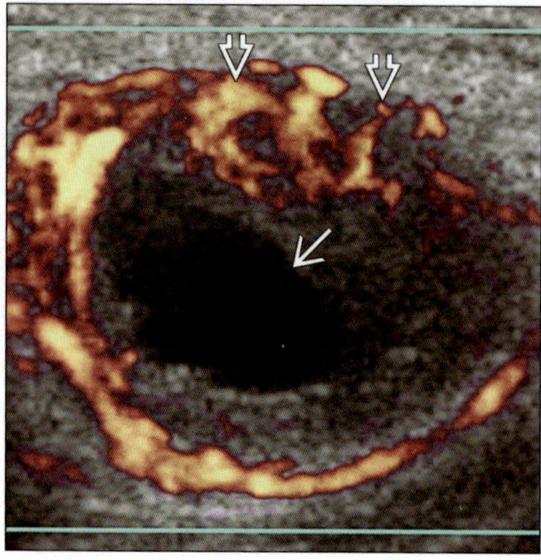

Metastatic Lymph Node, Squamous Cell Carcinoma (SCCa)

Transverse power Doppler ultrasound shows a necrotic ➡ neck node from squamous cell carcinoma. Note the marked, disorganized, peripheral vascularity ➡, reflecting tumor neovascularity.

NECROTIC NECK LYMPH NODE

Tuberculous Lymphadenitis

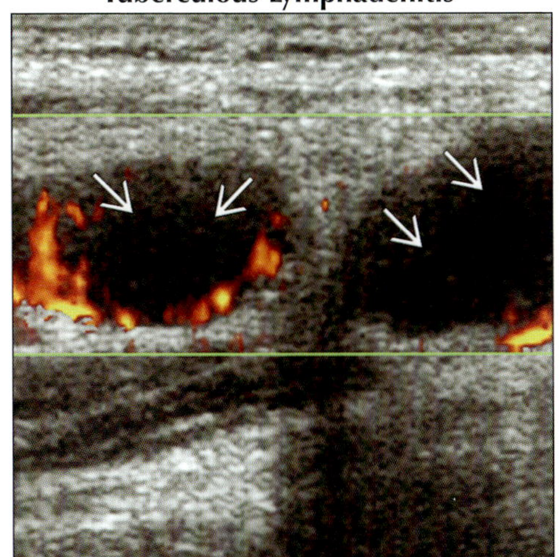

Tuberculous Lymphadenitis

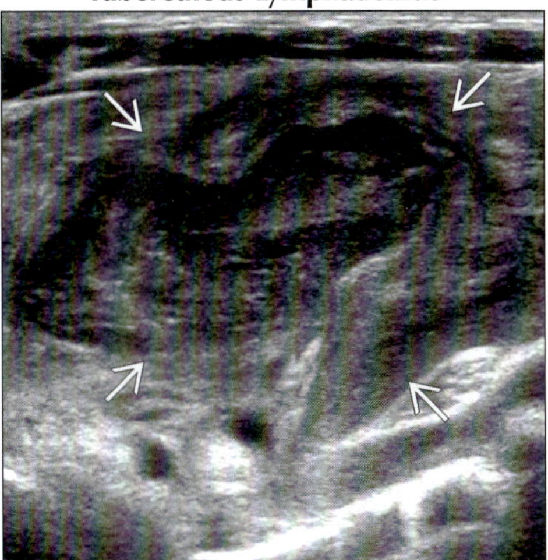

(Left) Longitudinal power Doppler ultrasound of a posterior triangle shows typical small TB lymph nodes. Note multiplicity of nodes, which are ill defined with necrotic, avascular, hypoechoic areas ➡. The vessels are displaced around the necrotic areas. (Right) Transverse ultrasound shows a large irregular TB abscess ➡ with thick walls and internal debris. The aspirated contents of such an abscess should be sent for PCR and AFB culture to confirm diagnosis.

Tuberculous Lymphadenitis

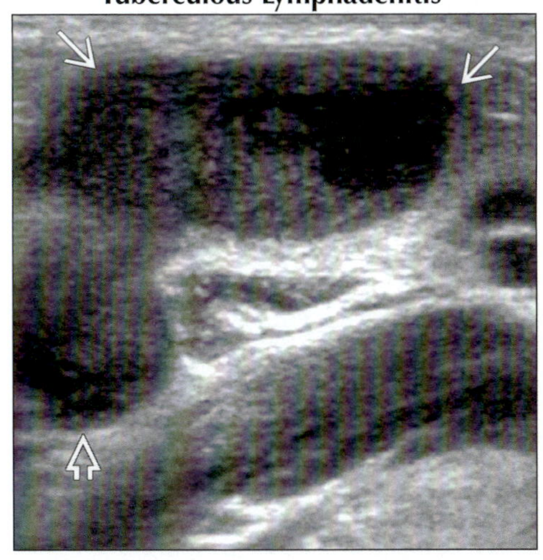

Tuberculous Lymphadenitis

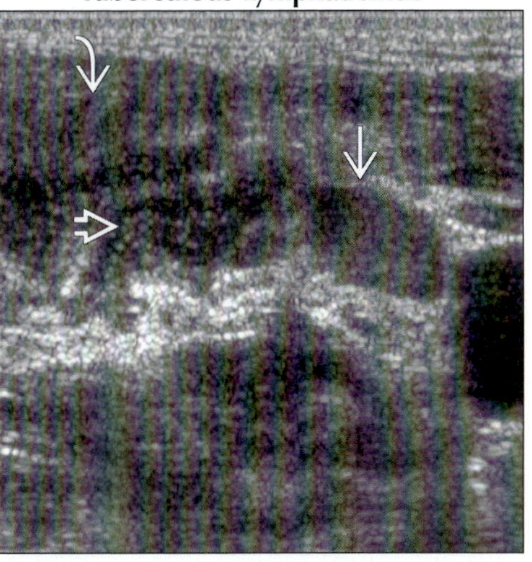

(Left) Transverse ultrasound of the right posterior triangle shows a characteristic "collar stud" abscess in TB lymphadenitis. Note that the necrotic node ➡ has discharged its contents into the subcutaneous tissues, forming an abscess ➡. (Right) Longitudinal ultrasound of the posterior triangle in a patient with TB lymphadenitis shows diffuse soft tissue edema ➡ with focal areas of abscess formation ➡ adjacent to an abnormal node ➡.

Metastatic Lymph Node, Papillary Thyroid Carcinoma

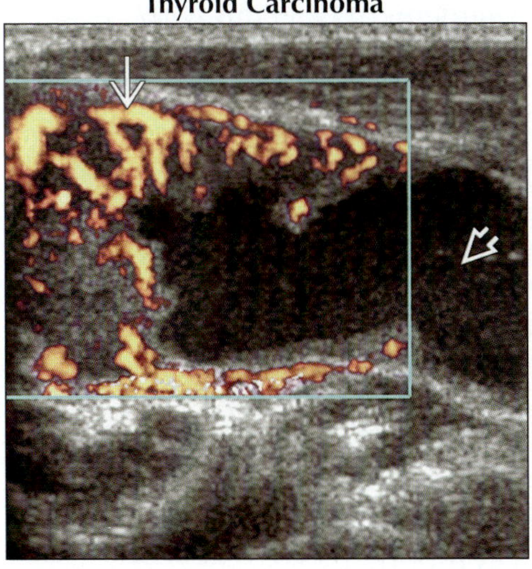

Metastatic Lymph Node, Papillary Thyroid Carcinoma

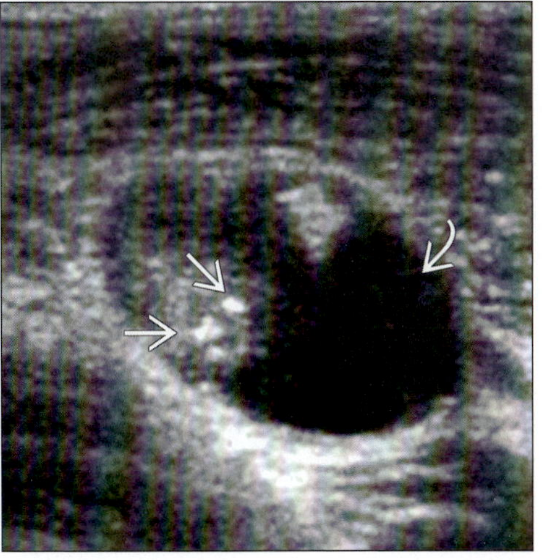

(Left) Longitudinal power Doppler ultrasound shows a well-defined, ovoid, metastatic neck node. Note the large cystic area ➡ and profuse vascularity ➡ in the solid component. (Right) Transverse ultrasound of a cervical lymph node shows a cystic area ➡ and a solid mural nodule with punctate calcifications ➡. The presence of punctate calcifications is very suggestive of a papillary thyroid carcinoma primary.

DIFFUSE SALIVARY GLAND ENLARGEMENT

DIFFERENTIAL DIAGNOSIS

Common
- Acute Sialadenitis
  - Calculus Sialadenitis
  - Infective Sialadenitis
- Chronic Sialadenitis

Less Common
- Sjögren Syndrome (SJS)
- Sarcoidosis
- Benign Lymphoepithelial Lesion (BLEL)
- Lymphangioma
- Hemangioma/Venous Vascular Malformation (VVM)
- Kuttner Tumor
- Kimura Disease

Rare but Important
- Metastasis
- Lymphoma

ESSENTIAL INFORMATION

Key Differential Diagnosis Issues
- Submandibular glands scanned in transverse, longitudinal, and oblique planes to demonstrate abnormality and anatomy
- For parotid glands, transverse scans define location of abnormality in relation to external carotid artery and retromandibular vein
  - Longitudinal scans help to evaluate parenchyma and parotid tail
- US does not evaluate pathology in deep lobe of parotid gland as gland is obscured by mandible
  - Consider CT or MR

Helpful Clues for Common Diagnoses
- **Acute Sialadenitis**
  - Diffusely hypoechoic, enlarged gland with hypervascularity ± abscess
  - ± ductal dilatation, ± echogenic ductal stone, ± posterior shadowing
    - Parotid calculi may be difficult to detect on US; NECT much more sensitive
  - Submandibular > parotid
    - Submandibular saliva is thicker, more mucinous, and alkaline than parotid
- **Chronic Sialadenitis**
  - Atrophic gland with heterogeneous, hypoechoic echopattern

---

  - Enlarged gland with cystic dilatation of ducts and parenchymal atrophy
    - Indistinguishable from SJS and BLEL
    - Sialadenitis often involves 1 gland rather than multiple (vs. SJS & BLEL)

Helpful Clues for Less Common Diagnoses
- **Sjögren Syndrome (SJS)**
  - Parotid > submandibular > sublingual ± lacrimal gland; bilateral involvement
  - Early phase
    - Normal-sized or diffusely enlarged glands, normal parenchymal pattern
  - Intermediate phase
    - Diffusely enlarged glands + multiple cysts of similar size and solid masses (representing parenchymal destruction & lymphoid aggregates)
    - Microcystic (cysts < 1 mm, may be missed) or macrocystic pattern
  - May be indistinguishable from BLEL on US, but tonsillar hyperplasia & reactive cervical LNs not features
  - Diagnosis is clinical, serological + confirmed with biopsy
  - Imaging to confirm/exclude salivary gland involvement and surveillance for lymphomatous change
- **Sarcoidosis**
  - Nonspecific US appearances
    - Affects submandibular > parotid glands
  - May be seen as diffuse hypoechogenicity with normal-sized or enlarged gland
- **Benign Lymphoepithelial Lesion (BLEL)**
  - Mainly involves parotid glands
  - 5% of HIV-positive patients develop BLEL of parotids
  - Diffuse enlargement of gland with multiple cysts, mixed cystic and solid lesions, &/or solid nodules
    - Cysts are thin walled ranging from a few mm up to 3.5 cm
    - Solid lesions: Ill-defined masses representing lymphoid aggregates
- **Lymphangioma**
  - Thin-walled, multiseptated cystic lesion ± debris, ± fluid level, hypo-/avascular
- **Hemangioma/Venous Vascular Malformation (VVM)**
  - US appearance reflects histology
    - Hemangioma: Small vessels with ↑ stromal component

DIFFUSE SALIVARY GLAND ENLARGEMENT

- ▪ VVM: Sinusoidal spaces with ↓ stroma
- Phleboliths may be seen; more in slow flow lesions such as VVM
- Doppler shows internal vascularity in medium to high flow vessels
  - ▪ Slow flow often better seen on grayscale as motion of debris/contents within VVM
- **Kuttner Tumor**
  - Chronic sclerosing sialadenitis
  - Submandibular > > > parotid gland
    - ▪ Bilateral involvement is common
  - Diffuse "cirrhotic" gland
    - ▪ Diffusely heterogeneous, hypoechoic parenchymal echopattern with lobulated contours
  - Focal "geographic" pattern
    - ▪ Focal, ill-defined, hypoechoic areas (simulating malignancy) in gland
  - Doppler US: Preserved architecture with hypervascularity in involved areas
    - ▪ No mass effect by hypoechoic "mass"
- **Kimura Disease**
  - Subcutaneous masses ± salivary gland (parotid > submandibular) masses ± lymphadenopathy in young Asian males
  - Masses may be ill/well defined and hypoechoic with variable vascularity on Doppler
  - Background glandular parenchyma may be heterogeneous

Helpful Clues for Rare Diagnoses
- **Metastasis**
  - Note: Parotid gland contains nodes and is, therefore, site of nodal metastases
  - Common 1° tumor: Malignant melanoma, squamous cell carcinoma in face, lateral scalp, & external auditory meatus
  - US: Solitary/multiple hypoechoic nodules, solid, ± ill-defined, ± skin/subcutaneous/extraparotid extension
  - Multiplicity and history of known head & neck malignant 1° should raise suspicion
- **Lymphoma**
  - Primary: More common in Sjögren syndrome, rheumatoid arthritis, & patients on immunosuppressants
  - Secondary: In 1-8% of patients with systemic lymphoma
  - 80% involve parotid glands (both 1° & 2°)
  - Nodal involvement: Enlarged lymph node + reticulated pattern or microcystic appearance + through transmission + central & peripheral vascularity
  - Parenchymal involvement: Diffuse, heterogeneous, hypoechoic pattern (mimicking sialadenitis) or as ill-defined, irregular, hypoechoic, hypervascular mass

Alternative Differential Approaches
- Cystic: Chronic sialadenitis, SJS, BLEL, lymphangioma ± hemangioma/VVM
- Diffuse hypoechoic infiltration: Acute calculus or infective sialadenitis ± metastasis
- Tumor-like: Hemangioma, Kimura disease, Kuttner tumor, metastasis, lymphoma

Acute Sialadenitis

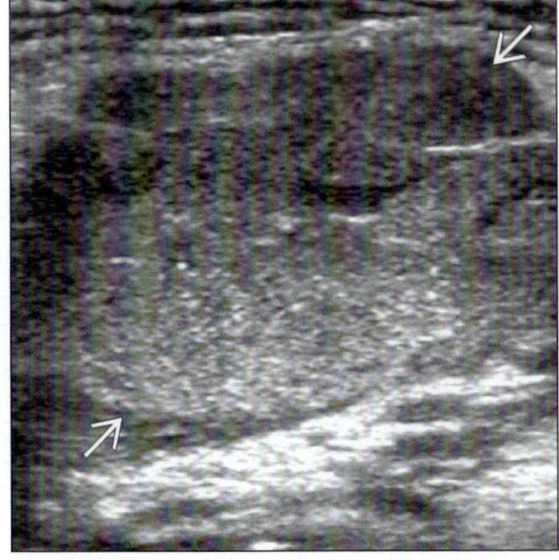

Transverse ultrasound shows a right submandibular gland ➡ that is diffusely enlarged and hypoechoic with a rounded contour. No focal lesion, stone, or duct dilatation is seen.

Acute Sialadenitis

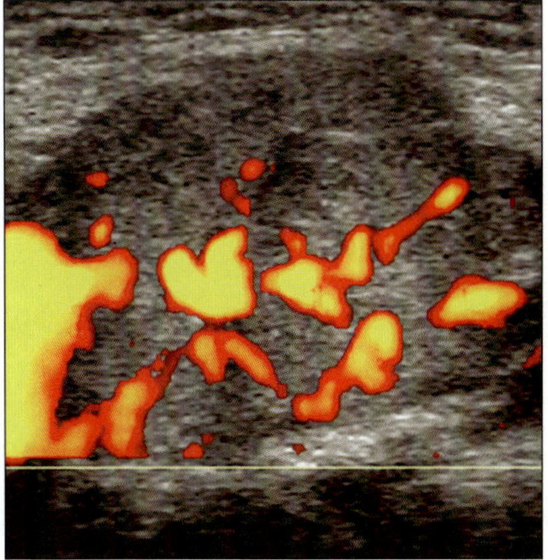

Transverse power Doppler ultrasound in the same patient with acute sialadenitis shows diffuse hypervascularity. Effort must be made to detect any duct dilatation or intraductal stone.

DIFFUSE SALIVARY GLAND ENLARGEMENT

(Left) Transverse ultrasound of the submental region in this patient with left submandibular sialadenitis shows a curvilinear echogenic focus ⇗ with strong posterior shadowing ⇨ at the termination site of the Wharton duct, representing salivary calculus as obstructive cause. (Right) Transverse power Doppler ultrasound shows an intraglandular ductal stone ⇨ & duct dilatation ⇨ in a patient with submandibular sialadenitis. Note posterior acoustic shadowing ⇨.

Calculus Sialadenitis

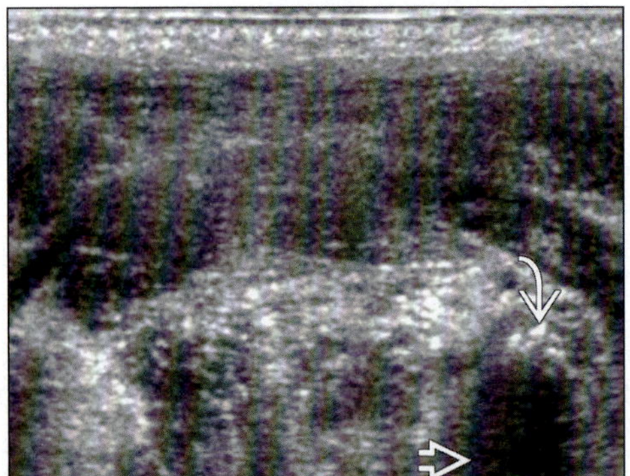

Calculus Sialadenitis

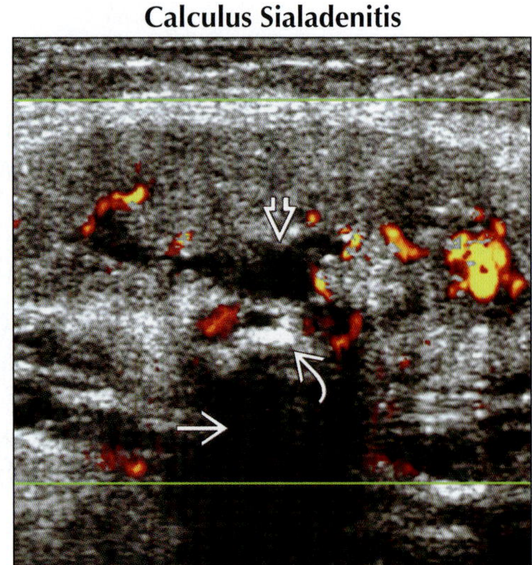

(Left) Transverse ultrasound shows an enlarged parotid gland with a multicystic ⇨ appearance. The cystic spaces are interconnecting ⇨, which would not be seen in SJS or BLEL. Note the parenchymal atrophy (mandible ⇨). (Right) Coronal T2WI MR with fat suppression (sialogram) in the same patient shows cystic spaces ⇨ along the branches of the parotid ducts ⇗, representing cystic dilatation of intraglandular ducts due to chronic sialadenitis.

Chronic Sialadenitis

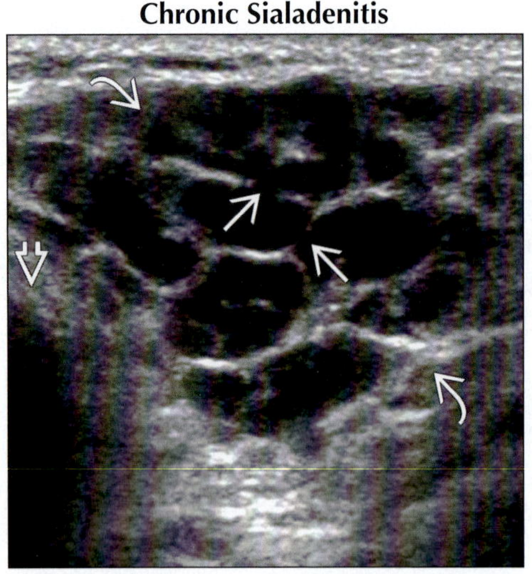

Chronic Sialadenitis

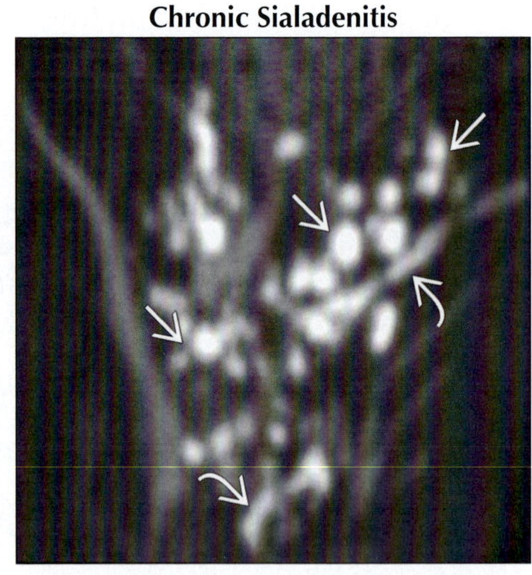

(Left) Transverse ultrasound shows an enlarged parotid gland with multiple cysts ⇨ and nodules ⇨ scattered throughout the gland, against a heterogeneous parenchymal background. (Right) Transverse ultrasound of the orbit in the same patient shows lacrimal gland ⇗ involvement. The gland is enlarged and heterogeneously hypoechoic with a similar appearance to that of the parotid gland. Lacrimal gland involvement is not seen in BLEL. Note the globe ⇨ and orbital rim ⇨.

Sjögren Syndrome (SJS)

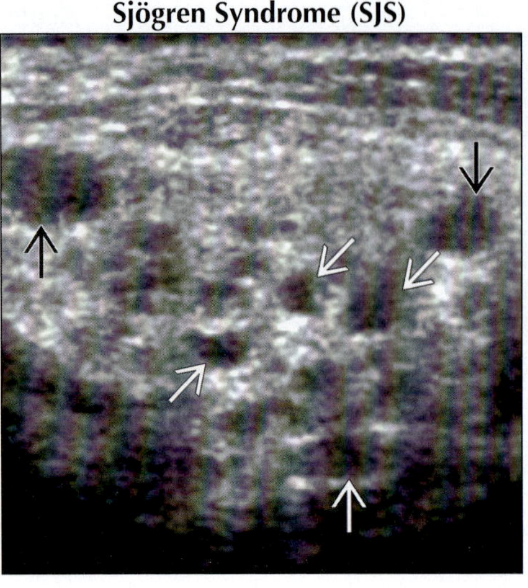

Sjögren Syndrome (SJS)

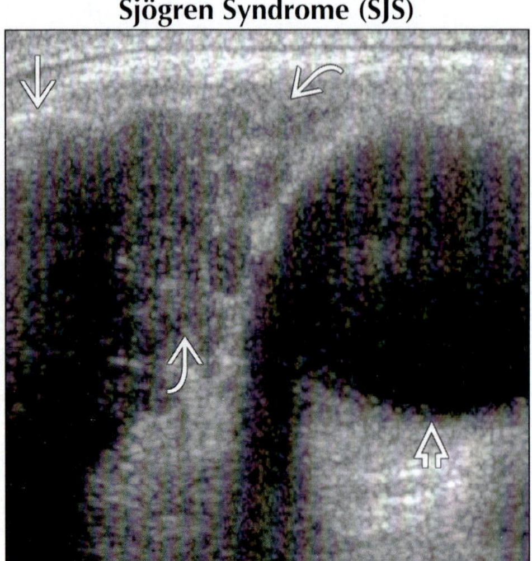

DIFFUSE SALIVARY GLAND ENLARGEMENT

Benign Lymphoepithelial Lesion (BLEL)

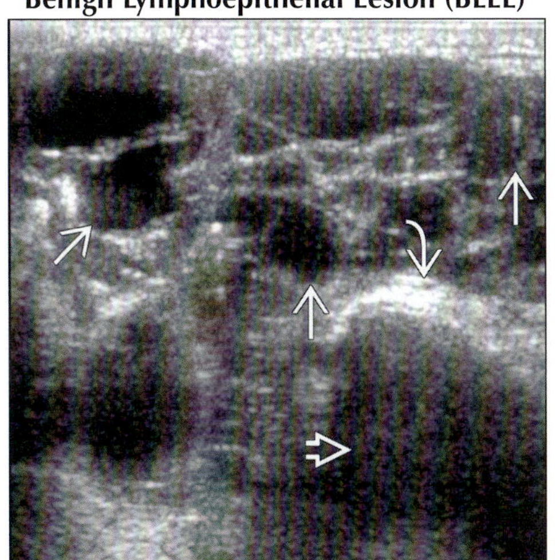

Benign Lymphoepithelial Lesion (BLEL)

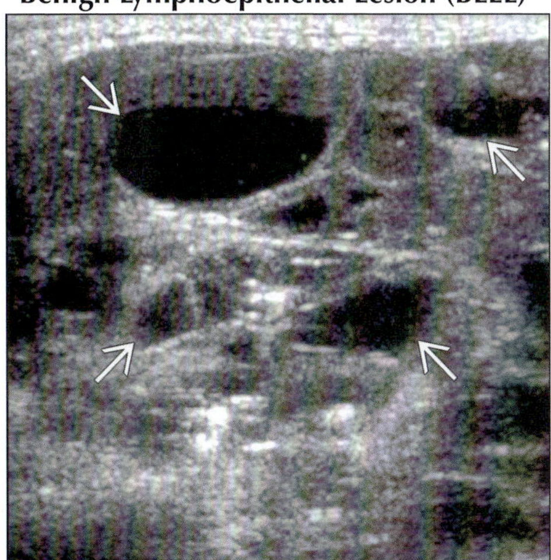

(Left) Transverse ultrasound shows diffuse enlargement of the parotid gland with a multicystic ➡ appearance. Cysts are of varying size. Note the mandibular ramus ➡, which causes posterior acoustic shadowing ➡. (Right) Longitudinal US in the same patient shows the multicystic ➡ appearance of the contralateral gland. BLEL mainly involves parotid glands and may be associated with solid lesions, representing lymphoid aggregates or salivary tumors.

Benign Lymphoepithelial Lesion (BLEL)

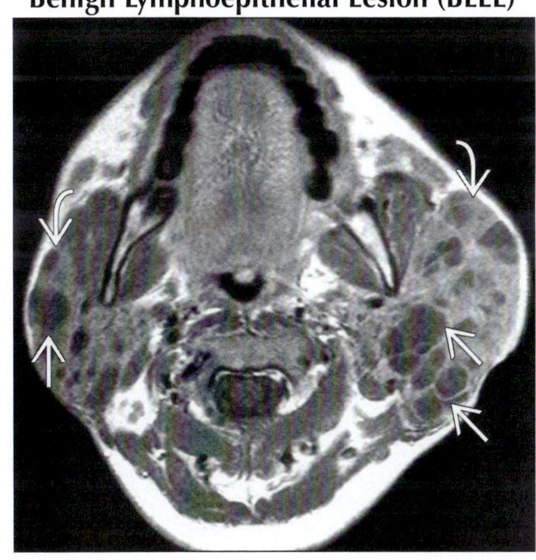

Benign Lymphoepithelial Lesion (BLEL)

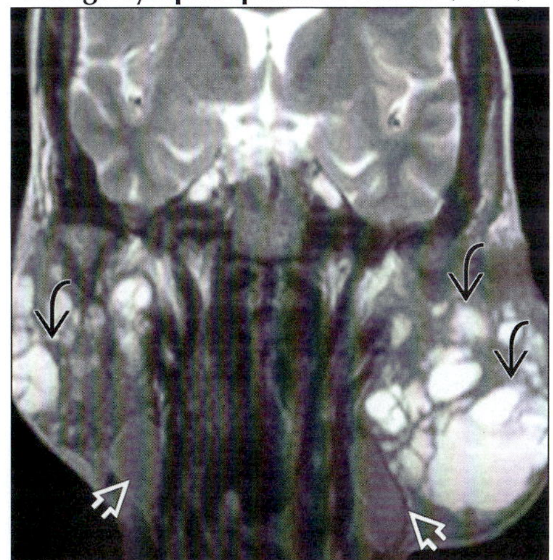

(Left) Axial T1WI C+ MR shows involvement of both parotid glands ➡. The multicystic ➡ areas do not enhance, and the cysts are of variable size. (Right) Coronal T2WI MR in the same patient shows hyperintense cystic spaces ➡ in both parotid glands. Note that the submandibular glands ➡ are not involved despite severe parotid disease, as compared with Sjögren syndrome. MR evaluates the deep lobe better than US.

Lymphangioma

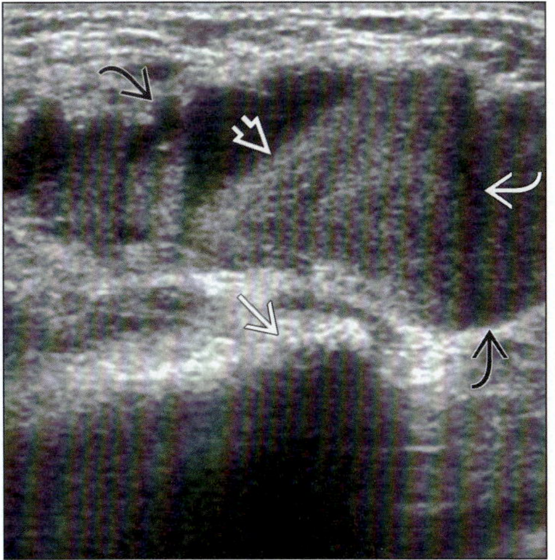

Lymphangioma

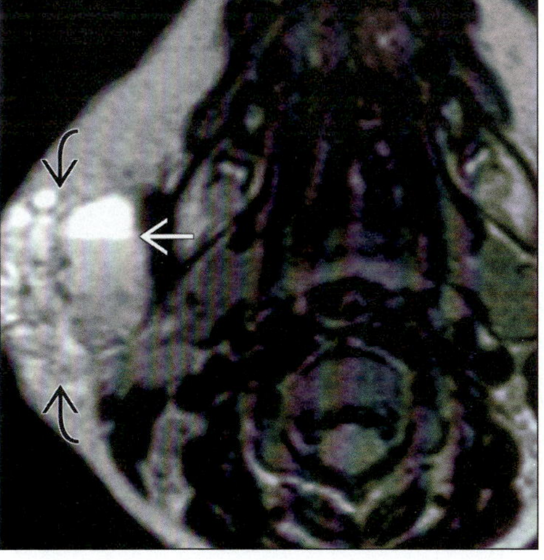

(Left) Longitudinal ultrasound shows a large cystic space ➡ in the parotid gland, representing a lymphangioma. The presence of internal debris ➡ and a fluid level ➡ is suggestive of previous infection/hemorrhage. Note the mandibular ramus ➡. (Right) Correlative T2WI MR shows the lymphangioma as a septated cystic lesion ➡ with a fluid level ➡. The other salivary glands were not involved.

DIFFUSE SALIVARY GLAND ENLARGEMENT

Hemangioma/Venous Vascular Malformation (VVM)

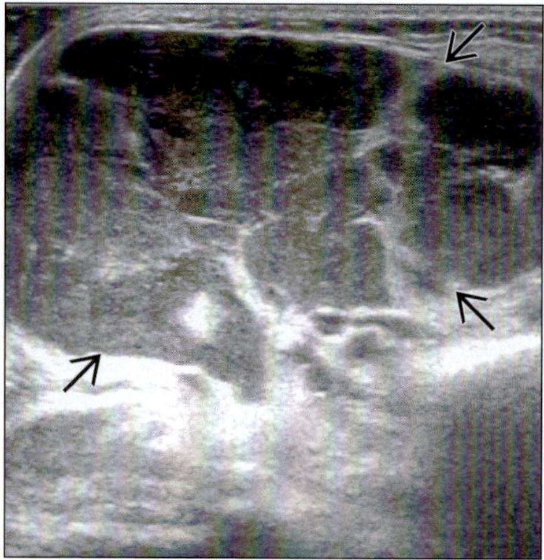

Hemangioma/Venous Vascular Malformation (VVM)

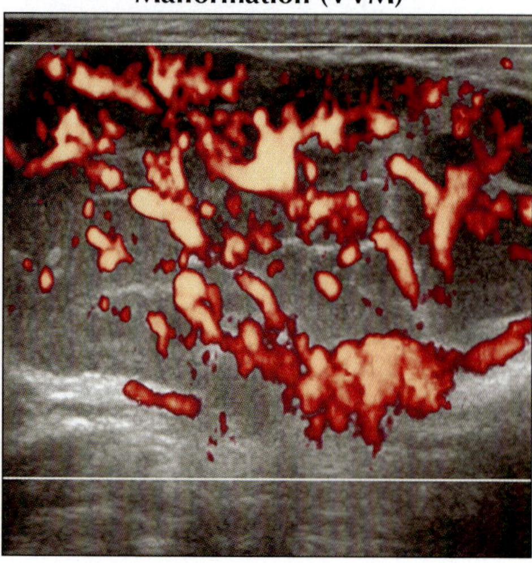

(Left) Transverse ultrasound shows a large, well-defined, hypoechoic mass ➡ in the parotid gland. It was soft on compression, there is a round contour, and the surrounding parotid glandular parenchyma was normal. *(Right)* Transverse power Doppler ultrasound in the same patient shows profuse internal vascularity. The appearance is typical of an intraparotid hemangioma. Such lesions usually regress as a child grows, and counseling often helps to reduce parental anxiety.

Kuttner Tumor

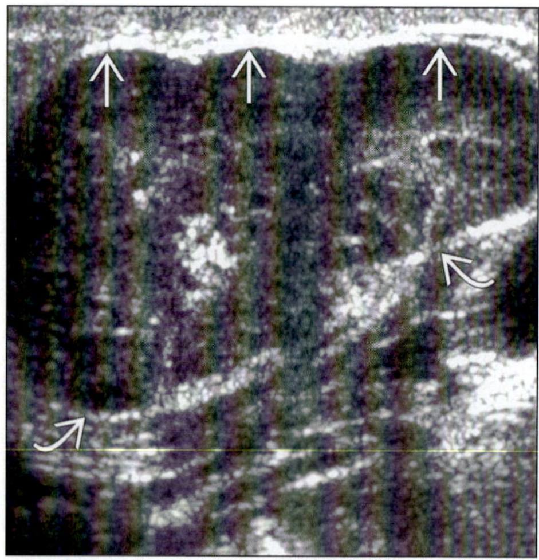

Kuttner Tumor

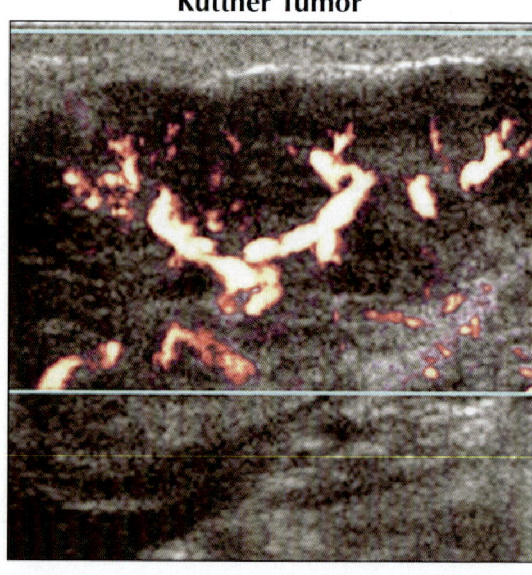

(Left) Transverse US shows an enlarged submandibular gland ➡ with lobulated contours ➡. The parenchyma is heterogeneous and hypoechoic, simulating a cirrhotic liver. The entire gland is involved. *(Right)* Transverse Power Doppler US in the same patient shows typical nondisplaced hypervascularity within the gland. These findings are characteristic of Kuttner tumor. The contralateral gland is usually also involved.

Kimura Disease

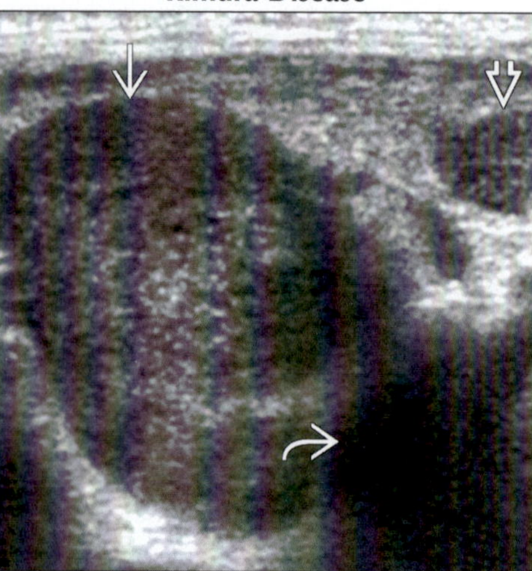

Kimura Disease

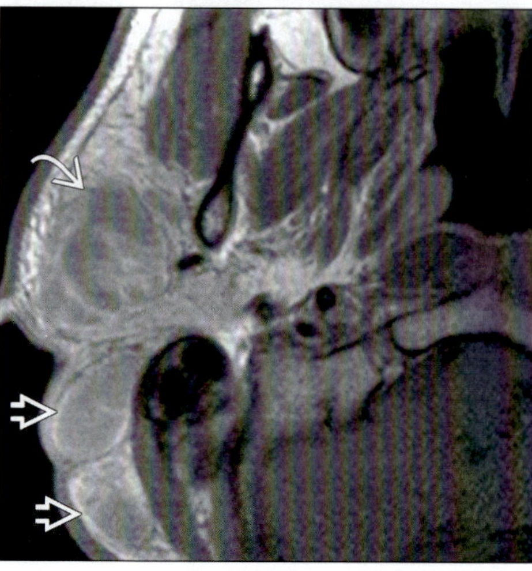

(Left) Transverse ultrasound shows a large, solid, fairly well-defined, hypoechoic mass ➡ in the parotid gland. Note the presence of a similar smaller mass ➡. Shadowing from the mandible ➡ is also visible. *(Right)* Axial T1WI C+ MR in the same patient shows the parotid mass ➡ and multiple subcutaneous soft tissue masses ➡ in the periparotid region. Biopsy confirmed Kimura disease in this young Chinese male.

DIFFUSE SALIVARY GLAND ENLARGEMENT

Kimura Disease

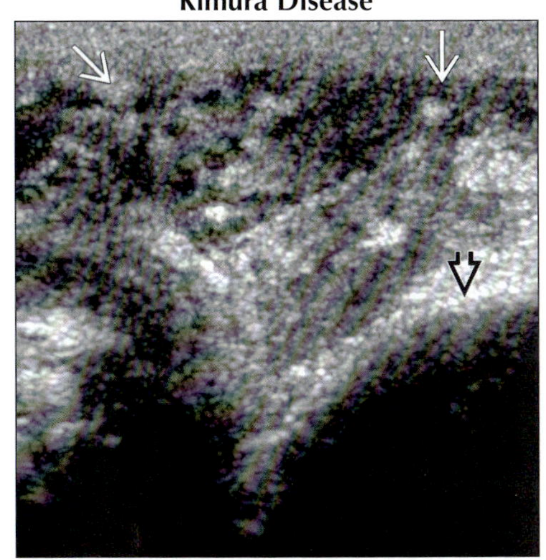

Kimura Disease

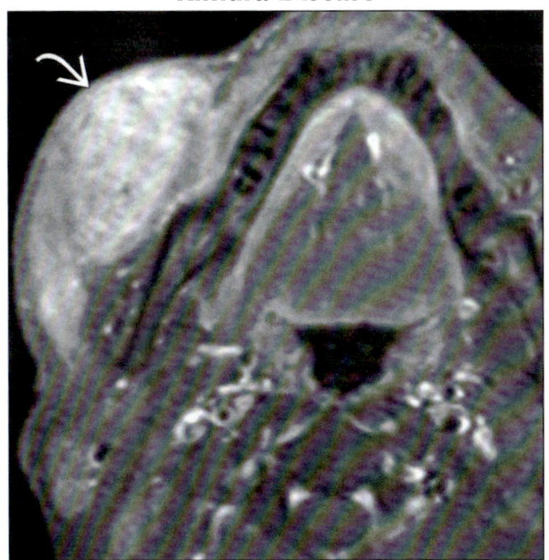

(Left) Transverse ultrasound shows a hypoechoic, heterogeneous, subcutaneous mass ➡ in the soft tissues anterior to the mandible ➡. (Right) Axial T1 C+ MR with fat suppression in the same patient shows avid enhancement of the subcutaneous mass ➡. Kimura disease may manifest as salivary masses (parenchymal mass or lymph nodes) or subcutaneous nodules and nodes in the vicinity of salivary glands in an Asian male.

Metastasis

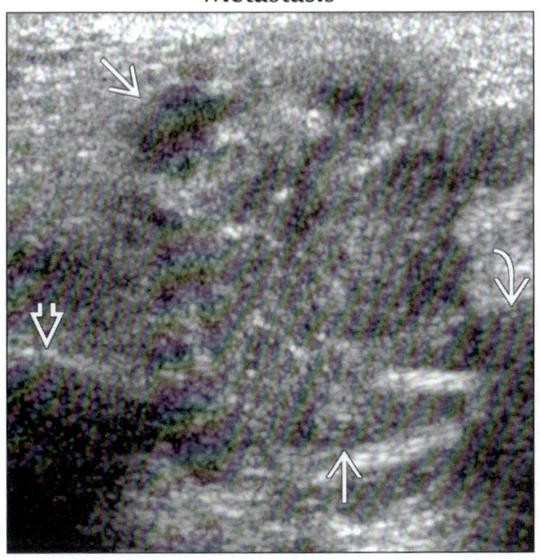

Metastasis

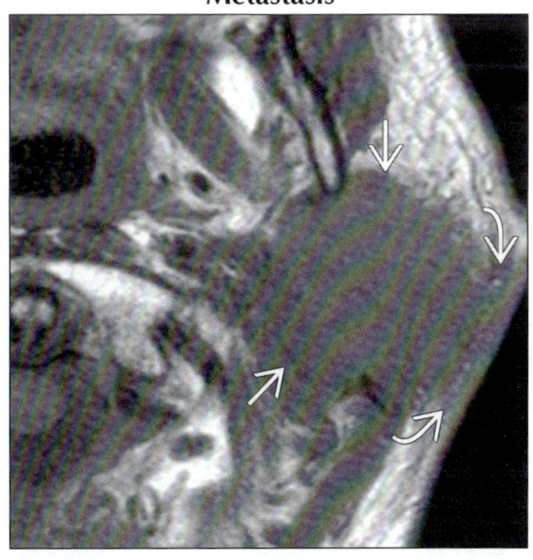

(Left) Transverse ultrasound shows a parotid metastasis ➡ in a patient with known squamous cell carcinoma of the external auditory canal. It is poorly defined, irregular, and heterogeneously hypoechoic. Note the mandible ➡ and mastoid ➡. (Right) Axial T1WI MR in the same patient shows the large parotid mass ➡ involving both the superficial and deep lobes. Its border is ill defined with infiltration of the overlying skin and subcutaneous tissue ➡.

Lymphoma

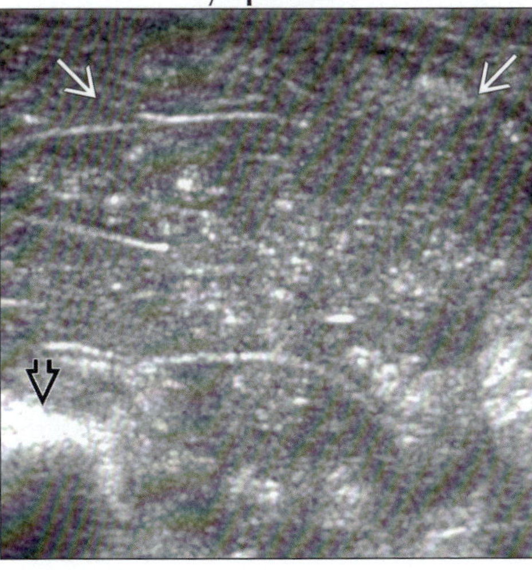

Lymphoma

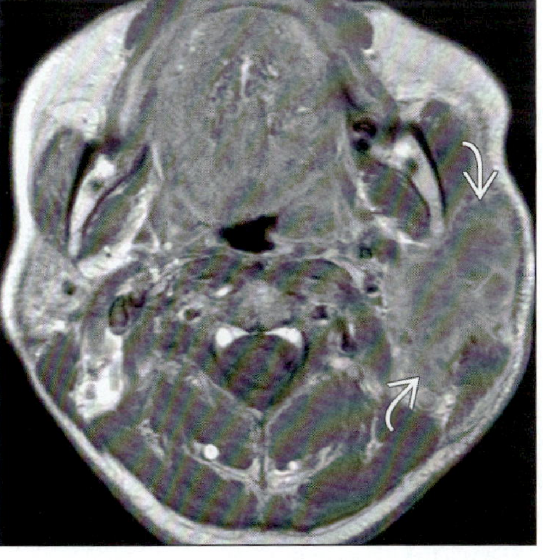

(Left) Transverse US shows primary lymphoma of the parotid gland in a patient on immunosuppressants. The parotid parenchyma is diffusely infiltrated ➡ with a hypoechoic and heterogeneous echopattern. Note the mandible ➡. (Right) Axial T1C+ MR in the same patient shows diffuse infiltration of the left parotid parenchyma ➡. Note the unilateral involvement. MR better delineates extent of disease.

FOCAL SALIVARY GLAND MASS

DIFFERENTIAL DIAGNOSIS

Common
- Benign Mixed Tumor (BMT)
- Warthin Tumor
- Intraparotid Lymph Node

Less Common
- Sialocele
- Lipoma
- Venous Vascular Malformation (VVM)
- Lymphangioma
- Abscess
- Tuberculous Infection
- Kuttner Tumor
- Salivary Gland Malignancy
  - Mucoepidermoid Carcinoma (MECa)
  - Adenoid Cystic Carcinoma
  - Adenocarcinoma
- Metastasis

Rare but Important
- Lymphoma
- Acinic Cell Carcinoma
- Pseudoaneurysm
- 1st Branchial Cleft Cyst

ESSENTIAL INFORMATION

Key Differential Diagnosis Issues
- US ideal to evaluate submandibular lesions due to their superficial location
  - Unable to evaluate parotid deep lobe lesions or deep lobe extension of superficial lobe abnormality
- Use high frequency (> 7.5 MHz) transducer
  - Benign tumors have well-defined edges, & malignant tumors have ill-defined edges
  - Internal architecture: Benign tumors are homogeneous; malignant tumors are heterogeneous (hemorrhage & necrosis)
    - Low-grade MECa may mimic benign tumor (homogeneous, well defined)
    - Warthin tumor often cystic with septa and heterogeneous architecture
  - Malignant tumors more likely to have adjacent soft tissue & nodal involvement
    - ± prominent intratumoral vessels and high resistance (RI > 0.8, PI > 2.0)
- US useful in identifying tumor, predicting malignancy, and guiding biopsy
  - CECT/MR best delineate tumor extent, perineural extension, & nodal disease

Helpful Clues for Common Diagnoses
- **Benign Mixed Tumor (BMT)**
  - US features: Well-defined, hypoechoic, lobulated, or bosselated surface, posterior acoustic enhancement, & intratumoral vascularity (mainly venous)
    - Cystic change and hemorrhage often seen in larger tumors (> 3 cm)
    - Dystrophic calcification seen occasionally in longstanding tumor
    - If left untreated, will undergo malignant transformation (9.5% for BMTs present more than 15 years)
  - Treatment by elective excision
- **Warthin Tumor**
  - Arise from intraparotid nodes
    - Typically seen in tail of parotid; rarely involves other salivary glands
    - Multiplicity of lesions, unilateral or bilateral (20%)
  - US features: Well-defined, heterogeneous hypoechoic mass, posterior acoustic enhancement, ± septa, & intratumoral vascularity ("hilar")
    - Cystic change more common than BMT
    - May look solid and mimic BMT
    - Malignant change (carcinoma or lymphoma) reported in < 1%
  - May be treated expectantly
- **Intraparotid Lymph Node**
  - Reactive intraparotid lymph nodes are common finding (particularly in children)
  - Echogenic hilar architecture and vascularity are preserved
  - Small lymph node with undetectable vascularity may be difficult to differentiate from small salivary tumor

Helpful Clues for Less Common Diagnoses
- **Sialocele**
  - Focal collection of saliva in glands
    - Leak from ductal system due to previous obstruction or inflammation
  - Unilocular, thin walled, with internal echogenic debris & no vascularity
  - Indistinguishable from 1st branchial cleft cyst (BCC)
    - Aspirated fluid sent for amylase (↑ in saliva vs. 1st BCC)
- **Lipoma**
  - 10% of all parotid tumors

FOCAL SALIVARY GLAND MASS

- Hypoechoic relative to surrounding parotid parenchyma
  - Linear hyperechoic "feathery" striation, parallel to transducer in both transverse & longitudinal planes
  - Avascular on Doppler
- **Venous Vascular Malformation (VVM)**
  - Sinusoidal thin-walled spaces with grayscale flow/motion ± phleboliths, ± slow flow on Doppler
- **Lymphangioma**
  - Multi-septated cystic mass, ± debris, ± fluid level, no intratumoral vascularity
- **Abscess, Tuberculous Infection**
  - Nodal &/or parenchymal involvement
  - Ill-defined mass (inflammatory phlegmon) ± abscess, ± involvement of other neck nodes
- **Kuttner Tumor**
  - Chronic sclerosing sialadenitis
  - Cirrhotic/geographic pattern, hypoechoic areas with nondisplaced hypervascularity
    - Submandibular > > > parotid involvement
- **Salivary Gland Malignancy**
  - Several histologic types: Adenoid cystic, mucoepidermoid, adenocarcinoma
  - Low-grade malignancy indistinguishable from benign tumors, so search carefully for features of malignancy
    - Ill-defined border, hypoechoic, necrosis
    - Abnormal vascularity,
    - Extrasalivary involvement, ± adjacent malignant nodes

- **Metastasis**
  - Hypoechoic mass(es) with malignant sonographic features
  - Multiplicity and history of known primary tumor raises suspicion

Helpful Clues for Rare Diagnoses

- **Lymphoma**
  - Nodal or parenchymal involvement
    - Parenchymal involvement may be seen as focal mass or diffuse enlargement
  - Note association with systemic lymphoma, Sjögren syndrome, rheumatoid arthritis, & immunosuppression
- **Acinic Cell Carcinoma**
  - Represents only 2-4% of all major salivary gland tumors; however, it is 2nd most common malignant parotid tumor
    - 80-90% occur in parotid gland
  - Middle-aged patients predominant, but it is also 2nd most frequent pediatric malignant salivary gland tumor
  - US appearance is similar to other salivary gland malignancies but tends to be multi-focal
- **Pseudoaneurysm**
  - Related to previous injury or infection
  - Exclude this diagnosis before biopsy; evaluate all salivary masses with Doppler
- **1st Branchial Cleft Cyst**
  - Seen in children; appearance similar to sialocele, but sinus tract may be seen
  - Evaluate temporal bone to exclude associated abnormality

Benign Mixed Tumor (BMT)

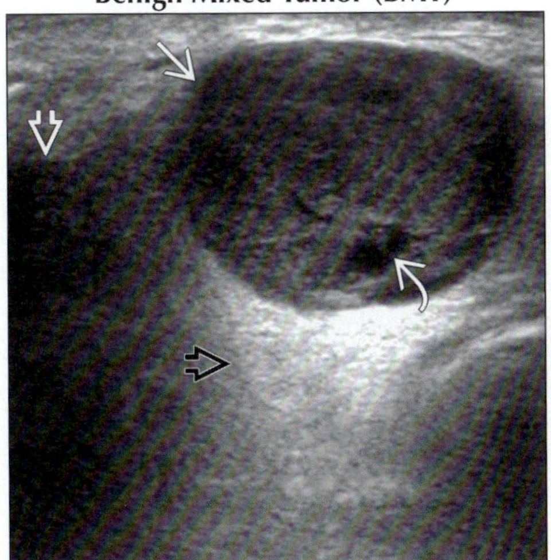

Transverse ultrasound shows a typical appearance of a parotid BMT ➡. It is well defined and hypoechoic, with posterior acoustic enhancement ➡. Internal cystic change ➡ may be seen. Note the mandible ➡.

Benign Mixed Tumor (BMT)

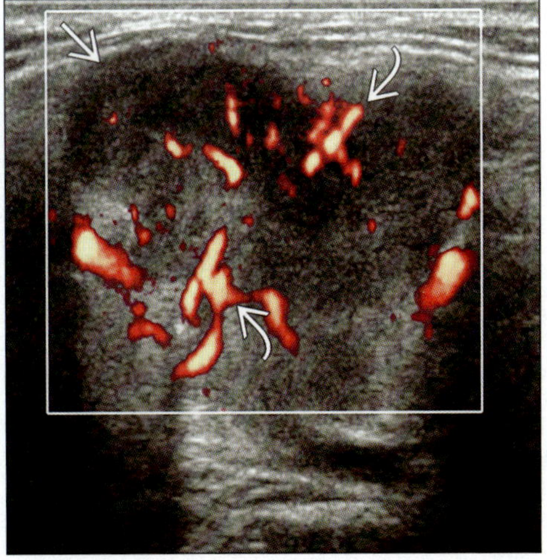

Transverse power Doppler ultrasound shows another parotid BMT ➡. Profuse intratumoral vascularity ➡ may be seen. Such vessels usually are of low resistance (RI < 0.8, PI < 2.0).

FOCAL SALIVARY GLAND MASS

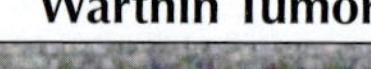

(Left) Transverse ultrasound shows a typical appearance of a Warthin tumor ➡ with a cystic portion ➡, septum ➡, and a solid component ➡, which is often vascular on Doppler. Note the posterior acoustic enhancement ➡. *(Right)* Longitudinal power Doppler ultrasound shows a Warthin tumor with the predominant peripheral vascularity ➡, often seen in larger Warthin tumors. Cystic change ➡ is also present.

Warthin Tumor

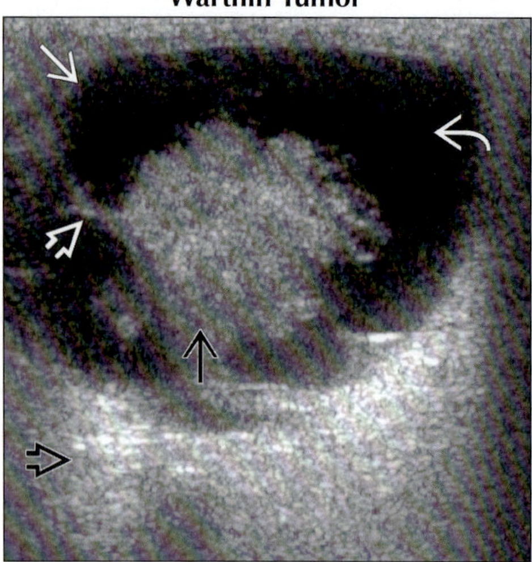

Warthin Tumor

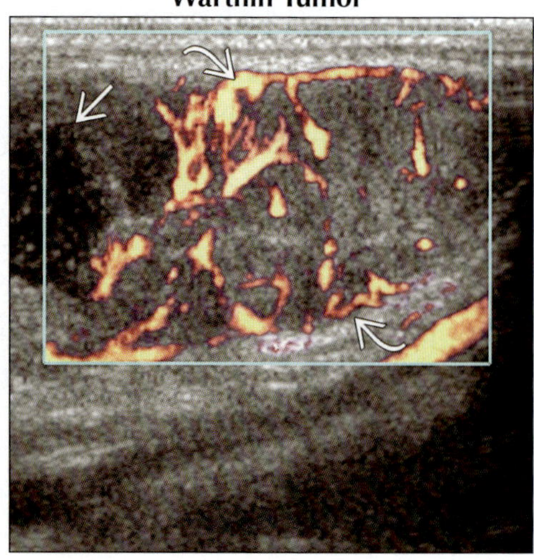

(Left) Transverse power Doppler ultrasound shows a solid-looking Warthin tumor ➡. The vascularity is central and peripheral ➡. Note the central "hilar" ➡ vascularity resembles vessels in a node. *(Right)* Longitudinal ultrasound shows that a Warthin tumor is often multiple ➡ (may be bilateral), most commonly seen in the tail of the parotid gland, and not in other salivary glands due to absence of an intraglandular lymph node. Note the internal cystic change ➡.

Warthin Tumor

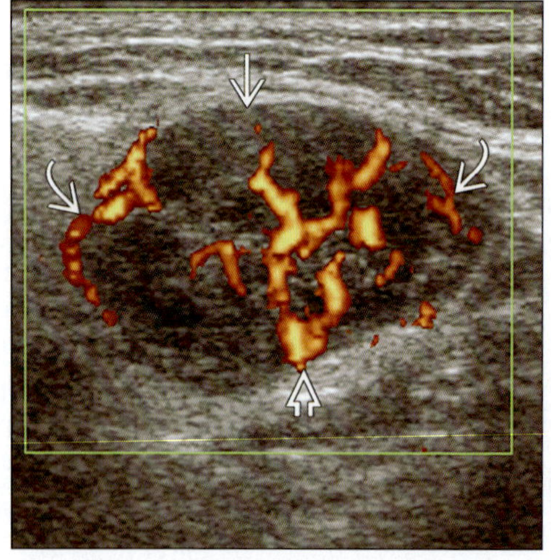

Warthin Tumor

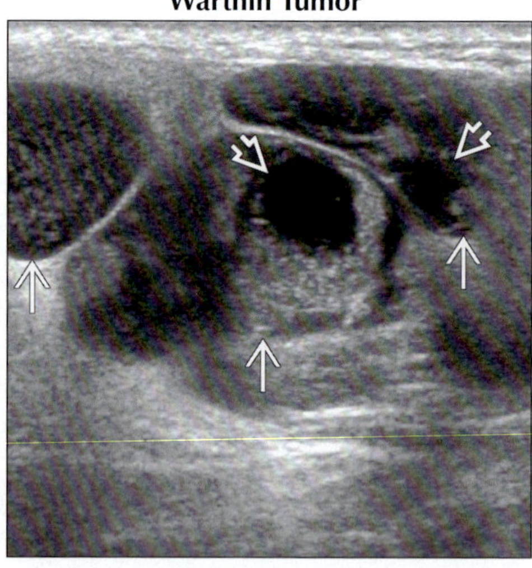

(Left) Longitudinal power Doppler ultrasound shows 2 intraparotid nodules. The smaller nodule has hilar vascularity ➡, suggestive of a LN. The larger nodule has profuse "intratumoral" vascularity ➡ & may be a Warthin tumor. US-guided FNAC helps to confirm diagnosis. *(Right)* Longitudinal ultrasound shows a parotid sialocele ➡ seen as a unilocular cyst. Multiple mobile echogenic foci ➡, representing debris, are typical. This could be confused with a 1st BCC.

Intraparotid Lymph Node

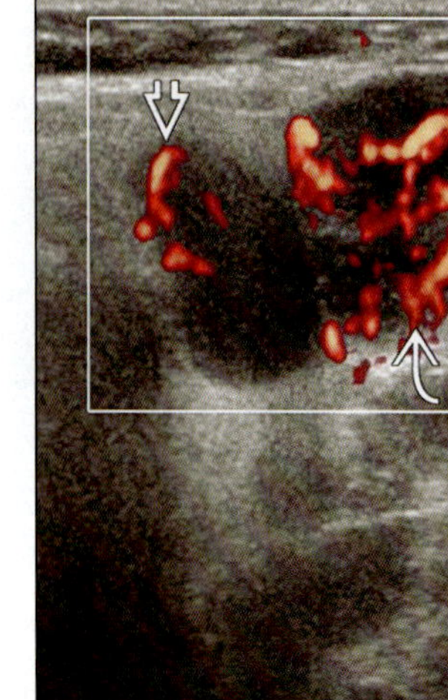

Sialocele

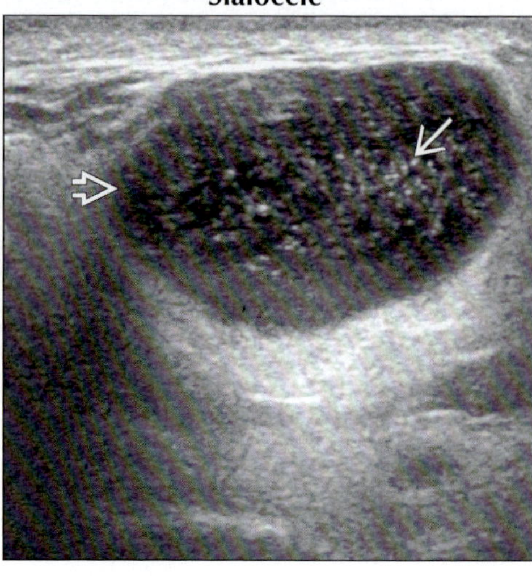

FOCAL SALIVARY GLAND MASS

Venous Vascular Malformation (VVM)

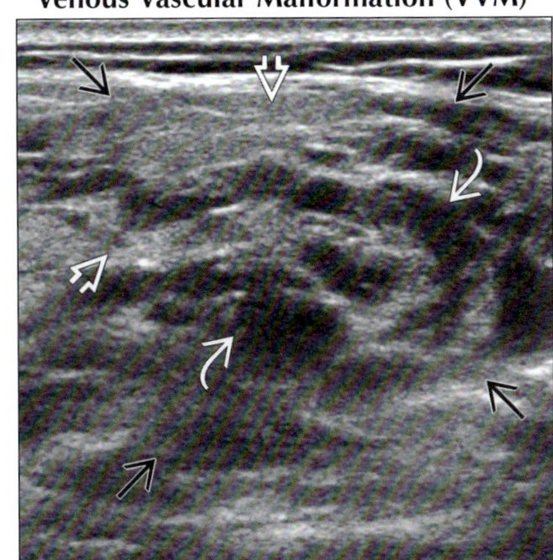

Venous Vascular Malformation (VVM)

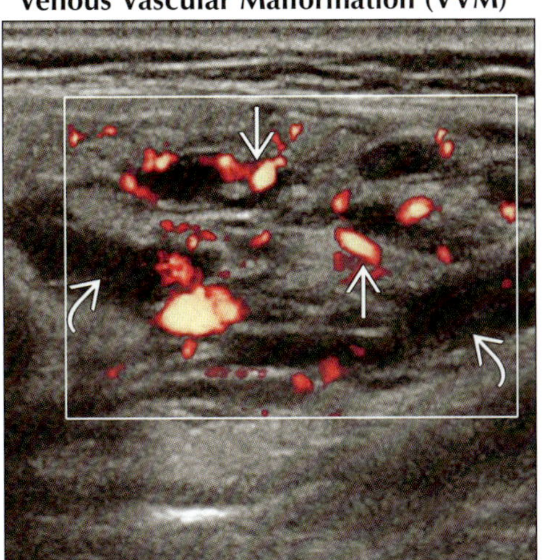

(Left) Longitudinal ultrasound shows a parotid VVM. The border ➡ is well defined and lobulated, and a soft tissue stromal component ➡ and sinusoidal vascular spaces ➡ are seen. (Right) Longitudinal power Doppler ultrasound in the same patient shows vascularity in smaller vessels ➡, though it is absent in the larger vascular spaces ➡ due to slow flow. Grayscale US better evaluates slow flow as motion/movement within the VVM.

Lipoma

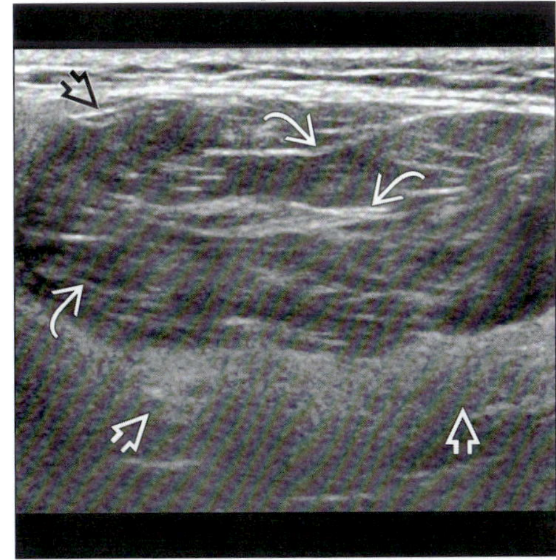

Abscess

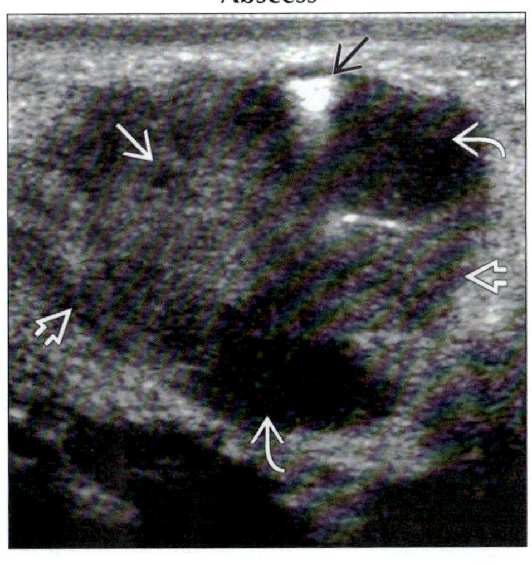

(Left) Longitudinal ultrasound shows a typical appearance of a lipoma ➡, in this case within the parotid gland ➡. The curvilinear horizontal stripes ➡ remain parallel to the transducer in both transverse and longitudinal planes. (Right) Transverse ultrasound shows an echogenic focus with a "comet tail" artifact ➡ representing gas within a parotid gland abscess ➡. Also note the presence of internal debris ➡ and necrosis ➡.

Tuberculous Infection

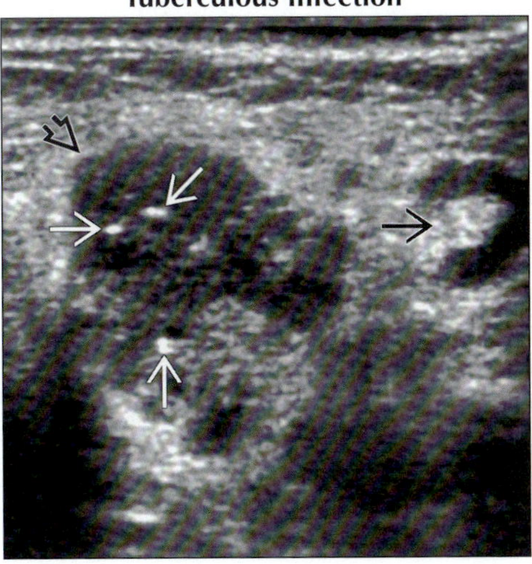

Kuttner Tumor

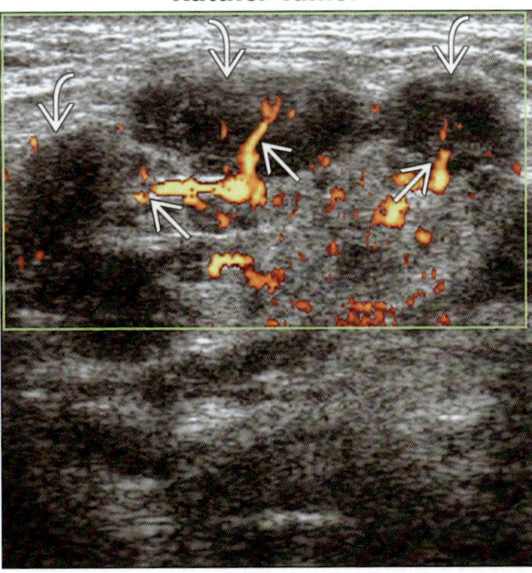

(Left) Oblique US shows an irregular, heterogeneously hypoechoic, tuberculous abscess ➡ in the submandibular gland. Note its ill-defined border and multiple echogenic foci ➡, representing gas. There is an adjacent prominent node ➡. (Right) Transverse power Doppler ultrasound shows geographic areas ➡ of hypoechoic submandibular parenchyma with round contours and internal nondisplaced vessels ➡, typical of a Kuttner tumor.

1

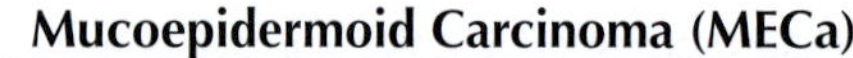

FOCAL SALIVARY GLAND MASS

(Left) Longitudinal ultrasound shows a low-grade MECa ➡ in the parotid gland. The appearance is similar to a benign salivary gland tumor, except for the soft sign of partly ill-defined edges ➡ and intratumoral cystic necrosis ➡. (Right) Transverse ultrasound shows ill-defined hypoechoic areas ➡ in the submandibular gland. The ill-defined margin & breach of capsule ➡ is suspicious for malignancy. FNAC confirmed an adenoid cystic carcinoma.

Mucoepidermoid Carcinoma (MECa)

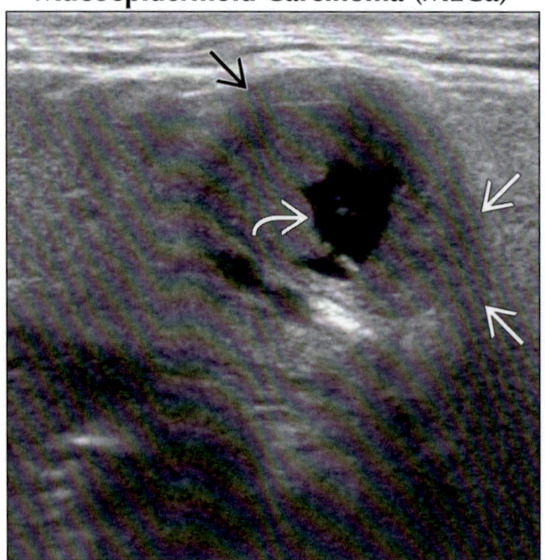

Adenoid Cystic Carcinoma

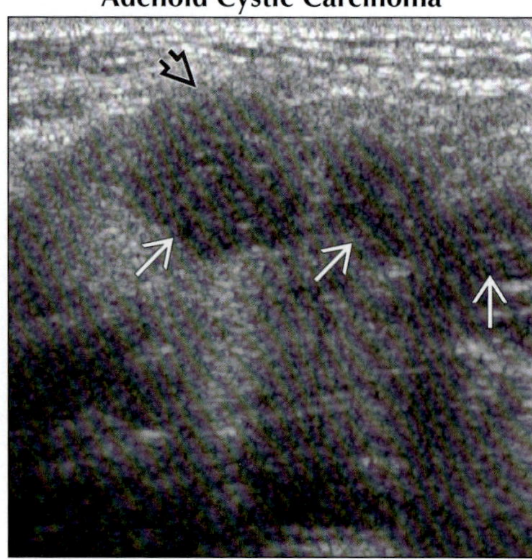

(Left) Transverse power Doppler ultrasound shows an adenocarcinoma ➡ in the parotid gland. The border is ill defined & the internal echoes are heterogeneous. The vascular pattern is nonspecific & does not differentiate a benign from a malignant salivary gland tumor. (Right) Axial T1 C+ MR in the same patient shows avid enhancement of the tumor ➡, internal necrosis ➡, and involvement of the deep lobe of the parotid gland. Note the intraparotid LN ➡.

Adenocarcinoma

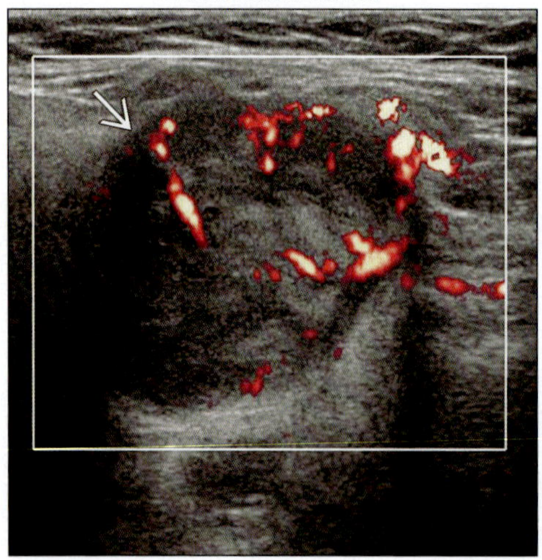

Adenocarcinoma

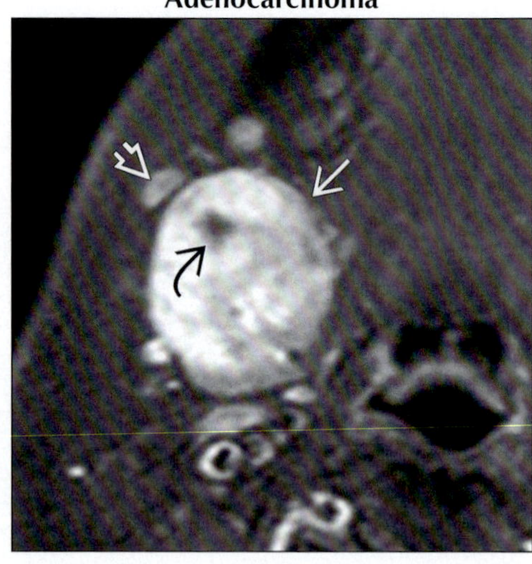

(Left) Transverse ultrasound shows metastases ➡ to the parotid gland. The sonographic features are nonspecific; the diagnostic clue is the history of a known primary tumor with draining lymphatics to an intraparotid node. (Right) Axial T1 C+ MR with fat suppression in the same patient shows avid contrast enhancement and an ill-defined border of the metastasis ➡. US-guided FNAC confirmed the diagnosis of intraparotid metastasis.

Metastasis

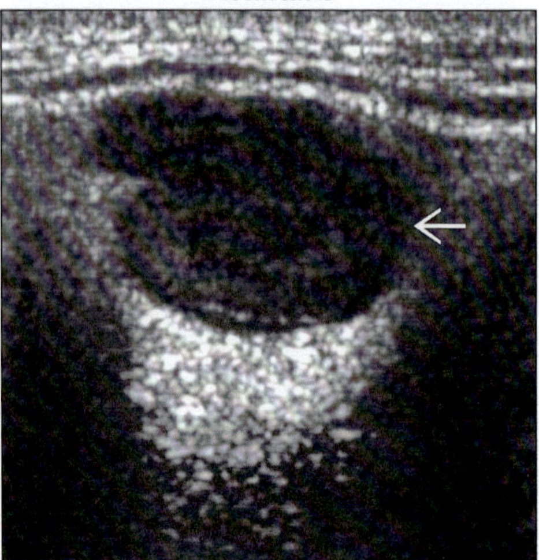

Metastasis

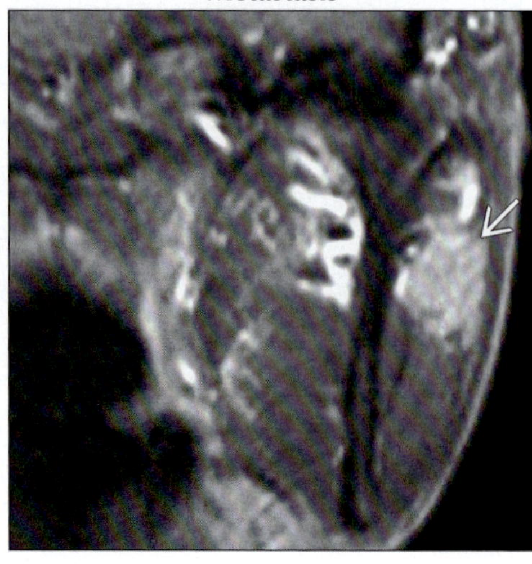

FOCAL SALIVARY GLAND MASS

Lymphoma

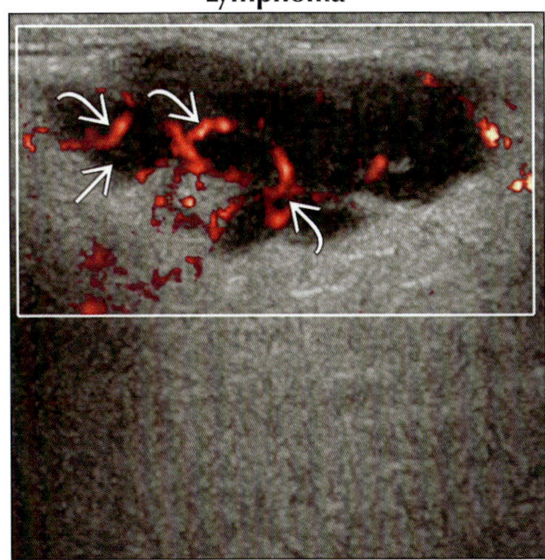

Acinic Cell Carcinoma

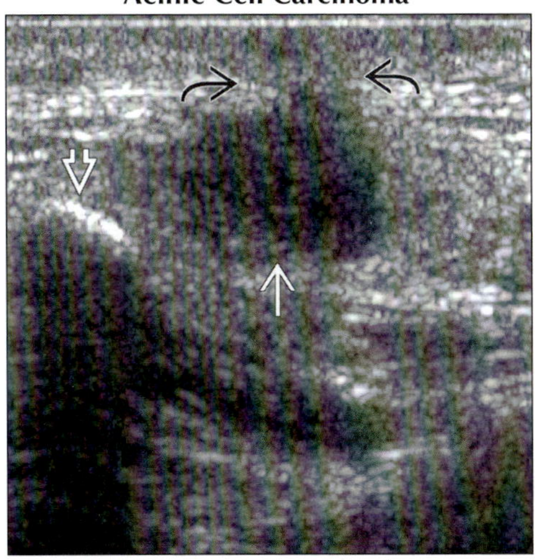

(Left) Transverse power Doppler ultrasound shows an irregular hypoechoic mass in the parotid gland, representing primary lymphoma ➡ of the parotid. Note intratumoral vascularity ➢. (Right) Longitudinal ultrasound shows an acinic cell carcinoma ➡ of the submandibular gland. The ill-defined margin, heterogeneous echopattern, and involvement of the subcutaneous tissue ➢ should raise the suspicion of malignancy. Note the mandible ➤.

Pseudoaneurysm

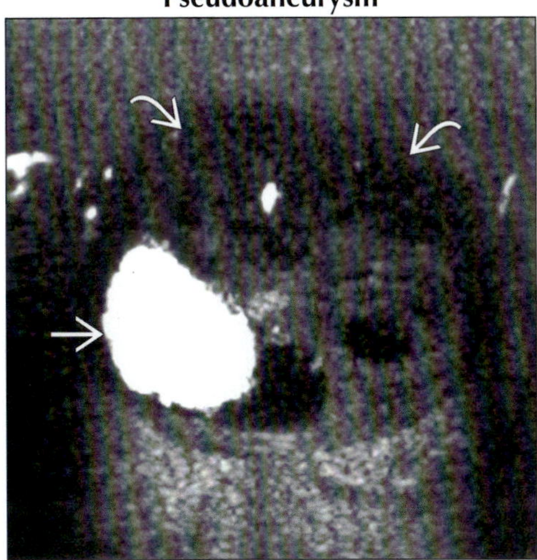

Pseudoaneurysm

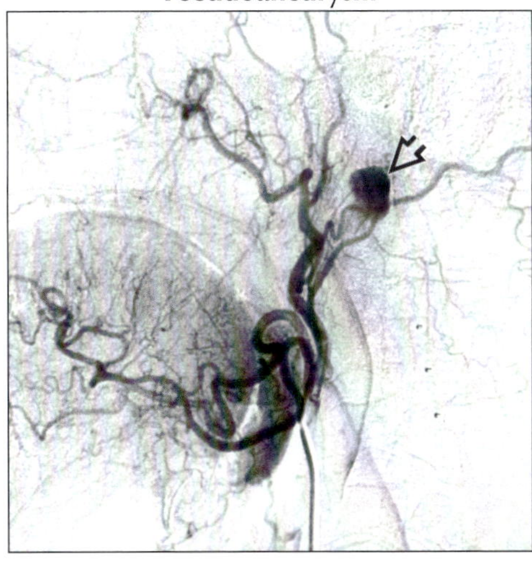

(Left) Transverse power Doppler ultrasound (shown in black & white) shows an intraparotid pseudoaneurysm ➡ arising from the external carotid artery. The majority of the lumen is thrombosed ➢. Color/power Doppler of a parotid mass should always be performed to avoid inadvertent biopsy of a pseudoaneurysm. (Right) Angiography of the ECA in the same patient confirms the pseudoaneurysm ➢ with residual lumen. The lesion was subsequently successfully embolized.

1st Branchial Cleft Cyst

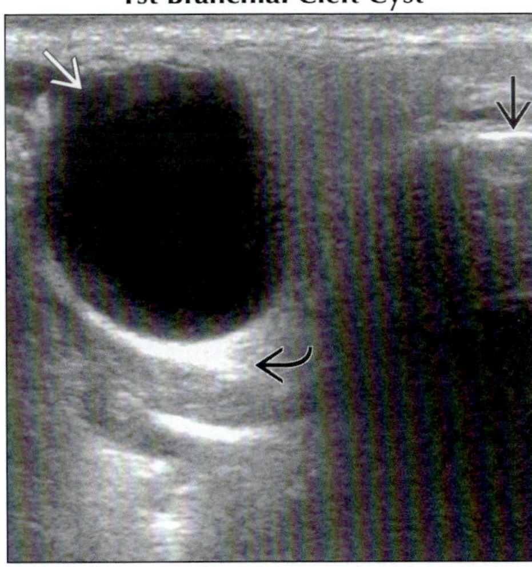

1st Branchial Cleft Cyst

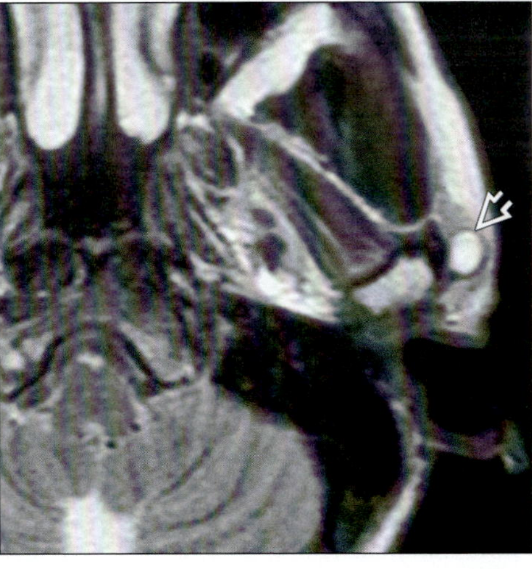

(Left) Transverse ultrasound shows a 1st BCC ➡, seen as a unilocular anechoic cystic lesion with posterior acoustic enhancement ➢. The appearance is indistinguishable from a sialocele. Clinical features and FNAC may help to differentiate them. Note the mandible ➡. (Right) Axial T2WI MR shows a unilocular cystic lesion ➡ in the preauricular region of the parotid gland, which was subsequently confirmed to be a 1st BCC.

SECTION 2
Thyroid/Parathyroid

DIFFERENTIAL DIAGNOSIS

Common
- Multinodular Goiter
- Graves Disease
- Hashimoto Thyroiditis

Less Common
- De Quervain Thyroiditis
- Acute Suppurative Thyroiditis
- Anaplastic Thyroid Carcinoma

Rare but Important
- Thyroid Metastasis
- Lymphoma
- Leukemia

ESSENTIAL INFORMATION

Key Differential Diagnosis Issues
- Most diagnoses are made clinically so ultrasound should be targeted to answer specific question
  - Is US done to confirm diagnosis, guide biopsy?
    - Will additional CT or MR help?
  - Is US done to evaluate associated abnormalities, complications?
    - In multinodular goiter (MNG), US done to identify presence of thyroid cancer; look for features of malignant nodule, ± lymph node
    - In Hashimoto thyroiditis, US done to look for any developing non-Hodgkin lymphoma (NHL) in gland or lymph nodes

Helpful Clues for Common Diagnoses
- **Multinodular Goiter**
  - Most common cause of diffuse thyroid enlargement (symmetric/asymmetric)
  - Typical MNG: Multiple heterogeneous nodules, cystic change, septation, internal debris, dense shadowing calcification
    - Solid nodules are often isoechoic with intranodular and perinodular vascularity
  - Look carefully for presence of malignant nodule against background of multinodularity
  - Features suggestive of malignancy

- Ill-defined, solid, hypoechoic, hypervascular, ± punctate calcification, extracapsular extension, ± associated malignant node
- **Graves Disease**
  - Moderately enlarged gland with hypoechoic spotty parenchymal echopattern and rounded contours
  - Heterogeneity may appear nodular, mimicking MNG
  - Diffuse parenchymal hypervascularity with high velocity on spectral Doppler
- **Hashimoto Thyroiditis**
  - Gradual painless enlargement of thyroid with euthyroid (majority), hypothyroid (20%), or hyperthyroid (5%) status
    - Atrophic gland at end stage
  - Diffuse, hypoechoic, heterogeneous, micronodular echopattern
  - Characteristic echogenic fibrous septa in chronic cases, seen as multiple echogenic horizontal lines
  - Avascular in acute focal/diffuse form, hypervascular when chronic, and hypothyroid (hypertrophic action of TSH)
    - Flow velocities within normal limits (↑ in Graves disease)
  - Always evaluate thyroid and lymph nodes (± FNAC) for known risk of developing NHL in chronic cases

Helpful Clues for Less Common Diagnoses
- **De Quervain Thyroiditis**
  - Typical history: Acute onset painful thyroid swelling preceded by upper respiratory tract infection 2-3 weeks prior
  - Transient hyperthyroidism (50%) but paradoxical low radioiodine uptake, due to severe glandular destruction
  - Mildly enlarged thyroid gland, with focal ill-defined hypoechoic heterogeneous area within gland initially
    - Mimics malignant nodule
  - Subsequently evolves to affect rest of gland, which becomes diffusely hypoechoic and heterogeneous
    - Mild to moderate hypervascularity; hypoechoic areas may be avascular due to severe glandular destruction
  - Clinical recovery correlates well with sonographic recovery
- **Acute Suppurative Thyroiditis**

DIFFUSE THYROID ENLARGEMENT

- ○ Clinical history of repeated neck/thyroid abscesses on left (95%)
- ○ Starts as perithyroidal abscess, subsequently involving thyroid gland, upper pole > lower pole
- ○ Ill-defined, hypoechoic, inflammatory thyroid "mass" ± liquefied center representing abscess
- ○ Must identify underlying fistula tract to pyriform fossa sinus after acute episode (barium, CECT, MR)
- • **Anaplastic Thyroid Carcinoma**
  - ○ Clinical diagnosis: Rapidly enlarging mass with obstructive symptoms in patient with known MNG
  - ○ Role of US is to confirm diagnosis, guide needle biopsy, evaluate extrathyroid spread, and identify malignant nodes
  - ○ Invasive hypoechoic heterogeneous thyroid mass, ± focal calcification (50%), ± necrosis against background of MNG
  - ○ ± extracapsular spread, malignant cervical lymph nodes, ± tumor thrombus in internal jugular vein
  - ○ Necrotic tumor may be avascular/hypovascular (vascular infiltration/occlusion)

Helpful Clues for Rare Diagnoses
- • **Thyroid Metastasis**
  - ○ Rapid onset goiter/hoarseness/dysphagia in patient with known malignancy
    - ▪ Breast, kidney, lung, colon most common
  - ○ Invariably associated with widely disseminated disease
  - ○ Nonspecific appearance
    - ▪ Cannot be differentiated from anaplastic carcinoma, other thyroid primary, lymphoma, or leukemia without biopsy
  - ○ Solitary/multiple, solid, hypoechoic nodules with intranodular vascularity or diffuse infiltration (mild goiter with heterogeneous hypoechoic parenchyma)
  - ○ Infiltrative type is easily missed; disseminated disease and neck nodes provide useful clues
- • **Lymphoma**
  - ○ Primary thyroid lymphoma is rare
    - ▪ Typically seen in patients with longstanding Hashimoto thyroiditis
  - ○ Rapidly enlarging thyroid mass
  - ○ Solid, ill-defined, hypoechoic, noncalcified mass
    - ▪ 80% solitary, often large (5-10 cm)
  - ○ Diffuse involvement: Goiter with heterogeneous echopattern or minimal change in echopattern (often missed)
  - ○ ± local infiltration, lymphomatous cervical nodes (hypoechoic with reticulated pattern/"pseudocystic" appearance)
  - ○ Color Doppler: Nonspecific, hypovascular, or chaotic intranodular vessels
- • **Leukemia**
  - ○ Thyroid lesion similar to lymphoma or metastatic involvement
  - ○ Lymphadenopathy does not show "reticulated" or "pseudocystic" appearance

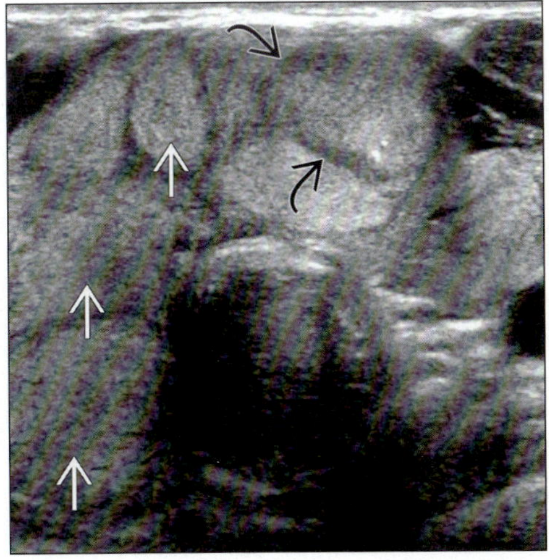

Multinodular Goiter

Transverse ultrasound shows diffuse thyroid enlargement with multiple solid, homogeneous, isoechoic nodules ➡ of varying size. Most nodules are surrounded by a complete hypoechoic halo ➡.

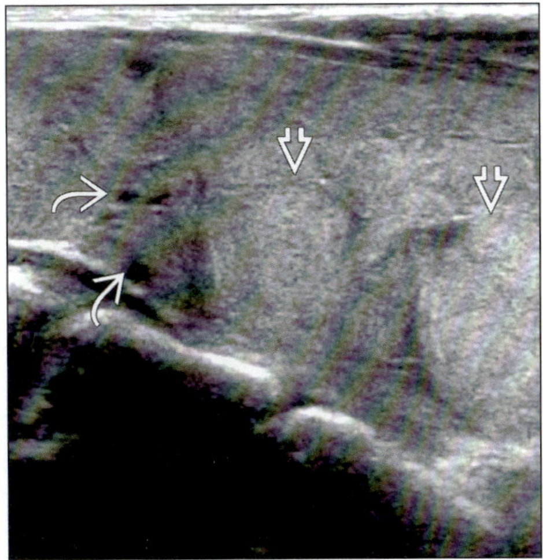

Multinodular Goiter

Longitudinal ultrasound shows multiple isoechoic nodules ➡ and 1 hypoechoic nodule with internal cystic change ➡. Cystic change & septation are often seen in hyperplastic nodules due to degeneration.

DIFFUSE THYROID ENLARGEMENT

(Left) Transverse ultrasound shows diffuse enlargement of the thyroid gland with a heterogeneous, "nodular," hypoechoic parenchymal pattern ➡, consistent with Graves disease. *(Right)* Transverse power Doppler ultrasound shows diffuse hypervascularity ➤ within the gland, the commonly described "thyroid inferno" of Graves disease. These vessels show high velocity on spectral Doppler (not shown), unlike the normal velocity seen in Hashimoto thyroiditis.

Graves Disease

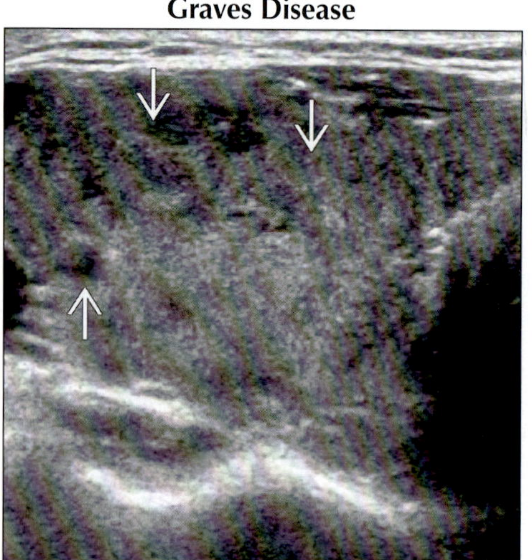

Graves Disease

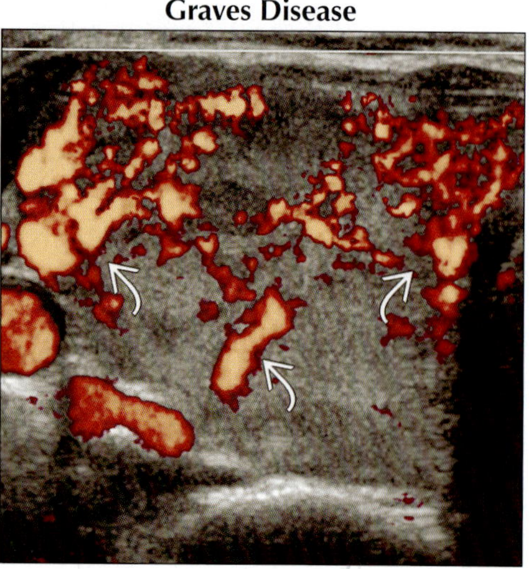

(Left) Coronal reformatted CT of the orbits shows hypertrophy of multiple extraocular muscles ➤, consistent with Graves ophthalmopathy. *(Right)* Coronal T2WI MR with fat suppression shows diffuse enlargement of the thyroid gland in a patient with Graves disease. The extent of the enlargement and absence of associated tracheal compression are clearly demonstrated. CT/MR are useful in evaluating a massively enlarged thyroid.

Graves Disease

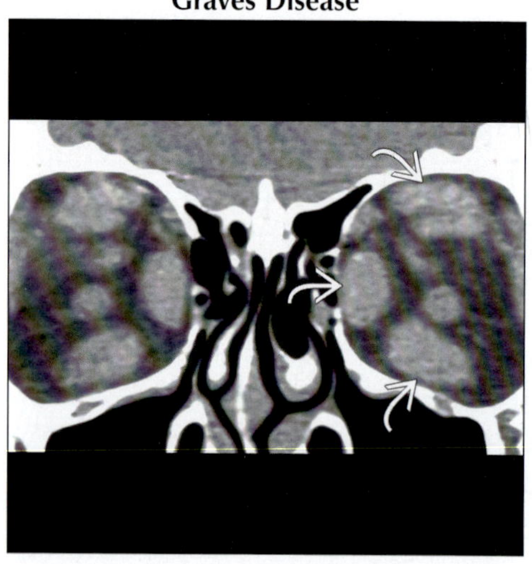

Graves Disease

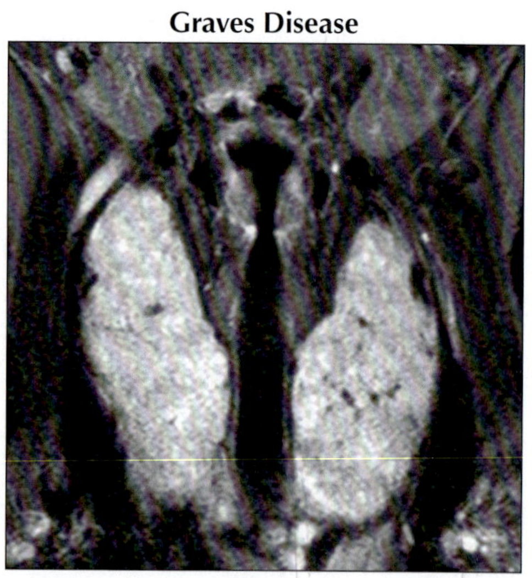

(Left) Transverse ultrasound shows mild thyroid enlargement ➡. Note that the parenchymal echoes are uniform, non-nodular, homogeneous, hypoechoic, and faintly "spotty." This is a common grayscale appearance of the thyroid in Graves disease. *(Right)* Longitudinal power Doppler shows the "thyroid inferno." If the gland is extremely vascular, one may have to use high pulse repetition frequency and filters to evaluate the vascularity and eliminate artifacts.

Graves Disease

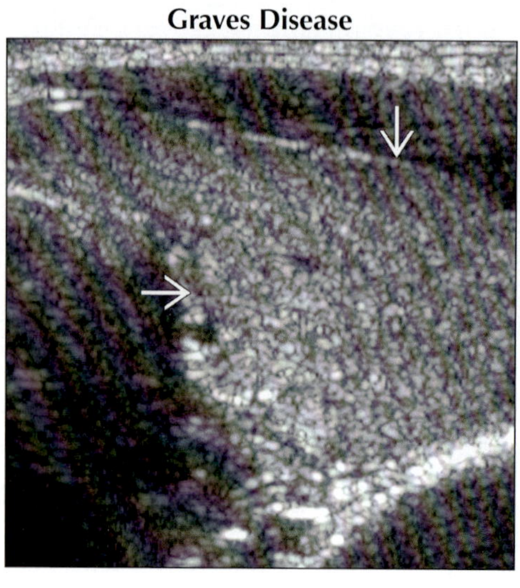

Graves Disease

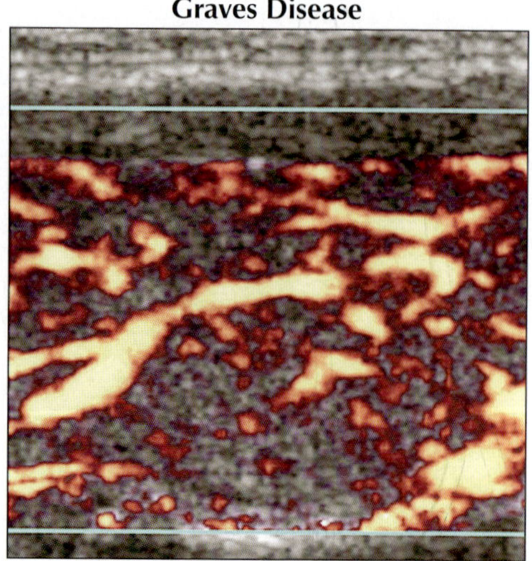

DIFFUSE THYROID ENLARGEMENT

Hashimoto Thyroiditis

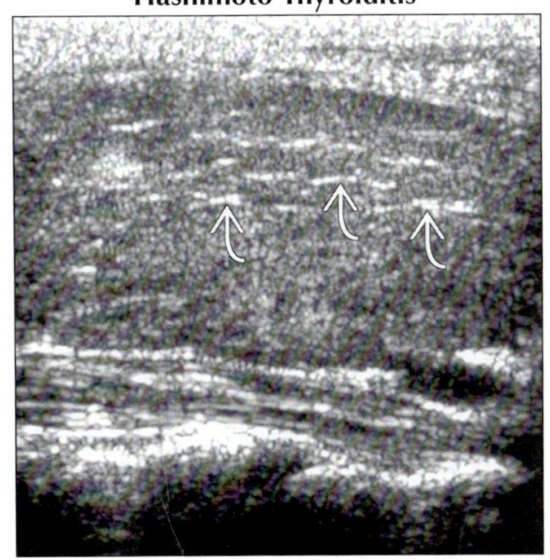

Hashimoto Thyroiditis

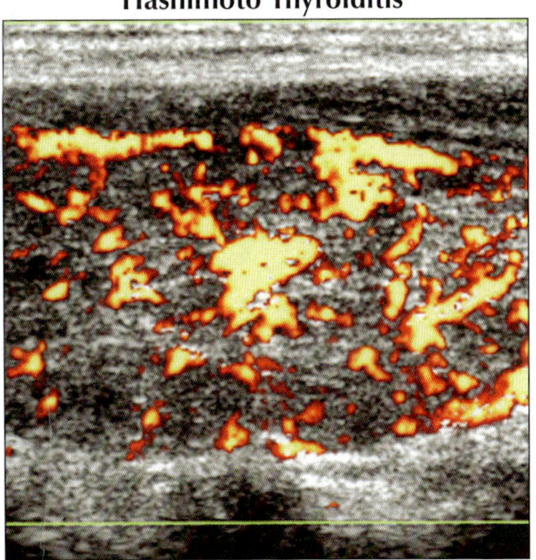

(Left) Longitudinal ultrasound of a thyroid gland shows multiple horizontal echogenic lines ➡, representing fibrous septae in Hashimoto thyroiditis. Rule out any suspicion of developing NHL in the thyroid and neck nodes in patients with chronic disease. (Right) Longitudinal power Doppler shows marked hypervascularity throughout the gland. Vessels show normal flow velocities compared to vessels with high velocities in Graves disease.

De Quervain Thyroiditis

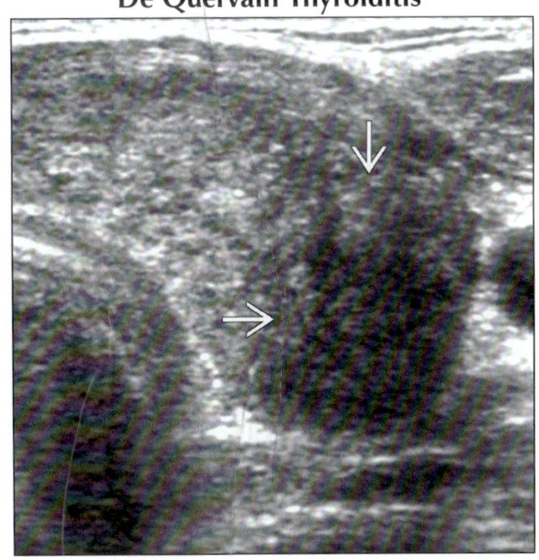

De Quervain Thyroiditis

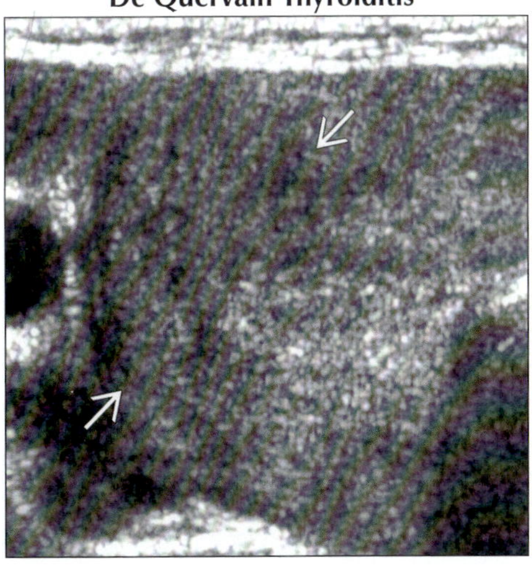

(Left) Transverse ultrasound shows diffuse thyroid enlargement with a focal, heterogeneous, hypoechoic area ➡ in this young patient with acute painful thyroid swelling, preceded by an upper respiratory tract infection. This appearance and history is consistent with de Quervain thyroiditis. (Right) Transverse ultrasound in the same patient a few days later shows ill-defined hypoechoic heterogeneity ➡ in the contralateral lobe.

Acute Suppurative Thyroiditis

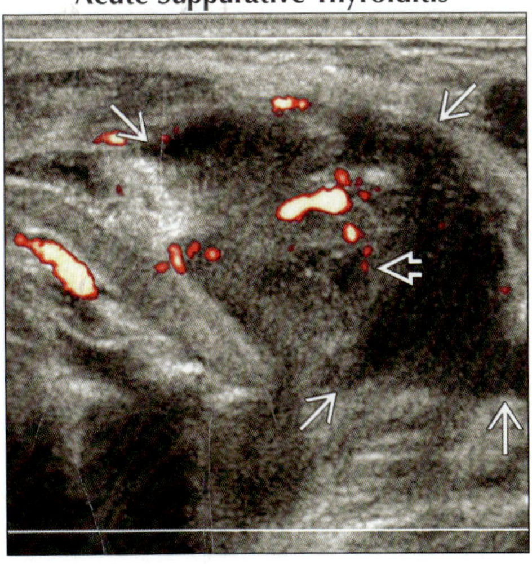

Acute Suppurative Thyroiditis

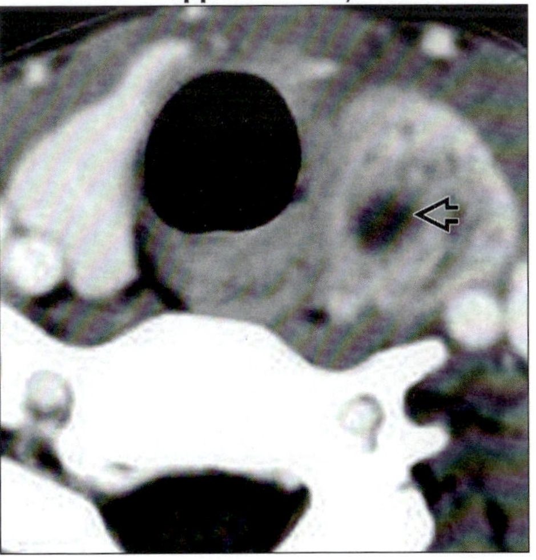

(Left) Transverse power Doppler ultrasound shows a perithyroidal abscess ➡ around the upper pole of the left lobe of the thyroid ➡. Acute suppurative thyroiditis is more common on the left side. (Right) Axial CECT in the same patient shows an enlarged left lobe of the thyroid with heterogeneous enhancement, suggesting inflammation. The low attenuation area ➡ corresponds to the abscess seen on US.

DIFFUSE THYROID ENLARGEMENT

(Left) Double contrast barium image of the pharynx shows the left pyriform sinus fistula ➡ in a patient with acute suppurative thyroiditis. The examination was performed after the acute episode subsided. (Right) Transverse ultrasound shows an anaplastic carcinoma in the left lobe of the thyroid. The tumor ➡ is poorly defined, solid, hypoechoic, and infiltrating most of the left lobe. It appears to have an extrathyroid extension posteriorly ➡.

Acute Suppurative Thyroiditis

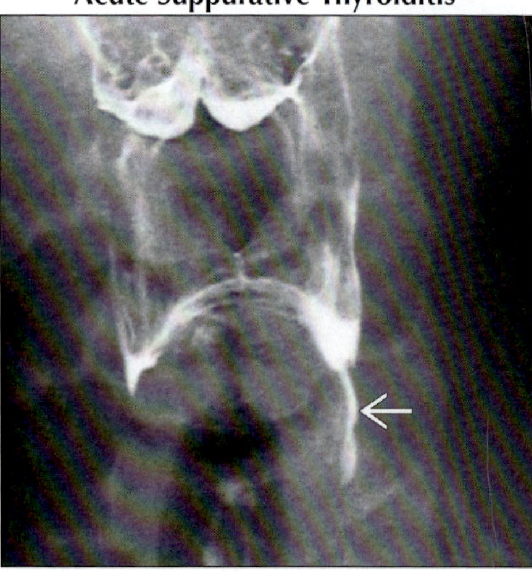

Anaplastic Thyroid Carcinoma

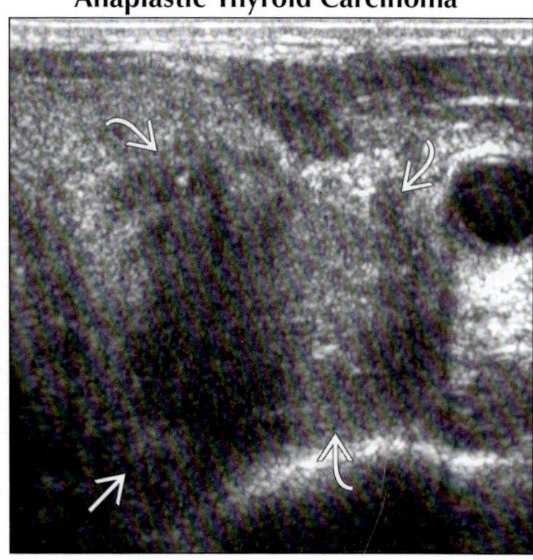

(Left) Transverse ultrasound in the same patient shows the tumor extending to the right thyroid bed ➡ via the prevertebral space and the tumor's association with multiple metastatic nodes ➡ in the contralateral neck. (Right) Axial CECT of the thyroid in the same patient clearly shows diffuse infiltration of the left lobe of the thyroid ➡ by the anaplastic carcinoma, with extrathyroid spread crossing the midline ➡ and encasing the left CCA ➡.

Anaplastic Thyroid Carcinoma

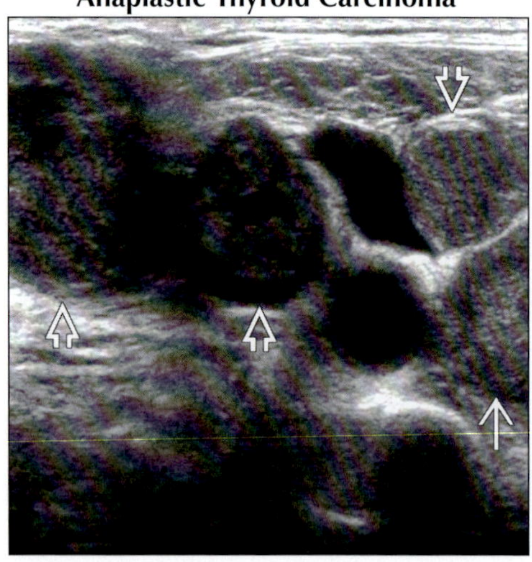

Anaplastic Thyroid Carcinoma

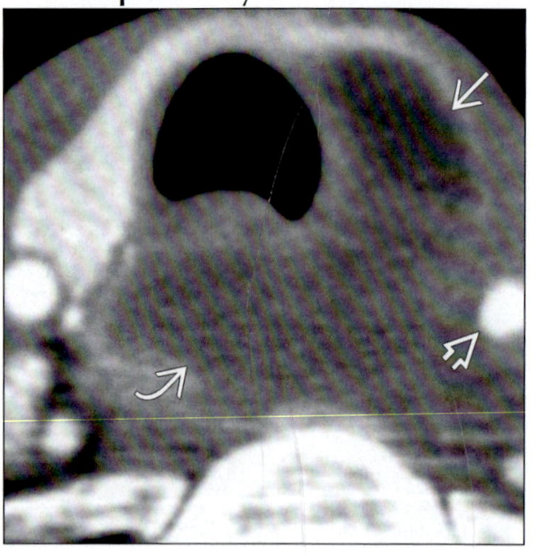

(Left) Transverse power Doppler ultrasound shows an ill-defined, hypoechoic, anaplastic carcinoma ➡ invading the trachea ➡. Extrathyroid extension is better evaluated with CT or MR (not shown). FNAC is best done using US. (Right) Transverse ultrasound of the right lobe of the thyroid shows mild diffuse enlargement with a focal ill-defined hypoechoic area ➡ in this patient with known disseminated carcinoma of breast. FNAC showed a metastasis.

Anaplastic Thyroid Carcinoma

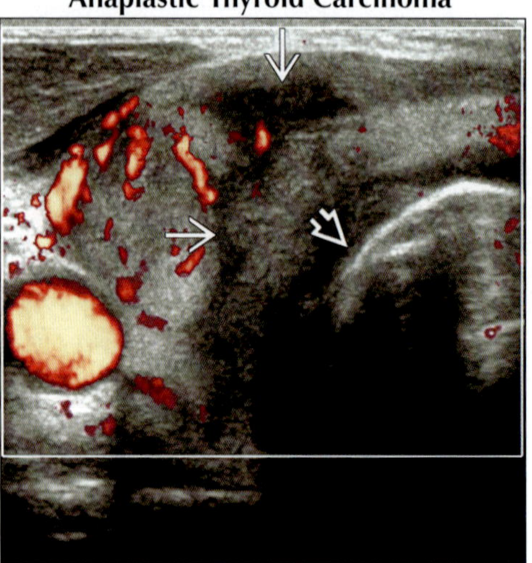

Thyroid Metastasis

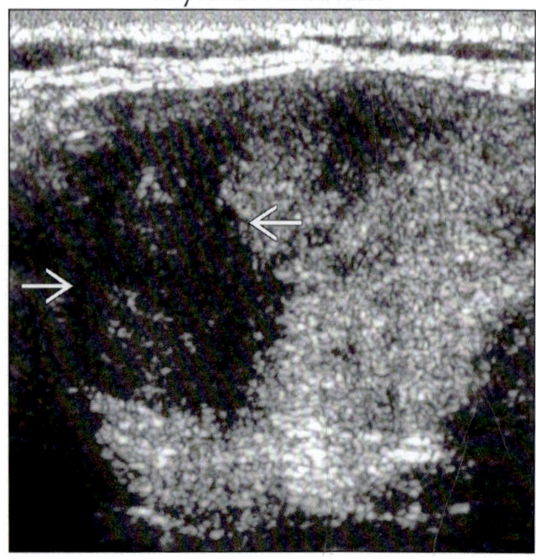

DIFFUSE THYROID ENLARGEMENT

Thyroid Metastasis

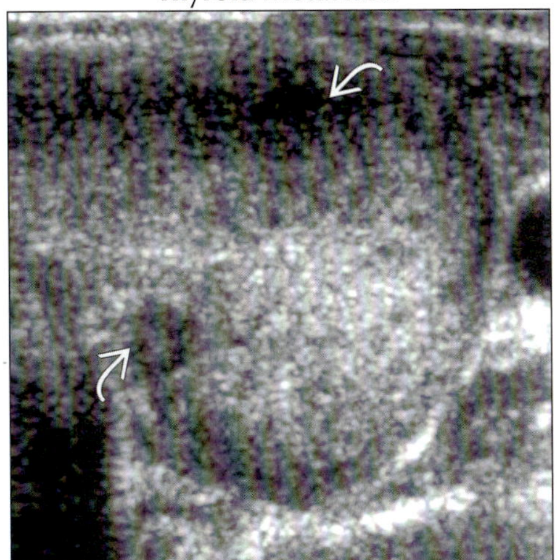

Thyroid Metastasis

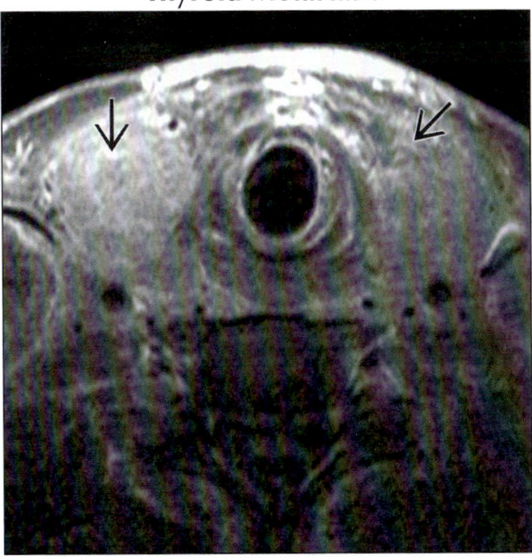

(Left) Transverse ultrasound in the same patient shows multiple hypoechoic nodules ➡ of the left lobe. Thyroid metastases are invariably associated with disseminated disease from lung, bone, liver, and lymph nodes. (Right) Axial T1 C+ MR in the same patient shows a goiter with mild heterogeneous thyroid parenchymal intensity ➡. Note that the metastatic lesions are subtle on MR, though clearly seen on the ultrasound.

Lymphoma

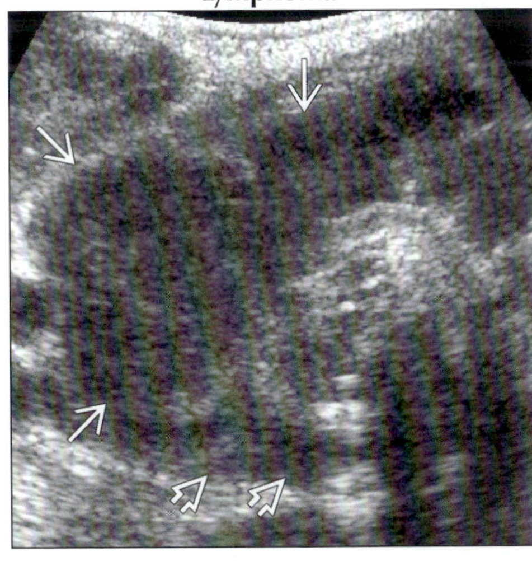

Lymphoma

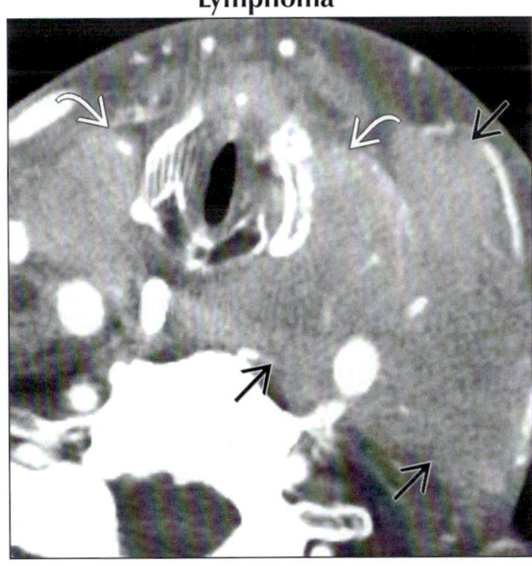

(Left) Transverse ultrasound shows a diffusely enlarged, heterogeneous, hypoechoic thyroid gland ➡. The thyroid capsule is interrupted with extrathyroid extension of the tumor ➡. (Right) Axial CECT in the same patient shows a hypoenhanced thyroid gland ➡ inseparable from the diffuse infiltrative abnormal soft tissue in the neck ➡. These findings are typical of lymphomatous involvement of the soft tissues of the neck and thyroid gland.

Leukemia

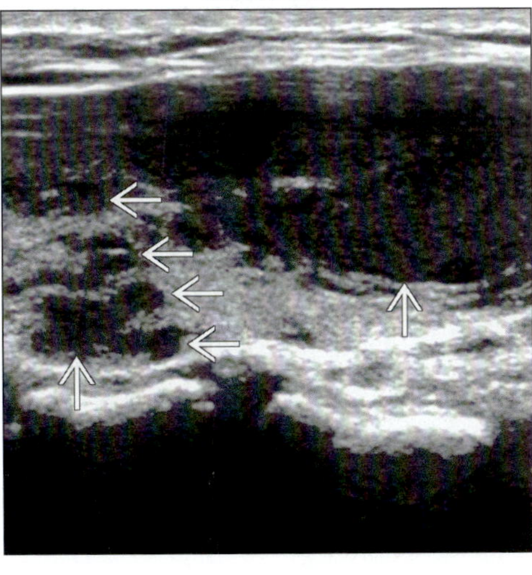

Leukemia

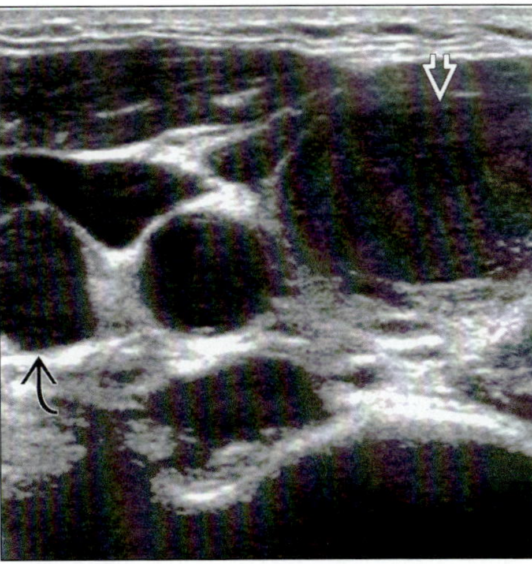

(Left) Longitudinal ultrasound shows thyroid involvement by chronic lymphocytic leukemia, seen as multiple ill-defined hypoechoic areas ➡ scattered in the gland. The appearance is nonspecific and mimics other thyroid malignancies. (Right) Transverse ultrasound in the same patient shows the mass ➡ in the right lobe of the thyroid and associated malignant lymph node ➡. Clinical correlation is crucial as US appearance is nonspecific.

ISO-/HYPERECHOIC THYROID NODULE

DIFFERENTIAL DIAGNOSIS

Common
- Multinodular Goiter
- Postoperative Hypertrophy

Less Common
- Follicular Lesion
  - Follicular Adenoma
  - Follicular Carcinoma
  - Hürthle Cell Neoplasm

ESSENTIAL INFORMATION

Key Differential Diagnosis Issues
- Likelihood of malignancy ↑ as echogenicity ↓
  - Review of malignant nodules shows 4% are hyperechoic, 26% isoechoic, and 63% hypoechoic
- Benign thyroid nodules very common; therefore, solitary hypoechoic nodule is statistically more likely to be benign

Helpful Clues for Common Diagnoses
- **Multinodular Goiter**
  - May show predominantly hyperplastic nodules, colloid nodules, or mixture
  - Hypoechoic halo and vascularity help to delineate hyperplastic nodules
- **Postoperative Hypertrophy**
  - Postoperative recurrence of multinodular goiter is common
  - Appearance is otherwise similar to multinodular goiter

- History of previous thyroid surgery should reveal diagnosis

Helpful Clues for Less Common Diagnoses
- **Follicular Lesion**
  - Imaging or fine-needle aspiration and cytology (FNAC) unable to differentiate benign follicular adenoma from follicular carcinoma
    - Differentiation made after surgery based on vascular and capsular invasion; therefore commonly lumped together
  - Ultrasound features of follicular adenoma
    - Well-defined oval solid nodule, iso-/hyperechoic, ± small area of cystic change
    - Calcification is rare
    - Perinodular > intranodular vascularity
  - Features more indicative of carcinoma
    - Ill-defined border, hypoechoic or hypoechoic portion of otherwise iso-/hyperechoic nodule, ± heterogeneous (necrotic, cystic areas)
    - Marked chaotic intranodular vascularity
  - **Hürthle Cell Neoplasm**
    - Adenoma or carcinoma, like follicular lesions, cannot be distinguished with imaging or FNAC
    - Association seen with Hashimoto thyroiditis, nodular goiter
    - Metastasize more often than follicular carcinoma
    - Sonographic appearance is similar to that of follicular lesion

Multinodular Goiter

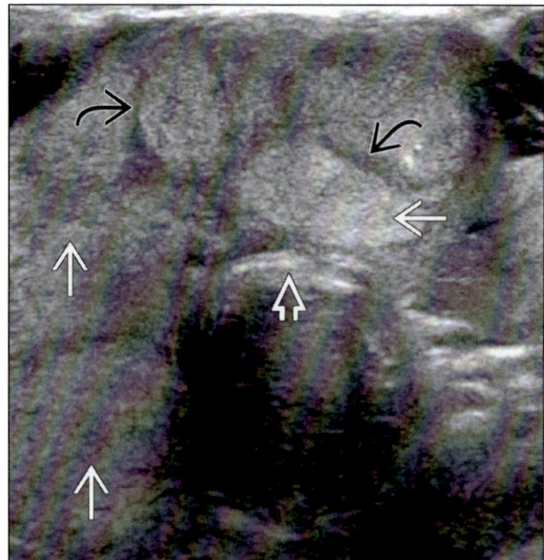

Transverse ultrasound shows diffuse thyroid enlargement. Multiple isoechoic nodules ➡ are delineated by the presence of a hypoechoic halo ➡. Note the trachea ➡.

Postoperative Hypertrophy

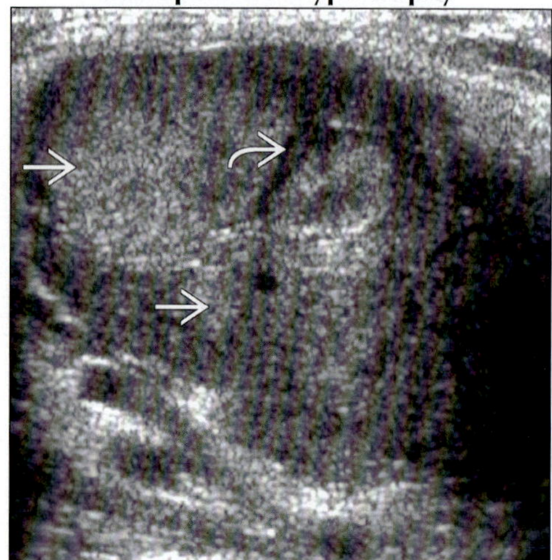

Longitudinal ultrasound shows a thyroid mass with lobulated contour. Note multiple isoechoic thyroid nodules ➡ & a hypoechoic halo ➡. The patient had history of hemithyroidectomy for multinodular goiter.

ISO-/HYPERECHOIC THYROID NODULE

Follicular Adenoma

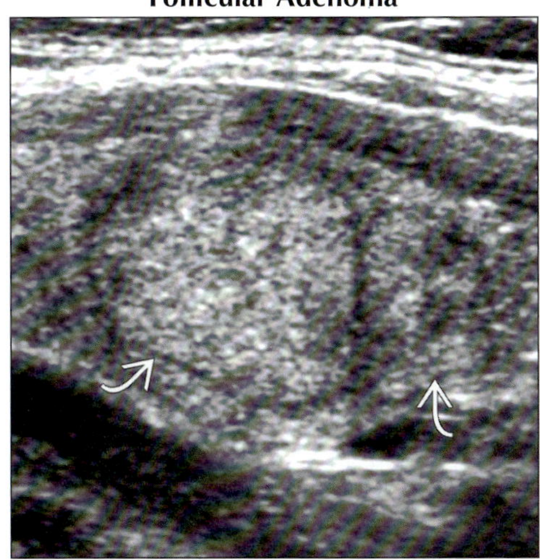

Follicular Adenoma

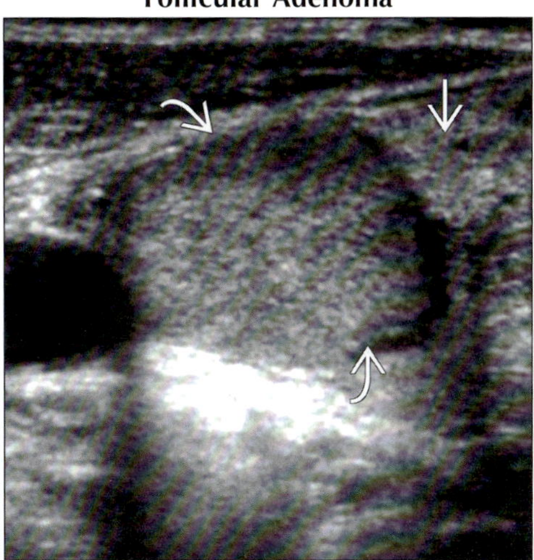

(Left) Longitudinal ultrasound shows well-defined, completely haloed, isoechoic nodules ➡ in the thyroid. They are solid, homogeneous, and without cystic change, colloid or punctate calcifications. The findings suggest a follicular lesion. (Right) Transverse ultrasound shows a nodule ➡ with similar characteristics, but it is slightly hypoechoic to the thyroid ➡. Surgery confirmed follicular adenomas in both cases.

Follicular Carcinoma

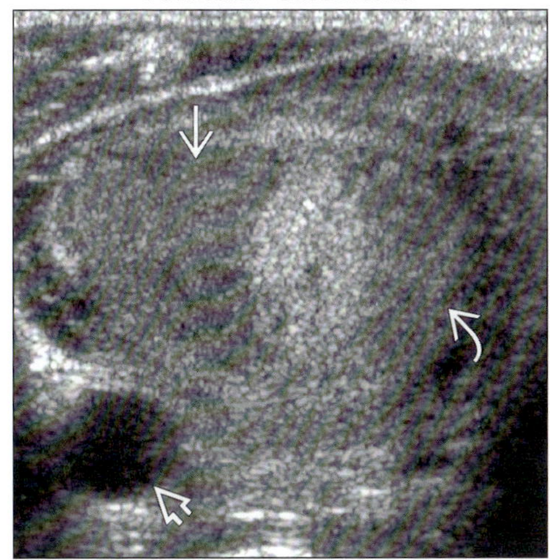

Follicular Carcinoma

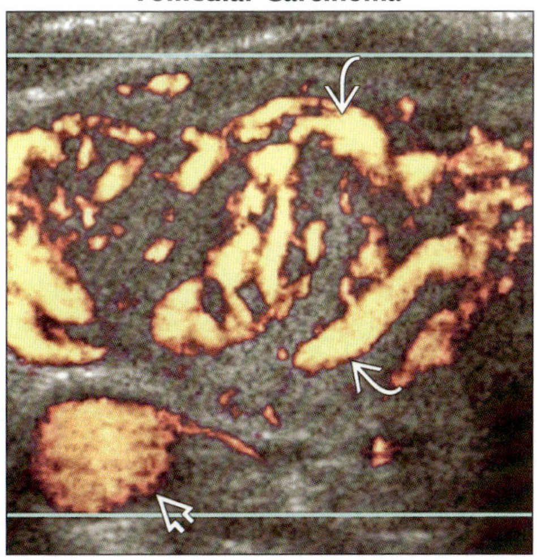

(Left) Transverse ultrasound shows a solid, heterogeneous thyroid nodule ➡ with indistinct borders. There is a hypoechoic component ➡, suspicious for follicular carcinoma. The common carotid artery (CCA) ➡ is also seen. (Right) Power Doppler ultrasound in the same patient shows profuse chaotic intratumoral vascularity ➡ (CCA ➡). Thyroidectomy showed follicular carcinoma. Imaging & FNAC are unable to differentiate benign from malignant follicular lesions.

Hürthle Cell Neoplasm

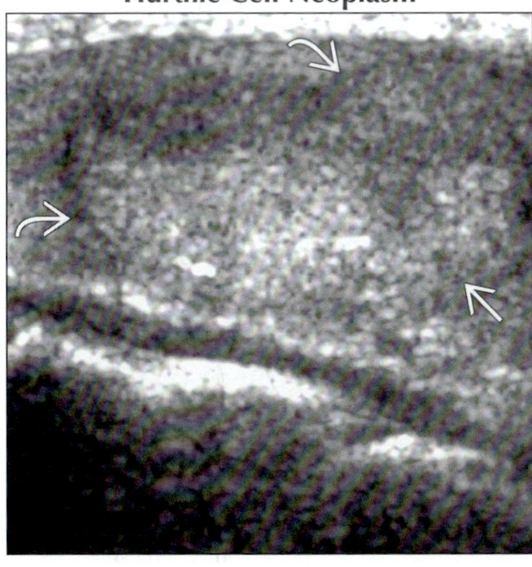

Hürthle Cell Neoplasm

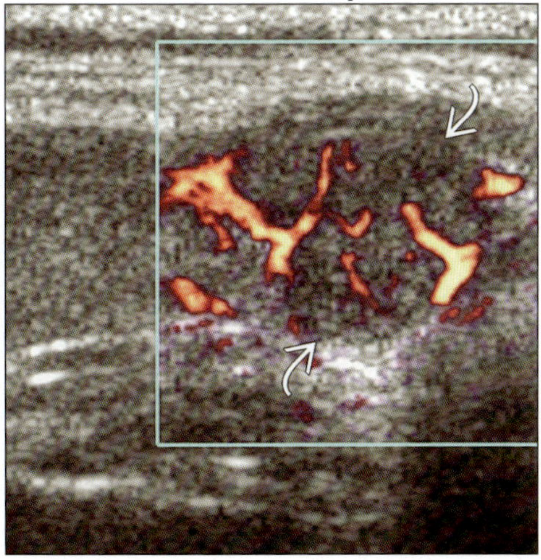

(Left) Longitudinal ultrasound shows a well-defined, solid, homogeneous, isoechoic nodule ➡ with a complete hypoechoic halo ➡. The appearance suggests a follicular lesion, and surgery showed Hürthle cell adenoma. (Right) Longitudinal power Doppler ultrasound shows another isoechoic Hürthle cell adenoma ➡. Moderate intratumoral vascularity is seen. Occasionally, Hürthle cell adenoma may be avascular (unlike follicular).

HYPOECHOIC THYROID NODULE

DIFFERENTIAL DIAGNOSIS

Common
- Multinodular Goiter

Less Common
- Papillary Carcinoma
- Follicular Carcinoma
- Medullary Carcinoma
- De Quervain Thyroiditis
- Acute Suppurative Thyroiditis

Rare but Important
- Anaplastic Carcinoma
- Lymphoma
- Metastasis

ESSENTIAL INFORMATION

Key Differential Diagnosis Issues
- In routine clinical practice, most common hypoechoic thyroid nodules are part of multinodular goiter (MNG)
  - Adenomatous, hyperplastic, colloid nodules
- However, many malignant nodules also seen against background of MNG
  - Main reason for US in MNG is to identify presence of malignancy in thyroid
  - Note: Anaplastic carcinomas, though rare, invariably occur against background of MNG
- Essential to be familiar with US appearance of thyroid cancers; papillary carcinoma is most common
- Crucial to identify malignant features in hypoechoic nodule & combine US with fine-needle aspiration and cytology (FNAC) for definitive diagnosis
- Overlap of features between benign and malignant thyroid nodules
  - Combination of sonographic features (grayscale & Doppler) will help identify malignant hypoechoic thyroid nodule
- Benign features
  - Well defined, completely haloed, cystic change, septation, presence of colloid, dense/dysmorphic calcification, predominant perinodular vascularity
- Malignant features
  - Ill defined, irregular, punctate calcification, necrosis, marked intranodular vascularity, local invasion, lymphadenopathy, internal jugular vein (IJV) thrombus

Helpful Clues for Common Diagnoses
- **Multinodular Goiter**
  - Degenerative nodules
    - Degenerative change in hyperplastic nodules
    - Cystic change → septation → entirely cystic ± colloid deposits
    - Well defined ± completely haloed
  - Colloid nodules
    - Thin walled, well defined, cystic
    - Echogenic foci with "comet tail" artifacts are characteristic
    - Thick septations ± aggregates of debris
  - Background parenchymal heterogeneity (± intranodular hemorrhage) may occur in both degenerative and colloid types
  - Other nodules/areas with dense/dysmorphic shadowing calcification may be present in both types
  - On Doppler, colloid nodules/septae are relatively avascular
    - Degenerative nodules with cystic change show predominant perinodular vascularity
    - Solid portions in hyperplastic nodules may be quite vascular

Helpful Clues for Less Common Diagnoses
- **Papillary Carcinoma**
  - Painless, enlarging thyroid/neck mass (lymphadenopathy) or incidental finding on thyroid ultrasound
  - Hypoechoic, ill defined, characteristic punctate calcification, ± cystic change
  - Hypervascular with disorganized intranodular vascularity
  - Metastatic nodes show features of primary: Punctate calcification, cystic change, & disorganized vascularity
- **Follicular Carcinoma**
  - Cannot be definitively differentiated from adenoma on either imaging or cytology
  - In most cases, develops from preexisting adenoma
  - Excision is required for definitive diagnosis (to detect any vascular or capsular invasion)

- Ultrasound features (suggestive of carcinoma)
  - Ill-defined border, hypoechoic areas in otherwise iso-/hyperechoic nodule, irregular thick walls, disorganized vascularity, extrathyroid extension
  - Metastatic disease in bones, lungs, less commonly in nodes
- **Medullary Carcinoma**
  - Multifocal & bilateral > solitary > diffusely infiltrative
  - Hypoechoic solid tumor, often well defined, frequently located in lateral upper 2/3 of gland in sporadic form
  - Echogenic foci (80-90%) = amyloid + Ca++
  - Hypoechoic lymph nodes with coarse shadowing calcification along mid & low IJV chain and superior mediastinum
  - Indistinguishable from papillary carcinoma (more common) on ultrasound; diagnosis made by FNAC
    - Differentiating clue: Coarser calcification and denser shadowing compared with punctate Ca++ in papillary carcinoma
- **De Quervain Thyroiditis**
  - Typical history + ill-defined hypoechoic noncalcified mass ± internal necrosis
  - Vascularity due to inflammatory hyperemia, avascular in necrotic region
- **Acute Suppurative Thyroiditis**
  - Acute onset painful thyroid swelling ± recurrent episodes, left (95%) > > right (5%)
  - Starts as perithyroidal inflammation/abscess
  - Late involvement of thyroid gland, typically left upper pole
  - Underlying pyriform fossa sinus

Helpful Clues for Rare Diagnoses
- **Anaplastic Carcinoma**
  - Rapidly enlarging lower neck mass (± obstructive symptoms) in elderly female with long history of goiter
  - Ultrasound features: Large ill-defined hypoechoic mass with background MNG
    - Necrosis (78%), dense amorphous/ring calcification (58%), abnormal intratumoral vascularity
    - Extracapsular spread with extensive local invasion with nodal (80%) and distant metastasis
  - US-guided FNAC to confirm diagnosis; CT for extent and extrathyroid involvement
- **Lymphoma**
  - Rapidly enlarging lower neck mass in longstanding Hashimoto thyroiditis
  - Ill-defined mass, often large or diffuse infiltration ± local invasion
  - Necrosis, calcification, and hemorrhage are rare; associated lymphomatous nodes
- **Metastasis**
  - Ill-defined hypoechoic mass; solitary > multifocal > diffuse infiltrative
  - Lack specific sonographic features, but most patients have known primary and disseminated disease

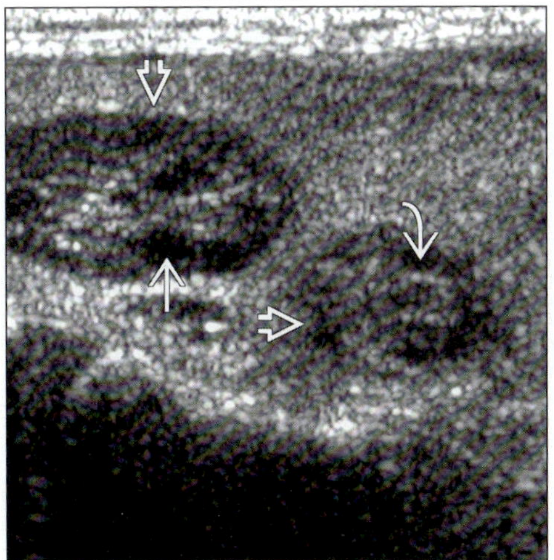

Multinodular Goiter

Longitudinal ultrasound shows multiple well-defined hypoechoic nodules ➔. The cystic change ➔ and early septation ➔ are characteristic of degenerative nodules, findings consistent with MNG.

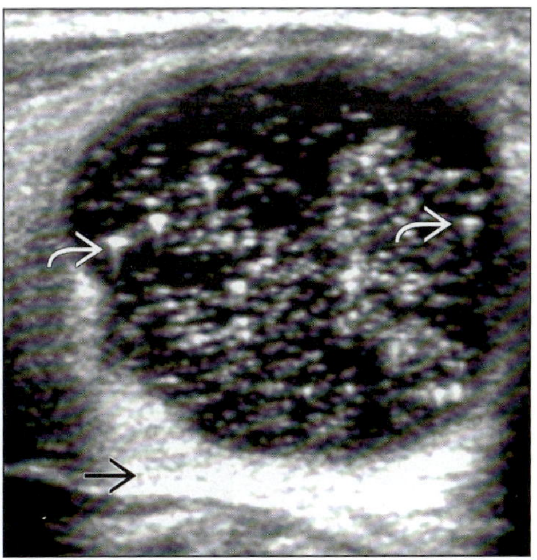

Multinodular Goiter

Longitudinal ultrasound shows a typical thin-walled colloid cyst with multiple dispersed/suspended echogenic foci and "comet tail" artifacts ➔. Note the posterior acoustic enhancement ➔.

HYPOECHOIC THYROID NODULE

(Left) Longitudinal ultrasound shows a fairly well-defined, solid, hypoechoic thyroid nodule ➡. Note the indistinct border ➡ and punctate calcifications ➡, suggesting a papillary carcinoma. *(Right)* Transverse ultrasound in the same patient shows a solid, hypoechoic, metastatic node ➡ from papillary carcinoma with punctate calcification ➡. Note that the appearance is very similar to the primary tumor ➡ in the thyroid. (CCA ➡ & IJV ➡.)

Papillary Carcinoma

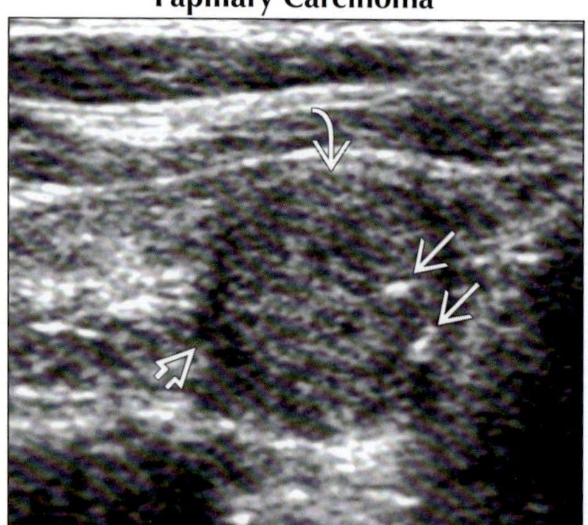

Papillary Carcinoma

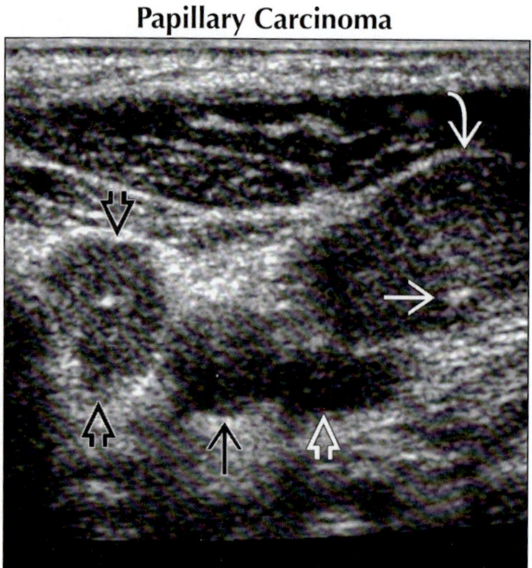

(Left) Transverse ultrasound shows a large, solid, hypoechoic, infiltrative papillary carcinoma with multiple punctate calcifications ➡. Note the irregular ill-defined border ➡ and extracapsular spread ➡. *(Right)* Transverse power Doppler ultrasound shows papillary carcinoma of the thyroid ➡ and an ipsilateral metastatic internal jugular chain lymph node ➡. Both show disorganized internal vascularity. Note the common carotid artery ➡ & IJV ➡.

Papillary Carcinoma

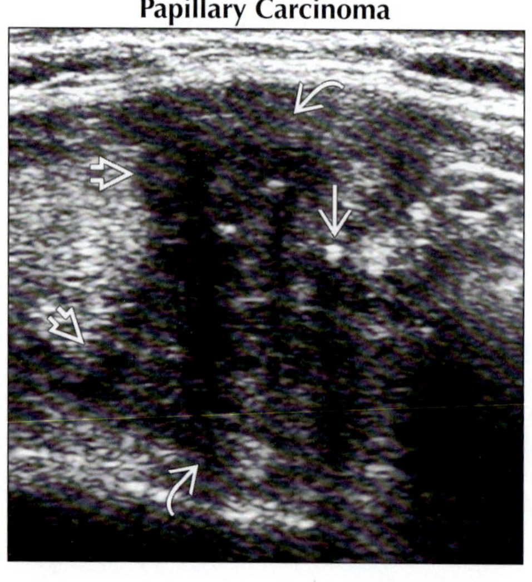

Papillary Carcinoma

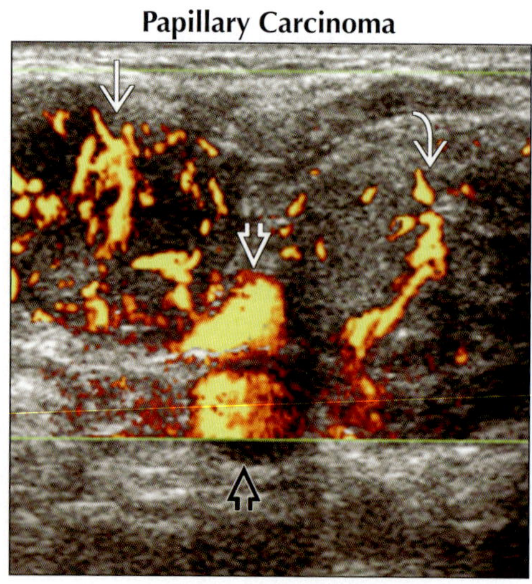

(Left) Longitudinal ultrasound shows an ovoid, solid, hypoechoic thyroid nodule. The homogeneous echopattern is suggestive of a follicular lesion. Partially indistinct border ➡ and hypoechogenicity are suspicious of malignant change. Excision showed follicular carcinoma. *(Right)* Axial NECT in the same patient shows multiple lung metastases ➡ from follicular carcinoma. Some patients with follicular carcinoma may 1st present with metastases.

Follicular Carcinoma

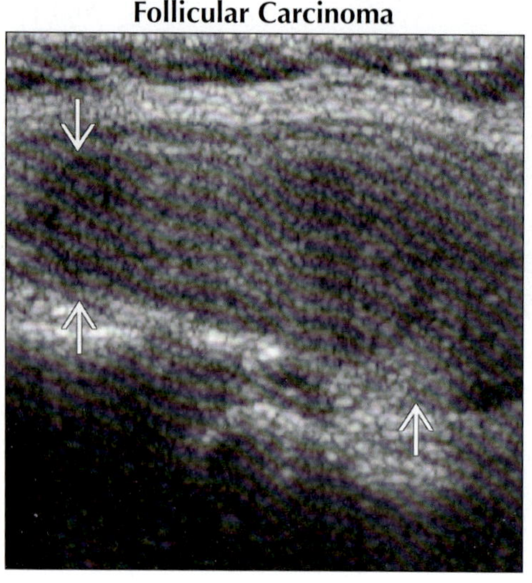

Follicular Carcinoma

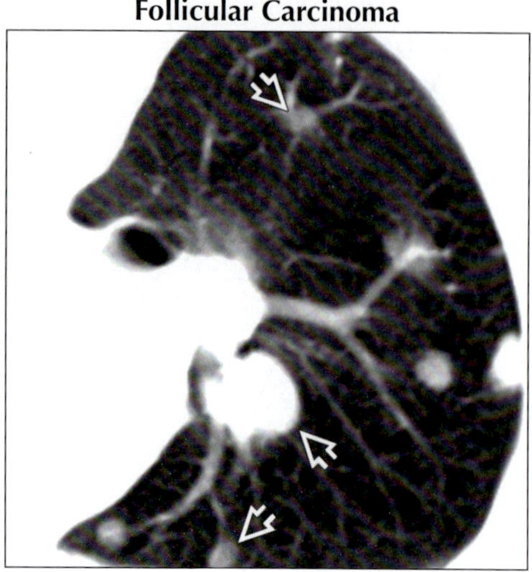

HYPOECHOIC THYROID NODULE

Follicular Carcinoma

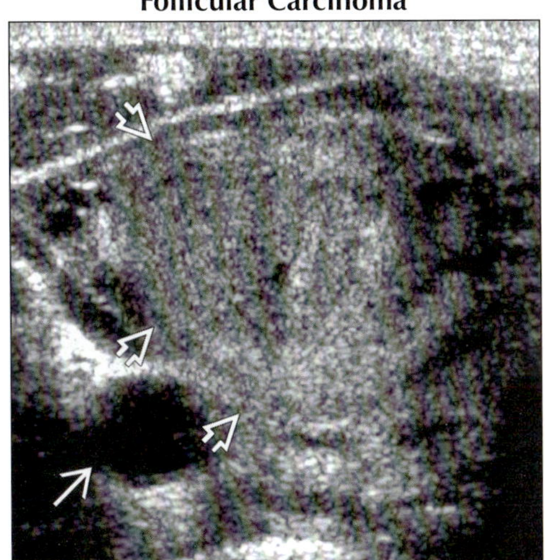

Follicular Carcinoma

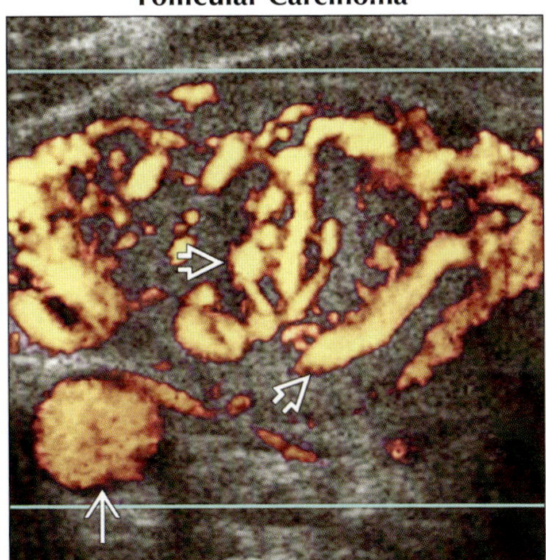

(Left) Transverse ultrasound shows a solid hypoechoic thyroid nodule. The ill-defined border ⮀ and heterogenicity are suspicious of malignant change in a follicular lesion. Note the CCA ➡. *(Right)* Transverse power Doppler ultrasound in the same patient shows profuse intratumoral vascularity ⮀ resembling a disrupted spoke wheel. The ill-defined hypoechogenicity and abnormal vascularity are clues to the malignant nature of the nodule. Note the CCA ➡.

Medullary Carcinoma

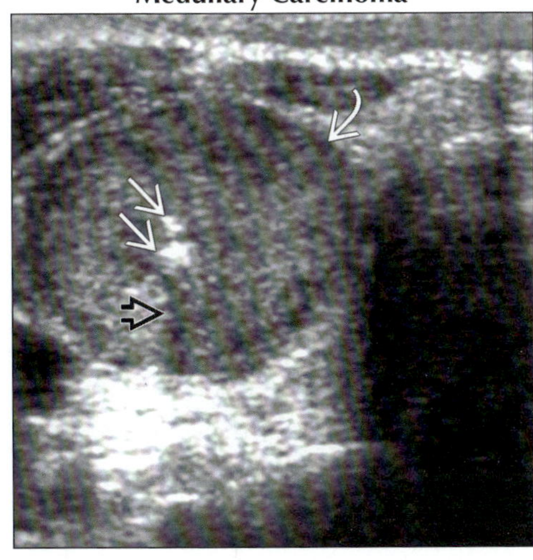

Medullary Carcinoma

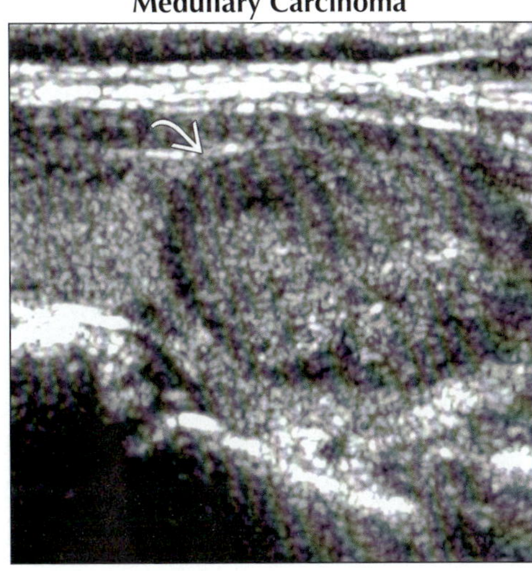

(Left) Transverse ultrasound shows a well-defined hypoechoic nodule ➡. It is solid with internal foci of dense calcifications ➡. Note its similarity to papillary carcinoma. Dense posterior shadowing ⮀ may be the only clue to suggest medullary carcinoma. *(Right)* Longitudinal ultrasound shows a solid, hypoechoic, well-defined, medullary carcinoma ➡ without calcification. A papillary or even follicular carcinoma may have a similar appearance.

De Quervain Thyroiditis

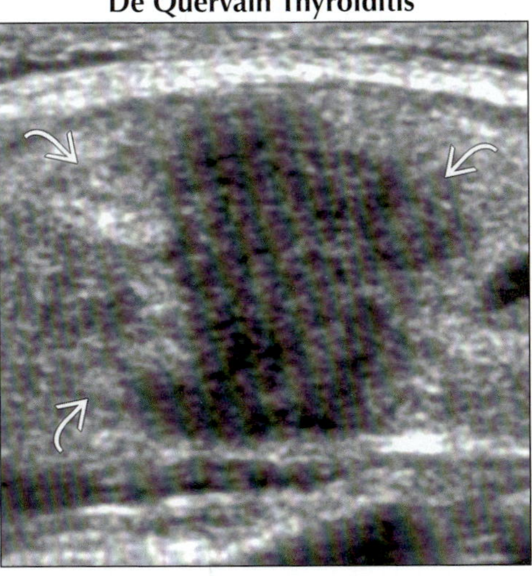

De Quervain Thyroiditis

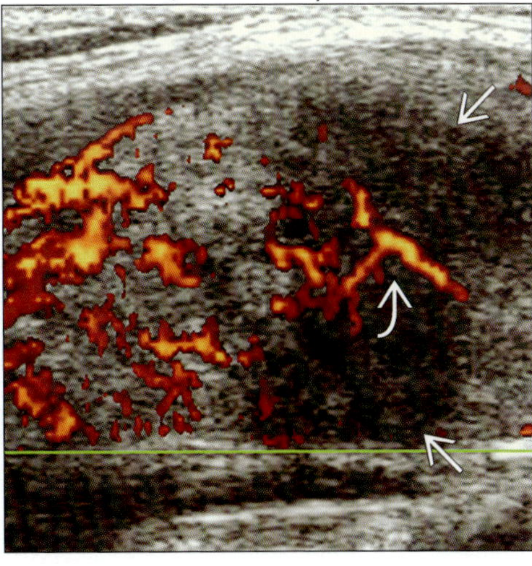

(Left) Longitudinal ultrasound shows an irregular, heterogeneously hypoechoic thyroid nodule ➡. The appearance is very similar to a malignant nodule. However, the patient had odynophagia and a fever, suggesting de Quervain thyroiditis. After a few days, the entire gland was involved. *(Right)* Longitudinal power Doppler ultrasound shows vascularity ⮀ in the hypoechoic area ➡, mimicking a malignant thyroid nodule.

HYPOECHOIC THYROID NODULE

(Left) Transverse ultrasound shows a large perithyroidal abscess ➡ with extension into the upper pole of the left lobe of the thyroid gland ⮞. Note the common carotid artery ⮞ and areas of internal necrosis within the abscess ➡. *(Right)* Axial CECT in the same patient shows a large multiloculated perithyroidal abscess ➡ with intrathyroid extension ➡. Note the common carotid artery ⮞, trachea ➡, and necrotic areas of the abscess ➡.

Acute Suppurative Thyroiditis

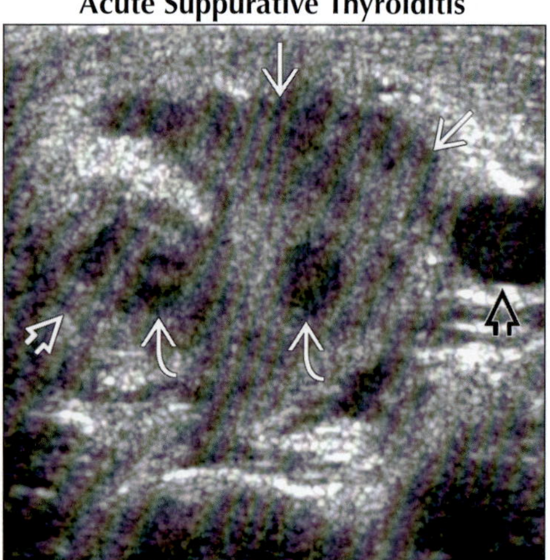

Acute Suppurative Thyroiditis

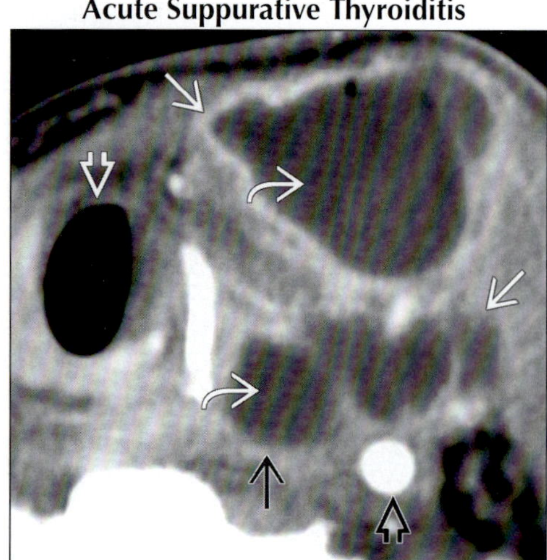

(Left) Transverse ultrasound shows an anaplastic carcinoma. Note the ill-defined border ⮞. The tissue plane with the trachea is lost, suspicious of tracheal invasion ➡. *(Right)* Transverse ultrasound shows an anaplastic carcinoma in the left lobe of the thyroid, seen as a large, ill-defined, hypoechoic mass ➡ with extracapsular spread ➡ invading the surrounding soft tissue. Note the CCA ⮞ and anterior cortex of the vertebral body ⮞.

Anaplastic Carcinoma

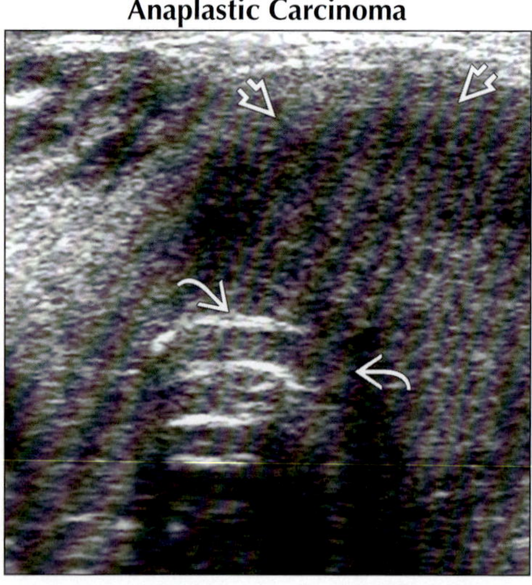

Anaplastic Carcinoma

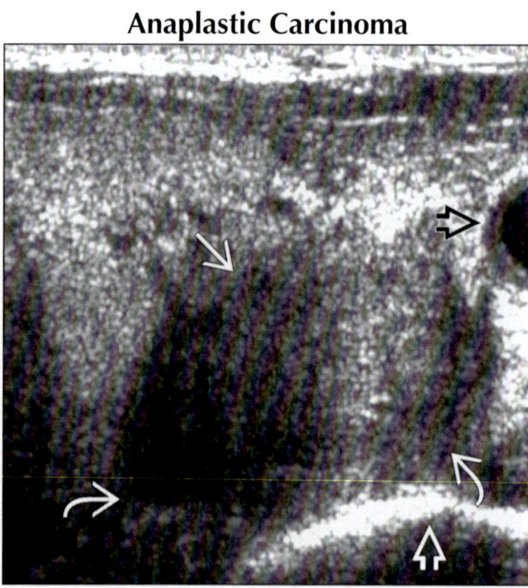

(Left) Axial CECT in the same patient shows extensive local infiltration by the tumor ➡, encasing the ipsilateral major vessels ➡, invading the ipsilateral prevertebral muscle, and crossing midline ➡. *(Right)* Transverse T2WI MR with fat suppression in the same patient shows an irregular hyperintense area representing intratumoral necrosis ➡. Invasion of the prevertebral muscle and crossing of the midline ➡ are seen.

Anaplastic Carcinoma

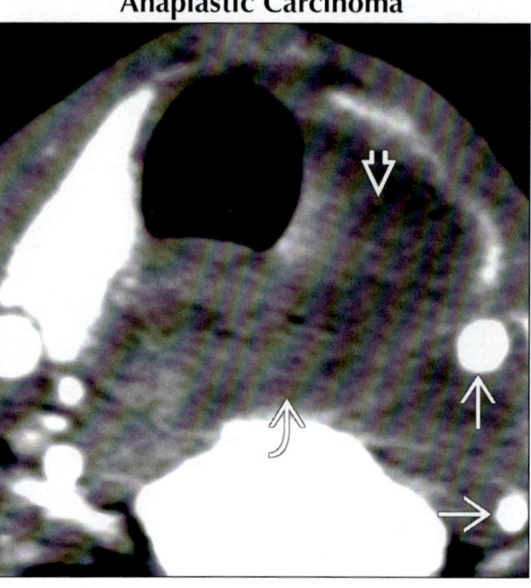

Anaplastic Carcinoma

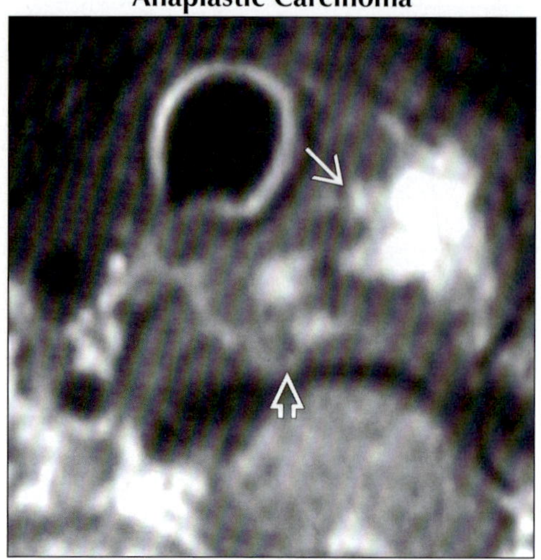

HYPOECHOIC THYROID NODULE

Lymphoma

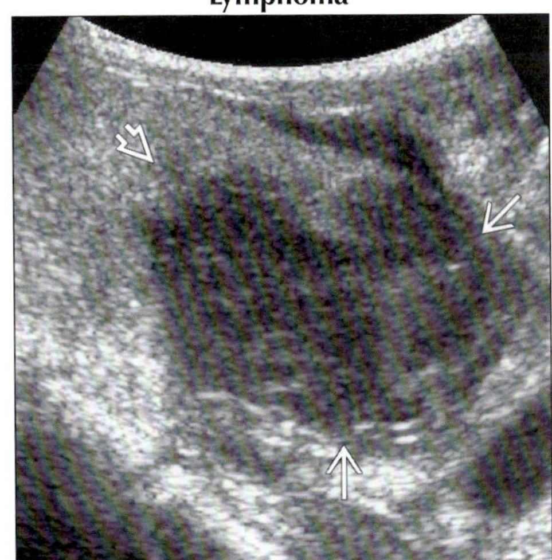

Lymphoma

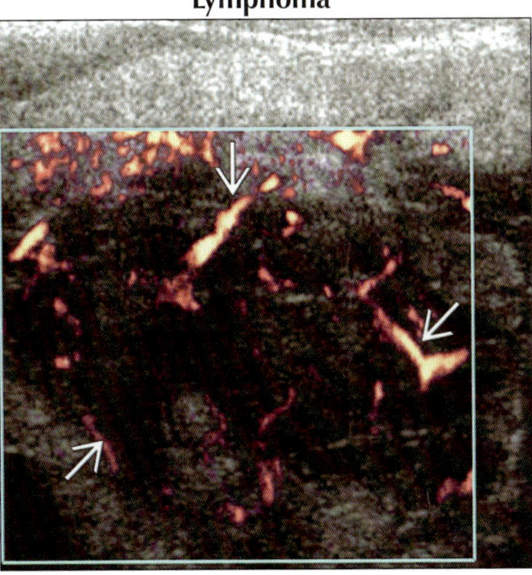

(Left) Longitudinal ultrasound shows an irregular hypoechoic mass infiltrating the lower pole of the thyroid ➡, representing a thyroid lymphoma. The ill-defined margin ➡ is suspicious of extracapsular spread. (Right) Longitudinal power Doppler ultrasound in the same patient shows disorganized internal vascularity ➡ scattered throughout the lesion. The presence of associated lymphomatous nodes (not shown) was a clue to the diagnosis.

Metastasis

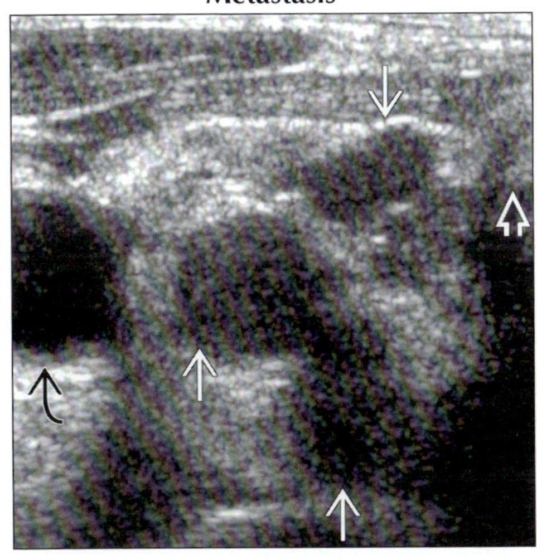

Metastasis

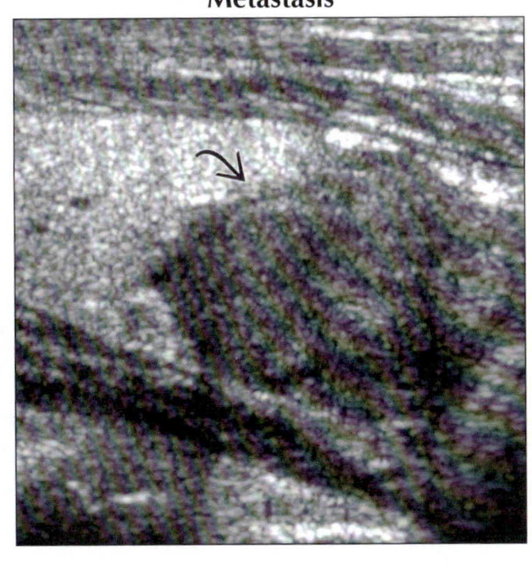

(Left) Transverse ultrasound shows multifocal thyroid metastases, seen as ill-defined, solid, hypoechoic nodules ➡. There is no internal calcification or cystic change. Note CCA ➡ and trachea ➡. (Right) Longitudinal ultrasound shows an ill-defined, hypoechoic, solid, noncalcified thyroid nodule with otherwise nonspecific features, representing a solitary metastasis ➡. The clue to the diagnosis is the history of a known primary and disseminated disease.

Metastasis

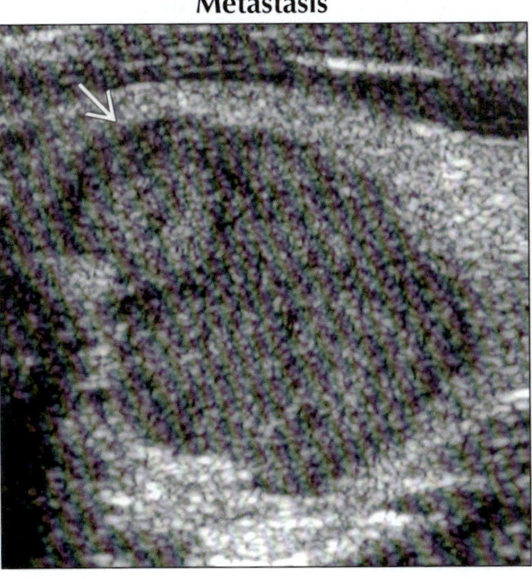

Metastasis

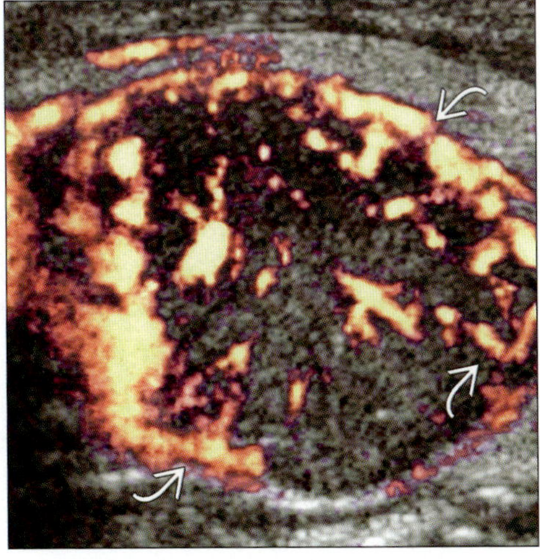

(Left) Transverse ultrasound shows an irregular, solid, heterogeneously hypoechoic, noncalcified nodule ➡ in the left lobe of the thyroid, representing a solitary metastasis. (Right) Transverse power Doppler ultrasound shows profuse, disorganized, peripheral, and intranodular vascularity ➡. Thyroid metastases are usually seen as part of disseminated disease in a patient with a known primary. The prognosis is usually poor.

CYSTIC THYROID NODULE

DIFFERENTIAL DIAGNOSIS

Common
- Colloid Cyst
- Hyperplastic Nodule
- Hemorrhagic Cyst

Less Common
- Papillary Carcinoma
- Acute Suppurative Thyroiditis

Rare but Important
- Follicular Carcinoma
- Congenital Cyst

ESSENTIAL INFORMATION

Key Differential Diagnosis Issues
- Thyroid cysts account for 15-25% of all thyroid nodules
- Most commonly seen in multinodular goiter (MNG) as combination of colloid cyst, hyperplastic nodule, hemorrhagic cyst
- Most thyroid cysts are macronodules, which undergo degeneration, with accumulation of serous fluid, colloid, or blood
  - "Solid" component of many cystic nodules is usually organized hemorrhage
  - Presence/absence of vascularity helps to differentiate avascular hemorrhage from vascular tissue in thyroid carcinoma and hyperplastic nodule
- Thyroid carcinomas, particularly papillary carcinoma, may have prominent cystic components

Helpful Clues for Common Diagnoses
- **Colloid Cyst**
  - Well-defined anechoic nodule with thick internal septae
  - Echogenic foci with "comet tail" artifacts may be adherent to septae/wall or dispersed in thick cystic content
  - "Comet tail" artifact due to reverberations from strong acoustic interface produced by inspissated colloid
    - When interrogating echogenic colloid foci, return to fundamental scanning mode to ensure "comet tails" are genuine artifacts
    - Need to differentiate from punctate calcifications seen in papillary carcinoma
  - Internal debris may aggregate to form echogenic nodule, mimicking neoplasm
    - Use Doppler to differentiate from solid tissue
  - Sonographic appearance may be specific enough to avoid fine-needle aspiration and cytology (FNAC), which is often inadequate due to viscus content
  - Symptomatic nodules are due to internal hemorrhage or superimposed infection
- **Hyperplastic Nodule**
  - Focal hyperplasia of thyroid tissue forms nodule
  - Incompletely encapsulated (vs. complete encapsulation in follicular adenoma)
  - Most commonly seen in background of hyperplasia in MNG
  - Cystic degeneration is common due to fluctuation in tissues' response to thyroid-related hormone
  - Appearances range from small cystic spaces to septated nodule to completely cystic nodule; frequently multiple
    - On Doppler, predominantly cystic nodule shows perinodular vascularity
    - However, marked intranodular vascularity is often seen in predominantly solid nodules
- **Hemorrhagic Cyst**
  - Hemorrhage into thyroid nodule, which may cause painful enlargement of thyroid nodule within hours or days
    - Rarely may cause pressure symptoms, dysphagia, or dyspnea
  - Seen as diffuse, mobile, echogenic particulate material or fluid level ± echogenic blood clots in thyroid nodule
    - Echogenic blood clots are avascular on Doppler
  - US-guided FNAC may be performed for symptomatic relief or cosmesis
  - Direct needle tip away from blood clots to facilitate aspiration of fluid

Helpful Clues for Less Common Diagnoses
- **Papillary Carcinoma**
  - Cystic change is not common in small tumors but often present in larger ones
  - Irregular ill-defined nodule with cystic change; often seen against background of MNG

- Eccentric solid portion may contain punctate calcification and is often hypervascular
  - Metastatic nodes more likely to also show cystic change; appearance mimics primary tumor
  - US-guided FNAC should direct needle tip to solid component (preferably calcified portion) for better yield
    - Aspirated fluid is high in thyroglobulin
- **Acute Suppurative Thyroiditis**
  - Children & adolescents: Left side involvement (95%) >> right side (5%)
  - Related to fistula tract extending from apex of pyriform sinus to lower anterior neck (4th branchial cleft anomaly)
  - Acutely present with fever, painful goiter, and odynophagia
    - History of recurrent episodes of left neck infection with incision & drainage
  - Perithyroidal abscess & soft tissue inflammation ± internal gas pockets
    - Subsequently involves upper pole of thyroid
    - Thyroiditis tends to be late occurrence due to inherent resistance of thyroid gland to infection (thick capsule & high iodine content)
  - CT/MR to exclude deep tissue and mediastinal involvement
  - Barium study after acute episode to demonstrate pyriform fossa fistula

Helpful Clues for Rare Diagnoses
- **Follicular Carcinoma**
  - US (+ FNAC) and core biopsy cannot differentiate follicular adenoma from carcinoma
  - Postoperative histology assesses capsular integrity and vascular invasion to establish diagnosis of follicular carcinoma
  - Therefore, on US, nodules are grouped as follicular lesions/neoplasms
    - Ovoid, solid, homogeneously iso-/hyperechoic
    - Hypoechoic nodule or hypoechoic portion in otherwise iso-/hyperechoic nodule raises possibility of malignancy
    - Border is well defined in less aggressive type and poorly defined in aggressive type
    - CT/MR help to evaluate extrathyroid extension of aggressive follicular carcinomas
    - Internal cystic area and coarse calcification are occasionally seen
    - Intranodular hypervascularity with "spoke-wheel" appearance on Doppler
- **Congenital Cyst**
  - True thyroid cysts lined with epithelium are rare; ≤ 1% of all thyroid nodules
  - Anechoic content ± fine cellular debris
  - Imperceptible walls & posterior acoustic enhancement

Colloid Cyst

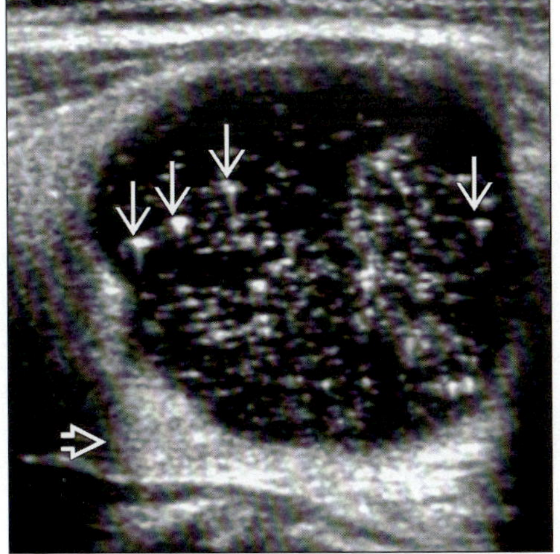

Longitudinal ultrasound shows the typical appearance of a colloid nodule with multiple "comet tail" artifacts ➡ scattered throughout the cyst. Note the thin walls and posterior acoustic enhancement ➡.

Colloid Cyst

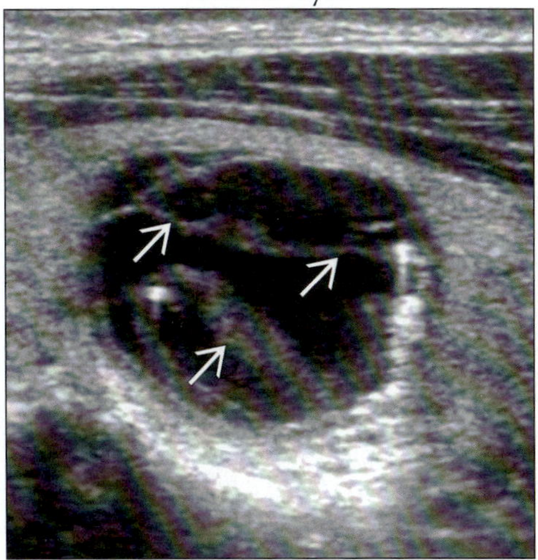

Longitudinal ultrasound shows a colloid nodule with "comet tail" artifacts. Note that the "comet tail" artifacts are adherent to the thick intranodular septae ➡, which are invariably avascular on Doppler.

CYSTIC THYROID NODULE

Hyperplastic Nodule

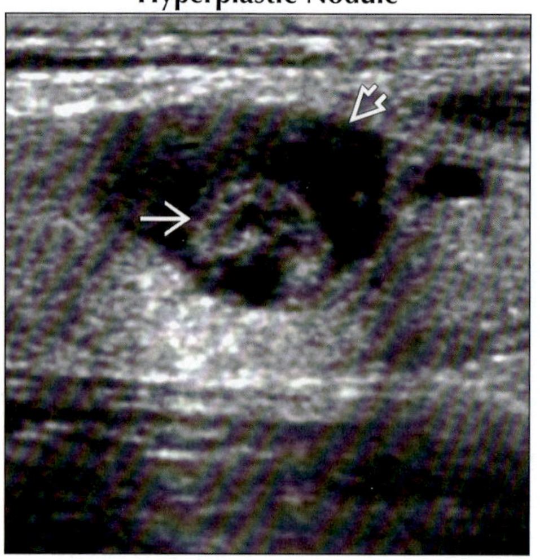

Hyperplastic Nodule

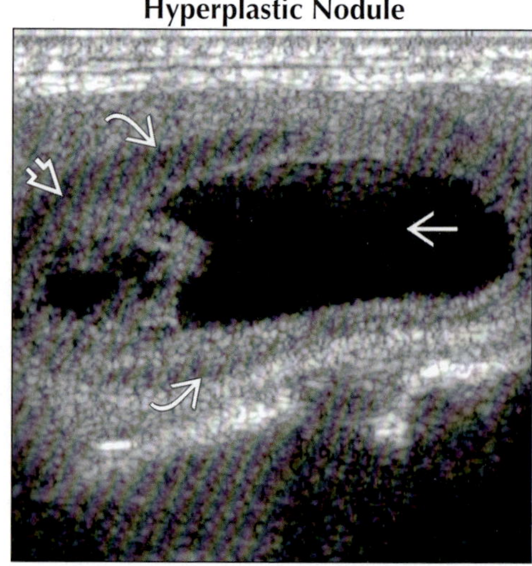

(Left) Longitudinal ultrasound shows a well-defined hyperplastic nodule ➡ with cystic change and internal debris ➡. The debris represents organized blood and is invariably avascular on Doppler. *(Right)* Longitudinal ultrasound shows a hyperplastic nodule ➡ with cystic degeneration ➡. Note the complete halo ➡ around the nodule. On Doppler, such nodules often have a predominantly peripheral vascularity with few vessels in the thick walls.

Hemorrhagic Cyst

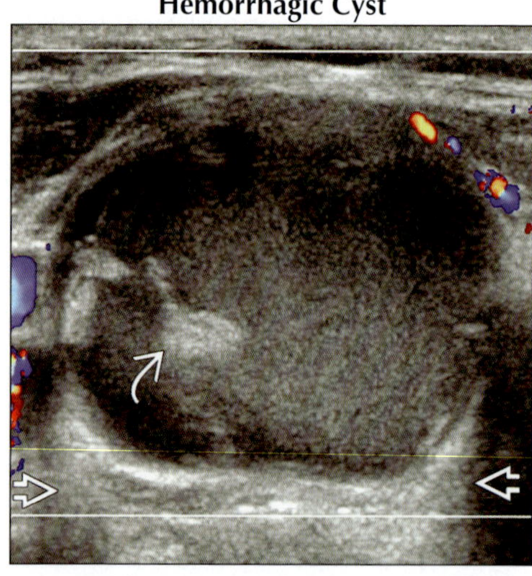

Hemorrhagic Cyst

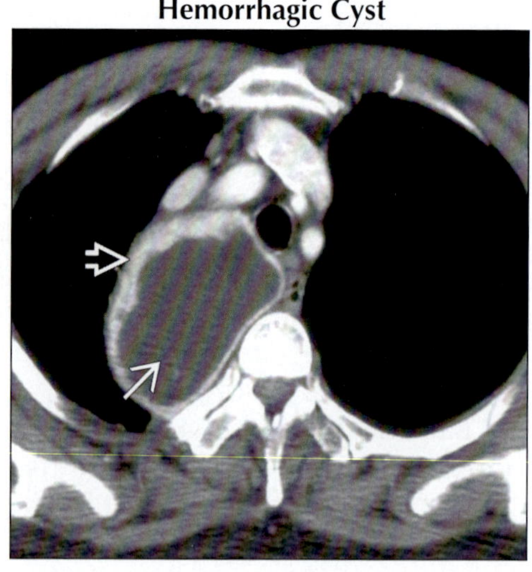

(Left) Transverse color Doppler ultrasound shows a thyroid nodule with dispersed fine internal debris (mobile on real-time scan). The avascular nature and posterior enhancement ➡ differentiate it from a solid nodule. Note debris/blood clot ➡. *(Right)* Axial CECT in the same patient shows cystic change ➡ within the nodule ➡, which extended into the mediastinum. CT better evaluates the inferior extent of the large nodules. Aspiration yielded degraded blood products.

Papillary Carcinoma

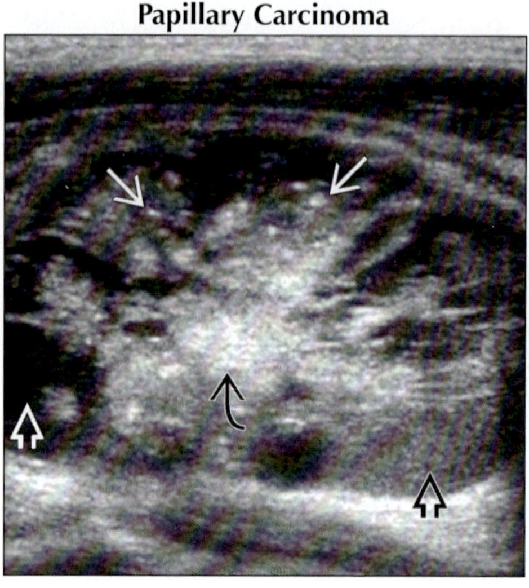

Papillary Carcinoma

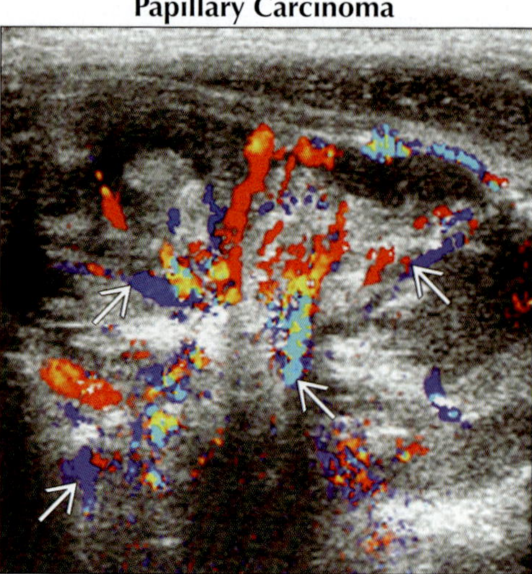

(Left) Longitudinal ultrasound shows a thyroid nodule with cystic change ➡, solid component ➡, and debris ➡. Multiple foci of punctate calcification ➡ are seen scattered in the solid component, suggestive of papillary carcinoma. *(Right)* Longitudinal color Doppler ultrasound in the same patient shows profuse internal vascularity ➡ in the solid component, consistent with papillary carcinoma. Biopsy should be directed to the solid portion.

2

CYSTIC THYROID NODULE

Papillary Carcinoma

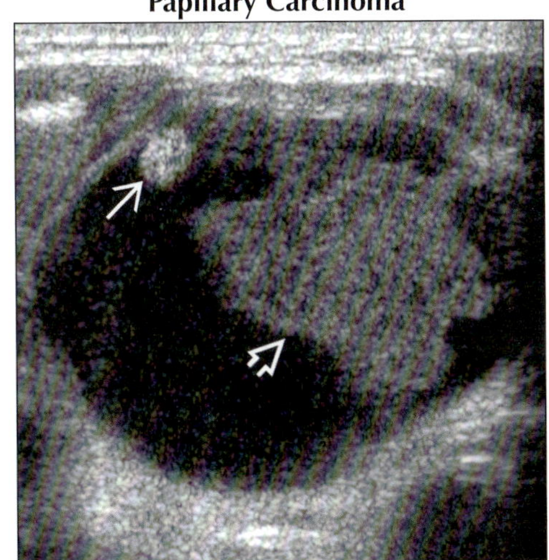

Papillary Carcinoma

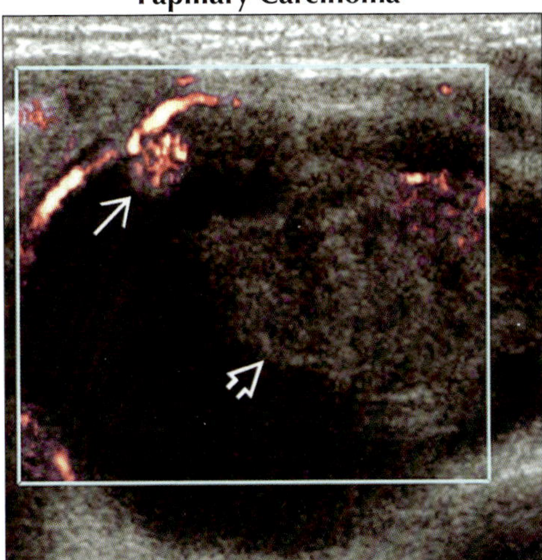

(Left) Transverse ultrasound shows a predominantly cystic nodule with 2 components of "solid" tissue: A small mural nodule ➡ and a large intranodular portion ➡. (Right) Transverse pulsed Doppler ultrasound in the same patient shows marked hypervascularity in the small solid portion ➡, but the larger one is avascular ➡. Guided biopsy of the smaller nodule confirmed papillary carcinoma, and the avascular component represents a blood clot.

Acute Suppurative Thyroiditis

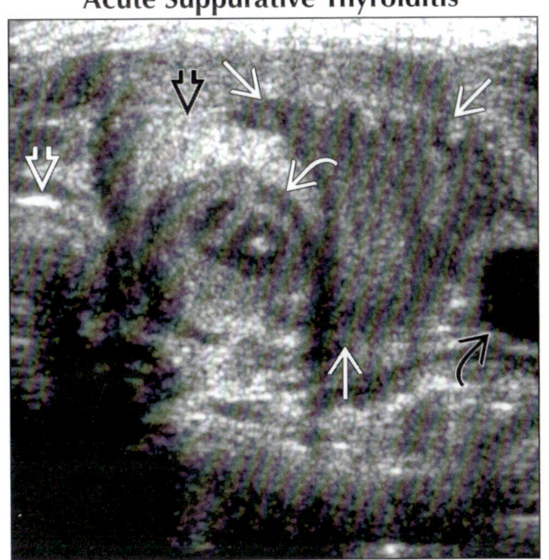

Acute Suppurative Thyroiditis

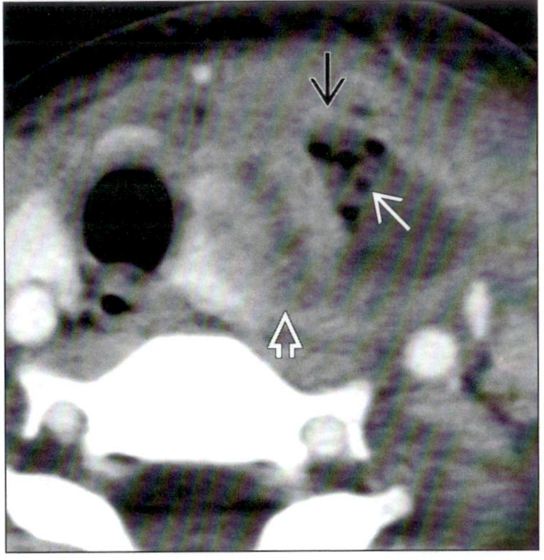

(Left) Transverse ultrasound shows a large perithyroidal abscess ➡ with intrathyroidal extension ➡ into the upper pole of the left lobe of the thyroid ➡ (trachea ➡, CCA ➡). (Right) Axial CECT in the same patient shows a perithyroidal abscess ➡ with internal gas ➡ and an associated abscess in the left lobe of the thyroid ➡. CECT evaluates extent of involvement and may demonstrate the sinus, seen as a track of air from the pyriform fossa.

Follicular Carcinoma

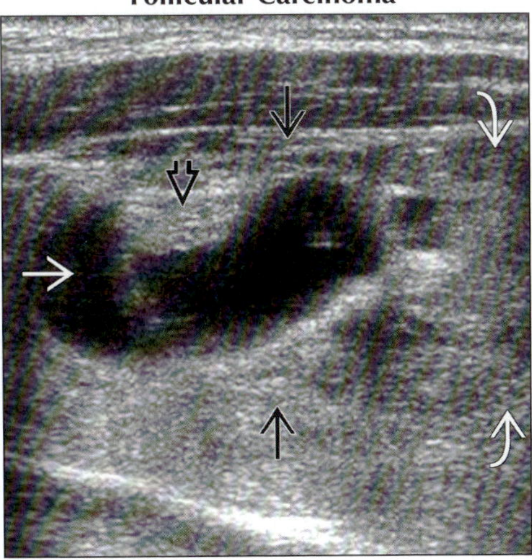

Follicular Carcinoma

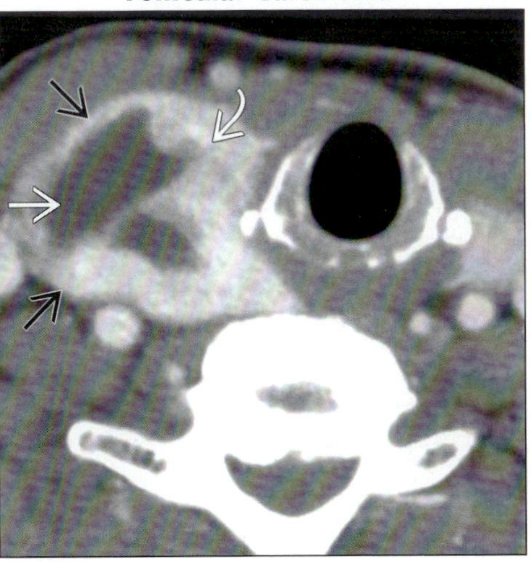

(Left) Transverse ultrasound shows an ill-defined thyroid nodule ➡, with an isoechoic solid component ➡ & cystic portion ➡. Note the ill-defined hypoechoic area ➡, which was hypervascular on Doppler (not shown). Surgery revealed follicular carcinoma. (Right) Axial CECT in the same patient shows corresponding follicular carcinoma ➡ in the right lobe of the thyroid gland. Note its ill-defined edges, cystic change ➡, and irregular solid tissue ➡.

CALCIFIED THYROID NODULE

DIFFERENTIAL DIAGNOSIS

Common
- Multinodular Goiter (MNG)

Less Common
- Papillary Carcinoma
- Anaplastic Carcinoma
- Follicular Carcinoma
- Medullary Carcinoma

ESSENTIAL INFORMATION

Key Differential Diagnosis Issues
- US is more sensitive than CT and MR in detecting punctate calcification
- Coarse shadowing calcification may obscure visualization of posterior part of lesion
  - Evaluating lesion from side or angling transducer may help
    - If this also fails, CT or MR may help
- Note: When using machines with image optimization software, "comet tail" artifact may mimic echogenic foci from punctate calcifications
  - Go back to scanning in fundamental mode, & thin shadowing from punctate calcification may be seen
  - Use grayscale image obtained during color/power Doppler
    - Automatically goes back to fundamental grayscale
  - On fundamental scans, raise scanning frequency, & fine shadowing from punctate calcification may be seen
    - As scanning frequency ↑, acoustic attenuation from calcification also ↑ and may show posterior shadowing
- For any lesion suspicious of malignancy, combine US with fine-needle aspiration and cytology (FNAC) for definitive diagnosis
  - Note: May be difficult to penetrate coarse dense calcification using fine needle

Helpful Clues for Common Diagnoses
- **Multinodular Goiter (MNG)**
  - Most common cause of calcified thyroid nodule
  - Thyroid enlargement due to multiple cysts (simple, colloid, or hemorrhagic) and nodules (hyperplastic or degenerative)
  - Nodules are well defined, haloed, iso- to hypoechoic

  - Early changes: Lower poles > > > upper poles
    - Background thyroid parenchymal echoes are heterogeneous
  - Calcification develops with time, coarse, amorphous, or ring-like
    - Most produce dense shadowing
  - Always search for presence of malignant nodule against background of MNG (papillary, anaplastic carcinoma)

Helpful Clues for Less Common Diagnoses
- **Papillary Carcinoma**
  - Presents as painless thyroid nodule or neck mass (lymph node)
    - May be incidentally detected during US of neck for other causes
  - Solitary, multifocal (10-20%), or diffusely infiltrative
  - Ill defined, hypoechoic (77-90%), solid nodule, ± cystic change, ± incomplete halo (15-30%)
  - Characteristic internal punctate calcification (psammoma bodies)
    - Fine discrete echogenic foci ± posterior acoustic shadowing
  - Metastatic lymph node
    - Ipsilateral > contralateral
    - May be very small (5 mm) but show characteristic appearance, such as round, hypoechoic/hyperechoic to muscle with punctate calcification
    - Large metastatic lymph nodes often show cystic change
  - Color Doppler ultrasound
    - Profuse disorganized intratumoral hypervascularity > > > hypovascularity
    - Disorganized intranodal vascularity in metastatic lymph node
- **Anaplastic Carcinoma**
  - Typically rapidly enlarging goiter in elderly woman with long history of goiter
    - ± dysphagia, ± dyspnea
  - Grayscale ultrasound
    - Large, ill-defined, hypoechoic, necrotic (78%), heterogeneous mass against background of MNG
    - Internal calcification (58%), typically ring-like, coarse, or amorphous, reflecting longstanding MNG
    - Often extracapsular spread with extensive local invasion

- Internal jugular vein (IJV) thrombus: Due to compression or invasion
- Nodal or distant metastases in 80% of patients
  - Color Doppler ultrasound
    - Necrotic tumor may be avascular/hypovascular (vascular infiltration/occlusion)
    - Vascularity in IJV thrombus suggests tumor thrombus & not bland thrombus
  - Ultrasound is ideal to characterize tumor, identify extracapsular spread/local invasion, & guide FNAC for diagnosis
  - CT/MR to delineate entire tumor extent, tracheal, prevertebral, vertebral, and mediastinal invasion
- **Follicular Carcinoma**
  - Differentiation of follicular adenoma and carcinoma cannot be made on imaging or biopsy
    - Therefore, called follicular lesion/neoplasm
  - Definitive diagnosis relies on excision, as follicular carcinoma is defined by presence of vascular or capsular invasion
    - Majority of follicular carcinomas develop from preexisting follicular adenoma
  - Sonographic features of follicular lesion
    - Well defined, oval, iso- to hyperechoic, homogeneous, solid, noncalcified
  - Features more suggestive of carcinoma than benign adenoma
    - Hypoechoic, focally ill-defined border

- Hypoechoic, hypervascular change in otherwise iso- to hyperechoic nodule
- Heterogeneous echopattern, disorganized intratumoral hypervascularity
- ± Internal cystic change, ± dense and coarse calcification
- **Medullary Carcinoma**
  - Middle-aged patient with lower neck mass or incidental finding in patient with family history of MEN syndrome
  - Uncommonly may present with paraneoplastic syndromes: Cushing or carcinoid syndromes
  - Bilateral in 2/3 of sporadic cases; familial type almost always multifocal and bilateral
  - Hypoechoic, solid tumor; well defined > ill defined
  - Solitary, multiple, or diffuse (familial)
  - Echogenic foci (80-90%) = amyloid deposition + calcification
    - Calcifications typically dense and coarse with posterior acoustic shadowing
  - 75% have lymphadenopathy at presentation
    - Mid & lower internal jugular chain and superior mediastinum
  - Color Doppler ultrasound
    - Disorganized intratumoral and intranodal vascularity
  - Nonfamilial form: Invariably mistaken for papillary carcinoma; diagnosis made by FNAC/biopsy
  - CT or MR necessary to detect mediastinal and distant metastases

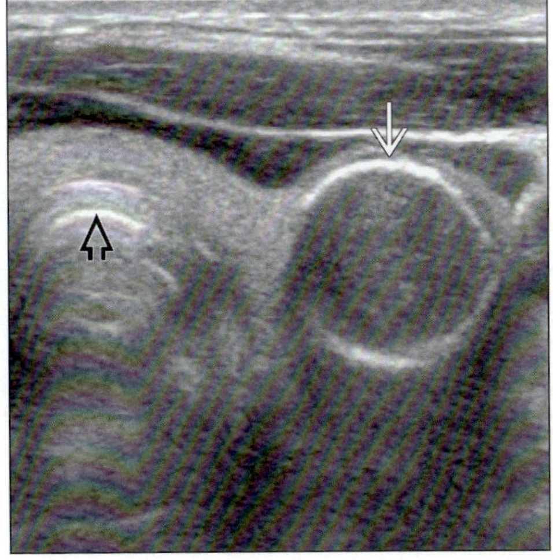

Multinodular Goiter (MNG)

Transverse ultrasound shows a well-defined nodule in the left lobe of the thyroid with a complete ring of calcification ➡, consistent with a longstanding nodular goiter. Note the trachea ⊵.

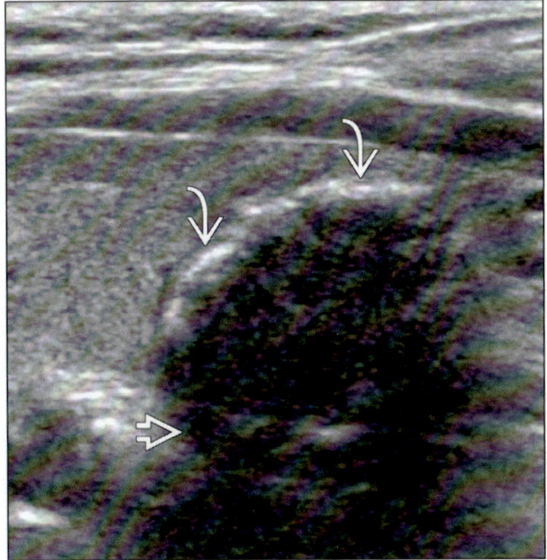

Multinodular Goiter (MNG)

Longitudinal ultrasound shows curvilinear calcification ➡ with a dense posterior acoustic shadow ⊵ in a nodule in a patient with MNG. The deep portion of the nodule is obscured by the shadowing.

CALCIFIED THYROID NODULE

(Left) Longitudinal US shows a nodule in a patient with MNG with internal dense calcification ➡ and strong posterior acoustic shadowing ⬌. Note the calcified echogenic rim ➡ of the nodule. *(Right)* Longitudinal US shows a thyroid nodule with both curvilinear peripheral calcification ➡ and central coarse calcification ➡. Note the posterior acoustic shadow ⬌. Extensive calcification and shadowing obscure large parts of the nodule, making US suboptimal.

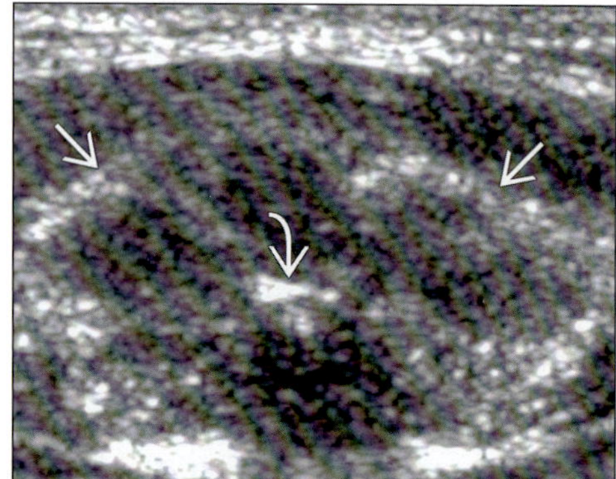

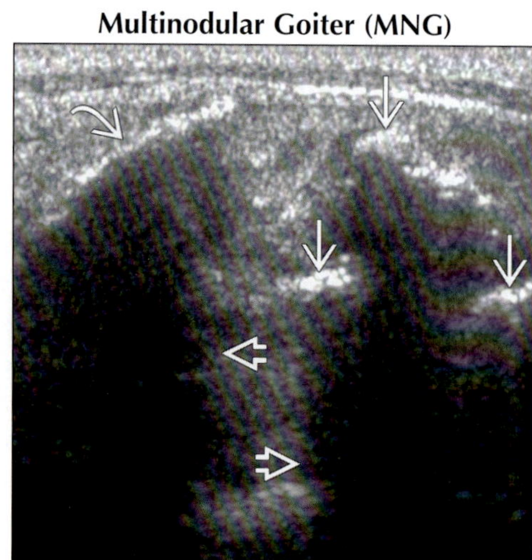

(Left) Longitudinal ultrasound shows multiple foci of punctate calcification ➡ diffusely scattered throughout the right lobe of the thyroid, some with acoustic shadow. Note that the change in parenchymal echogenicity is subtle. FNAC showed papillary carcinoma. *(Right)* Longitudinal ultrasound shows an ill-defined hypoechoic thyroid nodule ➡ with fine internal punctate calcifications ➡, casting a thin posterior acoustic shadow ⬌.

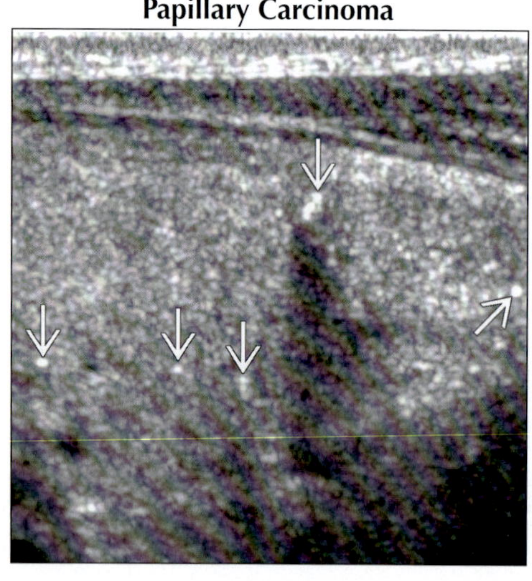

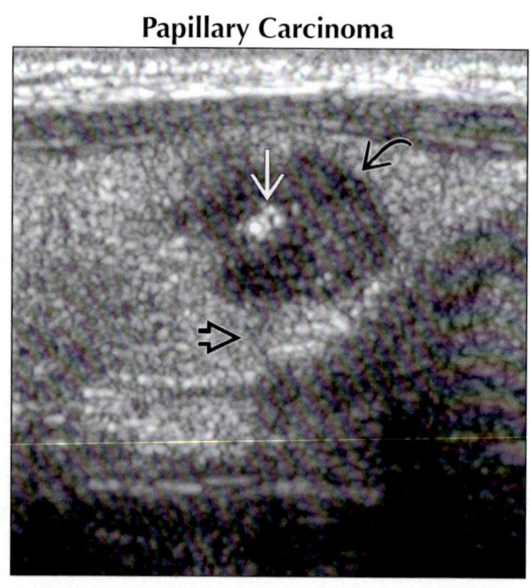

(Left) Transverse ultrasound shows a hypoechoic nodule ➡ with an indistinct border and characteristic internal punctate calcifications ➡. Note that small (5 mm) papillary carcinomas are frequently incidental findings. (Trachea ⬌, CCA ➡.) *(Right)* Longitudinal ultrasound shows a heterogeneous thyroid nodule with a large cystic area ➡ and an eccentric solid nodule ⬌ with internal punctate calcifications ➡, typical findings of papillary carcinoma.

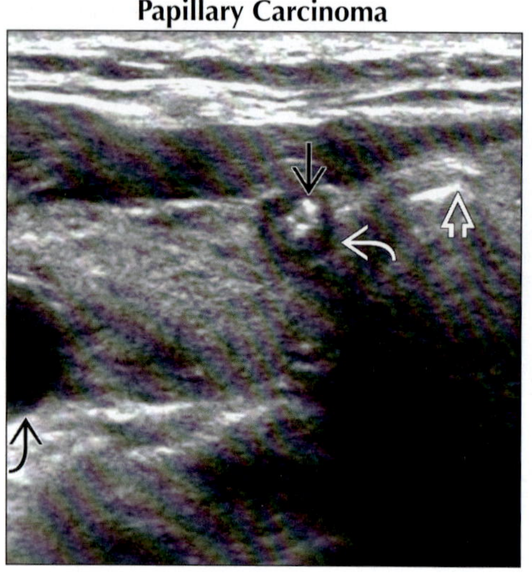

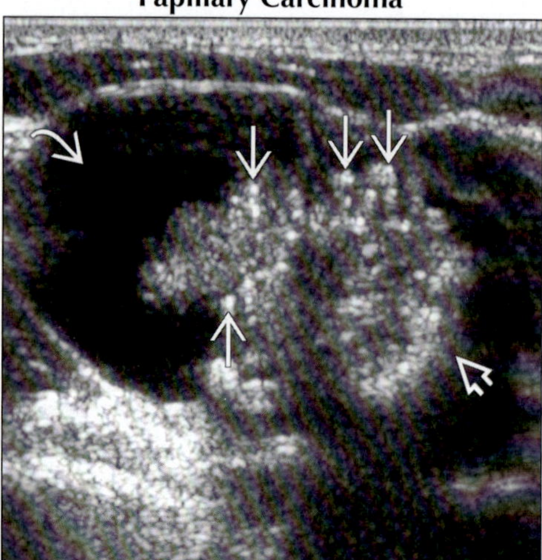

CALCIFIED THYROID NODULE

Anaplastic Carcinoma

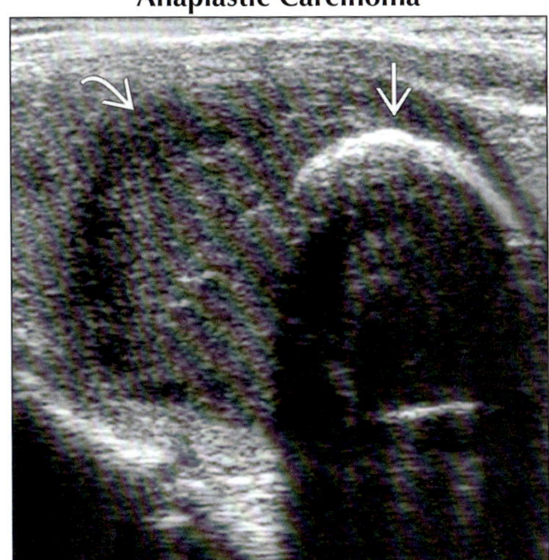

Anaplastic Carcinoma

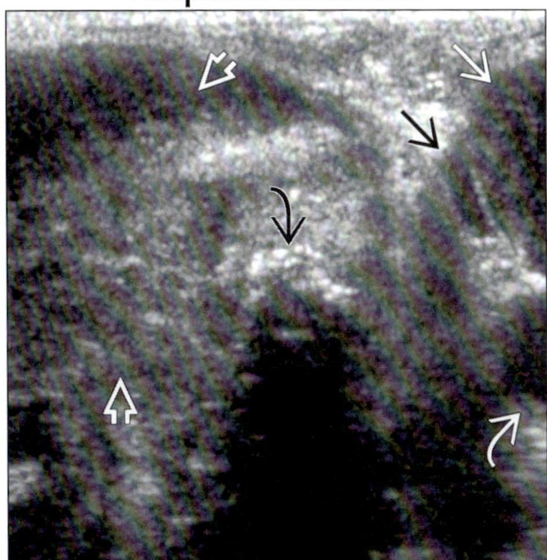

(Left) Longitudinal ultrasound shows a solid hypoechoic mass ➔ with an ill-defined border around a calcified nodule ➔ from a MNG. This appearance is typical for anaplastic carcinoma, which commonly develops in the setting of longstanding MNG. *(Right)* Transverse ultrasound shows a diffusely enlarged left lobe of the thyroid with a heterogeneous, infiltrating tumor ➔ and eccentric coarse calcification ➔. Note associated malignant lymph node ➔ (CCA ➔, IJV ➔).

Follicular Carcinoma

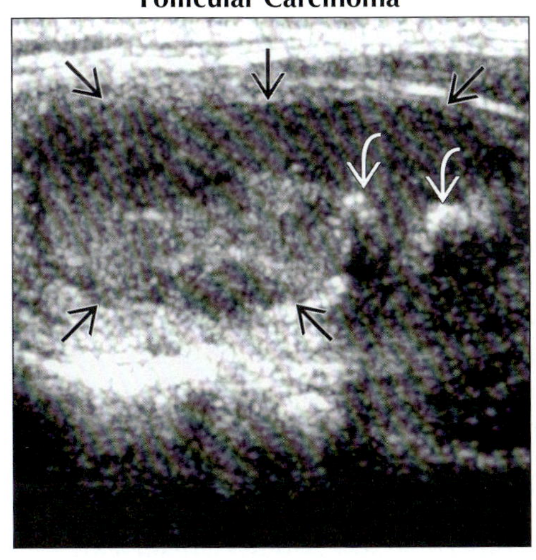

Follicular Carcinoma

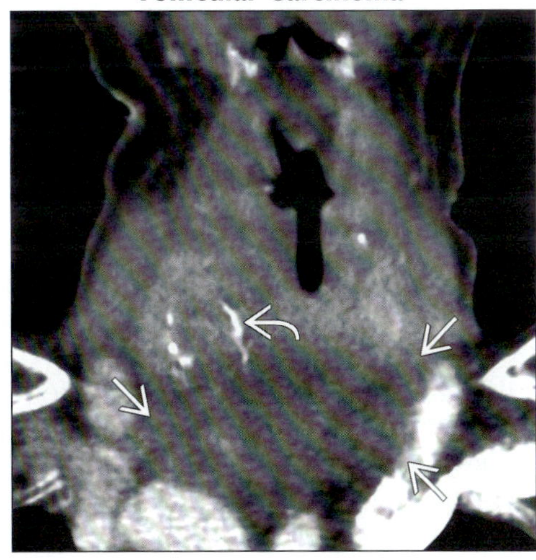

(Left) Longitudinal ultrasound shows an ill-defined, hypoechoic, heterogeneous thyroid nodule ➔ that was confirmed as a follicular carcinoma on excision. Foci of coarse calcification ➔ are occasionally seen in these tumors. *(Right)* Coronal reformatted CECT of the same patient shows extracapsular spread and extensive local invasion ➔. Note the calcification ➔, which was also seen on ultrasound.

Follicular Carcinoma

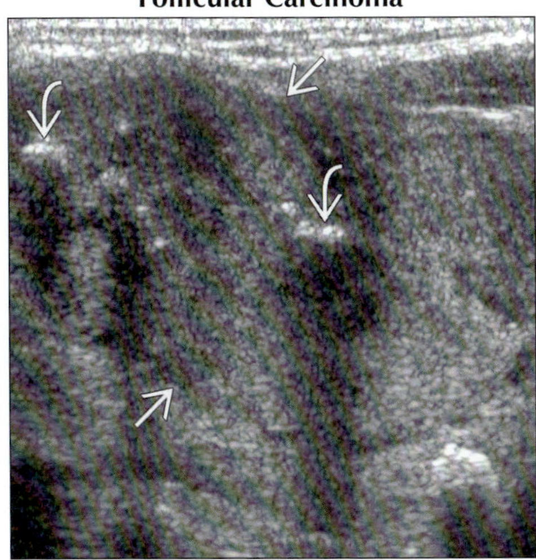

Medullary Carcinoma

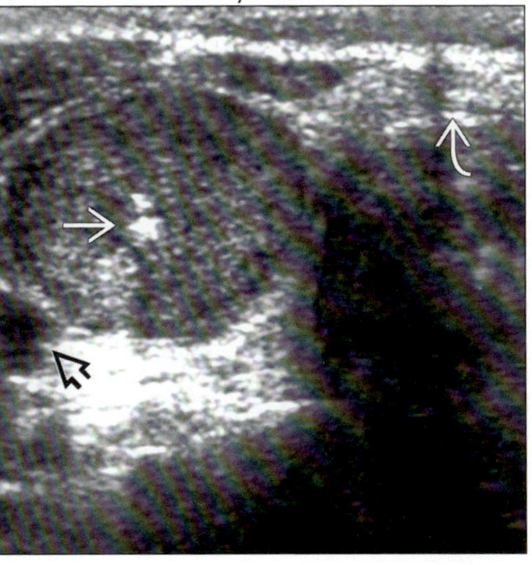

(Left) Longitudinal ultrasound shows an ill-defined, solid, hypoechoic nodule ➔ with infiltrative borders and areas of dense shadowing calcification ➔, confirmed as follicular carcinoma at surgery. *(Right)* Transverse ultrasound shows a well-defined, solid, hypoechoic nodule with small foci of calcification ➔. This appearance is suspicious for thyroid carcinoma, but histologic differentiation is not possible without FNAC (trachea ➔, CCA ➔).

ENLARGED PARATHYROID GLAND

DIFFERENTIAL DIAGNOSIS

Common
- Parathyroid Adenoma

Less Common
- Parathyroid Hyperplasia
- Parathyroid Cyst
- Parathyroid Carcinoma

ESSENTIAL INFORMATION

Key Differential Diagnosis Issues
- US accurately identifies parathyroid adenoma (PTA) in vicinity of thyroid gland
  - Scintigraphy best evaluates ectopic and intrathyroid PTA
- High frequency transducer: 9-12 MHz is essential
- Color Doppler increases diagnostic yield
- Irrespective of nature of lesion, abnormal parathyroid glands are hypoechoic (compared to thyroid)
- Enlarged parathyroid is quickly located on transverse scans, while longitudinal scans better evaluate vascularity
- Meticulous attention to technique and patient positioning yields better diagnostic results
  - Patient in supine position with extended neck to elevate low-lying PTA into neck
    - Neck extension is facilitated by putting small pillow/bolster under shoulder
    - Do not put patient in extended neck position for too long, as that may exacerbate postural hypotension
- US has limited use in obese patients with short necks and following failed surgery
- Parathyroid lesion must be differentiated from thyroid nodule and paratracheal lymph node
  - Thyroid nodule is within confines of thyroid capsule
    - Pedunculated thyroid nodule may create diagnostic difficulty
  - Paratracheal lymph nodes, especially when small, are easily confused with normal/enlarged parathyroid gland
    - If enlarged, lymphadenopathy tends to be multiple and arranged in chain
    - Lymph nodes have hilar architecture and vascularity
  - Normal longus colli muscle, blood vessels, and esophagus should not be mistaken for enlarged parathyroid
- US-guided fine-needle aspiration and cytology (FNAC) easily performed for definitive diagnosis

Helpful Clues for Common Diagnoses
- **Parathyroid Adenoma**
  - Primary hyperparathyroidism occurs in 0.14% of adult population
  - Parathyroid adenoma accounts for 75-85% of cases; single > > multiple
  - Upper parathyroid glands
    - Deep to upper-mid pole of thyroid
    - Rarely located posterior to pharynx or esophagus
  - Lower parathyroid glands
    - 65% inferior, lateral to lower pole of thyroid
    - 35% variably located along thymopharyngeal duct tract, extending from angle of mandible to lower anterior mediastinum
  - Common ectopic locations
    - Near hyoid bone, within carotid sheath, intrathyroidal, intrathymic, and mediastinal
  - Grayscale ultrasound
    - Well defined & hypoechoic with bright echogenic capsule, typically 1-3 cm
    - Deep to or in vicinity of thyroid glands, typically medial to common carotid artery (CCA)
    - Infrahyoid PTAs are usually spherical
    - Oval or flat if retrothyroid, as parathyroid glands in this position develop within longitudinally aligned fascial planes
    - "Arrowhead" appearance on longitudinal scan, with the "head" pointing superiorly
    - Bright echogenic line representing medulla may be seen in center
    - ± cystic change (multiple small cysts > solitary large cyst) or septa, representing cystic degeneration
    - Calcification is rare; more common in carcinoma or hyperplasia due to hyperparathyroidism
    - Hemorrhage may occur in larger lesions, causing cystic appearance with fluid level
  - Color or power Doppler

- PTAs are hypervascular with intraparenchymal vascularity; 10% are avascular (lesions < 1 cm)

Helpful Clues for Less Common Diagnoses
- **Parathyroid Hyperplasia**
  - Occurs as primary hyperparathyroidism or secondary/tertiary hyperparathyroidism in patient with chronic renal failure
  - Accounts for 10-15% of causes of primary hyperparathyroidism
    - Some are sporadic; others associated with MEN1, MEN2A, and familial hyperparathyroidism (autosomal dominant)
  - Clinical diagnosis, based on biochemical tests
  - Radiography shows typical bone changes
  - Main role of US is to identify glands when ethanol ablation is contemplated
  - Hyperplastic parathyroid glands are more spherical than with adenomas ± calcification
  - Treatment is medical or surgical removal
    - Surgery has high success rate
    - Usually 3.5 parathyroid glands are removed with portion of 1 gland implanted in forearm
  - Scintigraphy employed in patients with clinical evidence of recurrence when previous surgery fails to identify all 4 glands
    - Probably due to ectopic parathyroid
- **Parathyroid Cyst**
  - Most are nonfunctional and asymptomatic
    - M < F, 40-60 years old
  - 20-30% functional
    - M > F, with hyperparathyroidism (may be subclinical)
  - Ultrasound features
    - Solitary, unilocular, thin walled, anechoic with posterior acoustic enhancement
    - Septation and loculation are uncommon
    - Most are in lower neck near lower poles of thyroid gland but may be anywhere from angle of mandible to superior mediastinum
    - 65% involve inferior parathyroid glands
    - Cannot be definitely differentiated from branchial cleft cyst, thymic cyst
  - US-guided FNAC may be performed for diagnostic and therapeutic purposes
    - Fluid is typically "watery"; parathyroid hormone (PTH) level is higher than in serum, even in nonfunctioning cyst
- **Parathyroid Carcinoma**
  - Most are hyperfunctioning
    - Constitute 4% of patients with primary hyperparathyroidism
  - Ultrasound features
    - Similar appearance to parathyroid adenoma
    - ± invasion of adjacent structures, ± immobility on swallowing, ± calcification
  - 21-28% metastasize to cervical lymph nodes

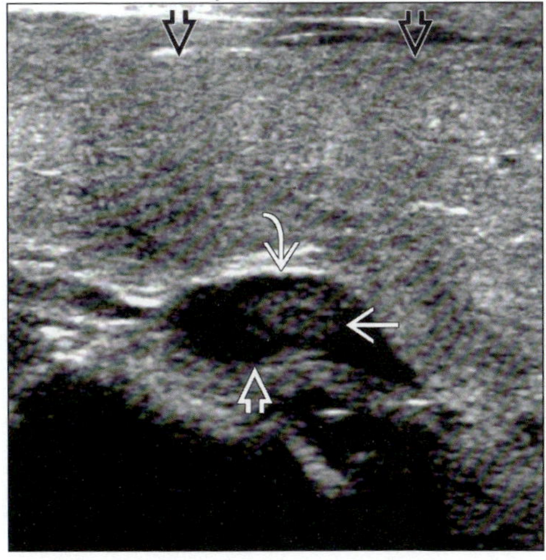

Parathyroid Adenoma

Longitudinal ultrasound shows a PTA ➔ behind the thyroid gland ➔. Note echogenic center ➔, representing the medulla, well-defined border, and a sharp echogenic line ➔ separating it from the thyroid.

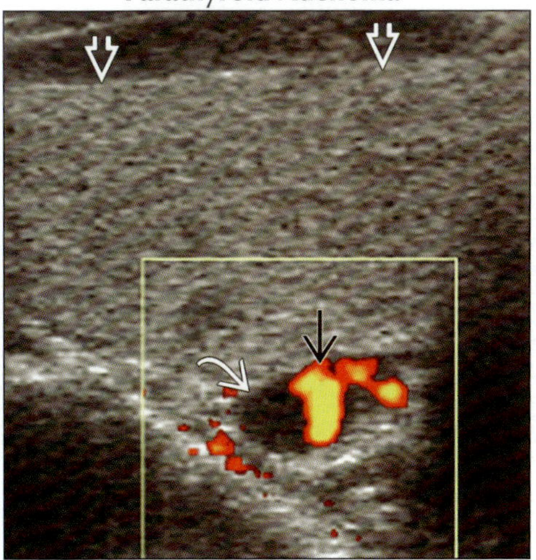

Parathyroid Adenoma

Transverse power Doppler ultrasound shows central vascularity ➔ in a small PTA ➔. Most PTAs are hypervascular with less than 10% being avascular on Doppler. Note the thyroid ➔.

ENLARGED PARATHYROID GLAND

(Left) Longitudinal ultrasound shows an "arrowhead" appearance of a PTA, with the "head" ➡ pointing cranially. Note the bright echogenic capsule ➡ and echogenic medulla ➡. *(Right)* Longitudinal power Doppler ultrasound in the same patient shows intraparenchymal hypervascularity ➡ in the parathyroid adenoma ➡, which is typical. Deep-seated lesions, < 1 cm, and those with cystic necrosis may be avascular.

Parathyroid Adenoma

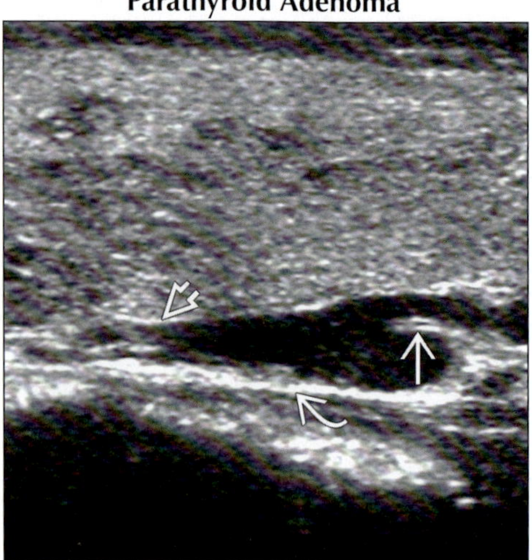

Parathyroid Adenoma

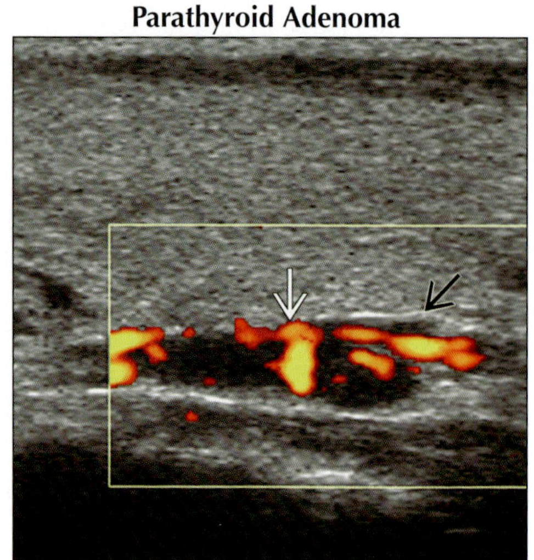

(Left) Longitudinal ultrasound shows a solid, well-defined, hypoechoic PTA ➡. Irrespective of the nature of the lesion, most PTAs are hypoechoic compared to the thyroid parenchyma ➡. This makes them conspicuous and readily visible when they are in the vicinity of the thyroid gland. *(Right)* Transverse power Doppler ultrasound in the same patient shows profuse parenchymal vascularity ➡ in the PTA. Note the thyroid ➡.

Parathyroid Adenoma

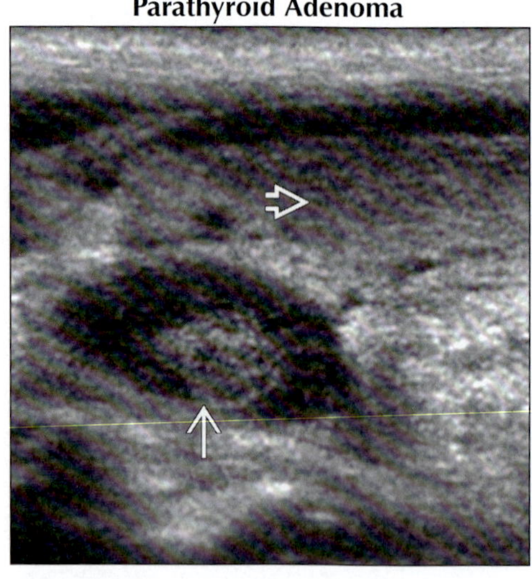

Parathyroid Adenoma

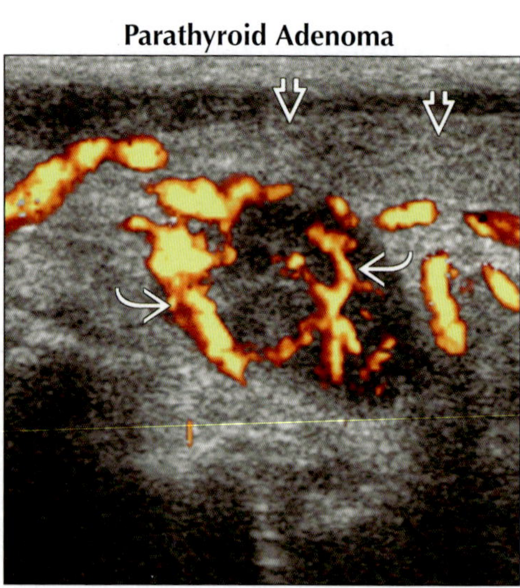

(Left) Transverse ultrasound shows a large PTA ➡ with a focal, well-defined, anechoic cystic area ➡. The appearance is consistent with cystic degeneration. Note the trachea ➡ and thyroid ➡. *(Right)* Longitudinal power Doppler ultrasound shows another PTA with 2 small cystic areas ➡ and intraparenchymal hypervascularity ➡. Multiple small cystic areas are more commonly seen than 1 large cystic area.

Parathyroid Adenoma

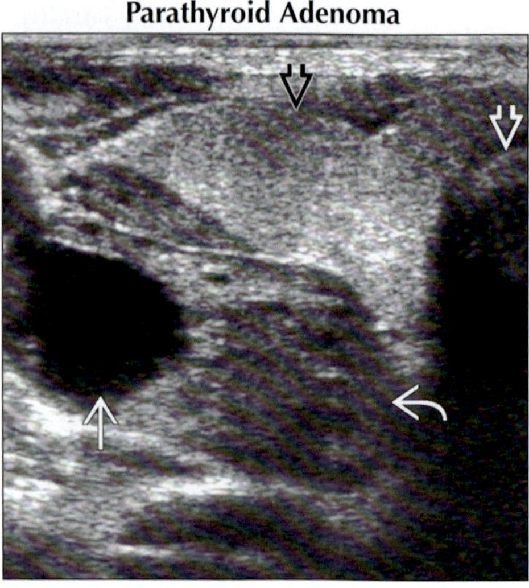

Parathyroid Adenoma

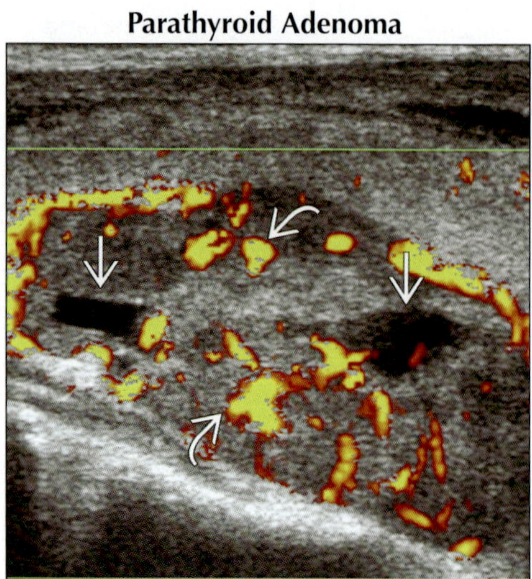

ENLARGED PARATHYROID GLAND

Parathyroid Adenoma

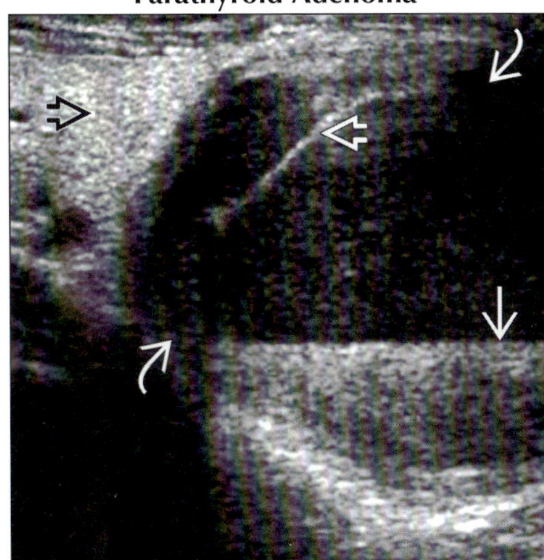

Parathyroid Adenoma

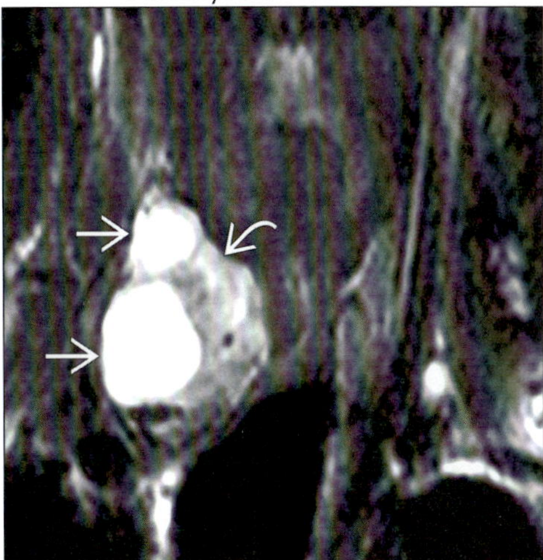

(Left) Transverse ultrasound shows a hemorrhagic PTA ➡. Note the internal fluid level ➡, septa ➡, and adjacent thyroid ➡. (Right) Coronal T2WI with fat suppression in the same patient shows the hemorrhagic PTA ➡. Note the cystic areas ➡ within. Such large lesions may compress the trachea, esophagus, and recurrent laryngeal nerve.

Parathyroid Adenoma

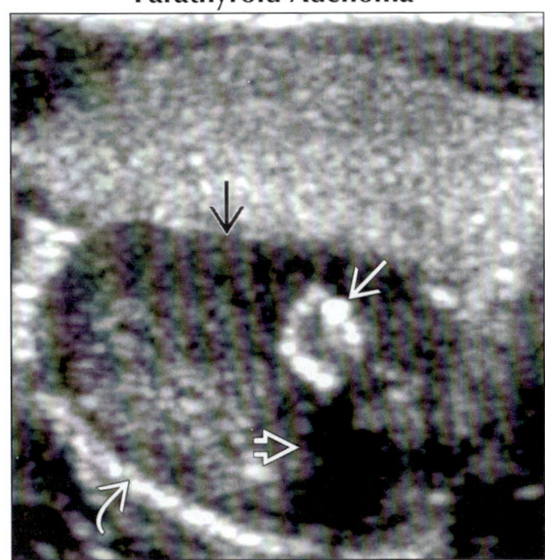

Parathyroid Hyperplasia

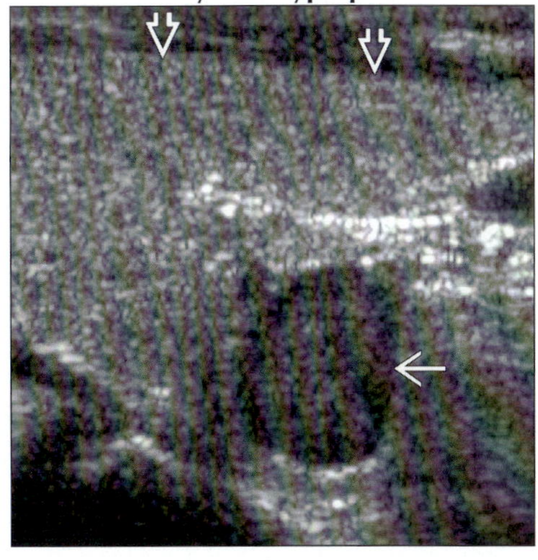

(Left) Transverse ultrasound shows a PTA ➡ behind the thyroid. Note calcification ➡ with acoustic shadowing ➡ & echogenic capsule ➡. Calcification is rare in a PTA & more commonly seen in hyperplasia due to hyperparathyroidism & parathyroid carcinoma. (Right) Longitudinal ultrasound shows an enlarged, well-defined, hypoechoic, noncalcified parathyroid gland ➡ in parathyroid hyperplasia. Note the thyroid ➡.

Parathyroid Cyst

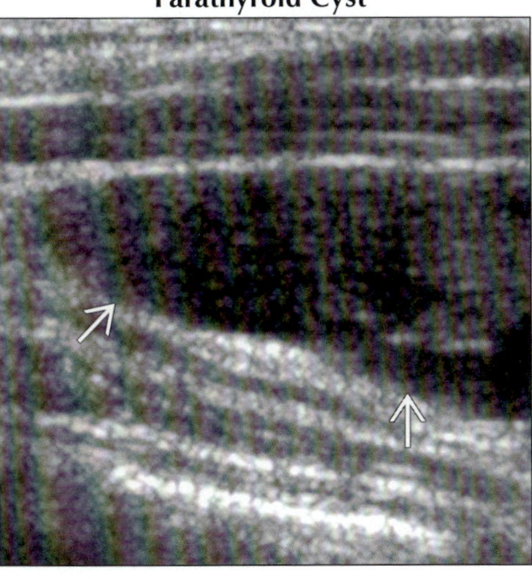

Parathyroid Cyst

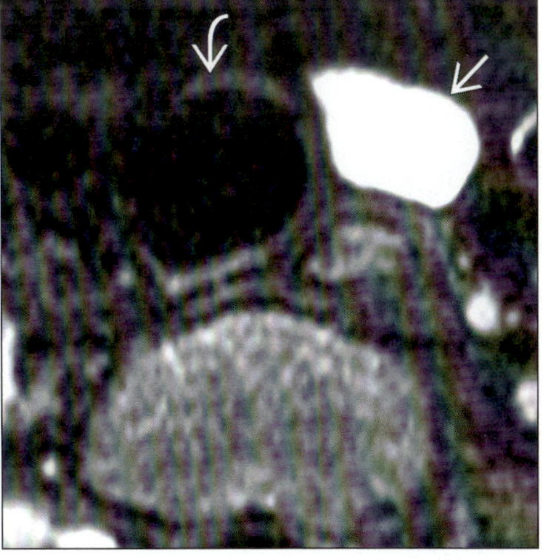

(Left) Longitudinal ultrasound shows a thin-walled parathyroid cyst ➡ inferior to the thyroid gland. (Right) Axial T2WI with fat suppression of the same patient shows the parathyroid cyst ➡, which is thin walled with homogeneous hyperintense fluid signal. Note the trachea ➡. Fluid aspirated from such cysts is usually clear and shows high parathyroid hormone levels compared to the serum.

SECTION 3
Liver

DIFFERENTIAL DIAGNOSIS

Common
- Congested Liver
  - Congestive Heart Failure
  - Budd-Chiari Syndrome
- Acute Viral Hepatitis
- Fatty Liver
- Steatohepatitis
- Fatty Cirrhosis
- Diffuse Neoplastic Infiltration
  - Hepatocellular Carcinoma
  - Lymphoma
  - Leukemia
  - Metastases

Less Common
- Glycogen Storage Disease

ESSENTIAL INFORMATION

Key Differential Diagnosis Issues
- More than 12 cm long on mid-clavicular line (± 3 cm)
  - Size varies depending on build of patient
  - Volumetric measurements are time consuming and may not be suitable for everyday practice
- Ancillary signs used to identify
  - Enlargement of caudate lobe (differential diagnosis of cirrhosis)
  - Extension of right lobe below right kidney (differential diagnosis of Riedel lobe)
  - Biconvex/rounded hepatic surface contour
  - Blunted, obtuse angle; rounded, inferior tip of right lobe
- Enlargement of left lobe (normally smaller than right)
  - Considered when left lobe is present between spleen and diaphragm

Helpful Clues for Common Diagnoses
- **Congested Liver**
  - **Congestive Heart Failure**
    - Dilated hepatic veins and inferior vena cava (IVC)
    - Venous "star" appearance at IVC-hepatic vein junction (instead of "rabbit ears")
    - Dilated hepatic veins may extend to periphery of liver
    - Venous flow shows turbulent appearance on color Doppler and pulsatile waveform on pulsed Doppler
    - Hypoechoic parenchyma, increased posterior enhancement, soft consistency (dynamic indentation by cardiac motion)
    - Ancillary findings: Ascites, pleural effusion, thickened visceral walls (gallbladder, bowel, stomach), splenomegaly
    - Cardiomegaly
  - **Budd-Chiari Syndrome**
    - Hepatic veins normal or distended (acute phase); narrowed or flattened (chronic phase)
    - Hepatic veins partially/completely filled with hypoechoic material
    - Hemorrhagic infarct
    - Color Doppler in acute phase: Aliasing or reversed flow in patent portions of IVC due to stenosis
- **Acute Viral Hepatitis**
  - Diffuse decrease in echogenicity
  - Echogenicity similar to renal cortex and spleen
  - "Starry sky" appearance
    - Increased echogenicity of portal triad walls against background hypoechoic liver
    - Nonspecific
  - Periportal hypoechoic/anechoic areas (hydropic swelling of hepatocytes)
- **Fatty Liver**
  - Increase in size of liver and change in shape as volume of infiltration increases
    - Inferior margin of right lobe has rounded contours
    - Left lobe becomes biconvex
  - Increased echogenicity; liver significantly more echogenic than kidney
    - Echogenicity may vary between segments (areas of focal fatty sparing)
  - Margins of hepatic veins are blurred due to increased refraction and scattering of sound
  - Vessels course through liver without distortion but may be spread apart secondary to expansion of liver parenchyma
  - Preservation of hepatic architecture
  - Hepatic veins not dilated or narrowed (compared to congested liver)
  - Posterior segments of liver not clearly seen due to acoustic attenuation

HEPATOMEGALY

- ○ Focal fatty sparing may simulate hypoechoic lesion
- ○ Soft consistency: Dynamic indentation by cardiac motion
- **Steatohepatitis**
  - ○ Characterized by inflammation accompanying fat accumulation
    - ▪ Definitive diagnosis made by liver biopsy
  - ○ May occur in alcoholic hepatitis and nonalcoholic steatohepatitis (NASH)
  - ○ Etiology of NASH unknown but frequently seen in following conditions
    - ▪ Obesity
    - ▪ Diabetes
    - ▪ Hyperlipidemia
    - ▪ Drugs and toxins
  - ○ Ultrasound findings
    - ▪ Signs of fatty liver
    - ▪ Firm consistency (due to inflammation) on dynamic scanning during cardiac cycle
    - ▪ Irregular borders of hepatic veins due to hepatic inflammation
    - ▪ Intermittent loss of visualization of hepatic veins
- **Fatty Cirrhosis**
  - ○ Enlarged left and caudate lobes and atrophic right lobe
  - ○ Hyperechoic but heterogeneous liver echopattern
  - ○ Irregular hepatic veins
  - ○ Portal venous collaterals
  - ○ Stiff consistency
  - ○ Ancillary signs of portal hypertension
    - ▪ Ascites, varices, hepatofugal flow, splenomegaly
- **Diffuse Neoplastic Infiltration**
  - ○ **Hepatocellular Carcinoma**
    - ▪ Background cirrhosis &/or portal hypertension
    - ▪ Infiltrative lesion with heterogeneous echogenicity, ± multifocal masses
    - ▪ Color Doppler may show chaotic tumor vascularity or portal venous thrombus vascularity (tumor thrombus)
  - ○ **Lymphoma**
    - ▪ Diffuse/infiltrative form presents as innumerable subcentimeter hypoechoic foci
    - ▪ Miliary pattern
    - ▪ Periportal location
    - ▪ Infiltrative pattern may be indistinguishable from normal liver
    - ▪ Also look for lymphadenopathy, splenomegaly or splenic lesions, bowel wall thickening, ascites
  - ○ **Metastases**
    - ▪ Discrete nodules and masses or infiltrative pattern
    - ▪ Infiltrative hepatic metastases commonly from lung or breast primary
    - ▪ Infiltrative pattern shows heterogeneous echotexture and simulates cirrhosis

Helpful Clues for Less Common Diagnoses
- **Glycogen Storage Disease**
  - ○ Indistinguishable from fatty liver
  - ○ Requires biopsy for diagnosis

Congestive Heart Failure

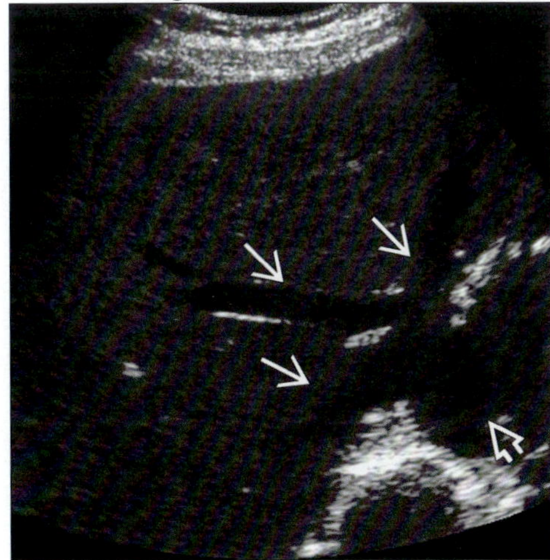

Oblique transabdominal ultrasound shows dilated hepatic veins ➡ and IVC ⧩ forming a star appearance in a patient with congestive heart failure. Note the diffuse decrease in echogenicity of liver parenchyma.

Congestive Heart Failure

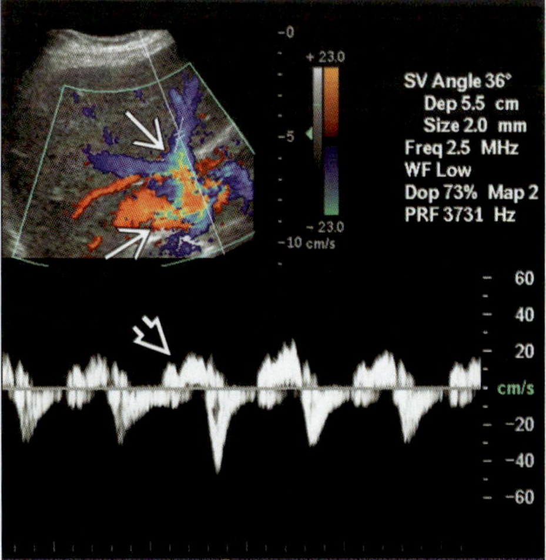

Pulsed Doppler ultrasound shows turbulent color flow ➡ in the hepatic veins and IVC. Pulsed Doppler tracing shows pulsatile waveform ⧩ due to back-transmission from cardiac contractions.

HEPATOMEGALY

(Left) Longitudinal transabdominal ultrasound shows a markedly dilated inferior vena cava 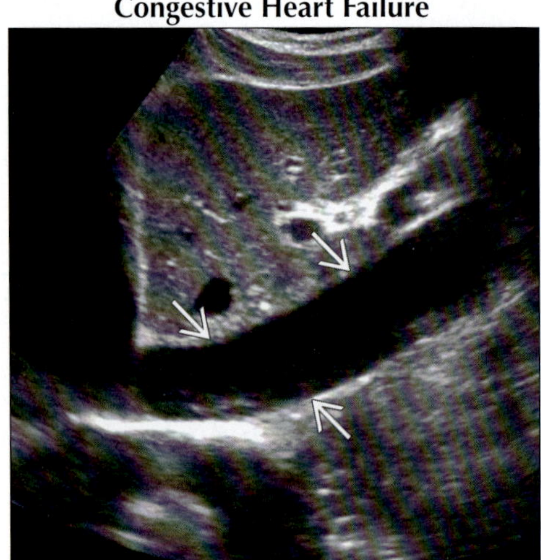 in a patient with congestive heart failure. *(Right)* Longitudinal color Doppler ultrasound in the same patient shows blood flow ➡ from the inferior vena cava and hepatic vein ➡ to the right heart. There is neither aliasing nor turbulence in this particular case.

Congestive Heart Failure

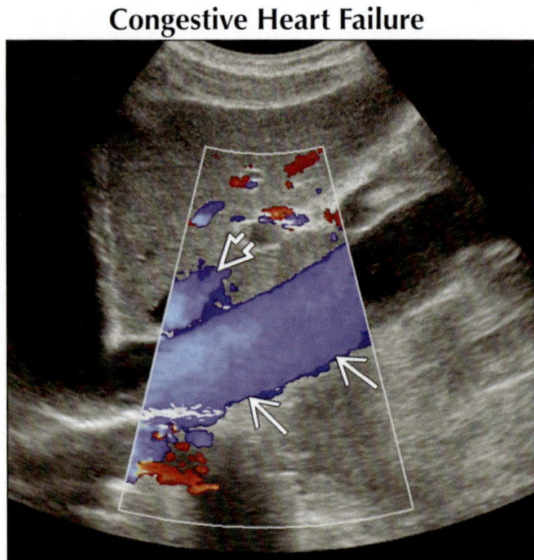

Congestive Heart Failure

(Left) Oblique transabdominal ultrasound shows a severely narrowed right hepatic vein ➡ and IVC ➡ in a patient with acute Budd-Chiari syndrome. The right hepatic vein is echogenic, suggesting slow flow or thrombosis. *(Right)* Longitudinal color Doppler ultrasound shows aliasing ➡ within the inferior vena cava in a patient with Budd-Chiari syndrome. This is due to increased resistance of flow in the narrowed vein.

Budd-Chiari Syndrome

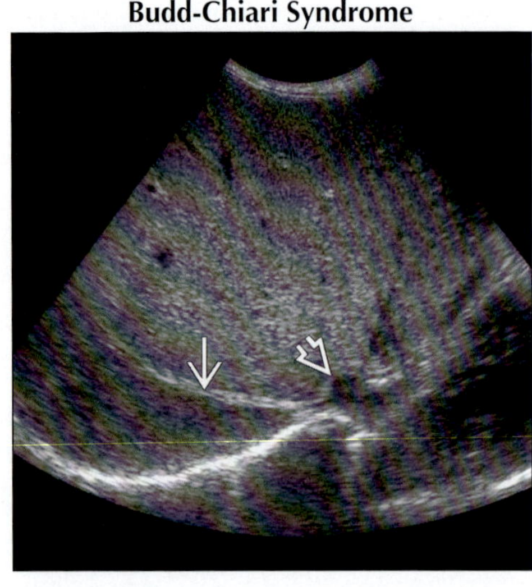

Budd-Chiari Syndrome

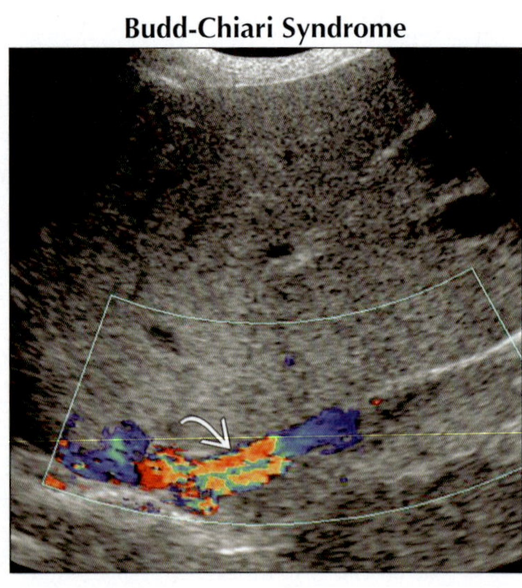

(Left) Oblique ultrasound shows a diffuse, hypoechoic, enlarged liver in a patient with acute hepatitis. Portal triads stand out as hyperechoic foci ➡, creating a "starry sky" pattern. *(Right)* Longitudinal ultrasound shows fatty steatosis. Note the diffuse increase in echogenicity ➡ compared to the hypoechoic renal cortex ➡. The inferior margin of the liver extends beyond that of the right kidney, and the contour is bulging ➡, suggesting hepatomegaly.

Acute Viral Hepatitis

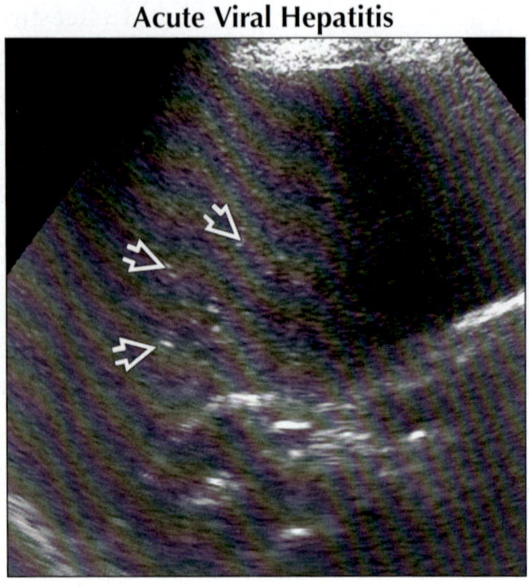

Fatty Liver

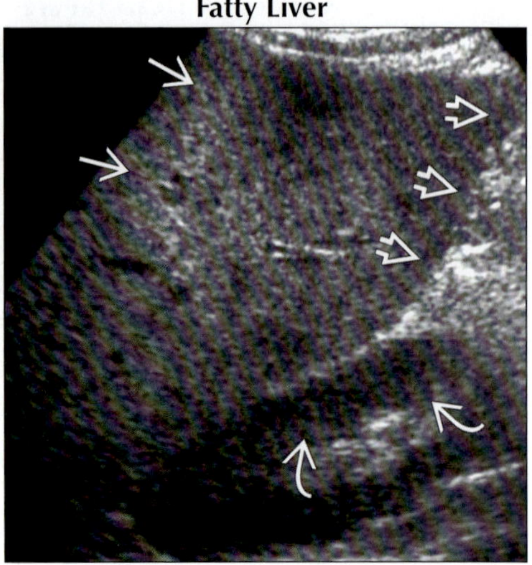

HEPATOMEGALY

Steatohepatitis

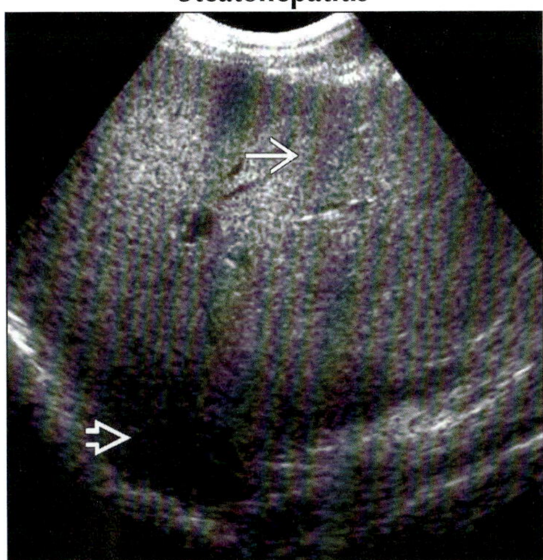

Fatty Cirrhosis

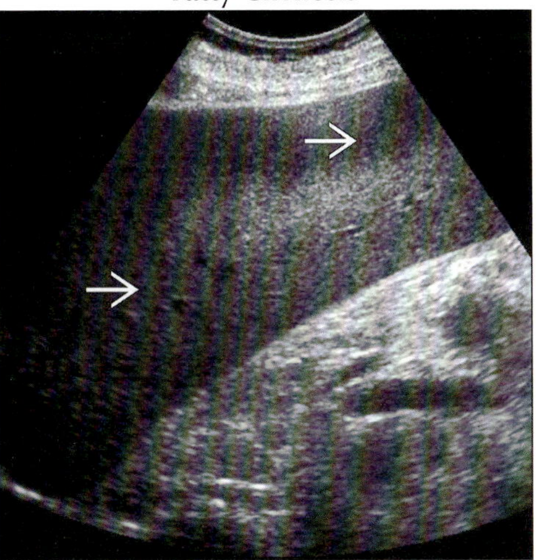

(Left) Oblique ultrasound shows diffuse hepatomegaly and fatty infiltration ➡ in acute alcoholic hepatitis. Note the decreased penetration/acoustic attenuation ➡ in the deep parts of the liver. (Right) Oblique ultrasound shows hepatomegaly with alcoholic cirrhosis and a coarsened hepatic echopattern ➡. Alcoholic cirrhosis tends to produce micronodular cirrhosis (nodules < 1 cm) compared to the macronodular cirrhosis seen in viral hepatitis.

Hepatocellular Carcinoma

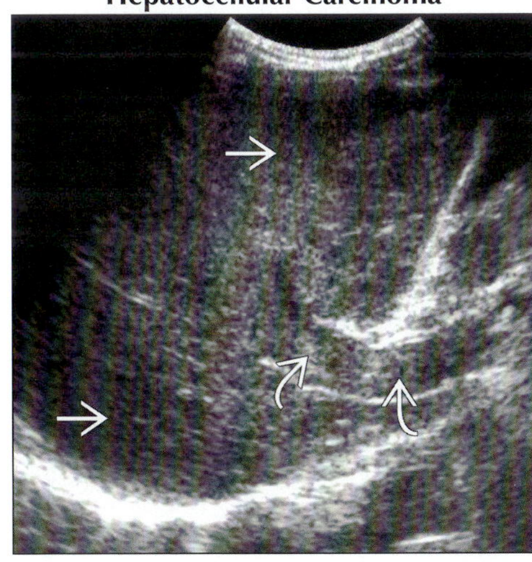

Leukemia

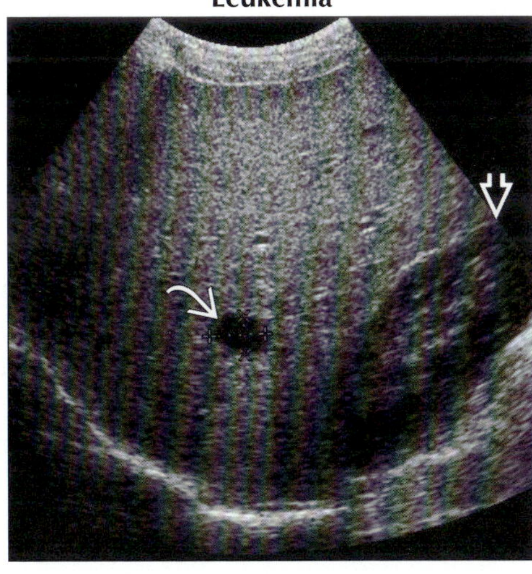

(Left) Oblique transabdominal ultrasound shows hepatomegaly in a patient with infiltrative hepatocellular carcinoma. Note the heterogeneous hepatic echopattern ➡ and tumor thrombus ➡ in the right portal vein. (Right) Oblique transabdominal ultrasound shows hepatomegaly in a patient with leukemia. The liver is enlarged, extending beyond the inferior margin of the right kidney ➡. A small simple hepatic cyst ➡ is incidentally seen.

Metastases

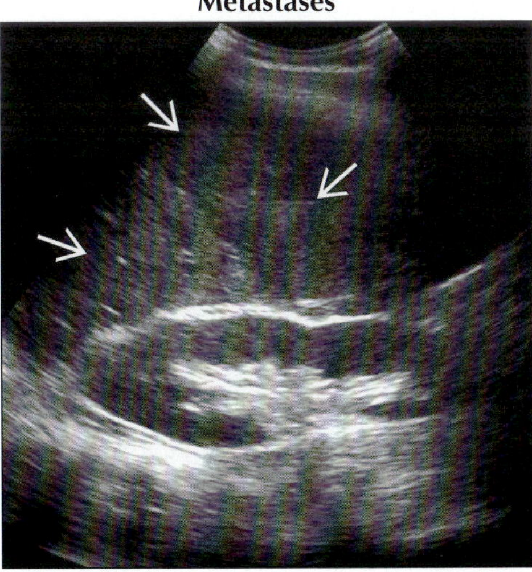

Glycogen Storage Disease

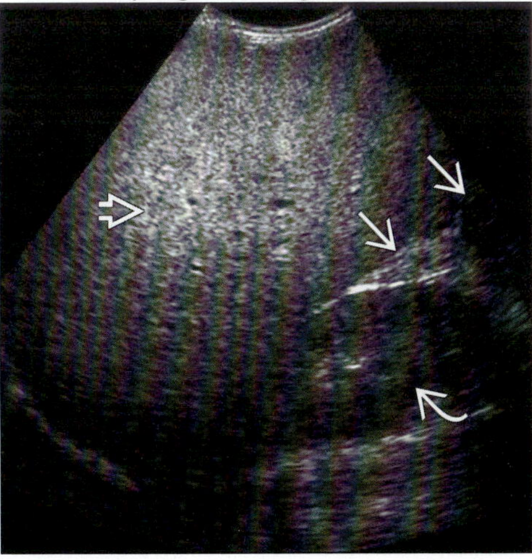

(Left) Longitudinal ultrasound shows hepatomegaly due to diffuse metastases. Note the heterogeneous and nodular hepatic echopattern ➡. Although the appearance is difficult to distinguish from cirrhosis, the history of a known primary tumor is helpful. (Right) Longitudinal transabdominal ultrasound shows hepatomegaly due to glycogen storage disease. Note the diffuse hepatic fatty infiltration ➡ and lower edge of the liver ➡ covering the entire right kidney ➡.

3

HYPERECHOIC LIVER, DIFFUSE

DIFFERENTIAL DIAGNOSIS

Common
- Steatosis (Fatty Liver)
- Cirrhosis
- Chronic Hepatitis
- Acute Alcoholic Hepatitis
- Metastases and Lymphoma
- Technical Artifact (Mimic)

Less Common
- Hepatocellular Carcinoma
- AIDS
- Hepatic Sarcoidosis
- Miliary Tuberculosis
- Schistosomiasis
- Biliary Hamartomas
- Mononucleosis
- Glycogen Storage Disease
- Wilson Disease

ESSENTIAL INFORMATION

Key Differential Diagnosis Issues
- Steatosis & cirrhosis account for most cases

Helpful Clues for Common Diagnoses
- **Steatosis (Fatty Liver)**
  - Diffuse increased echogenicity with acoustic attenuation
  - Liver often large with smooth contour
  - With increasing infiltration, vessels are pushed apart and hepatic veins take more curved course
- **Cirrhosis**
  - Increased echogenicity and heterogeneous background
- **Chronic Hepatitis**
  - Chronic viral or acute alcoholic hepatitis causes increased echogenicity
    - Acute viral hepatitis usually causes decreased echogenicity
- **Metastases and Lymphoma**
  - Most are hypoechoic, focal or diffuse
  - Mucinous and vascular metastases may be hyperechoic
- **Technical Artifact (Mimic)**
  - Improper transducer or gain setting

Helpful Clues for Less Common Diagnoses
- **Hepatocellular Carcinoma**
  - May be multifocal, diffuse, heterogeneous
  - Usually in cirrhotic liver
- **AIDS**
  - Opportunistic hepatic infections (Cytomegalovirus, mycobacterial, etc.)
- **Hepatic Sarcoidosis**
  - Diffuse heterogeneous echopattern
  - Granulomas seen as hypoechoic nodules
- **Miliary Tuberculosis**
  - Innumerable small echogenic granulomas
- **Schistosomiasis**
  - Diffuse periportal septal thickening causes increased echogenicity
- **Biliary Hamartomas**
  - Tiny (< 1.5 cm) echogenic nodules (due to fibrous tissue in walls)
  - When multiple or widespread results in ↑ echogenicity

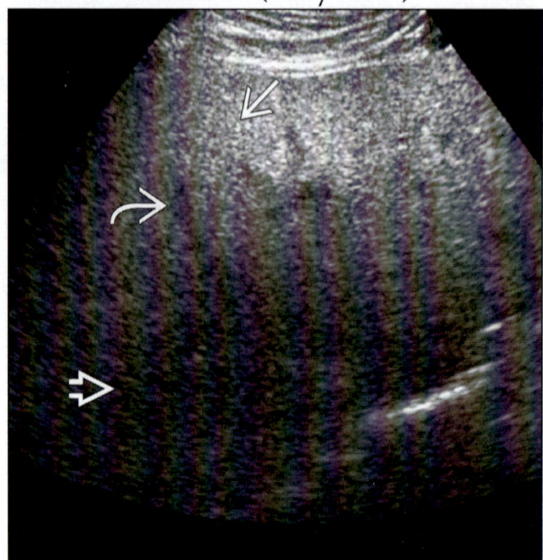

Steatosis (Fatty Liver)

Oblique transabdominal ultrasound shows moderate diffuse fatty infiltration with an increase in echogenicity ⮞, posterior acoustic attenuation ⮞, and impaired definition of intrahepatic vessels ⮞.

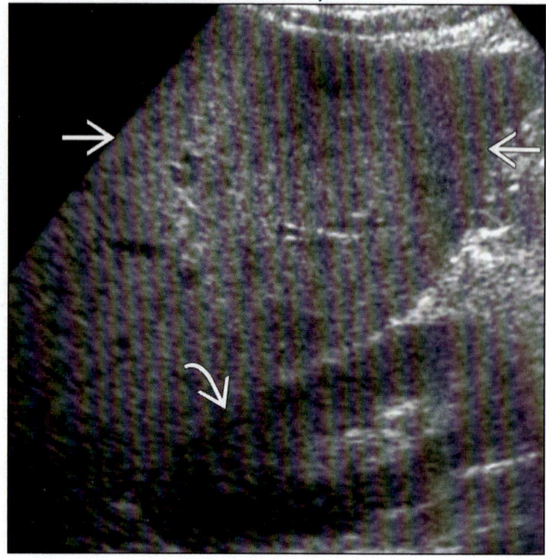

Steatosis (Fatty Liver)

Oblique transabdominal ultrasound shows mild fatty steatosis. Note the diffuse increase in echogenicity ⮞ compared to the hypoechoic renal cortex ⮞, an internal reference helpful for diagnosis.

HYPERECHOIC LIVER, DIFFUSE

Cirrhosis

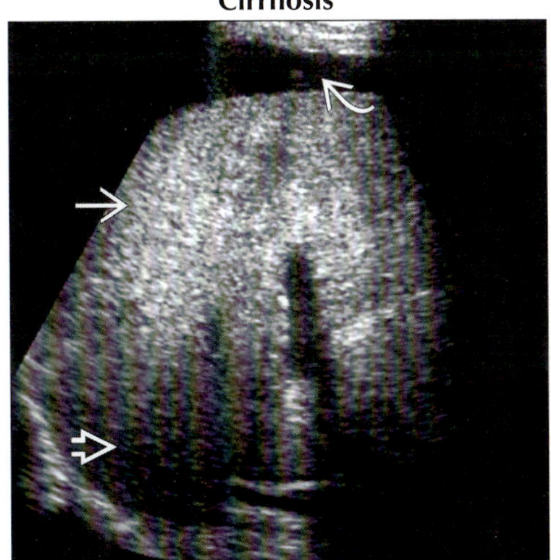

Acute Alcoholic Hepatitis

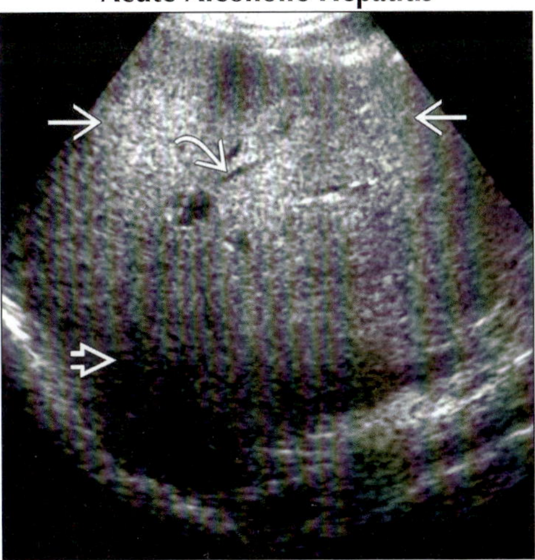

(Left) Oblique transabdominal ultrasound of a cirrhotic liver shows a small right lobe with increased echogenicity ➡, coarse architecture, and posterior acoustic attenuation ➡. Note the ascites ➡. (Right) Oblique transabdominal ultrasound in a patient with acute alcoholic hepatitis shows increased echogenicity ➡ and posterior attenuation ➡. The hepatic veins ➡ have a curved course.

Metastases and Lymphoma

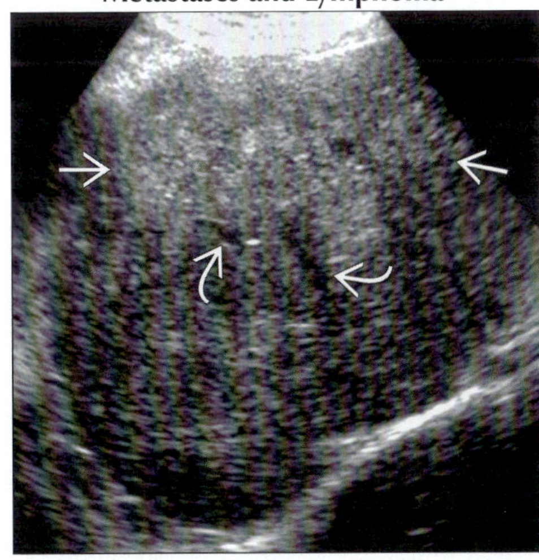

Technical Artifact (Mimic)

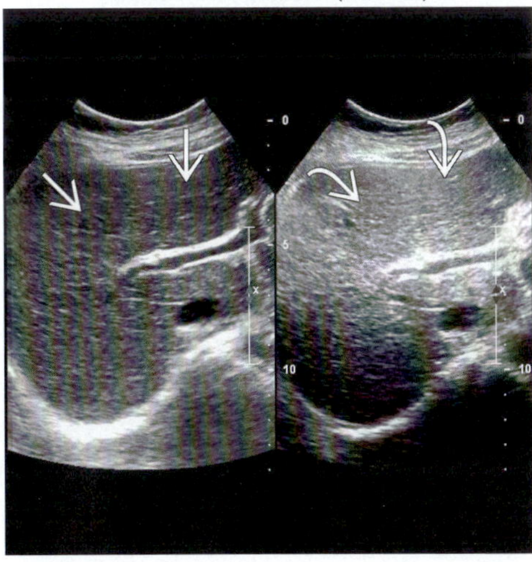

(Left) Oblique transabdominal ultrasound in a patient with diffuse infiltrative metastases shows heterogeneous increased echogenicity ➡ and distortion of the vascular architecture ➡. (Right) This composite image shows normal echogenicity of liver parenchyma ➡ on the left. Improper gain settings can cause an artifactually increased echogenicity ➡, as shown on the right.

Hepatocellular Carcinoma

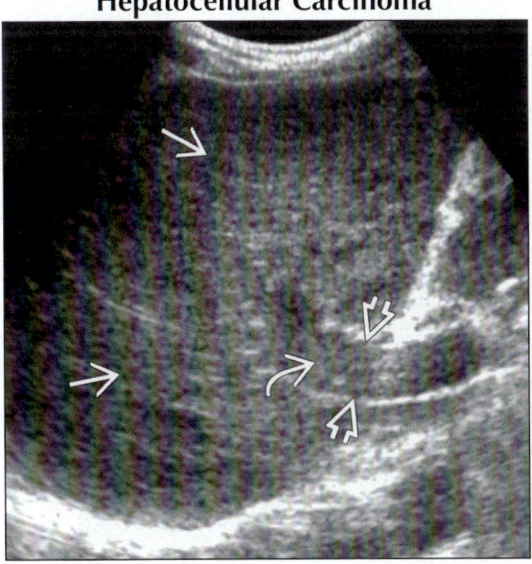

Schistosomiasis

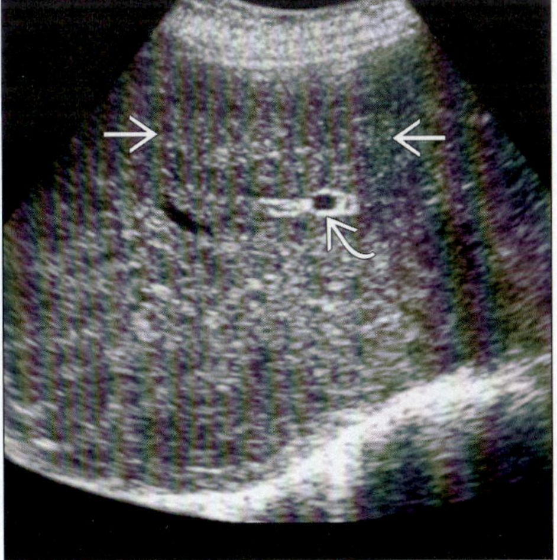

(Left) Oblique transabdominal ultrasound shows diffuse HCC, resulting in increased echogenicity ➡ and an echogenic thrombus ➡ in the portal vein ➡. Doppler is helpful for identifying tumor thrombus. (Right) Oblique transabdominal ultrasound shows an echogenic mottled appearance ➡ of the liver secondary to periportal fibrosis from schistosomiasis. Note the thickened and hyperechoic portal vein walls ➡.

DIFFERENTIAL DIAGNOSIS

Common
- Chronic Hepatitis
- Cirrhosis
- Infiltrative/Diffuse Hepatocellular Carcinoma
- Diffuse Metastasis

Less Common
- Schistosomiasis

ESSENTIAL INFORMATION

Helpful Clues for Common Diagnoses
- **Chronic Hepatitis**
  - Increased echogenicity of liver parenchyma
  - "Silhouetting" of portal vein walls (loss of definition of portal veins)
  - Heterogeneous parenchymal echopattern due to regenerating nodules
  - Hepatoduodenal or periportal adenopathy
- **Cirrhosis**
  - Nodular liver surface contour
  - Enlarged caudate lobe and lateral segment of left lobe plus atrophy of right lobe & medial segment of left lobe
  - Increased echogenicity of fissures and portal structures
  - Coarse echopattern, increased parenchymal echogenicity
  - Compression of hepatic veins
  - Signs of portal hypertension
    - Splenomegaly, ascites
- **Infiltrative/Diffuse Hepatocellular Carcinoma**
  - Heterogeneity more common in larger hepatocellular carcinoma and indicates tumor necrosis/fibrosis
  - Infiltrative growth makes borders difficult to separate from background cirrhotic liver
  - Invasion of portal vein and less commonly hepatic vein may occur
  - Color Doppler
    - Shows irregular hypervascularity within neoplasm
    - Tumor thrombus (portal vein) shows hypervascularity
- **Diffuse Metastasis**
  - Infiltrative/diffuse metastases may simulate cirrhosis
  - Most commonly lung or breast primary
  - Causes architectural/vascular distortion if large or numerous
  - Metastasis much less common than hepatocellular carcinoma in cirrhotic liver
  - Contrast-enhanced US increases conspicuity of hepatic metastases

Helpful Clues for Less Common Diagnoses
- **Schistosomiasis**
  - Echogenic periportal fibrotic bands most severe at porta hepatis
  - Mosaic network of echogenic septa outlining polygonal areas of normal-appearing liver
  - Irregular/notched liver surface
  - Hyperechoic gallbladder bed

Chronic Hepatitis

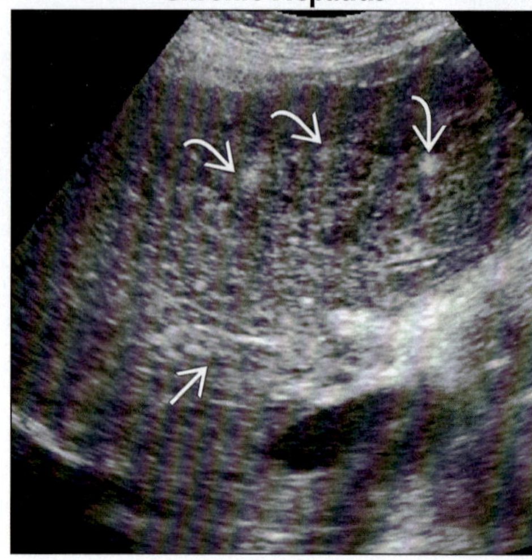

Oblique transabdominal ultrasound shows chronic active viral hepatitis with a heterogeneous increase in echogenicity ➡. The portal vein walls have lost their normal, sharp definition ➡.

Chronic Hepatitis

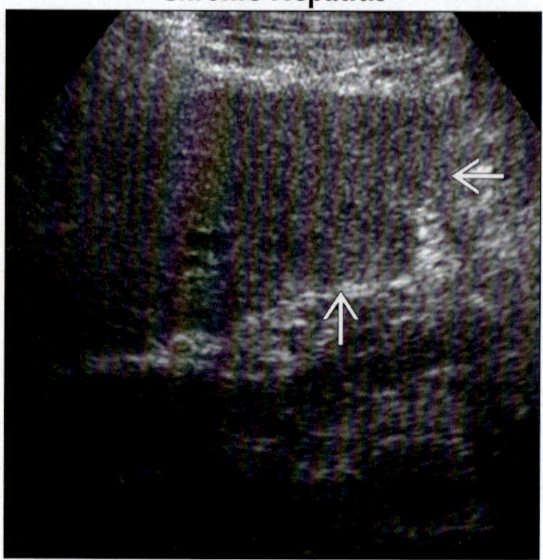

Oblique transabdominal ultrasound shows chronic alcoholic hepatitis with a diffuse, coarse, bright echopattern. A nodular surface ➡ is evident in advanced cases.

HETEROGENEOUS LIVER ECHOPATTERN

Cirrhosis

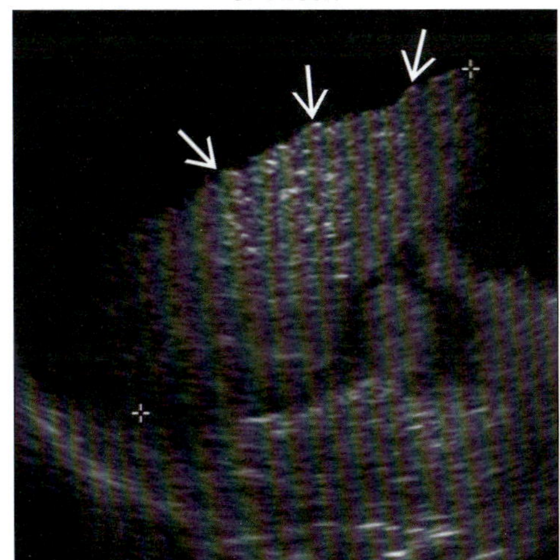

Cirrhosis

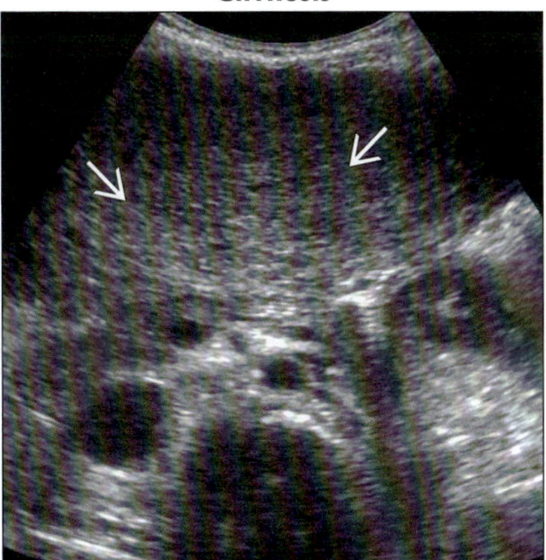

(Left) Oblique transabdominal ultrasound shows micronodular cirrhosis with ascites highlighting the nodular hepatic surface ➡. (Right) Oblique transabdominal ultrasound shows micronodular cirrhosis with a diffuse coarse hepatic echopattern ➡, but no obvious discrete nodule can be discerned (as compared to macronodular cirrhosis).

Diffuse Metastasis

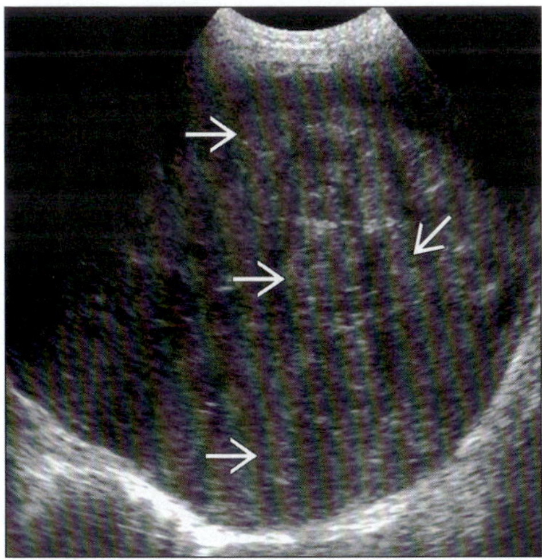

Diffuse Metastasis

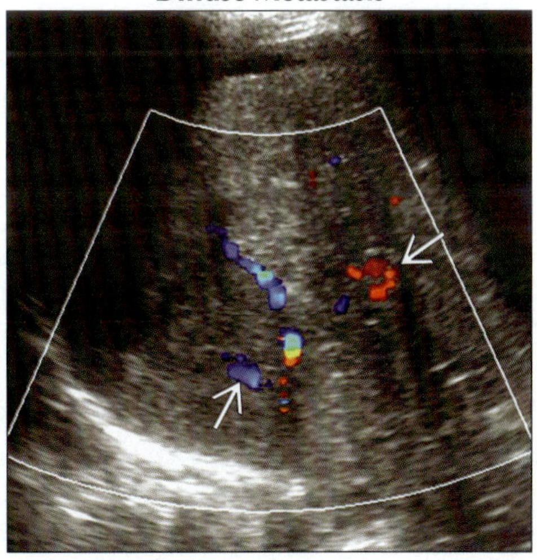

(Left) Oblique ultrasound shows numerous, diffuse, small metastases ➡ throughout the hepatic parenchyma giving it a coarse echopattern. (Right) Oblique color Doppler ultrasound in the same patient shows distortion of the normal vascular architecture ➡, suggesting the presence of infiltrative disease.

Infiltrative/Diffuse Hepatocellular Carcinoma

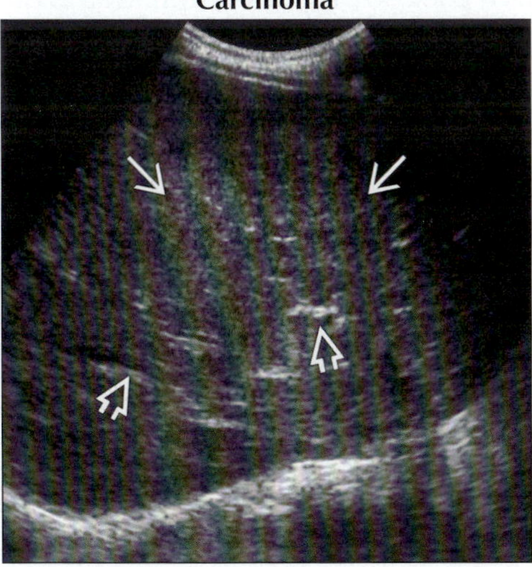

Schistosomiasis

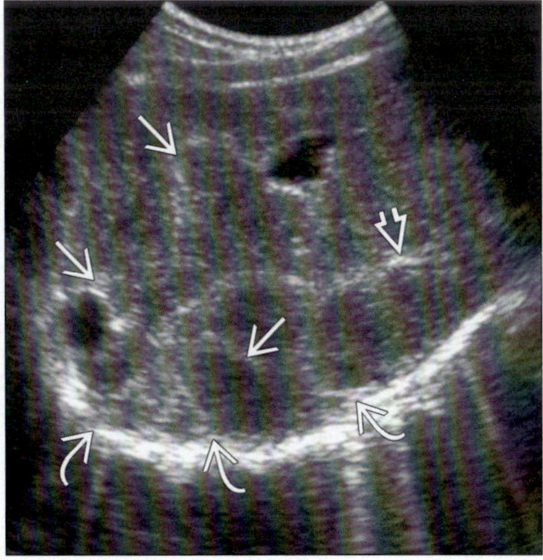

(Left) Oblique ultrasound shows an infiltrative hepatocellular carcinoma ➡. The borders cannot be separated from background cirrhosis. Displacement of the normal hepatic vessels ➡ gives a clue to the presence of a mass lesion. (Right) Oblique US shows a mosaic network of thickened interlobular septae ➡ in a patient with schistosomiasis. Note periportal fibrosis resulting in thickened portal tracts ➡. The liver surface is irregular ➡ from fibrotic retraction by the septae.

DIFFERENTIAL DIAGNOSIS

Common
- Hepatic Cyst
- Polycystic Liver Disease
- Pyogenic Hepatic Abscess
- Recent Hepatic Hemorrhage
- Biloma
- Vessels
- Dilated Bile Ducts
- Hepatic Echinococcal Cyst

Less Common
- Hepatic Lymphoma
- Hepatic Metastases

Rare but Important
- Caroli Disease

ESSENTIAL INFORMATION

Key Differential Diagnosis Issues
- Lesions have few to no echoes within them
- Termed "simple" when unilocular with no internal septae, no lobulated or irregular contour
- Anechoic lesions tend to be round or oval-shaped with smooth contour on all surfaces
- Degree of posterior acoustic enhancement or shadowing and thickness of wall may help limit differential diagnoses

Helpful Clues for Common Diagnoses
- **Hepatic Cyst**
  - Anechoic with strong posterior acoustic enhancement
  - Smooth borders but occasionally lobulated
  - Thin or imperceptible wall with no mural nodule
  - Often subcapsular and may bulge liver contour
  - Do not cross liver segments
  - Do not communicate with each other or bile ducts
  - No internal or mural vascularity but may distort adjacent vessels
  - May have increased echogenicity after hemorrhage or infection
- **Polycystic Liver Disease**
  - May have concomitant autosomal dominant polycystic kidney disease (less likely to have pancreatic cysts as well)
    - May make diagnosis of polycystic liver disease easier
  - Individual cysts look identical to simple hepatic cysts
  - Number of cysts increases with age
  - When cysts become numerous and sizable, liver architecture is distorted, making diagnosis easier
  - Some cysts may be complicated by hemorrhage and become hyperechoic or contain debris or septae
- **Pyogenic Hepatic Abscess**
  - Anechoic (50%), hyperechoic (25%), hypoechoic (25%)
  - Small or microabscesses closely simulate simple cyst; may have some echogenic debris when large
  - Variable in shape, thin or thick walls
  - Borders range from well defined to irregular
  - Tendency to cluster: Group of small pyogenic abscesses coalesce into single large cavity
  - May have adjacent hepatic parenchymal edema, which appears hypoechoic with coarse echopattern, ± vascularity
    - Vascularity may be seen in thick wall portion
  - Diagnosis is made based on combination of clinical and sonographic features
- **Recent Hepatic Hemorrhage**
  - May be due to direct trauma, coagulopathy, surgery/biopsy
  - Initially traumatic hematoma is usually echogenic and becomes anechoic after a few days
    - May have pseudowall of compressed liver parenchyma
  - Contour may be smooth or irregular
  - May be secondary hemorrhage into preexisting mass (adenoma, hepatocellular carcinoma, metastasis, etc.), usually not completely anechoic
- **Biloma**
  - Almost always secondary to trauma, making it difficult to differentiate from traumatic hematoma
    - Over time, hematomas show debris, septations
    - Bilomas remain anechoic
  - Round or oval in shape

SIMPLE ANECHOIC LIVER MASS

- ○ Fluid content may be anechoic with posterior acoustic enhancement, suggesting fresh biloma
- ○ Thin capsule wall usually not discernible
- ○ Larger lesions may compress adjacent liver surface/architecture
- ○ Communication with biliary tree usually too small to be visible
- ○ No vascularity within lesion
- **Vessels**
  - ○ Portal veins: Venectasia, varicosities, collaterals from portal hypertension
  - ○ Hepatic veins: Venectasia, Budd-Chiari, etc.
  - ○ Hepatic arteries: Aneurysms, shunts, vascular malformation
  - ○ Use color Doppler to confirm vascular nature and vessel type
- **Dilated Bile Ducts**
  - ○ Ducts may simulate anechoic nodules when viewed on cross-section
  - ○ Ducts follow periportal distribution; long axis orientation with hepatic artery and portal vein provide clues to its nature
- **Hepatic Echinococcal Cyst**
  - ○ May be solitary or multiple
  - ○ Large, well-defined, cystic liver mass with numerous peripheral daughter cysts
  - ○ Cyst-within-cyst appearance
  - ○ Floating membrane within cyst
  - ○ Unilocular anechoic cyst is classified as type 1 appearance by WHO
  - ○ Layered cyst wall is diagnostic: Thickness reduces posterior acoustic enhancement

Helpful Clues for Less Common Diagnoses
- **Hepatic Lymphoma**
  - ○ May be irregular or round/oval in shape
  - ○ ± posterior acoustic enhancement, "pseudocystic" appearance
  - ○ May have extrahepatic signs such as lymphadenopathy, splenomegaly (± splenic infiltration)
- **Hepatic Metastases**
  - ○ Anechoic hepatic metastasis are suspicious of low degree of differentiation and high degree of malignancy
  - ○ Usually no posterior acoustic enhancement
  - ○ May have debris, mural nodularity, &/or thick septations
  - ○ May have irregular margins and contour
  - ○ Wall vascularity

Helpful Clues for Rare Diagnoses
- **Caroli Disease**
  - ○ "Central dot" sign: Portal radicles within dilated intrahepatic bile ducts on color Doppler ultrasound

Technical Issues
- Important to make sure that gain settings are correct
- Gallbladder or inferior vena cava can be used as internal references for gain settings, as these anatomic structures should normally look anechoic

Hepatic Cyst

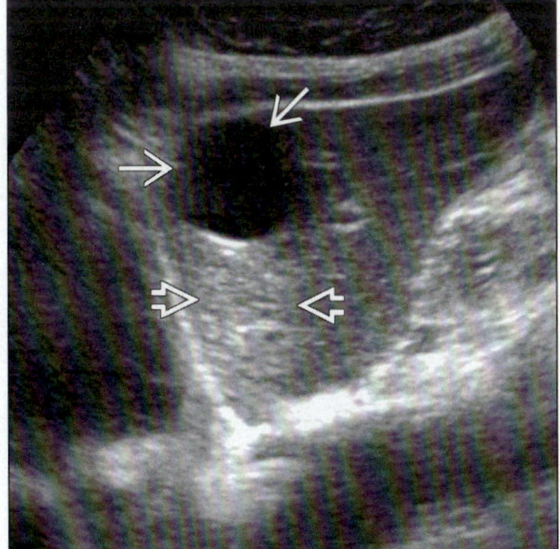

Longitudinal transabdominal ultrasound shows a simple anechoic cyst ➡ with a smooth contour and posterior acoustic enhancement ➡. Note the absence of septae, an appreciable wall, or a mural nodule.

Hepatic Cyst

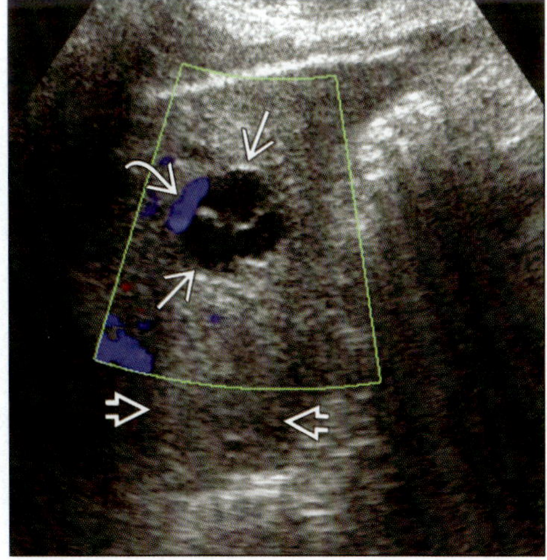

Longitudinal color Doppler ultrasound shows an anechoic hepatic cyst ➡ distorting the adjacent vein ➡. This is not mural vascularity. Note the thin septum within and the posterior acoustic enhancement ➡.

SIMPLE ANECHOIC LIVER MASS

(Left) Oblique transabdominal US shows polycystic liver disease with multiple anechoic cysts ➡ of varying size with irregular borders. Cysts become more irregular as they enlarge with age. **(Right)** Oblique US shows an anechoic abscess ➡ with posterior enhancement ➡ and no appreciable wall. This atypical anechoic appearance makes an abscess difficult to differentiate from a cyst. Clinical correlation is essential.

Polycystic Liver Disease

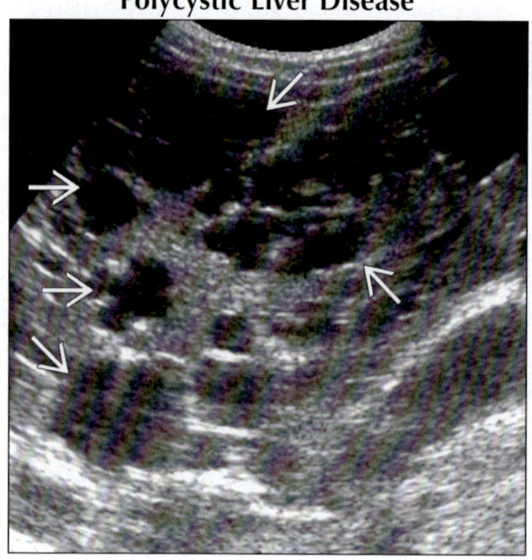

Pyogenic Hepatic Abscess

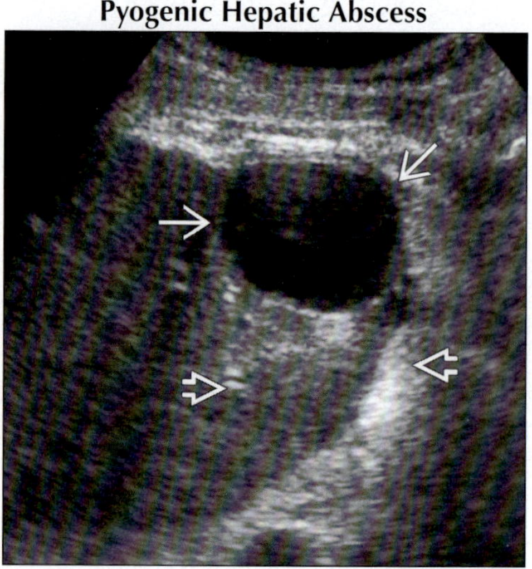

(Left) Oblique transabdominal ultrasound shows an anechoic hematoma ➡ appearing as a cystic lesion without internal echoes. Hematomas are initially echogenic and become hypoechoic after 4-5 days. **(Right)** Transverse transabdominal ultrasound shows an anechoic (sterile) biloma ➡ with no appreciable capsule. Its deep surface is in contact with the porta hepatis ➡. An infected biloma may have internal debris and septae.

Recent Hepatic Hemorrhage

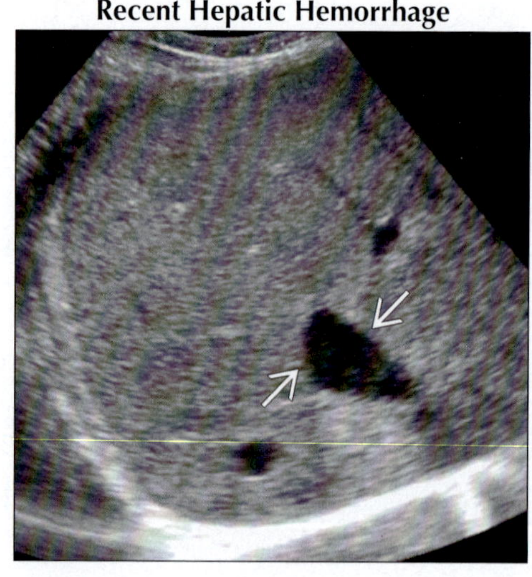

Biloma

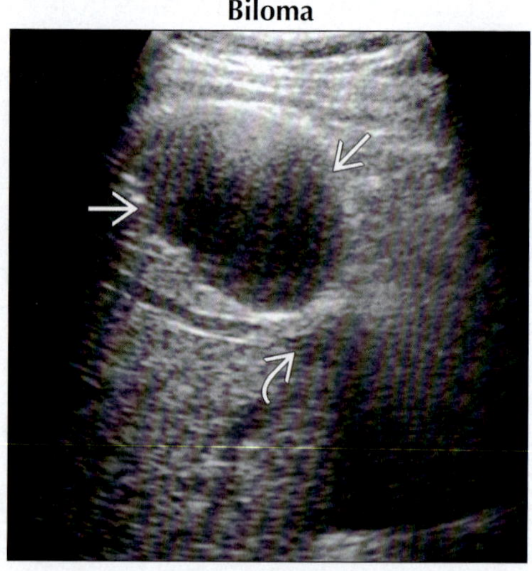

(Left) Oblique transabdominal ultrasound shows cross sections of anechoic masses ➡ representing varices from a portosystemic shunt. These show no appreciable wall. **(Right)** Oblique color Doppler ultrasound in the same patient shows color filling the lumen ➡ of the varices of the portosystemic shunt. Color flow also reveals smaller vessels and the extent of the lesion.

Vessels

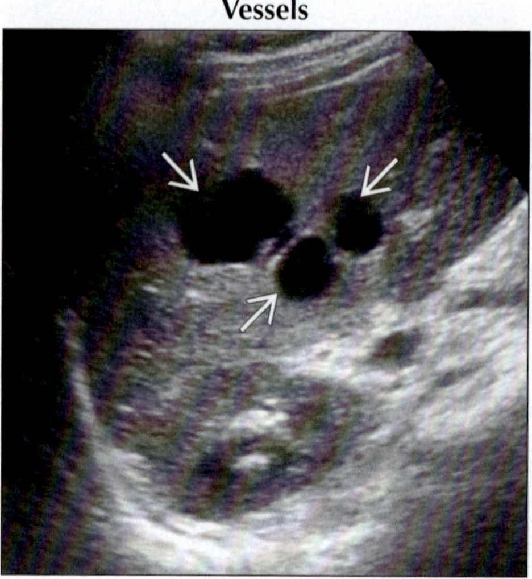

Vessels

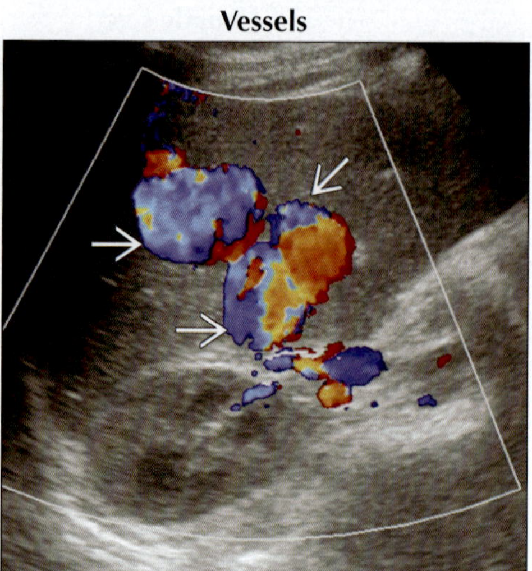

SIMPLE ANECHOIC LIVER MASS

Dilated Bile Ducts

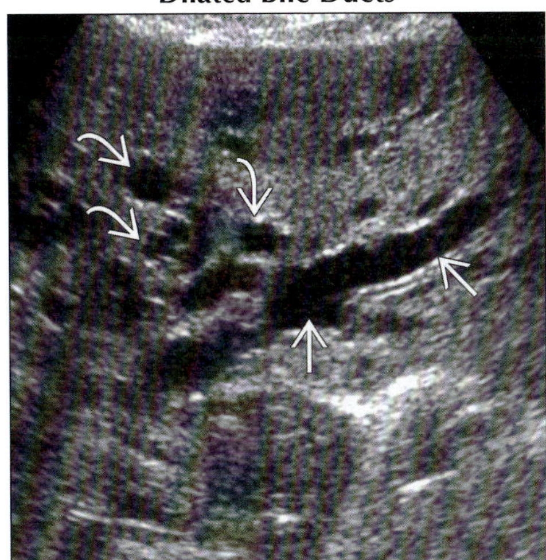

Hepatic Echinococcal Cyst

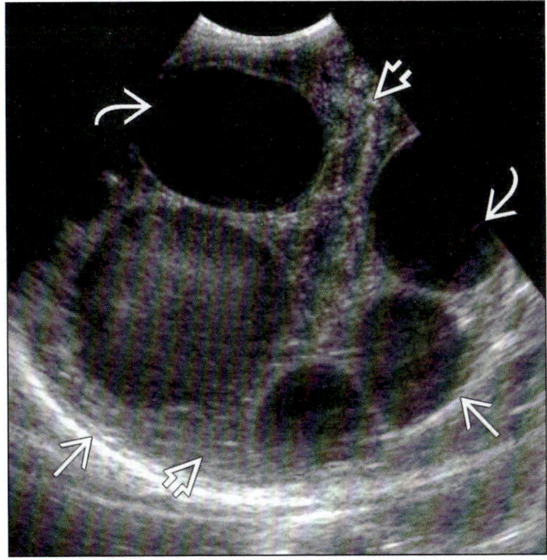

(Left) Transverse transabdominal ultrasound shows anechoic nodules and tubes representing ducts in longitudinal ➡ and transverse profile ➡. Color Doppler showed no flow, confirming these as ducts. (Right) Longitudinal transabdominal ultrasound shows a large echinococcal cyst in the right lobe of the liver, with an outer capsule (endocyst) ➡ containing anechoic daughter cysts ➡ and isoechoic debris (hydatid sand) ➡ between the cysts.

Hepatic Lymphoma

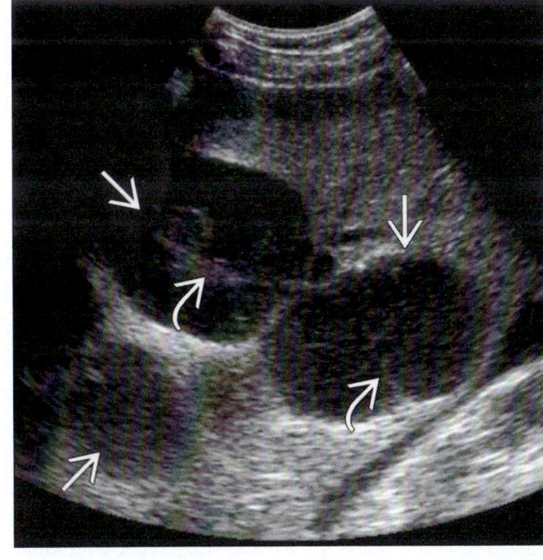

Hepatic Metastases

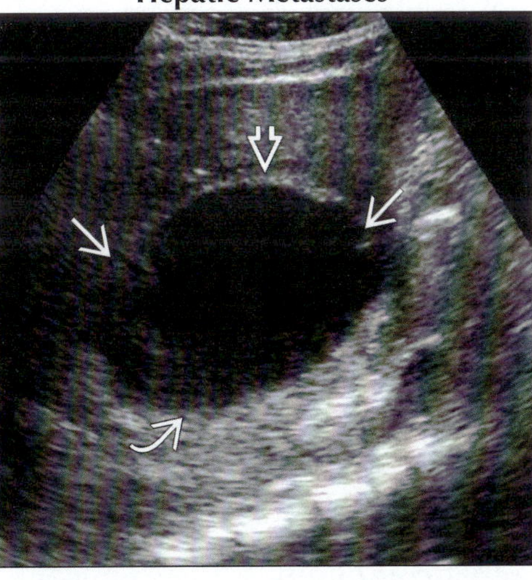

(Left) Oblique ultrasound shows multiple anechoic masses ➡ with internal septae ➡. Because they are homogeneous and anechoic, these lymphoma deposits appear "pseudocystic." (Right) Oblique ultrasound shows an anechoic metastasis ➡ with no appreciable wall at the posterior border ➡. There is a barely appreciable wall ➡ in the anterior aspect of this lesion, which suggests that this is not a hepatic cyst.

Hepatic Metastases

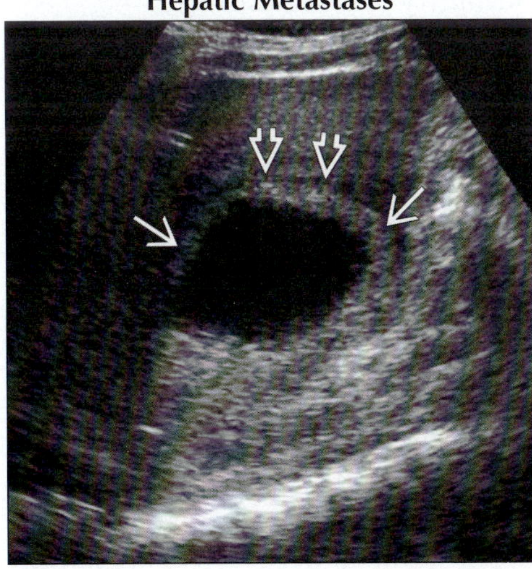

Caroli Disease

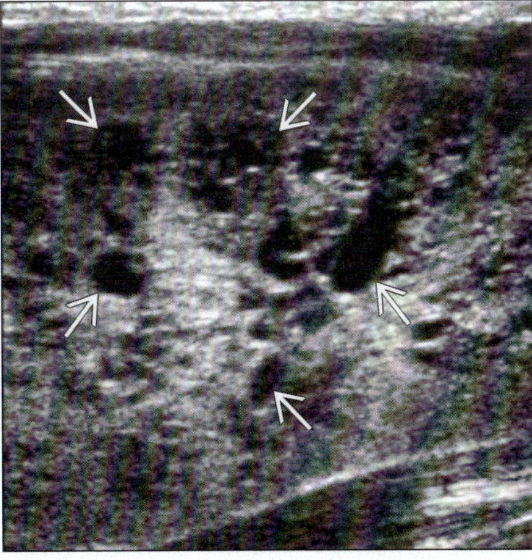

(Left) Oblique transabdominal ultrasound shows an anechoic lesion with a thick wall ➡. The presence of this wall makes the lesion suspicious for a metastasis. Note the thin hypoechoic halo ➡. (Right) Oblique transabdominal ultrasound shows multiple anechoic nodules and tubes ➡ diffusely involving the liver and representing dilated ducts in Caroli disease. Color Doppler interrogation may show small portal veins surrounded by ducts.

COMPLEX CYSTIC LIVER MASS

DIFFERENTIAL DIAGNOSIS

Common
- Complicated Benign Hepatic Cysts
- Hematoma
- Atypical Hemangioma
- Pyogenic Hepatic Abscess
- Hepatic Metastases

Less Common
- Cholangiocarcinoma
- Gallbladder Carcinoma (Mimic)
- Hepatic Echinococcus Cyst

ESSENTIAL INFORMATION

Key Differential Diagnosis Issues
- Masses with posterior acoustic enhancement
  - Lesion itself may be any combination of hyper-, iso-, or hypoechoic

Helpful Clues for Common Diagnoses
- **Complicated Benign Hepatic Cysts**
  - May contain thin septae, internal debris, or fluid-debris level
  - Septae may form after hemorrhage or infection, giving cyst a multiloculated appearance
  - Cyst wall may develop calcification
  - Posterior acoustic enhancement
  - May distort adjacent vessels and simulate mural vascularity
  - Color Doppler shows no mural or septal vascularity
- **Hematoma**
  - Due to hepatic trauma that commonly occurs in segments 6, 7, and 8
  - Intraparenchymal hematomas are usually round in shape
  - Parenchymal laceration
    - Irregularly shaped hematoma
    - May point toward capsular surface and show associated disruption of capsular surface
  - Echogenicity of hematoma evolves over time
    - Initially: Echogenic
    - After 4-5 days: Hypoechoic
    - After 1-4 weeks: Internal echoes and septations

- Rate of hematoma evolution depends on vascularity of region: Slower for intraperitoneal or subcapsular regions, faster for parenchymal hematomas
  - Ancillary signs of trauma may be present
    - Subcapsular hematoma
    - Hemoperitoneum
    - Renal or splenic laceration/hematoma
- **Atypical Hemangioma**
  - Large lesions more likely to have atypical appearance
    - Irregular rim
    - Heterogeneous/hypoechoic center (represents area of necrosis, hemorrhage, scarring)
    - Calcification
  - Posterior acoustic enhancement may be present
  - Color Doppler
    - May show vessels in periphery of tumor
    - No visible color Doppler flow in center of lesion (flow too slow to be detected)
    - Contrast-enhanced Doppler US demonstrates same filling-in phenomenon as seen on CECT
  - Power Doppler
    - May detect slow flow within hemangiomas
- **Pyogenic Hepatic Abscess**
  - Commonly ill-defined borders
  - Often multiple
  - "Cluster" sign: Aggregation of small abscesses, sometimes coalesce into single septate cavity
  - Thick and irregular wall
  - Thick or thin internal septae
  - Mural nodularity (± vascularity)
  - May contain gas within abscess
    - Seen as echogenic foci of air (with reverberation artifact) or air-fluid level
  - Changes to anechoic when center becomes necrotic as it enlarges
  - May have coarse, hypoechoic (inflamed, edematous) surrounding liver parenchyma
  - Periportal distribution suggests dissemination along biliary tree
  - Random distribution suggests hematogenous spread
  - Color Doppler
    - Vascularity may be seen in thick wall

3

COMPLEX CYSTIC LIVER MASS

- ▪ May show hypervascularity in surrounding inflamed liver parenchyma
  - ○ Amebic abscess
    - ▪ More likely to be peripherally located than pyogenic abscess, abutting liver capsule
    - ▪ Often solitary
    - ▪ Round or oval shaped
    - ▪ Sharply defined
- **Hepatic Metastases**
  - ○ Due to cyst-forming or necrotic metastases
    - ▪ Cystic: Cystadenocarcinoma of pancreas or ovary; colonic carcinoma
    - ▪ Necrotic: Treated metastasis, sarcoma, squamous cell carcinoma
  - ○ Commonly multiple
  - ○ ± posterior acoustic enhancement
  - ○ Internal debris
  - ○ Mural nodularity
  - ○ Thick irregular septae
  - ○ Color Doppler may show mural vascularity with chaotic/bizarre intratumoral vascularity
  - ○ ± associated lymphadenopathy

Helpful Clues for Less Common Diagnoses
- **Cholangiocarcinoma**
  - ○ Usually solid but can be cystic (rare)
    - ▪ Result of necrosis
  - ○ Usually large mass
  - ○ Mural nodule or papillary excrescence from wall
  - ○ May show fine mural or septal calcification
    - ▪ Rarely nonseptate

- ○ No surrounding inflammatory changes
- ○ Color Doppler may show mural/papillary vascularity
- **Hepatic Echinococcus Cyst**
  - ○ Commonly large lesion
  - ○ Peripheral daughter cysts
  - ○ Curvilinear or ring-like pericyst calcification
  - ○ Dilated intrahepatic bile ducts
    - ▪ Due to compression or rupture of cyst products into ducts
  - ○ *E. granulosa*
    - ▪ Anechoic cyst with double echogenic lines separated by hypoechoic layer
    - ▪ Honeycombed cyst, multiple septations between daughter cysts in mother cyst
    - ▪ Detachment of endocyst from pericyst results in undulating floating membrane within cyst or "water lily" sign
    - ▪ Anechoic cyst with internal debris, hydatid sand, "snowstorm" pattern
  - ○ *E. multilocularis*
    - ▪ Single/multiple echogenic lesions
    - ▪ Ill-defined, infiltrative, solid masses
    - ▪ Irregular necrotic regions and microcalcifications may give it cystic appearance
    - ▪ Tend to spread to liver hilum
    - ▪ Invasion of inferior vena cava and diaphragm

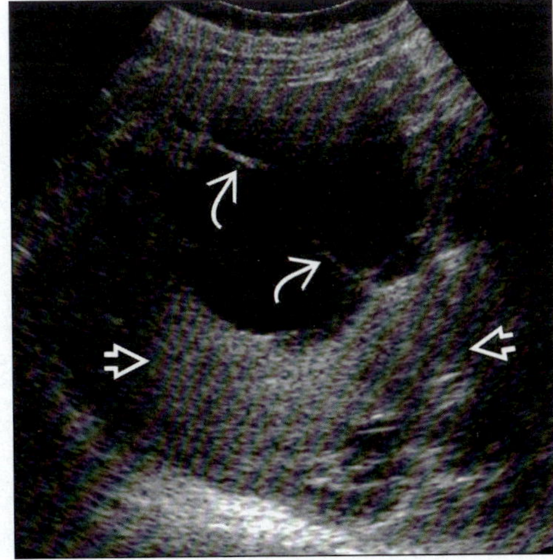

Complicated Benign Hepatic Cysts

Oblique transabdominal ultrasound shows thin septae ⮞ within this benign hepatic cyst. Note the posterior acoustic enhancement ⮞. The wall is thin and there is no mural nodularity.

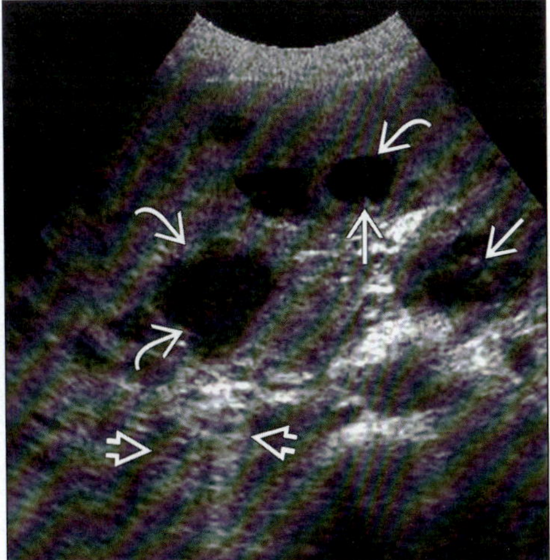

Complicated Benign Hepatic Cysts

Oblique transabdominal ultrasound shows several cysts with smooth wall contours ⮞, posterior enhancement ⮞, and internal septae ⮞. There is no thickened wall or mural nodule.

COMPLEX CYSTIC LIVER MASS

(Left) Oblique ultrasound shows polycystic liver disease with numerous cysts ➡ of varying sizes. As cysts become larger, their contours become more irregular, and the liver architecture is distorted. Note the posterior acoustic enhancement ➡. (Right) Oblique ultrasound shows a benign cyst with organizing hematoma ➡. Blood products and fibrin strands ➡ form septae and divide liquified compartments. Note the posterior acoustic enhancement ➡.

Complicated Benign Hepatic Cysts

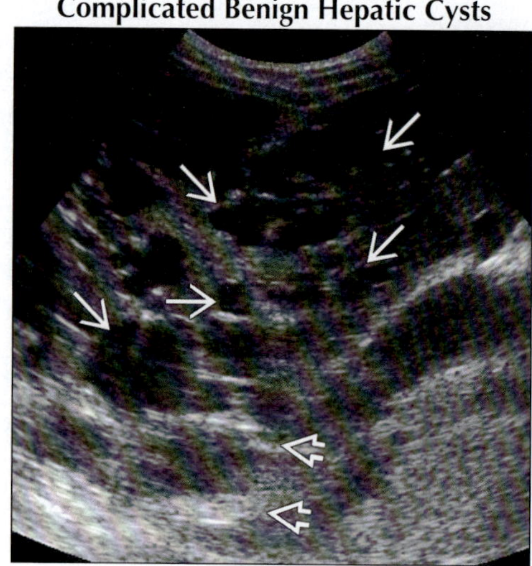

Hematoma

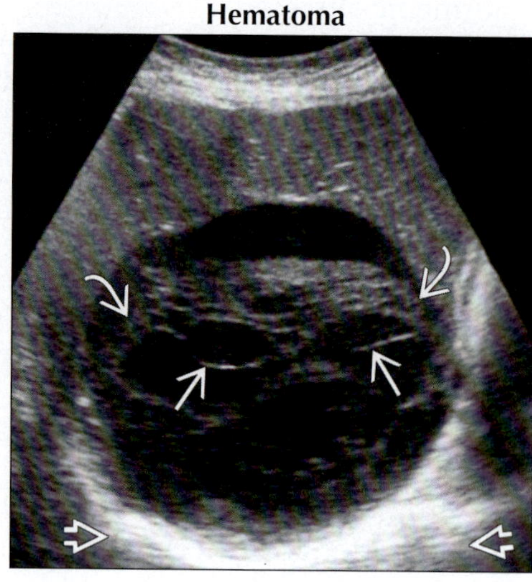

(Left) Oblique transabdominal ultrasound shows a benign cyst with a previous hemorrhage layering debris ➡, posterior enhancement ➡, and a smooth contour ➡. There is no wall thickening or mural nodule. (Right) Oblique transabdominal ultrasound shows atypical hemangioma ➡, which is hypoechoic (typical appearance is hyperechoic) with hyperechoic internal septae and low-level internal echoes (blood) ➡. Note the posterior enhancement ➡.

Hematoma

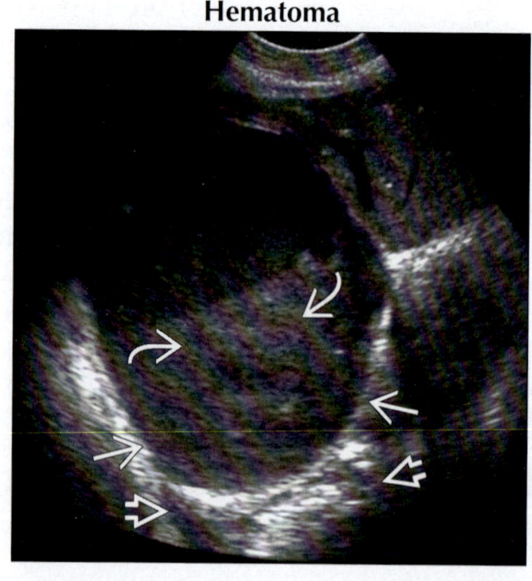

Atypical Hemangioma

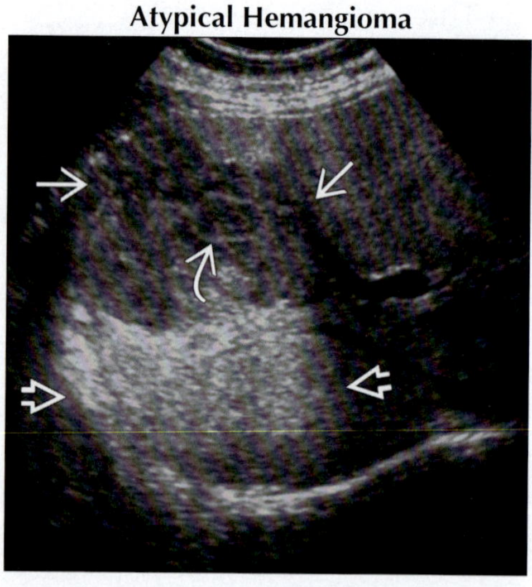

(Left) Oblique transabdominal ultrasound shows a cluster of coalescing pyogenic abscesses ➡ with thick septae, low-level internal echoes ➡, irregular contour, and posterior acoustic enhancement ➡. (Right) Oblique power Doppler ultrasound shows a pyogenic abscess with irregular contour ➡ and thick septae. There is prominent vascularity ➡ in a thick septum within the lesion.

Pyogenic Hepatic Abscess

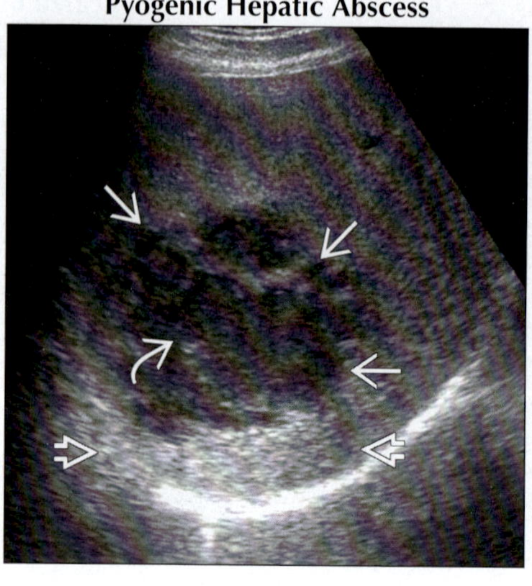

Pyogenic Hepatic Abscess

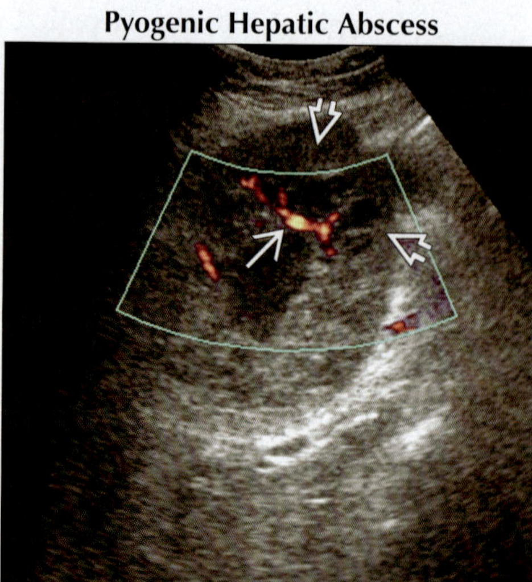

3

COMPLEX CYSTIC LIVER MASS

Hepatic Metastases

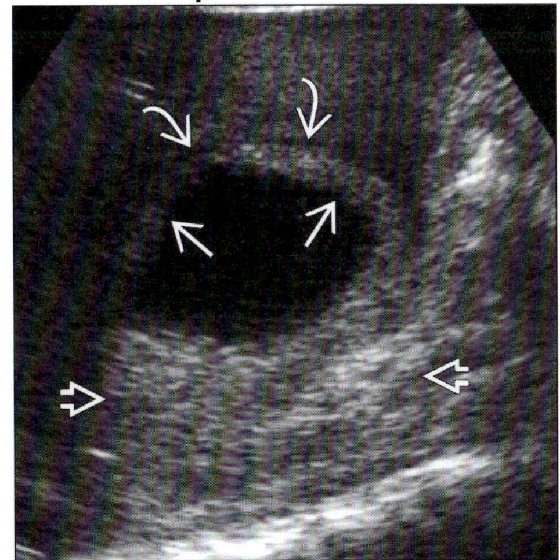

Hepatic Metastases

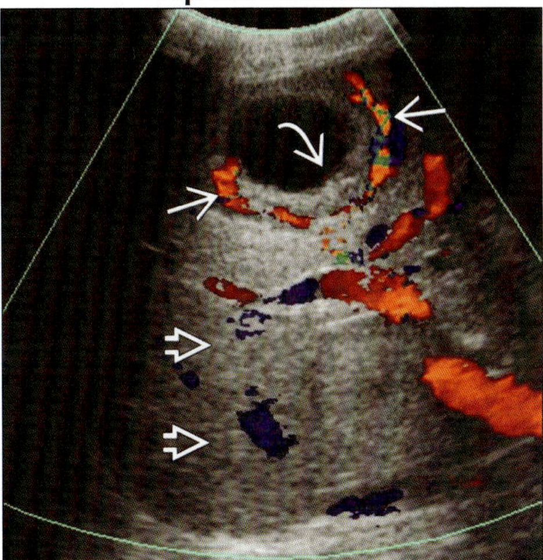

(Left) Oblique transabdominal ultrasound shows a thick-walled anechoic cystic metastasis ➡ in the liver. A thin hypoechoic halo can be seen around the wall of the metastasis ➡, representing compressed edematous liver parenchyma. Note the posterior enhancement ➡. (Right) Oblique color Doppler ultrasound shows prominent tumor vessels ➡ in the thick wall ➡ of a cystic metastasis of the liver. Note the posterior acoustic enhancement ➡.

Cholangiocarcinoma

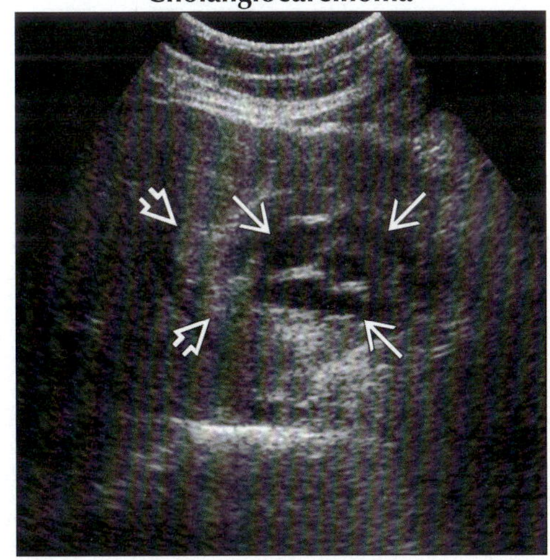

Cholangiocarcinoma

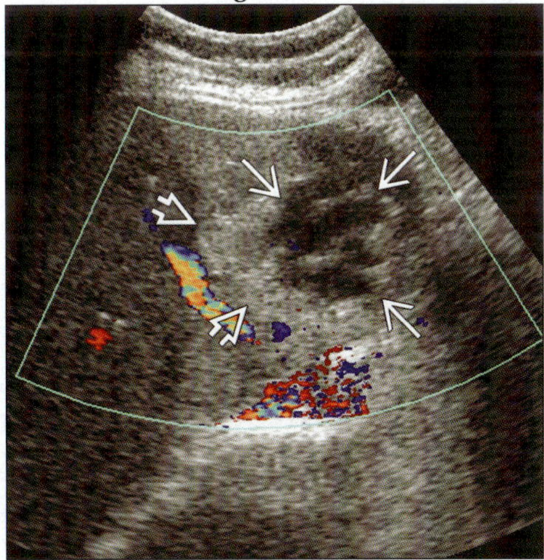

(Left) Transverse ultrasound shows marked intrahepatic duct dilatation ➡ in the periphery of the left lobe. This is caused by the poorly marginated, slightly hyperechoic cholangiocarcinoma ➡ in the more central aspect of the left lobe of the liver. (Right) Transverse color Doppler ultrasound in the same patient shows an absence of vascularity in the dilated intrahepatic ducts ➡. This cholangiocarcinoma ➡ is hypovascular.

Gallbladder Carcinoma (Mimic)

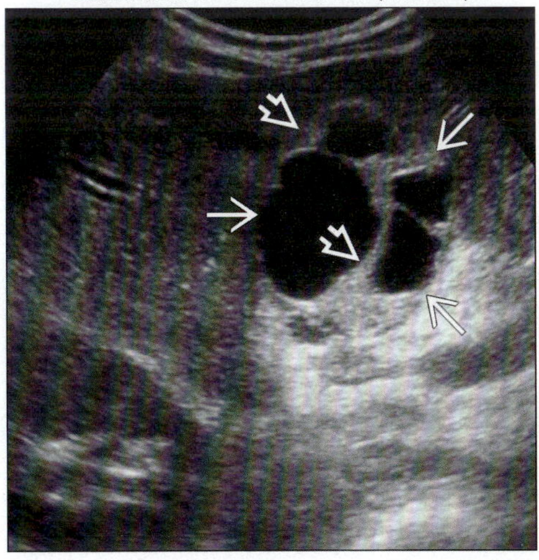

Hepatic Echinococcus Cyst

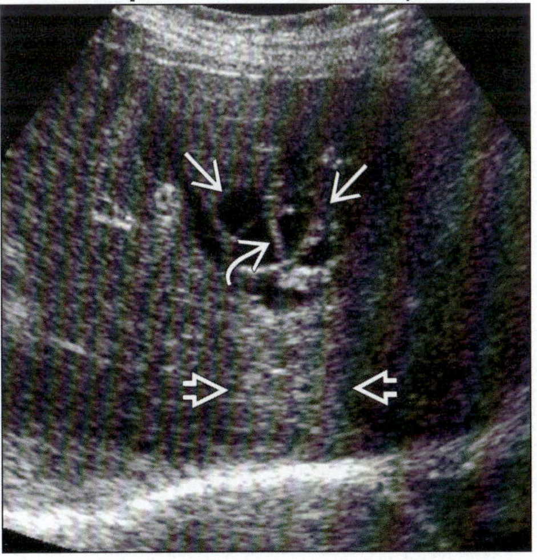

(Left) Transverse ultrasound shows a multiloculated cystic carcinoma ➡ of the gallbladder, filling the gallbladder fossa and extending into the liver, giving the appearance of a hepatic mass. Note the thick irregular septae and walls ➡. (Right) Oblique ultrasound shows a "honeycomb" appearance ➡ of an echinococcal cyst. There are thick and irregular septae ➡ separating the daughter cysts. Note the posterior acoustic enhancement ➡.

DIFFERENTIAL DIAGNOSIS

Common
- Complicated Benign Hepatic Cyst
- Hepatic Metastases
- Infection
  - Pyogenic Hepatic Abscess
  - Amebic Hepatic Abscess
- Focal Fatty Sparing

Less Common
- Hepatic Lymphoma
- Hepatic Adenoma
- Focal Nodular Hyperplasia
- Atypical Hemangioma
- Hepatocellular Carcinoma
- Hepatic Hematoma
- Abnormal Bile Ducts
- Abnormal Vessels

ESSENTIAL INFORMATION

Key Differential Diagnosis Issues
- Lesions of lower echogenicity than liver parenchyma with some low-level internal echogenicity (compared to purely anechoic lesions)

Helpful Clues for Common Diagnoses
- **Complicated Benign Hepatic Cyst**
  - Superimposed hemorrhage or infection in hepatic cyst
  - Septation/thickened wall ± mural calcification
  - Posterior acoustic enhancement
  - Solid-appearing if internal debris (clots or fibrin strands) dispersed within cyst
  - Fluid-debris level if debris settles under influence of gravity
  - No mural nodule
  - Color Doppler shows absence of internal or mural vascularity
    - Adjacent vessels distorted by large cyst
- **Hepatic Metastases**
  - Hypoechoic metastases tend to be numerous and small
    - Larger lesions tend to have heterogeneous echogenicity
  - May have irregular or ill-defined borders
  - Hypoechogenicity may reflect poor cellular differentiation, active growth
  - Suggest hypovascular and hypercellular tumor origin
    - Lung, breast, lymphoma
  - No posterior acoustic enhancement
  - Causes architectural distortion if large or numerous
  - Color Doppler may show no vascularity as most are hypovascular
  - Metastases are difficult to differentiate from lymphoma without history of known primary lesion
- **Pyogenic Hepatic Abscess**
  - Cystic mass with irregular border and debris
  - Posterior acoustic enhancement
  - Multiple thick or thin septations
  - Mural nodularity & vascularity
  - Adjacent parenchyma may be coarse & hypoechoic due to inflammation
  - "Cluster sign": Coalescence of group of abscesses
  - May contain gas within abscess
    - Reverberation artifact or air-fluid level
  - Changes to anechoic when center becomes necrotic as center enlarges
  - Periportal distribution suggests dissemination along biliary tree
  - Random distribution suggests hematogenous spread
- **Amebic Hepatic Abscess**
  - Abuts liver capsule, under diaphragm
  - Amebic abscess is more likely to be round or oval-shaped than pyogenic abscess (82% vs. 60%)
  - Hypoechoic with fine internal echoes is more common in amebic than pyogenic abscess (58% vs. 36%)
  - Internal septae may be present
  - Posterior acoustic enhancement
  - No vascularity seen in wall or septa of amebic abscess
  - Sub-diaphragmatic rupture in presence of adjacent hepatic abscess suggests amebic nature of abscess
- **Focal Fatty Sparing**
  - Typical locations
    - Gallbladder fossa
    - Inferior aspect of segment 4b
    - Around hepatic veins
    - Near bifurcation of portal vein
  - Geographic hypoechoic area within echogenic liver
  - No architectural distortion

HYPOECHOIC LIVER MASS

- Vessels course through mass undistorted, no mass effect
  - Does not cross segments

Helpful Clues for Less Common Diagnoses

- **Hepatic Lymphoma**
  - Hypoechoic mass with irregular margins
  - Low echogenicity probably due to high cellular density and lack of background stroma
  - Large/conglomerate masses may appear to contain septae and mimic abscesses
  - Other sites of involvement commonly seen
    - Lymphadenopathy, splenomegaly ± focal splenic lesions provide clues to diagnosis
- **Hepatic Adenoma**
  - Only slightly hypoechoic compared to normal liver parenchyma
    - May be isoechoic
  - May have hypoechoic rim
  - Complications including hemorrhage, central necrosis, and rupture may be present and may make lesion more conspicuous
  - Color Doppler shows distinct venous vascularity at borders
- **Focal Nodular Hyperplasia**
  - Distinctly heterogeneous, coarse echotexture, hypo-/isoechoic
  - Central hypoechoic stellate scar with radiating fibrous septa
  - Doppler shows hypervascularity
- **Atypical Hemangioma**
  - < 10% of hemangiomas are hypoechoic to liver parenchyma
  - May appear hypoechoic in fatty liver
    - Background hyperechoic liver
  - Hypoechoic areas within large lesions may represent necrosis, hemorrhage, scar, or vessels
  - Smooth, well-defined borders
  - May see posterior acoustic enhancement
  - Occasionally hypoechoic center with hyperechoic rim
  - No visible color Doppler flow (flow too slow to be detected)
    - May be detected with power Doppler
- **Hepatocellular Carcinoma**
  - Ill-defined borders, ± multifocal
  - Background of cirrhotic liver
  - Irregular hypervascularity
  - Invasion of portal vein with portal venous thrombosis and portal hypertension
    - Arterial Doppler signal in portal vein thrombus
- **Hepatic Hematoma**
  - Appearance varies with age from hyperechoic to hypoechoic
- **Abnormal Bile Ducts**
  - Dilated duct with sludge or tumor
  - Interrogate in perpendicular plane to show its tubular nature
- **Abnormal Vessels**
  - Dilated portal or hepatic vein with hypoechoic thrombus
  - Interrogate in perpendicular plane to show its tubular nature

Complicated Benign Hepatic Cyst

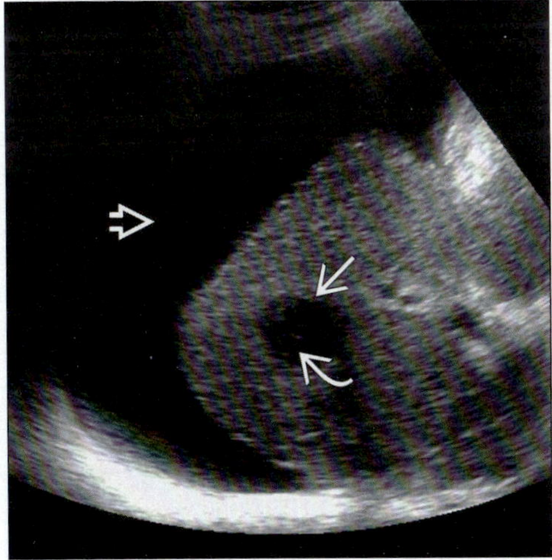

Oblique transabdominal ultrasound of a cirrhotic liver shows a small benign hepatic cyst ➡ with internal debris ➡. Note the low-level echoes within the cyst, especially as compared to the anechoic ascites ➡.

Complicated Benign Hepatic Cyst

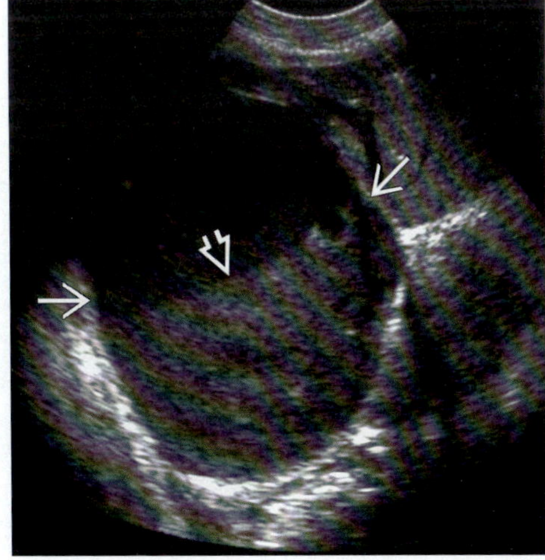

Oblique transabdominal ultrasound shows a large benign hepatic cyst ➡ with previous hemorrhage. It is filled with internal debris, producing low-level internal echoes and fluid-debris level ➡.

HYPOECHOIC LIVER MASS

(Left) Oblique transabdominal ultrasound shows a well-defined, hypoechoic metastasis ➡ in the right lobe of the liver. Note the slightly irregular contour ➡ and the lack of posterior acoustic enhancement. *(Right)* Longitudinal ultrasound shows a cluster of pyogenic abscesses ➡ with a lobulated contour. There are multiple, thick, irregular internal septae ➡ and echogenic foci ➡ of gas.

Hepatic Metastases

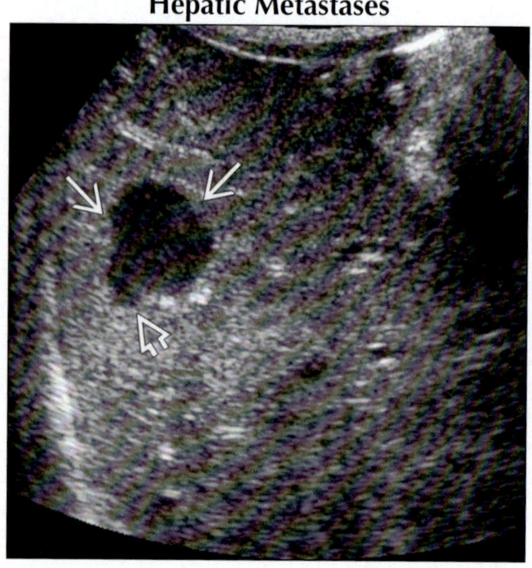

Pyogenic Hepatic Abscess

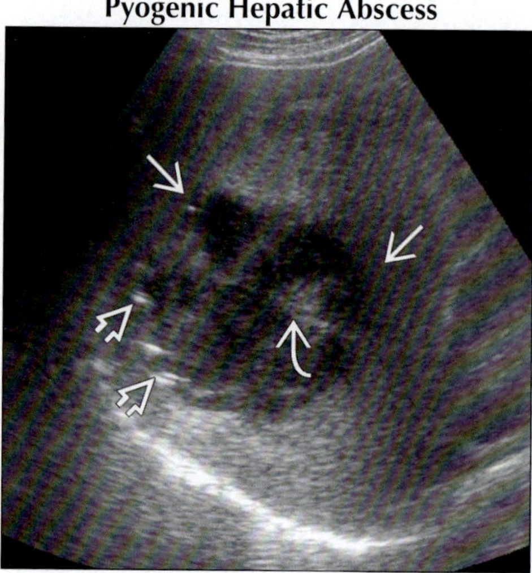

(Left) Longitudinal transabdominal ultrasound shows a geographic area of focal fatty steatosis ➡ affecting the superior part of the liver. This borders an area of normal (spared) liver, which appears relatively hypoechoic ➡. *(Right)* Transverse transabdominal ultrasound shows 2 hypoechoic lymphomatous deposits ➡ in the liver. Note the internal low-level echoes ➡ within the lesions.

Focal Fatty Sparing

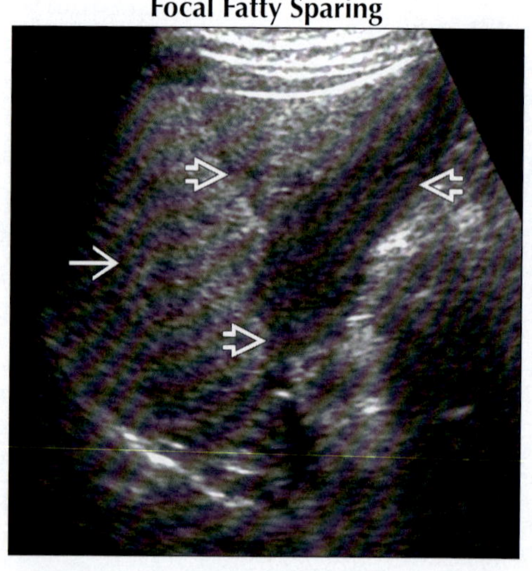

Hepatic Lymphoma

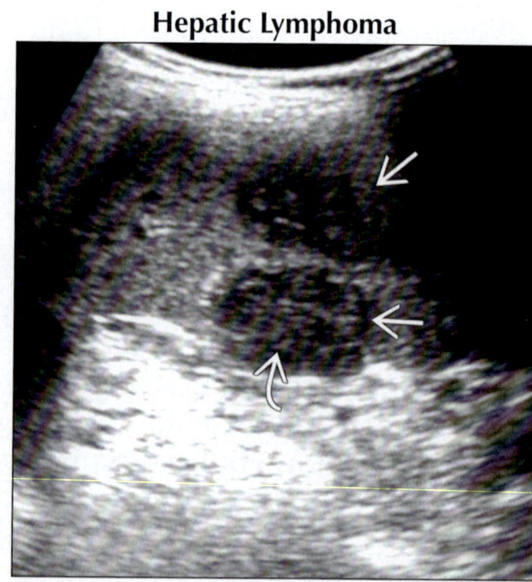

(Left) Oblique transabdominal ultrasound shows a well-circumscribed, hypoechoic, hepatic adenoma ➡ close to the gallbladder ➡. The liver is fatty (hyperechoic), highlighting the hypoechoic adenoma. *(Right)* Transverse transabdominal ultrasound shows a well-defined, hypoechoic focal nodular hyperplasia ➡ in the left lobe of the liver. A central scar is helpful for the diagnosis but is not always present as in this case.

Hepatic Adenoma

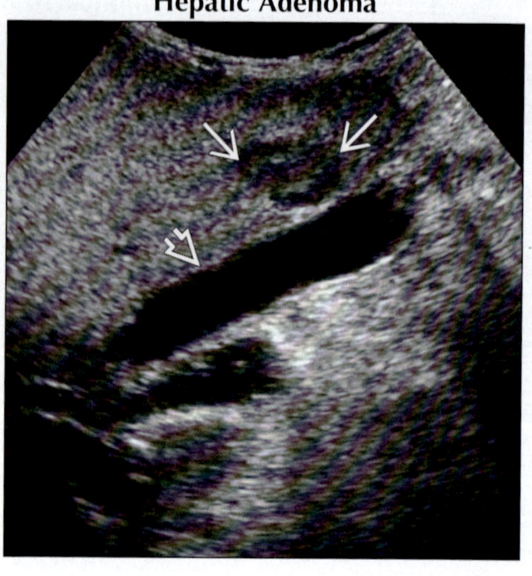

Focal Nodular Hyperplasia

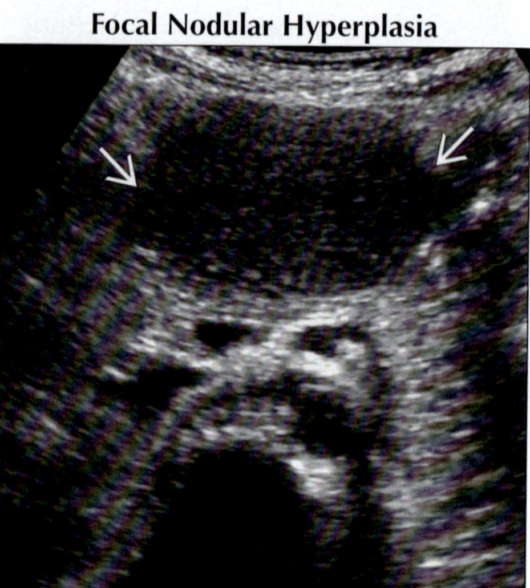

HYPOECHOIC LIVER MASS

Atypical Hemangioma

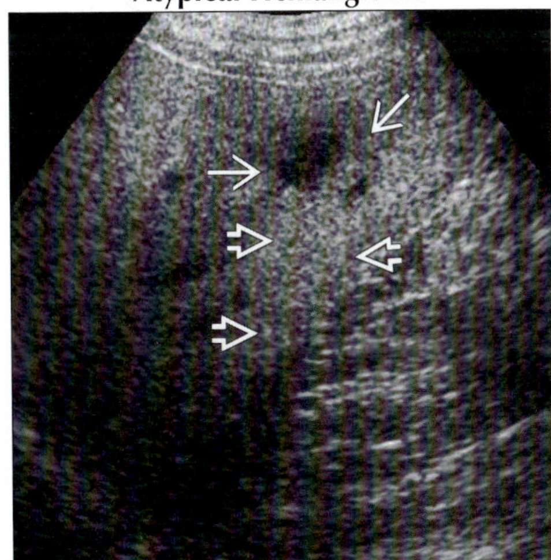

Atypical Hemangioma

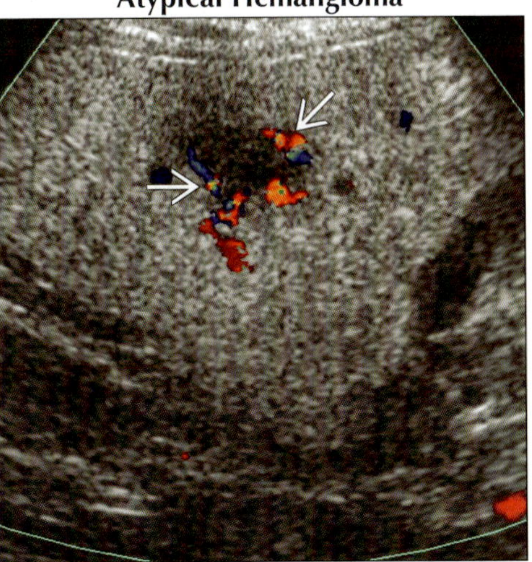

(Left) Oblique ultrasound shows an atypical hypoechoic hemangioma ➡ (typically hyperechoic) in the right lobe of the liver. Note the subtle posterior acoustic enhancement ⮞. (Right) Oblique color Doppler ultrasound in the same patient shows prominent peripheral vascularity ➡ in the margins of the mass. Slow flow in the center of the hemangioma is not detected on color Doppler, though it may be seen on power Doppler.

Hepatocellular Carcinoma

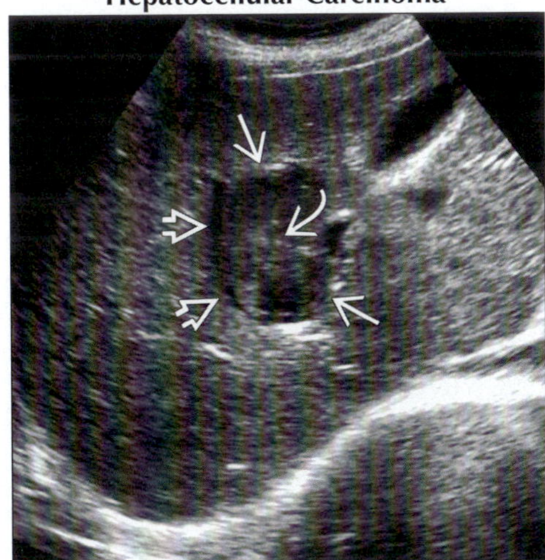

Hepatocellular Carcinoma

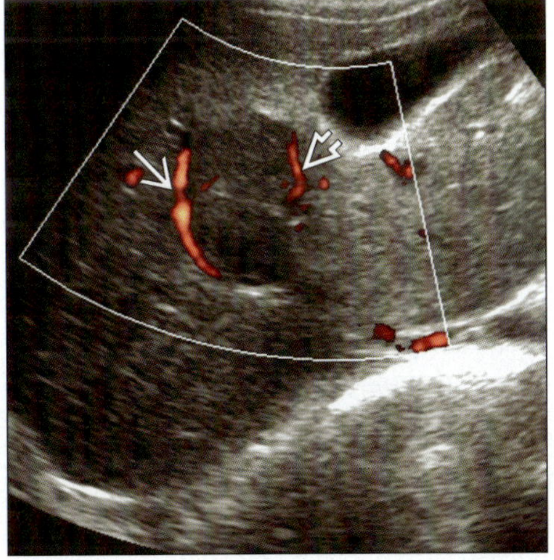

(Left) Oblique ultrasound shows a well-circumscribed, hypoechoic, hepatocellular carcinoma ➡ in the right lobe of the liver, displacing the adjacent vein ⮞. Some increase in internal echogenicity ➡ may represent necrosis or fibrosis. (Right) Oblique power Doppler ultrasound in the same patient shows flow within displaced vessels ➡ and in the periphery ⮞ of the hepatocellular carcinoma. In this case, there is little flow within the central portion of the tumor.

Abnormal Vessels

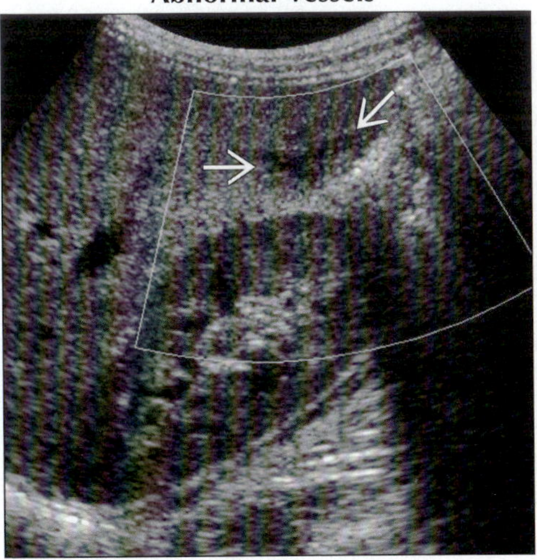

Abnormal Vessels

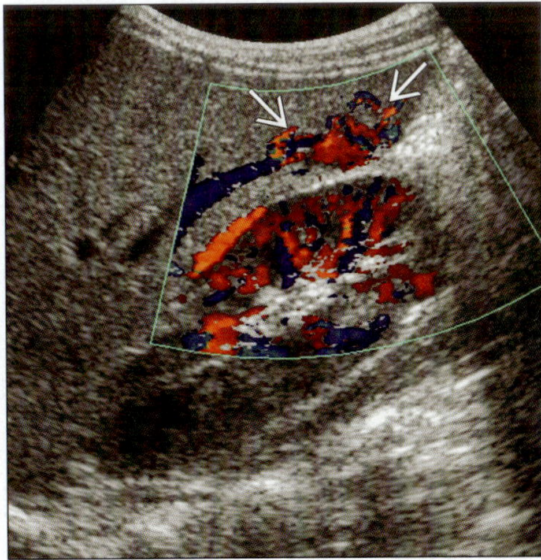

(Left) Longitudinal ultrasound shows a small arteriovenous malformation ➡ in segment 6 of the liver, which appears as an irregular hypoechoic mass. The lesion is slightly flattened but does not appear serpiginous. (Right) Longitudinal color Doppler ultrasound in the same patient shows complete filling-in with color of the small arteriovenous malformation ➡. The turbulent flow (mixed red and blue colors) suggests high flow.

3

DIFFERENTIAL DIAGNOSIS

Common
- Hepatocellular Carcinoma
- Hepatic Metastases
- Hematoma
- Focal Nodular Hyperplasia
- Atypical Hemangioma
- Cholangiocarcinoma
- Hepatic Adenoma
- Hepatic Lymphoma
- Biliary Sludge

Less Common
- Hepatized Gallbladder
- Abnormal Vessels

ESSENTIAL INFORMATION

Key Differential Diagnosis Issues
- Isoechoic masses may be difficult to detect as they appear similar to rest of liver parenchyma
- Key to detection is mass effect with distortion of hepatic surface contour or displacement/compression of vasculature to help detect lesion
- Subtle difference in echopattern of lesion compared to rest of liver may be present
- Color Doppler may show abnormal vascular supply or peripheral abnormal vasculature

Helpful Clues for Common Diagnoses
- **Hepatocellular Carcinoma**
  - Infiltrative hepatocellular carcinomas are not uncommonly isoechoic with cirrhotic liver
  - Distortion of vessels may be only clue to presence of HCCs
  - Color Doppler may show abnormal vessels supplying tumor
  - Portal venous thrombus may be present
  - Arterial flow in portal venous thrombus is virtually diagnostic of tumor thrombus and hepatocellular carcinoma
- **Hepatic Metastases**
  - Infiltrative/diffuse lesions without background cirrhotic liver
  - No posterior acoustic enhancement
  - Most commonly from lung or breast primary
  - Color Doppler may show distorted vessels and provide clue to diagnosis
  - Contrast-enhanced ultrasound increases detectability of hepatic metastases
- **Hematoma**
  - Appearances vary with age of hematoma from hyperechoic to hypoechoic to septate with internal debris
  - Other signs of abdominal trauma and history are helpful
- **Focal Nodular Hyperplasia**
  - Usually homogeneous and isoechoic, occasionally hypoechoic or hyperechoic
  - Mass effect with displacement of normal hepatic vessels and ducts
  - May simulate normal liver, making detection difficult if there is no significant mass effect or bulge in liver contour
  - Central scar may be only clue: Hypoechoic or less commonly hyperechoic; may contain calcification
  - Prominent draining veins seen as hypoechoic "nodules" around lesion
  - Color Doppler may show large central feeding artery with multiple small vessels radiating peripherally, i.e., "spoke-wheel" pattern
  - High-velocity Doppler signal due to increased blood flow or arteriovenous shunts
  - When small (≤ 3 cm), focal nodular hyperplasia without scar may be indistinguishable from adenoma
- **Atypical Hemangioma**
  - Rare for hemangioma to be isoechoic
  - Echogenicity dependent on plane of scanning, direction, and angle of insonation: Presumably due to septal interfaces within hemangioma
  - Echogenicity of hemangioma may also be different at different times of scanning: Presumably due to change in flow within hemangioma
  - Posterior acoustic enhancement may be present
  - Color Doppler may show vessels in periphery of mass
  - No visible color Doppler flow in center of lesion (flow too slow to be detected)
  - Power Doppler (more sensitive to slow flow) may detect flow within lesion
  - Contrast-enhanced Doppler ultrasound or CT show these lesions better

ISOECHOIC LIVER MASS

- **Cholangiocarcinoma**
  - Intrahepatic duct dilatation without dilatation of common hepatic or common bile duct
  - Usually hyperechoic, but may be heterogeneous or isoechoic
  - Ill-defined mass with heterogeneous echopattern
  - Polypoidal isoechoic intraluminal mass within bile duct
  - Invasion of portal vein (much less common than hepatocellular carcinoma) or hepatic artery may be present
  - Absence of choledocholithiasis is important negative finding
- **Hepatic Adenoma**
  - Heterogeneity makes mass stand out (due to fat, hemorrhage, necrosis, or calcification)
  - Without hemorrhage or other signs, mass may appear identical to hepatic parenchyma
  - When large, hypoechoic halo of compressed liver tissue with multiple vessels may be present
  - Color Doppler may show intratumoral veins, which are absent in focal nodular hyperplasia (distinguishing feature)
- **Hepatic Lymphoma**
  - Diffuse or infiltrative form may show innumerable sub-centimeter hypoechoic foci, miliary in pattern and periportal in location
  - Infiltrative pattern may be indistinguishable from normal liver; many cases only diagnosed on autopsy
  - May have other signs of lymphoma
    - Splenomegaly, splenic lesions, lymphadenopathy, bowel wall thickening
- **Biliary Sludge**
  - Sludge in bile duct changes its normal hypoechoic appearance to isoechoic
  - Tracing along biliary tree helps to make diagnosis

Helpful Clues for Less Common Diagnoses
- **Hepatized Gallbladder**
  - Filled with sludge
  - Nonvisualization of gallbladder without history of cholecystectomy may be a clue
  - Color Doppler will show lack of vascularity in this "mass"
- **Abnormal Vessels**
  - Slow flow or thrombus in abnormal vessels may make them appear isoechoic
  - Color Doppler will show flow in abnormal vessels and allow characterization of lesion (arterial/venous)
  - Power Doppler is better at demonstrating slow flow
  - Pulsed Doppler used to differentiate systemic veins from portal veins and to characterize arterial resistance

Hepatocellular Carcinoma

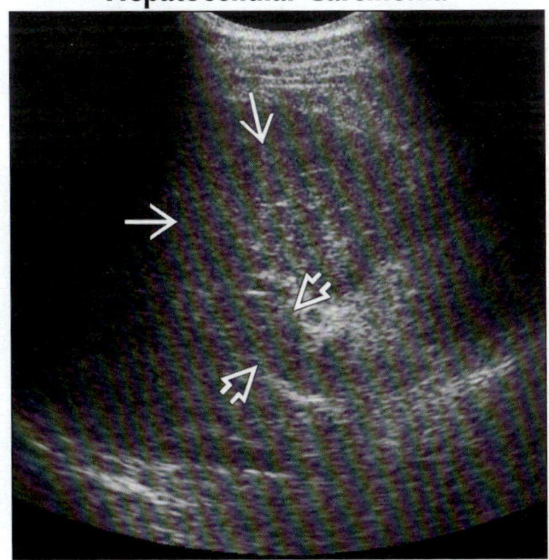

Oblique transabdominal ultrasound shows an isoechoic infiltrative hepatocellular carcinoma ➡, which is indistinguishable from the surrounding cirrhotic liver. The portal vein thrombus ⇛ suggests the diagnosis.

Hepatocellular Carcinoma

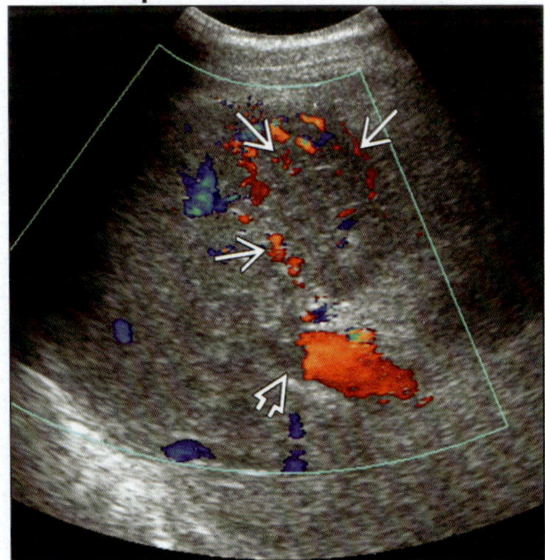

Oblique color Doppler ultrasound shows chaotic color flow ➡ within and around an isoechoic infiltrative hepatocellular carcinoma. Note the abrupt cessation of portal venous flow due to thrombus ⇛.

ISOECHOIC LIVER MASS

(Left) Oblique transabdominal ultrasound shows multiple, small, isoechoic metastases ➡, which are difficult to distinguish from the background hepatic parenchyma. (Right) Oblique transabdominal ultrasound shows a large isoechoic hematoma ➡ within a large hemorrhagic cyst ⇨ in the right lobe of the liver. The hematoma has retracted slightly, allowing some fluid ➡ to show the hematoma's separation from the wall of the cyst.

Hepatic Metastases

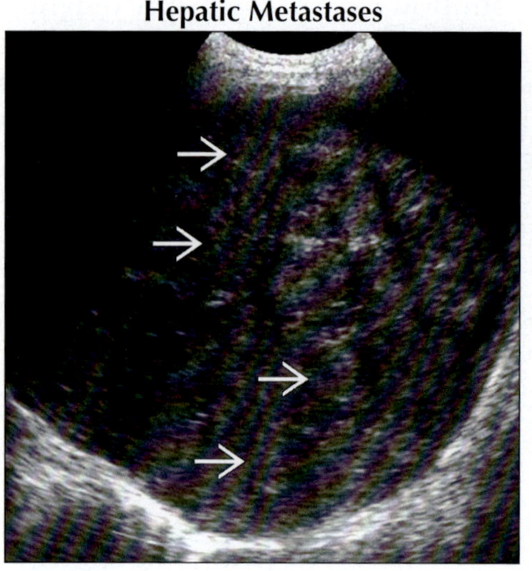

Hematoma

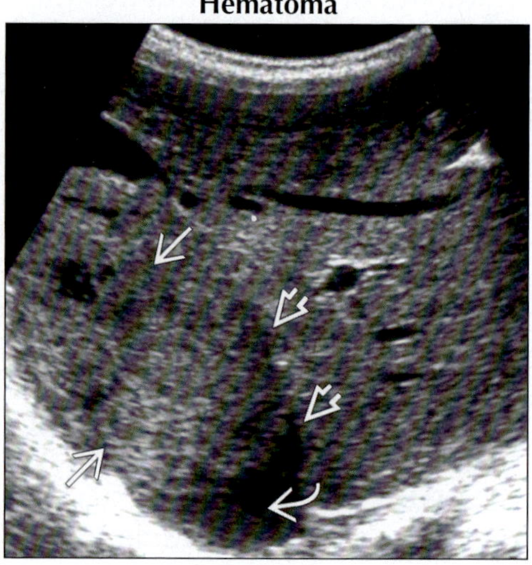

(Left) Longitudinal ultrasound shows an isoechoic focal nodular hyperplasia ➡ in the inferior edge of the right lobe of the liver, identified by its focal bulging appearance. There is a subtle central scar ⇨ in this mass. (Right) Correlative longitudinal power Doppler ultrasound in the same patient shows the feeding artery ➡ within the central scar of focal nodular hyperplasia ➡, with vessels emanating from it in a centripetal fashion ➡.

Focal Nodular Hyperplasia

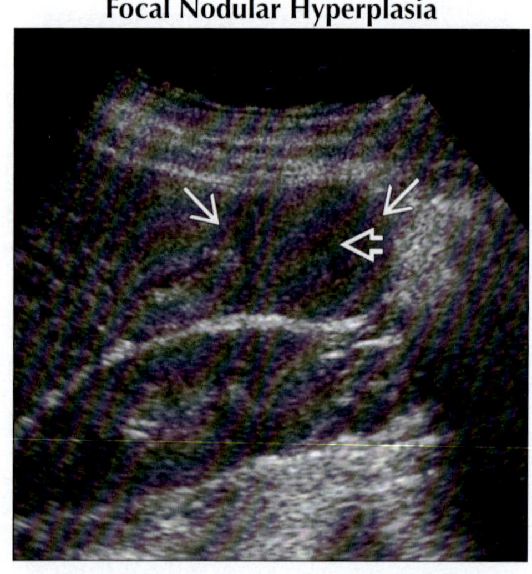

Focal Nodular Hyperplasia

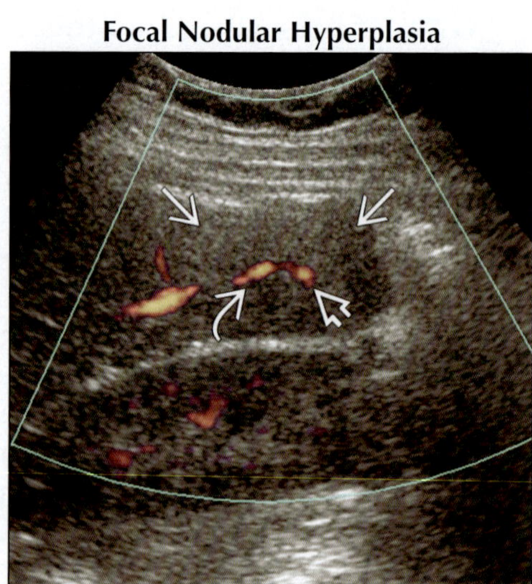

(Left) Transverse US shows 2 atypical isoechoic hemangiomas ➡ in the left lobe of the liver, which blend almost imperceptively with surrounding parenchyma. Typical hemangiomas are hyperechoic and easy to detect. (Right) Axial CECT in the same patient shows the 2 hemangiomas ➡ in the left lobe of the liver. Note the nodular contrast enhancement of both lesions during the portal venous phase. Contrast US (not shown) appeared similar.

Atypical Hemangioma

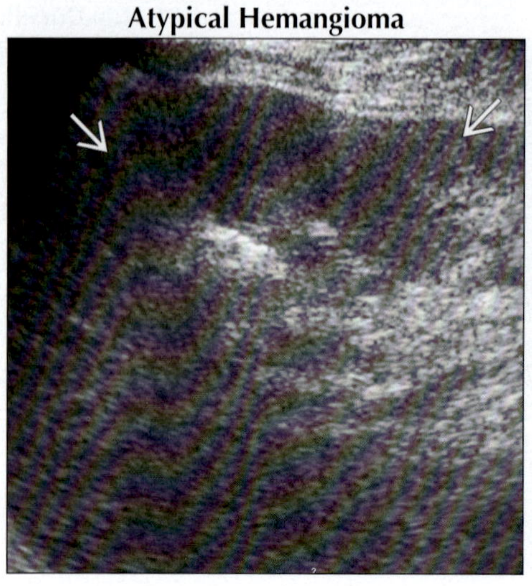

Atypical Hemangioma

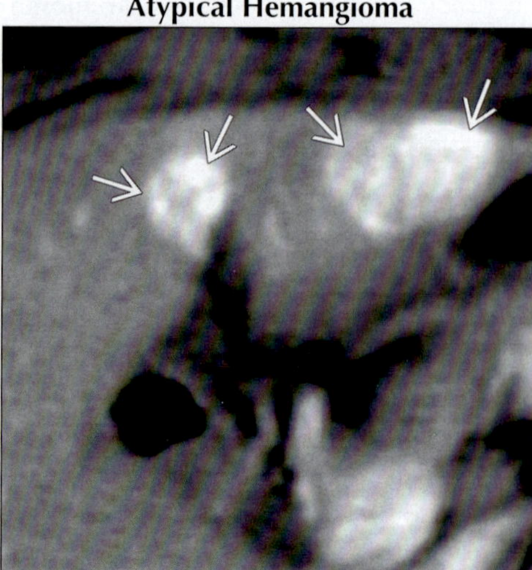

3

ISOECHOIC LIVER MASS

Cholangiocarcinoma

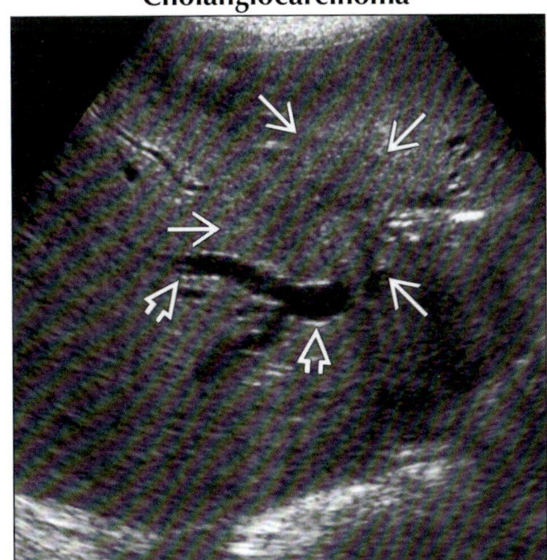

Hepatic Adenoma

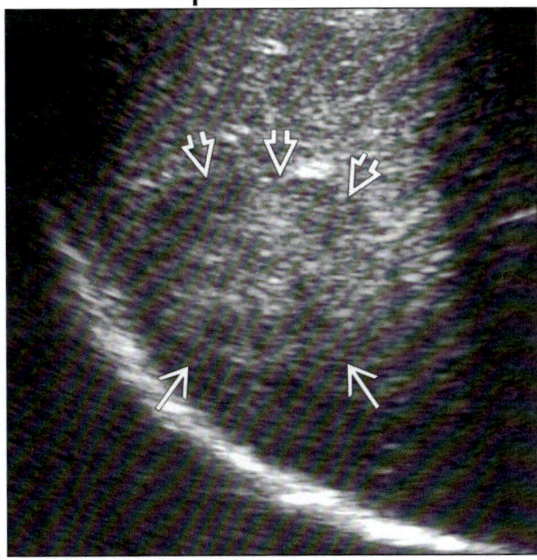

(Left) Oblique ultrasound shows an ill-defined, isoechoic cholangiocarcinoma ➡ at the porta hepatis. The mass is causing associated right intrahepatic ductal dilatation ➡. *(Right)* Oblique ultrasound shows an isoechoic adenoma ➡ in the right lobe of the liver, adjacent to the diaphragm. There is an incomplete hypoechoic halo of compressed liver tissue and veins ➡, distinguishing part of the lesion from the rest of the liver.

Biliary Sludge

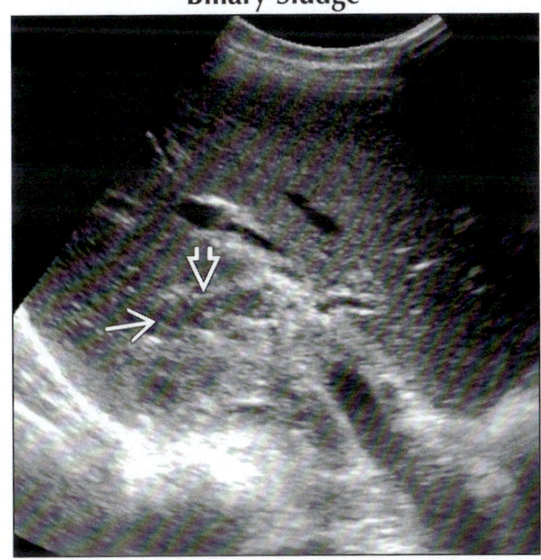

Hepatized Gallbladder

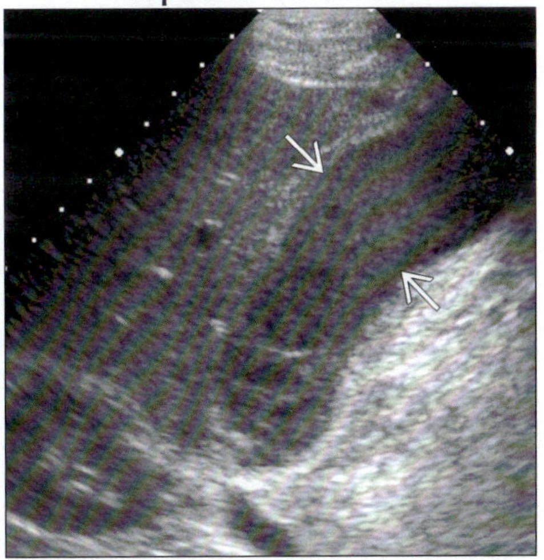

(Left) Oblique ultrasound shows isoechoic sludge ➡ within a dilated intrahepatic duct ➡. Biliary sludge is often isoechoic to liver parenchyma. The wall of the bile duct provides a clue to the diagnosis. A thrombosed vein looks similar but may show some color Doppler signal. *(Right)* Transverse ultrasound of a patient in the intensive care unit shows a gallbladder ➡ completely filled with sludge. Note the echogenicity is very similar to the adjacent liver.

Abnormal Vessels

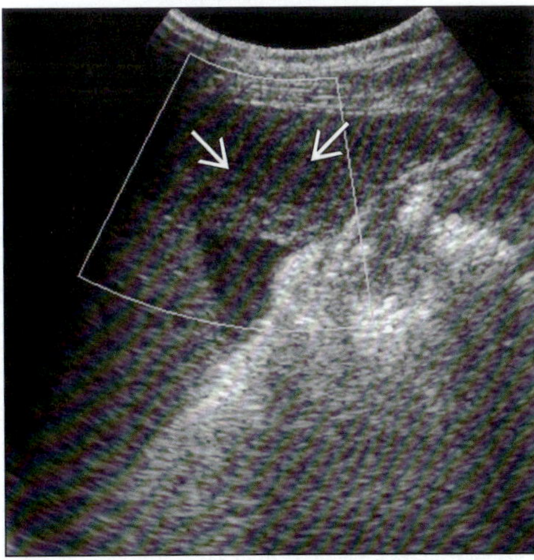

Abnormal Vessels

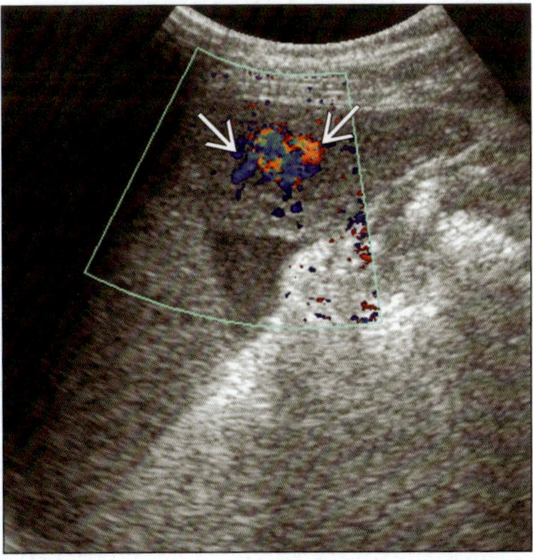

(Left) Transverse transabdominal ultrasound shows an isoechoic vascular malformation ➡ in the left lobe of the liver, which is difficult to distinguish from the normal hepatic parenchyma. *(Right)* Correlative transverse color Doppler ultrasound in the same patient shows color filling of the vascular malformation ➡. The color flow is chaotic, suggesting fast and turbulent flow, which in turn suggests an arteriovenous malformation.

DIFFERENTIAL DIAGNOSIS

Common
- Focal Steatosis
- Calcified Granuloma
- Hepatic Cavernous Hemangioma
- Hepatic Metastases
- Pneumobilia
- Intrahepatic Biliary Calculi
- Pyogenic Hepatic Abscess
- Surgical Devices
- Portal Vein Gas
- Normal Anatomic Pitfalls
  - Hepatic Ligaments and Fissures
  - Diaphragmatic Leaflets
  - Refractile Artifact

Less Common
- Hepatocellular Carcinoma (HCC)
- Fibrolamellar Carcinoma
- Cholangiocarcinoma
- Hepatic Adenoma
- Amebic Hepatic Abscess
- Hepatic Hydatid Cyst
- Hepatic Infarction
- Biliary Hamartoma
- Hemangioendothelioma
- Hepatic Angiomyolipoma
- Postoperative State
- Hepatic Trauma

ESSENTIAL INFORMATION

Key Differential Diagnosis Issues
- Is echogenic lesion a mass (usually spherical) vs. echogenic focus (often linear such as TIPS shunt or gas in bile ducts)?
- Significant overlap in many of these entities
  - CT and MR may be needed for further evaluation of echogenic masses

Helpful Clues for Common Diagnoses
- **Focal Steatosis**
  - Typically caudate, right lobe, perihilar region
  - No mass effect, with vessels running undisplaced through lesion
  - Varied appearances
    - Hyperechoic nodule/confluent hyperechoic lesions (may simulate metastases)
    - Fan-shaped lobar/segmental distribution
  - CT or MR are good problem-solving tools

- **Calcified Granuloma**
  - Histoplasmosis, TB, etc.; usually small (few mm) and multiple
  - Spleen also usually involved
- **Hepatic Cavernous Hemangioma**
  - > 2/3 are hyperechoic
    - Large lesions more heterogeneous
  - May have acoustic enhancement (due to fluid content)
- **Hepatic Metastases**
  - Hyperechoic metastases most commonly from GI tract (especially colon)
    - Others include vascular metastases from neuroendocrine tumors, melanoma, choriocarcinoma, renal cell carcinoma
  - "Target" metastases or "bull's eye" in aggressive primary tumors
    - Bronchogenic carcinoma classic example
- **Pneumobilia**
  - Echogenic shadowing foci in center of liver (biliary gas flows toward porta hepatis)
- **Intrahepatic Biliary Calculi**
  - Majority appear as highly echogenic foci with posterior acoustic shadowing
  - May have associated dilated ducts
- **Pyogenic Hepatic Abscess**
  - Gas within abscess may be echogenic
  - Most pyogenic abscesses are hypoechoic
- **Surgical Devices**
  - Clips, drains, shunts, catheters
  - Scan in multiple planes to appreciate linear shape
- **Portal Vein Gas**
  - Echogenic shadowing foci in periphery of liver; portovenous gas flows away from porta hepatis (vs. biliary gas)
  - Very obvious on real-time imaging
- **Normal Anatomic Pitfalls**
  - **Hepatic Ligaments and Fissures, Diaphragmatic Leaflets**
    - Infolding of fat along these normal structures creates echogenic focus near surface of liver
    - In short axis section, "lesions" can appear spherical and resemble masses
    - Turn US beam perpendicular to show linear shape of "lesion"
  - **Refractile Artifact**
    - At junction of vessels & gallbladder neck

Helpful Clues for Less Common Diagnoses
- **Hepatocellular Carcinoma (HCC)**

○ Small lesion more likely to be hyperechoic
○ May simulate hemangioma or focal steatosis
  ▪ Look for background cirrhotic liver, portal vein thrombosis
  ▪ Generally irregular intratumoral hypervascularity
- **Fibrolamellar Carcinoma**
  ○ Large heterogeneous mass in adolescent or young adult
  ○ Look for central scar (may be hypo- or hyperechoic)
- **Cholangiocarcinoma**
  ○ Mass with ill-defined margin, mostly hyperechoic (75%) and heterogeneous
  ○ Causes proximal bile duct obstruction
- **Hepatic Adenoma**
  ○ Hypervascular mass ± hemorrhage in young woman on birth-control pills
- **Amebic Hepatic Abscess**
  ○ Usually homogeneous and hypoechoic
  ○ Hyperechoic if complicated by bacterial superinfection or fistula to bowel
- **Hepatic Hydatid Cyst**
  ○ Often cystic-appearing but may see hyperechoic areas
    ▪ "Hydatid sand," parenchymal invasion, calcified rim
- **Biliary Hamartoma**
  ○ Heterogeneous, hyperechoic foci on US
  ○ Better evaluated on CT/MR (multiple, predominately cystic, < 15 mm)
- **Hemangioendothelioma**

○ Infantile type: Well-defined large hypervascular mass
○ Epithelioid (adult) type: Multiple peripheral confluent masses
- **Hepatic Angiomyolipoma**
  ○ Variable echogenicity, CT/MR better for showing fat
- **Postoperative State**
  ○ Any procedure that introduces fat or gas into liver can create echogenic, shadowing lesion

Alternative Differential Approaches
- Vascular masses
  ○ Cavernous hemangioma, HCC, hemangioendothelioma
- Fat-containing masses
  ○ Focal fatty infiltration, hepatic adenoma, HCC, lipid-containing metastases, angiomyolipoma, liposarcoma, teratoma (primary or metastatic to liver)
- Gas-containing masses
  ○ Abscess, infarction, treated hepatic tumors with resulting sudden necrosis
- Solid masses
  ○ Primary liver tumors, metastases, cholangiocarcinoma
- Masses with calcified rim
  ○ Chronic cystic masses
- Masses with calcified scar
  ○ Fibrolamellar, HCC, cavernous hemangioma (large ones)

Focal Steatosis

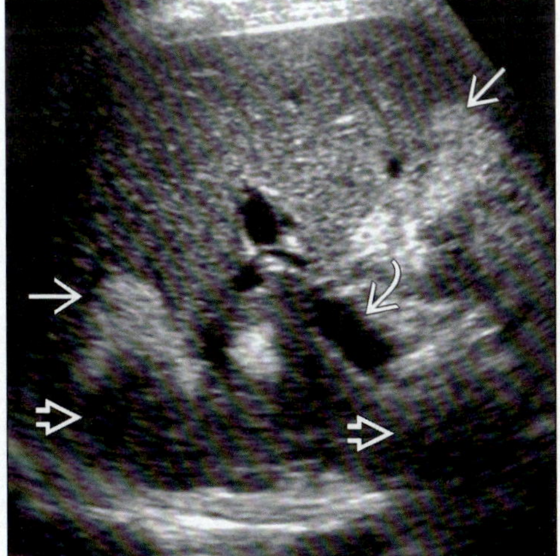

Transverse transabdominal ultrasound shows multiple hyperechoic areas ➡ with posterior acoustic attenuation ➡. Note the lack of mass effect on the hepatic vessels ➡.

Calcified Granuloma

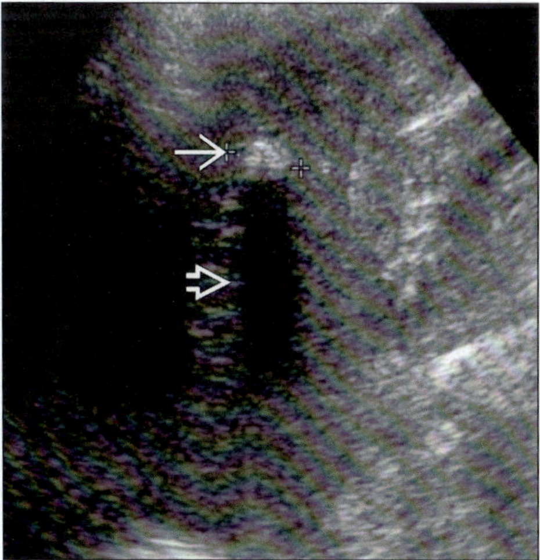

Transverse transabdominal ultrasound shows a coarsely calcified liver granuloma ➡ with posterior acoustic shadowing ➡. Note the amorphous nature of the calcification.

ECHOGENIC LIVER MASS

(Left) *Oblique US shows multiple echogenic metastases* ➡️ *from a colonic primary. Other hyperechoic metastases include neuroendocrine tumor, choriocarcinoma, and melanoma. (Right) Longitudinal transabdominal ultrasound shows "target" lesions in the liver representing metastases from lung carcinoma. The center* ➡️ *is hyperechoic with a thick hypoechoic rim* ➡️.

Hepatic Metastases

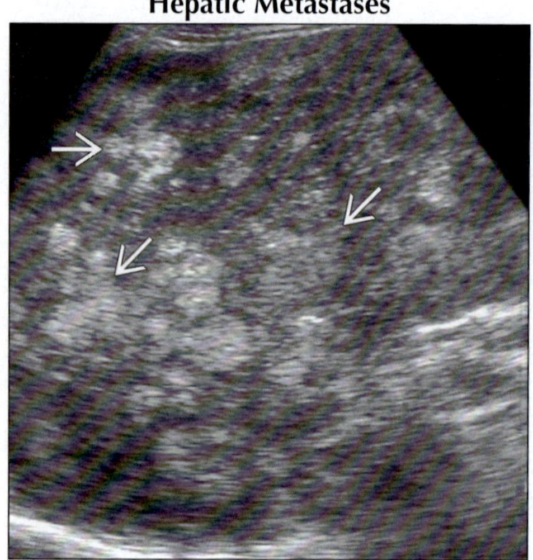

Hepatic Metastases

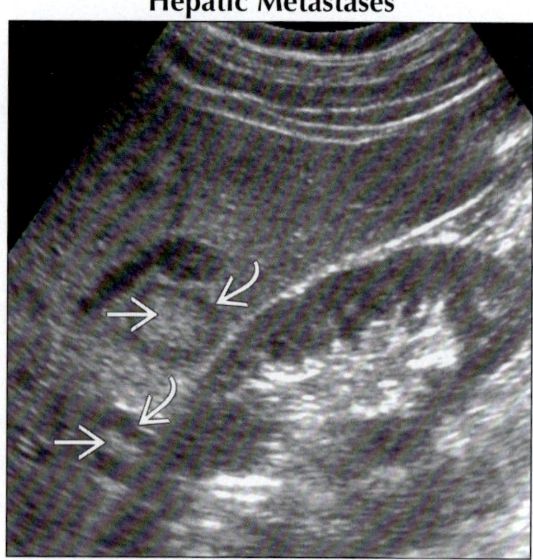

(Left) *Oblique transabdominal ultrasound shows a markedly dilated intrahepatic duct* ➡️ *containing gas* ➡️ *in a patient with Caroli disease. Note the echogenic linear reverberation artifact* ➡️ *posterior to the gas. (Right) Longitudinal transabdominal ultrasound shows linear hyperechoic structures* ➡️ *that indicate pneumobilia in the intrahepatic ducts. Note the associated reverberation artifact* ➡️.

Pneumobilia

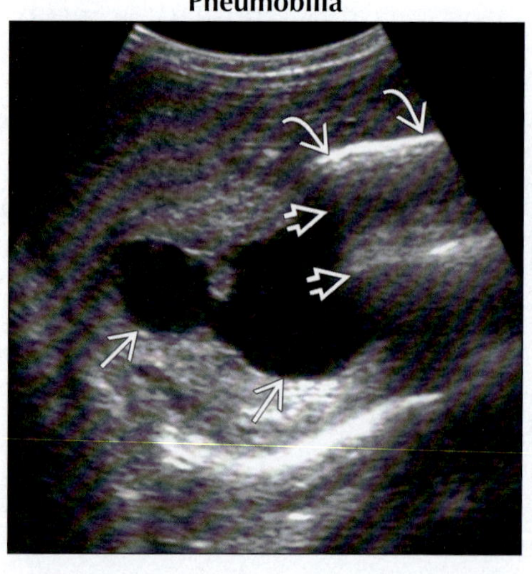

Pneumobilia

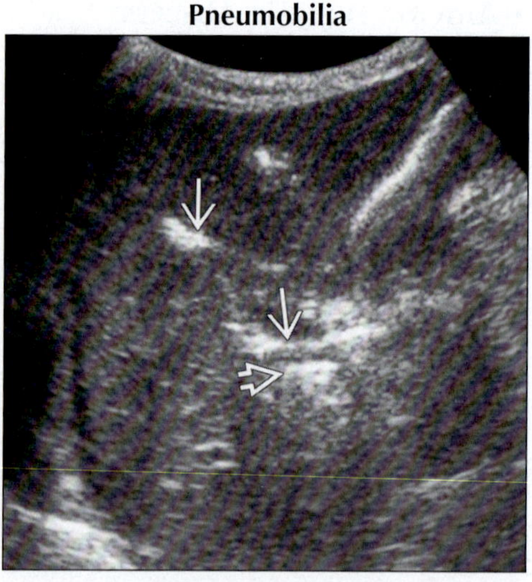

(Left) *Oblique US shows 2 hemangiomas* ➡️ *seen as well-defined, homogeneous, hyperechoic, rounded lesions. The appearance is typical (seen in 2/3 of hemangiomas) but is nonspecific. Follow-up is usually required. (Right) Oblique transabdominal ultrasound shows multiple, intrahepatic, biliary calculi in a patient with recurrent pyogenic cholangitis. The echogenic stones* ➡️ *show acoustic shadowing* ➡️. *Also note the pneumobilia* ➡️ *in the intrahepatic duct.*

Hepatic Cavernous Hemangioma

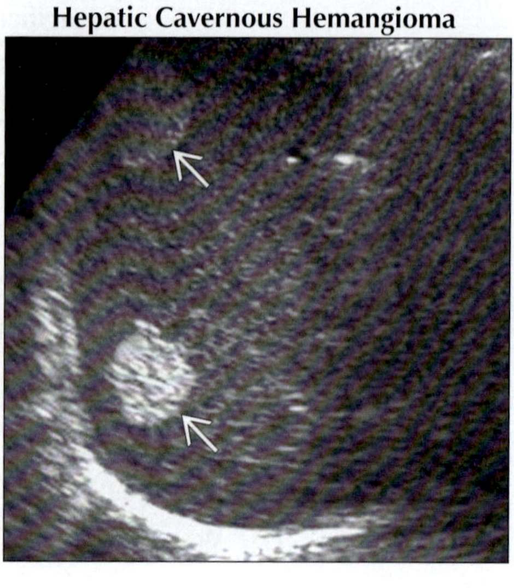

Intrahepatic Biliary Calculi

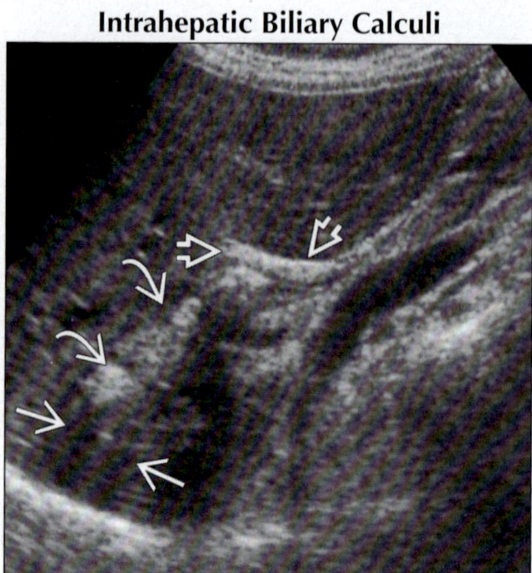

ECHOGENIC LIVER MASS

Pyogenic Hepatic Abscess

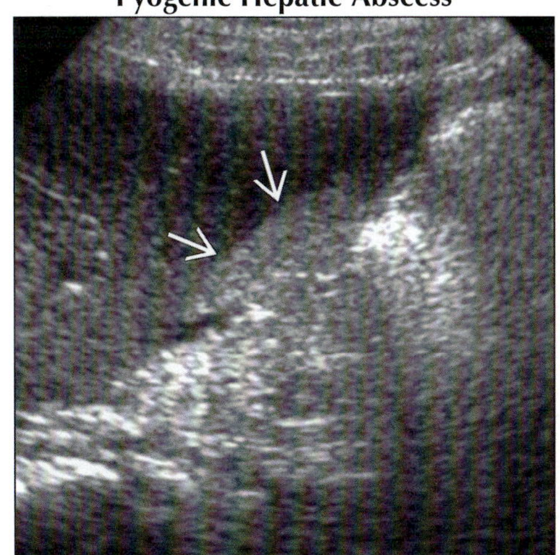

Portal Vein Gas

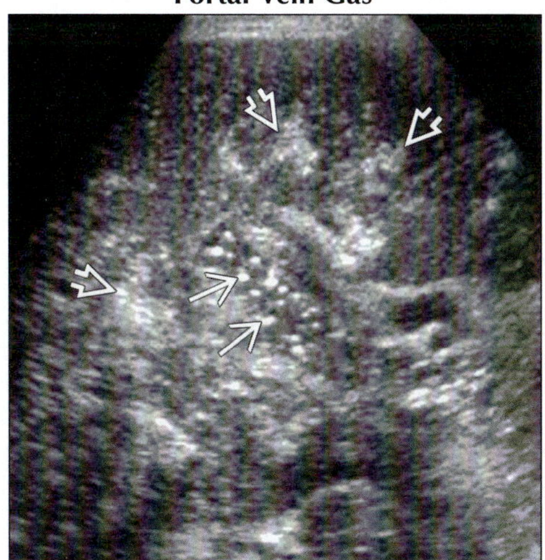

(Left) Oblique transabdominal ultrasound shows a hyperechoic perihepatic abscess ➡ indenting the surface of the liver and simulating an intrahepatic mass. (Right) Oblique transabdominal ultrasound shows tiny echogenic foci of gas ➡ within the portal vein. There are also echogenic patches of parenchymal gas ➡.

Hepatic Ligaments and Fissures

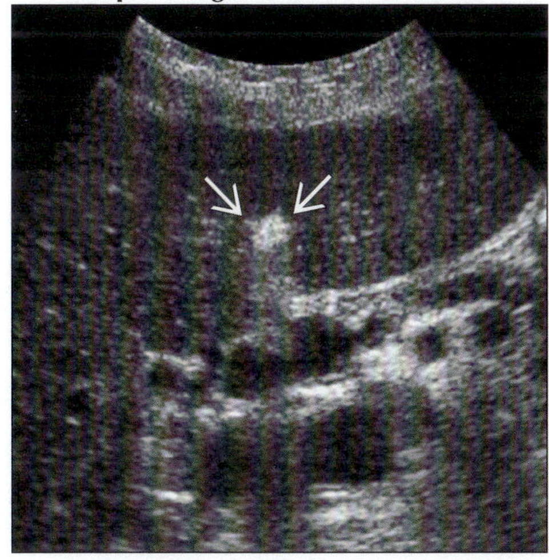

Hepatic Ligaments and Fissures

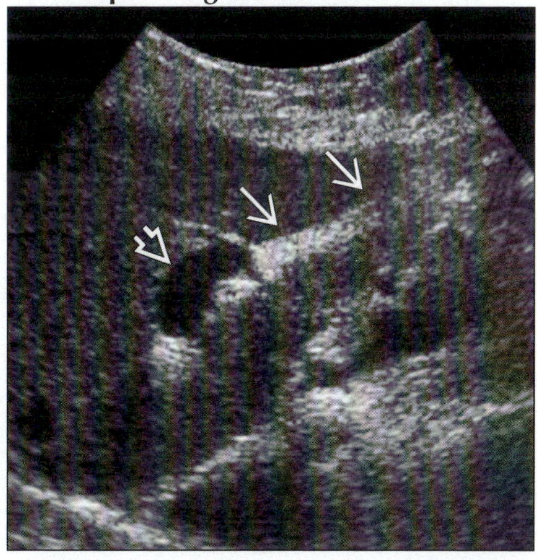

(Left) Transverse transabdominal ultrasound shows a cross section of the ligamentum teres ➡, which appears as a round echogenic focus in the left lobe of the liver. Its echogenicity increases with age. It may mimic a focal echogenic hepatic tumor. (Right) Longitudinal ultrasound in the same patient shows the ligamentum teres lengthwise ➡, confirming that it is not a mass. It runs from the left portal vein ➡ to the inferior tip of the left lobe.

Diaphragmatic Leaflets

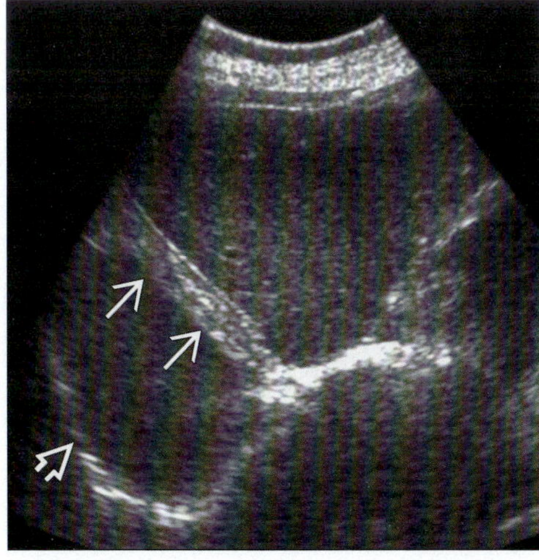

Hepatocellular Carcinoma (HCC)

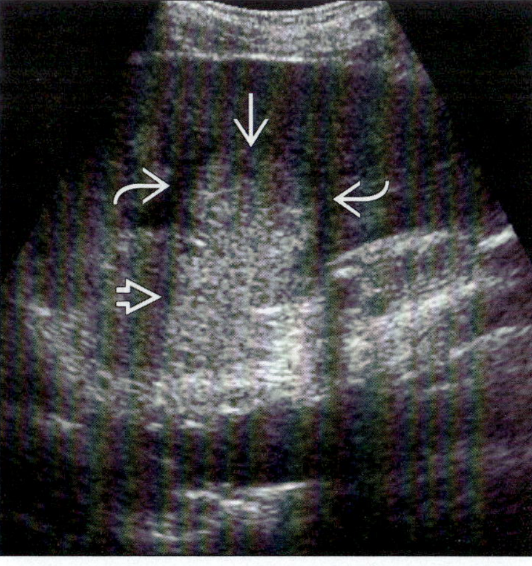

(Left) Oblique US shows a tubular, echogenic, diaphragmatic leaflet ➡. This is seen when the transducer is angled cephalad towards the diaphragm ➡. (Right) Oblique US shows a small hyperechoic HCC ➡. Small HCCs have a homogeneous echopattern. There is even posterior enhancement ➡ in this case, making differentiation from a hemangioma difficult. Note the thin hypoechoic halo ➡, which is generally not seen in hemangiomas.

ECHOGENIC LIVER MASS

Hepatocellular Carcinoma (HCC)

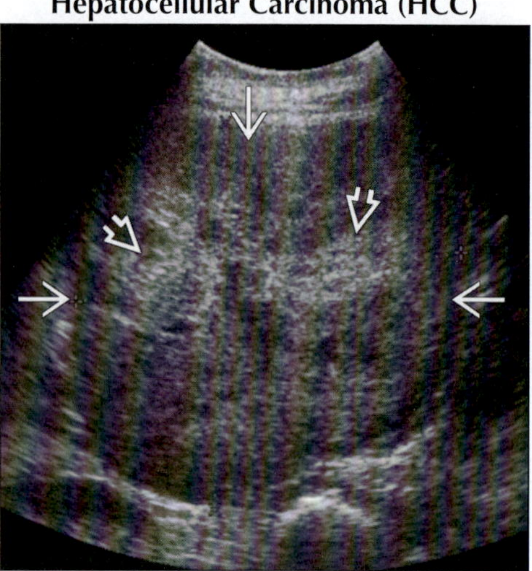

Fibrolamellar Carcinoma

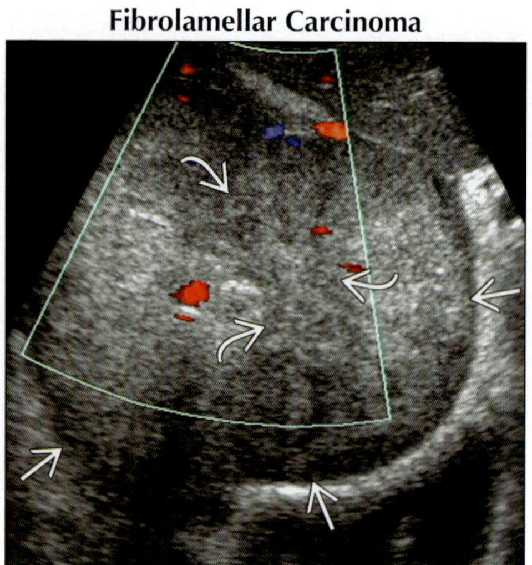

(Left) Transverse ultrasound shows the heterogeneous echopattern of a large hepatocellular carcinoma ➜ with hyperechoic areas ➛.
(Right) Oblique color Doppler US shows a large echogenic mass ➜ representing a fibrolamellar hepatocellular carcinoma. Note the central hypoechoic scar ➜, which is typically seen in fibrolamellar HCC but not specific to it.

Cholangiocarcinoma

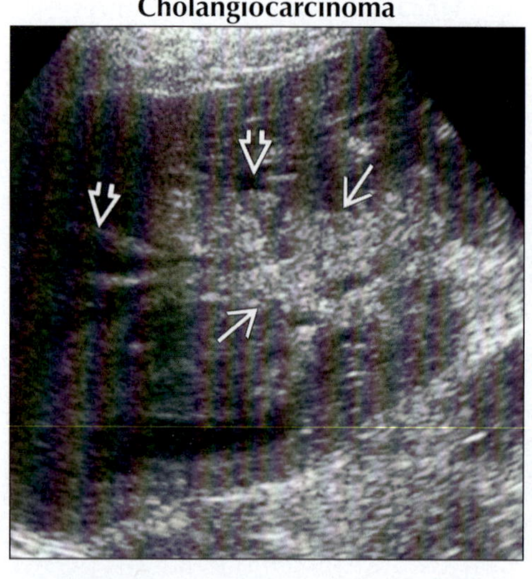

Amebic Hepatic Abscess

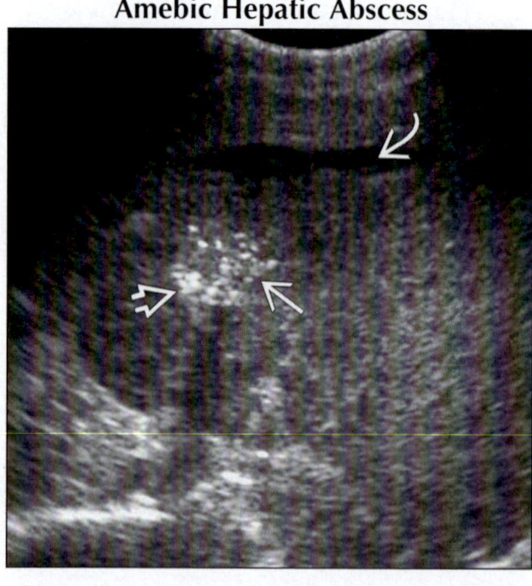

(Left) Oblique transabdominal ultrasound shows an echogenic Klatskin tumor ➜ causing intrahepatic biliary duct obstruction in both lobes of the liver. Note the enlarged intrahepatic ducts ➛.
(Right) Oblique transabdominal ultrasound shows a ruptured amebic abscess ➜, which has fistulized with the colon. Note the hyperechoic gas locules ➛ within the abscess and the small amount of ascites ➜.

Hepatic Hydatid Cyst

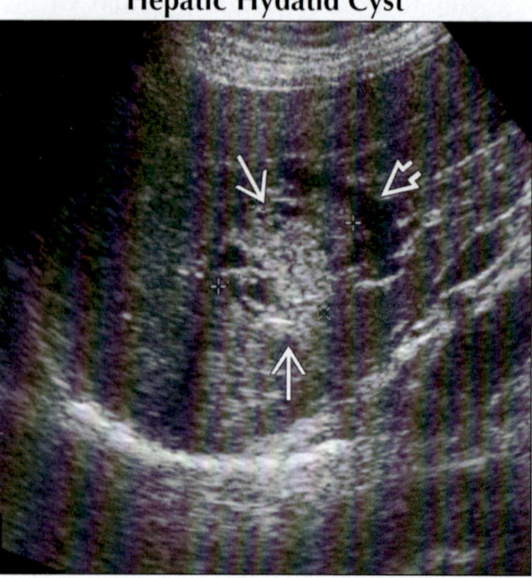

Hepatic Hydatid Cyst

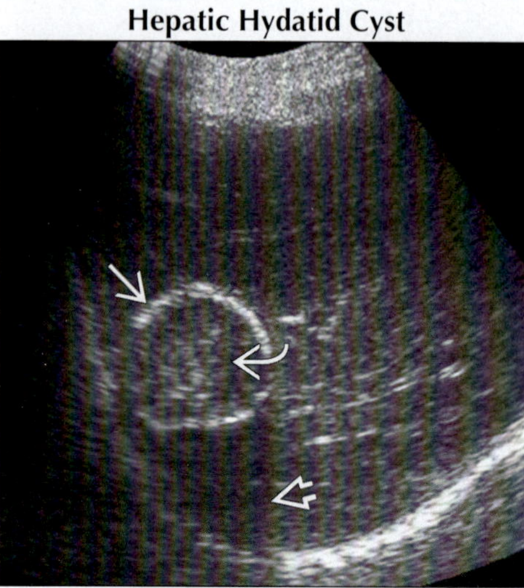

(Left) Oblique transabdominal ultrasound shows a ruptured hepatic echinococcal cyst ➛. There is echogenic "hydatid sand" ➜ within and around the cyst. (Right) Oblique transabdominal ultrasound shows the echogenic calcified wall ➜ of a hydatid cyst of the liver with posterior acoustic shadowing ➛. Note the echogenic content ➜, representing "hydatid sand."

ECHOGENIC LIVER MASS

Hepatic Angiomyolipoma

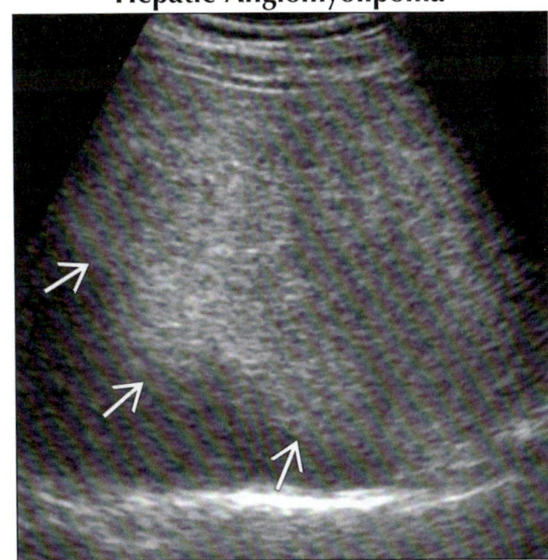

Hepatic Trauma

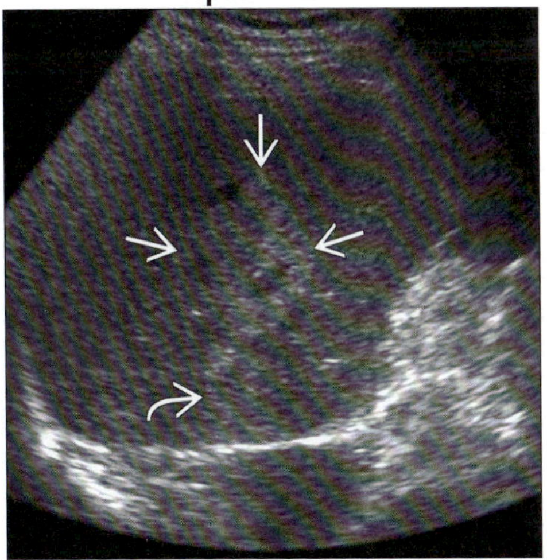

(Left) Oblique transabdominal ultrasound shows a large hepatic angiomyolipoma, which is hyperechoic and shows lobulated geographic borders ➡. (Right) Oblique ultrasound shows a hyperechoic area of hemorrhage ➡ after hepatic trauma. The hematoma extends to the posterior surface of the liver ➡, demonstrating the tract of laceration.

Hemangioendothelioma

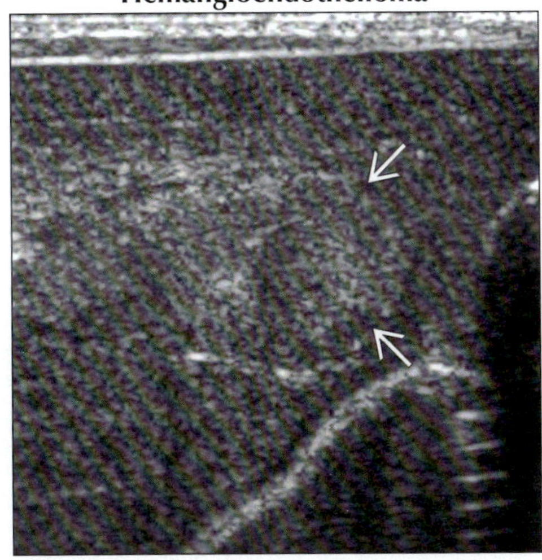

Hemangioendothelioma

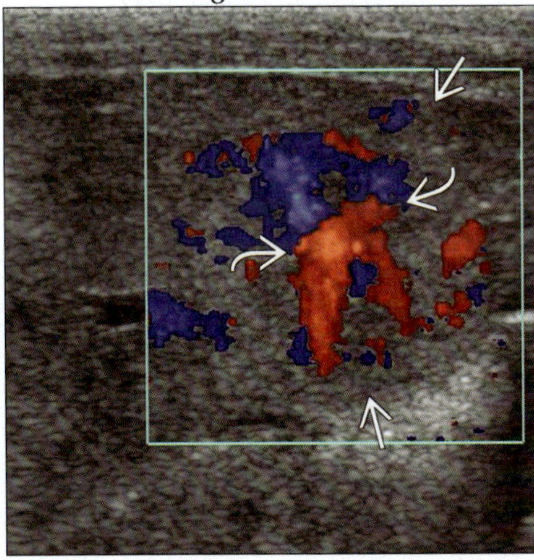

(Left) Oblique transabdominal ultrasound shows an infantile hemangioendothelioma as a moderate-sized, mildly hyperechoic, homogeneous mass ➡. (Right) Oblique color Doppler ultrasound shows vascularity within the same infantile hemangioendothelioma ➡. Note the large cavernous vascular channels ➡ filled by color flow. This is due to significant arteriovenous shunting.

Postoperative State

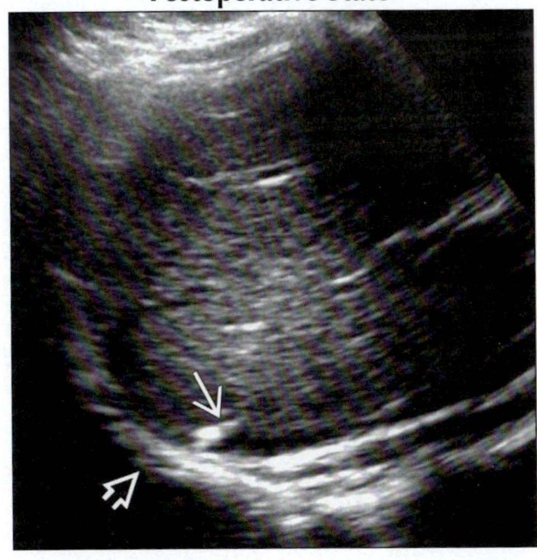

Postoperative State

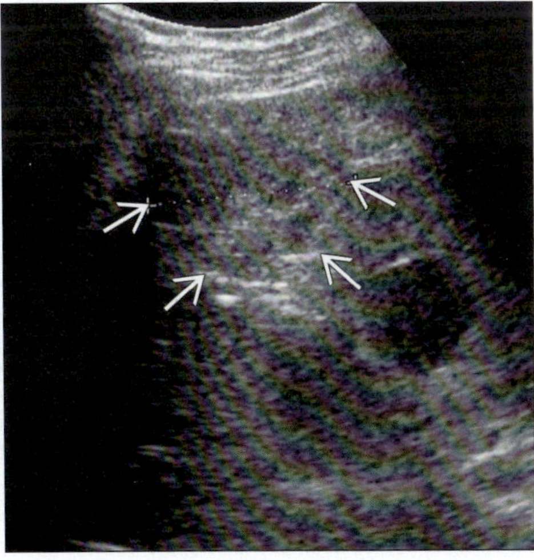

(Left) Oblique transabdominal ultrasound shows an echogenic surgical clip ➡ near the dome of the diaphragm ➡ in the right lobe of the liver. (Right) Oblique ultrasound shows the postsurgical appearance of the liver after subsegmental resection for hepatocellular carcinoma. The resected area is packed with fat ➡, giving it a heterogeneous echogenic appearance.

3

DIFFERENTIAL DIAGNOSIS

Common
- Hepatic Metastases
- Hepatocellular Carcinoma (HCC)
- Hepatic Lymphoma
- Hepatic Adenoma
- Fungal Hepatic Abscess
- Amebic Hepatic Abscess
- Pyogenic Hepatic Abscess

Less Common
- Hepatic Atypical Hemangioma
- Hepatic Hematoma

Rare but Important
- Sarcoidosis
- Kaposi Sarcoma
- Candidiasis

ESSENTIAL INFORMATION

Key Differential Diagnosis Issues
- Also known as "bull's-eye" lesions
- Malignancy far outnumbers other causes

Helpful Clues for Common Diagnoses
- **Hepatic Metastases**
  - Usually from aggressive primary tumor, e.g., bronchogenic carcinoma
  - Solid central tumor with hypoechoic halo or necrotic center with viable surrounding wall of tumor
- **Hepatocellular Carcinoma (HCC)**
  - Background of cirrhosis, portal hypertension, ascites
  - Rare for cirrhotic livers to develop metastases from nonhepatic primary
    - Any mass in a cirrhotic liver is more likely HCC than metastasis
- **Hepatic Lymphoma**
  - Vast majority uniformly hypoechoic
  - Splenomegaly or splenic lesions, lymphadenopathy, thickened bowel wall provide clues toward diagnosis
- **Hepatic Adenoma**
  - Usually isoechoic or slightly hypoechoic
  - Complications such as hemorrhage, central necrosis make center echogenic
  - Occasional hypoechoic rim to form target-like lesion
- **Fungal Hepatic Abscess**
  - Often multiple lesions
  - Typically in immunocompromised patient
- **Amebic Hepatic Abscess**
  - Iso- to mildly hyperechoic center with hypoechoic halo
  - Abuts liver capsule
- **Pyogenic Hepatic Abscess**
  - Central hyperechoic inflammatory nodule surrounded by hypoechoic halo of fibrosis
  - Lobulated or irregular contour

Helpful Clues for Less Common Diagnoses
- **Hepatic Atypical Hemangioma**
  - Power Doppler may show slow flow in center of hemangioma
- **Hepatic Hematoma**
  - May have laceration tract leading to hepatic surface, other organs involved

Hepatic Metastases

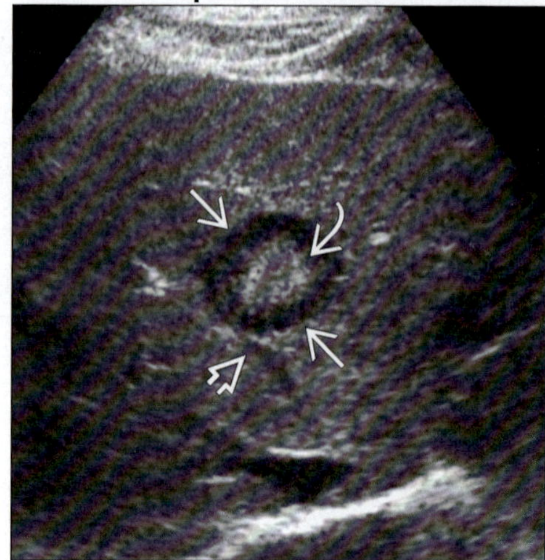

Transverse transabdominal ultrasound shows a target lesion representing a metastasis. The echogenic core ➡ is surrounded by a thick hypoechoic rim ➡. The middle hepatic vein ➡ is mildly displaced by the mass.

Hepatocellular Carcinoma (HCC)

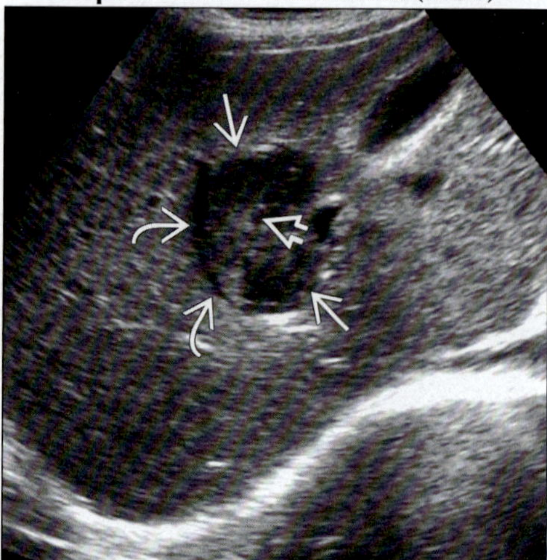

Transverse transabdominal ultrasound shows a hypoechoic HCC ➡ in the right anterior segment, displacing the adjacent vessel ➡. It has a mildly echogenic center ➡, producing a target appearance.

TARGET LESIONS IN LIVER

Hepatic Lymphoma

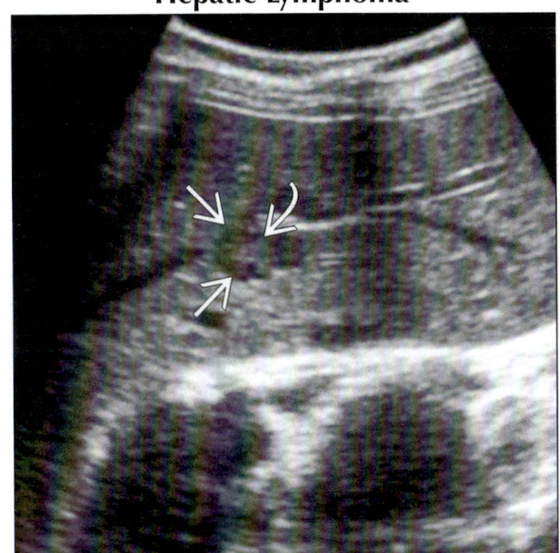

Hepatic Adenoma

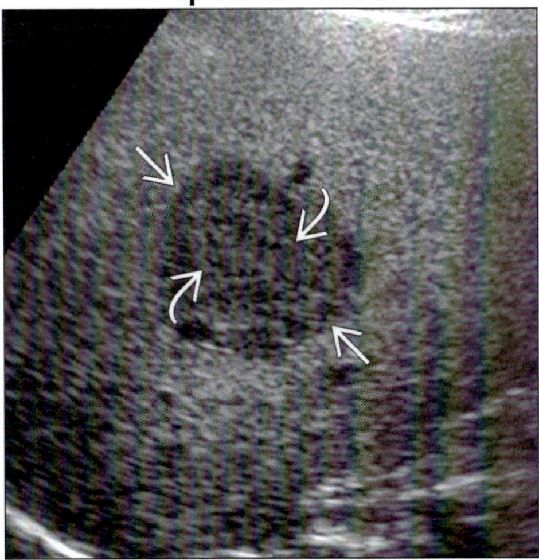

(Left) Oblique transabdominal ultrasound shows a small, hypoechoic, periportal, lymphomatous deposit. Note the slightly hyperechoic core ➡ surrounded by the hypoechoic rim ➡, giving it a target appearance. *(Right)* Oblique transabdominal ultrasound shows a hepatic adenoma ➡ with a slightly hyperechoic center ➡.

Amebic Hepatic Abscess

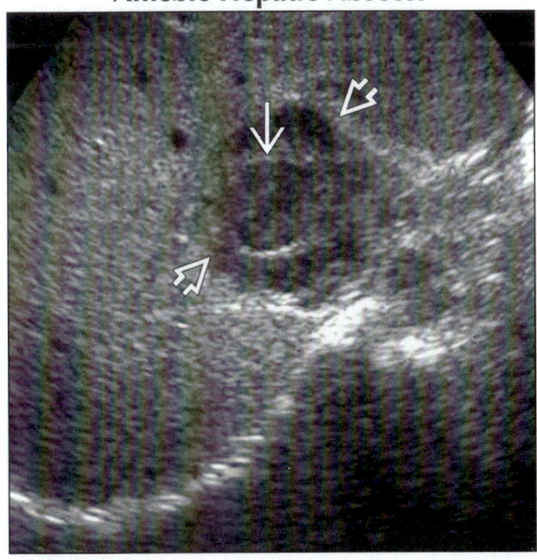

Pyogenic Hepatic Abscess

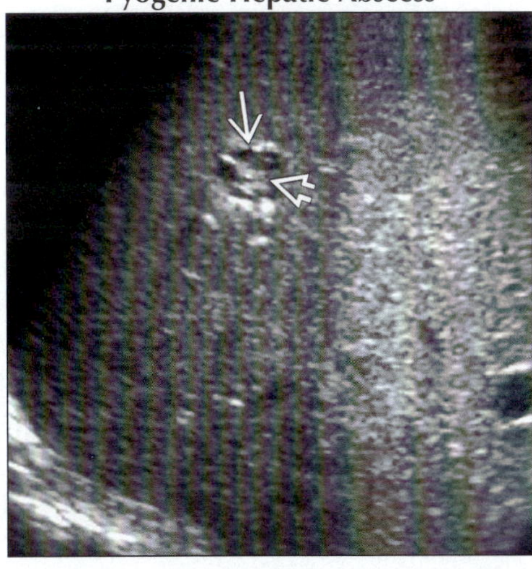

(Left) Transverse transabdominal ultrasound shows a round, hypoechoic, amebic abscess ➡ abutting the posterior hepatic surface. Note the low-level internal echoes and septum ➡, which gives it a target appearance. *(Right)* Oblique transabdominal ultrasound shows a pyogenic microabscess ➡ with a central echogenic core ➡ surrounded by fibrosis, giving it a target appearance.

Hepatic Atypical Hemangioma

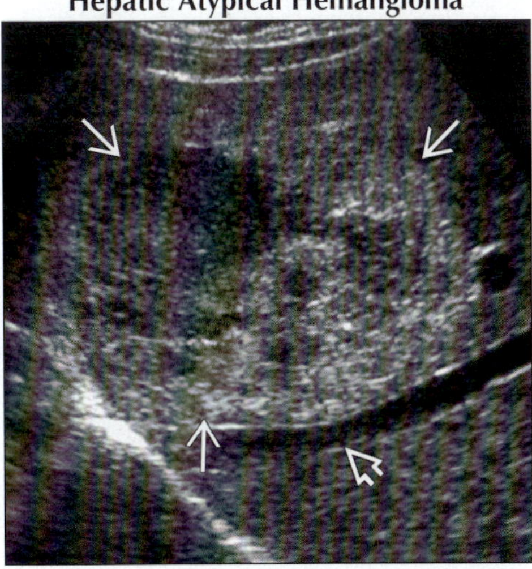

Hepatic Hematoma

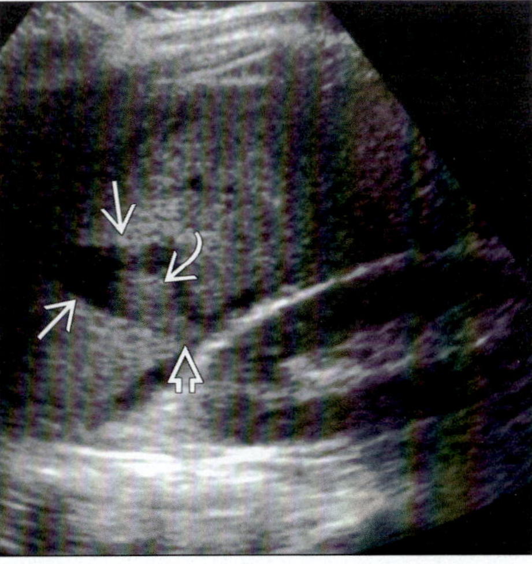

(Left) Oblique transabdominal US shows an atypical hemangioma ➡ with both hyperechoic and hypoechoic components, which gives the appearance of multiple target lesions. The adjacent vessel ➡ is mildly displaced. *(Right)* Oblique transabdominal US shows an acute hematoma ➡ with a tract extending posteriorly to the liver capsule ➡. Note the echogenic contracting clot ➡. This is a typical configuration for a hepatic laceration.

IRREGULAR BORDER LIVER MASS

DIFFERENTIAL DIAGNOSIS

Common
- Hepatic Metastases
- Hepatocellular Carcinoma
- Cholangiocarcinoma
- Hepatic Cyst
- Focal Fatty Replacement/Sparing
- Pyogenic Hepatic Abscess
- Subphrenic Abscess
- Postsurgical Change

Less Common
- Atypical Hemangioma
- Hematoma
- Echinococcus Cyst
- Lymphoma

ESSENTIAL INFORMATION

Helpful Clues for Common Diagnoses
- **Hepatic Metastases**
  - Mimic nodular or multifocal hepatocellular carcinoma (HCC)
  - Infiltrative border by single lesion or irregular border by multiple diffuse metastases
  - Common primary lesions with this pattern: Lung and breast
  - Lower incidence in cirrhotic livers
    - Irregular border mass in cirrhotic liver is more likely to be HCC than metastasis
  - Much less likely to invade portal veins (compared to HCC)
  - Color Doppler shows no significant vascularity
    - Most metastases are hypovascular, except those from neuroendocrine tumors
    - Contrast-enhanced US increases detectability of hepatic metastases
- **Hepatocellular Carcinoma**
  - Background changes of cirrhosis and portal hypertension: Ascites, splenomegaly, portosystemic collaterals
  - Irregular borders usually in larger lesions
  - Large masses tend to be heterogeneous, indicating tumor necrosis/fibrosis
  - Heterogeneous mass with irregular borders blending with background cirrhosis may make detection difficult
  - Calcification is rare unless the HCC is treated
    - Portal vein invasion is strongly suggestive of HCC
    - Hepatic vein is less commonly invaded
    - Color Doppler shows irregular hypervascularity within tumor
    - Portal venous thrombus may show vascularity (tumor thrombus)
    - Pulsed Doppler of tumor mass shows high velocity (arterial type) flow and low resistance (tumor vessels)
- **Cholangiocarcinoma**
  - Intrahepatic duct dilatation without common bile duct dilatation
  - Mass with ill-defined margins, ± hepatic parenchymal infiltration
  - Mostly hyperechoic (75%)
  - Heterogeneous architecture
  - May cause capsular retraction and local hepatic volume loss
  - Less likely to invade portal vein than hepatocellular carcinoma
  - Enlarged lymph nodes in cystic duct, porta hepatis, periceliac groups
- **Hepatic Cyst**
  - Uncomplicated simple cysts may be lobulated, posterior acoustic enhancement
  - Cysts in polycystic liver disease are more irregular in shape, especially when they get bigger
  - Complicated cysts (hemorrhagic or infected) may have thickened and irregular walls
  - May appear solid if there is internal debris dispersed within cyst
  - Color Doppler shows no vascularity in uncomplicated or complicated cysts
- **Focal Fatty Replacement/Sparing**
  - Focal fatty sparing: Hypoechoic normal area in hyperechoic fatty liver
  - Focal fatty infiltration: Focal hyperechoic area (commonly segment 4 around porta hepatis, subcapsular, or gallbladder fossa)
  - Geographic borders
  - Vessels may pass through lesion without distortion
  - No mass effect on adjacent portal or hepatic veins or contour deformity
  - Posterior acoustic shadowing behind fatty area and acoustic enhancement behind fatty sparing
- **Pyogenic Hepatic Abscess**

- Variable in shape and echogenicity
- Anechoic (50%), hyperechoic (25%), hypoechoic (25%)
- Fluid level or debris ± gas (reverberation artifact)
- Internal septae, thick or thin walls
- Posterior acoustic enhancement
- Pyogenic abscesses may coalesce to form conglomerate lesion ("cluster" sign)
- Color Doppler may show vascularity in thick wall
- **Subphrenic Abscess**
  - Extends along liver surface
  - Variable shape and echogenicity
  - Wall may be visible
  - Color Doppler may show vascularity on hepatic side
- **Postsurgical Change**
  - History of previous surgery is most important
  - Surgical resection frequently segmental
  - Surgical margin may contain sutures, clips, fat, and bowel, making interrogation difficult
  - Altering plane and location of interrogation may help

Helpful Clues for Less Common Diagnoses
- **Atypical Hemangioma**
  - Uncommon to have irregular borders, which tend to occur in larger lesions
  - Usually hyperechoic but may be iso-/hypoechoic

- Heterogeneous echogenicity is more likely in large lesions
- Posterior acoustic enhancement
- Color Doppler may show vessels in periphery of tumor
  - No visible color Doppler flow in center of lesion (flow too slow to be detected)
- Power Doppler may detect slow flow within hemangiomas
- **Hematoma**
  - Parenchymal laceration usually irregularly shaped
  - May point toward capsular surface or show tract
  - History of trauma, ± evidence of other associated injuries
- **Echinococcus Cyst**
  - *E. multilocularis*
    - Single or multiple lesions
    - Ill-defined infiltrative margins
    - Mass with irregular necrotic regions ± microcalcification
    - Tend to spread to liver hilum
    - May invade inferior vena cava or diaphragm
- **Lymphoma**
  - Diffuse form may show innumerable subcentimeter hypoechoic foci, miliary in pattern and usually periportal in location
  - Infiltrative pattern may be indistinguishable from normal liver

Hepatic Metastases

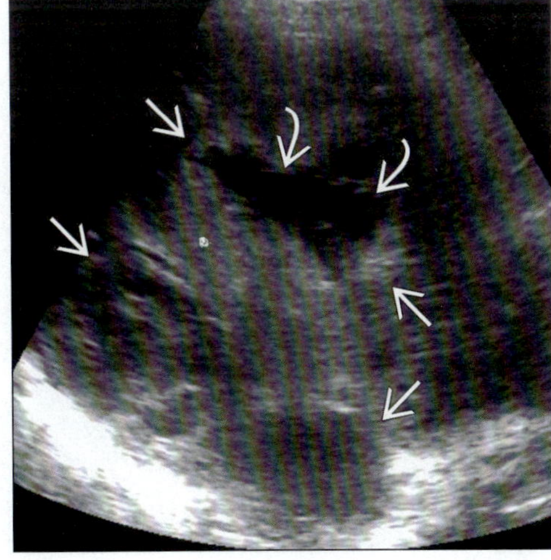

Oblique transabdominal ultrasound shows 2 metastases ➡, both with irregular borders. The more anterior lesion has a thick wall with a central hypoechoic center ➡, representing necrosis.

Hepatocellular Carcinoma

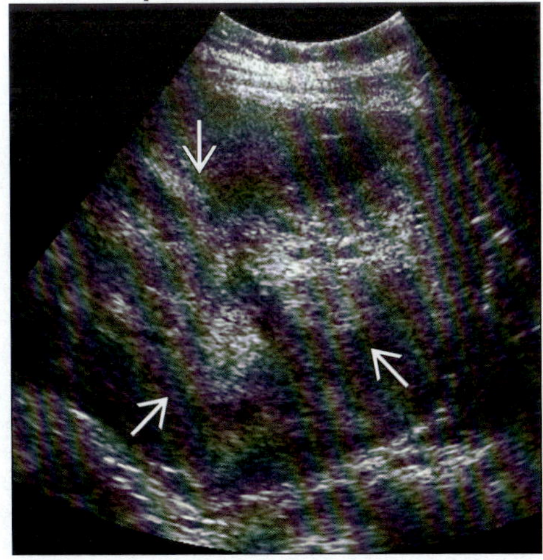

Oblique transabdominal ultrasound shows a large infiltrative and heterogeneous hepatocellular carcinoma ➡. The margins of this mass are ill defined and irregular, blending with the cirrhotic liver.

IRREGULAR BORDER LIVER MASS

Cholangiocarcinoma

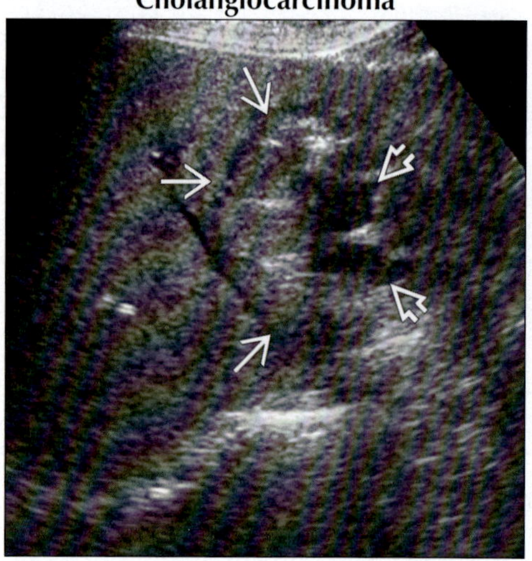

Cholangiocarcinoma

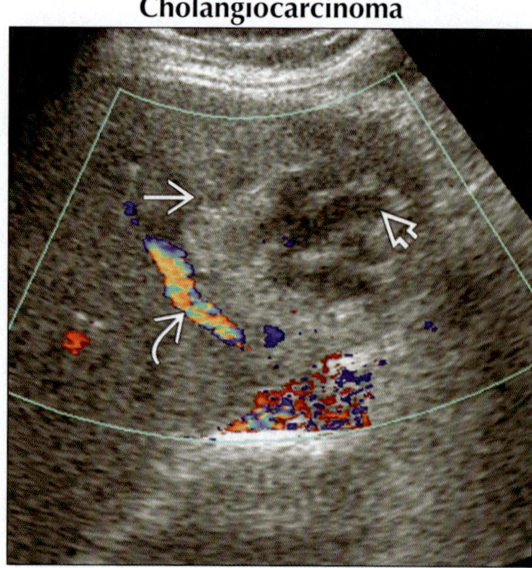

(Left) Transverse transabdominal ultrasound shows a heterogeneous cholangiocarcinoma ➡ in the left lobe of the liver. There is dilatation of the more peripheral intrahepatic ducts ⮞. Note the ill-defined margins of the cholangiocarcinoma. *(Right)* Correlative transverse color Doppler US in the same patient shows a lack of color flow in the cholangiocarcinoma ➡ and duct dilatation ⮞. Note the displaced and distorted hepatic vein ➚.

Hepatic Cyst

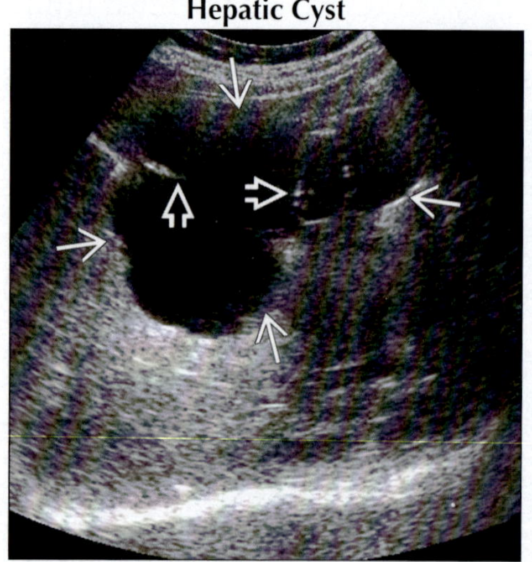

Hepatic Cyst

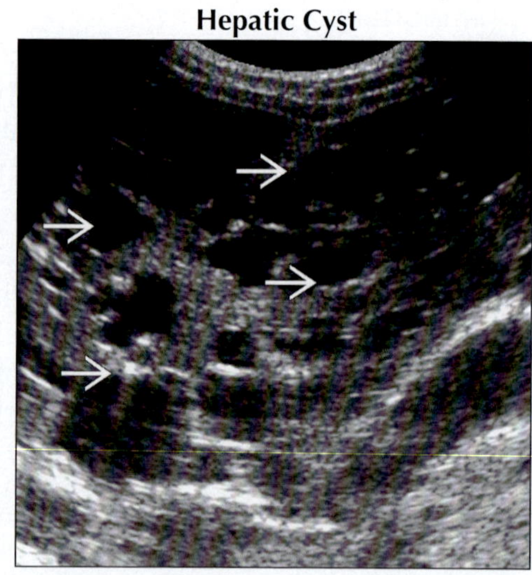

(Left) Oblique transabdominal ultrasound shows a large, benign, hepatic cyst. The cyst has irregular lobulated borders ➡, which are well defined. There are irregular internal septae ⮞ within. *(Right)* Oblique transabdominal ultrasound shows multiple cysts with irregular borders ➡ in a patient with polycystic liver disease. As the cysts enlarge, they become more irregular and distort the hepatic architecture.

Focal Fatty Replacement/Sparing

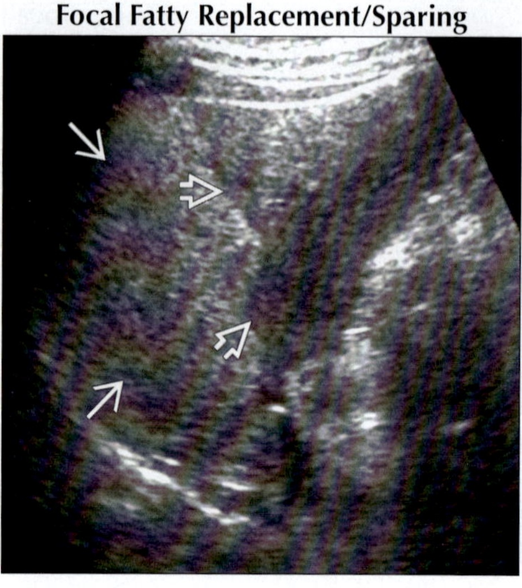

Pyogenic Hepatic Abscess

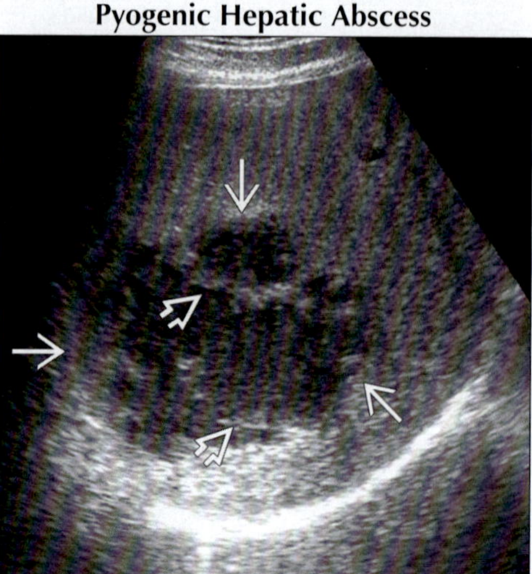

(Left) Longitudinal transabdominal ultrasound shows a large area of fatty infiltration, causing an increase in echogenicity ➡. The area has a geographic border ⮞ with the normal liver. *(Right)* Oblique transabdominal ultrasound shows a large hepatic abscess with irregular borders ➡ and multiple, thick internal septae ⮞. There are also low-level internal echoes that indicate debris.

IRREGULAR BORDER LIVER MASS

Subphrenic Abscess

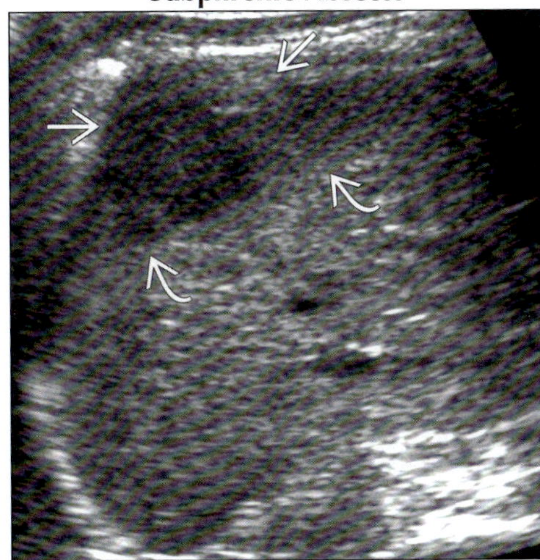

Postsurgical Change

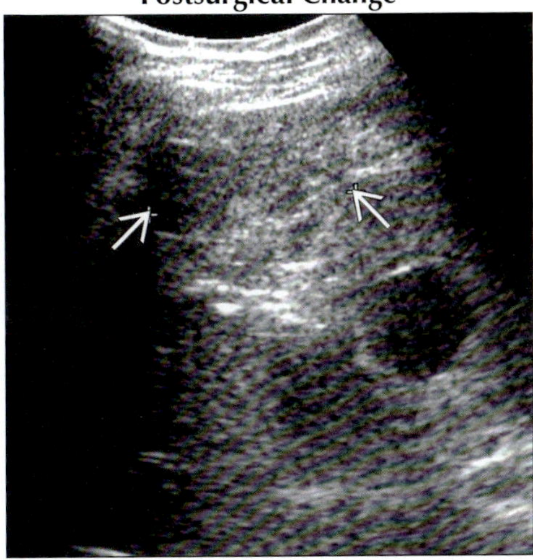

(Left) Oblique ultrasound shows a triangular-shaped, hypoechoic subphrenic abscess ➡ compressing the hepatic surface. The abscess wall produces an irregular border ➡ with the hepatic parenchyma. (Right) Oblique ultrasound shows a postsurgical change after a hepatic resection for hepatocellular carcinoma. The defect has been packed with fat ➡. Note the underlying cirrhotic liver and the irregular border of this area due to scarring.

Atypical Hemangioma

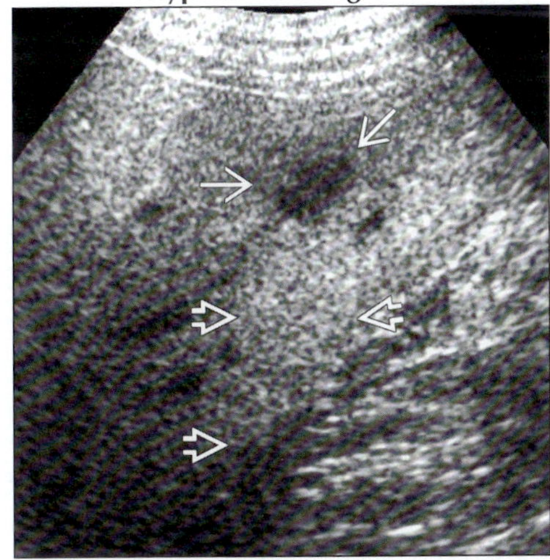

Atypical Hemangioma

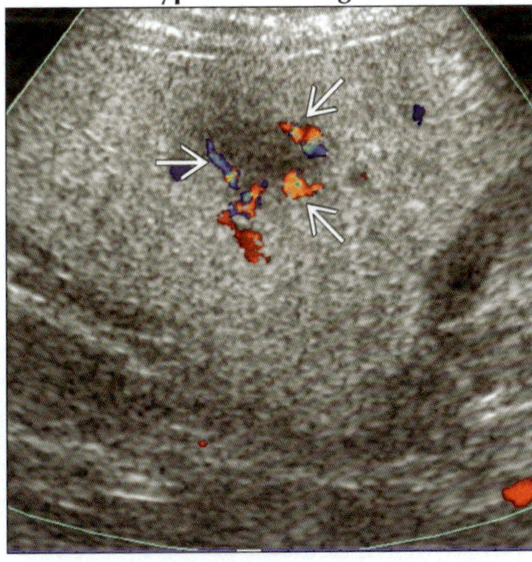

(Left) Oblique ultrasound shows an atypical hypoechoic hemangioma (typical hemangioma is usually hyperechoic). The mass shows irregular borders ➡. Note the posterior acoustic enhancement ➡. (Right) Transverse color Doppler ultrasound in the same patient shows prominent vessels ➡ in the periphery of this atypical hypoechoic hemangioma.

Hematoma

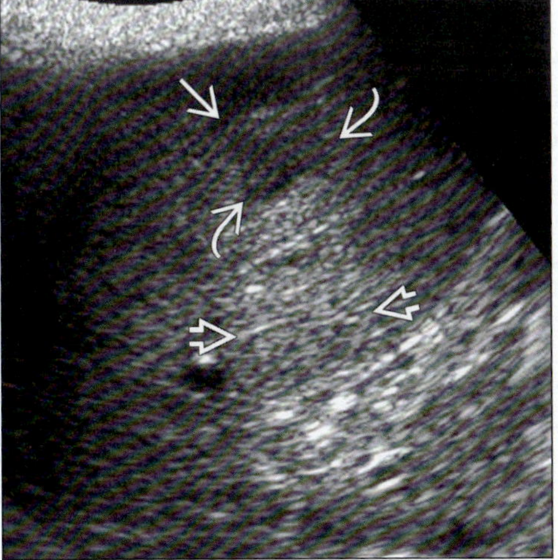

Echinococcus Cyst

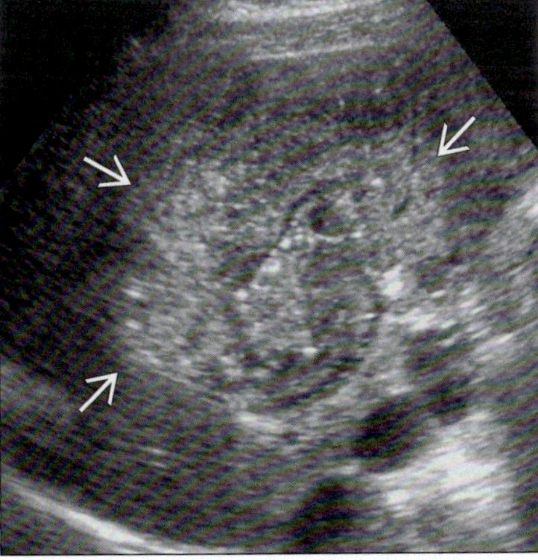

(Left) Oblique transabdominal ultrasound shows an irregularly shaped hypoechoic hematoma ➡. Note the tract of laceration leading from the hepatic surface ➡ and the posterior acoustic enhancement ➡. (Right) Transverse transabdominal ultrasound shows an echinococcal cyst (E. multilocularis) with an irregular border ➡. Note that the mass has an infiltrative echogenic border, which indicates its invasiveness.

3

MULTIPLE HEPATIC MASSES

DIFFERENTIAL DIAGNOSIS

Common
- Hepatic Cysts
- Hepatic Metastases
- Hepatic Steatosis (Multifocal)
- Hepatic Hemangioma
- Hepatic Lymphoma (Discrete Form)
- Cirrhosis with Regenerative &/or Dysplastic Nodules
- Multifocal Hepatocellular Carcinoma
- Pyogenic Hepatic Abscess
- Diffuse Hepatic Microabscesses
- Cholangitis
- Vessels

Less Common
- Hepatic Echinococcus Cyst
- Hepatic Hematoma

Rare but Important
- Caroli Disease

ESSENTIAL INFORMATION

Helpful Clues for Common Diagnoses
- **Hepatic Cysts**
  - Consider polycystic liver disease if numerous (> 10, usually hundreds ± renal cysts)
  - Thin-walled anechoic mass with posterior acoustic enhancement
  - Smooth or lobulated borders without septae or mural nodules
  - Do not communicate with each other or biliary tract
  - Do not demonstrate saccular configuration (vs. Caroli disease)
  - Not associated with biliary duct dilatation (vs. hydatid cysts or Caroli disease)
- **Hepatic Metastases**
  - Hypoechoic necrotic metastases may simulate cysts or abscesses
    - Abnormal intratumoral vascularity contains debris, mural nodules, or septae
  - Hyperechoic metastases simulate hemangioma or focal steatosis
    - Distort vessels and bile ducts
- **Hepatic Steatosis (Multifocal)**
  - Focal fatty infiltration
    - Location: Right lobe, caudate lobe, perihilar
    - Hyperechoic/confluent nodules
  - Focal fatty sparing
    - Location: Gallbladder bed, segment 4 anterior to portal bifurcation
    - Hypoechoic areas within echogenic liver
  - Lesions extend to edge of liver
  - No mass effect, vessels run undisplaced through lesion
- **Hepatic Hemangioma**
  - Well-defined margins + mass effect
  - Hyperechoic mass, typically homogeneous
  - Posterior acoustic enhancement
  - Atypical features
    - Hypoechoic, heterogeneous, calcification, irregular borders
- **Hepatic Lymphoma (Discrete Form)**
  - Well-defined nodule(s)/mass(es)
  - Hypoechoic or anechoic (low echogenicity due to high cellular density)
  - Large/conglomerate masses may appear to contain septae and mimic abscesses
  - Background vascular architecture ± distortion
  - Lymphoma more common in immunocompromised patients, e.g., AIDS patients and organ transplant recipients
- **Cirrhosis with Regenerative &/or Dysplastic Nodules**
  - Coarse echopattern, increased parenchymal echogenicity, and other signs of hepatic cirrhosis
  - Regenerating nodules (siderotic)
    - Iso-/hypoechoic nodules (regenerating nodules)
    - Hyperechoic rim (surrounding fibrosis)
  - Dysplastic nodules
    - Hypoechoic nodule > 1 cm diameter
    - Smooth or irregular borders
    - Difficult to differentiate from small hepatocellular carcinoma
- **Multifocal Hepatocellular Carcinoma**
  - Most commonly hypoechoic
  - May be surrounded by thin hyperechoic halo (capsule), cirrhotic background
  - Irregular hypervascularity within mass
  - Can invade portal vein
- **Pyogenic Hepatic Abscess**
  - "Cluster" sign: Aggregation of small abscesses, sometimes coalesces into single septated cavity
  - Complex cyst with septae and debris
  - ± ill-defined borders

MULTIPLE HEPATIC MASSES

- o Mural nodularity and vascularity
- o May contain gas within abscess: Seen as echogenic foci of air or air-fluid level
- o Adjacent parenchyma may be coarse and hypoechoic
- o Color Doppler may show hypervascularity in inflamed surrounding liver parenchyma
- **Diffuse Hepatic Microabscesses**
  - o Multiple small hypo-/iso-/hyperechoic lesions
  - o Central hypoechoic area of necrosis within hyperechoic lesion
  - o "Target" sign: Central hyperechoic inflammation surrounded by hypoechoic halo of fibrosis
  - o Similar lesions may be found in spleen
- **Cholangitis**
  - o Circumferential bile duct wall thickening
  - o Dilatation of intra- and extrahepatic ducts
  - o Periportal hypo-/hyperechogenicity due to periductal edema/inflammation
  - o Ascending cholangitis
    - Obstructing calculus in extrahepatic duct
  - o Recurrent pyogenic cholangitis
    - Biliary calculi: Cast-like (unlike Caroli disease) and often fill duct lumen
    - Atrophy of affected lobe/segment
- **Vessels**
  - o Portal veins
    - Venectasia, varicosities, collaterals from portal hypertension
  - o Hepatic veins
    - Venectasia, Budd-Chiari, etc.
  - o Hepatic arteries

- Aneurysms, shunts, vascular malformation
- o Use color Doppler to confirm vascular nature and vessel type

Helpful Clues for Less Common Diagnoses

- **Hepatic Echinococcus Cyst**
  - o Large well-defined hypoechoic masses
  - o Numerous peripheral daughter cysts
  - o Intrahepatic duct dilatation may be seen
  - o May show curvilinear or ring-like pericyst calcification
- **Hepatic Hematoma**
  - o Lesions commonly in segments 6, 7, 8
  - o Round hyper- or hypoechoic foci
  - o Initially echogenic; hypoechoic after 4-5 days; internal echoes with septae after 1-4 weeks
  - o Ancillary signs: Subcapsular hematoma, hemoperitoneum, renal or splenic laceration

Helpful Clues for Rare Diagnoses

- **Caroli Disease**
  - o Hypoechoic masses
  - o Saccular or fusiform shape
  - o "Central dot" sign: Small portal venous branches partially or completely surrounded by dilated ducts
  - o May contain calculi, which do not form casts of ducts (vs. recurrent pyogenic cholangitis)

Hepatic Cysts

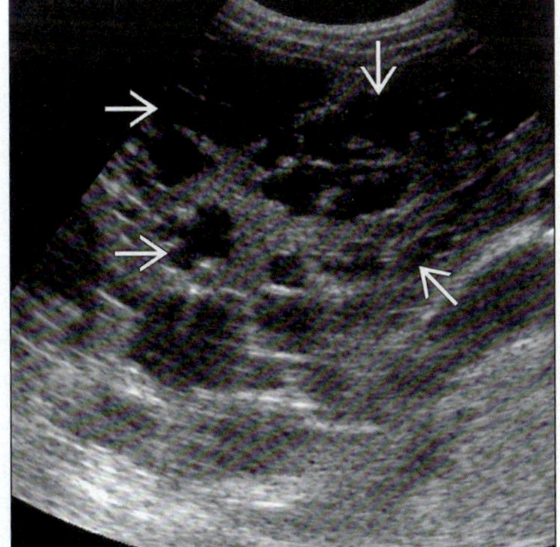

Oblique transabdominal ultrasound shows numerous cysts ➡ of varying size with irregular walls in a patient with polycystic liver disease. The cysts do not communicate with the biliary tree or with each other.

Hepatic Metastases

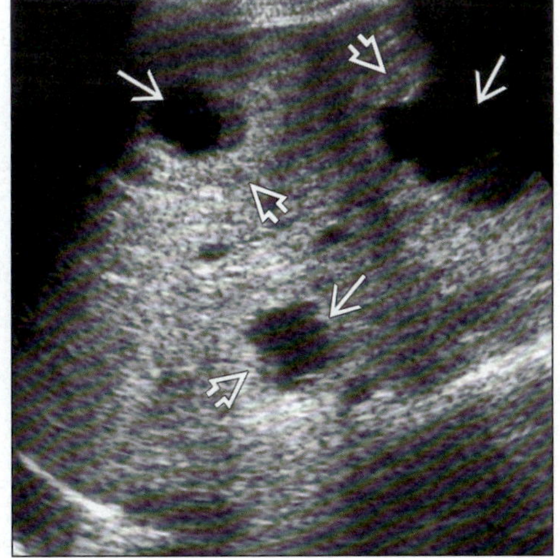

Transverse transabdominal ultrasound shows multiple cystic/necrotic metastases ➡ from nasopharyngeal carcinoma. Note the thick irregular walls ➡ and mural nodularity.

3

MULTIPLE HEPATIC MASSES

(Left) *Oblique power Doppler ultrasound shows multiple hypoechoic metastases ➡. Abnormal vascularity ➡ is detected in these lesions. Color/power Doppler helps differentiate benign from neoplastic lesions by showing the distribution and character of vascularity.* **(Right)** *Transverse ultrasound shows typical, multiple, hyperechoic metastases ➡ from colon carcinoma. The lesions are of varying size, and the larger ones show irregular nodular borders ➡.*

Hepatic Metastases

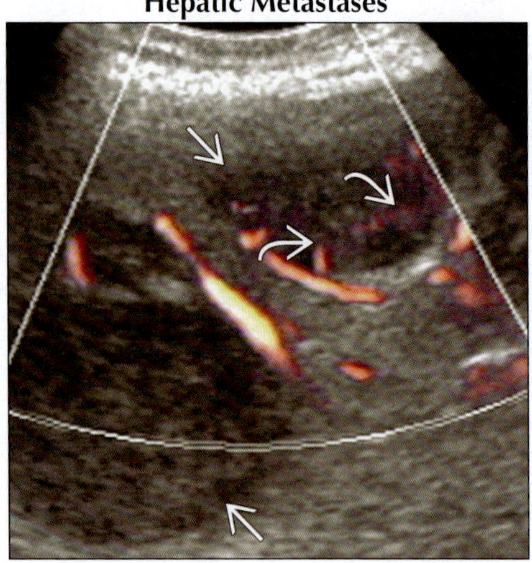

Hepatic Metastases

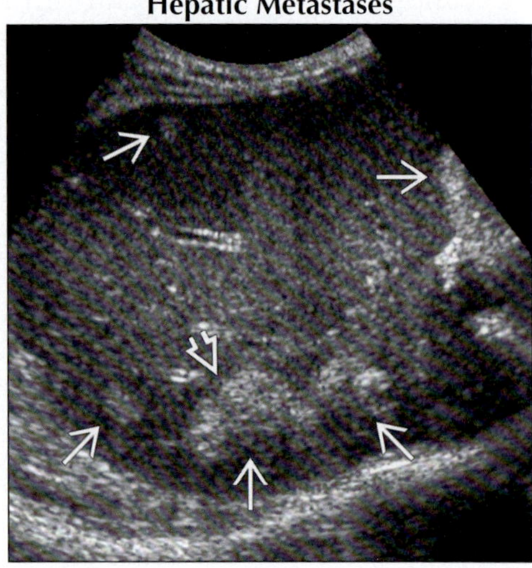

(Left) *Oblique ultrasound shows multiple areas of focal hyperechoic steatosis ➡ in the right lobe of the liver. Note that the surrounding architecture is not distorted. Normal hepatic vessels can pass undisturbed through these lesions.* **(Right)** *Transverse ultrasound shows multiple hyperechoic hemangiomata ➡ in the right lobe of the liver. Note the smooth borders of the lesions and weak posterior acoustic enhancement ➡, with slight displacement of the intrahepatic vessels ➡.*

Hepatic Steatosis (Multifocal)

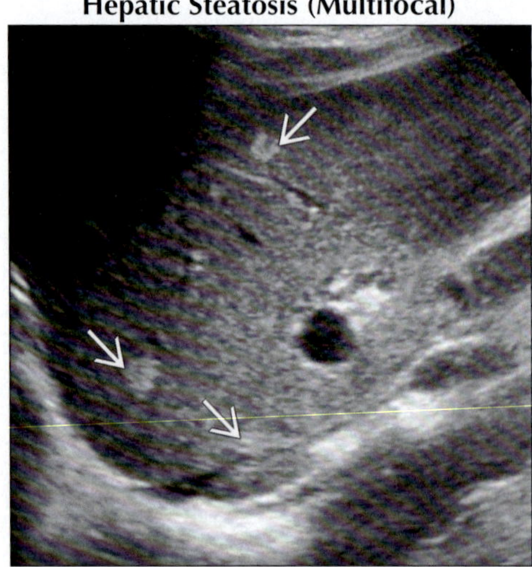

Hepatic Hemangioma

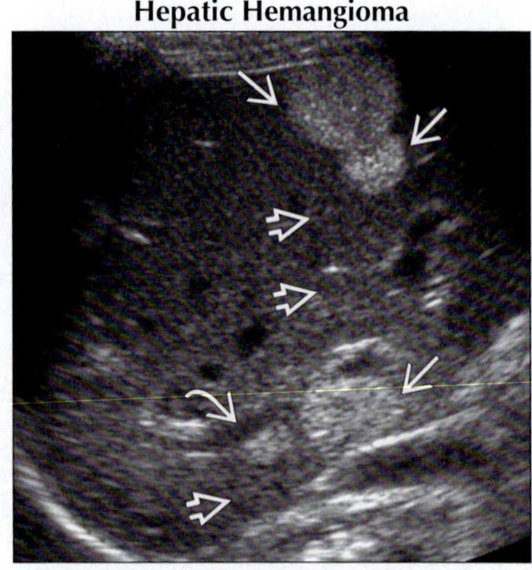

(Left) *Oblique transabdominal ultrasound shows multiple, hypo-/anechoic, lymphomatous deposits ➡, some with septae ➡. Such nodules are often referred to as "pseudocystic."* **(Right)** *Oblique transabdominal ultrasound shows multiple, hypoechoic, regenerating nodules ➡ with well-defined round borders. Note the coarse echopattern ➡ and nodular surface ➡ of background hepatic cirrhosis.*

Hepatic Lymphoma (Discrete Form)

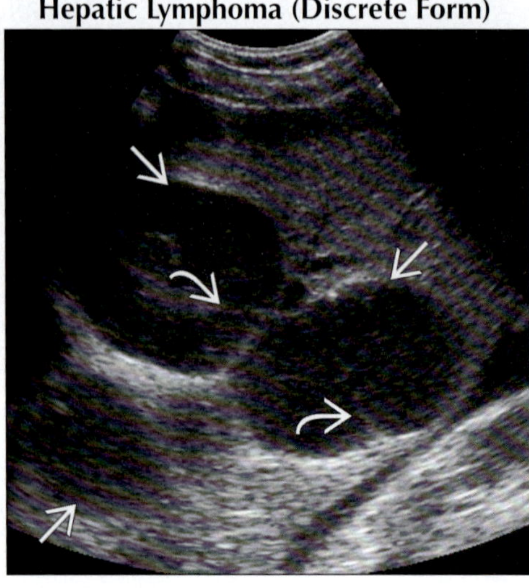

Cirrhosis with Regenerative &/or Dysplastic Nodules

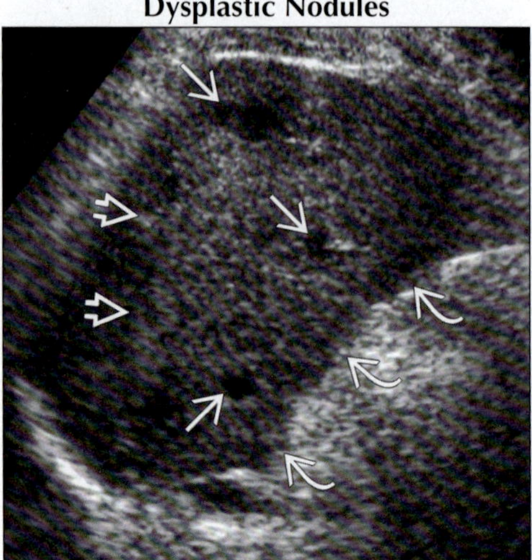

3

MULTIPLE HEPATIC MASSES

Multifocal Hepatocellular Carcinoma

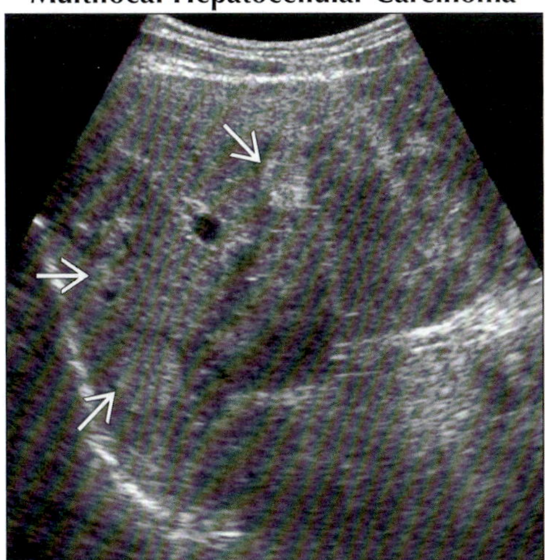

Pyogenic Hepatic Abscess

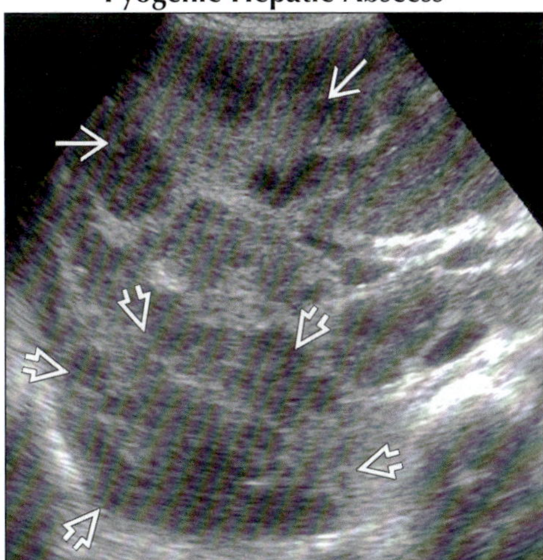

(Left) Transverse ultrasound shows multiple mixed echogenicity hepatic masses ➡ in multifocal hepatocellular carcinoma. Masses show irregular borders. Note the background cirrhosis. Metastases from nonhepatic primaries are less common than multifocal HCC in cirrhotic livers. *(Right)* Transverse ultrasound shows multiple abscesses ➡ in the right lobe of the liver, with low-level internal echoes, irregular walls, and a "cluster" sign ➡.

Diffuse Hepatic Microabscesses

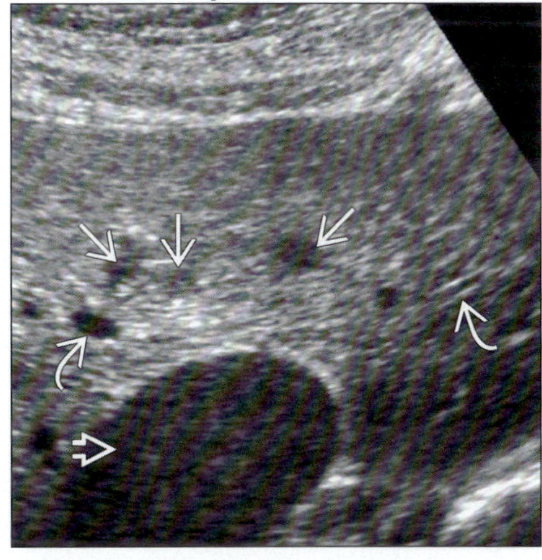

Hepatic Echinococcus Cyst

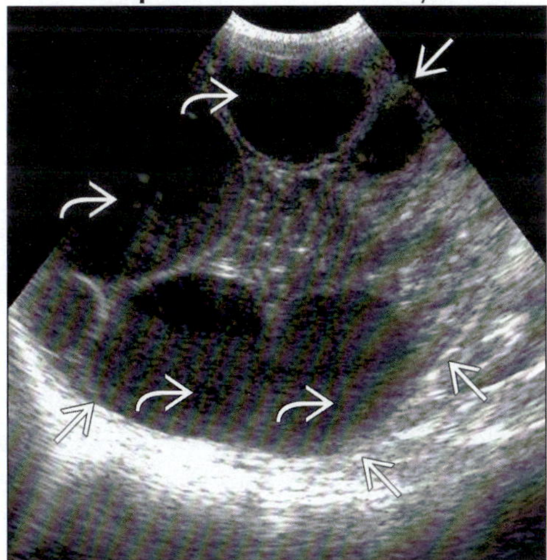

(Left) Oblique transabdominal ultrasound shows multiple, hypoechoic microabscesses ➡ with echogenicity similar to the gallbladder ➡. In comparison to the vessels ➡, the borders of these abscesses are not well defined due to adjacent inflammation and edema. *(Right)* Longitudinal transabdominal ultrasound shows a large echinococcal cyst ➡ containing multiple hypoechoic daughter cysts ➡ in the right lobe of the liver.

Hepatic Hematoma

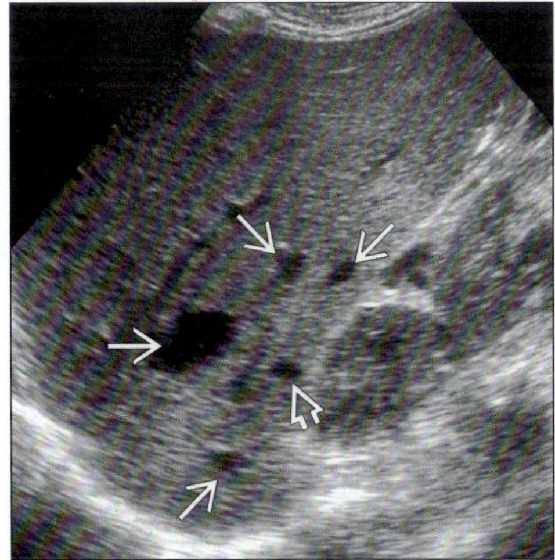

Caroli Disease

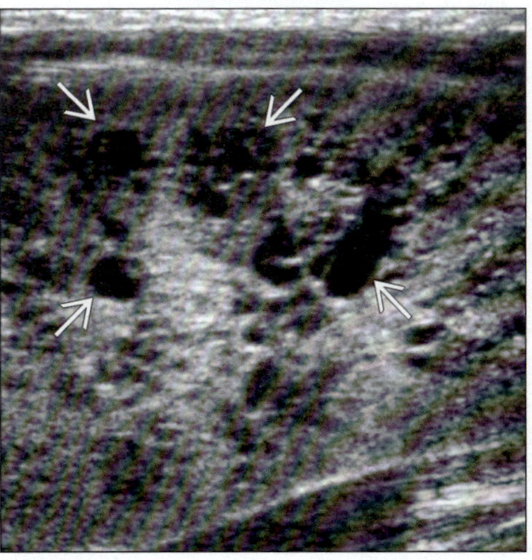

(Left) Oblique transabdominal US shows multiple, well-defined, hypoechoic hematomas ➡ in segment 6, a common location for injury. There is evidence of a laceration ➡ on the surface of liver. *(Right)* Oblique transabdominal US shows multiple anechoic nodules and tubular structures ➡ diffusely involving the liver. These represent dilated ducts in Caroli disease. Color Doppler interrogation may reveal small portal veins surrounded by ducts.

3

HEPATIC MASS WITH CENTRAL SCAR

DIFFERENTIAL DIAGNOSIS

Common
- Focal Nodular Hyperplasia
- Fibrolamellar Hepatocellular Carcinoma
- Hepatocellular Carcinoma
- Hepatic Adenoma
- Hepatic Metastases

Less Common
- Atypical Hemangioma
- Hepatic Echinococcus Cyst

ESSENTIAL INFORMATION

Helpful Clues for Common Diagnoses
- **Focal Nodular Hyperplasia**
  - Hypoechoic central scar (18% hyperechoic)
  - Central scar contains central feeding artery ± calcification
  - Color Doppler may show prominent central feeding artery with multiple small vessels radiating peripherally in "spoke-wheel" pattern
- **Fibrolamellar Hepatocellular Carcinoma**
  - Presents in otherwise healthy young adults
  - Well-defined, partially/completely encapsulated, large mass
  - Prominent central fibrous scar ± calcification
  - Vascular, biliary, and nodal invasion may be present
- **Hepatocellular Carcinoma**
  - Nonfibrolamellar type
    - Background cirrhosis ± signs of portal hypertension
    - Central tumor necrosis/fibrosis produces apparent central scar
    - Color Doppler may show irregular tumor hypervascularity &/or tumor thrombus in portal vein
- **Hepatic Adenoma**
  - Well-defined round or mildly lobulated contour
  - Can have central fat, hemorrhage, necrosis, and calcification, which may simulate central scar
  - Color Doppler shows hypervascular tumor supplied by hepatic artery
- **Hepatic Metastases**
  - Necrotic or treated metastases with necrotic center simulating central scar
  - Color Doppler usually does not show vascularity as most metastases are hypovascular

Helpful Clues for Less Common Diagnoses
- **Atypical Hemangioma**
  - Occasionally see hypoechoic center with hyperechoic rim simulating central scar
  - Posterior acoustic enhancement
  - No visible color Doppler flow in center of lesion (flow too slow to be detected)
- **Hepatic Echinococcus Cyst**
  - Honeycombed cyst; multiple septations between daughter cysts in mother cyst
  - "Spoke-wheel" appearance of septa simulating central scar

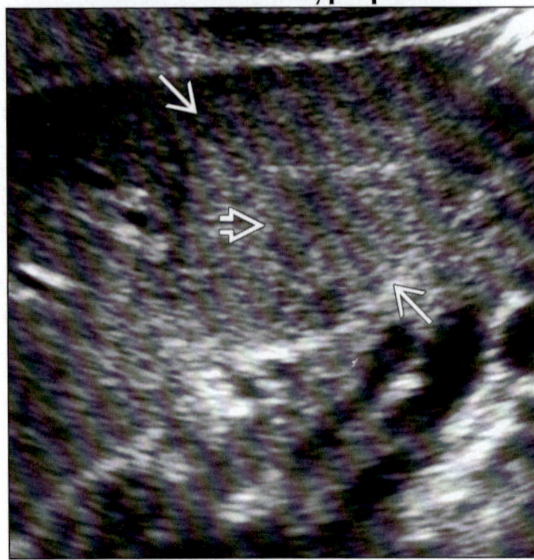

Focal Nodular Hyperplasia

Oblique transabdominal ultrasound shows a hypoechoic central scar ➡ in an isoechoic focal nodular hyperplasia ➡.

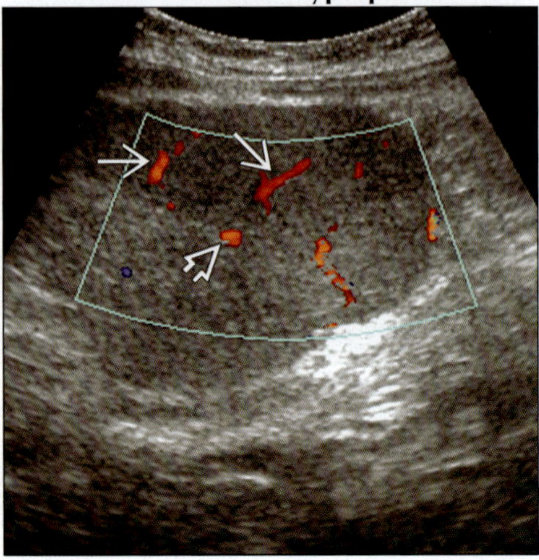

Focal Nodular Hyperplasia

Transverse color Doppler ultrasound shows centrifugal blood flowing away ➡ from the central feeding artery ➡ of the focal nodular hyperplasia. This gives the blood flow a partial "spoke-wheel" appearance.

HEPATIC MASS WITH CENTRAL SCAR

Fibrolamellar Hepatocellular Carcinoma

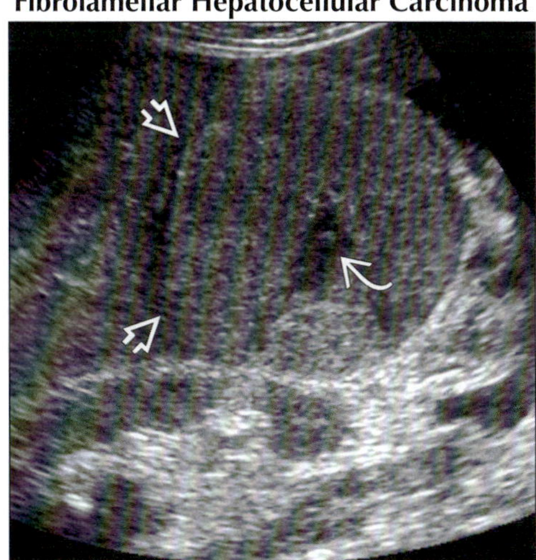

Fibrolamellar Hepatocellular Carcinoma

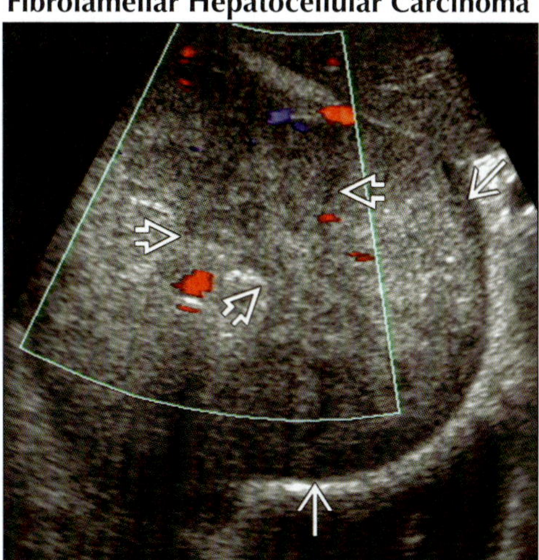

(Left) Transverse transabdominal ultrasound shows an isoechoic hepatocellular carcinoma with a thin halo ⮕ and central necrosis ➔, simulating a scar. (Right) Oblique transabdominal ultrasound shows a large fibrolamellar hepatocellular carcinoma with a bulging surface contour ➔ and slightly echogenic central scar ⮕. Note the irregular tumor vascularity and lack of a "spoke-wheel" appearance.

Hepatocellular Carcinoma

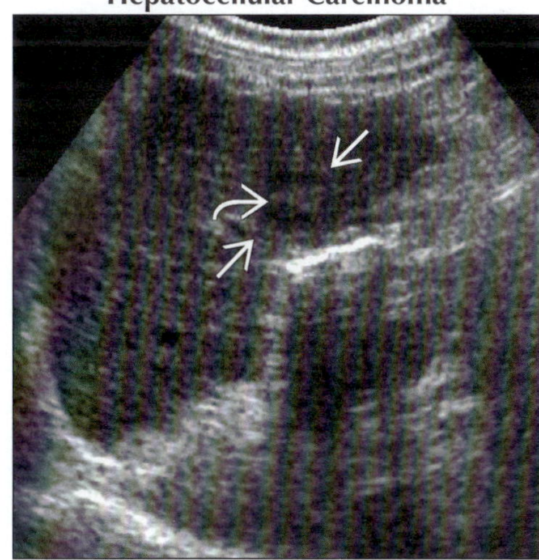

Hepatic Adenoma

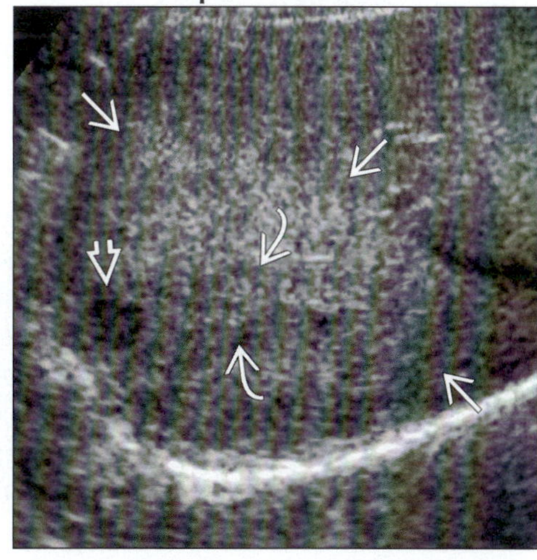

(Left) Oblique transabdominal ultrasound shows a small, nonfibrolamellar hepatocellular carcinoma ➔ with a central scar ⮕. Small lesions, such as this one, have a target appearance. (Right) Oblique transabdominal ultrasound shows a large hyperechoic adenoma ➔ containing a central scar ⮕ from necrosis and hemorrhage. There is also a more discrete hypoechoic focus ⮕, which may represent focal hematoma/necrosis.

Hepatic Metastases

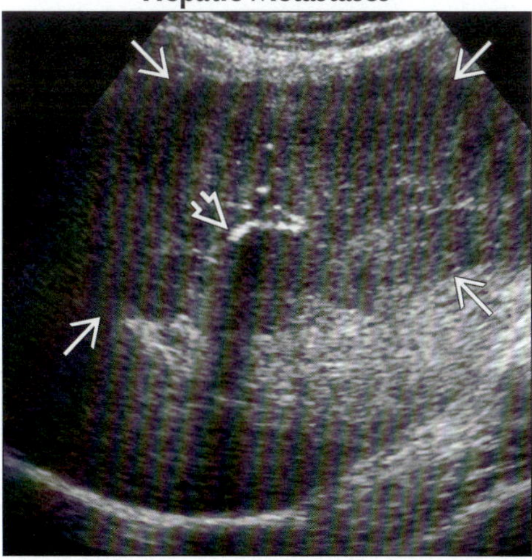

Atypical Hemangioma

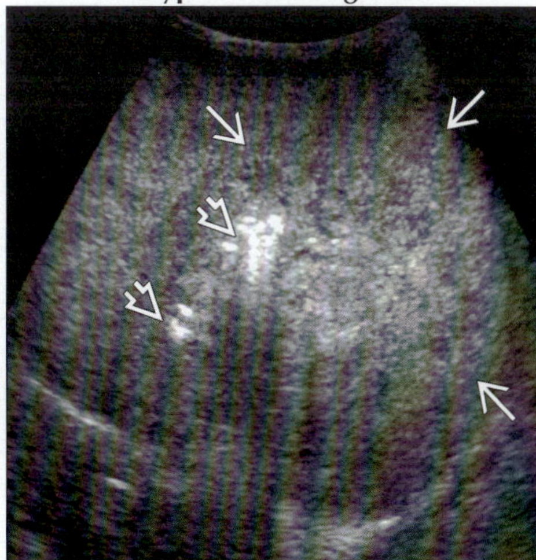

(Left) Oblique transabdominal ultrasound shows a large hypoechoic metastasis ➔ in the liver with central calcification ⮕ simulating a central scar. (Right) Oblique transabdominal ultrasound shows a large cavernous hemangioma ➔ with internal calcifications ⮕ and posterior acoustic shadowing. The calcifications suggest a central scar.

HEPATIC LESION WITH POSTERIOR SHADOWING

DIFFERENTIAL DIAGNOSIS

Common
- Small Calcified Granulomas
- Biliary Calculi
- Metastases
- Vascular Calcification
- Hepatocellular Carcinoma
- Hematoma
- Cavernous Hemangioma
- Pyogenic Hepatic Abscess
- Pneumobilia
- Portal Vein Gas
- Postoperative
  - Scar, Clips, Stents, Coils
- Focal Fatty Infiltration
- Echinococcus Cyst

ESSENTIAL INFORMATION

Key Differential Diagnosis Issues
- Curvilinear reflection: Suggests cyst wall
- Lobulated reflection: Nonspecific
- Indistinct reflection: Amorphous/soft intralesional calcification
- Posterior reverberation: Suggests gas

Helpful Clues for Common Diagnoses
- **Small Calcified Granulomas**
  - From TB, histoplasmosis, or fungal diseases
  - Well-defined, densely calcified nodules
- **Biliary Calculi**
  - Intrahepatic calculi calcify much less often than stones in gallbladder or common bile duct
    - Calcification may also be from remains of previous infestation (e.g., *Ascaris*)
- **Metastases**
  - Multiple lesions with different degrees of calcification
  - Mucinous/calcific/ossific primaries or treated metastases
- **Vascular Calcification**
  - Mural calcification of arterial wall
  - Intraluminal calcification: Chronic portal vein thrombosis
- **Hepatocellular Carcinoma**
  - Rarely calcifies unless treated
- **Hematoma**
  - Chronic hematoma may calcify
- **Cavernous Hemangioma**
  - Unusual to have central calcification with posterior shadowing
- **Pyogenic Hepatic Abscess**
  - May form cluster
  - For amebic abscess, presence of gas indicates fistula with bowel
- **Pneumobilia**
  - Ring-down artifact ("dirty shadow") posterior to gas
  - History of instrumentation of biliary tree or passage of stone
- **Focal Fatty Infiltration**
  - No mass effect: Vessels running undisplaced through lesion
- **Echinococcus Cyst**
  - Circumferential calcification usually indicates infection is no longer active

Small Calcified Granulomas

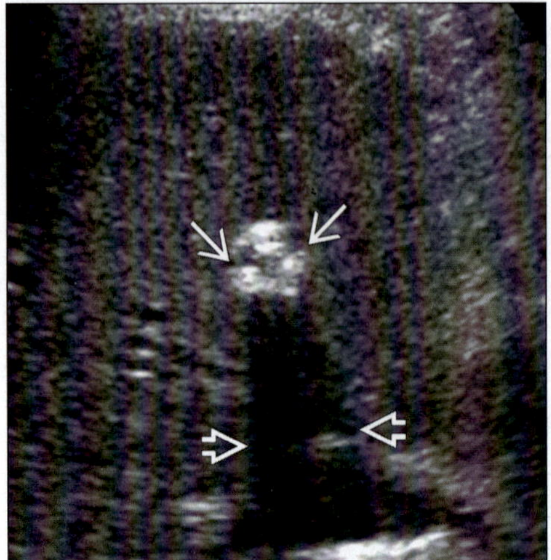

Oblique transabdominal ultrasound shows a small calcified granuloma ➡ in the right lobe of the liver with strong posterior shadowing ⇨. Note the highly echogenic calcification despite its small size.

Metastases

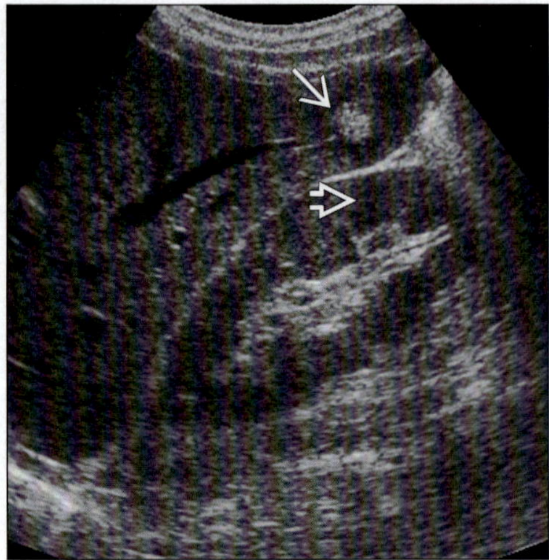

Oblique ultrasound of a hepatic metastasis shows soft amorphous calcification ➡ with mild posterior shadowing ⇨. History is important as treated and untreated metastases can have similar appearances.

Cavernous Hemangioma

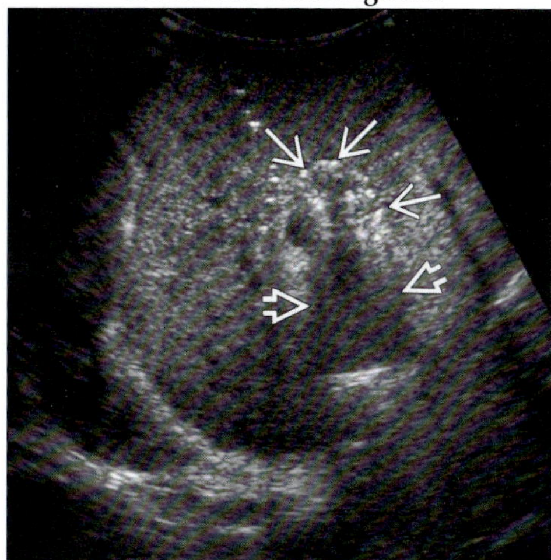

Pyogenic Hepatic Abscess

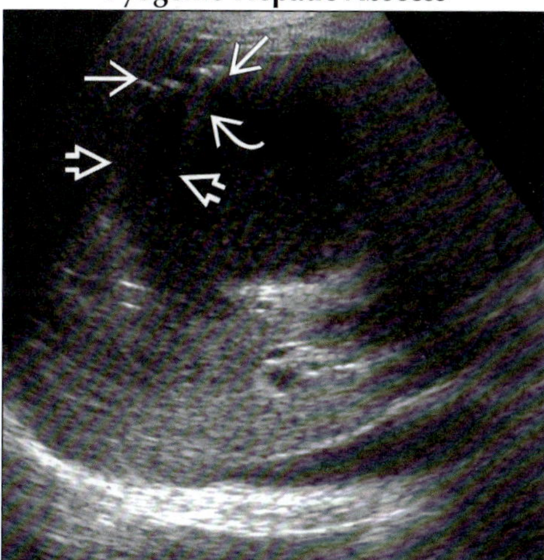

(Left) Oblique ultrasound shows multiple small specks of calcification ➡ with posterior acoustic shadowing ⮞ in a hepatic hemangioma. Note that noncalcified hemangiomas usually have posterior acoustic enhancement. *(Right)* Transverse transabdominal ultrasound shows gas ➡ with shadowing ⮞ and reverberation artifacts ➡ in the nondependent portion of a pyogenic hepatic abscess. Note the low-level internal echoes within the abscess.

Pneumobilia

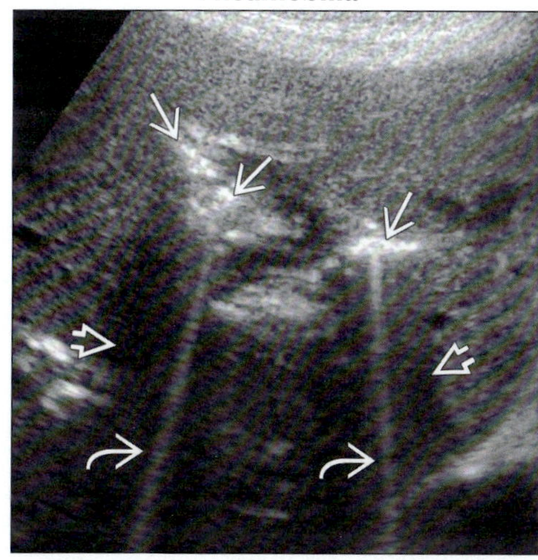

Postoperative

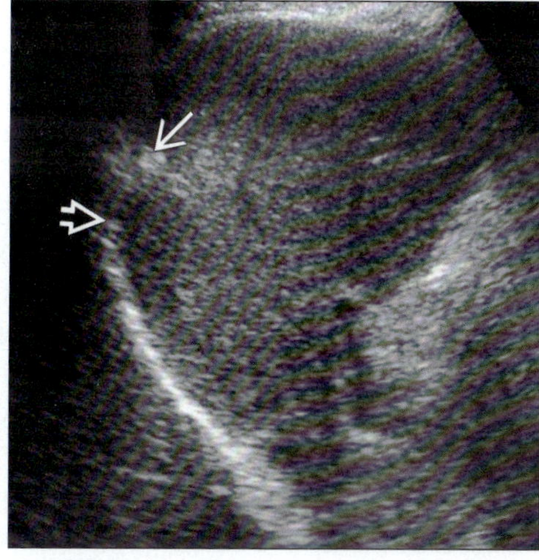

(Left) Transverse transabdominal ultrasound shows multiple echogenic foci ➡ with posterior acoustic shadowing ⮞ and associated reverberation artifacts ➡ adjacent to the left portal vein in a patient with pneumobilia. *(Right)* Oblique transabdominal ultrasound shows focal hepatic scarring ➡ with posterior acoustic shadowing ⮞. This patient had a previous surgery in this area.

Postoperative

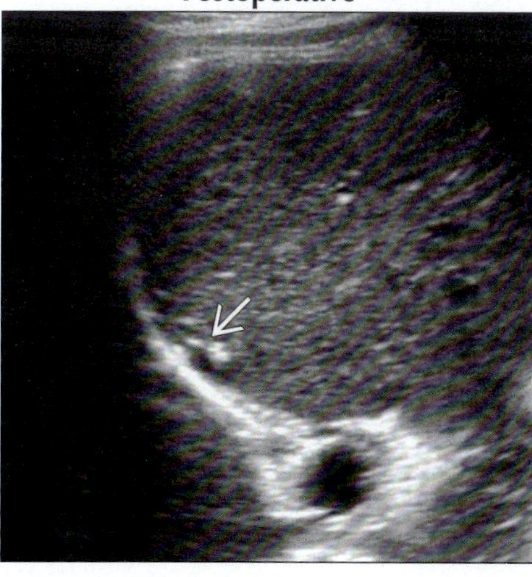

Echinococcus Cyst

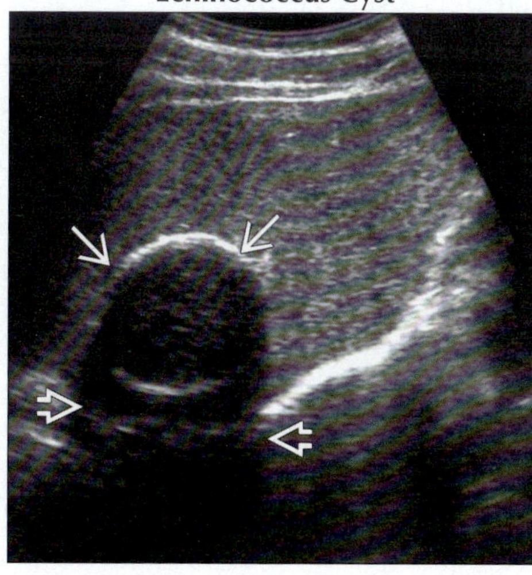

(Left) Oblique transabdominal ultrasound shows an echogenic surgical clip ➡ in the right lobe of the liver. Note that this does not cause significant posterior acoustic shadowing, which may be due to its small size. *(Right)* Oblique transabdominal ultrasound shows a curvilinear, specular, echogenic interface ➡ with strong posterior acoustic shadowing ⮞ of a calcified echinococcal cyst.

DIFFERENTIAL DIAGNOSIS

Common
- Ascending Cholangitis
- Cavernous Transformation of Portal Vein
- Portosystemic Collaterals
- Hepatic Trauma
- Acute Viral Hepatitis
- Fatty Sparing, Liver
- Diffuse/Infiltrative Hepatic Lymphoma
- Pneumobilia
- Choledocholithiasis

Less Common
- Hepatic Schistosomiasis
- Recurrent Pyogenic Cholangitis
- Iatrogenic Material
- Caroli Disease

ESSENTIAL INFORMATION

Helpful Clues for Common Diagnoses
- **Ascending Cholangitis**
  - Periportal hypo- or hyperechogenicity adjacent to dilated intrahepatic ducts, due to periductal edema/inflammation
  - Dilatation of intrahepatic bile ducts
  - Purulent bile/sludge as intraluminal echogenic material in dilated ducts
  - Circumferential thickening of bile duct wall: Hypoechoic layer
  - Obstructing stone in common bile duct
- **Cavernous Transformation of Portal Vein**
  - Collateralization due to portal vein occlusion
  - Usually in subacute or chronic portal hypertension/vein obstruction
  - Serpiginous tubular channels along course of portal vein
  - Color Doppler shows hepatopetal flow
  - Signs of portal vein occlusion
    - Acute: Enlarged portal vein
    - Chronic: Small/imperceptible portal vein
    - Color Doppler: Lack of flow in portal vein (except if occlusion due to tumor thrombus)
- **Portosystemic Collaterals**
  - Serpiginous hypoechoic channels in or around portal triad
  - Location

- Intrahepatic: Portal to portal veins, portal to hepatic veins, portal to systemic veins
    - Umbilical vein (recanalization)
    - Gastroesophageal: Coronary and right gastric, left gastric and splenogastric
    - Lienorenal/mesenteric/retroperitoneal
  - Color Doppler
    - Shows hepatofugal flow in vessels (opposite to cavernous transformation)
    - Extent of collaterals
  - Background changes of cirrhosis/portal hypertension/portal vein thrombosis
- **Hepatic Trauma**
  - Lesions are commonly located in segments 6, 7, 8
  - Initially echogenic; becomes hypoechoic after 4-5 days; internal echoes with septae may develop after 1-4 weeks
  - Hematoma tracking along portal triad
    - Linear, focal, or diffuse periportal lesion
  - Ancillary signs of trauma: Subcapsular hematoma; hemoperitoneum, renal, or splenic laceration/hematoma
  - Better evaluated by MDCT
- **Acute Viral Hepatitis**
  - Increased echogenicity of fat in periportal tissues, ligamentum venosum, and falciform ligament
  - Hepatomegaly with diffuse decrease in echogenicity
  - "Starry sky" appearance: Increased echogenicity of portal triad walls against background of hypoechoic liver
  - Periportal hypo-/anechoic area due to hydropic swelling of hepatocytes
- **Fatty Sparing, Liver**
  - Focal hypoechoic area within otherwise echogenic liver
  - No mass effect (vessels run undisplaced through lesion)
  - Due to direct drainage of hepatic blood into systemic circulation
  - Typical location
    - Next to gallbladder (drained by cystic vein)
    - Segment 4/anterior to portal bifurcation (drained by aberrant gastric vein)
- **Diffuse/Infiltrative Hepatic Lymphoma**
  - Subcentimeter periportal hypoechoic foci, miliary in pattern

- Other evidence of lymphoma
  - Lymphadenopathy, splenomegaly/splenic lesions, bowel wall thickening, ascites
- **Pneumobilia**
  - Highly echogenic linear foci in portal triad
  - Rises to nondependent portion of liver (left lobe if patient lying supine)
  - Change in position of gas with change in patient position
  - Posterior acoustic shadowing
  - Reverberation artifact deep to lesion
  - Due to recent passage of stone from or instrumention of biliary tree, choledochoenteric fistula, biliary infection by gas-forming organism
- **Choledocholithiasis**
  - Multiple echogenic foci along portal triad
  - Posterior acoustic shadowing
    - Small (< 5 mm) or soft pigmented stones may not produce posterior shadowing
  - Large stones may cause biliary obstruction, resulting in focal bile duct dilatation

Helpful Clues for Less Common Diagnoses
- **Hepatic Schistosomiasis**
  - Periportal fibrosis
    - Hyperechoic and thickened walls of portal venules, described as "clay-pipestem" fibrosis
    - Widened portal tracts
    - "Bull's-eye" lesion describes anechoic portal vein surrounded by echogenic mantle of fibrous tissue

- Most severe at porta hepatis
  - Mosaic pattern
    - Network of echogenic septa outlining polygonal areas of normal-appearing liver
    - Represents septal fibrosis (inflammation & fibrosis in reaction to embolized eggs)
    - May be discontinuous and appear mottled, nodular, or sieve-like (partial septal fibrosis or calcification)
- **Recurrent Pyogenic Cholangitis**
  - Early disease with active biliary sepsis
    - Periportal hypo- or hyperechogenicity due to periductal edema/inflammation
    - Biliary duct wall thickening due to edema
    - Floating echoes within dilated ducts due to inflammatory debris
  - Late-stage disease
    - Severe atrophy of affected segment/lobe
    - Crowded stone-filled ducts (may appear as single heterogeneous mass)
    - Stones may form casts of duct
- **Iatrogenic Material**
  - Shunts, embolization material, drainage tubes, staples, etc.
  - Echogenic material with strong reflective surface or smooth outline
- **Caroli Disease**
  - Hypoechoic mass(es): Saccular or fusiform shape
  - "Central dot" sign: Small portal venous branches partially or completely surrounded by dilated ducts

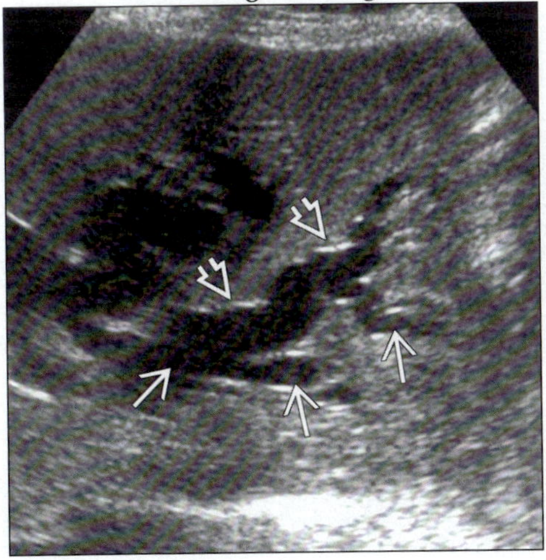

Ascending Cholangitis

Transverse transabdominal ultrasound shows markedly dilated intrahepatic ducts ➡ in ascending cholangitis. Note the irregular fusiform contour with a mild degree of wall thickening ➡ of the ducts.

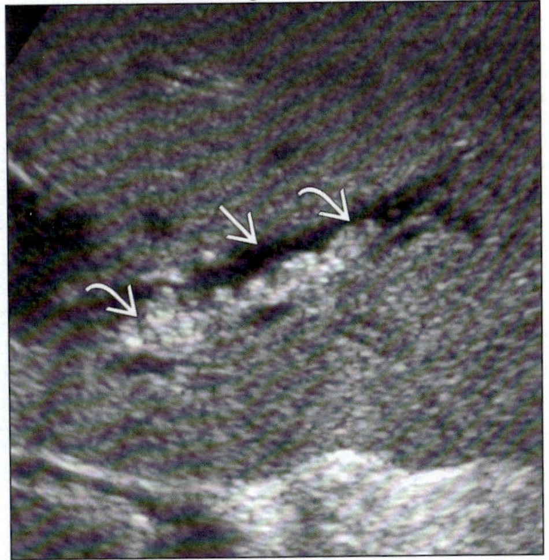

Ascending Cholangitis

Oblique transabdominal US of ascending cholangitis shows dilatation of the intrahepatic duct ➡ in the left lobe of the liver. Note echogenic material within the dilated duct ➡, representing infected biliary sludge.

(Left) Transverse transabdominal ultrasound shows cavernous transformation in a patient with portal hypertension. Note the multiple, fusiform, hypoechoic, tubular structures ➾ around the left portal vein ➾. *(Right)* Transverse color Doppler ultrasound shows hepatopetal (toward liver parenchyma and away from porta hepatis) color flow within the cavernous transformation ➾ with lack of flow in the portal vein ➾.

Cavernous Transformation of Portal Vein

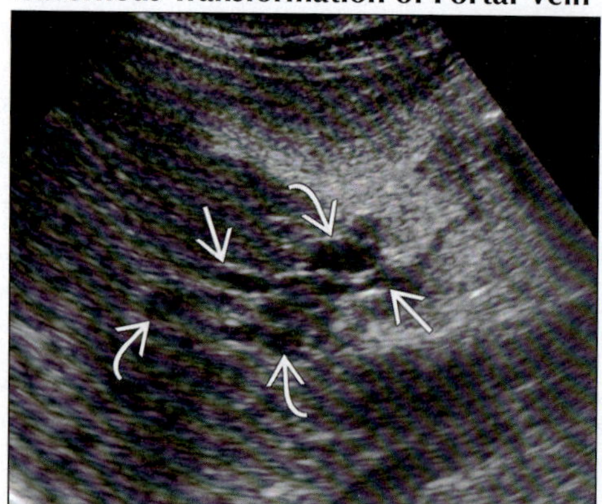

Cavernous Transformation of Portal Vein

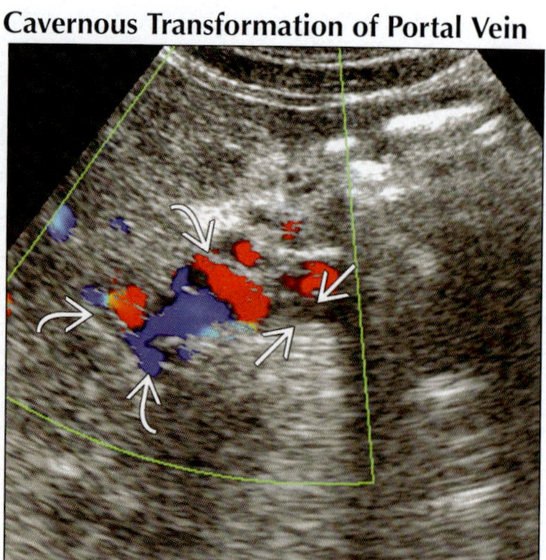

(Left) Oblique transabdominal ultrasound shows an irregularly shaped, hypoechoic hematoma ➾ tracking along the portal triads in segment 5. Note the nearby portal vein ➾. *(Right)* Longitudinal transabdominal ultrasound shows the diffusely enlarged hypoechoic liver with echogenic portal triads ➾ in this patient with acute viral hepatitis. This produces a "starry sky" appearance.

Hepatic Trauma

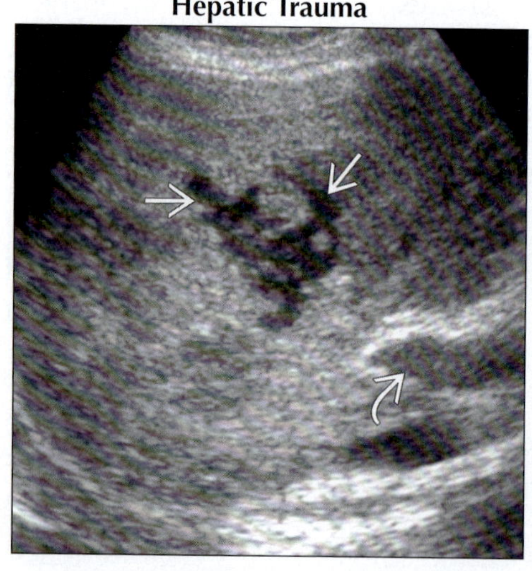

Acute Viral Hepatitis

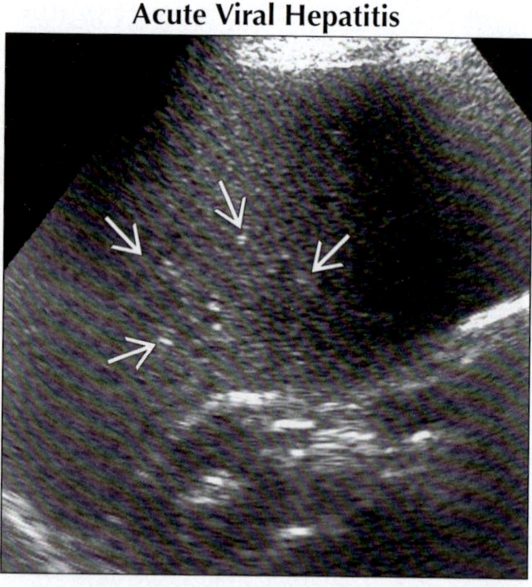

(Left) Transverse transabdominal ultrasound shows focal fatty sparing as a periportal hypoechoic area ➾, in which a portal vein ➾ courses through without deviation or distortion. *(Right)* Oblique ultrasound shows small, hypoechoic, lymphomatous deposits ➾ around the portal vein ➾. Those deposits can be anechoic and may be mistaken for cysts. Such deposits are often referred to as "pseudocystic."

Fatty Sparing, Liver

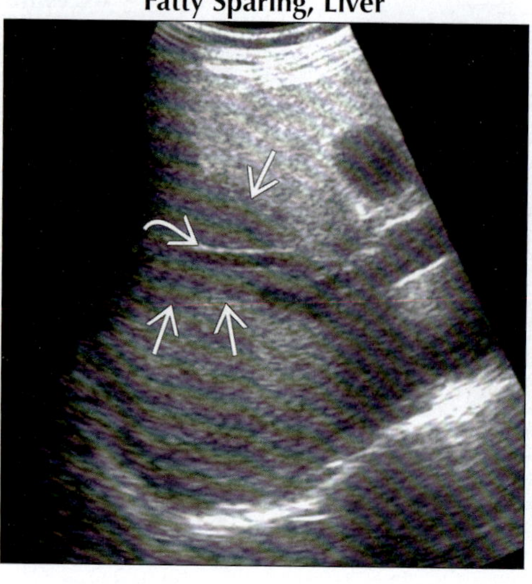

Diffuse/Infiltrative Hepatic Lymphoma

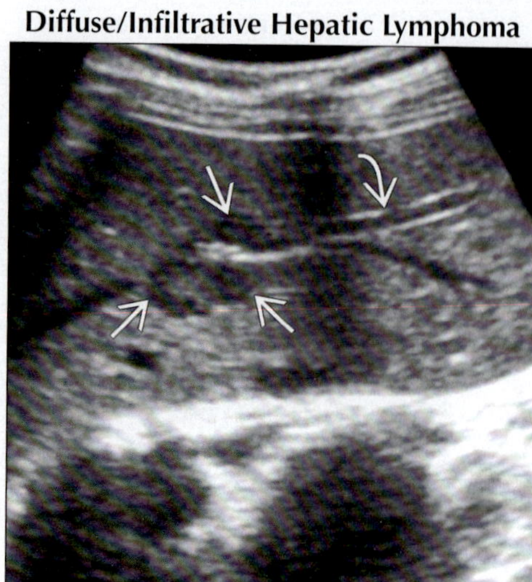

Choledocholithiasis

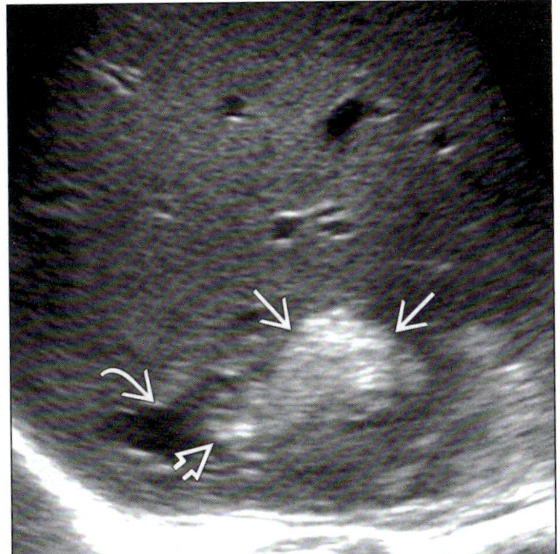

Choledocholithiasis

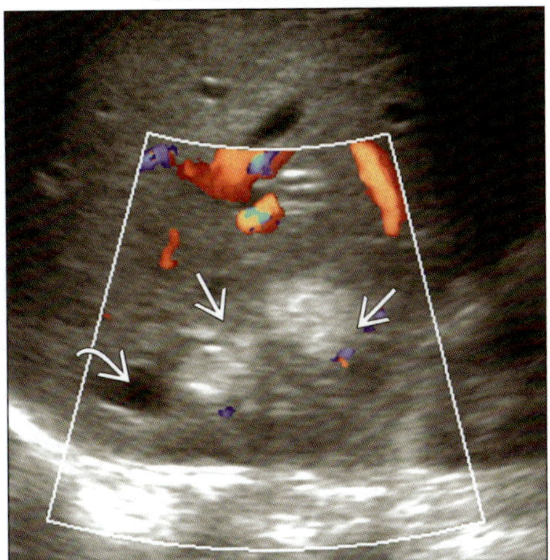

(Left) Oblique transabdominal ultrasound shows a cluster of intrahepatic duct stones as a hyperechoic periportal mass ➡ within a dilated intrahepatic duct ➡. Note the margin of stone within the duct ➡. *(Right)* Oblique transabdominal color Doppler ultrasound in the same patient shows absence of color within the dilated intrahepatic duct ➡ and the echogenic duct stones ➡.

Pneumobilia

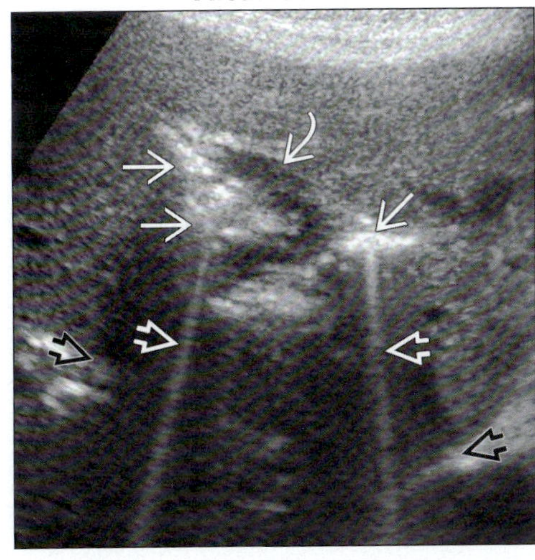

Hepatic Schistosomiasis

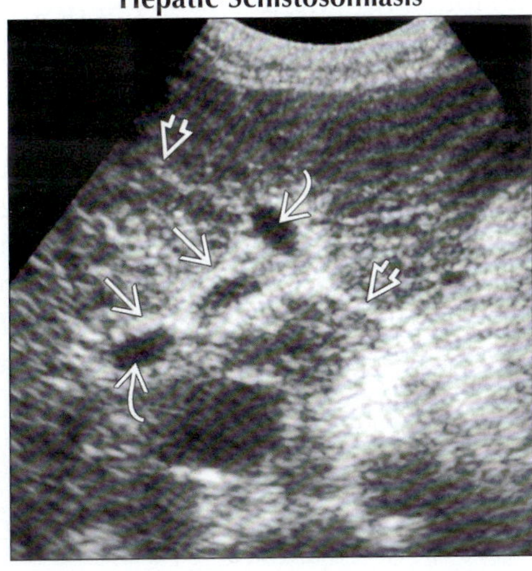

(Left) Transverse US shows biliary duct gas as periportal, highly hyperechoic, linear foci ➡ adjacent to the left portal vein ➡, casting posterior acoustic shadows ➡ with associated reverberation artifacts ➡. *(Right)* Oblique transabdominal US shows a thick layer of hyperechoic periportal fibrosis ➡ around the left portal vein ➡ in schistosomiasis, described as "clay-pipestem" fibrosis. Note septal fibrosis ➡ (inflammation & fibrosis in reaction to embolized eggs).

Recurrent Pyogenic Cholangitis

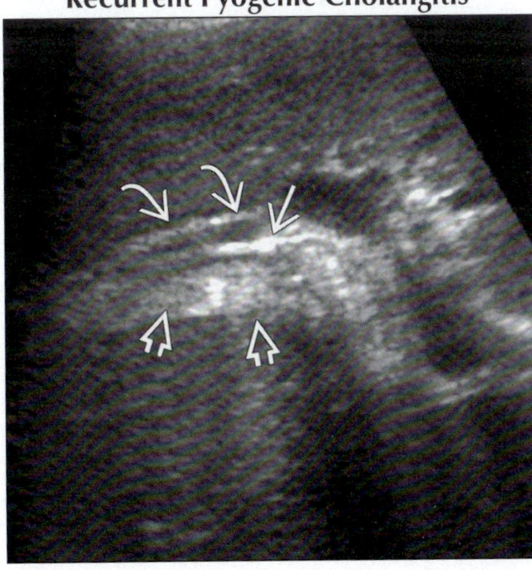

Caroli Disease

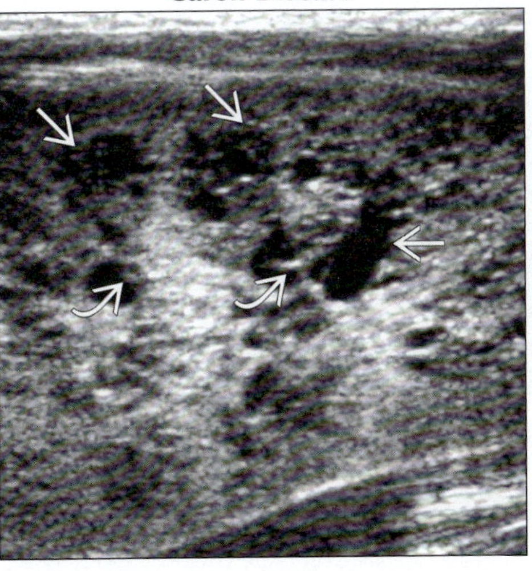

(Left) Oblique ultrasound shows recurrent pyogenic cholangitis with the presence of intrahepatic duct stones ➡, thickening of intrahepatic duct walls ➡, and increased periportal echogenicity ➡ due to inflammation. *(Right)* Transverse transabdominal ultrasound shows multiple, dilated, hypoechoic, intrahepatic ducts ➡ in a patient with Caroli disease. Note the portal veins surrounded by dilated ducts in a "central dot" sign ➡.

DIFFERENTIAL DIAGNOSIS

Common
- Cirrhosis
- Capsular Hepatic Metastasis
- Subcapsular Hepatic Neoplasm
- Postsurgical Hepatic Resection

Less Common
- Ruptured Hepatocellular Carcinoma
- Schistosomiasis

ESSENTIAL INFORMATION

Helpful Clues for Common Diagnoses
- **Cirrhosis**
  - Nodular surface contour
    - Micronodular (< 1 cm diameter): Due to alcoholism
    - Macronodular: Due to viral hepatitis
  - Hypertrophy of caudate lobe and lateral segment of left lobe
  - Atrophy of right lobe and medial segment of left lobe
  - Coarse/nodular parenchymal echopattern
- **Capsular Hepatic Metastasis**
  - Commonly due to gastric, ovarian, or pancreatic primary
  - Sign of peritoneal metastatic disease
  - Commonly associated with ascites
- **Subcapsular Hepatic Neoplasm**
  - Primary or secondary subcapsular neoplasm may distort surface contour when large or numerous
  - Lesions cause architectural distortion of liver parenchyma
  - Treated metastases (e.g., from breast) may shrink and fibrose, simulating nodular contour of cirrhotic liver
- **Postsurgical Hepatic Resection**
  - Combination of surgical defect and surrounding scarring causes irregularity of contour
  - Surgical material ± fat in surgical defect causes further heterogeneity of surgical site

Helpful Clues for Less Common Diagnoses
- **Ruptured Hepatocellular Carcinoma**
  - Echogenic blood clot on surface of liver
  - May see breach of hepatic capsule or irregularity of capsular surface from hepatocellular carcinoma
  - Hemoperitoneum may be present
    - More echogenic than ascites
- **Schistosomiasis**
  - Irregular/notched, liver surface
  - Echogenic periportal fibrotic bands (most severe at porta hepatis)
  - Mosaic pattern: Network of echogenic septa outlining polygonal areas of normal-appearing liver
    - Represents complete septal fibrosis (inflammation and fibrosis as reaction to embolized eggs)

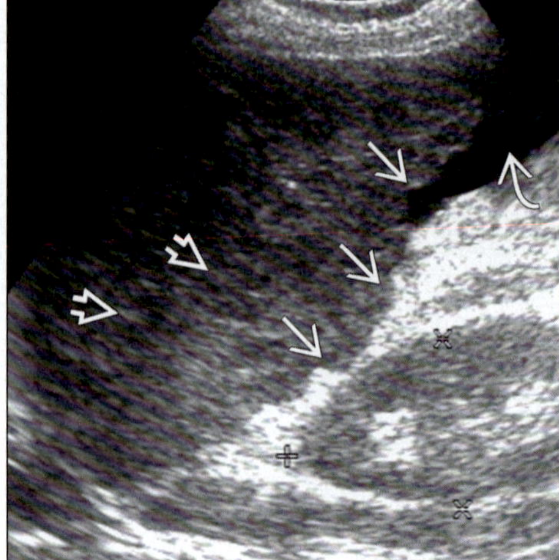

Cirrhosis

Oblique transabdominal ultrasound shows an irregular, nodular, hepatic surface ➡ in macronodular cirrhosis. Note the internal, coarse, nodular echogenicity ➡ and small amount of ascites ➡.

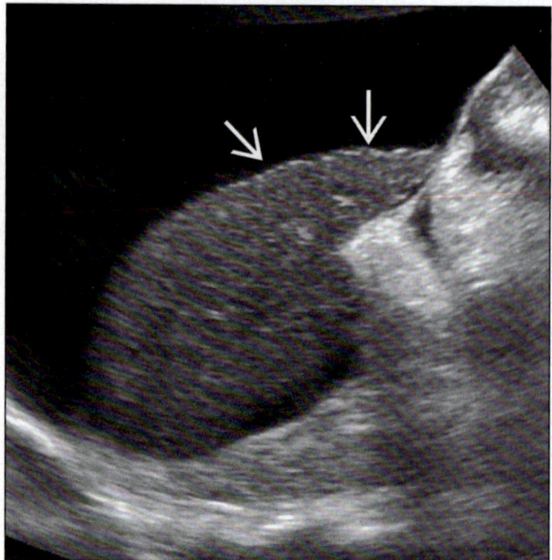

Cirrhosis

Oblique transabdominal ultrasound shows a subtle, nodular, hepatic surface ➡ in micronodular cirrhosis, which is highlighted by the presence of ascites. Note the coarse but not nodular echogenicity of liver.

IRREGULAR HEPATIC SURFACE

Capsular Hepatic Metastasis

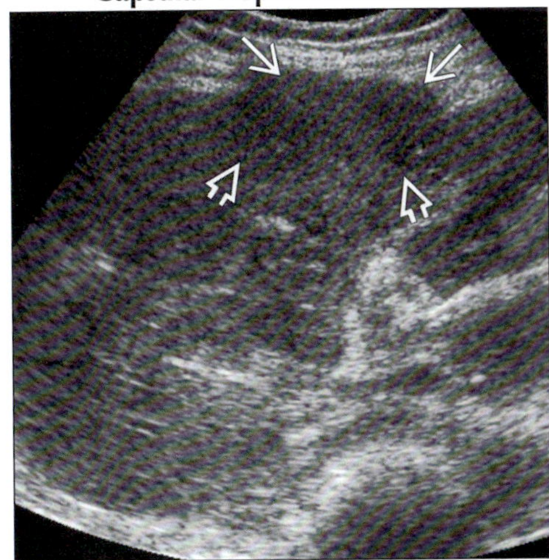

Postsurgical Hepatic Resection

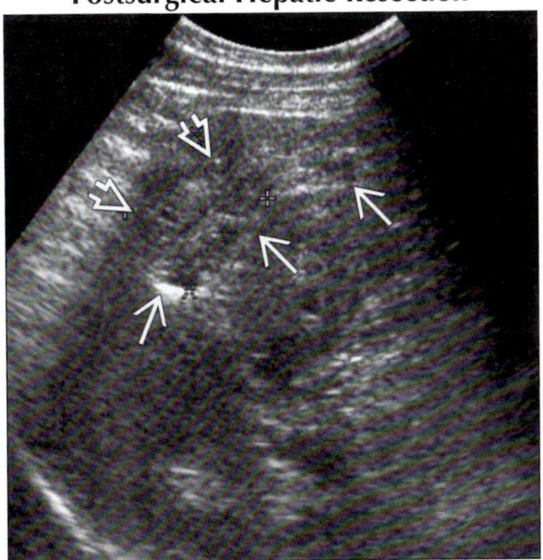

(Left) Oblique transabdominal ultrasound shows an isoechoic metastasis ⇨ on the surface of the right lobe of the liver, causing a lobulated anterior hepatic surface. The mass has infiltrated into the liver ⇨. (Right) Oblique transabdominal ultrasound shows the site of previous resection of hepatocellular carcinoma. Note the adipose tissue ⇨ used for filling the surgical defect and the irregular surface and borders ⇨ it has created.

Subcapsular Hepatic Neoplasm

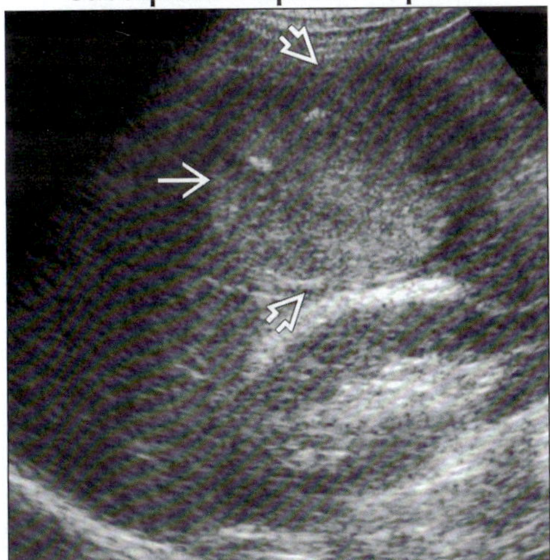

Subcapsular Hepatic Neoplasm

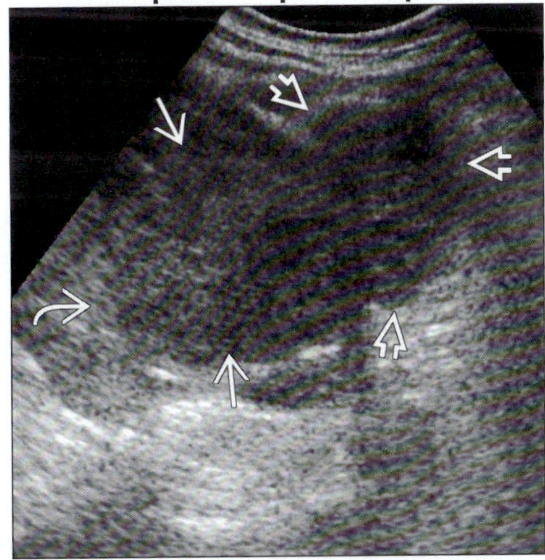

(Left) Oblique transabdominal ultrasound shows a hyperechoic hepatocellular carcinoma ⇨ at inferior right lobe, causing a bulging surface contour ⇨ and expanding the free edge (normally there is a sharp edge of liver over the right kidney). (Right) Oblique transabdominal ultrasound shows a large hepatocellular carcinoma ⇨ with extension through the hepatic capsule, producing a surface protrusion ⇨. Note the irregular border of cirrhotic liver ⇨.

Ruptured Hepatocellular Carcinoma

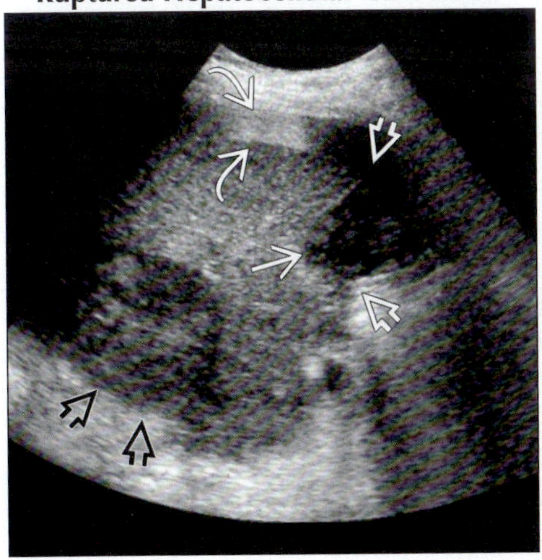

Schistosomiasis

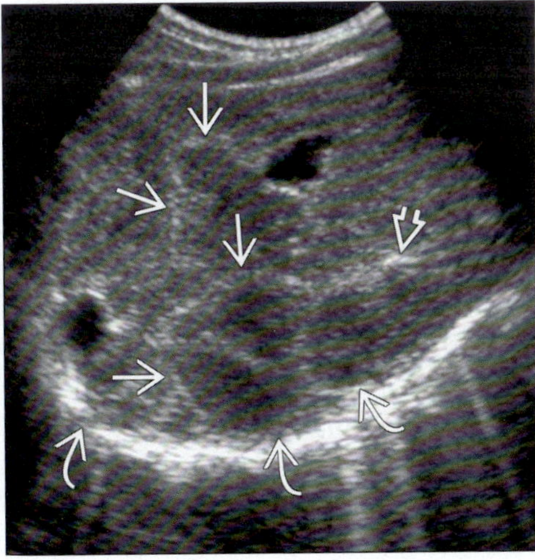

(Left) Oblique transabdominal US shows a break in the hepatic capsule ⇨ in a ruptured hepatocellular carcinoma ⇨. Note the layer of hyperechoic (acute) blood ⇨ on the anterior hepatic surface. A 2nd HCC ⇨ is also seen. (Right) Oblique transabdominal US shows a mosaic network of thickened interlobular septae ⇨ in schistosomiasis. There is also periportal fibrosis ⇨. The hepatic surface is irregular ⇨ due to fibrosis.

3

DIFFERENTIAL DIAGNOSIS

Common
- Complicated Ascites
- Pyogenic Perihepatic Abscess
- Biloma
- Hematoma
- Exophytic Hepatic Cyst
- Perihepatic Seroma/Lymphocele

Less Common
- Pancreatic Pseudocyst
- Gallbladder Carcinoma
- Peritoneal Metastasis
- Ruptured Hepatocellular Carcinoma

ESSENTIAL INFORMATION

Helpful Clues for Common Diagnoses
- **Complicated Ascites**
  - Noncomplicated ascites is freely mobile, homogeneously anechoic, and compressible by transducer pressure
  - Complicated ascites shows loculation and internal septae
    - Exerts mass effect
    - Displaces surrounding structures or depresses/distorts liver contour
    - Usually found in peritoneal recesses
    - Rounded margins
  - Malignant ascites may have thickened interfaces between fluid and adjacent structures
    - Evaluate peritoneal lining, omentum
  - Anechoic content
    - Transudative due to liver disease, congestive cardiac failure, or renal failure
  - Echogenic content
    - Exudative due to infection, inflammation, blood, or neoplasm
- **Pyogenic Perihepatic Abscess**
  - Usual locations
    - Subphrenic (superior to coronary ligament)
    - Subhepatic (inferior to coronary ligament)
    - Bare area (confined within attachment of coronary ligament)
  - Crescentic/ovoid fluid collection on liver surface
  - Echogenic content due to internal debris
  - May contain gas mixed with fluid

- Gas appears as echogenic foci with posterior ring-down artifact
  - Subphrenic abscess may be associated with pleural effusion/basal lung atelectasis
  - Thick and irregular wall
  - Peripheral/rim vascularity may be seen on color Doppler
- **Biloma**
  - Focal fluid collection close to biliary tree
    - Round or oval-shaped
    - Thin/nondiscernible wall
    - Posterior acoustic enhancement
    - Usually unilocular
  - Large lesion may compress liver
  - Fresh biloma
    - Anechoic fluid
    - No vascularity on color Doppler
  - Infected biloma
    - Debris or septae
    - May show increased vascularity in adjacent tissue
- **Hematoma**
  - Lentiform or curvilinear collection on surface of liver
  - History of trauma
    - Commonly involves segments 6, 7, or 8
  - Rupture of hepatic capsule may be seen as gap in hepatic contour (laceration)
  - Hepatic fracture defined as laceration extending across 2 surfaces
  - Echogenicity of contents dependent on age of hemorrhage
    - Initially: Echogenic
    - After 4-5 days: Hypoechoic
    - After 1-4 weeks: Internal echoes and septation may develop within hematoma
  - Rate of hematoma evolution depends on vascularity of region
    - Slower for intraperitoneal or subcapsular regions
    - Faster for parenchymal hematoma
  - Other signs of trauma
    - Hemoperitoneum
    - Right renal or splenic laceration/hematoma
  - CT is modality of choice in patients with suspected liver trauma
- **Exophytic Hepatic Cyst**
  - Anechoic if cyst is sterile
  - Smooth borders (occasionally lobulated)
  - Thin or nondetectable wall

PERIHEPATIC CYST/FLUID COLLECTION

- o No or few septations
- o No mural nodule or wall calcification
- o Normal adjacent hepatic parenchyma
- o Internal debris or septae if infected or hemorrhagic
- o Posterior acoustic enhancement
- o Color Doppler shows no internal or mural vascularity
- **Perihepatic Seroma/Lymphocele**
  - o May be anechoic or contain debris or septae and loculations
  - o Thick and irregular wall may be present
  - o Difficult to distinguish from biloma
    - Aspiration biopsy may be required for accurate diagnosis

Helpful Clues for Less Common Diagnoses
- **Pancreatic Pseudocyst**
  - o History of pancreatitis usually elicited
    - Pseudocyst develops > 4 weeks after acute pancreatitis
  - o Amylase rich
  - o May extend into lesser sac, mediastinum, lower quadrant of abdomen
    - Often see multiple cysts in various locations
  - o Uncomplicated pseudocyst
    - Smooth walled
    - Unilocular
    - Anechoic
    - Posterior acoustic enhancement
  - o Complicated pseudocyst
    - Multilocular or with septae
    - Internal echoes ± fluid-debris level

- Wall calcification
- **Gallbladder Carcinoma**
  - o Asymmetrical gallbladder wall thickening
  - o Internal masses or thick septae
  - o Distortion of gallbladder contour
  - o Irregularity of gallbladder wall
  - o Gallstones, wall calcification, tumoral calcification
  - o Infiltration of adjacent liver
  - o Associated lymphadenopathy
    - Porta hepatis, celiac
- **Peritoneal Metastasis**
  - o More rounded in contour (rather than crescentic)
  - o Associated with ascites (complicated)
  - o Thick irregular wall ± vascularity
- **Ruptured Hepatocellular Carcinoma**
  - o Collection associated with hypoechoic heterogeneous mass close to liver surface
  - o Hemoperitoneum: Fluid collection with fine echogenic debris/echoes
  - o Color Doppler shows irregular hypervascularity within hepatocellular carcinoma
  - o Tumor thrombus within portal veins may be present, ± thrombus vascularity
  - o Signs of cirrhosis, portal hypertension

Complicated Ascites

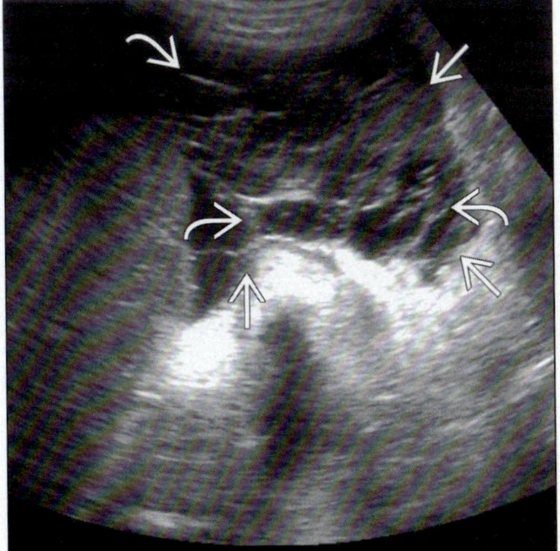

Longitudinal transabdominal ultrasound shows loculated ascites ➡ with multiple internal fibrin strands ➡ inferior to the right lobe of the liver. Noncomplicated ascites moves freely and is anechoic.

Complicated Ascites

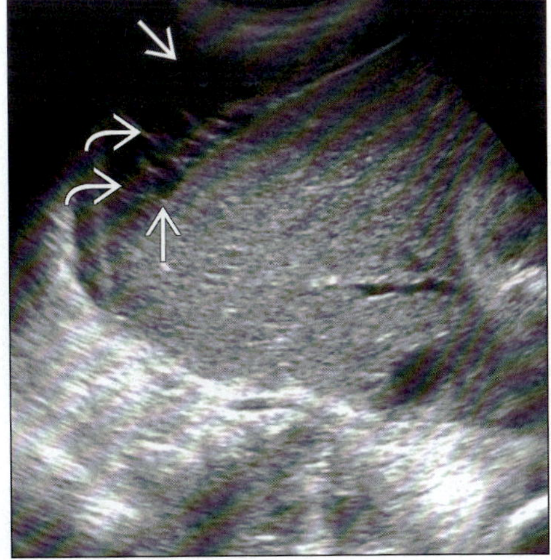

Oblique transabdominal ultrasound shows loculated ascites ➡ with multiple internal fibrin strands ➡ in the subphrenic space.

3

PERIHEPATIC CYST/FLUID COLLECTION

(Left) Longitudinal transabdominal ultrasound shows malignant ascites ➡ with multiple internal septations ➡ inferior to the liver surface. Note that the presence of septae is not specific to malignancy. *(Right)* Oblique transabdominal ultrasound shows ascites ➡ which was loculated in the posterior subdiaphragmatic recess. Note the cirrhotic change in the liver ➡.

Complicated Ascites

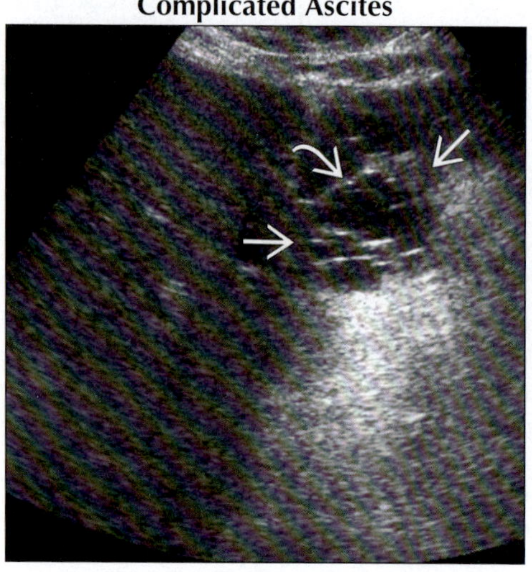

Complicated Ascites

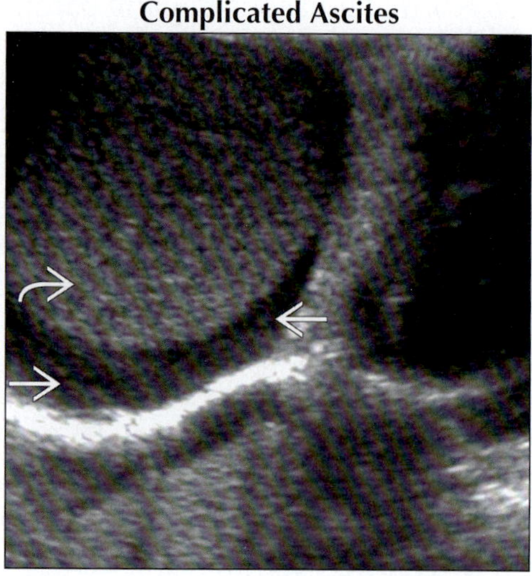

(Left) Oblique transabdominal ultrasound shows a hypoechoic subphrenic abscess ➡ with low-level echogenic debris ➡ and lobular indentation on the liver surface ➡. *(Right)* Oblique transabdominal ultrasound shows a subphrenic abscess ➡ and pleural effusion ➡. Note the diaphragm ➡. An abscess at this location is frequently associated with pleural effusion and atelectasis.

Pyogenic Perihepatic Abscess

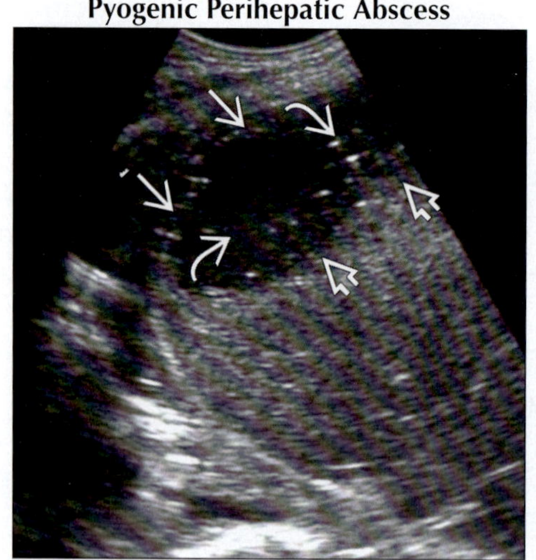

Pyogenic Perihepatic Abscess

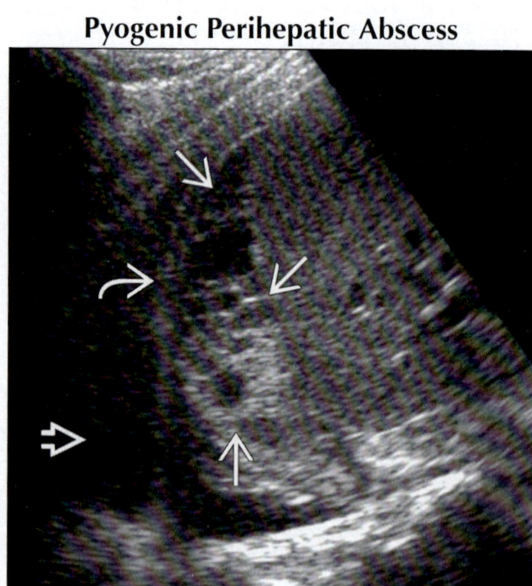

(Left) Oblique ultrasound shows an anechoic abscess ➡ in the bare area of the liver (mainly the posterior surface of the right lobe). The lack of echoes and a thick wall make this similar to an anechoic collection of ascites. *(Right)* Transverse ultrasound shows an infected subhepatic biloma ➡ inferior to the left hepatic lobe surface. Note the presence of internal septae ➡ and posterior acoustic enhancement ➡. Sterile bilomas tend to be anechoic.

Pyogenic Perihepatic Abscess

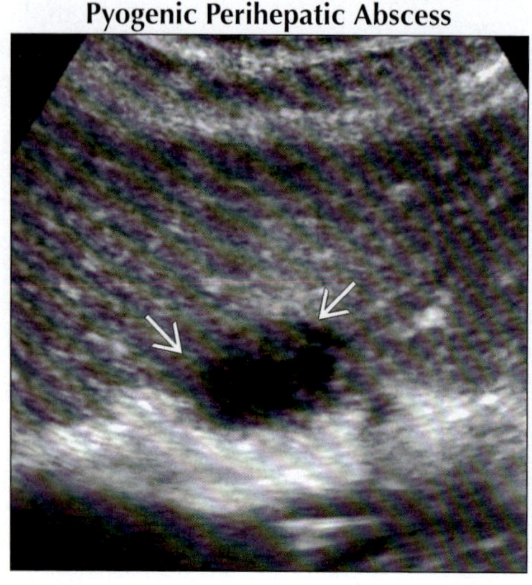

Biloma

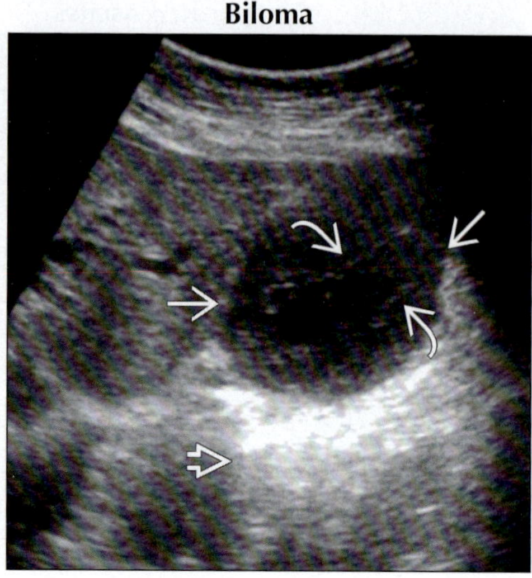

PERIHEPATIC CYST/FLUID COLLECTION

Hematoma

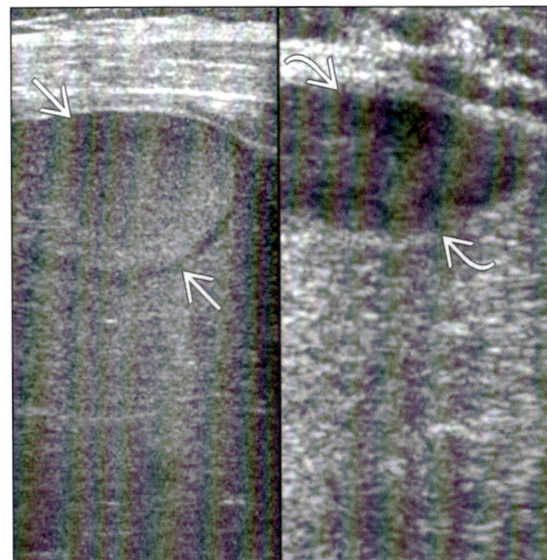

Exophytic Hepatic Cyst

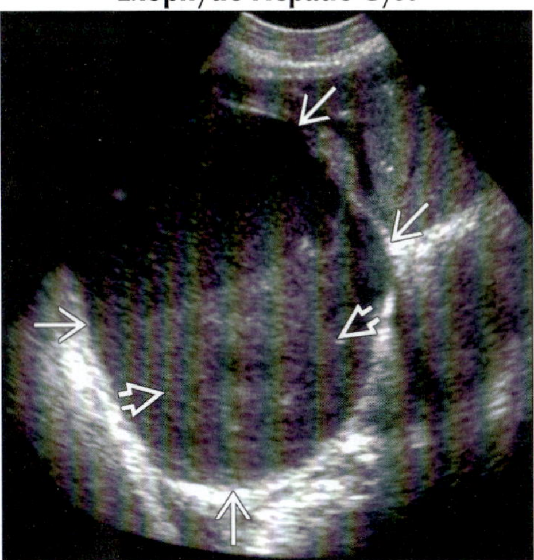

(Left) Composite image shows a subcapsular hematoma indenting the liver surface and its evolution from isoechoic ➡ (left) to hypoechoic ➡ (right) over a 2-week period. Note the contraction of the hematoma and the formation of fibrin strands. *(Right)* Longitudinal ultrasound shows a large, exophytic, hepatic cyst ➡ with debris ➡ gravitating posteriorly. The debris was from a previous hemorrhage.

Pancreatic Pseudocyst

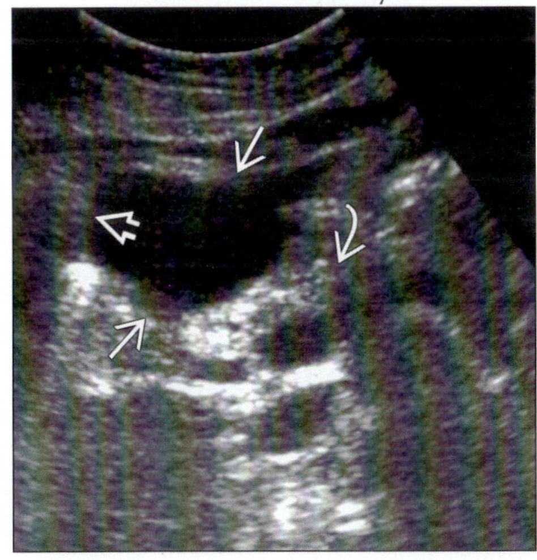

Gallbladder Carcinoma

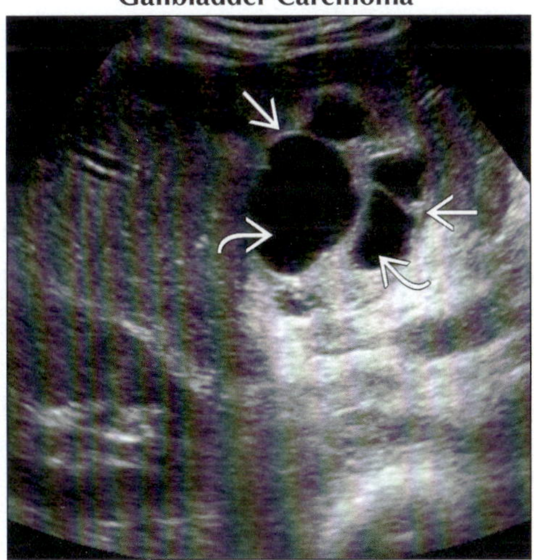

(Left) Transverse transabdominal ultrasound shows a well-circumscribed unilocular pseudocyst ➡ in contact with the inferior liver surface ➡ and anterior to the pancreatic head ➡. *(Right)* Transverse transabdominal ultrasound shows a multiloculated, cystic, gallbladder carcinoma ➡ at the edge of the liver. Note the lack of internal echoes ➡ in the cystic components.

Peritoneal Metastasis

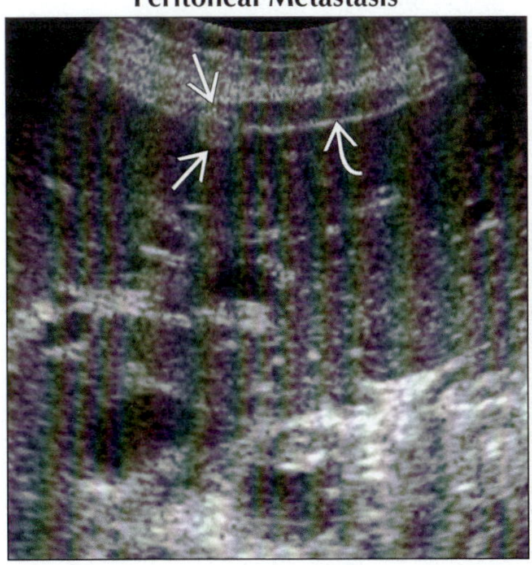

Ruptured Hepatocellular Carcinoma

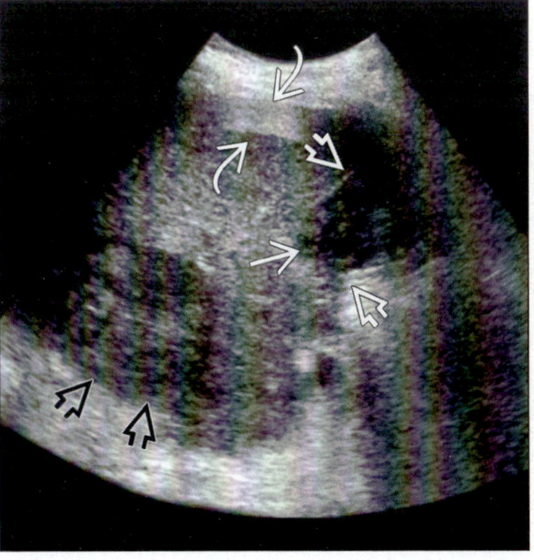

(Left) Transverse ultrasound shows a small, hyperechoic, peritoneal deposit ➡ at the anterior liver surface. There is a thin layer of loculated ascitic fluid ➡ adjacent to the deposit. The appearance suggests peritoneal metastasis. *(Right)* Oblique transabdominal ultrasound shows a break in the hepatic capsule ➡ in a ruptured hepatocellular carcinoma ➡. Note a layer of hyperechoic (acute) blood ➡ on the anterior hepatic surface and the presence of a 2nd HCC ➡ in the liver.

DIFFERENTIAL DIAGNOSIS

Common
- Portal Hypertension
- Portosystemic Collaterals
- Bland Portal Vein Thrombosis
- Portal Vein Tumor Thrombus

Less Common
- Portal Vein Gas

ESSENTIAL INFORMATION

Helpful Clues for Common Diagnoses
- **Portal Hypertension**
  - Portal venous pressure is 10 mmHg or greater than inferior vena cava pressure
  - Portal vein may be dilated (not sensitive sign)
  - Color Doppler shows decreased hepatopetal flow or reversed (hepatofugal) flow in main portal vein/splenic vein
  - Pulsed Doppler shows lack of respiratory phasicity
  - Decreased portal vein flow velocity
  - Background cirrhosis, splenomegaly, ascites, thickened bowel wall
  - Development of portosystemic shunts
- **Portosystemic Collaterals**
  - Common locations
    - Inferior hepatic margin via gastroepiploic vein
    - Gastroesophageal junction via left gastric vein
    - Anterior abdominal wall via ligamentum teres
    - Lienorenal ligament via lienorenal collaterals
  - Color Doppler shows low velocity hepatofugal flow
- **Bland Portal Vein Thrombosis**
  - Echogenic material within portal vein
  - Poor/no visualization of portal vein (filled with isoechoic thrombus)
  - Cavernous transformation of portal vein
  - Color Doppler shows interrupted/irregular flow in portal vein
  - Pulsed Doppler shows decreased or absent flow in portal vein
  - Signs of liver dysfunction or portal hypertension: Cirrhosis, ascites, splenomegaly
- **Portal Vein Tumor Thrombus**
  - Majority arise from hepatocellular carcinoma
  - Echogenic material within portal vein
  - Suspect tumor thrombus if there is adjacent hepatic tumor
  - Color Doppler may show tumor vessels or abnormal flow within thrombus

Helpful Clues for Less Common Diagnoses
- **Portal Vein Gas**
  - Echogenic foci in portal vein
  - Moves to periphery of liver (opposite to biliary gas, which moves to liver hilum)

Portal Hypertension

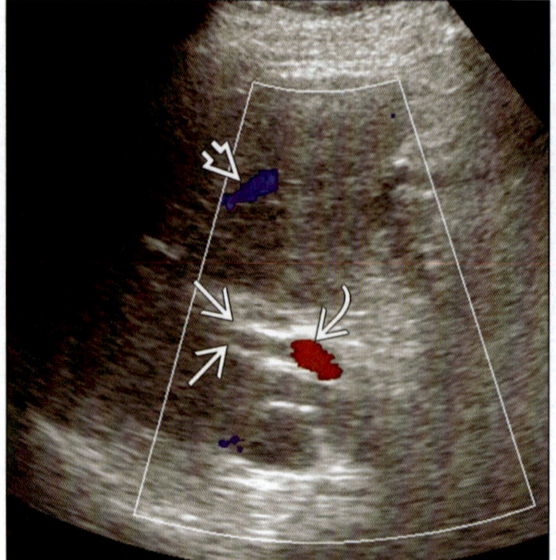

Oblique color Doppler ultrasound shows decreased portal vein ➡ flow in portal hypertension. Note that the flow direction ➡ remains hepatopetal, opposite to the flow direction of the hepatic vein ➡.

Portal Hypertension

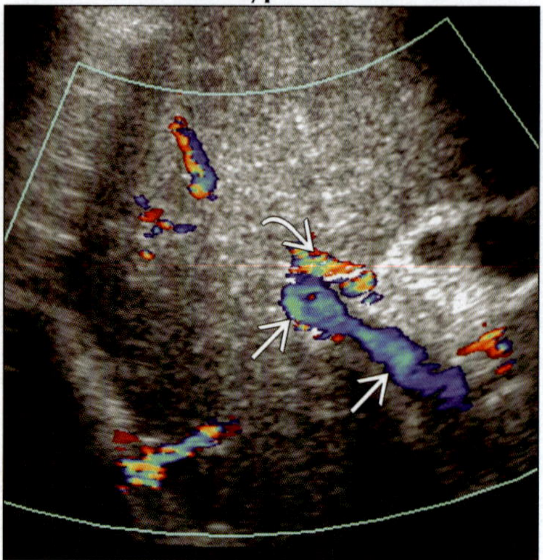

Oblique transabdominal US shows hepatofugal flow ➡ in this case of cirrhosis with portal hypertension. The adjacent hepatic artery ➡ is hypertrophied and shows aliasing artifact on the venous Doppler flow setting.

PORTAL VEIN ABNORMALITY

Portosystemic Collaterals

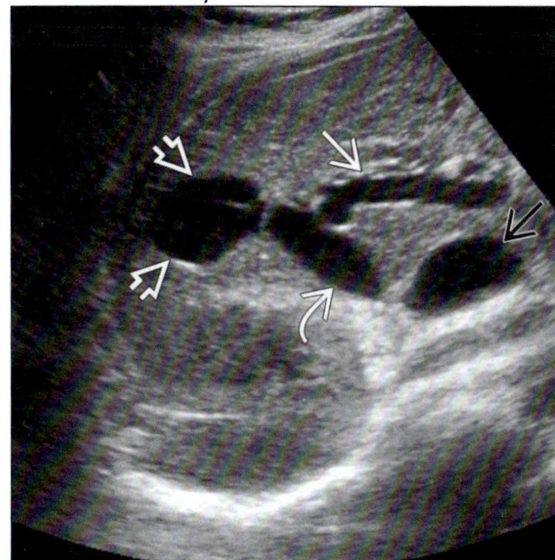

Portosystemic Collaterals

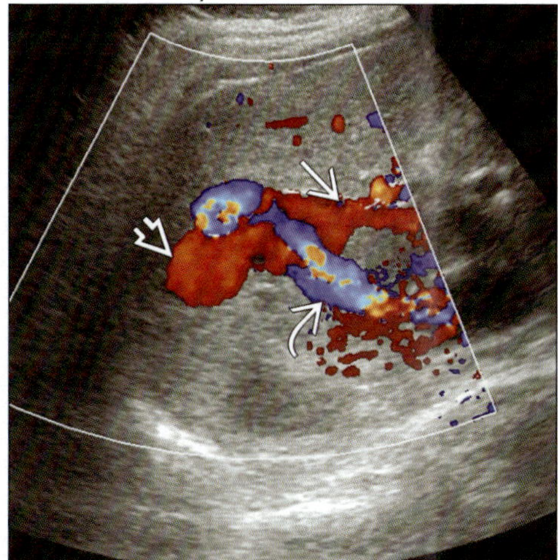

(Left) Transverse transabdominal ultrasound shows an intrahepatic portosystemic shunt ⊟ between the portal vein ⊟ and a dilated branch of the hepatic vein ⊟ and inferior vena cava ⊟ in the right lobe of the liver. *(Right)* Transverse color Doppler ultrasound in the same patient shows the portosystemic shunt ⊟ draining blood flow from the portal vein ⊟ to the dilated branch of the hepatic vein ⊟.

Bland Portal Vein Thrombosis

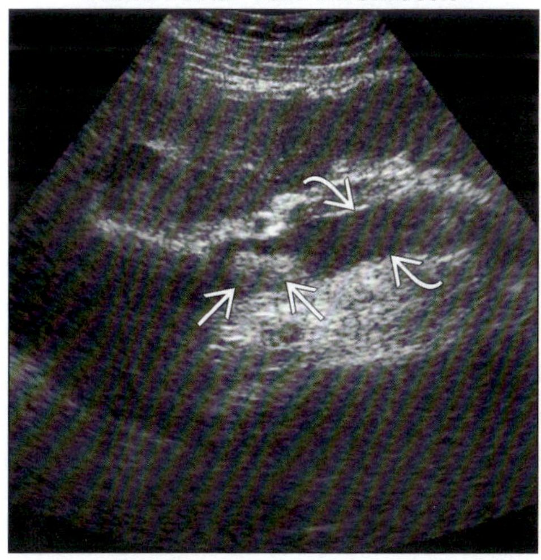

Bland Portal Vein Thrombosis

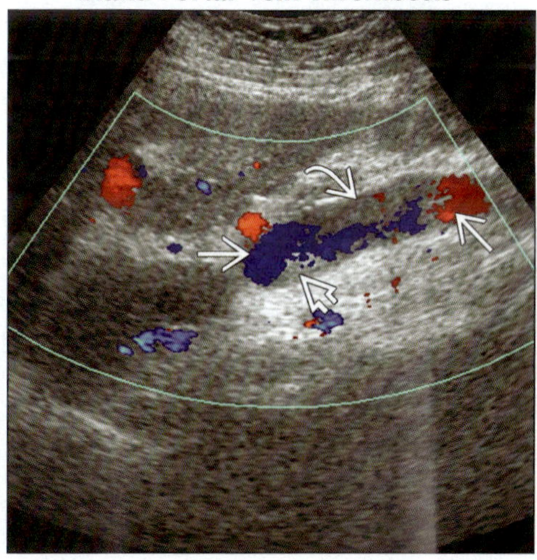

(Left) Oblique transabdominal US shows a nonocclusive echogenic thrombus ⊟ in the main portal vein ⊟. *(Right)* Oblique color Doppler US shows the presence of color flow ⊟ in the residual lumen of the main portal vein in nonocclusive portal vein thrombosis ⊟. Note the lack of color seen in part of the patent lumen ⊟ due to the angling effect of Doppler US. It is important to evaluate the portal vein from multiple angles to confirm thrombosis.

Portal Vein Tumor Thrombus

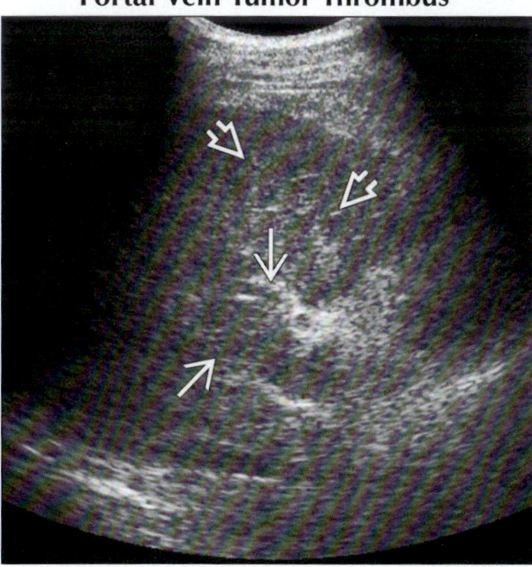

Portal Vein Tumor Thrombus

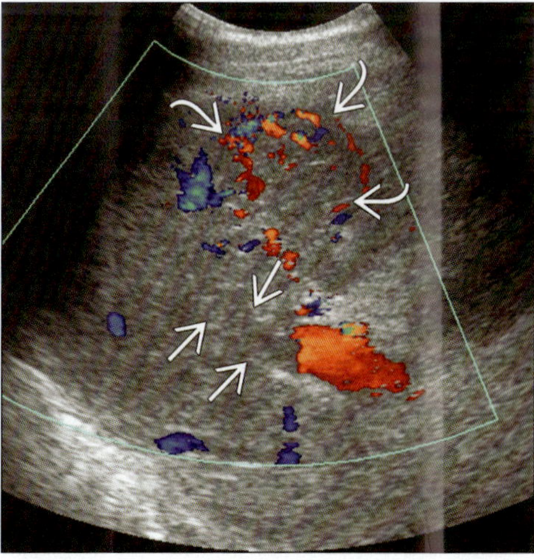

(Left) Oblique transabdominal ultrasound shows an occlusive portal vein tumor thrombus ⊟ in a cirrhotic patient with a heterogeneous liver echopattern ⊟. and isoechoic hepatocellular carcinoma. *(Right)* Oblique color Doppler ultrasound shows an occlusive portal vein invasion with absence of color flow ⊟. Note the chaotic vascularity ⊟ in the heterogeneous hepatic parenchyma, indicating the presence of infiltrative hepatocellular carcinoma.

3

DIFFERENTIAL DIAGNOSIS

Common
- Porta Hepatis Lymph Node
- Porta Hepatis Lymphomatous Node
- Gallstones
- Gallbladder Carcinoma
- Klatskin Tumor
- Biloma
- Pancreatic Pseudocyst
- Pancreatic Neoplasm
- Porta Hepatis Metastases
- Gastric Neoplasm
- Amebic Hepatic Abscess

Less Common
- Choledochal Cyst
- Varices

Rare but Important
- Hepatic Artery Aneurysm

ESSENTIAL INFORMATION

Helpful Clues for Common Diagnoses
- **Porta Hepatis Lymph Node**
  - Hypoechoic nodule(s) of small size (< 1 cm short axis) suggests inflammatory node
  - Large node (> 1 cm short axis) suggests neoplastic infiltration
  - Hypoechoic center may indicate central necrosis
    - Suggestive of TB or necrotic metastasis
  - Fatty hilum difficult to discern; size is main criterion for distinguishing reactive from malignant nodes
  - Color or power Doppler for vascularity assessment usually not practical as lesions are deep and small
- **Porta Hepatis Lymphomatous Node**
  - Hypoechoic/anechoic "pseudocystic" nodule(s)
  - Low echogenicity due to high cellular density and lack of background stroma
  - May form conglomerate mass when nearby lymph nodes fuse (mimics abscess)
  - Other signs of lymphoma
    - Lymphadenopathy: Hepatogastric, celiac, paraaortic, mesenteric, etc.
    - Hepatomegaly: Diffuse infiltration usually as secondary site in Hodgkin and non-Hodgkin lymphoma

  - Hepatic hypoechoic masses: Discrete lesions more likely to be primary non-Hodgkin lymphoma or AIDS-associated lymphoma
  - Splenomegaly, bowel wall thickening, ascites
- **Gallstones**
  - Highly reflective foci within gallbladder lumen
  - Posterior acoustic shadowing
  - Reverberation artifact
  - Gravitates to dependent part of gallbladder on movement
    - Not useful when gallbladder not visualized due to contraction or packed with stones
  - No color flow on Doppler
- **Gallbladder Carcinoma**
  - Echogenic mass
  - Polypoidal or irregular shape
  - Distortion or thickening of remaining gallbladder wall
  - Biliary dilatation if carcinoma infiltrates into hepatic confluence
  - Large carcinoma may extend into liver
  - Calcified gallbladder wall (porcelain gallbladder)
  - Associated lymphadenopathy: Cystic duct, porta hepatis, celiac
  - Color Doppler: Areas of increased vascularity within carcinoma
- **Klatskin Tumor**
  - Cholangiocarcinoma at confluence of left and right hepatic ducts
  - Dilatated intrahepatic ducts without dilatation of common hepatic or common bile duct
  - Nonunion of dilated left and right hepatic ducts
  - Primary tumor may be difficult to visualize; infiltrative and isoechoic to liver
  - Nodular or polypoidal mass in/around confluence of ducts
  - May invade portal vein or hepatic artery
- **Biloma**
  - Well-circumscribed anechoic (fresh biloma) collection of fluid
  - Usually unilocular
  - Fine internal septae/debris suggest infected biloma
  - Posterior acoustic enhancement

○ Round or oval-shaped
○ Larger lesions may compress adjacent liver structure/distort architecture
○ No vascularity on color Doppler for simple biloma
○ Vascularity may be present in surrounding inflamed tissue in infected biloma
- **Pancreatic Pseudocyst**
  ○ 1/3 of pseudocysts occur in extrapancreatic location
  ○ Develops 4-6 weeks after onset of acute pancreatitis
  ○ Well circumscribed, smooth walled
  ○ Unilocular anechoic mass
  ○ May contain fluid-debris level, internal echoes, and septations from hemorrhage or infection
  ○ Posterior acoustic enhancement
  ○ Wall may calcify
  ○ May compress common bile duct and cause biliary duct dilatation
- **Pancreatic Neoplasm**
  ○ Serous more common in pancreatic head, & mucinous more common in body & tail
  ○ Serous cystadenoma
    - Well-demarcated mass with external lobulations
    - Slightly echogenic (solid-appearing) mass
    - Amorphous central calcification (with posterior acoustic shadowing)
    - Rarely causes bile duct dilatation because of its soft consistency
    - Increased vascularity in peripheral portion of mass or in septae

○ Mucinous cystic neoplasm
  - Well-demarcated, thick-walled, cystic mass; thick septae
  - Cysts may be anechoic or contain echogenic debris
  - Solid nodule protruding into cyst suggests malignancy
  - Hypovascular on color Doppler
○ Ductal carcinoma
  - Poorly defined mass
  - Hypoechoic to rest of pancreatic parenchyma
  - Diffuse pancreatic involvement may make it difficult to differentiate from acute pancreatitis
- **Porta Hepatis Metastases**
  ○ May represent transcelomic intraperitoneal metastasis (from gastric, pancreatic, ovarian primary lesions)
  ○ Lymph node metastasis from hepatocellular carcinoma, cholangiocarcinoma, gallbladder carcinoma, etc.
- **Gastric Neoplasm**
  ○ Mass continuous with gastric wall or pylorus
  ○ Slightly echogenic mass with irregular borders
  ○ Vascularity demonstrable on color Doppler
- **Amebic Hepatic Abscess**
  ○ More likely than pyogenic abscess to occur in liver periphery (or porta hepatis) than pyogenic abscess

Porta Hepatis Lymph Node

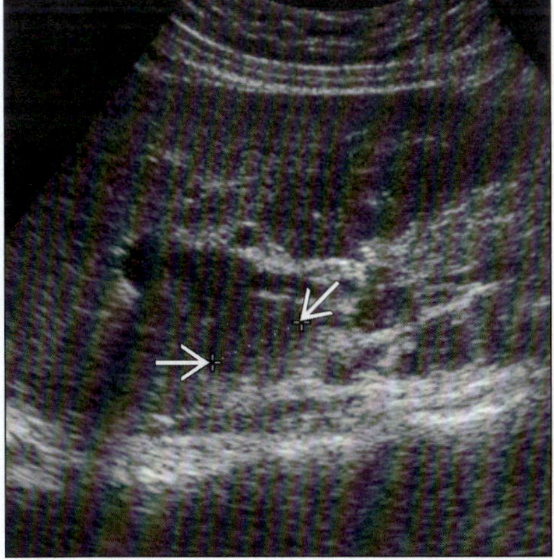

Oblique transabdominal ultrasound shows an enlarged, hypoechoic, inflammatory lymph node ➡ *at the porta hepatis. This patient was suffering from chronic active hepatitis.*

Gallstones

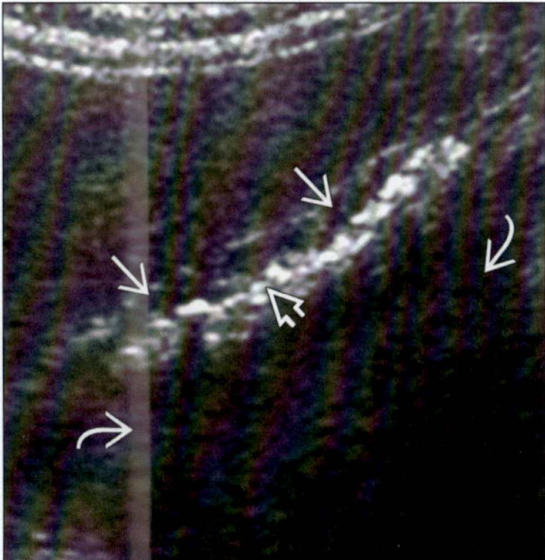

Oblique transabdominal ultrasound shows a contracted gallbladder ➡ *filled with echogenic gallstones* ➡ *at the gallbladder fossa. Note the posterior acoustic shadow cast by the whole gallbladder* ➡.

MASS IN PORTA HEPATIS

(Left) Oblique transabdominal ultrasound shows enlarged (> 1 cm) lymph nodes ➡ at the porta hepatis in a patient with lymphoma. Note the hypoechoic mass differs, mainly in size, when compared to inflammatory nodes. *(Right)* Oblique transabdominal ultrasound shows multiple, well-defined, hypoechoic lymphomatous deposits ➡ in the right lobe of the liver, extending centrally to the porta hepatis.

Porta Hepatis Lymphomatous Node

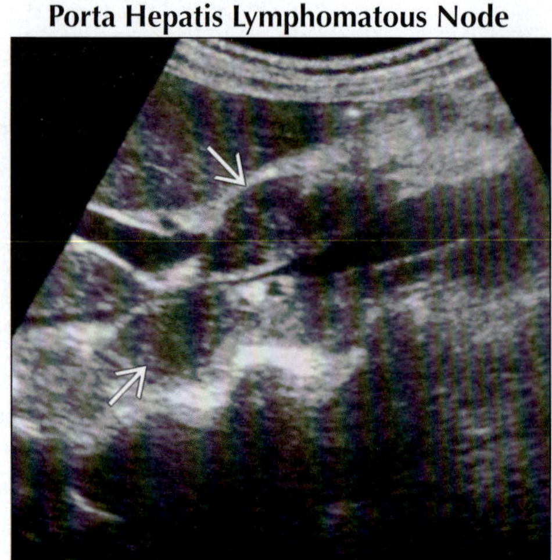

Porta Hepatis Lymphomatous Node

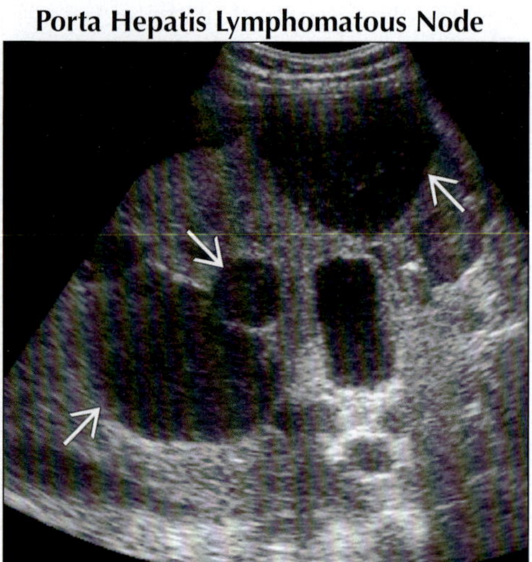

(Left) Oblique transabdominal ultrasound shows an irregular gallbladder carcinoma ➡ at the porta hepatis, infiltrating the common bile duct ➡ and adjacent hepatic parenchyma, causing biliary duct dilatation ➡. *(Right)* Transverse transabdominal ultrasound shows a multiloculated, cystic gallbladder carcinoma ➡. Note that this large, irregular, thick-walled mass in the gallbladder fossa has extended to the porta hepatis ➡.

Gallbladder Carcinoma

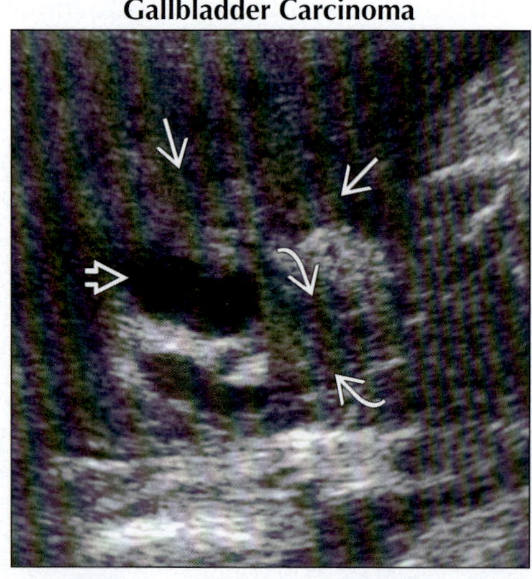

Gallbladder Carcinoma

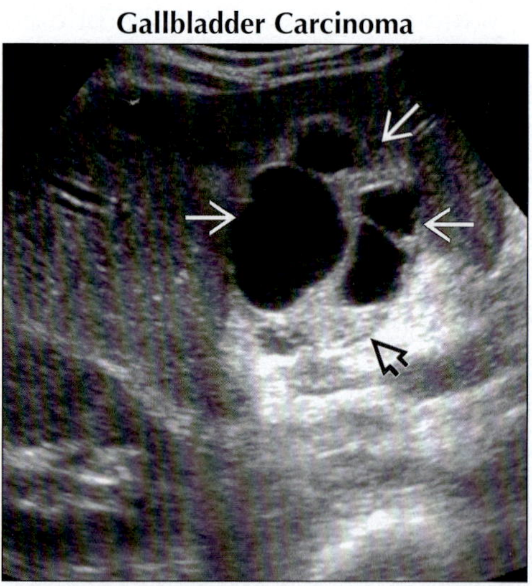

(Left) Transverse transabdominal ultrasound shows an ill-defined, isoechoic mass ➡ at the porta hepatis, causing left and right intrahepatic duct dilatation ➡. This was biopsied and confirmed to be cholangiocarcinoma (Klatskin tumor). *(Right)* Oblique transabdominal ultrasound shows an anechoic mass ➡ representing a sterile biloma. Its neck ➡ extends to the porta hepatis, giving a clue to the diagnosis.

Klatskin Tumor

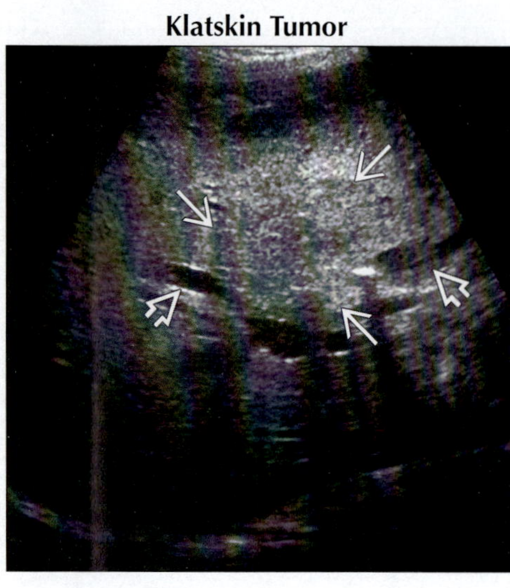

Biloma

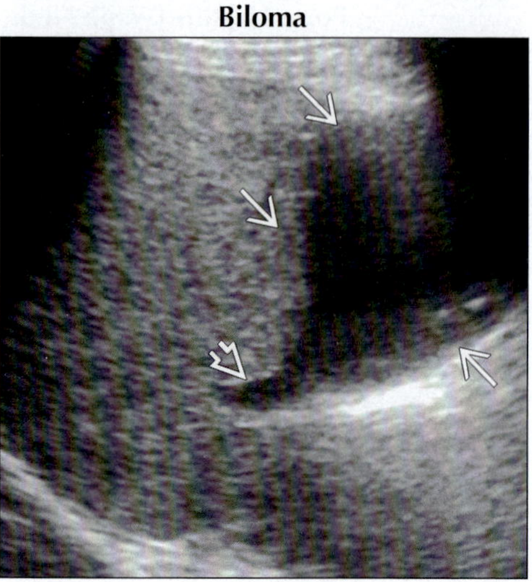

MASS IN PORTA HEPATIS

Pancreatic Pseudocyst

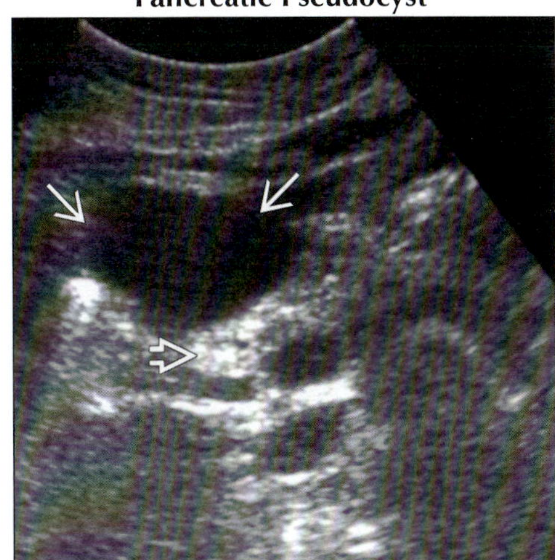

Pancreatic Neoplasm

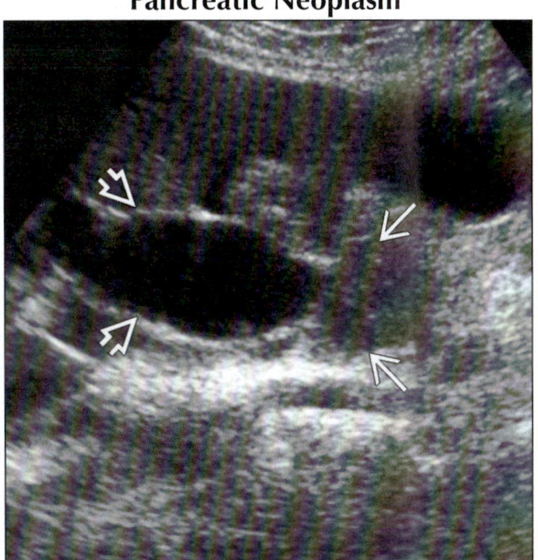

(Left) Transverse transabdominal US shows a well-defined anechoic mass ➡ representing a pancreatic pseudocyst, which is in contact with the pancreatic head ➡ and extends to the porta hepatis. (Right) Oblique transabdominal US shows an ill-defined, hypoechoic mass ➡ in the pancreatic head, causing truncation of the distal common bile duct and associated proximal duct dilatation ➡. This mass was a ductal pancreatic carcinoma.

Gastric Neoplasm

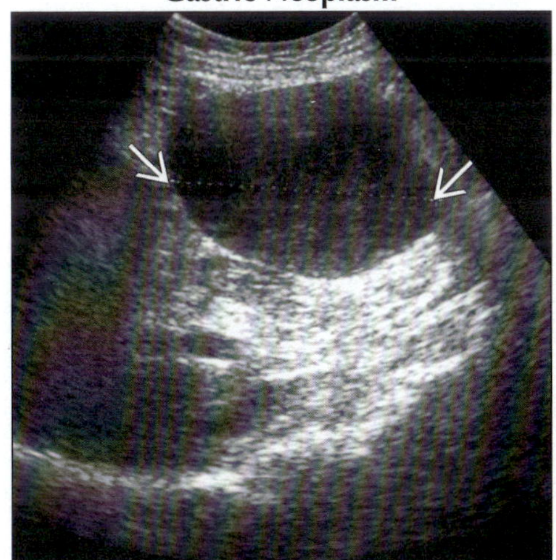

Amebic Hepatic Abscess

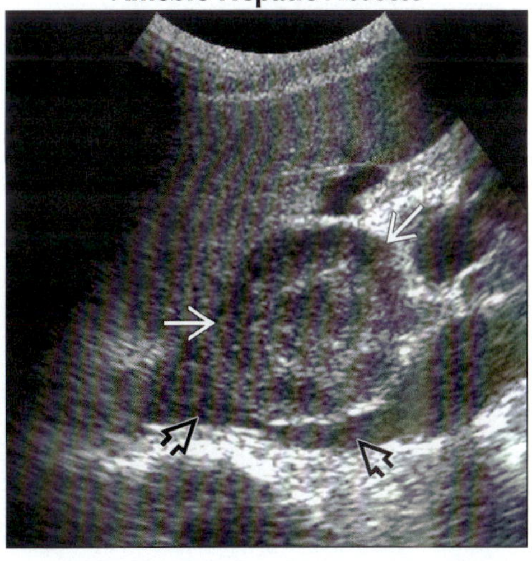

(Left) Oblique transabdominal ultrasound shows a large, well-circumscribed, hypoechoic gastric leiomyoma ➡ inferior to the hepatic surface, adjacent to the porta hepatis region. (Right) Oblique transabdominal ultrasound shows an amebic abscess ➡ at the porta hepatis region compressing the adjacent inferior vena cava ➡.

Choledochal Cyst

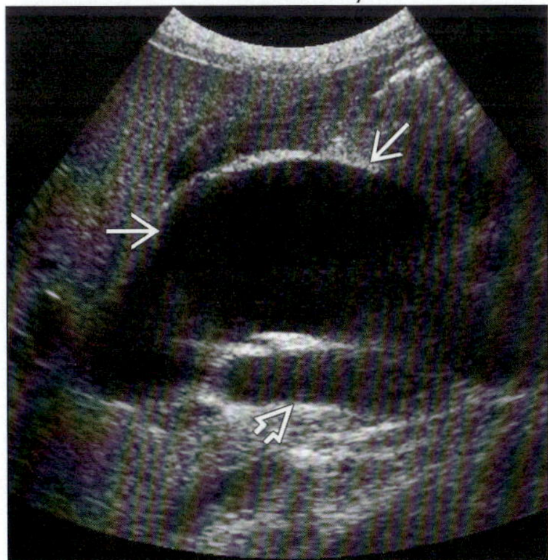

Choledochal Cyst

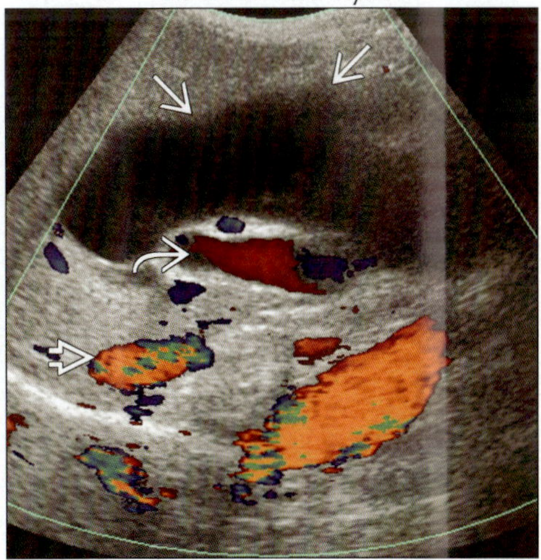

(Left) Oblique transabdominal ultrasound shows a large, anechoic, fusiform, tubular dilatation of the extrahepatic common bile duct ➡, anterior to the main portal vein ➡. This tubular structure shows a smooth contour and thin wall. This is a type 1 choledochal cyst. (Right) Oblique color Doppler ultrasound in the same patient shows absence of color flow within the choledochal cyst ➡. Note the flow in the portal vein ➡ and inferior vena cava ➡.

SECTION 4
Biliary System

Gallbladder

Bile Ducts

HYPOECHOIC GALLBLADDER WALL THICKENING

DIFFERENTIAL DIAGNOSIS

Common
- Acute Calculous Cholecystitis
- Chronic Cholecystitis
- Hyperplastic Cholecystosis
- Wall Thickening due to Systemic Diseases
  - Congestive Heart Failure
  - Renal Failure
  - Hepatic Cirrhosis
  - Hypoalbuminemia

Less Common
- Acute Acalculous Cholecystitis
- Acute Hepatitis
- Perforated Peptic Ulcer
- Acute Pancreatitis
- Gallbladder Carcinoma
- Lymphoma
- AIDS-Related Cholangiopathy

ESSENTIAL INFORMATION

Key Differential Diagnosis Issues
- Clinical information is important in formulating possible differential diagnosis
  - Presence of sepsis and RUQ pain favor acute cholecystitis
  - Presence of known systemic diseases: Congestive heart failure, renal failure

Helpful Clues for Common Diagnoses
- **Acute Calculous Cholecystitis**
  - Clinical: RUQ pain, fever, positive Murphy sign
  - Acute GB inflammation secondary to calculus obstructing cystic duct
  - Gallstones ± impaction in GB neck
  - Diffuse GB wall thickening (> 4 mm)
    - Striated appearance: Several alternating, irregular, discontinuous lucent and echogenic bands within GB wall
    - GB wall lucency "halo" sign: Sonolucent middle layer due to edema
  - Distended GB (GB hydrops)
  - Positive sonographic Murphy sign
  - Presence of pericholecystic fluid
  - Complicated cholecystitis
    - GB perforation: Pericholecystic abscess
    - Gangrenous cholecystitis: Asymmetric wall thickening, marked wall irregularities, intraluminal membrane
    - Emphysematous cholecystitis: Gas in GB wall/lumen
    - Empyema of GB: Intraluminal echoes, purulent exudate/debris
- **Chronic Cholecystitis**
  - Mostly asymptomatic
  - Diffuse GB wall thickening
    - Mean thickness ~ 5 mm
    - Smooth/irregular contour
  - Contracted GB
    - GB lumen may be obliterated in severe cases
  - Presence of gallstones in nearly all cases
  - Xanthogranulomatous cholecystitis
    - Rare form of chronic cholecystitis
    - Diffuse irregular wall thickening, may appear infiltrative; mimics GB carcinoma
- **Hyperplastic Cholecystosis**
  - Adenomyomatosis of GB
  - Clinically asymptomatic, usually incidental US finding
  - Focal or diffuse GB wall thickening
  - Tiny echogenic foci in GB wall producing "comet tail" artifacts
  - Presence of cystic spaces within GB wall
  - Fundal adenomyomatosis: Smooth thickening of fundal region
  - Hourglass GB: Affecting mid-portion of GB with transverse septum
- **Wall Thickening due to Systemic Diseases**
  - Clinical correlation is key to explain presence of GB wall thickening
  - Appearance of wall thickening is nonspecific
  - Other ancillary US findings
    - **Congestive Heart Failure**: Engorged hepatic veins and IVC, diffuse hypoechoic liver echopattern
    - **Renal Failure**: Small kidneys with increased parenchymal echogenicity
    - **Hepatic Cirrhosis**: Coarse liver echopattern, irregular/nodular liver contour, signs of portal hypertension (e.g., ascites, splenomegaly, varices)
    - **Hypoalbuminemia**: Presence of ascites, diffuse bowel wall thickening

Helpful Clues for Less Common Diagnoses
- **Acute Acalculous Cholecystitis**
  - More commonly seen in critically ill patients (e.g., post major surgery, severe trauma, sepsis, etc.)

HYPOECHOIC GALLBLADDER WALL THICKENING

- ○ US features are similar to acute calculous cholecystitis except for absence of impacted gallstone
    - ■ GB wall thickening: Hypoechoic, layered/striated appearance
    - ■ GB distension: Often filled with sludge
    - ■ Positive sonographic Murphy sign
    - ■ Pericholecystic fluid
- • **Acute Hepatitis**
  - ○ Clinical history: General malaise, vomiting, deranged liver function test with hepatitic pattern
  - ○ Hepatomegaly with diffuse decrease in echogenicity
  - ○ "Starry sky" appearance: Increased echogenicity of portal triad walls against hypoechoic liver parenchyma
  - ○ Periportal hypo-/anechoic area
- • **Perforated Peptic Ulcer**
  - ○ Penetrating ulcer in duodenal wall causes sympathetic GB wall thickening
  - ○ Presence of extraluminal fluid/gas
- • **Acute Pancreatitis**
  - ○ Spread of inflammation to GB fossa
  - ○ Nonspecific GB wall thickening
  - ○ Diffuse/focal, swollen, hypoechoic pancreas
- • **Gallbladder Carcinoma**
  - ○ Asymmetric GB wall thickening
  - ○ Diffuse GB infiltration with locally advanced tumor
  - ○ Presence of gallstones
  - ○ Invasion of adjacent structures (e.g., liver, duodenum)
  - ○ Regional nodal and liver metastases
- • **Lymphoma**
  - ○ Rare involvement of GB by secondary lymphoma
  - ○ Nonspecific diffuse GB wall thickening
  - ○ Presence of intraabdominal lymphomatous lymph nodes
- • **AIDS-Related Cholangiopathy**
  - ○ Biliary inflammatory lesions caused by AIDS-related opportunistic infections leading to biliary stricture/obstruction or cholecystitis
  - ○ Diffuse GB wall thickening
  - ○ Bile duct wall thickening/inflammation
    - ■ Periductal hyper-/hypoechoic areas
  - ○ Focal biliary stricture and dilatation

Alternative Differential Approaches

- • Etiology of GB wall thickening
  - ○ Inflammatory conditions
    - ■ Acute calculous cholecystitis
    - ■ Acute acalculous cholecystitis
    - ■ Chronic cholecystitis
    - ■ AIDS-related cholangiopathy
    - ■ Secondary causes: Acute hepatitis, perforated peptic ulcer, pancreatitis
  - ○ Systemic diseases
    - ■ Congestive heart failure
    - ■ Renal failure
    - ■ Liver cirrhosis
    - ■ Hypoalbuminemia
  - ○ Neoplastic infiltration
    - ■ Gallbladder carcinoma
    - ■ Leukemic/lymphomatous infiltration

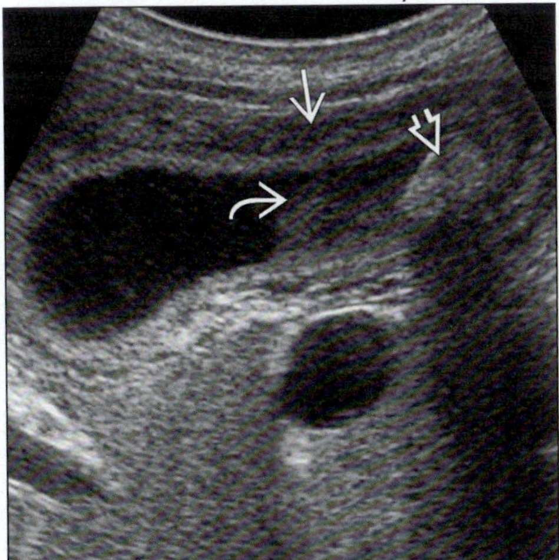

Acute Calculous Cholecystitis

Oblique transabdominal ultrasound shows a distended gallbladder with wall thickening ➡, a stone ⇒, and sludge ➡. This patient had a positive sonographic Murphy sign.

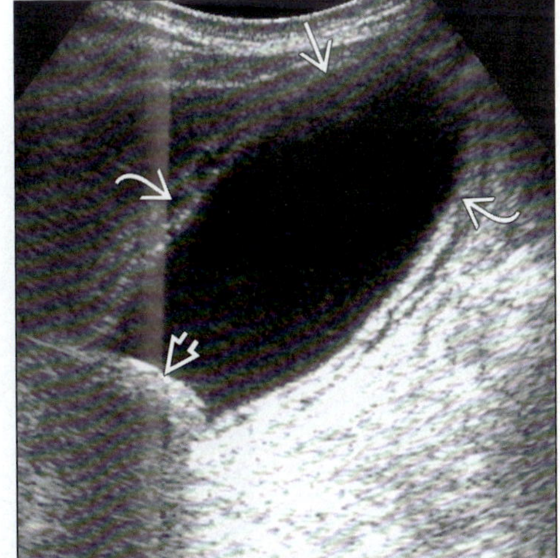

Acute Calculous Cholecystitis

Oblique transabdominal ultrasound shows a distended gallbladder ➡ with an impacted gallstone ⇒ at the neck and diffuse wall thickening ➡.

HYPOECHOIC GALLBLADDER WALL THICKENING

(Left) Oblique transabdominal ultrasound shows marked hypoechoic wall thickening ➡ with a striated appearance. There was a large gallstone impacted in the gallbladder neck (not shown). Sonographic Murphy sign was positive in this febrile patient. *(Right)* Transverse transabdominal ultrasound shows a contracted gallbladder with diffuse wall thickening ➡; the gallbladder contains an echogenic sludge ball and gallstone ⇨.

Acute Calculous Cholecystitis

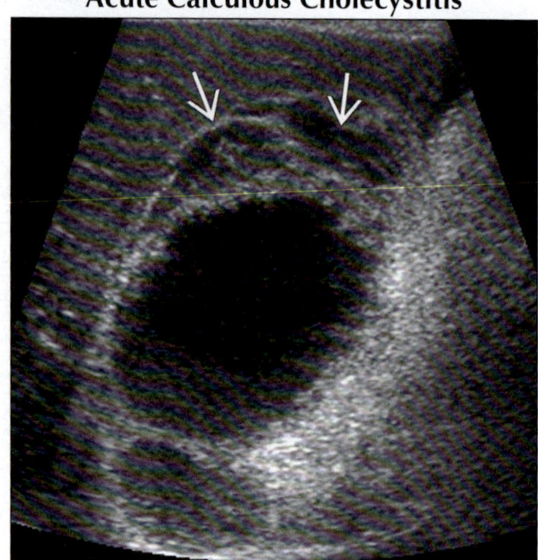

Chronic Cholecystitis

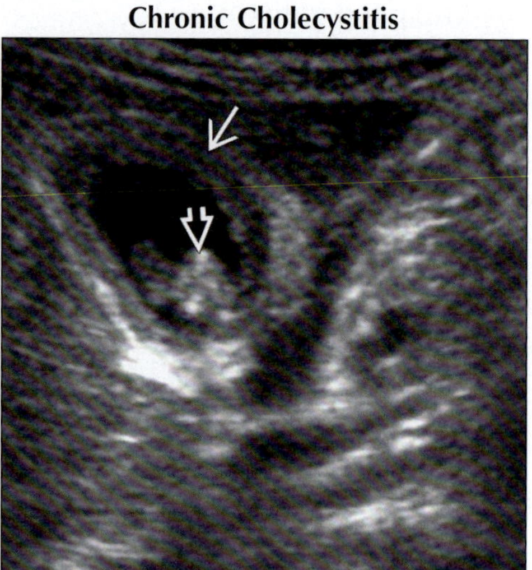

(Left) Oblique transabdominal ultrasound shows diffuse wall thickening ➡ in a contracted gallbladder. This patient was asymptomatic. *(Right)* Oblique transabdominal ultrasound shows eccentric gallbladder wall thickening ➡, mainly involving the fundus. Note the presence of echogenic sludge ⇨ within the gallbladder.

Chronic Cholecystitis

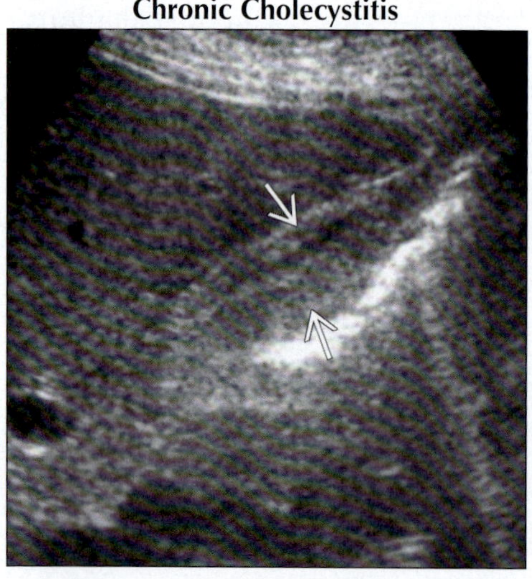

Hyperplastic Cholecystosis

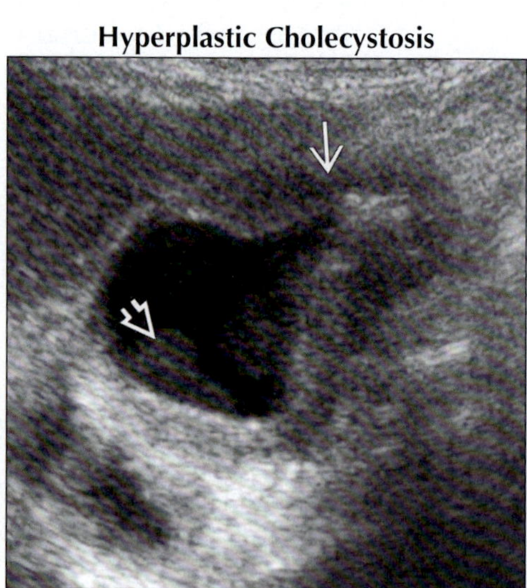

(Left) Oblique transabdominal ultrasound shows marked, diffuse wall thickening ➡ in a contracted gallbladder due to underlying congestive heart failure. Note the absence of a gallstone. *(Right)* Oblique transabdominal ultrasound shows a diffusely thickened gallbladder wall ➡ with a small gallstone ⇨ at the gallbladder neck. Note the presence of ascites ➡ due to underlying liver cirrhosis.

Congestive Heart Failure

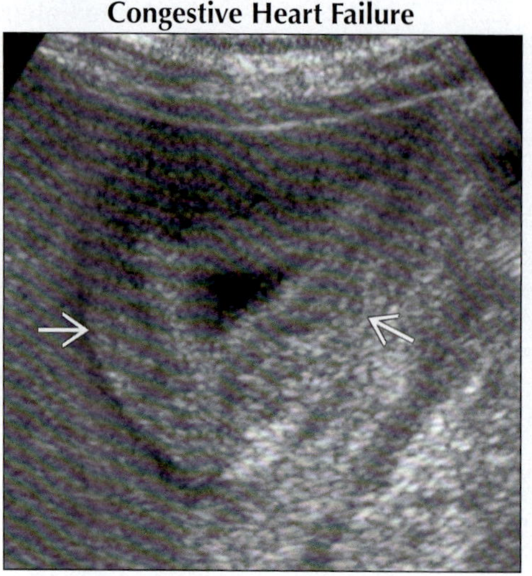

Hepatic Cirrhosis

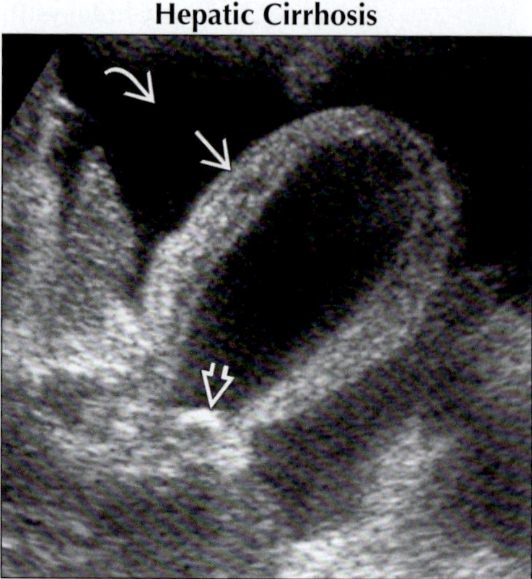

HYPOECHOIC GALLBLADDER WALL THICKENING

Hypoalbuminemia

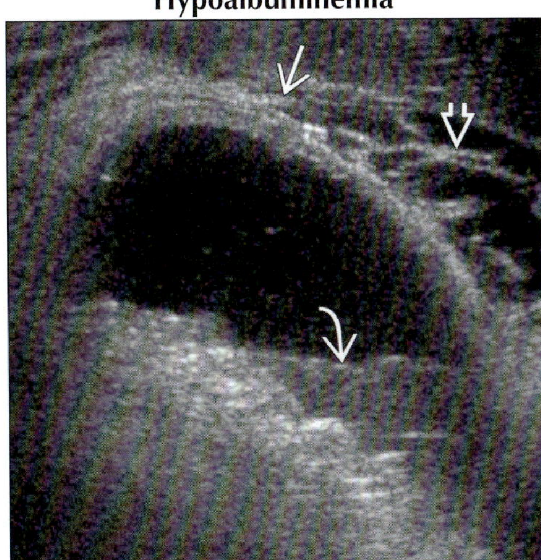

Acute Acalculous Cholecystitis

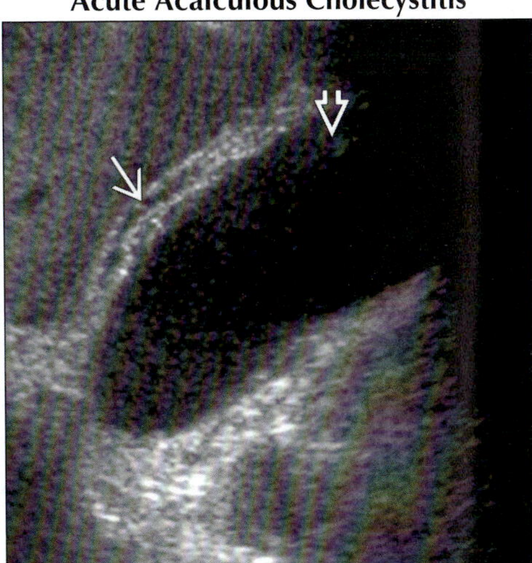

(Left) Oblique transabdominal ultrasound shows diffuse wall thickening ➡ with echogenic striations ➡. Note the presence of biliary sludge ➡ within the gallbladder lumen. (Right) Oblique transabdominal ultrasound shows a distended gallbladder ➡ with diffuse wall thickening and a striated hypoechoic appearance ➡. Sonographic Murphy sign was positive. Note the absence of an impacted gallstone within the gallbladder.

Acute Hepatitis

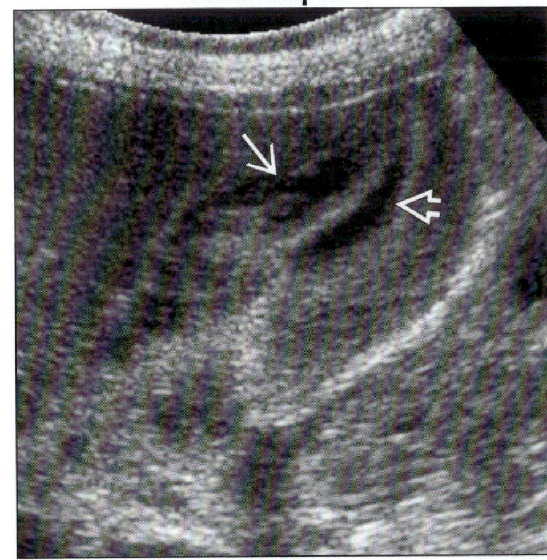

Gallbladder Carcinoma

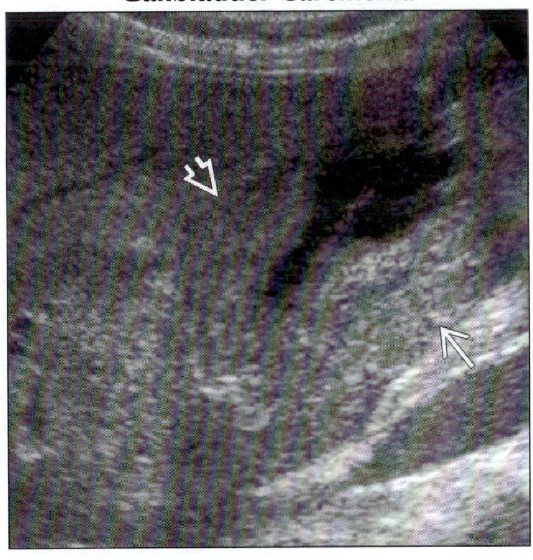

(Left) Oblique transabdominal ultrasound shows marked, diffuse, hypoechoic, gallbladder wall thickening ➡ obliterating the gallbladder lumen ➡ in a patient with acute hepatitis. (Right) Oblique transabdominal ultrasound shows diffuse wall thickening with an irregular margin ➡ involving the gallbladder wall. The tumor infiltrates into the adjacent liver parenchyma ➡. Color/power Doppler should be used to evaluate for flow.

Lymphoma

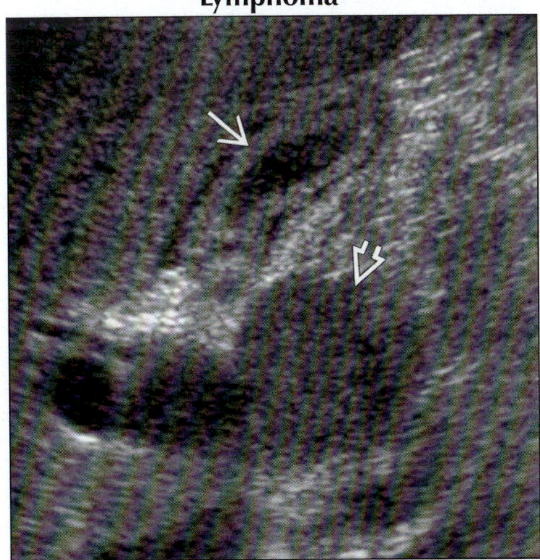

AIDS-Related Cholangiopathy

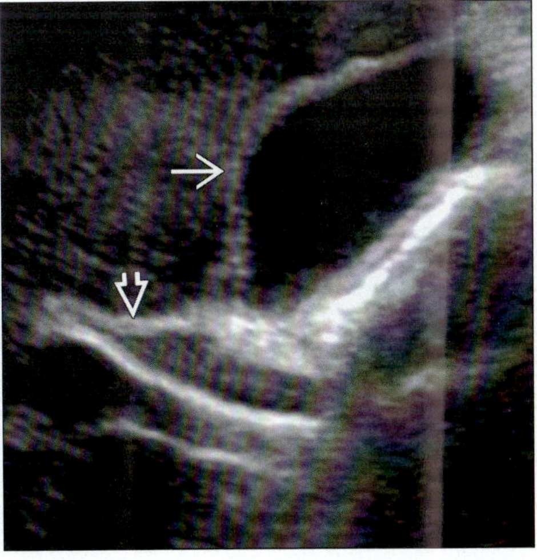

(Left) Oblique transabdominal ultrasound shows a diffusely thickened gallbladder wall ➡ due to lymphomatous infiltration. Note the abnormal lymph node ➡ in the adjacent porta hepatis region. (Right) Oblique transabdominal ultrasound in an HIV-infected patient shows diffuse wall thickening involving the gallbladder ➡ and common bile duct ➡ due to a Cytomegalovirus infection of the biliary tree.

4

HYPERECHOIC GALLBLADDER WALL

DIFFERENTIAL DIAGNOSIS

Common
- Gas-Filled Duodenal Bulb
- Porcelain Gallbladder
- Large Gallstone
- Contracted Gallbladder with Gallstones

Less Common
- Hyperplastic Cholecystosis
- Adherent Gallstones
- Emphysematous Cholecystitis

ESSENTIAL INFORMATION

Key Differential Diagnosis Issues
- Need to exclude echogenic gas-filled bowel loops in/near gallbladder fossa
  - Especially in patient with previous cholecystectomy
  - Relevant clinical information is essential

Helpful Clues for Common Diagnoses
- **Porcelain Gallbladder**
  - Diffuse form
    - Diffuse gallbladder wall calcification
    - Echogenic curvilinear line in gallbladder fossa
    - Dense posterior acoustic shadowing
  - Segmental form
    - Coarse echogenic foci in GB wall with posterior acoustic shadowing
    - Interrupted echogenic line on anterior GB wall; scattered irregular echogenic clumps within GB wall

- **Large Gallstone**
  - Anterior edge of large gallstone touching inner GB wall; strong acoustic impedance at wall-stone interface
  - Wall-echo-shadow complex appearance
  - Mobile on changing patient's position
- **Contracted Gallbladder with Gallstones**
  - Multiple, closely packed echogenic stones mimic echogenic GB wall
  - Thickened gallbladder wall
  - Gallstones mobile on changing patient's position

Helpful Clues for Less Common Diagnoses
- **Hyperplastic Cholecystosis**
  - Focal/diffuse GB wall thickening
  - Tiny echogenic foci in GB wall with "comet tail" artifacts
  - Fundal adenomyoma: Smooth sessile mass or thickening in GB fundus
  - Hourglass GB: Wall thickening in mid-portion of GB with transverse septum
- **Adherent Gallstones**
  - Not curvilinear in configuration
  - Not mobile
- **Emphysematous Cholecystitis**
  - Complicated form of acute cholecystitis
  - Clinical evidence of fulminant biliary sepsis is usually present
  - Gas in GB wall/lumen
    - Echogenic crescent in GB with reverberation artifacts ("dirty" shadowing)

Gas-Filled Duodenal Bulb

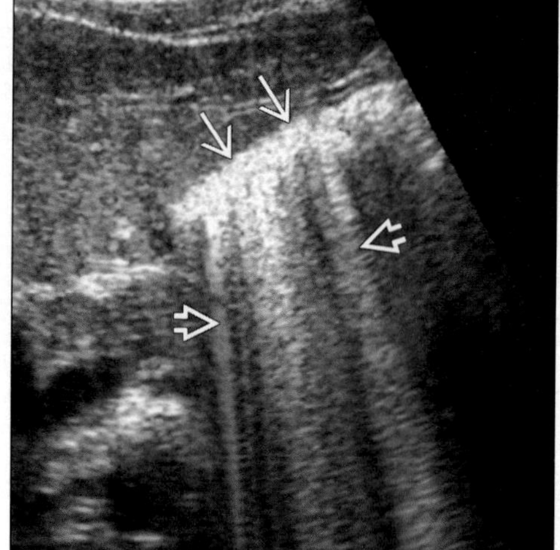

Oblique transabdominal ultrasound shows marked hyperechogenicity ➡ in the gallbladder fossa producing reverberation artifacts ➡. A gas-filled duodenal bulb occupies the empty GB fossa.

Porcelain Gallbladder

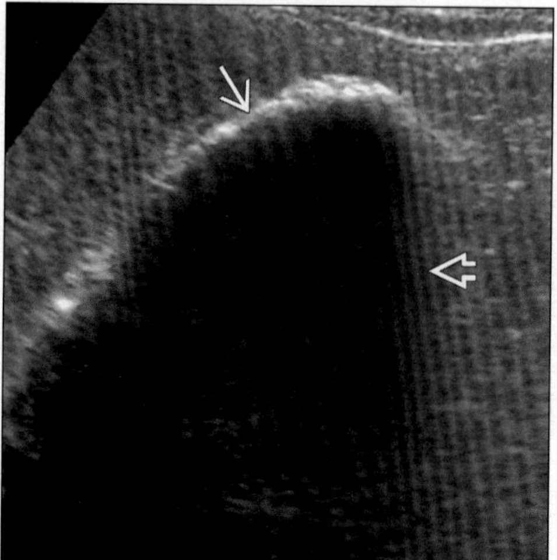

Oblique transabdominal ultrasound shows a curvilinear echogenicity ➡ in the gallbladder wall casting dense posterior acoustic shadowing ➡. Absence of wall-echo-shadow sign suggests porcelain gallbladder.

HYPERECHOIC GALLBLADDER WALL

Porcelain Gallbladder

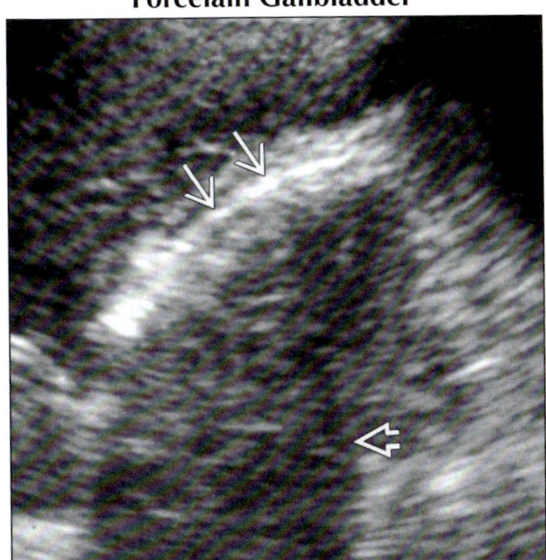

Porcelain Gallbladder

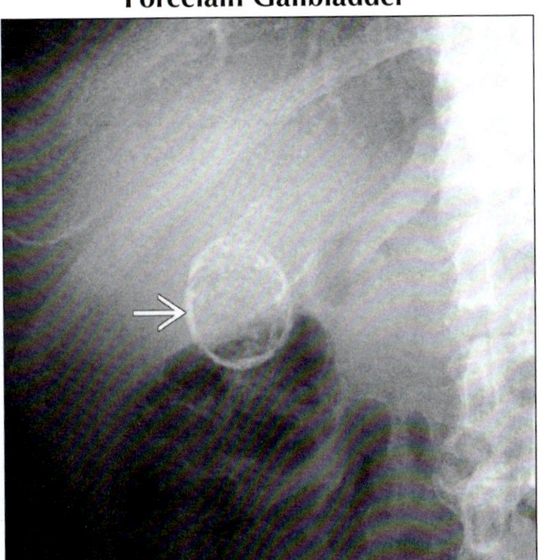

(Left) Oblique transabdominal ultrasound shows diffuse gallbladder wall calcification, which appears as an echogenic band ➡ *with posterior acoustic shadowing* ➡. *(Right) Corresponding plain abdominal radiograph shows a globular curvilinear calcification* ➡ *projected over the right upper abdomen, findings consistent with a porcelain gallbladder.*

Large Gallstone

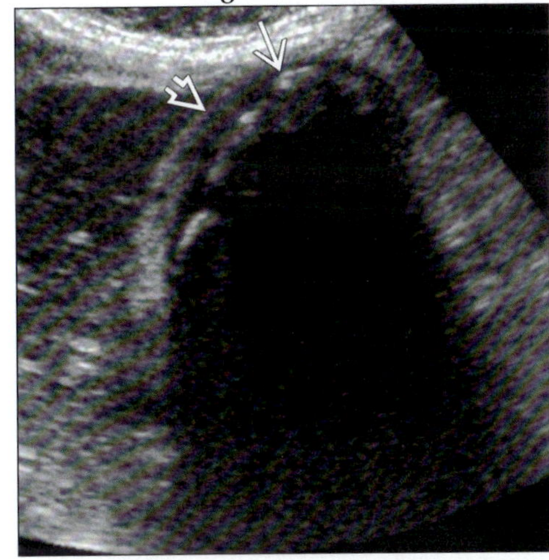

Contracted Gallbladder with Gallstones

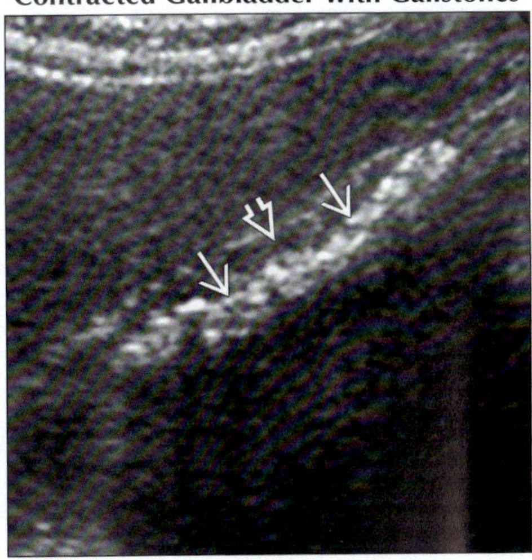

(Left) Oblique transabdominal ultrasound shows a large echogenic focus ➡ *within the gallbladder, casting a dense posterior acoustic shadow. The gallbladder wall* ➡ *is seen separately. This is the wall-echo-shadow sign, which suggests a large gallstone rather than porcelain gallbladder. (Right) Oblique transabdominal ultrasound shows numerous small shadowing echogenic gallstones* ➡ *filling a contracted gallbladder* ➡.

Hyperplastic Cholecystosis

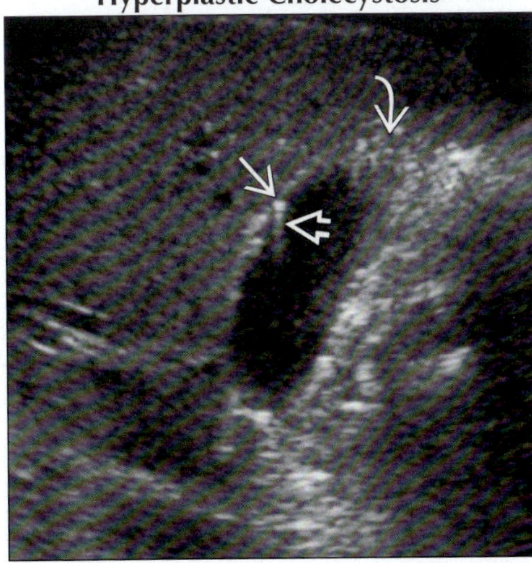

Emphysematous Cholecystitis

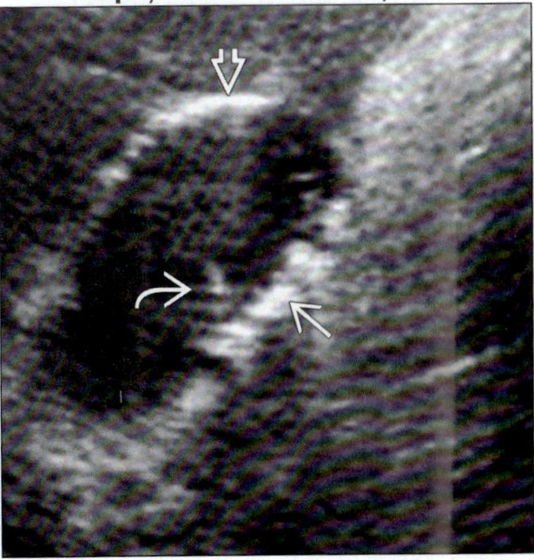

(Left) Oblique transabdominal ultrasound shows a tiny echogenic focus ➡ *with a "comet tail" artifact* ➡ *within the wall of the gallbladder. Note the presence of GB wall thickening* ➡ *in the region of the GB fundus. (Right) Oblique transabdominal ultrasound shows curvilinear echogenicity within the wall of the gallbladder* ➡ *and in its nondependent portion* ➡. *Note the presence of reverberation artifacts* ➡.

FOCAL GALLBLADDER WALL THICKENING/MASS

DIFFERENTIAL DIAGNOSIS

Common
- Gallbladder Cholesterol Polyp
- Hyperplastic Cholecystosis
- Adenomatous Polyp
- Adherent Gallstone
- Gallbladder Carcinoma

Less Common
- Parasitic Granuloma
- Intramural Epithelial Cyst
- Leiomyosarcoma
- Metastases

Rare but Important
- Xanthogranulomatous Cholecystitis

ESSENTIAL INFORMATION

Key Differential Diagnosis Issues
- Most lesions are benign; key is to identify gallbladder carcinoma
  - Large irregular lesion
  - Ill-defined margin, infiltration of adjacent liver parenchyma
  - Presence of regional nodal/liver metastases

Helpful Clues for Common Diagnoses
- **Gallbladder Cholesterol Polyp**
  - Usually 2-10 mm in size
  - Multiple, small, nonshadowing lesions with soft tissue echogenicity
  - Smooth in contour, sometimes multilobulated in outline
  - Round or ovoid shape; broad base is attached to gallbladder wall
  - Nonmobile on decubitus positioning
  - Overlying gallbladder wall is intact and normal
- **Hyperplastic Cholecystosis**
  - Fundal form more common
    - Smooth sessile mass/thickening in fundal region
  - Diffuse form with hourglass appearance
    - Wall thickening affecting mid-portion with transverse septum
  - Tiny echogenic foci within gallbladder wall with "comet tail" artifacts
- **Adenomatous Polyp**
  - Larger size (> 10 mm), solitary lesion
  - Usually pedunculated in appearance
- **Gallbladder Carcinoma**
  - Asymmetric gallbladder wall thickening
  - Intramural mass protruding into gallbladder lumen
  - Ill-defined infiltrative mass in GB fossa
  - Invasion of adjacent liver parenchyma: Indistinct separation between gallbladder mass and liver capsule
  - Presence of regional nodal/liver metastases ± intratumoral vascularity

Helpful Clues for Rare Diagnoses
- **Xanthogranulomatous Cholecystitis**
  - Rare form of chronic cholecystitis
  - Irregular gallbladder wall thickening with infiltrative margin and calculi
  - Mimics gallbladder carcinoma

Gallbladder Cholesterol Polyp

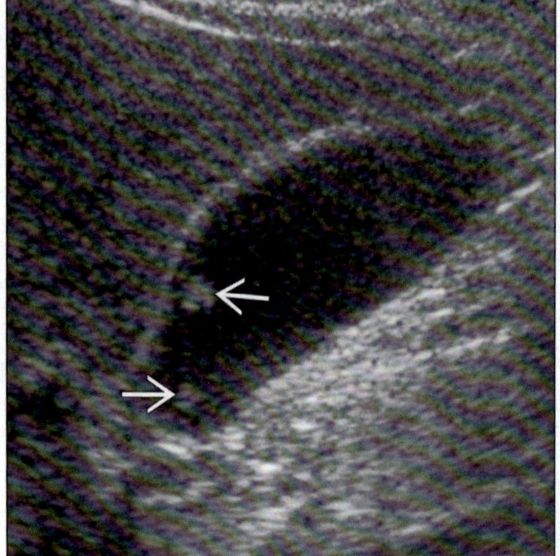

Oblique transabdominal ultrasound shows small, nonshadowing, well-defined, round nodules ➡ adherent to the gallbladder wall, suggestive of gallbladder polyps.

Gallbladder Cholesterol Polyp

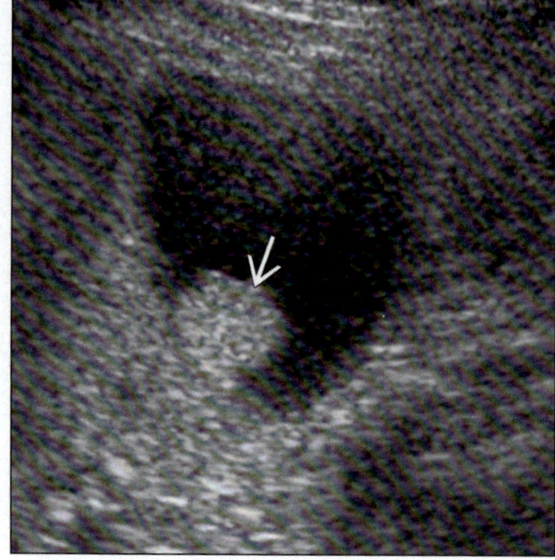

Oblique transabdominal ultrasound shows a small well-circumscribed homogeneous mass ➡ with a smooth margin arising from the gallbladder wall, compatible with a gallbladder polyp.

FOCAL GALLBLADDER WALL THICKENING/MASS

Hyperplastic Cholecystosis

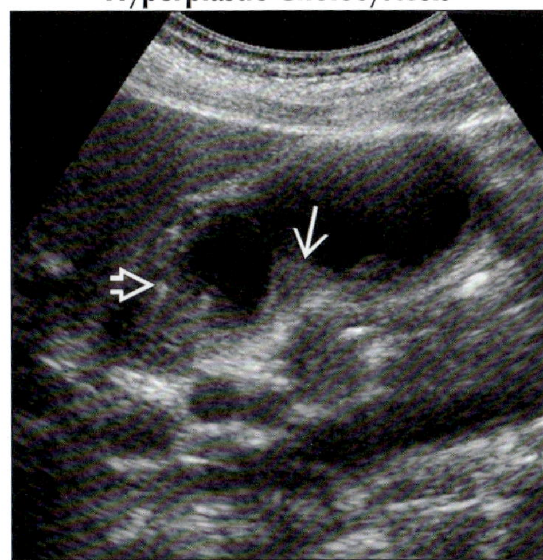

Hyperplastic Cholecystosis

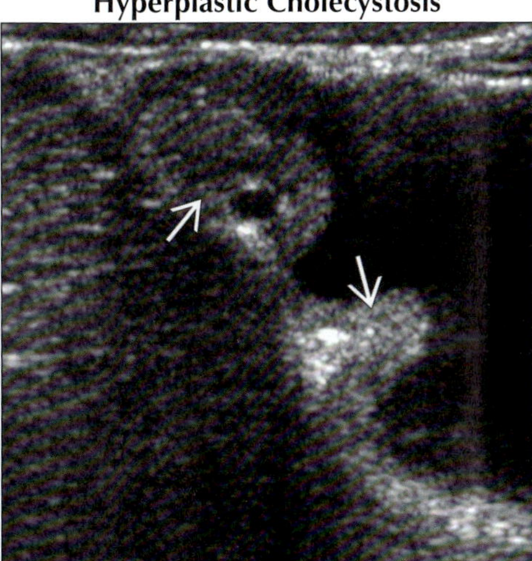

(Left) Oblique transabdominal ultrasound shows a thickened gallbladder wall, with "comet tail" artifacts ➡ and focal mid-wall constriction ➡ (hourglass appearance). *(Right)* Oblique transabdominal ultrasound shows focal wall thickening ➡ involving the fundus of the gallbladder. "Comet tail" artifacts were present in the body of the gallbladder (not shown). These are all typical features of hyperplastic cholecystosis.

Adenomatous Polyp

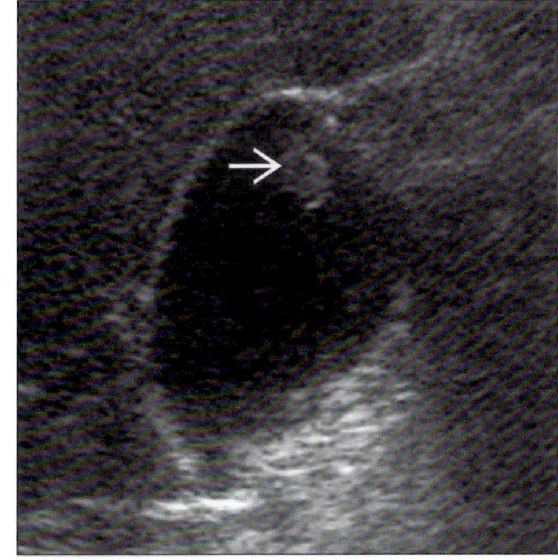

Adherent Gallstone

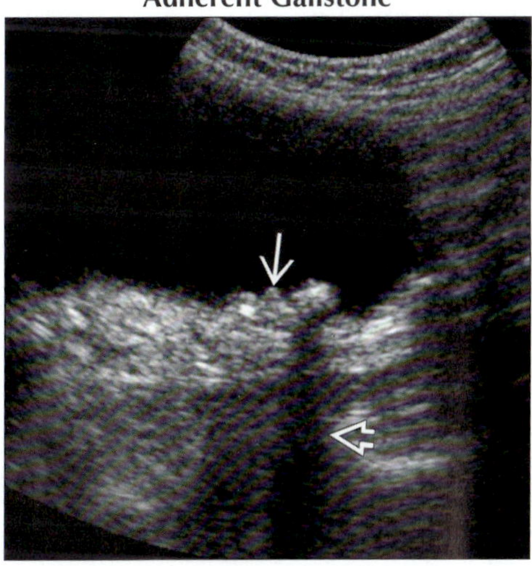

(Left) Oblique transabdominal ultrasound shows a solitary, well-defined, solid nodule ➡ with a smooth lobulated margin adherent to the gallbladder wall. Pathology determined this was an adenomatous polyp. *(Right)* Oblique transabdominal ultrasound shows echogenic gallstones ➡ casting posterior acoustic shadowing ➡. The gallstones adhere to the gallbladder wall and were therefore not mobile upon changing the patient's position.

Gallbladder Carcinoma

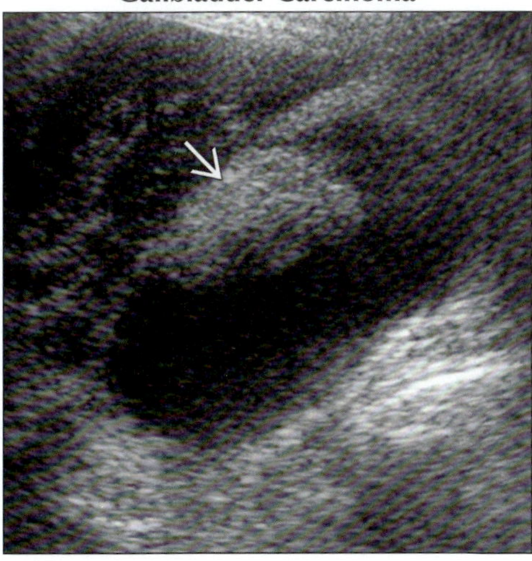

Xanthogranulomatous Cholecystitis

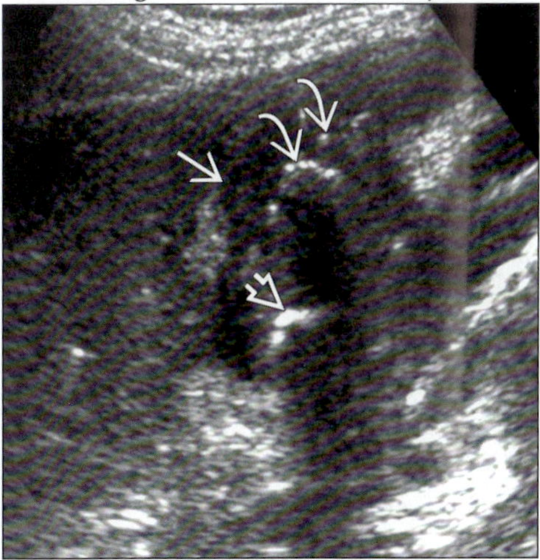

(Left) Oblique transabdominal ultrasound shows focal eccentric wall thickening ➡ with an irregular inner margin arising from the anterior wall of the gallbladder. *(Right)* Oblique transabdominal ultrasound shows an ill-defined thickening of the gallbladder wall ➡, which contains echogenic foci ➡. A gallstone ➡ is also present. The indistinct margin with adjacent liver parenchyma mimics gallbladder carcinoma.

4

ECHOGENIC MATERIAL IN GALLBLADDER

DIFFERENTIAL DIAGNOSIS

Common
- Cholelithiasis
- Sludge/Sludge Ball

Less Common
- Blood Clot
- Echogenic Bile
- Gas within Gallbladder
- Parasitic Infestation

Rare but Important
- Gangrenous Cholecystitis

ESSENTIAL INFORMATION

Helpful Clues for Common Diagnoses
- **Cholelithiasis**
  - Highly reflective echogenic focus within gallbladder lumen
  - Prominent posterior acoustic shadowing
  - Gravity-dependent movement on change of patient position
  - Variant ultrasound features
    - Nonshadowing gallstones, usually small (< 5 mm) in size
    - Immobile adherent/impacted gallstones
    - Nonvisualization of gallbladder with large collection of bright echoes with posterior acoustic shadowing in gallbladder fossa
    - Wall-echo-shadow appearance for large gallstone
  - Superimposed complications
    - Acute calculous cholecystitis: GB wall thickening, GB hydrops, sonographic Murphy sign, pericholecystic fluid
- **Sludge/Sludge Ball**
  - Intraluminal material of medium echogenicity
    - Sludge ball: Well-defined round contour
  - Mobile on changing patient's position
  - Absence of posterior acoustic shadowing

Helpful Clues for Less Common Diagnoses
- **Blood Clot**
  - Echogenic/mixed echoes within gallbladder
  - Occasionally retractile and conforms to gallbladder shape
  - Blood-fluid level within gallbladder
- **Echogenic Bile**
  - Amorphous, mid/high level echoes within gallbladder
  - Sediment in dependent portion
  - "Hepatization" of gallbladder: Sludge-filled gallbladder with same echotexture as liver
- **Parasitic Infestation**
  - Tubular, parallel echogenic lines
  - Active movement in viable worm; gravity-dependent movement in dead worm

Helpful Clues for Rare Diagnoses
- **Gangrenous Cholecystitis**
  - Complicated form of acute cholecystitis
  - Asymmetric wall thickening, marked wall irregularities, intraluminal echogenic debris and membrane

Cholelithiasis

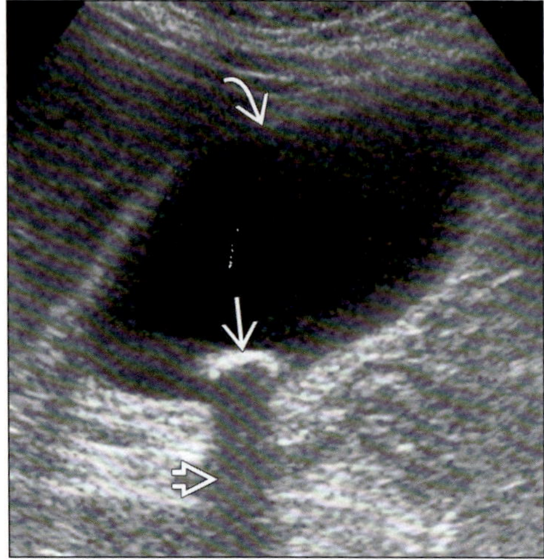

Oblique transabdominal ultrasound shows a dense echogenic focus ➡ with marked posterior acoustic shadowing ➡ within the dependent portion of a nondistended gallbladder ➡.

Cholelithiasis

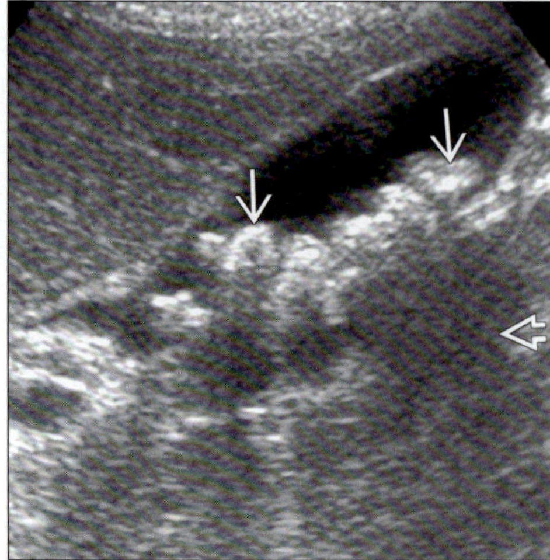

Oblique transabdominal ultrasound shows multiple echogenic foci ➡ within the gallbladder, representing gallstones. Note the posterior acoustic shadowing ➡. The stones were mobile.

ECHOGENIC MATERIAL IN GALLBLADDER

Cholelithiasis

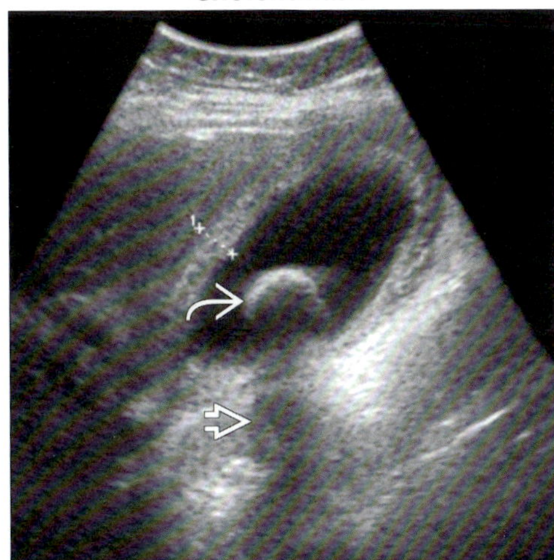

Sludge/Sludge Ball

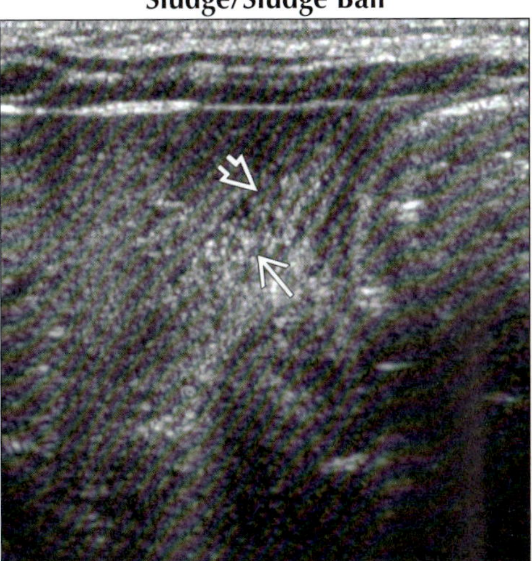

(Left) Longitudinal ultrasound shows a thick-walled GB (cursors) that was tender to palpation and contains an echogenic stone ➡ with acoustic shadowing ➡ in this patient with cholecystitis. (Right) Oblique transabdominal ultrasound shows echogenic material ➡ filling the partially contracted gallbladder ➡ due to the presence of biliary sludge in a patient with prolonged fasting.

Sludge/Sludge Ball

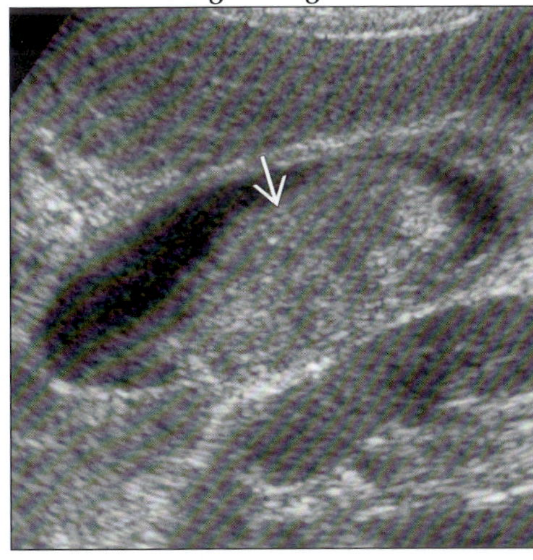

Echogenic Bile

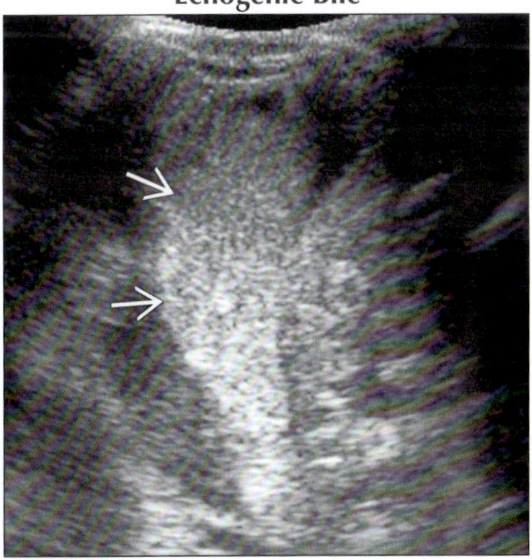

(Left) Oblique transabdominal ultrasound shows a mobile echogenic "lesion" ➡ within the gallbladder, consistent with a sludge ball. Note the absence of posterior acoustic shadowing. (Right) Oblique transabdominal ultrasound shows markedly echogenic material ➡ almost filling the gallbladder lumen (hepatization of gallbladder). Note the lack of posterior acoustic shadowing.

Parasitic Infestation

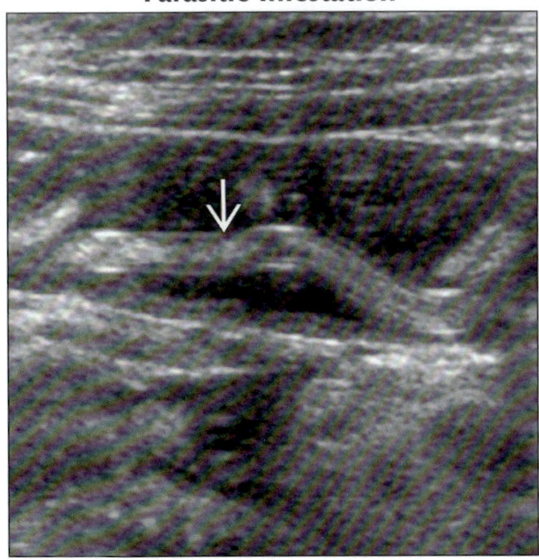

Gangrenous Cholecystitis

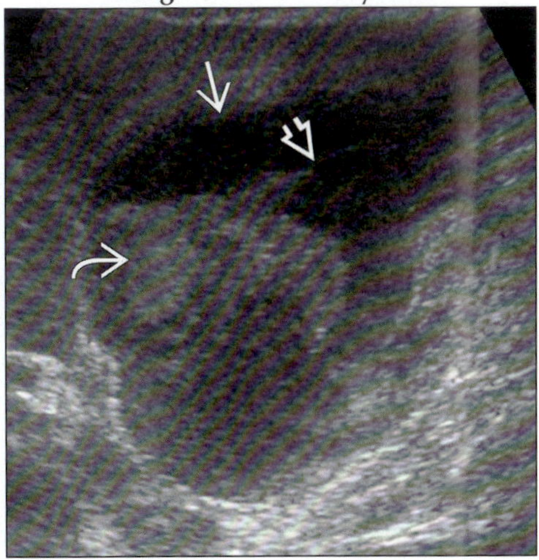

(Left) Oblique transabdominal ultrasound shows a tubular structure ➡ with parallel echogenic lines and a sonolucent center within the gallbladder, suggestive of parasitic infestation by Ascaris lumbricoides. (Right) Oblique transabdominal ultrasound shows a distended gangrenous gallbladder ➡ containing echogenic debris ➡, an irregular wall, and an intraluminal membrane ➡ due to sloughing of the mucosa.

"SOFT TISSUE" MATERIAL IN GALLBLADDER

DIFFERENTIAL DIAGNOSIS

Common
- Sludge/Sludge Ball
- Inflammatory Debris
- Gallbladder Polyp
- Hyperplastic Cholecystosis
- Gallbladder Carcinoma

Less Common
- Blood Clot
- Gallbladder Empyema

ESSENTIAL INFORMATION

Helpful Clues for Common Diagnoses
- **Sludge/Sludge Ball**
  - Clinically asymptomatic
  - Medium-level echogenicity
  - Mobile on changing patient position
  - No posterior acoustic shadowing
  - Fluid-sediment level
  - Sludge ball
    - Discrete, round contour
- **Inflammatory Debris**
  - Seen in acute cholecystitis
    - Inflammatory exudate from gallbladder (GB) wall inflammation
  - Floating low-level echoes within GB lumen
  - GB wall thickening, distended GB, impacted gallstones
- **Gallbladder Polyp**
  - Cholesterol polyp small (< 10 mm in size), often multiple
  - Adenomatous polyp larger (> 10 mm), usually solitary
  - Pedunculated polyp may appear as luminal lesion
  - No posterior acoustic shadowing
  - Not mobile on changing patient position
- **Hyperplastic Cholecystosis**
  - Focal adenomyomatosis
    - Most common at GB fundus
    - Mass-like abnormality arising from GB fundal wall
  - Associated features of adenomyomatosis in rest of GB (e.g., echogenic foci with "comet tail" artifacts)
- **Gallbladder Carcinoma**
  - May appear as irregular mass protruding into GB lumen
  - Ill-defined margin with GB wall
  - ± regional nodal/liver metastases
  - Increased vascularity on color Doppler US

Helpful Clues for Less Common Diagnoses
- **Blood Clot**
  - Fresh blood clot may appear hypoechoic
  - Blood-fluid level within GB
  - Most common following biliary instrumentation/intervention
- **Gallbladder Empyema**
  - Complicated form of acute cholecystitis
  - Clinically septic with localized peritoneal signs in right upper quadrant
  - Intraluminal heterogeneous floating echo
  - Irregular GB wall thickening
  - Distended GB

Sludge/Sludge Ball

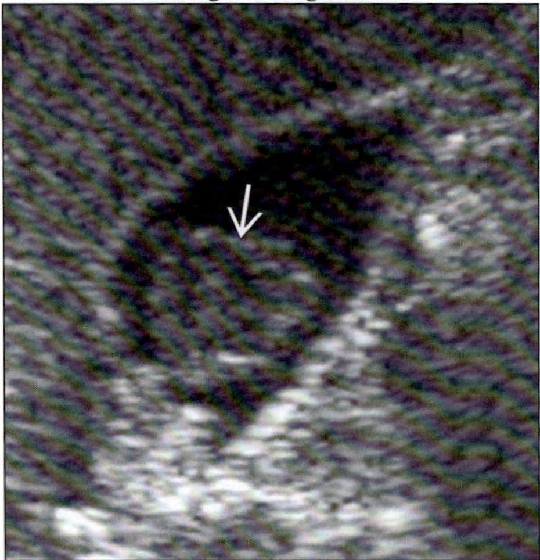

Oblique transabdominal ultrasound shows a sludge ball ➡ with a well-defined round contour within the gallbladder. Note the absence of posterior acoustic shadowing.

Sludge/Sludge Ball

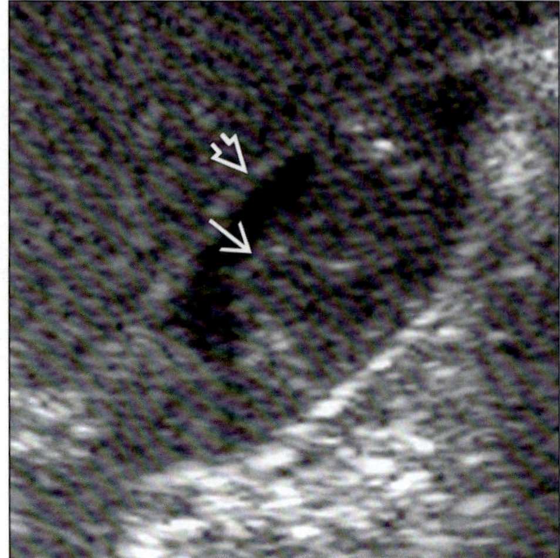

Oblique transabdominal ultrasound shows sludge ➡ nearly filling up the lumen of the gallbladder. The gallbladder wall ➡ is not thickened.

"SOFT TISSUE" MATERIAL IN GALLBLADDER

Sludge/Sludge Ball

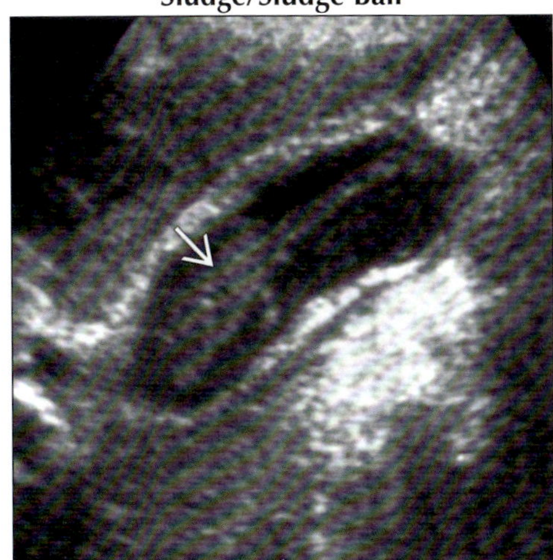

Inflammatory Debris

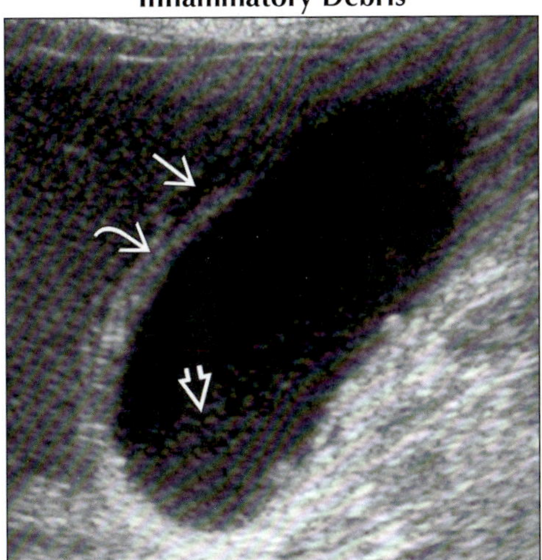

(Left) Oblique transabdominal ultrasound shows echogenic debris ➡ within the gallbladder. Note the lack of posterior acoustic shadowing. There is no evidence of cholecystitis such as gallbladder wall thickening or pericholecystic fluid. *(Right)* Oblique transabdominal ultrasound shows low-level internal echoes ➡ within the lumen of a distended gallbladder. Note the presence of diffuse wall thickening ➡ with a thin rim of pericholecystic fluid ➡.

Gallbladder Polyp

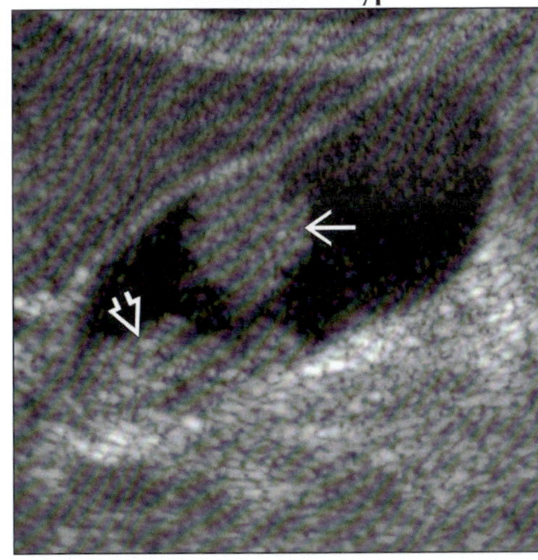

Hyperplastic Cholecystosis

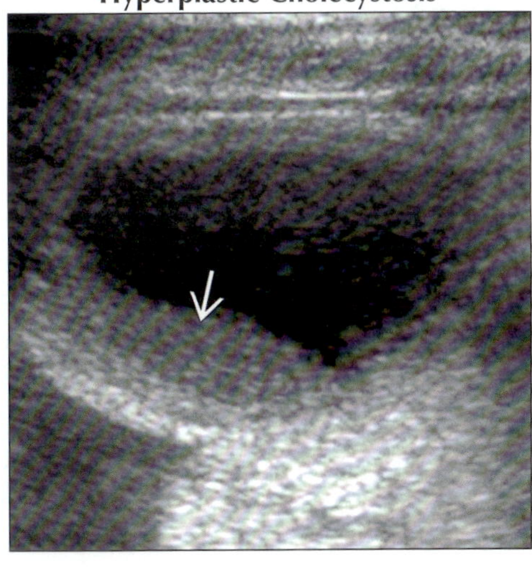

(Left) Oblique transabdominal ultrasound shows a large polypoid growth ➡ with a slightly lobulated contour arising from the anterior wall of the gallbladder. A similar lesion with a sessile appearance ➡ is present on the posterior gallbladder wall. *(Right)* Transverse transabdominal ultrasound shows focal thickening ➡ at the fundal region of the gallbladder. Note the absence of posterior acoustic shadowing.

Blood Clot

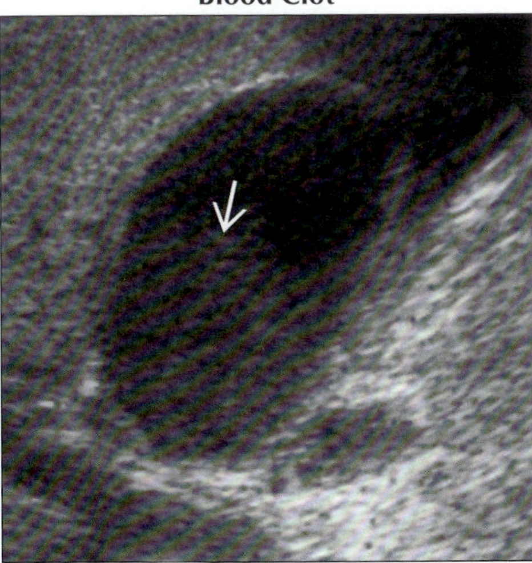

Gallbladder Empyema

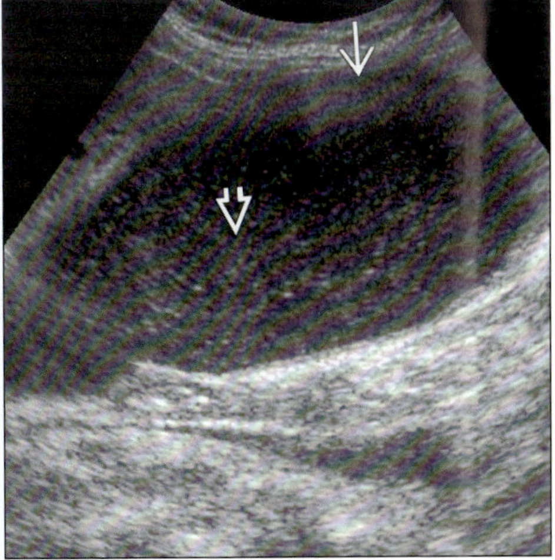

(Left) Oblique transabdominal ultrasound shows heterogeneous material with low echogenicity ➡ in the dependent portion of the gallbladder lumen due to a blood clot following percutaneous transhepatic biliary drainage. *(Right)* Oblique transabdominal ultrasound shows marked gallbladder distension ➡ with mild wall thickening and floating low-level echoes ➡ due to gallbladder empyema.

4

OBSTRUCTIVE JAUNDICE

DIFFERENTIAL DIAGNOSIS

Common
- Choledocholithiasis
- Ascending Cholangitis
- Recurrent Pyogenic Cholangitis
- Pancreatic Ductal Carcinoma
- Cholangiocarcinoma
- Postoperative Biliary Stricture

Less Common
- Parasitic Infestation
- Biliary Sludge
- Sclerosing Cholangitis
- Periampullary Tumor
- Gallbladder Carcinoma
- Hepatocellular Carcinoma
- Hepatic Metastases
- Enlarged Periportal Lymph Node

ESSENTIAL INFORMATION

Key Differential Diagnosis Issues
- Role of US in patients with obstructive jaundice
  - Differentiate biliary obstruction from liver parenchymal disease
  - Determine presence, level, and possible cause of biliary obstruction
- Level of biliary obstruction
  - Intrahepatic
  - Hepatic confluence/porta hepatis
  - Extrahepatic
- Criteria for malignant obstruction
  - Abrupt transition from dilatation to narrowing
  - Eccentric duct wall thickening with contour irregularities
  - Mass in/around duct
  - Presence of enlarged regional lymph nodes, liver metastases, or vascular invasion

Helpful Clues for Common Diagnoses
- **Choledocholithiasis**
  - Extrahepatic biliary stones
    - Most commonly seen within common bile duct (CBD)
    - Round echogenic intraluminal focus with posterior acoustic shadowing
    - Extrahepatic and intrahepatic biliary dilatation
  - Intrahepatic biliary stones
    - Echogenic foci in region of portal triad with posterior acoustic shadowing
    - If affected duct is completely filled with stones, it appears as linear echogenic structure with posterior acoustic shadowing
    - Large stones cause focal intrahepatic biliary dilatation distal to obstructing stone
    - Small or soft pigmented stones may not produce acoustic shadowing
- **Ascending Cholangitis**
  - Clinical symptoms of Charcot triad (RUQ pain, fever, jaundice)
  - Presence of obstructing CBD stone
  - Dilatation of intra- and extrahepatic bile ducts (in ~ 75% of cases)
    - In early cholangitis or intermittent CBD obstruction, bile ducts may not be dilated
  - Circumferential bile duct wall thickening
  - Periportal hypo-/hyperechogenicity adjacent to dilated intrahepatic ducts
  - Multiple small intrahepatic cholangitic abscesses
    - Hypoechoic cystic lesions with internal echoes and debris
- **Recurrent Pyogenic Cholangitis**
  - Clinical history: Recurrent attacks of RUQ pain, fever, and jaundice
  - Early disease
    - Dilated intra- and extrahepatic bile ducts
    - Echogenic sludge/stones
    - Periportal hypo-/hyperechogenicity due to periductal inflammation
    - Bile duct wall thickening ± cholangitic abscesses
  - Late-stage disease
    - Severe atrophy of affected liver lobe/segment
    - Development of biliary cirrhosis with portal hypertension
- **Pancreatic Ductal Carcinoma**
  - 60-70% affect head of pancreas
  - Ill-defined infiltrative, solid pancreatic head mass
  - Intra- and extrahepatic biliary dilatation
  - Dilatation of pancreatic duct
  - Vascular encasement
  - Regional lymph node and liver metastases
- **Cholangiocarcinoma**

- Extrahepatic cholangiocarcinoma
  - Dilatation of both intra- and extrahepatic bile ducts
  - Ill-defined, solid, heterogeneous mass within or surrounding extrahepatic bile duct
- Klatskin tumor
  - Infiltrative iso-/hypoechoic mass in hilar region
  - Dilatation of intrahepatic ducts in both lobes sparing extrahepatic bile ducts
  - Noncommunication between right and left hepatic ducts
- Intrahepatic cholangiocarcinoma
  - Mass with ill-defined margin, mostly hyperechoic and heterogeneous
  - Isolated intrahepatic duct dilatation

- **Postoperative Biliary Stricture**
  - Stricture of previous biliary-enteric anastomosis (e.g., hepatojejunostomy)
  - Dilatation of intrahepatic and residual extrahepatic bile duct
  - No associated mass
  - History of surgery

Helpful Clues for Less Common Diagnoses

- **Parasitic Infestation**
  - Most common infestations: *Ascaris*, *Clonorchis*, ruptured hydatid cyst
  - Parallel echogenic tubular structures with sonolucent center within bile duct
  - Active movement of parasite
- **Biliary Sludge**
  - Low-level echoes without posterior acoustic shadowing
  - Mobile on change of patient position
- **Sclerosing Cholangitis**
  - Idiopathic or autoimmune reaction or genetic
  - Intra- and extrahepatic bile duct segmental dilatation and strictures
- **Hepatic Metastases**
  - Extrinsic intrahepatic biliary obstruction by hepatocellular carcinoma, liver metastases
  - Isolated duct dilatation of involved lobe/segment distal to obstructing tumor

Alternative Differential Approaches

- Level of obstruction vs. possible diagnoses
  - Intrahepatic
    - Recurrent pyogenic cholangitis
    - Intrahepatic choledocholithiasis
    - Intrahepatic cholangiocarcinoma
    - Hepatic tumor with extrinsic biliary compression
  - Porta hepatis/hepatic confluence
    - Cholangiocarcinoma
    - Choledocholithiasis
    - Extrinsic compression by primary tumor (e.g., GB carcinoma) or metastatic lymph nodes
  - Extrahepatic
    - Choledocholithiasis in CBD
    - Ascending cholangitis
    - Cholangiocarcinoma
    - Pancreatic head/periampullary tumor

Choledocholithiasis

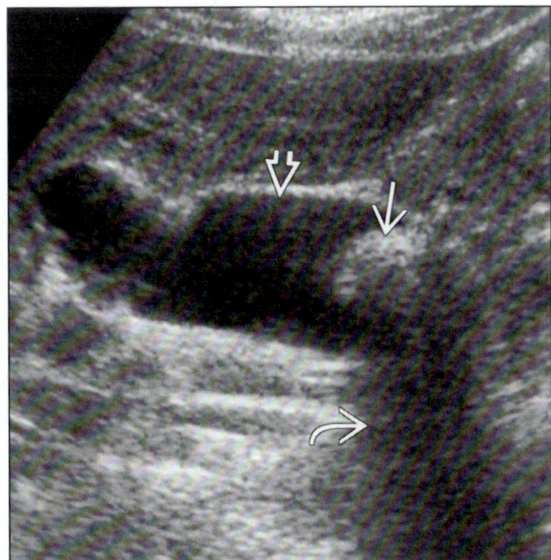

Oblique transabdominal ultrasound shows an echogenic focus ➡ within the distal portion of the dilated common bile duct ⏩, with posterior acoustic shadowing ➡ in extrahepatic choledocholithiasis.

Choledocholithiasis

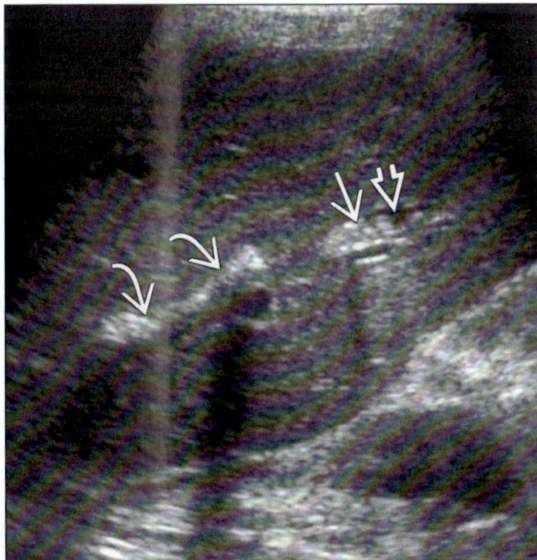

Oblique ultrasound shows intrahepatic duct stones ➡ with dilated intrahepatic ducts ⏩ in the right liver lobe. Note hyperechogenicity along the portal triad ➡ from an intrahepatic duct packed with stones.

4

OBSTRUCTIVE JAUNDICE

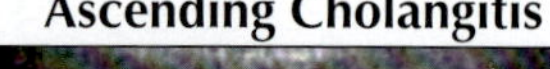

(Left) Oblique transabdominal ultrasound shows a grossly dilated intrahepatic duct ➡ in the right lobe of the liver, containing echogenic debris ⇨ due to infected biliary sludge. *(Right)* Transverse transabdominal ultrasound in a patient with recurrent pyogenic cholangitis shows echogenic foci ➡ within the dilated intrahepatic ducts ⇨ of the lateral segment of the left lobe of the liver.

Ascending Cholangitis

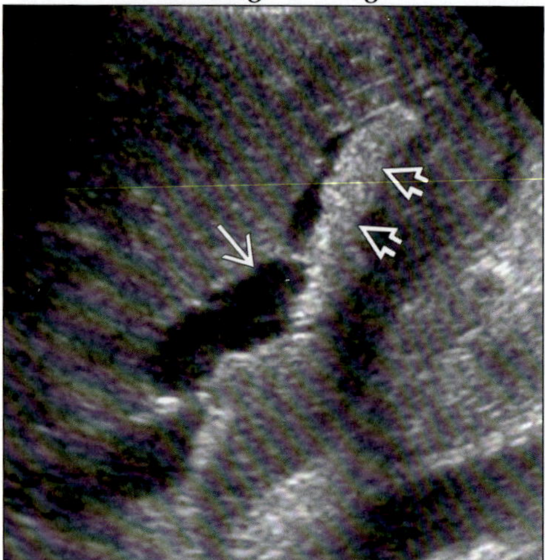

Recurrent Pyogenic Cholangitis

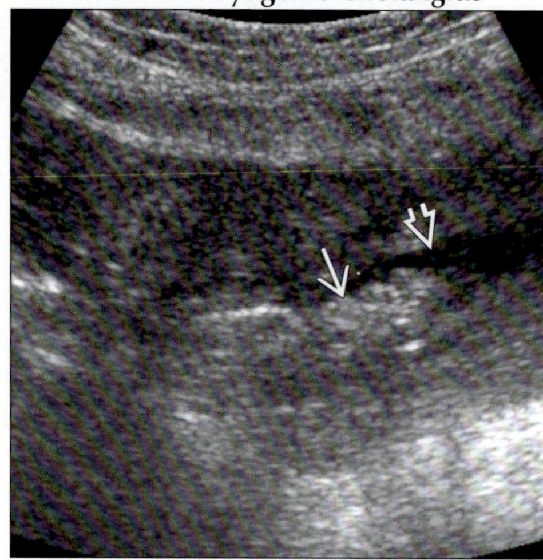

(Left) MRCP shows changes from recurrent pyogenic cholangitis in a patient with previous right segmentectomy and hepatojejunostomy. Note the presence of signal void filling defects ➡ within the dilated intrahepatic ducts ⇨ in the left lateral segment. *(Right)* Oblique transabdominal ultrasound shows an ill-defined, solid, hypoechoic mass ➡ in the pancreatic head, causing truncation of the terminal portion of the common bile duct with proximal dilatation ⇨.

Recurrent Pyogenic Cholangitis

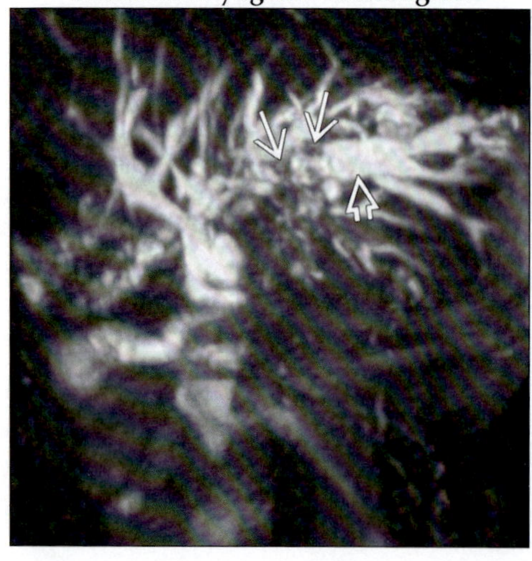

Pancreatic Ductal Carcinoma

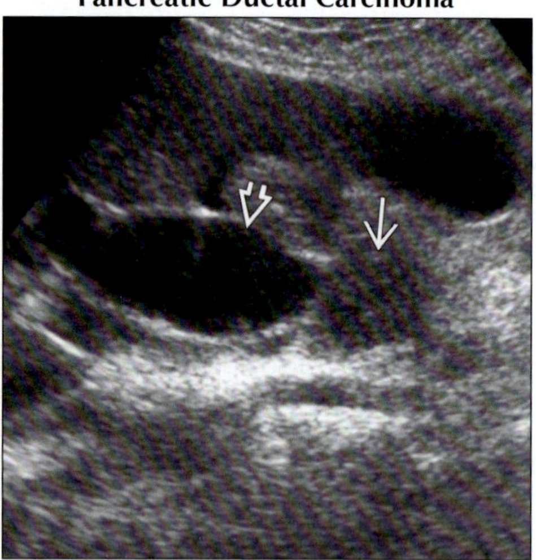

(Left) Oblique transabdominal ultrasound of the right lobe of the liver shows marked dilatation of the intrahepatic bile ducts ➡. There was a malignant biliary obstruction in the proximal extrahepatic bile duct. *(Right)* Transverse transabdominal ultrasound shows an ill-defined isoechoic mass ➡ at the hepatic confluence, which is associated with marked dilatation of intrahepatic bile ducts ⇨, compatible with an intrahepatic cholangiocarcinoma.

Cholangiocarcinoma

Cholangiocarcinoma

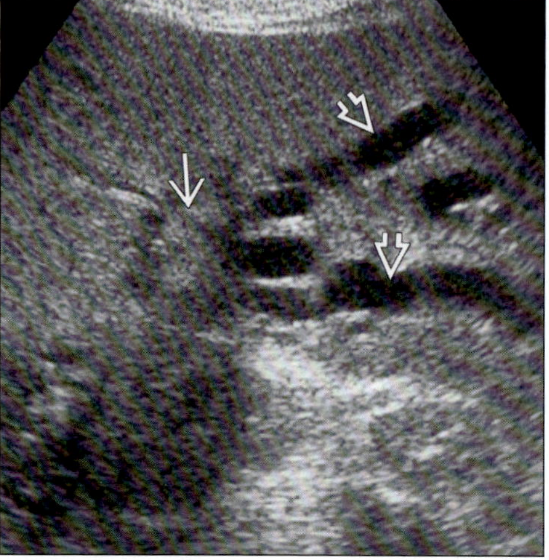

OBSTRUCTIVE JAUNDICE

Parasitic Infestation

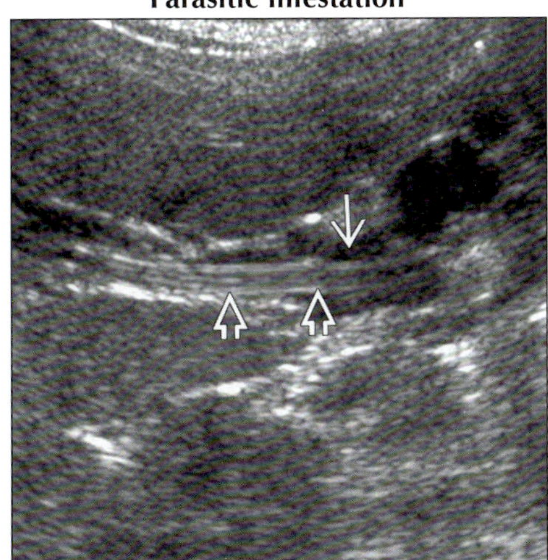

Parasitic Infestation

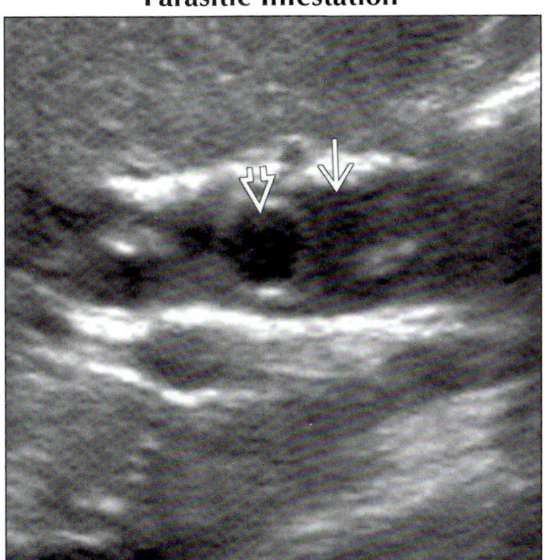

(Left) Oblique transabdominal ultrasound shows a long tubular structure ➡ with parallel echogenic lines within the dilated common bile duct ➡. It showed active movement on real-time ultrasound, compatible with a viable worm. (Right) Oblique transabdominal ultrasound shows a daughter cyst ➡ within the dilated common bile duct ➡ due to a rupture of a hepatic hydatid cyst into the biliary tree.

Biliary Sludge

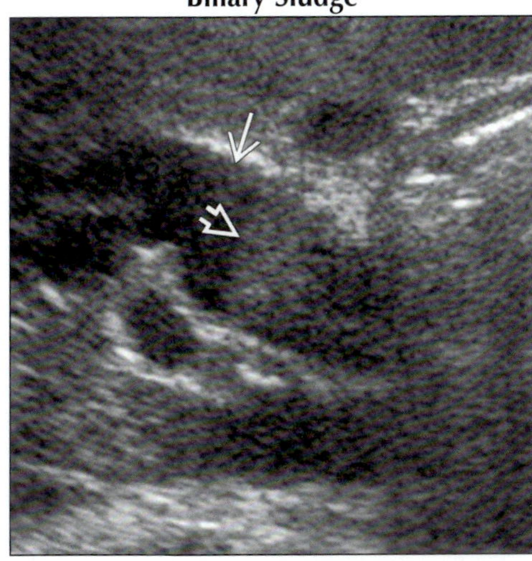

Gallbladder Carcinoma

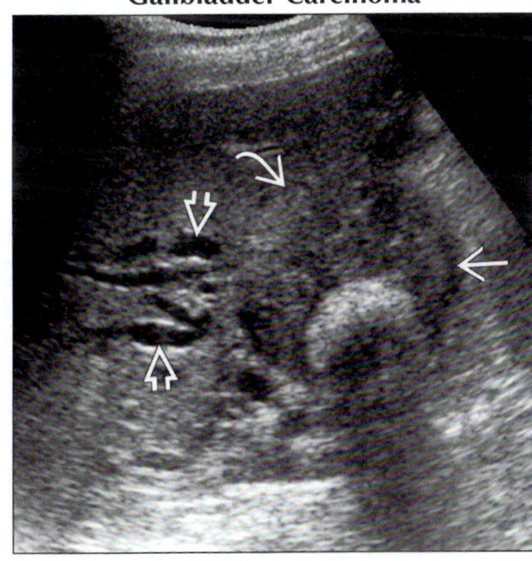

(Left) Oblique transabdominal ultrasound shows a dilated CBD ➡ with a thickened wall and echogenic debris ➡ in its distal portion due to infected biliary sludge in ascending cholangitis. (Right) Oblique transabdominal ultrasound shows an ill-defined gallbladder mass ➡ surrounding a large gallstone. Note the tumor infiltration of the adjacent liver parenchyma ➡ with extrinsic compression and dilatation of the intrahepatic bile ducts ➡.

Hepatocellular Carcinoma

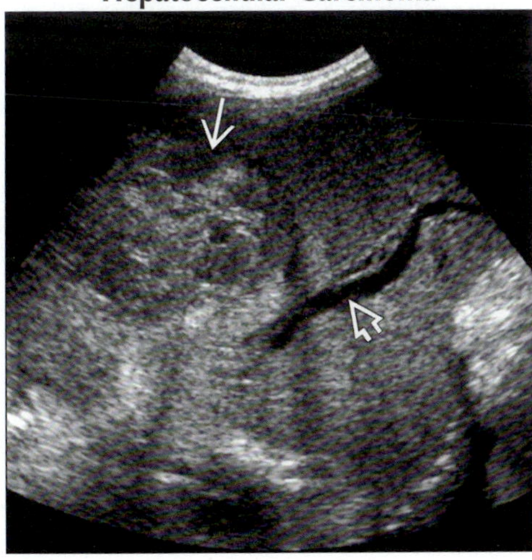

Hepatic Metastases

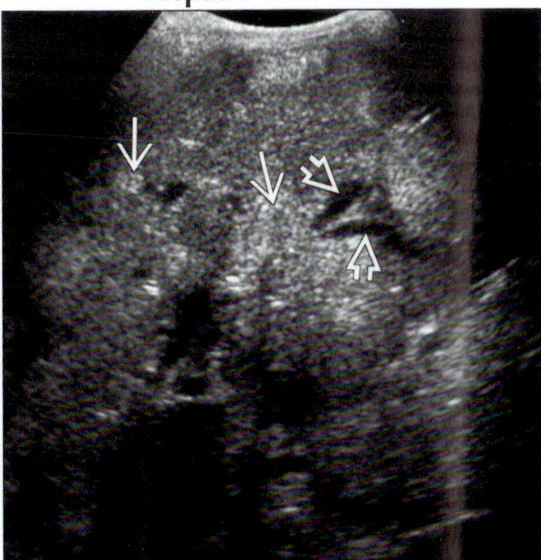

(Left) Transverse transabdominal ultrasound shows a large, heterogeneous, hyperechoic liver mass ➡ that causes compression and dilatation of the intrahepatic bile ducts ➡. (Right) Oblique transabdominal ultrasound shows multiple, ill-defined, hyperechoic liver metastases ➡, causing extrinsic compression and dilatation of the intrahepatic bile ducts ➡.

4

INTRAHEPATIC & EXTRAHEPATIC DUCT DILATATION

DIFFERENTIAL DIAGNOSIS

Common
- Choledocholithiasis
- Ascending Cholangitis
- Recurrent Pyogenic Cholangitis
- Pancreatic Ductal Carcinoma
- Cholangiocarcinoma
- Choledochal Cyst

Less Common
- Parasitic Infestation
- Sludge
- Periampullary Tumor
- Sclerosing Cholangitis
- AIDS-Related Cholangiopathy

ESSENTIAL INFORMATION

Helpful Clues for Common Diagnoses
- **Choledocholithiasis**
  - Most common in common bile duct (CBD)
  - Round echogenic focus with marked posterior acoustic shadowing
    - Small soft stones may lack posterior acoustic shadowing
- **Ascending Cholangitis**
  - Obstructing CBD stone
  - Biliary duct wall thickening
  - Periportal inflammatory hypo-/hyperechogenicity
- **Recurrent Pyogenic Cholangitis**
  - Stones in both intrahepatic and extrahepatic bile ducts
    - Densely packed intrahepatic stones: Appear as echogenic masses, serpiginous in configuration, along portal triads
  - Atrophy of involved lobe/segment of liver in later stages
- **Pancreatic Ductal Carcinoma**
  - Ill-defined solid mass in pancreatic head
  - Pancreatic duct dilatation
  - Vascular encasement ± regional nodal/liver metastases
- **Cholangiocarcinoma**
  - Extrahepatic cholangiocarcinoma causing intra- and extrahepatic biliary dilatation
  - Ill-defined, infiltrative, iso-/hyperechoic mass
  - Irregular soft tissue thickening of extrahepatic bile duct
  - Polypoidal mass within CBD
- **Choledochal Cyst**
  - Congenital biliary malformation characterized by fusiform duct dilatation
  - Most commonly involves CBD
  - Cystic extrahepatic mass separated from gallbladder and communicating with CHD or intrahepatic ducts
  - Fusiform dilatation of extra- ± intrahepatic bile ducts
  - Abrupt change in caliber at junction of dilated segment to normal ducts

Helpful Clues for Less Common Diagnoses
- **Sclerosing Cholangitis**
  - Multiple intra- and extrahepatic biliary strictures + dilatation

Choledocholithiasis

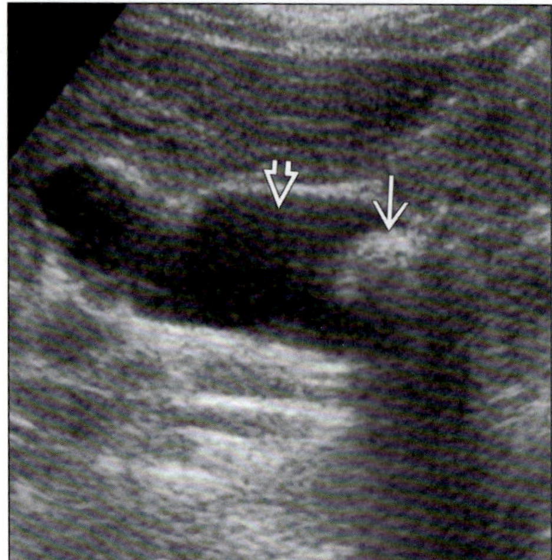

Oblique transabdominal ultrasound shows a large echogenic stone ➜ with posterior acoustic shadowing within the distal portion of a dilated common bile duct ➜, causing biliary obstruction.

Choledocholithiasis

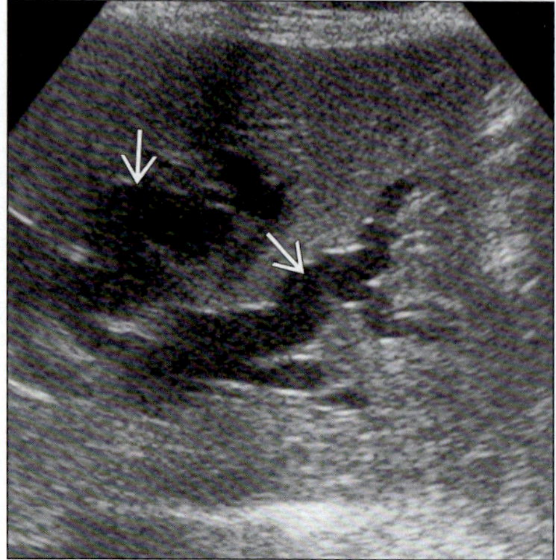

Oblique transabdominal ultrasound shows a tortuous dilatation of left intrahepatic ducts ➜ due to a large stone impacted at the distal common bile duct. The right intrahepatic ducts (not shown) were also dilated.

INTRAHEPATIC & EXTRAHEPATIC DUCT DILATATION

Ascending Cholangitis

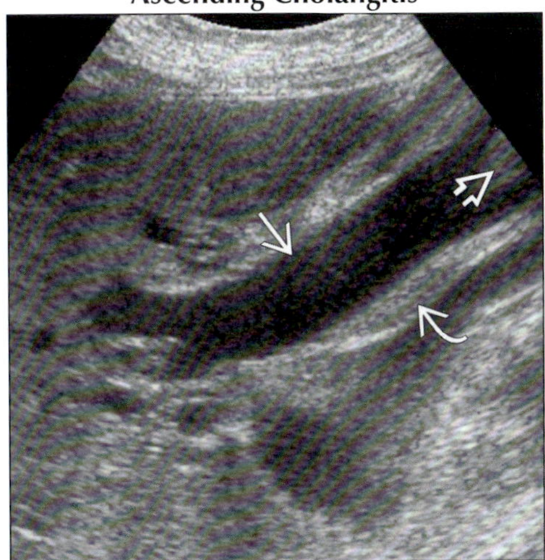

Recurrent Pyogenic Cholangitis

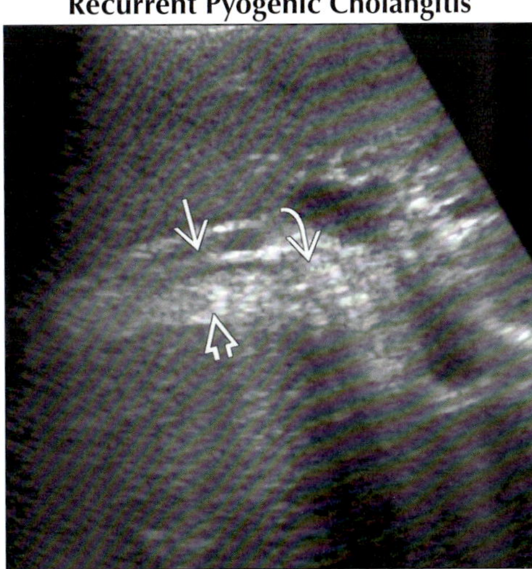

(Left) Oblique transabdominal ultrasound shows a dilated common bile duct ➡ with a distal obstructing stone ⮞ and markedly thickened wall ➡ in a patient with acute ascending cholangitis. *(Right)* Oblique transabdominal ultrasound shows thickening of the intrahepatic ducts ➡ and stones ➡ in the right lobe of the liver. There is increased periportal echogenicity ⮞ due to periductal inflammation.

Pancreatic Ductal Carcinoma

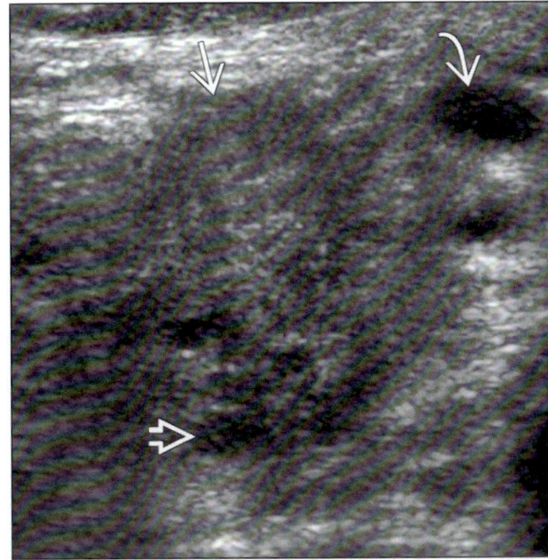

Cholangiocarcinoma

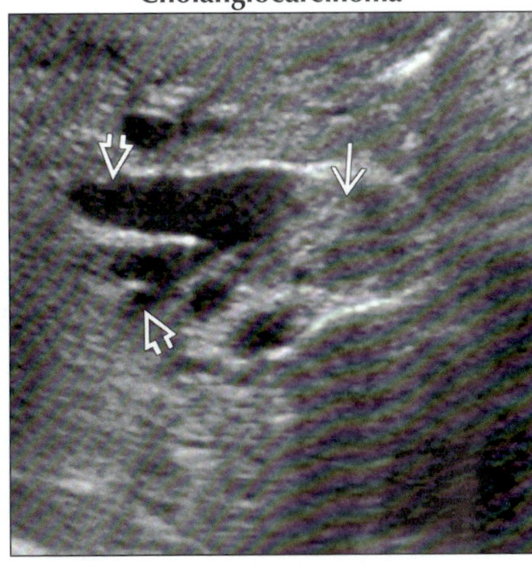

(Left) Transverse transabdominal ultrasound shows a large, heterogeneous, hypoechoic, solid mass ➡ in the pancreatic head. The distal common bile duct ⮞ and pancreatic duct ➡ are dilated. *(Right)* Oblique transabdominal ultrasound shows an intraluminal nodular growth ➡ within the proximal extrahepatic bile duct. Note the presence of intrahepatic biliary duct dilatation ⮞.

Choledochal Cyst

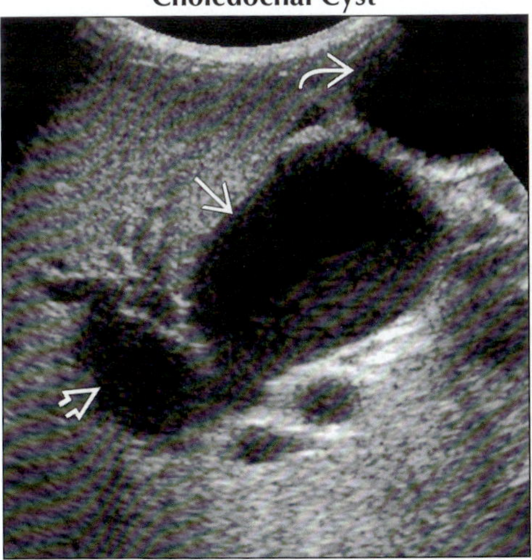

Sludge

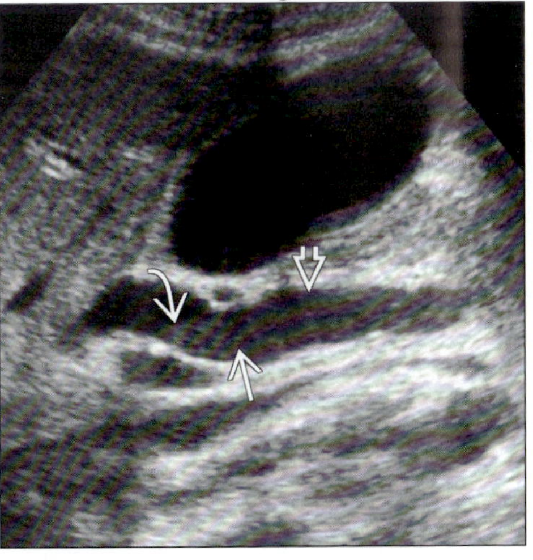

(Left) Oblique transabdominal ultrasound shows fusiform dilatation of the common bile duct ➡ and proximal intrahepatic bile duct ⮞ in a patient with a choledochal cyst. Note the extrahepatic portion of the choledochal cyst is separated from the gallbladder ➡. *(Right)* Oblique transabdominal ultrasound shows the presence of medium-level echogenic material ➡ within a dilated CBD ⮞ causing biliary obstruction. Note presence of bile-sludge level ➡.

ISOLATED INTRAHEPATIC DUCT DILATATION

DIFFERENTIAL DIAGNOSIS

Common
- Choledocholithiasis
- Cholangiocarcinoma
- Recurrent Pyogenic Cholangitis

Less Common
- Caroli Disease
- Extrinsic Compression by Liver Mass
  - Metastases, GB Carcinoma, etc
- Postoperative/Inflammatory Biliary Stricture
- Blocked Internal Biliary Stent

ESSENTIAL INFORMATION

Helpful Clues for Common Diagnoses
- **Choledocholithiasis**
  - Intrahepatic stones may cause intrahepatic duct dilatation
  - Most calculi appear as highly echogenic foci with posterior acoustic shadowing
    - Located in region of portal triad; parallel to course of intrahepatic portal veins
  - Small (< 5 mm) or soft pigmented stones may not produce shadowing
  - Linear echogenic lesion with shadowing if duct is completely packed with stones
- **Cholangiocarcinoma**
  - Intrahepatic cholangiocarcinoma
    - Mass with ill-defined margin
    - Mostly hyperechoic and heterogeneous
  - Klatskin tumor
    - Tumor at hepatic confluence
    - Noncommunication between left and right hepatic ducts
    - Primary tumor may not be discernible on US as it may be isoechoic to liver
    - May appear as small infiltrative iso-/hyperechoic mass in hilar region or nodular/polypoid mass in central bile duct
- **Recurrent Pyogenic Cholangitis**
  - Clinical history: Recurrent attacks of RUQ pain, fever, and jaundice
  - Presence of both intra- and extrahepatic stones
  - Multiple intrahepatic bile duct strictures and dilatation
  - Associated with biliary parasitic infection
    - *Clonorchis sinensis* &/or *Ascaris lumbricoides*

Helpful Clues for Less Common Diagnoses
- **Caroli Disease**
  - Congenital cystic dilatation of intrahepatic bile duct
  - Saccular or fusiform dilatation of intrahepatic duct
  - Lobar or segmental in distribution
  - May contain calculus or sludge within dilated duct
- **Blocked Internal Biliary Stent**
  - Usually deployed for palliation of malignant biliary stricture
  - Dilatation of ducts in stented lobe if blocked by tumor cast, blood clot, or inspissation

Choledocholithiasis

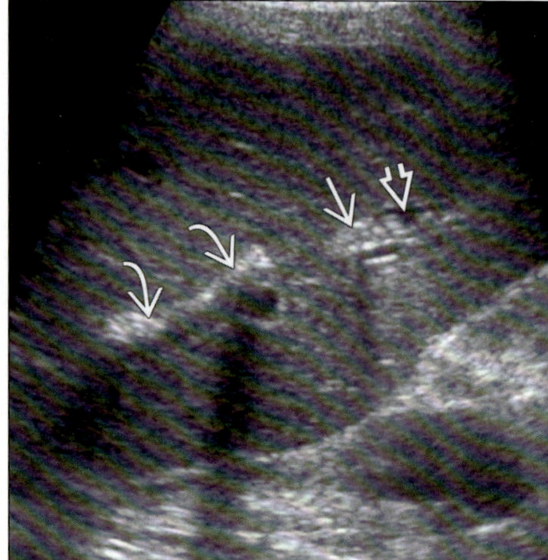

Oblique transabdominal ultrasound shows intrahepatic duct stones ➡ in a dilated intrahepatic duct ➡. Note hyperechogenicity along portal triad ➡, representing an intrahepatic duct packed with stones.

Recurrent Pyogenic Cholangitis

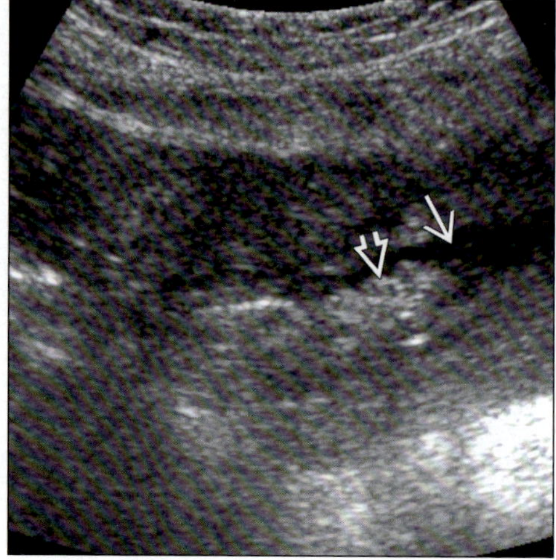

Transverse transabdominal ultrasound shows a dilated intrahepatic duct ➡ in the lateral segment of left lobe of the liver, containing echogenic stones ➡ in a patient with known recurrent pyogenic cholangitis.

ISOLATED INTRAHEPATIC DUCT DILATATION

Cholangiocarcinoma

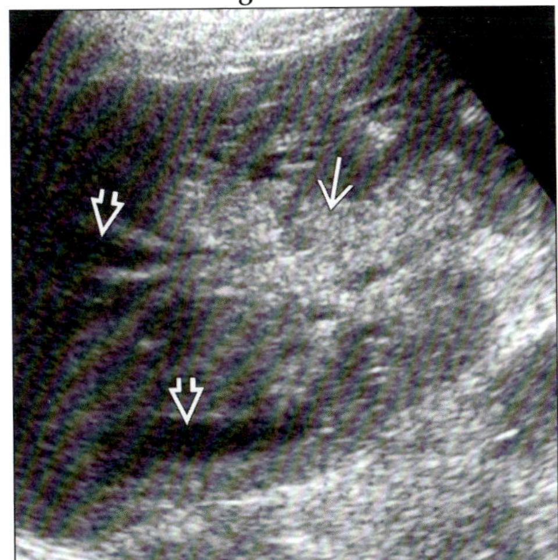

Cholangiocarcinoma

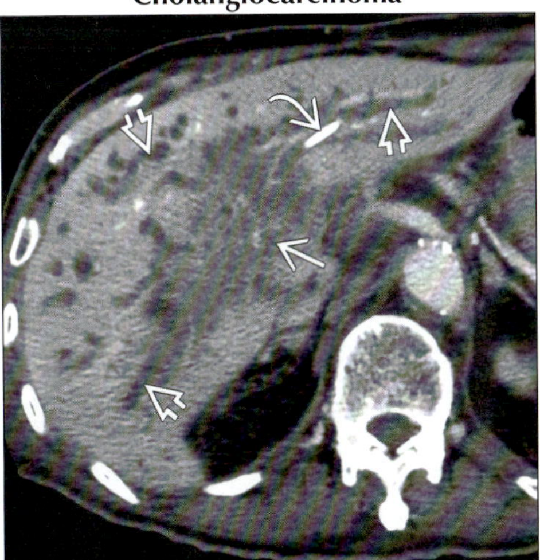

(Left) Oblique transabdominal ultrasound shows an ill-defined hyperechoic tumor ➡ at the hepatic confluence, causing marked dilatation of the intrahepatic ducts ➡ in both lobes of the liver. (Right) Corresponding CECT shows an ill-defined, heterogeneously enhancing, central cholangiocarcinoma ➡ (Klatskin tumor) with associated dilatation of intrahepatic bile ducts ➡. Note the presence of a stent ➡ in the left-sided duct system.

Caroli Disease

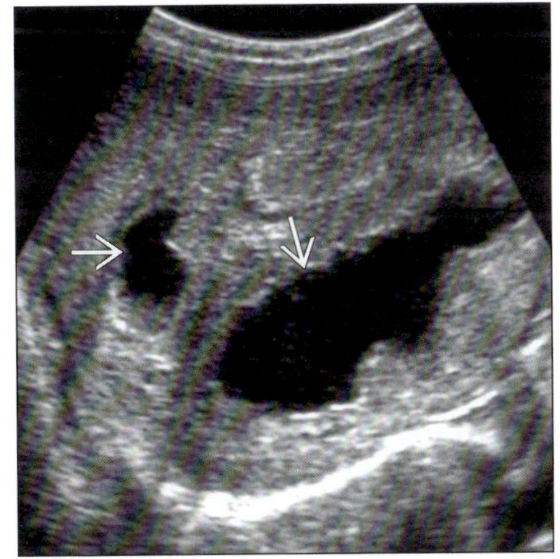

Extrinsic Compression by Liver Mass

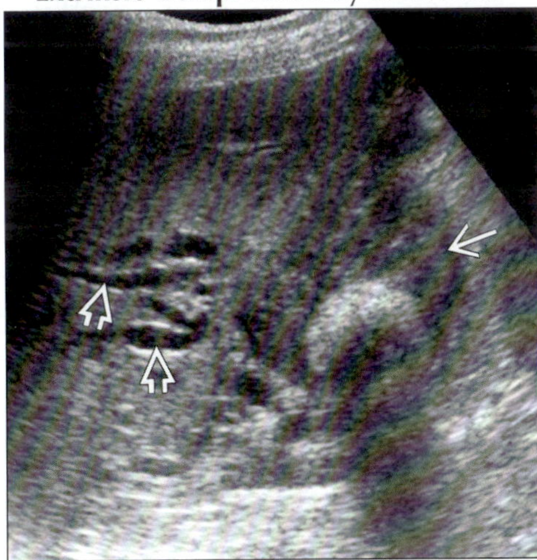

(Left) Transverse transabdominal ultrasound shows fusiform dilatation of intrahepatic ducts ➡ along the portal tract in the right posterior segment of the liver. No internal debris or intraductal calculi are seen. The features suggest Caroli disease. (Right) Oblique transabdominal ultrasound shows an ill-defined gallbladder carcinoma ➡ with adjacent liver infiltration at the hepatic confluence, causing intrahepatic duct compression and dilatation ➡.

Extrinsic Compression by Liver Mass

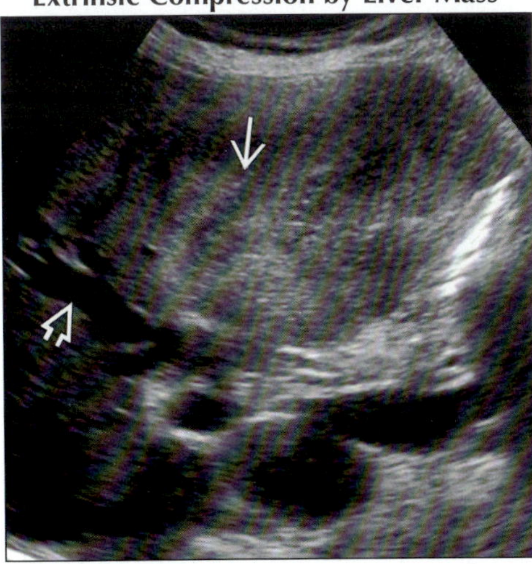

Blocked Internal Biliary Stent

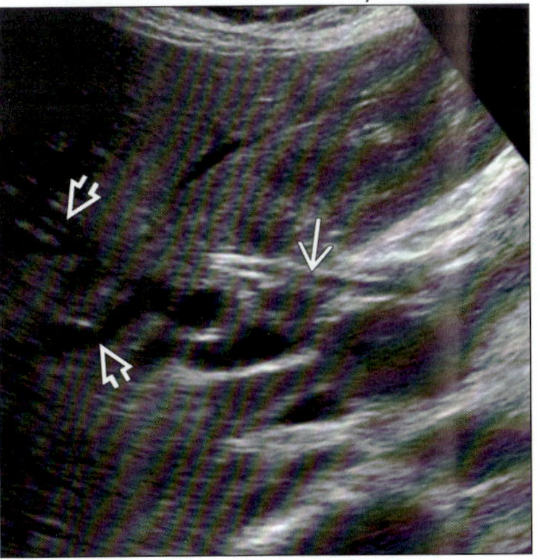

(Left) Oblique transabdominal ultrasound shows a large, mildly hyperechoic, metastatic tumor ➡ in the left lobe of the liver compressing the hepatic confluence, resulting in intrahepatic biliary ductal dilatation ➡. (Right) Oblique transabdominal ultrasound shows dilatation of the intrahepatic bile ducts ➡ in the right lobe of the liver due to blockage of the internal biliary stent ➡ within the common bile duct.

4

DIFFERENTIAL DIAGNOSIS

Common
- Choledocholithiasis
- Sludge/Sludge Ball
- Ascending Cholangitis
- Recurrent Pyogenic Cholangitis
- Cholangiocarcinoma

Less Common
- Parasitic Infestation
- Biliary Duct Gas
- Blood Clot
- Tumor Cast
- Biliary Stent/Drainage Catheter

ESSENTIAL INFORMATION

Helpful Clues for Common Diagnoses
- **Choledocholithiasis**
  - Highly reflective echogenic focus
  - Posterior acoustic shadowing
    - Small or soft stones may not produce posterior shadowing
    - Sometimes difficult to differentiate from sludge ball
- **Sludge/Sludge Ball**
  - Low- to medium-level echoes
  - Sludge-fluid level
  - Discrete round contour for sludge ball
  - Absence of posterior acoustic shadowing
- **Ascending Cholangitis**
  - Obstructing common bile duct stone
  - Intra- and extrahepatic biliary dilatation
  - Bile duct wall thickening
  - Inflammatory periportal hypo-/hyperechogenicity
- **Recurrent Pyogenic Cholangitis**
  - Presence of intra- and extrahepatic stones
  - Multiple sites of biliary strictures and associated duct dilatation
  - Atrophy lobe/segment in later stages
- **Cholangiocarcinoma**
  - Polypoid irregular mass/soft tissue thickening in bile duct
  - Associated biliary dilatation; distribution depends on level of primary tumor
  - May have increased vascularity on color Doppler US

Helpful Clues for Less Common Diagnoses
- **Parasitic Infestation**
  - Most common: *Ascaris, Clonorchis,* ruptured hydatid cyst
  - Parallel echogenic tubular structures with sonolucent center
  - Active movement in viable worm
  - Lack of posterior acoustic shadowing
- **Biliary Duct Gas**
  - Bright echogenic foci linear in configuration, following portal triads
  - In nondependent position: Left lobe with patient in supine position
  - "Dirty" posterior acoustic shadow ± reverberation artifacts
  - Movement of gas following change in patient's position

Choledocholithiasis

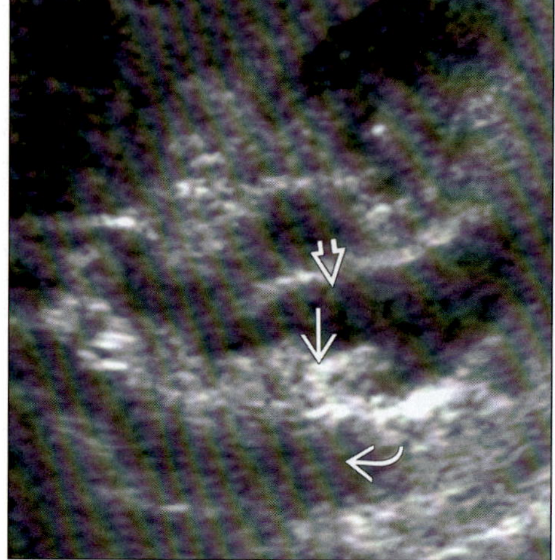

Oblique transabdominal ultrasound shows multiple echogenic masses ➡ in the dependent portion of the common bile duct ➡, which is dilated. Note the presence of mild posterior acoustic shadowing ➡.

Choledocholithiasis

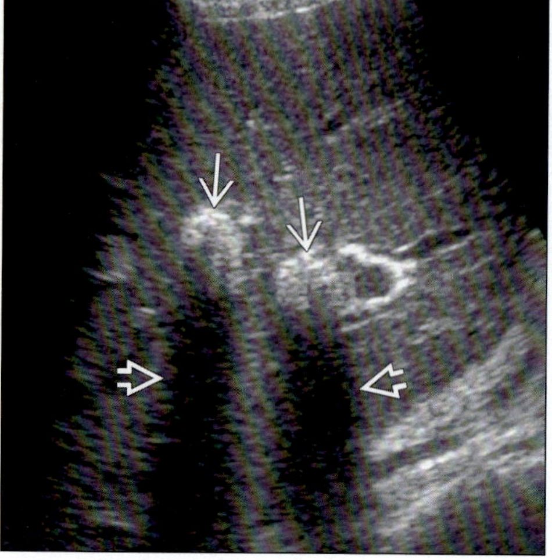

Oblique transabdominal ultrasound shows large intrahepatic duct stones ➡ with strong posterior acoustic shadowing ➡ in the right lobe of the liver.

INTRALUMINAL ECHOES IN BILIARY DUCT

Sludge/Sludge Ball

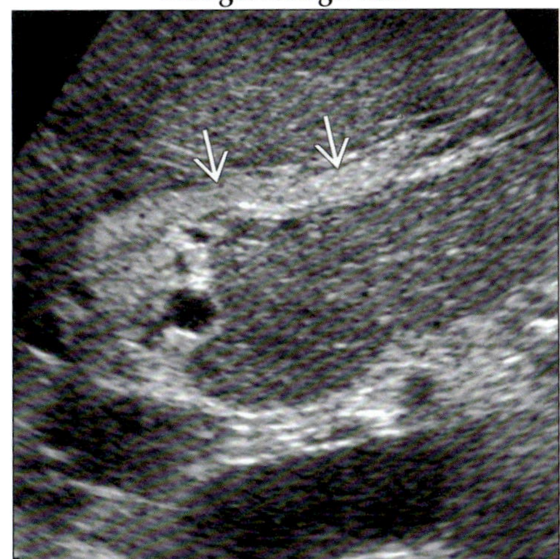

Cholangiocarcinoma

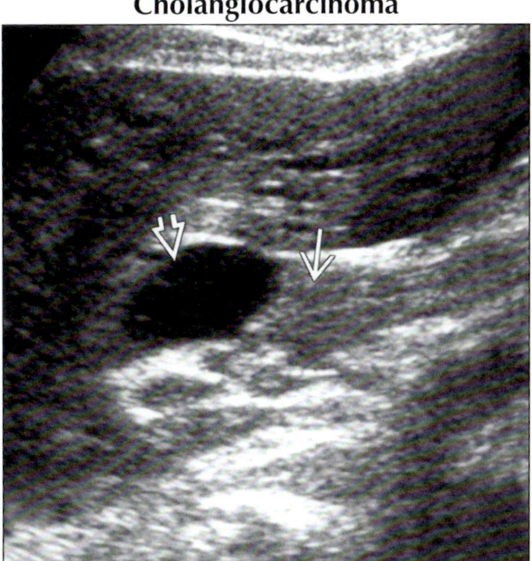

(Left) Oblique transabdominal ultrasound shows linear echogenic material ➡ along the portal triad, involving the left lobe of the liver & representing a sludge-filled intrahepatic duct. Note absence of posterior acoustic shadowing. (Right) Oblique transabdominal ultrasound shows soft tissue of medium echogenicity ➡ filling the distal portion of the common bile duct, causing proximal duct dilatation ➡. Color Doppler revealed vascular flow within.

Parasitic Infestation

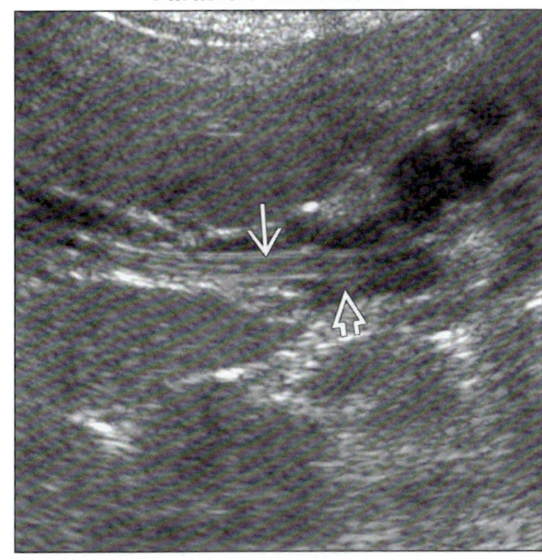

Biliary Duct Gas

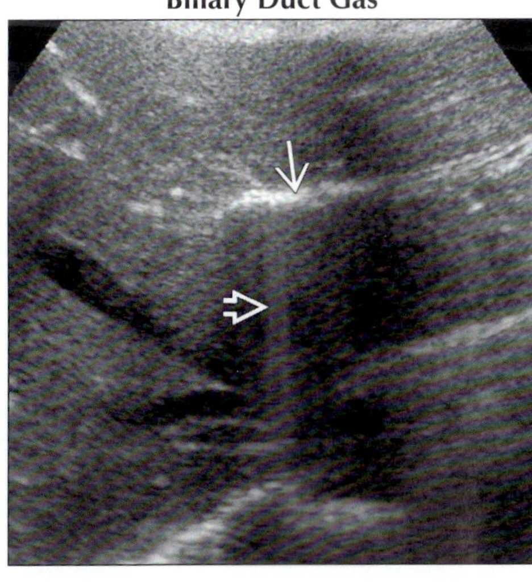

(Left) Oblique transabdominal ultrasound shows a tubular structure ➡ with parallel echogenic lines and a sonolucent center within the dilated common bile duct ➡. It showed active movement on real-time ultrasound, compatible with a viable worm. (Right) Transverse transabdominal ultrasound shows linear hyperechogenicity in the portal triad ➡ with "dirty" shadowing and reverberation artifacts ➡.

Tumor Cast

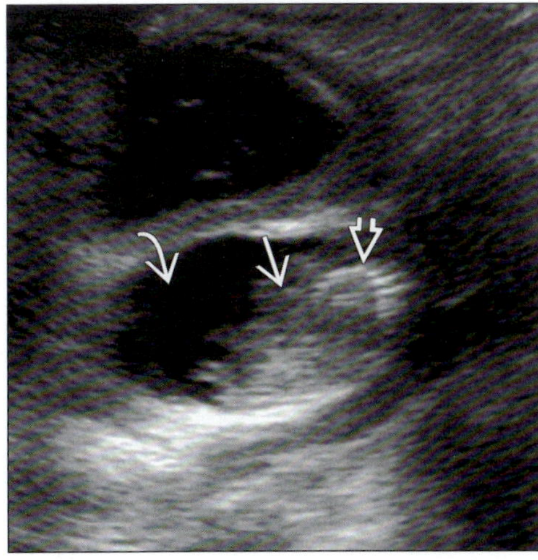

Biliary Stent/Drainage Catheter

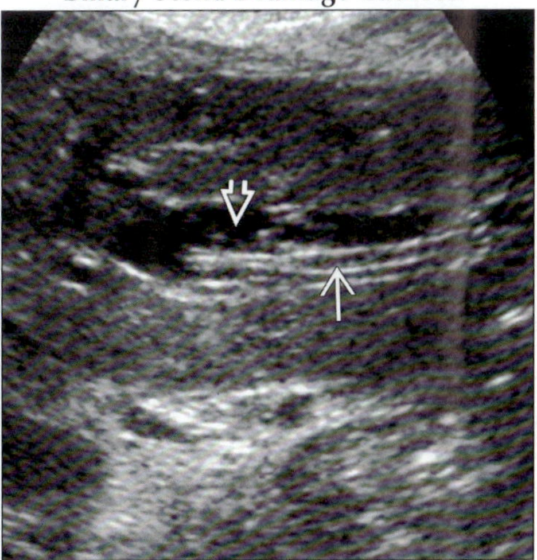

(Left) Oblique transabdominal ultrasound shows a polypoidal mass ➡ of medium echogenicity within a CBD, closely related to the proximal end of a metallic internal biliary stent ➡. The internal stent is blocked by a tumor cast, causing biliary obstruction. Note dilatation of proximal CBD ➡. (Right) Transverse transabdominal ultrasound shows echogenic parallel lines ➡ within a dilated left intrahepatic duct ➡, representing a percutaneous biliary drainage catheter.

4

BILIARY DUCT WALL THICKENING +/- PERIPORTAL CHANGE

DIFFERENTIAL DIAGNOSIS

Common
- Ascending Cholangitis
- Recurrent Pyogenic Cholangitis
- Cholangiocarcinoma

Less Common
- Sclerosing Cholangitis
- AIDS-Related Cholangiopathy
- Periportal Fibrosis

ESSENTIAL INFORMATION

Key Differential Diagnosis Issues
- Smooth duct wall thickening more common in inflammatory disease
  - Suspect malignancy if irregular contour, more bulky soft tissue
- Hypo- or hyperechoic periportal changes suggest presence of periductal inflammation or fibrosis

Helpful Clues for Common Diagnoses
- **Ascending Cholangitis**
  - Obstructing CBD stone
  - Dilatation of intra- and extrahepatic bile duct
    - May contain purulent bile/sludge: Presence of intraluminal echogenic material
  - Circumferential thickening of bile duct wall
    - May extend to involve gallbladder, causing GB wall thickening
  - Periportal hypo-/hyperechogenicity adjacent to dilated intrahepatic ducts
- **Recurrent Pyogenic Cholangitis**
  - Presence of intra- and extrahepatic biliary stones
  - Multiple biliary strictures + dilatation
  - In superimposed acute infective exacerbation
    - Bile duct wall thickening
    - Periportal hypo-/hyperechoic changes due to periductal inflammation
- **Cholangiocarcinoma**
  - Focal/asymmetric bile duct wall thickening with irregular contour
  - Associated biliary duct dilatation
  - Regional nodal/liver metastases

Helpful Clues for Less Common Diagnoses
- **Sclerosing Cholangitis**
  - Diffuse thickening of CBD ± intrahepatic bile ducts
  - Multiple intrahepatic strictures and dilatation
  - Associated with inflammatory bowel disease
- **AIDS-Related Cholangiopathy**
  - Wall thickening may involve both intra- and extrahepatic bile ducts
  - Mild biliary duct dilatation + periductal hyper-/hypoechoic areas
  - Diffuse GB wall thickening
- **Periportal Fibrosis**
  - Biochemical profile of cirrhosis
  - Diffuse periportal hyperechogenicity

Ascending Cholangitis

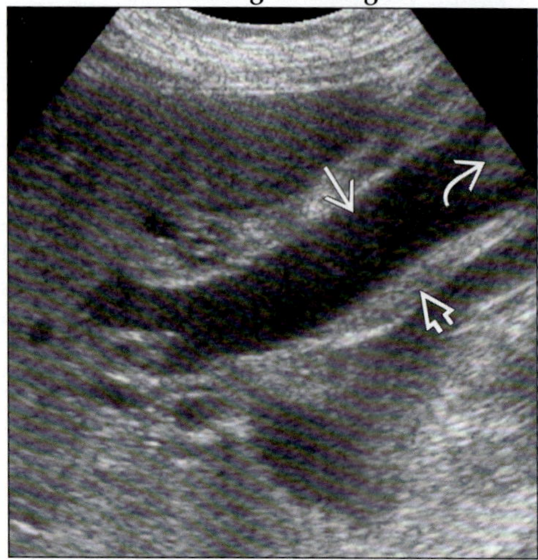

Oblique transabdominal ultrasound shows a dilated common bile duct ➡ with a markedly thickened wall ⇉. Note the presence of a distal obstructing stone ⇊. Features are consistent with ascending cholangitis.

Ascending Cholangitis

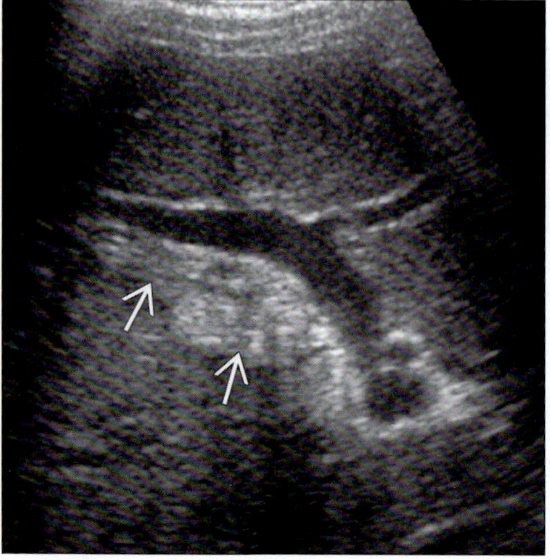

Oblique transabdominal ultrasound in a patient with ascending cholangitis shows marked periportal hyperechogenicity ➡ adjacent to a right portal venous radicle due to periductal inflammation.

BILIARY DUCT WALL THICKENING +/- PERIPORTAL CHANGE

Recurrent Pyogenic Cholangitis

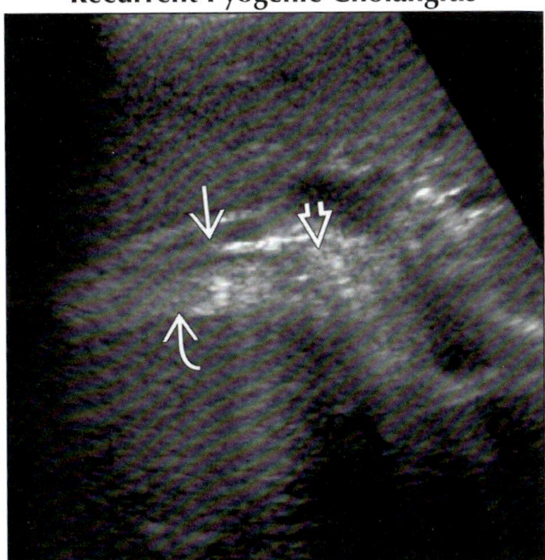

Recurrent Pyogenic Cholangitis

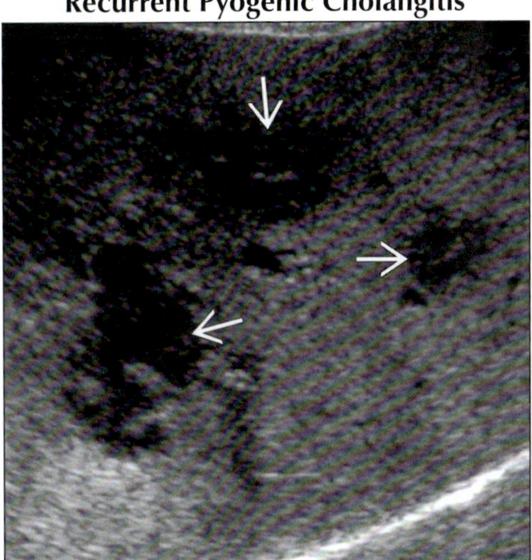

(Left) Oblique transabdominal ultrasound shows wall thickening ➡ of dilated intrahepatic bile ducts with stones ➡ in the right lobe of the liver. Note the presence of increased periportal echogenicity ➡ due to active periductal inflammation. (Right) Oblique transabdominal ultrasound shows multiple cystic liver masses ➡ with low-level internal echoes compatible with cholangitic abscesses in a patient with recurrent pyogenic cholangitis.

Cholangiocarcinoma

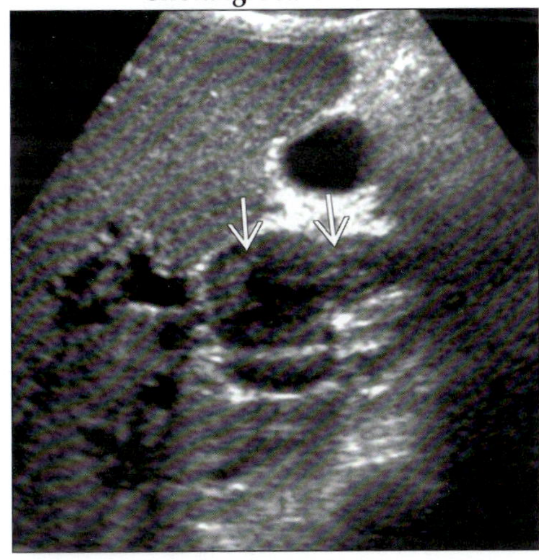

Sclerosing Cholangitis

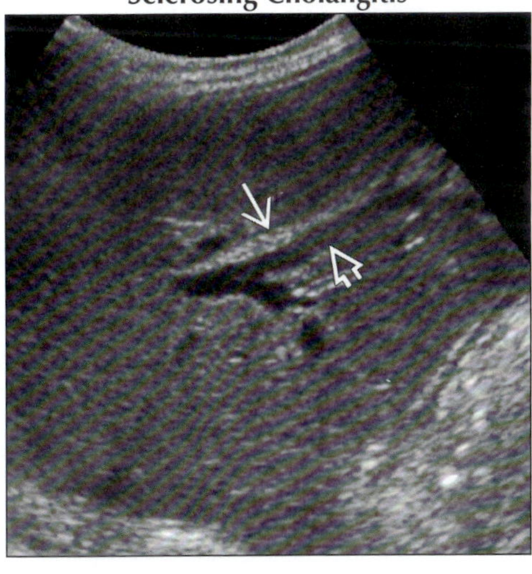

(Left) Oblique transabdominal ultrasound shows an ill-defined circumferential tumor ➡ along the proximal extrahepatic bile duct with extension to the hepatic confluence. (Right) Oblique transabdominal ultrasound shows wall thickening and periportal increased echogenicity ➡ adjacent to a dilated intrahepatic duct ➡ in the left lateral segment. Similar changes were also noted in other parts of both lobes of the liver.

AIDS-Related Cholangiopathy

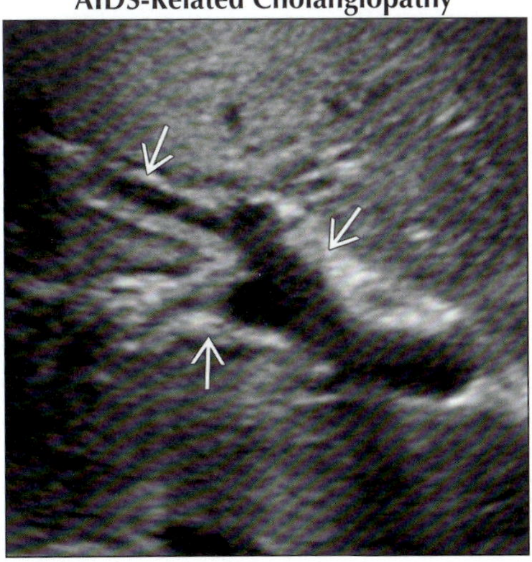

Periportal Fibrosis

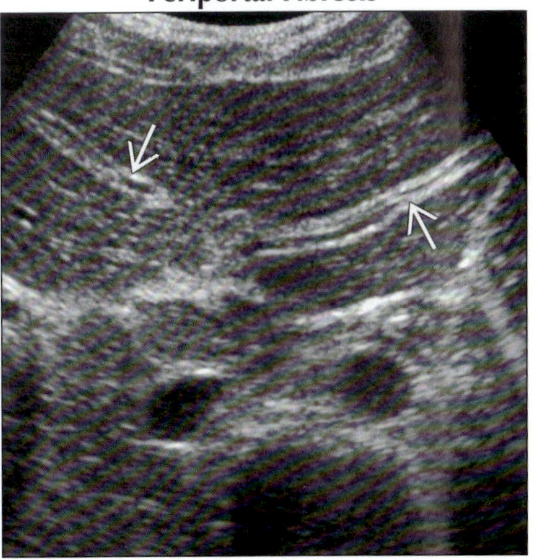

(Left) Oblique transabdominal ultrasound in an HIV-infected patient with impaired liver function shows mild intrahepatic duct dilatation with diffuse echogenic wall thickening ➡. (Right) Transverse transabdominal ultrasound shows diffuse increase in periportal hyperechogenicity ➡ involving both the left and right (not shown) lobes of the liver. The patient has a history of biliary atresia with development of periportal fibrosis years after Kasai operation.

SECTION 5
Pancreas

CYSTIC PANCREATIC LESION

DIFFERENTIAL DIAGNOSIS

Common
- Pancreatic Pseudocyst
- Serous Cystadenoma of Pancreas
- Mucinous Cystic Neoplasm
- Necrotic Pancreatic Ductal Carcinoma

Less Common
- Congenital Cyst
- Solid and Papillary Neoplasm
- Intraductal Papillary Mucinous Tumor (IPMT)
- Cystic Islet Cell Tumor
- Lymphangioma
- Cystic Metastases/Lymphoma

ESSENTIAL INFORMATION

Key Differential Diagnosis Issues
- Pancreatic pseudocysts account for most cystic pancreatic lesions
  - Consider cystic neoplasm if "cystic" lesion contains solid component/large internal septations/vascularity

Helpful Clues for Common Diagnoses
- **Pancreatic Pseudocyst**
  - Common late complication of pancreatitis
    - Develops 4-6 weeks after onset of acute pancreatitis
    - Seen in ~ 15% of patients
  - Generally well circumscribed, smooth walled, unilocular, anechoic with posterior acoustic enhancement
    - May be complicated in appearance
      - Multilocular (~ 6%)
      - Fluid-debris level, internal echoes, septations if previous hemorrhage or infection
      - Wall calcification
- **Serous Cystadenoma of Pancreas**
  - Benign pancreatic tumor from acinar cells
  - Most frequently seen in pancreatic head
  - Solid mass with small cystic areas
    - Cysts vary from 1-20 mm in size
  - Central echogenic scar with "sunburst" calcification
- **Mucinous Cystic Neoplasm**
  - More common in pancreatic tail
  - Multiloculated thick-walled cystic mass
  - Solid components/echogenic septae
  - May be indistinguishable from pseudocyst

Helpful Clues for Less Common Diagnoses
- **Congenital Cyst**
  - True epithelial-lined cyst
  - Associated with von Hippel-Lindau and adult polycystic kidney disease (ADPKD)
- **Solid and Papillary Neoplasm**
  - Well-defined, large mass pancreatic tail with solid and cystic areas
  - Most commonly seen in young African-American females
- **Intraductal Papillary Mucinous Tumor (IPMT)**
  - Dilated main pancreatic duct
  - "Multicystic" mass in pancreatic head/uncinate process

Pancreatic Pseudocyst

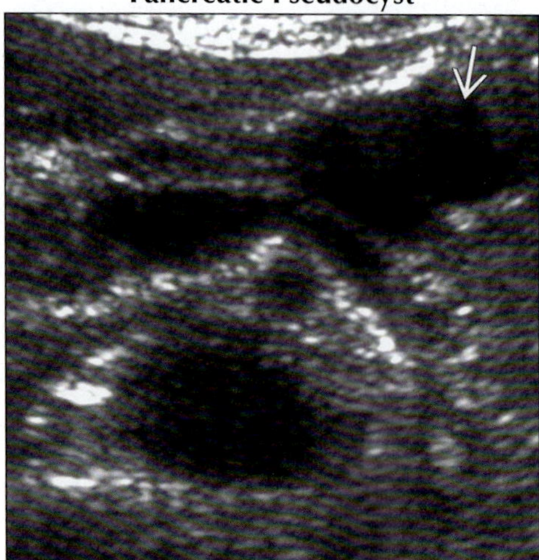

Transverse transabdominal ultrasound shows a well-circumscribed unilocular pseudocyst ➡ in the pancreatic body. In this case there is no pancreatic parenchymal calcification or duct dilatation.

Pancreatic Pseudocyst

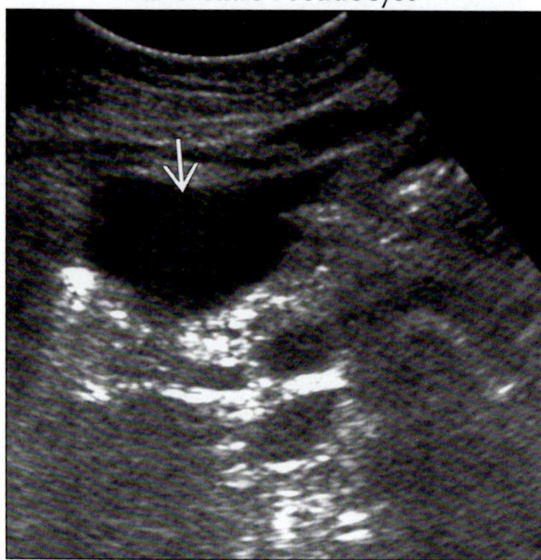

Transverse transabdominal ultrasound shows a round, well-defined, anechoic, cystic lesion ➡ in the head of the pancreas, consistent with a pseudocyst. No internal solid component or septa is seen.

CYSTIC PANCREATIC LESION

Pancreatic Pseudocyst

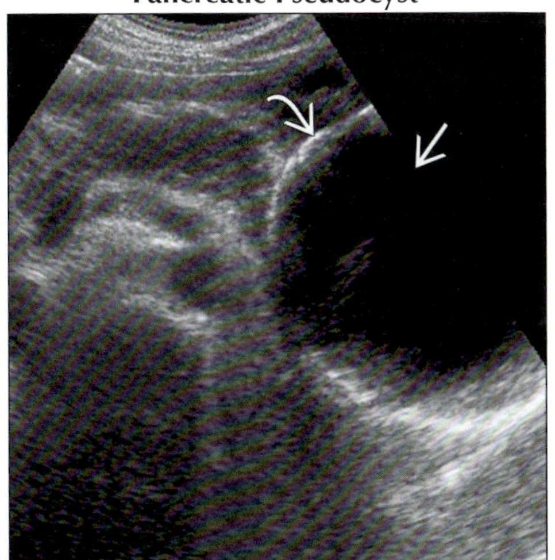

Pancreatic Pseudocyst

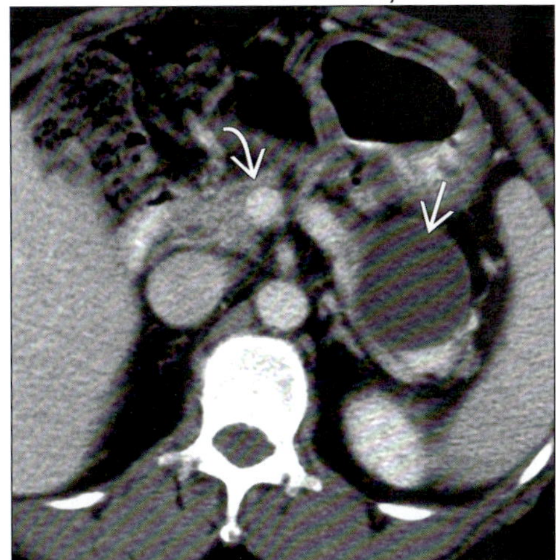

(Left) Transverse transabdominal ultrasound shows a large, well-circumscribed, unilocular pseudocyst ➡ in the pancreatic tail. Note the presence of smooth calcification ➡ of the cyst wall, suggesting that the pseudocyst is longstanding. *(Right)* Axial CECT shows a well-defined unilocular pseudocyst ➡ in the pancreatic tail. Note that the pancreas ➡ appears atrophic.

Serous Cystadenoma of Pancreas

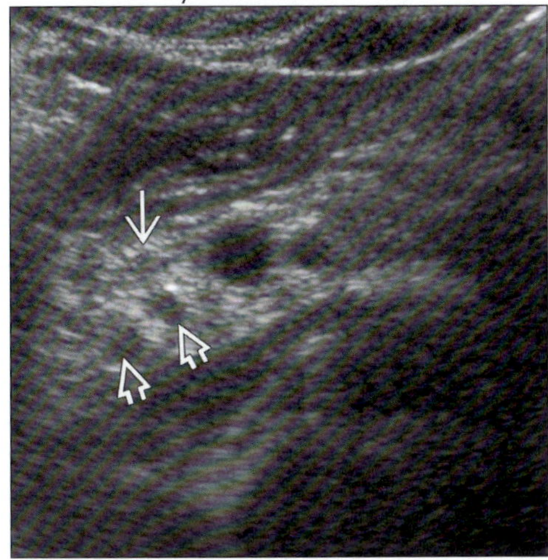

Mucinous Cystic Neoplasm

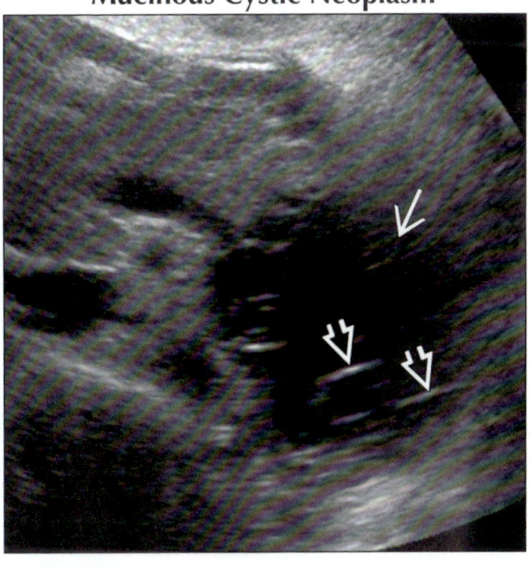

(Left) Transverse transabdominal ultrasound shows a well-defined, predominantly solid, slightly hyperechoic mass ➡ in the pancreatic head. Note the presence of microcysts ➡ within the lesion. The pancreatic duct is not dilated. *(Right)* Transverse transabdominal ultrasound shows a well-circumscribed cystic mass ➡ with multiple thin septations ➡ in the tail of the pancreas. The location and appearances are consistent with a mucinous cystic pancreatic tumor.

Congenital Cyst

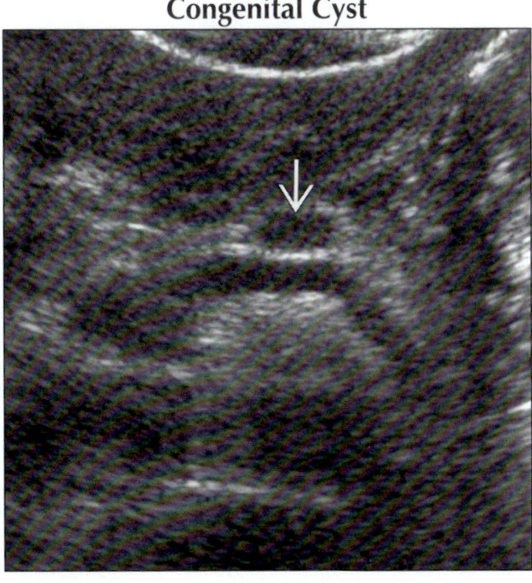

Intraductal Papillary Mucinous Tumor (IPMT)

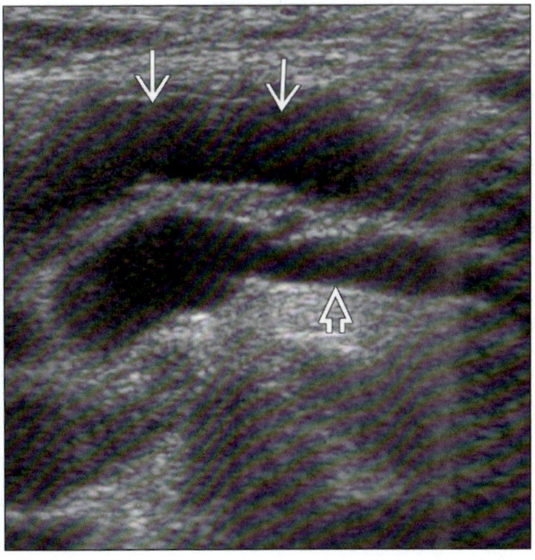

(Left) Transverse transabdominal ultrasound in a patient with ADPKD shows a small, well-circumscribed, cystic lesion ➡ in the body of the pancreas. Note the absence of an internal solid component, calcification, or septation. *(Right)* Transverse transabdominal ultrasound shows a markedly dilated pancreatic duct ➡ within an atrophic pancreas. This should not be confused with the splenic vein ➡. Note the absence of pancreatic parenchymal calcification or ductal calculus.

SOLID PANCREATIC LESION

DIFFERENTIAL DIAGNOSIS

Common
- Pancreatic Ductal Carcinoma
- Serous Cystadenoma of Pancreas
- Pancreatic Islet Cell Tumor
- Focal Acute Pancreatitis
- Chronic Pancreatitis

Less Common
- Solid and Pseudopapillary Neoplasm
- Mucinous Cystic Pancreatic Neoplasm
- Metastasis
- Lymphoma

ESSENTIAL INFORMATION

Key Differential Diagnosis Issues
- Correlate with clinical information (e.g., evidence of acute/chronic pancreatitis)
- Pancreatic duct dilatation favors diagnosis of pancreatic ductal carcinoma
  - Biliary dilatation present as well in pancreatic head ductal carcinoma
- Other ancillary findings to look for include
  - Presence of intralesional calcification
  - Cystic component
  - Internal septation
  - Regional lymph node and liver metastases
  - Vascular encasement
- Clues to detection of small tumor
  - Focal contour irregularity
  - Subtle pancreatic duct/bile duct dilatation
- CECT helps to detect and characterize solid pancreatic lesions
  - Aids in detection of vascular encasement

Helpful Clues for Common Diagnoses
- **Pancreatic Ductal Carcinoma**
  - Pathology: Scirrhous infiltrative adenocarcinoma with dense cellularity and sparse vascularity
  - Arises from ductal epithelium of exocrine pancreas
  - Location: Head of pancreas (60-70%), body (20%), diffuse (15%), tail (5%)
  - Average size ~ 2-3 cm
  - Typical US findings
    - Poorly defined, homogeneous or heterogeneous, hypoechoic mass
    - Pancreatic duct dilatation distal to tumor with abrupt tapering at site of obstruction

- Bile duct dilatation seen in pancreatic head tumor
- Necrosis/cystic component is rarely seen
- Displacement/encasement of adjacent vascular structures (e.g., superior mesenteric vessels, splenic artery, hepatic artery, gastroduodenal artery)
- Presence of liver and regional nodal metastases
- Ascites due to peritoneal metastases
- **Serous Cystadenoma of Pancreas**
  - More common in pancreatic head
  - US appearance depends on size of individual cysts
    - Slightly echogenic, solid-appearing mass (small cysts provide multiple acoustic interfaces)
    - Partly solid-looking mass with anechoic cystic areas; cysts usually at periphery
    - Multicystic mass with septae and solid component
  - Amorphous central calcification
    - Echogenic foci with "sunburst" appearance
    - Dense posterior acoustic shadowing distal to pancreatic mass
  - Central echogenic stellate scar
    - Characteristic feature
    - Present in up to ~ 20% of cases
  - No pancreatic duct dilatation
- **Pancreatic Islet Cell Tumor**
  - Detection of islet cell tumor is difficult due to small tumor size
  - Endoscopic US detects tumors in pancreatic head and body
  - Intraoperative US is useful for tumor localization
  - Usually small, solid, hypoechoic mass
  - Occasionally isoechoic in appearance; seen as focal bulge of contour
  - Usually lack of calcification or necrosis
  - Liver and regional lymph node metastases seen in 60-90% at clinical presentation
    - Hyperechoic liver metastases more suggestive of islet cell tumors than ductal carcinoma
  - Hypervascular on power Doppler US, CT, and angiography
- **Focal Acute Pancreatitis**
  - Clinical information very important for correct imaging interpretation

SOLID PANCREATIC LESION

- Acute onset of epigastric pain, fever, and vomiting
- Raised serum amylase and lipase
- Presence of underlying predisposing factors: Biliary stone, alcoholism, drugs (e.g., steroid), trauma, etc.
  - Focal, ill-defined, hypoechoic enlargement of pancreatic parenchyma
    - Heterogeneous appearance in cases with intrapancreatic necrosis/hemorrhage
  - Blurred pancreatic outline/margin
  - Presence of peri-pancreatic fluid collection
  - Lack of pancreatic duct dilatation
  - No parenchymal calcification
- **Chronic Pancreatitis**
  - Longstanding clinical symptoms, recurrent attacks of epigastric pain, typically radiates to back
  - Most common US features
    - Diffuse atrophic pancreas with calcification/ductal calculus and pancreatic duct dilatation
  - Focal mass/enlargement in 40%
    - Pancreatic parenchymal calcification
    - Pancreatic duct dilatation
  - Some cases of chronic pancreatitis and pancreatic cancer impossible to differentiate without surgical excision and histology

Helpful Clues for Less Common Diagnoses
- **Solid and Pseudopapillary Neoplasm**
  - Most common in pancreatic tail
  - Well-demarcated, large, heterogeneous mass
  - Small cystic component often present
  - Dystrophic calcification occasionally seen
  - No pancreatic duct dilatation or calcification
  - Liver metastases seen in ~ 4% of patients with a solid and papillary neoplasm
  - Color Doppler: Hypervascular pattern
- **Mucinous Cystic Pancreatic Neoplasm**
  - More common in pancreatic tail
  - Well-demarcated, thick-walled, cystic mass
  - Uni-, multilocular cysts
  - Separated by thick echogenic septae
  - Solid papillary tissue protruding into tumor suggests malignancy
  - Liver metastases appear as thick-walled cystic hepatic lesions
- **Metastasis**
  - Nonspecific imaging findings
  - Focal or diffuse involvement
  - History of known primary malignancy, disseminated disease
    - Common sites of primary: Lung, breast, melanoma, ovary, liver, kidney
- **Lymphoma**
  - Secondary lymphoma more common than primary lymphoma
    - Known clinical history of systemic lymphomatous involvement
  - Large, homogeneous, solid mass
  - Presence of peri-pancreatic nodal masses
  - Peri-pancreatic vessels displaced or stretched

Pancreatic Ductal Carcinoma

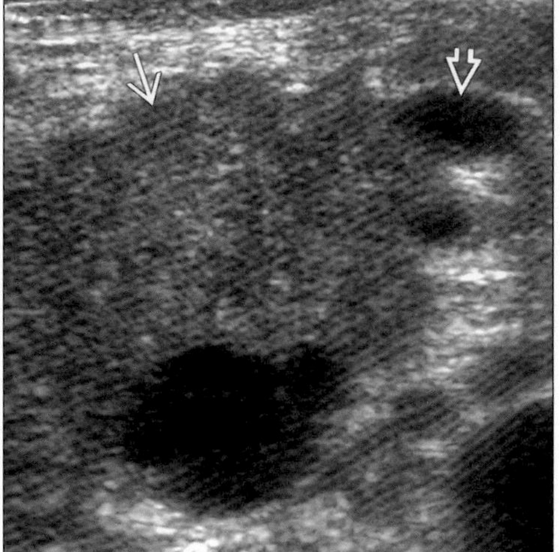

Transverse transabdominal ultrasound shows an infiltrative, solid, hypoechoic mass ➡ in the pancreatic head and uncinate process associated with pancreatic duct dilatation ➡, compatible with ductal carcinoma.

Pancreatic Ductal Carcinoma

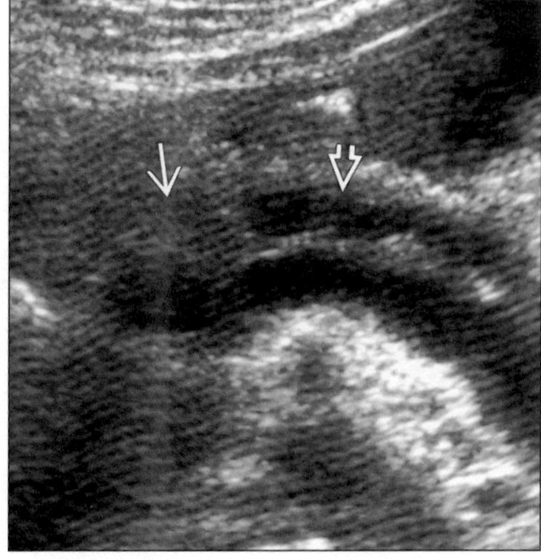

Transverse transabdominal ultrasound shows an ill-defined, solid, isoechoic mass ➡ in the head of the pancreas. Note the presence of pancreatic duct dilatation ➡ in the body and tail of the pancreas.

SOLID PANCREATIC LESION

(Left) Transverse transabdominal ultrasound shows an ill-defined, solid, hypoechoic mass ➡ in the head of the pancreas with associated distal pancreatic duct dilatation ➡, compatible with pancreatic ductal carcinoma. (Right) Oblique transabdominal ultrasound shows a round, ill-defined, solid, hypoechoic mass ➡ in the pancreatic head, causing truncation of the terminal portion of the common bile duct and proximal extrahepatic biliary duct dilatation ➡.

Pancreatic Ductal Carcinoma

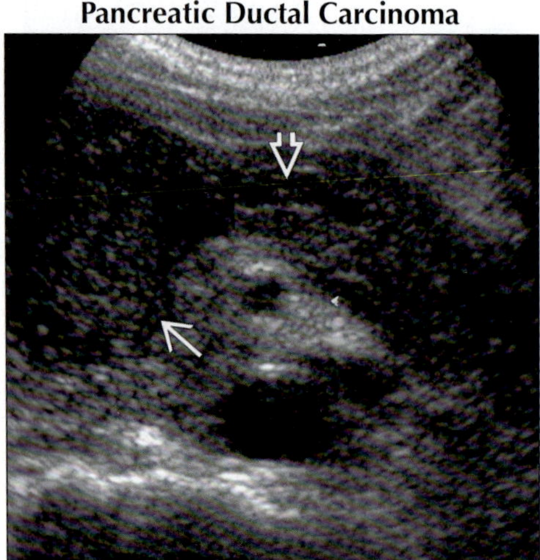

Pancreatic Ductal Carcinoma

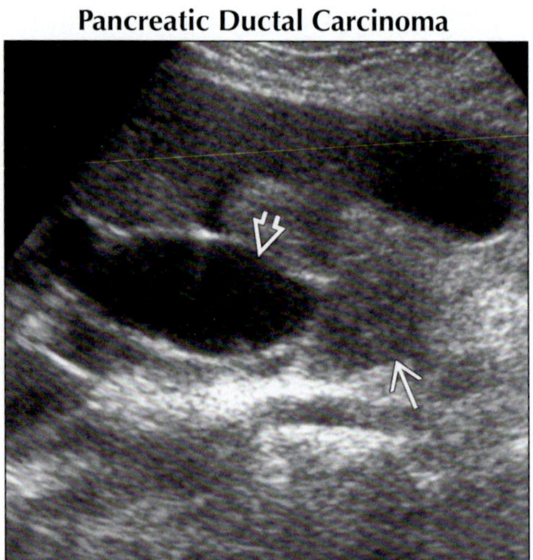

(Left) Transverse transabdominal ultrasound shows a well-circumscribed, solid, slightly hyperechoic mass ➡ in the pancreatic tail. Note the absence of pancreatic duct dilatation, cystic component, or internal calcification. The ultrasound appearance is difficult to differentiate from that of other solid pancreatic neoplasms. (Right) Longitudinal transabdominal ultrasound shows small cystic components ➡ within a solid pancreatic tail mass ➡.

Serous Cystadenoma of Pancreas

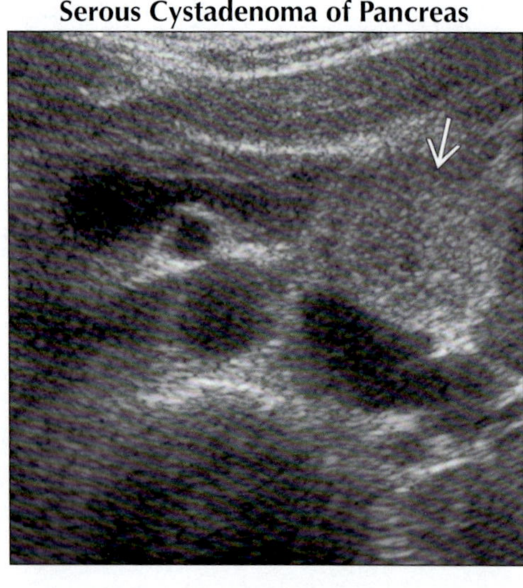

Serous Cystadenoma of Pancreas

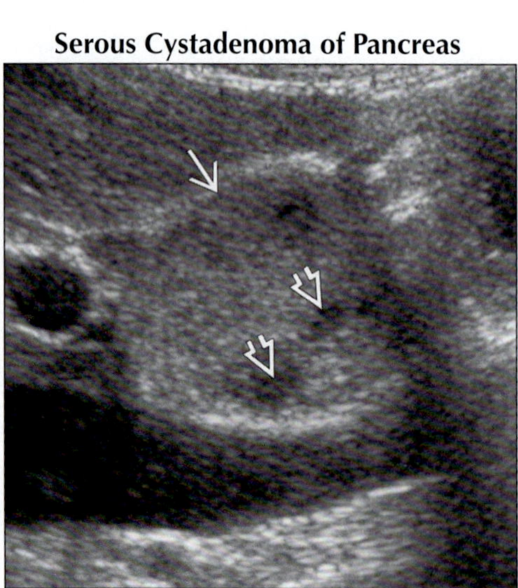

(Left) Transverse transabdominal ultrasound shows a well-circumscribed, solid, hypoechoic mass ➡ in the tail of the pancreas. (Right) Axial CECT of the same patient shows a well-defined hypervascular mass ➡ on arterial phase in the pancreatic tail. This patient presented with recurrent hypoglycemia. Surgery confirmed a pancreatic insulinoma.

Pancreatic Islet Cell Tumor

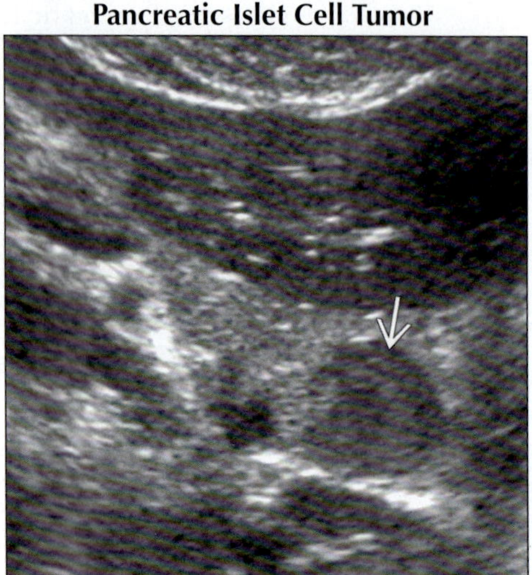

Pancreatic Islet Cell Tumor

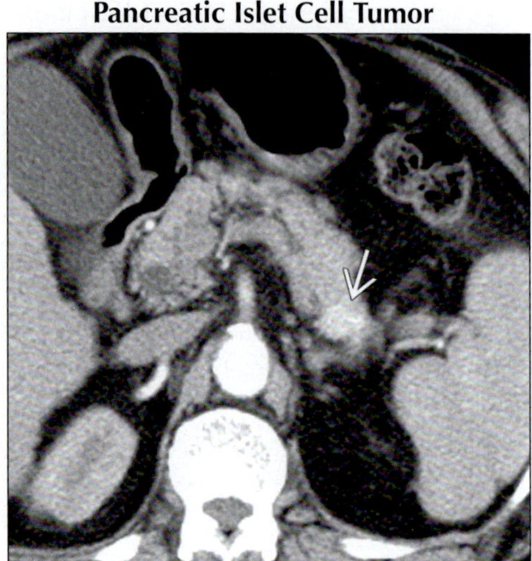

5

SOLID PANCREATIC LESION

Focal Acute Pancreatitis

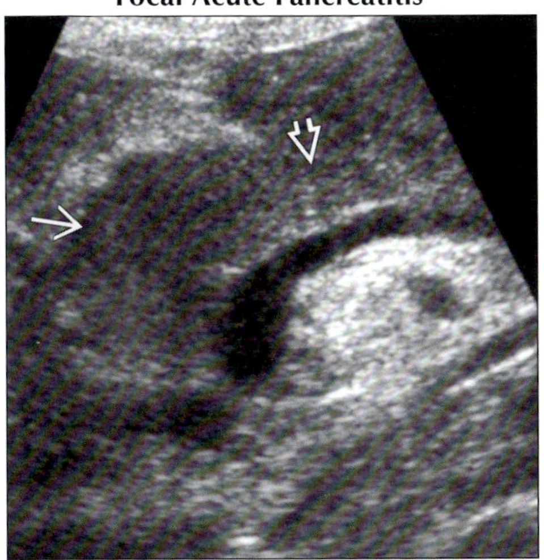

Focal Acute Pancreatitis

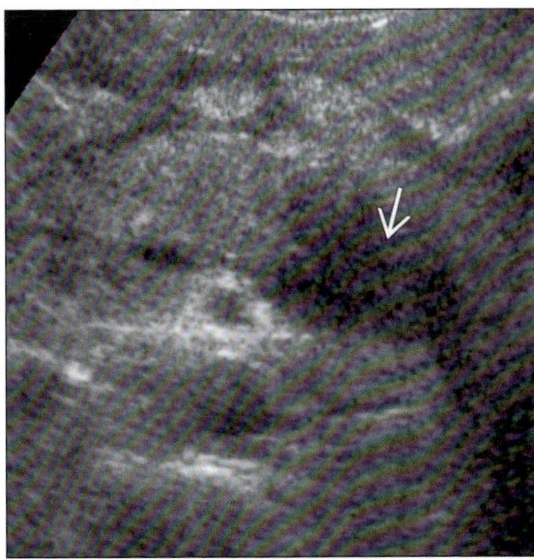

(Left) Transverse transabdominal ultrasound shows focal enlargement of the pancreatic head ➔ with a homogeneous hypoechoic echopattern in a patient with focal acute pancreatitis. Note the normal echopattern of the pancreatic body ➔ and lack of pancreatic duct dilatation. *(Right)* Transverse transabdominal ultrasound shows swelling with a hypoechoic echopattern ➔ in the pancreatic tail, compatible with focal acute pancreatitis.

Chronic Pancreatitis

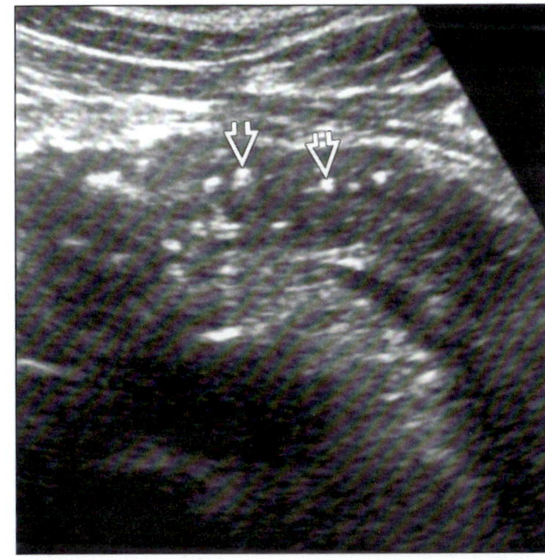

Solid and Pseudopapillary Neoplasm

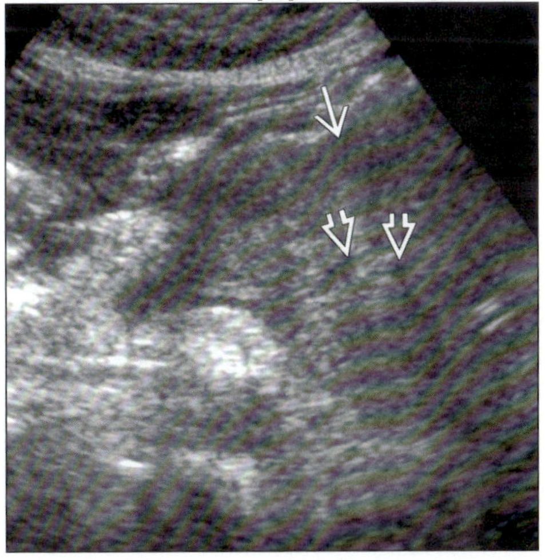

(Left) Transverse ultrasound shows multiple, small, parenchymal calcifications ➔ in the pancreatic body, compatible with chronic pancreatitis. Note the blurred pancreatic outlines. *(Right)* Transverse ultrasound shows a large, ill-defined, heterogeneous, hypoechoic, solid mass ➔ occupying the pancreatic body and tail. Note the presence of small cysts ➔ within the mass. The pancreatic tail is the most common location for this tumor.

Metastasis

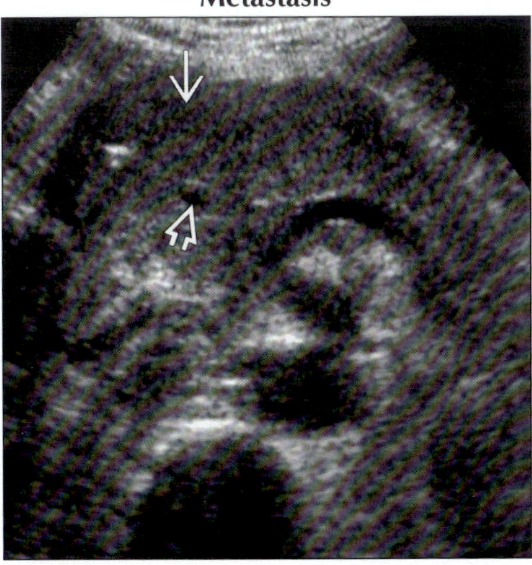

Lymphoma

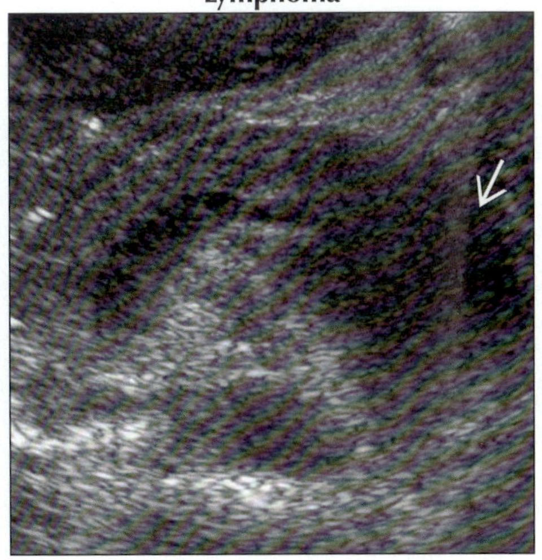

(Left) Transverse transabdominal ultrasound shows an ill-defined, solid, hypoechoic mass ➔ involving the head and body of the pancreas. The common hepatic artery is encased ➔. Note the absence of pancreatic duct dilatation. *(Right)* Transverse transabdominal ultrasound shows an ill-defined, solid, hypoechoic mass ➔ in the tail of the pancreas, compatible with lymphomatous involvement, in this patient with known disseminated lymphoma.

PANCREATIC DUCT DILATATION

DIFFERENTIAL DIAGNOSIS

Common
- Chronic Pancreatitis
- Pancreatic Ductal Carcinoma
- Periampullary Tumor

Less Common
- Acute Pancreatitis
- Obstructing Distal Common Bile Duct Stone
- Intraductal Papillary Mucinous Tumor (IPMT)

ESSENTIAL INFORMATION

Key Differential Diagnosis Issues
- Pancreatic ductal dilatation is present on US
  - Pancreatic duct > 3 mm in diameter
  - Loses its parallel nature
  - Tortuous in configuration
  - Abrupt tapering at site of obstruction
- Presence of pancreatic duct dilatation should prompt careful search for focal pancreatic lesion

Helpful Clues for Common Diagnoses
- **Chronic Pancreatitis**
  - Clinical history of longstanding recurrent attacks of epigastric pain; typically radiates to back
  - Atrophic pancreas with irregular outline and heterogeneous, hypo-/hyperechoic echopattern
  - Pancreatic calcification
    - Intraductal calculus: Due to deposition of calcium carbonate within intraductal protein plugs
    - Parenchymal calcification
- **Pancreatic Ductal Carcinoma**
  - Causes pancreatic duct obstruction as tumor arises from ductal epithelium of exocrine pancreas
  - Irregular, heterogeneous, solid, hypoechoic mass
  - Pancreatic duct dilatation distal to tumor
  - Bile duct dilatation with tumor in pancreatic head
  - Lack of pancreatic calcification or ductal calculus
  - ± liver and regional lymph node metastases

Helpful Clues for Less Common Diagnoses
- **Acute Pancreatitis**
  - Diffuse or focal hypoechoic enlargement of pancreas, blurred margins
  - Mild ductal dilatation sometimes seen due to obstruction by pancreatic edema
- **Obstructing Distal Common Bile Duct Stone**
  - Obstructive jaundice and epigastric pain
  - Presence of bile duct dilatation
- **Intraductal Papillary Mucinous Tumor (IPMT)**
  - Low-grade malignancy arises from main or branch pancreatic duct
  - Dilated main pancreatic duct and parenchymal atrophy

Chronic Pancreatitis

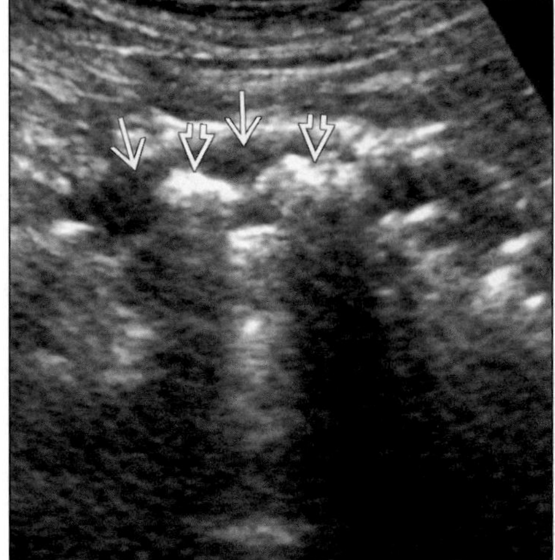

Transverse transabdominal ultrasound shows atrophic pancreatic parenchyma with multiple intraductal stones ⇨ within a markedly dilated pancreatic duct ➡. These are classic features of chronic pancreatitis.

Chronic Pancreatitis

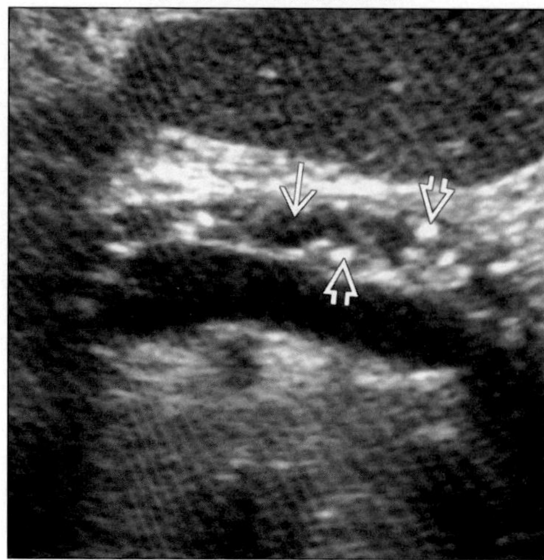

Transverse transabdominal ultrasound shows an atrophic pancreas with pancreatic duct dilatation ➡ and parenchymal calcifications ⇨, compatible with chronic pancreatitis.

PANCREATIC DUCT DILATATION

Pancreatic Ductal Carcinoma

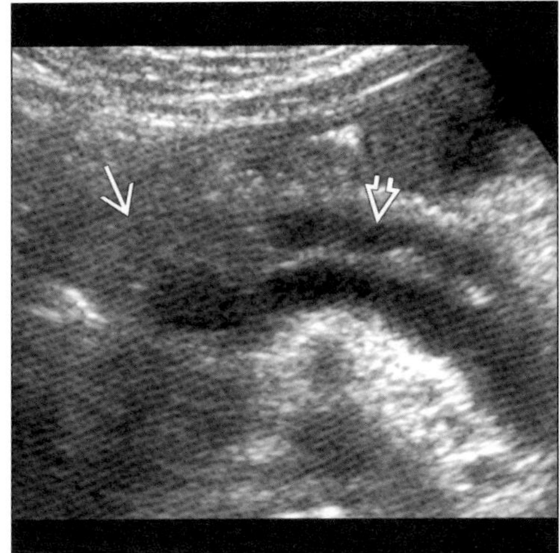

Pancreatic Ductal Carcinoma

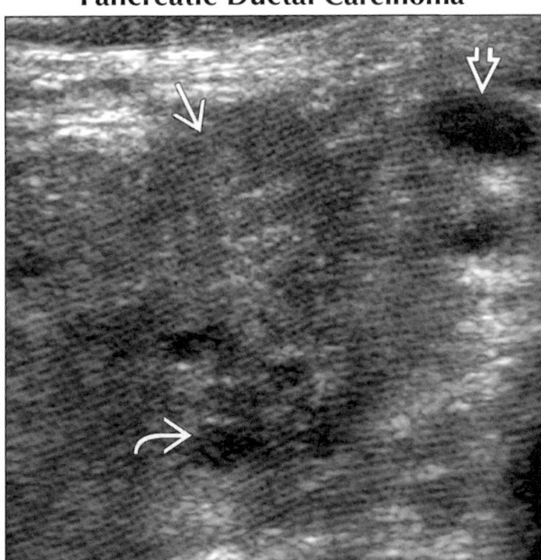

(Left) Transverse transabdominal ultrasound shows an ill-defined solid isoechoic mass ➡ in the head of the pancreas with dilatation of the pancreatic duct ➡ in the body and tail. (Right) Transverse transabdominal ultrasound shows a large, heterogeneous, hypoechoic, solid mass ➡ in the pancreatic head. The distal common bile duct ➡ and pancreatic duct ➡ are dilated due to compression by the large pancreatic head ductal carcinoma.

Periampullary Tumor

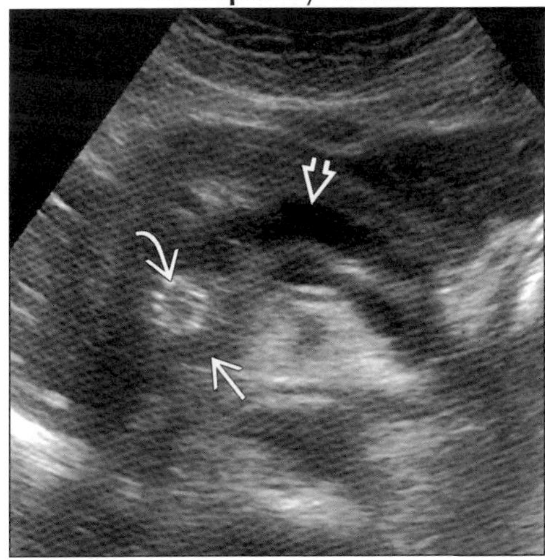

Acute Pancreatitis

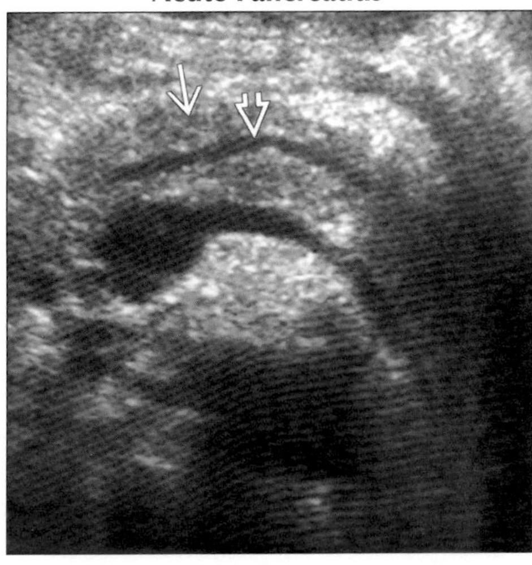

(Left) Transverse US shows a periampullary hypoechoic mass ➡ causing obstruction of the pancreatic duct ➡ and extrahepatic bile duct. Note the proximity of the tumor to a metallic internal biliary stent ➡. (Right) Transverse US shows diffuse hypoechoic enlargement of the pancreas ➡ with mild pancreatic duct dilatation ➡. Pancreatic duct dilatation, due to compression by an edematous pancreas, is an uncommon finding in acute pancreatitis.

Obstructing Distal Common Bile Duct Stone

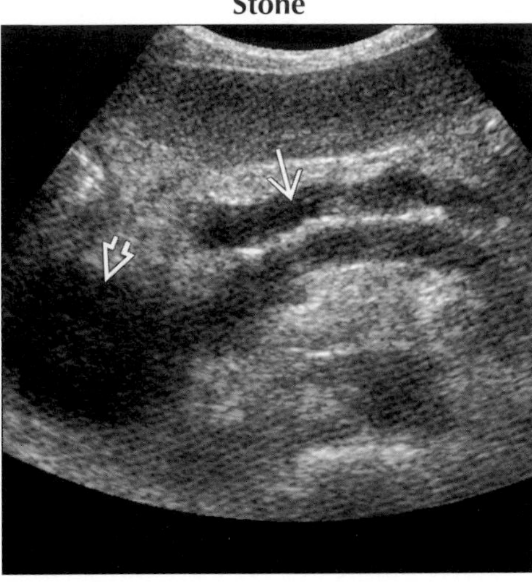

Intraductal Papillary Mucinous Tumor (IPMT)

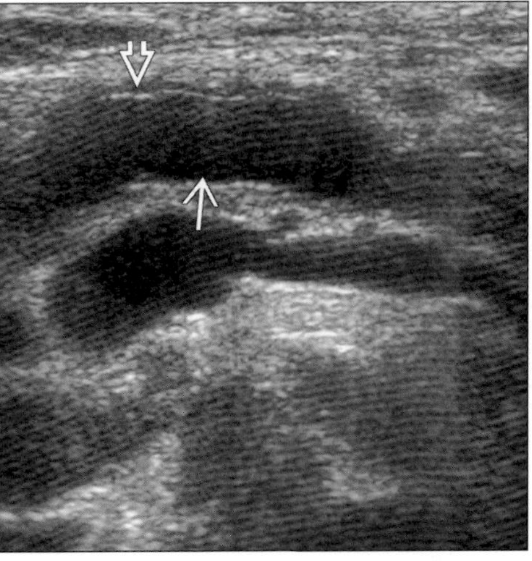

(Left) Transverse ultrasound shows dilatation of the pancreatic duct ➡ caused by a distal obstructing common bile duct stone (not shown). This patient has a type 1 choledochal cyst ➡, which are predisposed to stone formation. (Right) Transverse transabdominal ultrasound shows a markedly dilated pancreatic duct ➡ in an atrophic pancreas ➡. Note the absence of parenchymal calcification or ductal calculus.

5

DIFFUSE/FOCAL PANCREATIC ENLARGEMENT

DIFFERENTIAL DIAGNOSIS

Common
- Acute Pancreatitis
- Pancreatic Ductal Carcinoma

Less Common
- Chronic Pancreatitis, Early Stage
- Perforated Duodenal Ulcer
- "Shock" Pancreas
- Solid and Pseudopapillary Neoplasm
- Metastases
- Lymphoma

ESSENTIAL INFORMATION

Helpful Clues for Common Diagnoses
- **Acute Pancreatitis**
  - Clinical history of sudden onset of epigastric pain and vomiting
  - Lab data: Raised amylase and lipase
  - Diffuse/focal hypoechoic enlargement of pancreas
  - Blurred pancreatic outline/margin
  - Heterogeneous pancreas in cases with pancreatic necrosis/hemorrhage
  - Peripancreatic fluid, pleural effusion
- **Pancreatic Ductal Carcinoma**
  - Diffuse glandular involvement in ~ 15%
  - Diffuse, solid, hypoechoic enlargement of involved parenchyma
  - Pancreatic duct dilatation
  - Regional nodal and liver metastases

Helpful Clues for Less Common Diagnoses
- **Chronic Pancreatitis, Early Stage**
  - ± calcification/calculus
  - Pancreatic duct dilatation
  - Enlargement may be focal or diffuse
  - History of recurrent abdominal pain
- **Perforated Duodenal Ulcer**
  - Penetrating ulcers may infiltrate anterior pararenal space
  - Hypoechoic enlargement of pancreatic head
  - ± extraluminal gas/fluid collection
- **"Shock" Pancreas**
  - Infiltration of peripancreatic and mesenteric fat planes following hypotensive episode
  - Looks normal or appears as diffuse hypoechoic pancreatic enlargement
- **Solid and Pseudopapillary Neoplasm**
  - Well-defined, large, heterogeneous mass
  - Solid with small cystic component
  - No pancreatic duct dilatation
- **Metastases**
  - May present as multiple focal masses or diffuse involvement of pancreas
  - Known diagnosis of primary tumor with disseminated disease
- **Lymphoma**
  - Rare involvement of pancreas
  - Nodular, bulky, enlarged pancreas due to infiltration
  - Presence of enlarged regional lymph nodes ± other evidence of disease

Acute Pancreatitis

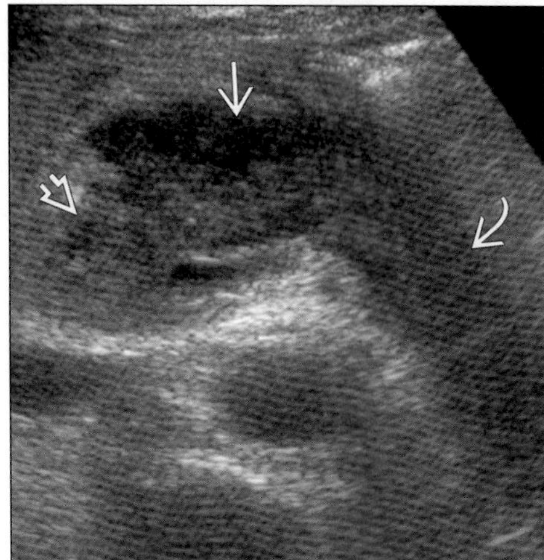

Transverse transabdominal ultrasound shows a swollen pancreatic body ➡ with an ill-defined, heterogeneous, hypoechoic echopattern. The pancreatic head ➡ and tail ➡ are less severely affected.

Acute Pancreatitis

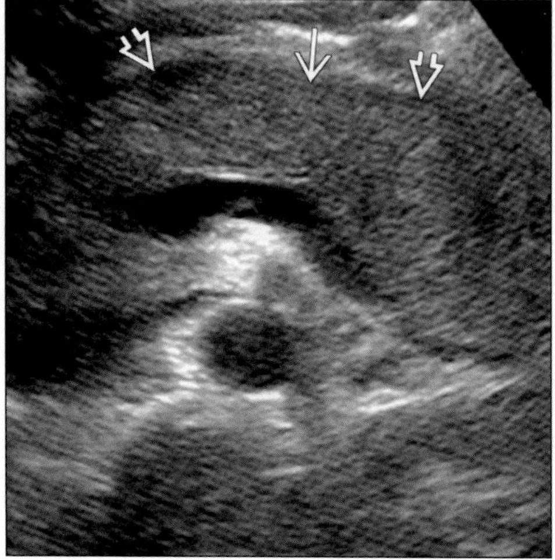

Transverse transabdominal ultrasound shows diffuse hypoechoic enlargement of the entire pancreas ➡. Note the presence of a thin rim of peripancreatic fluid ➡ due to inflammatory exudate.

DIFFUSE/FOCAL PANCREATIC ENLARGEMENT

Acute Pancreatitis

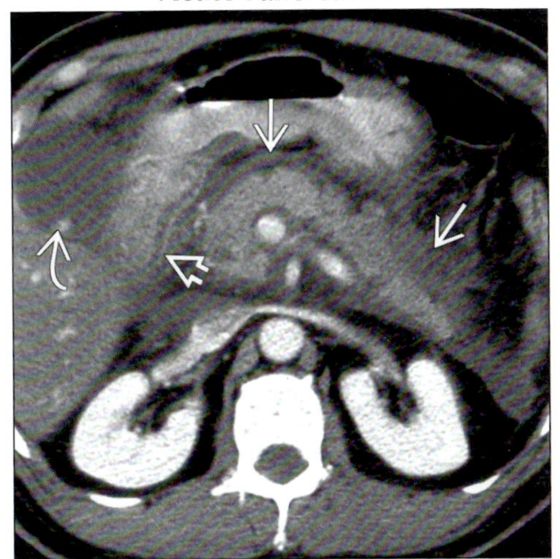

Acute Pancreatitis

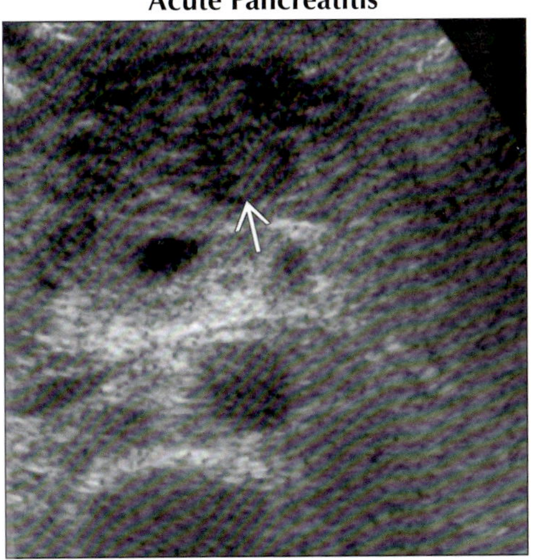

(Left) Axial CECT shows an inflamed pancreas with peripancreatic stranding and fluid collection ➡. The adjacent duodenum appears inflamed with an edematous wall ➡. Note the presence of a small calculus in the gallbladder ➡. (Right) Transverse transabdominal ultrasound shows a large heterogeneous collection of fluid ➡ involving the pancreatic head and body, compatible with abscess formation resulting from an infected phlegmon.

Pancreatic Ductal Carcinoma

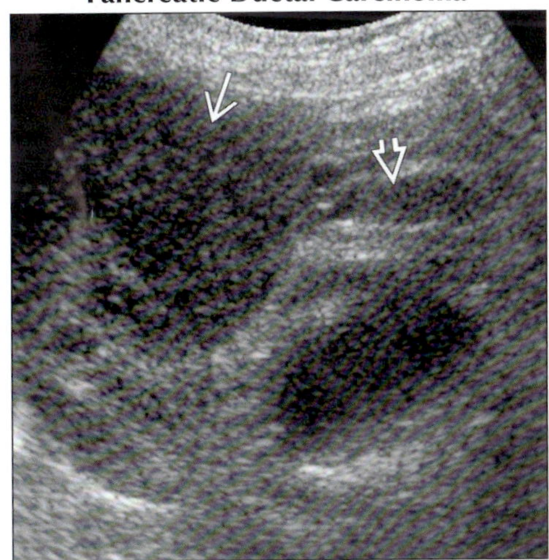

Pancreatic Ductal Carcinoma

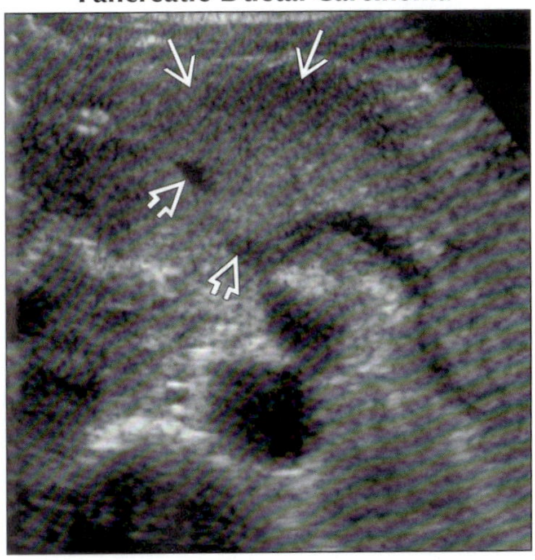

(Left) Transverse transabdominal ultrasound shows a large, ill-defined, heterogeneous, hypoechoic, solid mass ➡ in the head of the pancreas. The pancreatic duct ➡ distal to the mass is dilated. (Right) Transverse transabdominal ultrasound shows an ill-defined, solid, slightly hypoechoic mass ➡ that diffusely involves the head and body of the pancreas. Note the vascular encasement of the common hepatic artery ➡.

Solid and Pseudopapillary Neoplasm

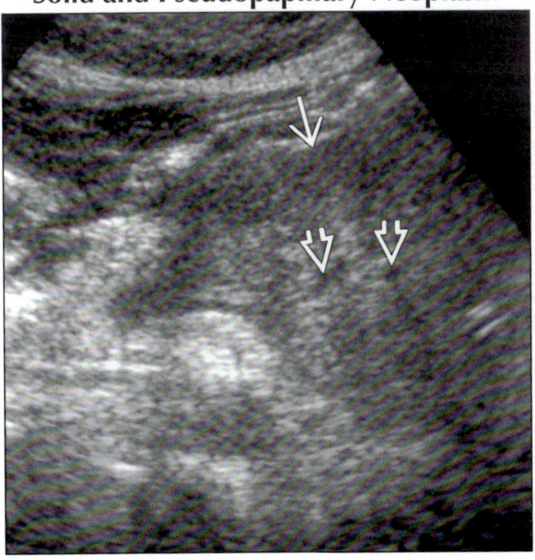

Lymphoma

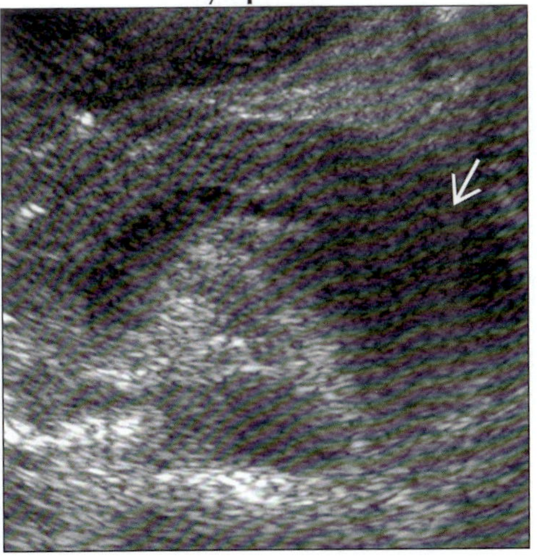

(Left) Transverse transabdominal ultrasound shows a large, ill-defined, heterogeneous, hypoechoic mass ➡ occupying and enlarging the pancreatic tail. Note the presence of a small cystic component ➡ within the tumor. (Right) Transverse transabdominal ultrasound shows an ill-defined hypoechoic enlargement of the pancreatic tail ➡ in a patient with known disseminated lymphoma. These findings are compatible with lymphomatous involvement.

DIFFERENTIAL DIAGNOSIS

Common
- Chronic Pancreatitis
- Vascular Calcification (Mimic)
- Serous Cystadenoma of Pancreas

Less Common
- Biliary/Pancreatic Stent (Mimic)
- Pancreatic Ductal Carcinoma
- Metastases
- Cavernous Lymphangioma/Hemangioma
- Hyperparathyroidism
- Cystic Fibrosis
- Hemochromatosis
- Tropical Pancreatitis

ESSENTIAL INFORMATION

Key Differential Diagnosis Issues
- Exclude calcifications from adjacent structures, particularly vascular calcifications (e.g., splenic artery)
- Evaluate distribution of calcification
  - Random distribution + intraductal calculus = chronic pancreatitis

Helpful Clues for Common Diagnoses
- **Chronic Pancreatitis**
  - Recurrent attacks of severe epigastric pain, longstanding history
  - Most common cause of pancreatic calcification
    - Intraductal calculus: Due to deposition of calcium carbonate within intraductal protein plugs
    - Parenchymal calcifications: Irregular, amorphous, coarse calcifications of varying sizes
    - Atrophic parenchyma
    - Dilated pancreatic duct
- **Vascular Calcification (Mimic)**
  - Calcification of adjacent vessels mimics pancreatic calcification
  - Most common: Splenic artery
  - Curvilinear calcification
  - Vascular flow on color Doppler US
- **Serous Cystadenoma of Pancreas**
  - Well-demarcated mass with microcystic component
  - "Sunburst" calcifications
    - Dense calcifications with posterior acoustic shadowing distal to mass
  - Central, stellate, echogenic scar
  - Pancreatic duct dilatation is rare

Helpful Clues for Less Common Diagnoses
- **Pancreatic Ductal Carcinoma**
  - Rarely (~ 2%) contains calcifications
  - Pancreatic duct dilatation
  - ± biliary dilatation with pancreatic head tumor
- **Metastases**
  - Metastasis from colorectal primary may contain calcification
- **Cavernous Lymphangioma/Hemangioma**
  - Multiple phleboliths

Chronic Pancreatitis

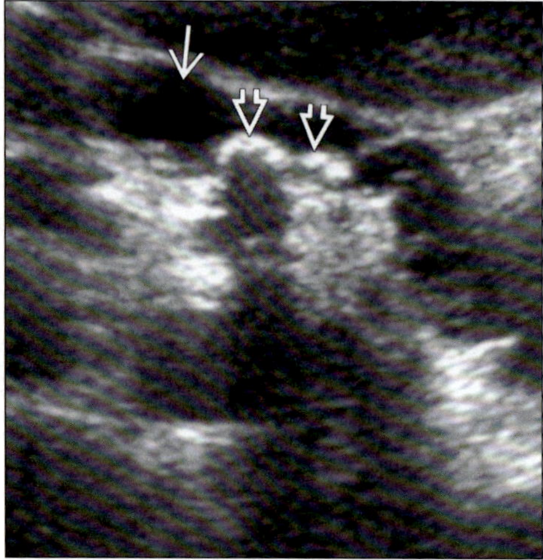

Transverse transabdominal ultrasound shows multiple echogenic intraductal stones ➡ within a dilated pancreatic duct ➡ casting a posterior acoustic shadow. Note the atrophic pancreatic parenchyma.

Chronic Pancreatitis

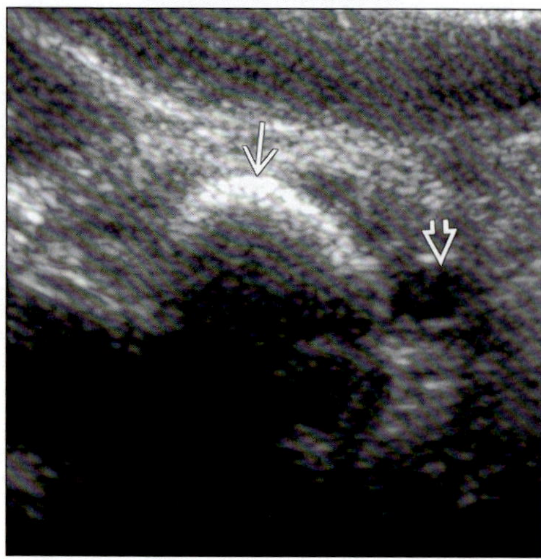

Transverse transabdominal ultrasound shows a large focus of calcification ➡ within an atrophic pancreas. Also note a small cystic lesion ➡ in the pancreatic tail due to a pancreatic pseudocyst.

PANCREATIC CALCIFICATION

Chronic Pancreatitis

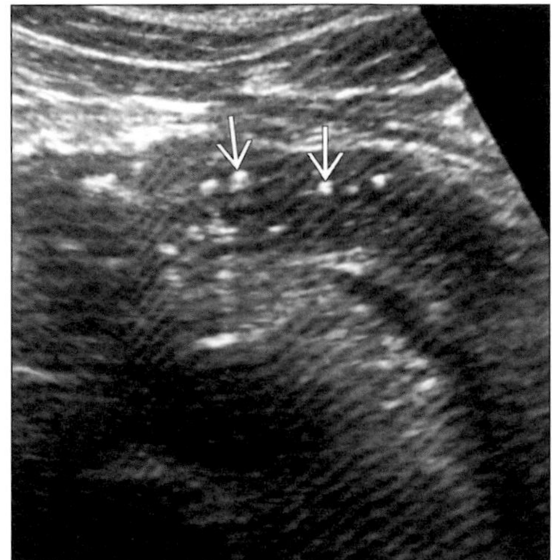

Chronic Pancreatitis

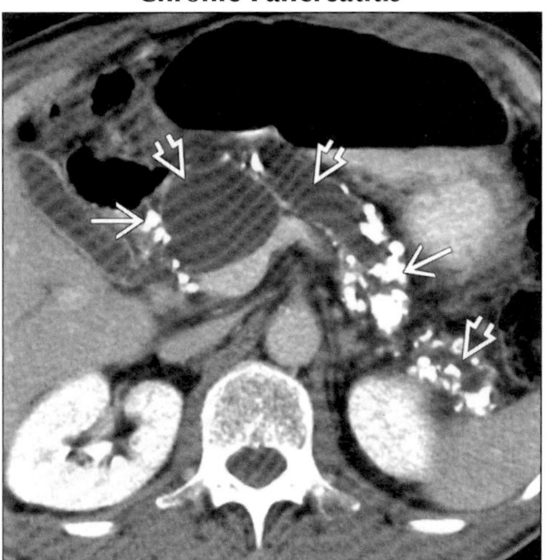

(Left) Transverse transabdominal ultrasound shows multiple small parenchymal calcifications ➡ in the pancreatic body in a patient with chronic pancreatitis. *(Right)* Corresponding axial CECT shows an atrophic pancreas with multiple parenchymal calcifications ➡. Note the dilatation of the pancreatic duct ➡ in the head, body, and tail of the pancreas.

Vascular Calcification (Mimic)

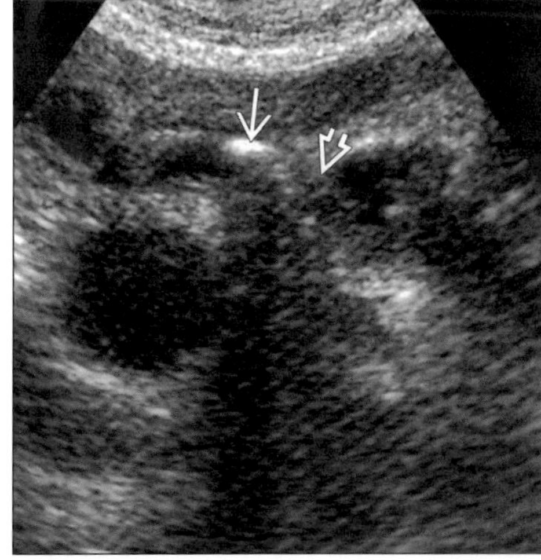

Biliary/Pancreatic Stent (Mimic)

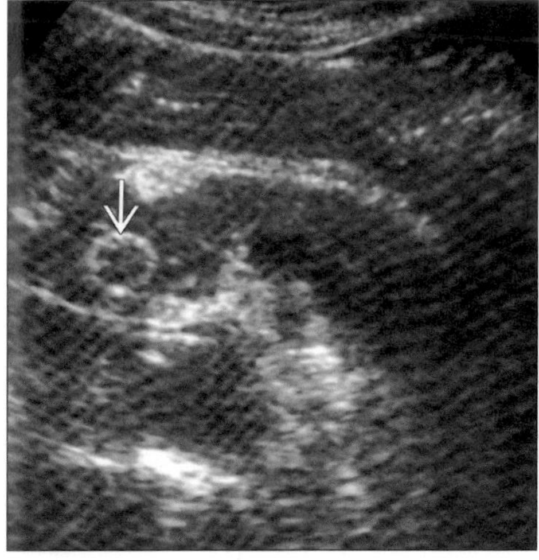

(Left) Transverse transabdominal ultrasound shows a linear echogenic focus ➡ with posterior acoustic shadowing due to splenic artery calcification. This appearance mimics pancreatic calcification due to its location near pancreatic parenchyma ➡. *(Right)* Transverse transabdominal ultrasound shows a metallic internal biliary stent (cross-section) ➡ in the head of the pancreas meant to relieve biliary obstruction due to a cholangiocarcinoma.

Serous Cystadenoma of Pancreas

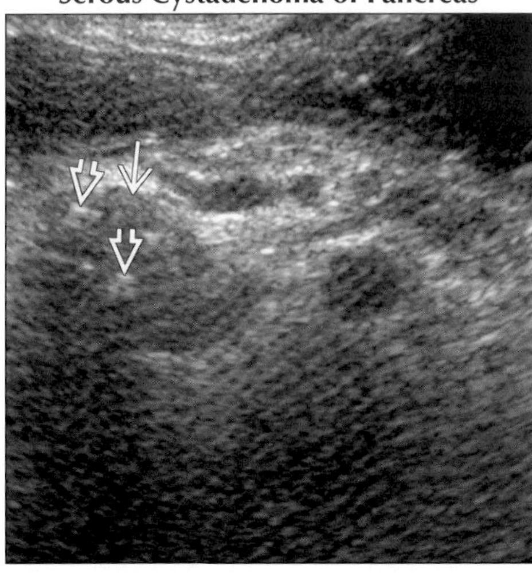

Serous Cystadenoma of Pancreas

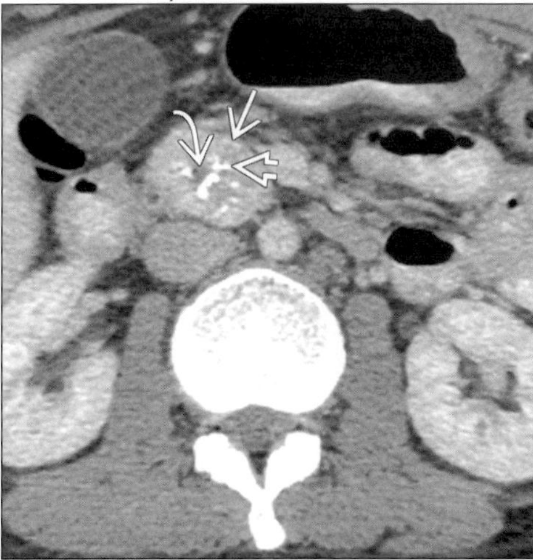

(Left) Transverse transabdominal ultrasound shows a well-defined, solid, hypoechoic mass ➡ in the pancreatic head. Note the presence of tiny echogenic calcifications ➡ within the lesion. The pancreatic duct is not dilated. *(Right)* Corresponding axial CECT shows a well-defined, enhancing, soft tissue mass ➡ in the pancreatic head. Foci of calcifications ➡ and a hypodense center ➡ (scar/cystic component) are noted.

5

SECTION 6
Spleen

DIFFERENTIAL DIAGNOSIS

Common
- Congestive
  - Portal Hypertension
  - Splenic Vein Thrombosis
- Infection
  - Viral, Bacterial, or Protozoa
- Neoplastic
  - Lymphoma
  - Leukemia
  - Myelodysplastic Syndrome
  - Metastasis
  - Langerhans Cell Histiocytosis
  - Mesenchymal Tumor
- Subcapsular Hematoma

Less Common
- Collagen Vascular Disease and Inflammatory Conditions
  - Rheumatoid Arthritis
  - Felty Syndrome
  - Sarcoidosis

Rare but Important
- Infiltrative
  - Metabolic Diseases
    - Gaucher Disease
    - Glycogen Storage Disease
    - Niemann-Pick Disease
  - Amyloidosis
- Hyperplastic
  - Hemoglobinopathies
  - Extramedullary Hematopoiesis
  - Thrombotic Thrombocytopenic Purpura

ESSENTIAL INFORMATION

Key Differential Diagnosis Issues
- Length > 12 cm, width > 7 cm, depth > 4 cm
- 1.25x longer than adjacent kidney in children
- Splenic index: Normal range 120-480 cm³ (product of length, breadth, & depth of spleen)
- 1st determine if spleen is diffusely enlarged (splenomegaly) or enlarged by splenic mass
  - Massive splenomegaly
    - Chronic myelogenous leukemia, myelofibrosis, malaria, schistosomiasis, leishmaniasis, Gaucher disease
  - Look for sonographic features of cause of splenomegaly

Helpful Clues for Common Diagnoses
- **Portal Hypertension**
  - Siderotic Gamna-Gandy nodules (13%)
    - Multiple scattered hyperechoic foci
    - Faint calcifications on CT
  - Evidence of portal hypertension
    - Monophasic portal venous flow
    - ↓ mean portal vein velocities to 7-12 cm/sec
    - Bi-directional/hepatofugal flow (< 10%)
    - Portal systemic shunt: Esophageal, gastric varices, etc.
    - Splenic varices
    - Ascites and lower limb edema
  - Possible causes of portal hypertension
    - Prehepatic: Portal vein thrombosis, portal vein compression
    - Hepatic: Cirrhosis (nodular contour with coarse echopattern ± regenerative nodules)
    - Schistosomiasis (periportal fibrosis, capsular "turtle back" or "tortoise shell" calcification)
    - Posthepatic: Congestive heart failure (dilated hepatic vein, ascites)
    - Budd-Chiari syndrome (hepatic vein narrowing with intrahepatic venous collaterals)
- **Splenic Vein Thrombosis**
  - May be sequelae of pancreatitis, hypercoagulable state, blunt trauma, etc.
- **Infection**
  - Viral infection (acute hepatitis, infectious mononucleosis), bacterial infection, protozoa
  - Viral infection usually associated with hepatosplenomegaly
  - Massive splenomegaly in malaria, schistosomiasis (with characteristic features), leishmaniasis
  - Indicative clinical features
- **Neoplastic**
  - **Leukemia, Lymphoma, Myelodysplastic Syndrome**
    - All may show diffuse enlargement of variable echogenicity
    - Multiple nodules may be seen in lymphoma (typically hypoechoic), less commonly present in leukemia
  - **Metastasis**

- Multiple hypoechoic nodules of varying sizes
- Most common primary sources in cases of multivisceral metastases: Ovarian, lung, colorectal, breast
- Most common primary sources of solitary splenic metastasis: Ovarian, colorectal, lung, and stomach carcinomas
  - ○ **Langerhans Cell Histiocytosis**
    - Splenomegaly ± multiple hypoechoic nodules (less often)
- **Subcapsular Hematoma**
  - ○ When isoechoic, may be difficult to visualize against background of splenic parenchyma
    - Mass effect with vascular displacement is important clue

Helpful Clues for Less Common Diagnoses
- **Collagen Vascular Disease and Inflammatory Conditions**
  - ○ **Rheumatoid Arthritis**
    - 1-5% of patients have splenomegaly ± lymphadenopathy
  - ○ **Felty Syndrome**
    - Rheumatoid arthritis + splenomegaly + neutropenia
  - ○ **Sarcoidosis**
    - 60% of patients have splenomegaly
    - ± multiple hypoechoic nodules (2-3 cm)
    - ± necrotic mass with focal Ca++

Helpful Clues for Rare Diagnoses
- **Infiltrative**
  - ○ **Gaucher Disease**
    - Splenomegaly + lymphadenopathy
    - Multiple hypoechoic/hyperechoic nodules represent clusters of reticuloendothelial cells laden with glucosylceramide
    - Splenic infarcts → fibrosis, in massive splenomegaly
  - ○ **Glycogen Storage Disease**
    - Excess deposition of glycogen in organs
    - Increased echogenicity of organs due to glycogen/fat content
  - ○ **Niemann-Pick Disease**
    - Lipid storage disease
    - May have only moderate hepatosplenomegaly
    - Neural impairment may be extensive
  - ○ **Amyloidosis**
    - 4-13% splenomegaly, discrete masses
- **Hyperplastic**
  - ○ **Hemoglobinopathies**
    - Sickle cell anemia, thalassemia
  - ○ **Extramedullary Hematopoiesis**
    - Myelofibrosis, osteopetrosis, autoimmune lymphoproliferative syndrome
  - ○ **Thrombotic Thrombocytopenic Purpura**
    - Rare condition causing clots to form in small vessels throughout body

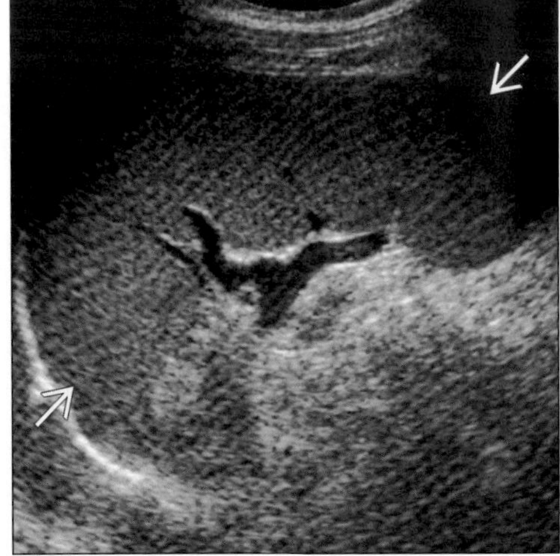

Portal Hypertension

Longitudinal transabdominal ultrasound shows splenomegaly ➡, which was associated with liver cirrhosis in this patient.

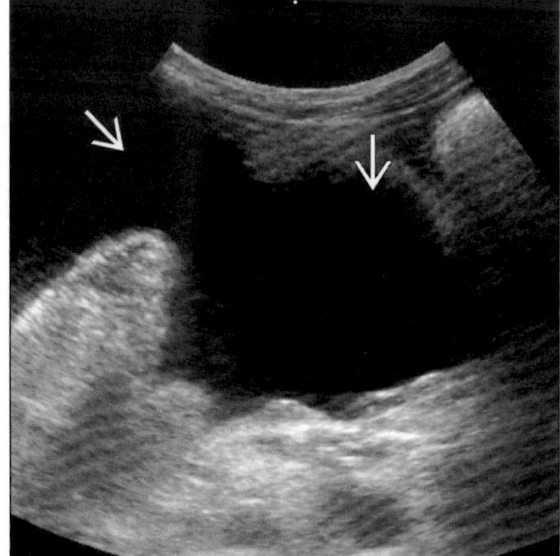

Portal Hypertension

Longitudinal transabdominal ultrasound shows marked ascites ➡ secondary to portal hypertension in a patient with splenomegaly.

(Left) Oblique color Doppler ultrasound shows color flow and Doppler spectrum ➤ of splenorenal collaterals ⇒ at the hilum of an enlarged spleen ➡. *(Right)* Longitudinal color Doppler ultrasound shows recanalization of the umbilical vein ➡ in the left lobe of the liver, another finding of portal hypertension. Note flow from left portal vein ⇒ to umbilical vein. When splenomegaly is seen, look for other findings to diagnose portal hypertension.

Portal Hypertension

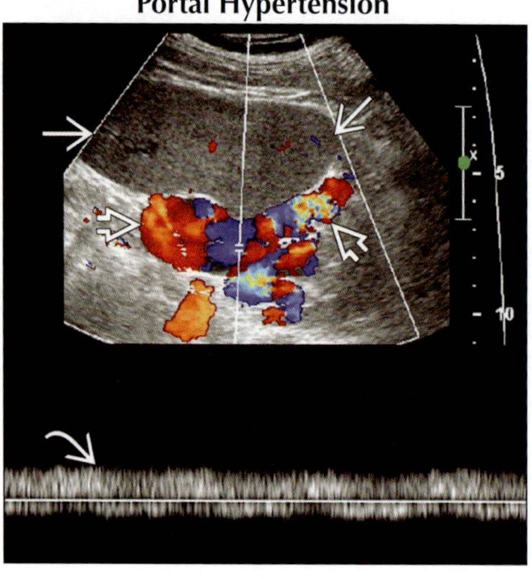

Portal Hypertension

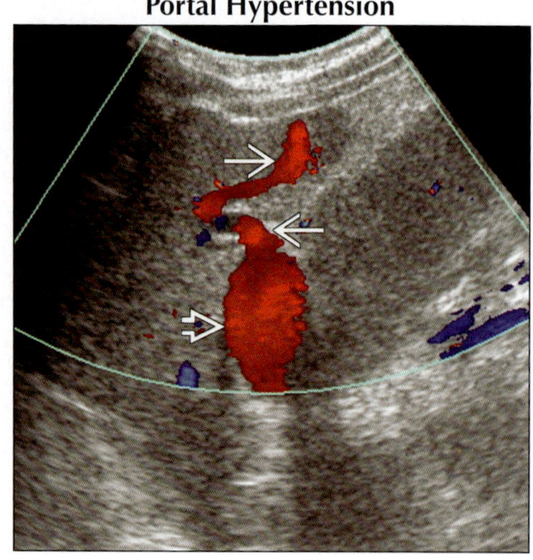

(Left) Transverse transabdominal ultrasound shows schistosomiasis with multiple echogenic linear fibrous septae ➡ in the right lobe of the liver. This patient has associated splenomegaly. *(Right)* Longitudinal transabdominal ultrasound shows diffuse enlargement of the spleen ➡ in a patient with chronic malaria. The appearance itself is nonspecific, and the diagnosis relies on relevant clinical history and serology.

Infection

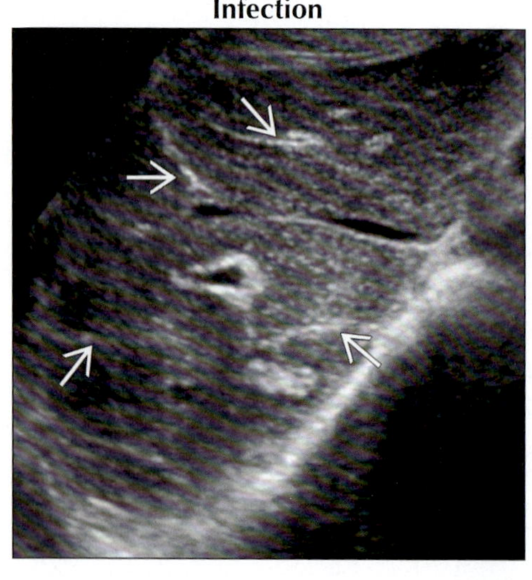

Infection

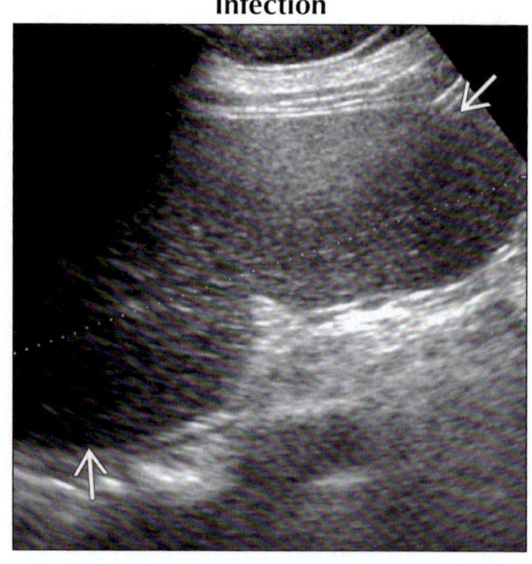

(Left) Longitudinal transabdominal ultrasound shows diffuse splenic enlargement ➡ in a patient with lymphoma. *(Right)* Transverse transabdominal ultrasound in the same patient shows enlarged lymph nodes ➡ in the hepatoduodenal ligament.

Lymphoma

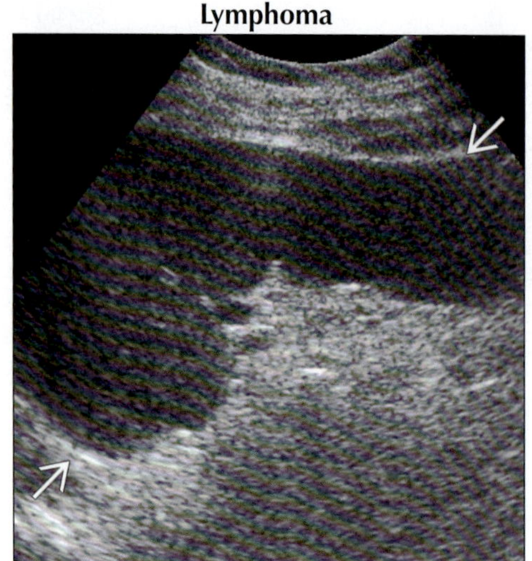

Lymphoma

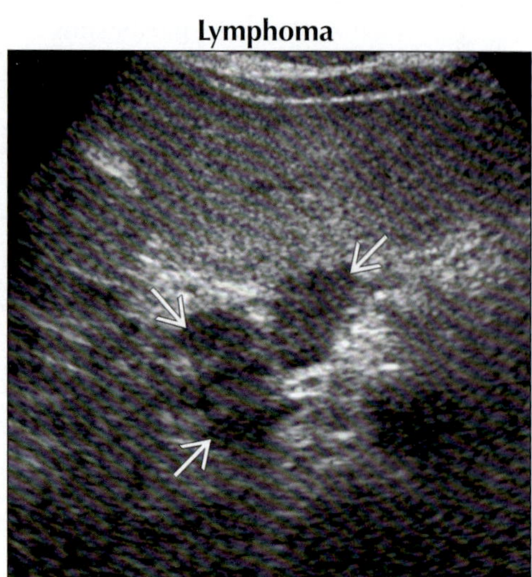

SPLENOMEGALY

Leukemia

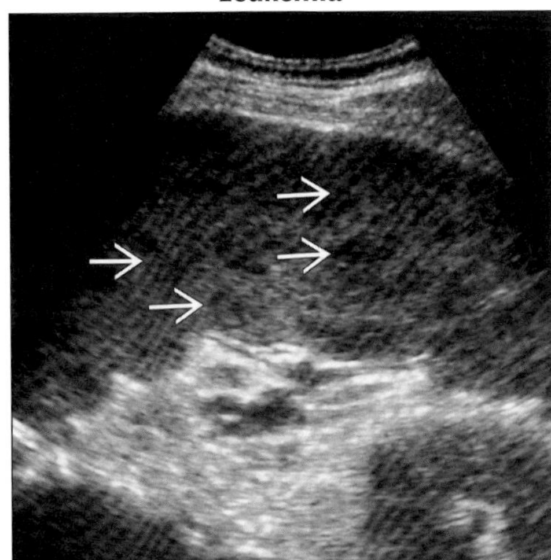

Infiltrative

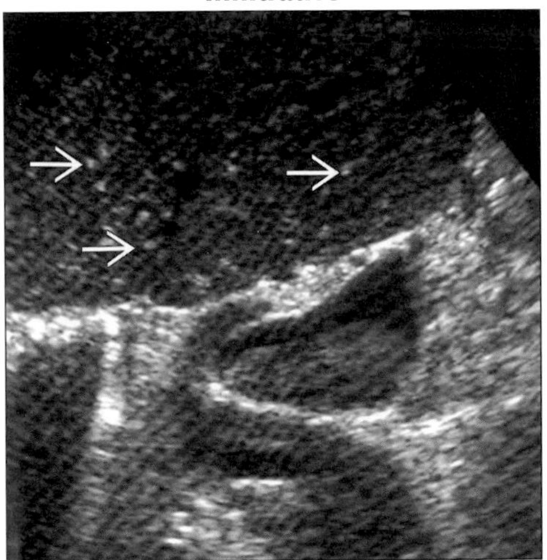

(Left) Longitudinal transabdominal ultrasound shows splenomegaly with multiple, ill-defined, hypoechoic nodules scattered throughout the spleen ➡, representing leukemic infiltration. (Right) Oblique transabdominal ultrasound shows splenomegaly with multiple small siderotic nodules ➡, known as Gamna-Gandy bodies.

Glycogen Storage Disease

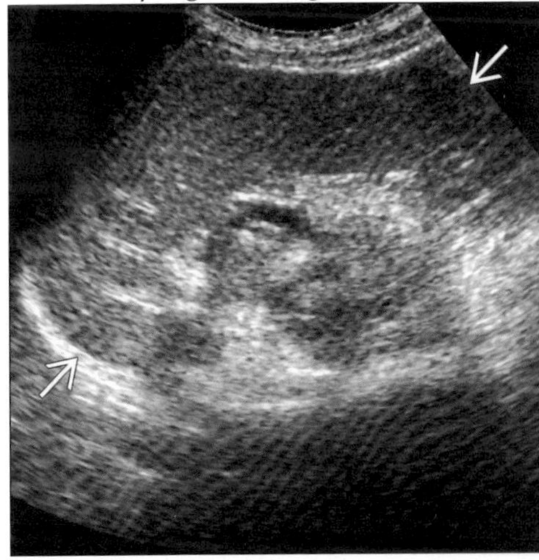

Glycogen Storage Disease

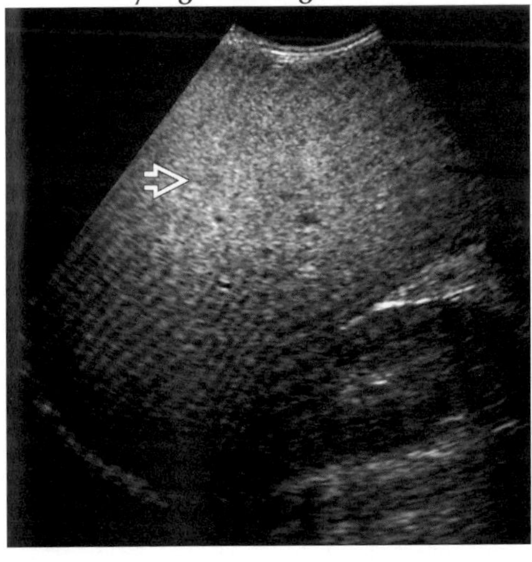

(Left) Longitudinal transabdominal ultrasound shows mild diffuse splenomegaly ➡. The appearance is otherwise nonspecific. (Right) Longitudinal transabdominal ultrasound of the liver shows gross hepatomegaly with fatty infiltration ➡, suggestive of underlying metabolic derangement in this child with glycogen storage disease. Splenomegaly was also present.

Hemoglobinopathies

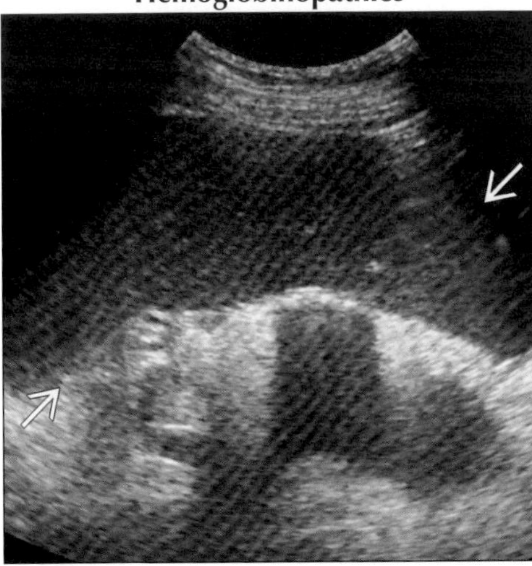

Hemoglobinopathies

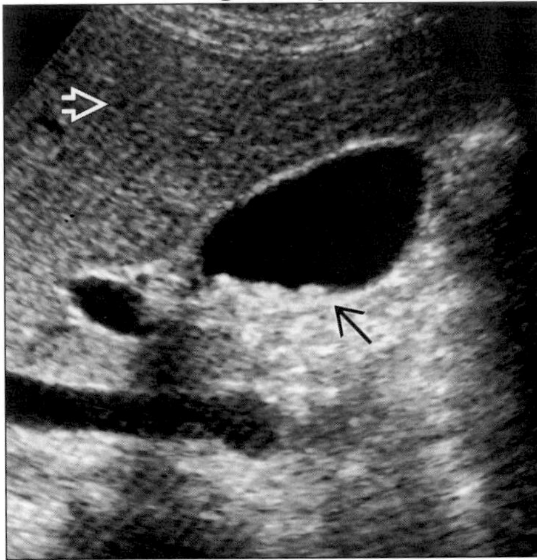

(Left) Longitudinal transabdominal ultrasound shows mild diffuse splenomegaly ➡ in a patient with hemoglobin H disease. (Right) Longitudinal transabdominal ultrasound in the same patient shows multiple small gallstones ➡ and a fatty liver ➡, findings also seen with hemoglobinopathy.

CYSTIC SPLENIC LESION

DIFFERENTIAL DIAGNOSIS

Common
- Acquired Splenic Cyst

Less Common
- Infective Cyst/Abscess
  - Pyogenic Abscess
  - Fungal Abscess
  - Parasitic Abscess
- Neoplastic
  - Lymphangioma
  - Hemangioma
  - Lymphoma
  - Cystic Metastasis

Rare but Important
- Congenital (Epidermoid) Cyst
- Peliosis
- Intrasplenic Pseudocyst

ESSENTIAL INFORMATION

Key Differential Diagnosis Issues
- Differentiate cystic from hypoechoic solid or vascular lesion
  - Clear fluid content is anechoic
  - Thick fluid content (proteinaceous fluid, hemorrhage, abscess) shows low-level internal echoes, mimics solid lesion
    - Grayscale movement of internal echoes and fluid level suggest fluid nature
    - Doppler study to exclude high flow vascular space, e.g., aneurysm
    - Internal vascularity suggests solid nature rather than thick fluid content
- Unilocular cystic lesion
  - False cysts (80%) > neoplasm with unilocular cystic appearance
    - Hemangioma > lymphangioma > metastases > lymphoma > congenital cyst
- Multilocular cystic lesion
  - Septated false cyst, infective cysts, organizing hematoma, lymphangioma
- Multiple cystic lesions
  - Abscesses > lymphangioma, hemangioma > cystic metastases (e.g., ovarian metastases) > > peliosis
- Solid lesion with internal cystic spaces
  - Early abscess formation in inflammatory phlegmon
  - Hemangioma (well-defined, rounded, cystic spaces)
  - Malignant tumor (irregular internal necrosis)

Helpful Clues for Common Diagnoses
- **Acquired Splenic Cyst**
  - = false cyst (80% of splenic cysts)
  - Due to liquefactive necrosis with cystic degeneration within lesions
    - Previous hematoma, laceration, old infarction, abscess
    - Remote history of LUQ injury can often be obtained (80% are post-traumatic)
  - Echogenic thick fibrous capsule without epithelial lining
  - Curvilinear wall calcification in 38-50%

Helpful Clues for Less Common Diagnoses
- **Infective Cyst/Abscess**
  - **Pyogenic Abscess**
    - Solitary or multiple
    - Mobile low-level internal echoes to anechoic with posterior acoustic enhancement
    - Irregular wall, no capsule or pseudocapsule, ± internal gas
    - Rim enhancement on CT is less frequently seen than in hepatic abscesses
  - **Fungal Abscess**
    - 26% of all splenic abscesses
    - Most common in immunocompromised patients
    - Multiple, small (few mm to 2 cm), hypoechoic foci representing microabscesses
    - Typically "target" appearance: Hypoechoic center = central necrotic hyphae, hyperechoic ring = concentric band of viable fungal element, outermost hypoechoic rim = inflammation
  - **Parasitic Abscess**
    - Hydatid cysts rarely involves spleen (less than 2% of patients with echinococcosis)
    - Usually due to systemic dissemination and intraperitoneal spread from ruptured liver cyst
    - Appearances similar to hepatic hydatid cysts; majority are anechoic with thin wall ± septae
    - Occasionally internal daughter cyst seen
    - Rarely echogenic hydatid cysts reported, due to infolded intracystic membrane and debris
- **Neoplastic**

- ○ **Lymphangioma**
  - ▪ Single or multiple; well-defined hypoechoic mass ± internal septations
  - ▪ Anechoic or hypoechoic content, depends on density of lymphatic content
  - ▪ Peripheral curvilinear calcification may be present
- ○ **Hemangioma**
  - ▪ Most common primary tumor of spleen
  - ▪ Most look solid (homogeneously hyperechoic similar to hepatic hemangioma)
  - ▪ May have discrete cystic spaces or be entirely cystic
  - ▪ Cystic content may be anechoic or echogenic (hemorrhagic)
  - ▪ Curvilinear or specks of calcification may be present
  - ▪ May occur as part of generalized angiomatosis, e.g., Klippel-Trenaunay-Weber syndrome
  - ▪ CECT shows peripheral nodular enhancement of vascular channels as in hepatic hemangioma
  - ▪ Progressive fill-in seen but often does not fill center entirely
- ○ **Lymphoma**
  - ▪ Most common malignant tumor of spleen
  - ▪ May contain internal irregular cystic area representing necrosis
  - ▪ Can have predominantly cystic appearance secondary to massive internal necrosis
  - ▪ Occasionally, markedly hypoechoic lymphoma infiltrate has "pseudocystic" appearance
  - ▪ Evidence of disease elsewhere in liver, splenic hilar adenopathy
- ○ **Cystic Metastasis**
  - ▪ Usually hypoechoic; irregular cystic area can be seen secondary to internal necrosis
  - ▪ Occasionally, entirely hyperechoic, e.g., from melanoma
  - ▪ Other evidence of disseminated disease

Helpful Clues for Rare Diagnoses

- • **Congenital (Epidermoid) Cyst**
  - ○ Only true congenital splenic cyst, lined by epithelium
  - ○ Developmental peritoneal mesothelial cell trapped in splenic sulcus
  - ○ Thin-walled, anechoic, unilocular ± internal debris due to cholesterol crystal deposits; occasional septae
- • **Peliosis**
  - ○ Rare, idiopathic; associated with malignant hematologic disease, disseminated metastases, tuberculosis, etc.
  - ○ Widespread blood-filled cystic spaces of varying size ± endothelial lining
  - ○ Thrombosis within blood-filled spaces may occur
- • **Intrasplenic Pseudocyst**
  - ○ Pancreatic pseudocyst (1-5% of patients with pancreatitis)

Acquired Splenic Cyst

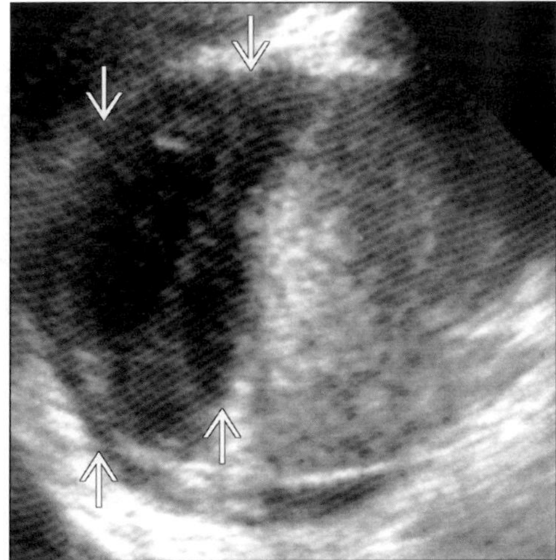

Longitudinal transabdominal ultrasound shows cystic change ➡ in a splenic hematoma. Note that part of the hematoma remains echogenic, representing acute component.

Acquired Splenic Cyst

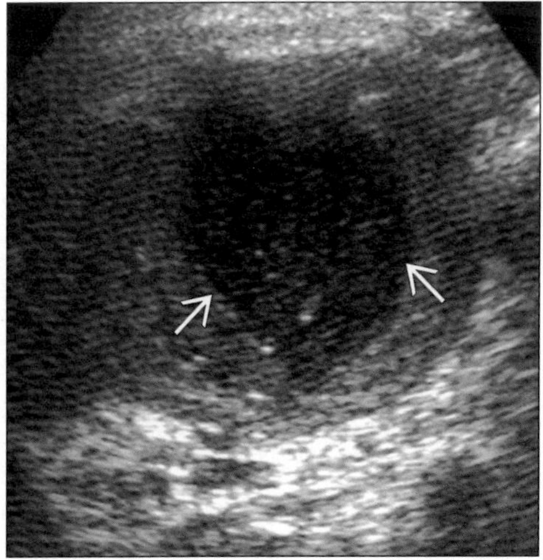

Longitudinal transabdominal ultrasound shows liquefactive necrosis with cystic change ➡ in the subacute stage of a splenic laceration.

6

(Left) Oblique ultrasound shows a small spleen an with irregular contour. Multiple cystic areas ➡ with internal septae are present in the subcapsular region, consistent with liquefactive necrosis from previous splenic infarcts. *(Right)* Longitudinal US shows dense curvilinear calcification of a longstanding splenic cyst ➡ in a patient with a remote history of LUQ injury. CT (not shown) revealed clear cystic content. The features are suggestive of a calcified pseudocyst.

Acquired Splenic Cyst

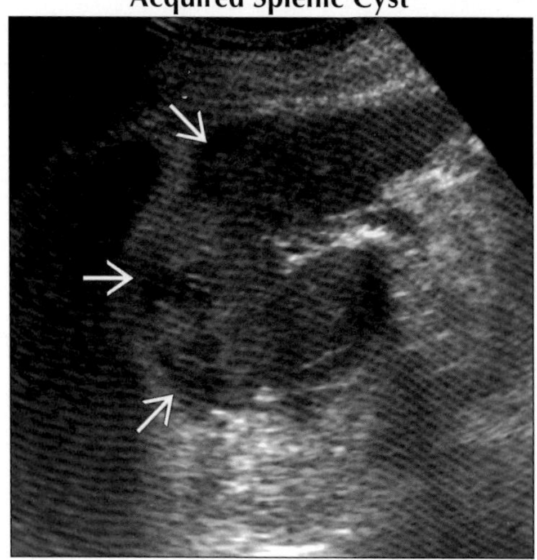

Acquired Splenic Cyst

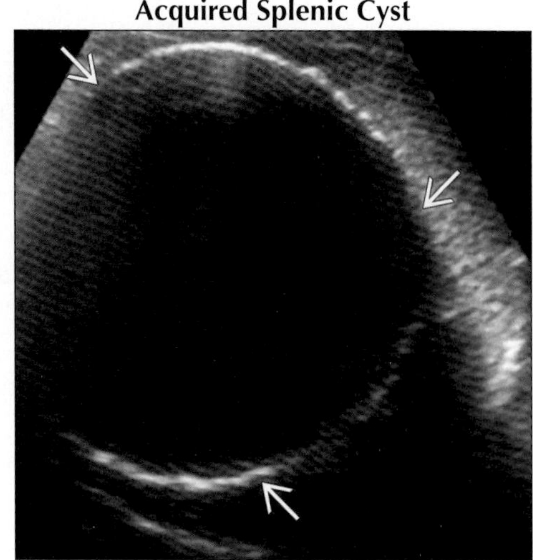

(Left) Longitudinal transabdominal ultrasound shows an early splenic abscess ➡ with nonspecific, rounded, well-defined, hypoechoic appearance. *(Right)* Longitudinal transabdominal ultrasound of the spleen shows multifocal splenic abscesses ➡. They are irregular, some with surrounding hypoechoic areas, suggestive of inflammatory edema.

Pyogenic Abscess

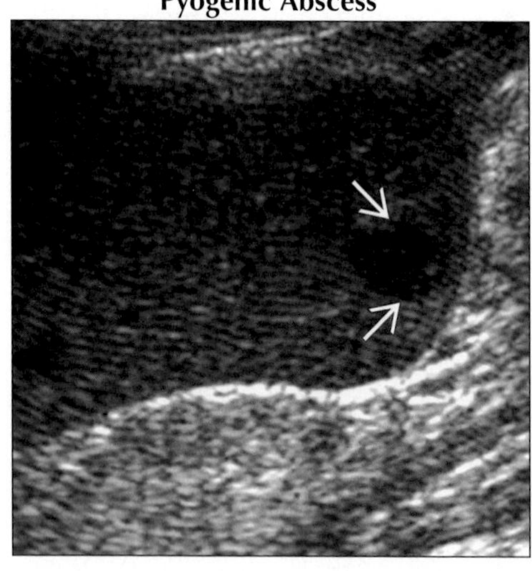

Pyogenic Abscess

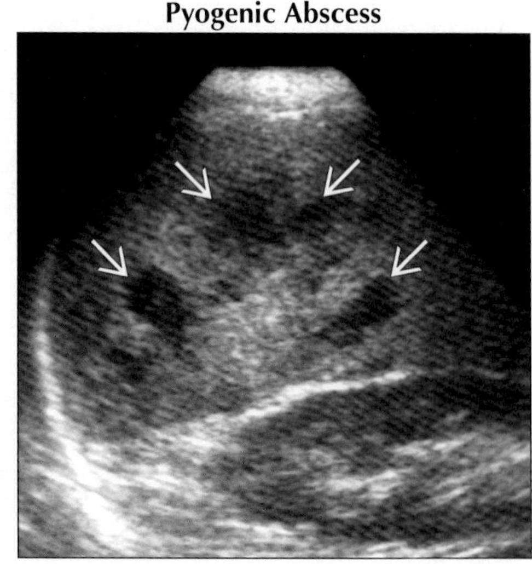

(Left) Longitudinal transabdominal ultrasound of the spleen shows a rounded splenic abscess with partial liquefaction ➡. A thick irregular rim of inflammatory tissue ➡ remains in the periphery. *(Right)* Longitudinal transabdominal ultrasound shows a large, almost completely liquefied splenic abscess ➡ with internal debris ➡, forming a fluid level.

Pyogenic Abscess

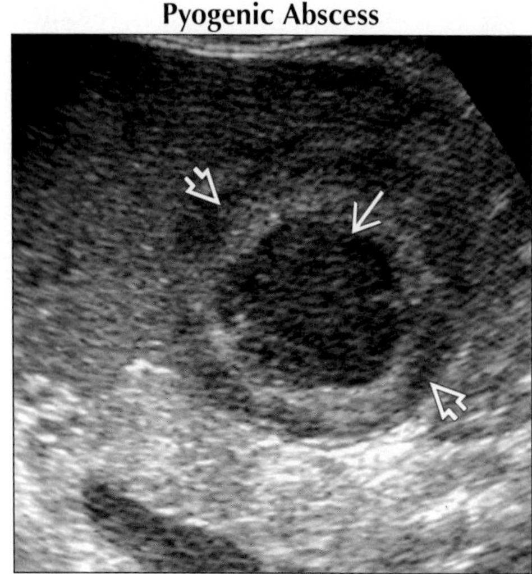

Pyogenic Abscess

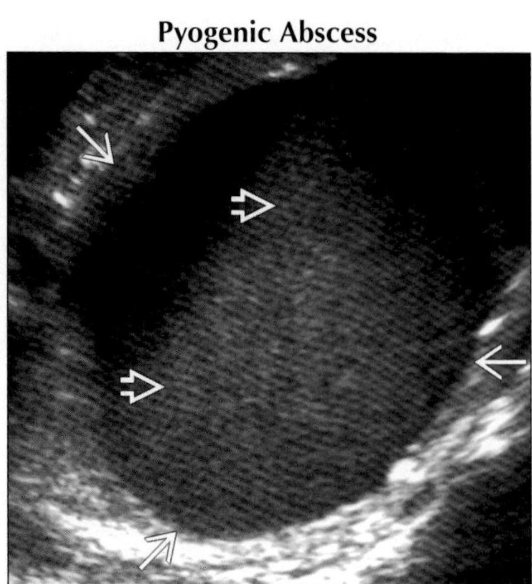

CYSTIC SPLENIC LESION

Parasitic Abscess

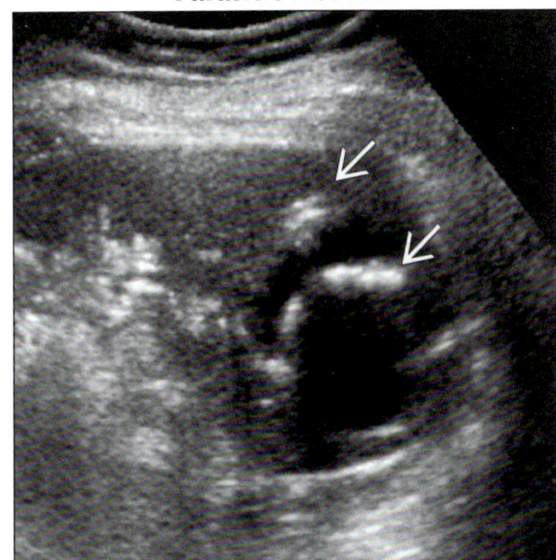

Lymphangioma

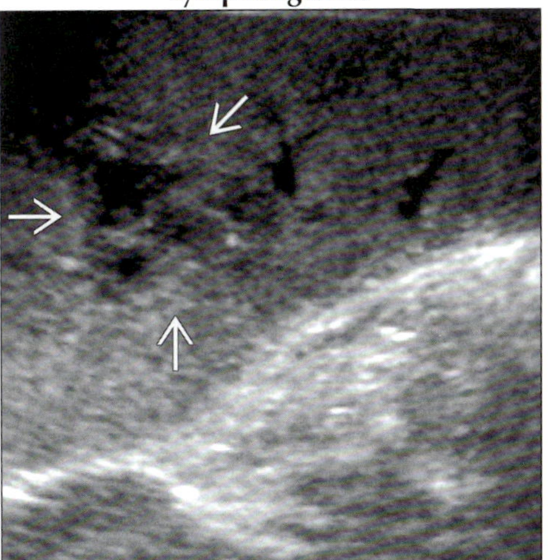

(Left) Transverse ultrasound of the spleen shows a multiloculated, thin-walled, anechoic cyst with a cyst-within-cyst appearance. Partial curvilinear calcification ➡ is seen in the cyst wall. This appearance represents a chronic healed hydatid cyst. *(Right)* Longitudinal ultrasound of the spleen shows a splenic lymphangioma ➡. Note its multiloculated, thin-walled, cystic appearance and the normal surrounding parenchyma.

Hemangioma

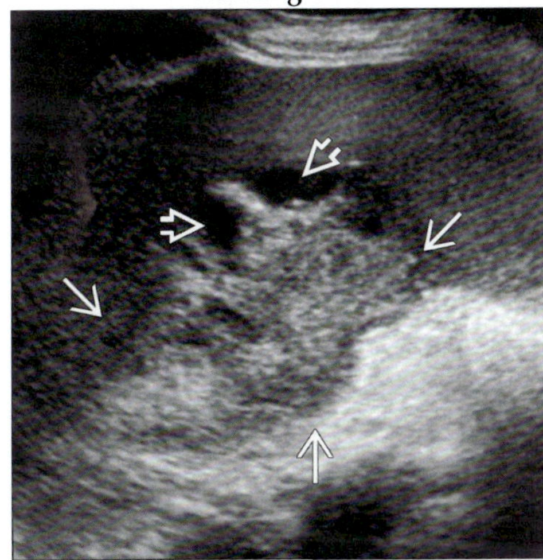

Hemangioma

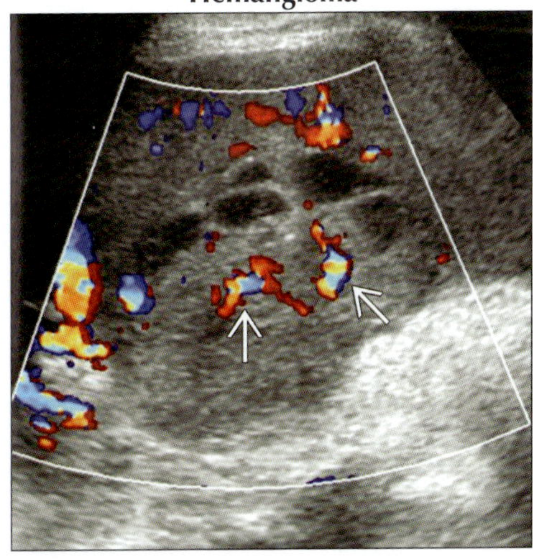

(Left) Longitudinal transabdominal ultrasound shows the typical appearance of a large splenic hemangioma ➡. Note the discrete cystic spaces ➡ in the periphery. The cystic areas may be as large as the entire lesion, giving the lesion a predominantly cystic appearance. *(Right)* Longitudinal color Doppler ultrasound in the same patient shows prominent internal vascularity ➡ in the solid portion of the splenic hemangioma.

Lymphoma

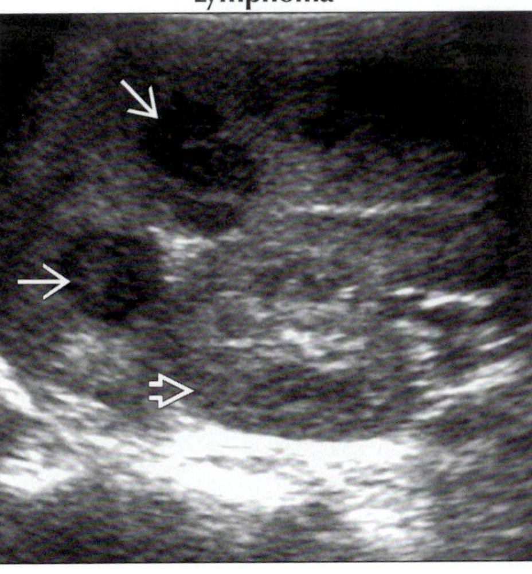

Congenital (Epidermoid) Cyst

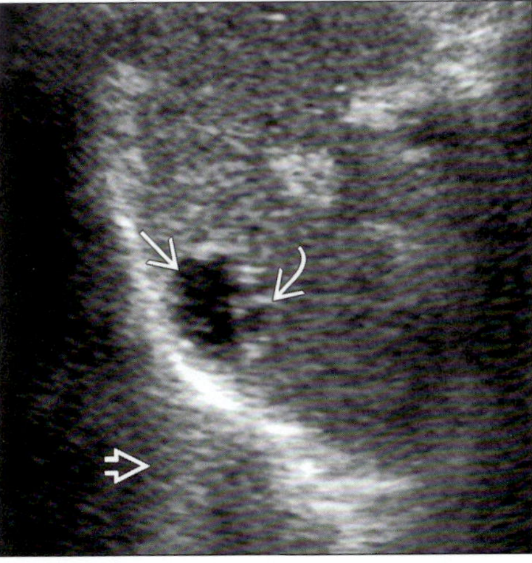

(Left) Transverse ultrasound shows lymphomatous deposits ➡ in the spleen. The markedly hypoechoic appearance may be confused with cystic lesions (left kidney ➡). *(Right)* Longitudinal ultrasound of the spleen shows a thin-walled anechoic cyst ➡ with thin internal septa ➡ and posterior enhancement ➡. This appearance is nonspecific. At histology, an epidermoid cyst has an epithelial lining, distinguishing it from other splenic cysts.

6

HYPOECHOIC SPLENIC LESION

DIFFERENTIAL DIAGNOSIS

Common
- Splenic Infarction
- Splenic Trauma

Less Common
- Splenic Metastases
- Splenic Lymphoma
- Infection/Abscess
- Hemangioma
- Lymphangioma
- Sarcoidosis

Rare but Important
- Primary Splenic Tumors
  - Angiosarcoma
  - Hemangiopericytoma
  - Hemangioendothelioma
  - Littoral Cell Angioma

ESSENTIAL INFORMATION

Key Differential Diagnosis Issues
- Primary benign splenic tumors are unusual; of these, hemangioma is most common
- Malignant splenic tumor is also rare; most common is lymphoma
- CT or MR provides additional information about tumor/disease
- Splenectomy may be required for definitive evaluation of splenic mass with atypical features

Helpful Clues for Common Diagnoses
- **Splenic Infarction**
  - Most common source of focal splenic defects
  - Causes: Parenchyma outgrows vascular supply in splenomegaly, local thrombosis, embolic, vasculitic, compromised splenic artery
  - Left upper quadrant (LUQ) pain, fever, elevated sedimentation rate and LDH
  - Single or multiple, ill-defined, wedge-shaped, hypoechoic areas in acute phase
  - Over time, increasingly well defined and echogenic with fibrosis ± Ca++ due to healing
- **Splenic Trauma**
  - Spleen: Most frequently injured intraabdominal organ in blunt abdominal trauma
  - MDCT is modality of choice for evaluation
  - Laceration: Linear hypoechoic area with shaggy border extending to capsule ± subcapsular hematoma
  - Hematoma: Varies in echogenicity with time
    - Ill-defined, hypoechoic in hyperacute stage
    - Heterogeneously hypoechoic with cystic area during organizing phase

Helpful Clues for Less Common Diagnoses
- **Splenic Metastases**
  - Most are seen with disseminated metastatic disease
    - Primary tumor: Ovarian, breast, lung, colorectal, and melanoma
  - Solitary splenic metastasis is extremely rare
    - Primary tumor: Ovarian, large intestine, lung, stomach
  - Majority are seen as multiple hypoechoic masses
  - Some appear as "target" lesions
  - May be cystic with irregular internal necrosis or entirely cystic, e.g., from ovarian primary
  - Occasionally entirely hyperechoic, e.g., from melanoma
  - Evidence of associated disseminated disease in body: Lung, liver, bone, lymph nodes
- **Splenic Lymphoma**
  - Nonspecific clinical symptoms; may mimic infective cause with fever, LUQ pain, and splenomegaly
  - Multiple small nodules, hypoechoic > hyperechoic
  - Large masses may have central necrosis
  - Majority associated with splenic hilar adenopathy and hepatic involvement
  - Homogeneous, diffuse, splenic enlargement itself is less specific for lymphomatous involvement
- **Infection/Abscess**
  - Pyogenic, fungal, or protozoal (hydatid disease)
    - Early infective focus (inflammatory phlegmon) may be seen as ill defined, hypo- or hyperechoic area

6

HYPOECHOIC SPLENIC LESION

- Central necrosis and liquefaction may develop
- Single to several foci in pyogenic infection
- Multiple microabscesses in fungal infection, usually in immunocompromised patients
- Hydatid disease in endemic areas; ill-defined hypoechoic mass in early phase with subsequent characteristic appearance of hydatid cysts, ± calcification
- **Hemangioma**
  - Most common benign neoplasm of spleen
  - Variable appearance
    - Majority are well defined, solid, echogenic ± internal discrete cystic spaces
    - Occasionally predominantly cystic
    - Heterogeneous complex appearance if it contains large cavernous component or is complicated with internal necrosis or fibrosis (usually in large tumors)
- **Lymphangioma**
  - Multiple splenic cysts (few millimeters to centimeters) ± septations ± tiny echogenic calcification
  - May be hypoechoic with debris due to proteinaceous material
- **Sarcoidosis**
  - Multiple hypoechoic nodules
  - 60% with splenic involvement have splenomegaly

Helpful Clues for Rare Diagnoses

- **Primary Splenic Tumors**
  - Majority are vascular tumors
  - Mostly hypoechoic
  - **Angiosarcoma**
    - Extremely rare but most common nonhematolymphoid malignant tumor of spleen
    - In older patients, M = F
    - Poor prognosis, mortality within 1 year
    - Disseminated metastases common at diagnosis
    - Most common appearance is complex heterogeneous mass + necrotic degeneration (common) ± hemoperitoneum (30%)
    - Cystic areas represent intratumoral necrosis and hemorrhage
    - Scattered calcification occasionally seen
    - Massive calcification in radial pattern has also been reported
  - **Hemangiopericytoma**: Relatively high malignant potential
  - **Hemangioendothelioma**: Variable malignant potential, nonspecific features
  - **Littoral Cell Angioma**
    - Benign ± malignant features
    - Clinical hypersplenism almost always present
    - Typically multiple small foci
    - Hypoattenuating on late portal phase CT
    - MR shows hemosiderin products (low intensity on both T1WI and T2WI)

Splenic Infarction

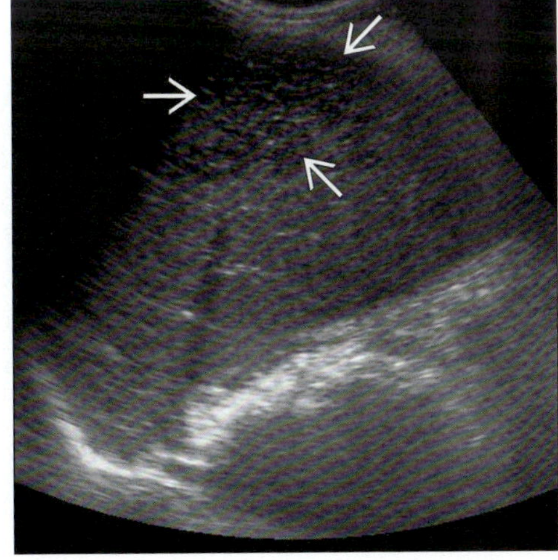

Oblique transabdominal ultrasound shows a wedge-shaped, peripherally located, hypoechoic area ➡, consistent with an acute splenic infarct.

Splenic Infarction

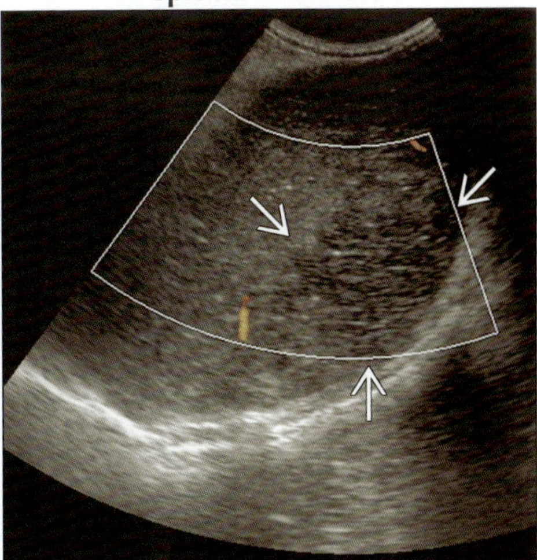

Transverse power Doppler ultrasound in the same patient shows absence of vascularity in the infarcted area ➡.

HYPOECHOIC SPLENIC LESION

Splenic Trauma

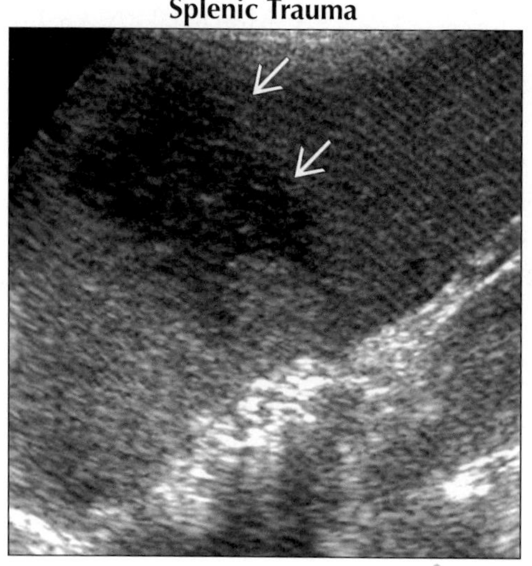

Splenic Trauma

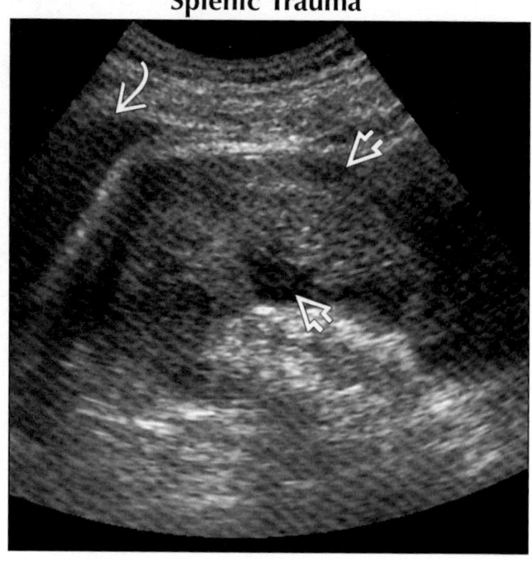

(Left) Oblique transabdominal ultrasound shows a splenic laceration ➡. The internal content is close to fluid echogenicity with mobile echoes, representing acute blood. (Right) Longitudinal transabdominal ultrasound shows a ruptured spleen. The irregular splenic parenchyma represents a large fragment with a disrupted splenic capsule. It is associated with hemoperitoneum ➡ and hemothorax ➡.

Splenic Metastases

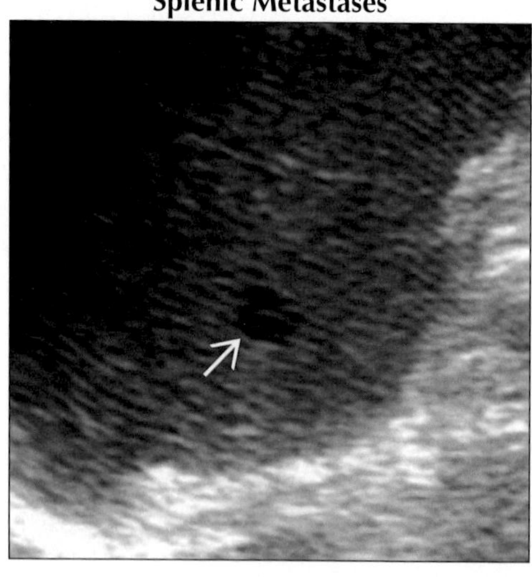

Splenic Metastases

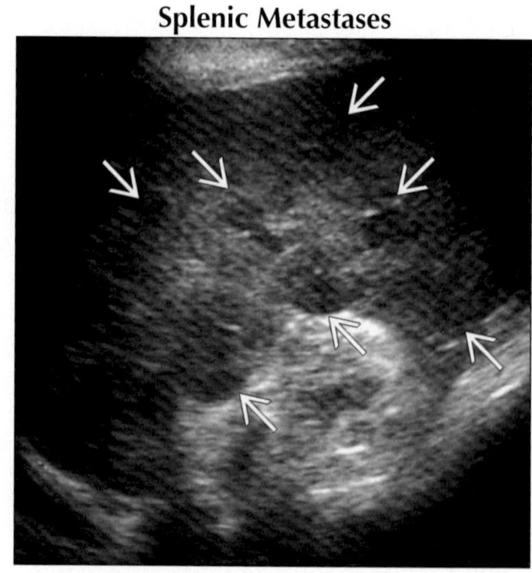

(Left) Oblique transabdominal ultrasound shows a small hypoechoic metastasis ➡ from nasopharyngeal carcinoma. Sonographically, it cannot be differentiated from a splenic tumor or abscess at this small size. (Right) Oblique transabdominal ultrasound shows multiple hypoechoic nodules ➡ of varying size, representing metastases. Stomach cancer is a primary tumor that causes isolated splenic metastasis before involving other organs.

Splenic Lymphoma

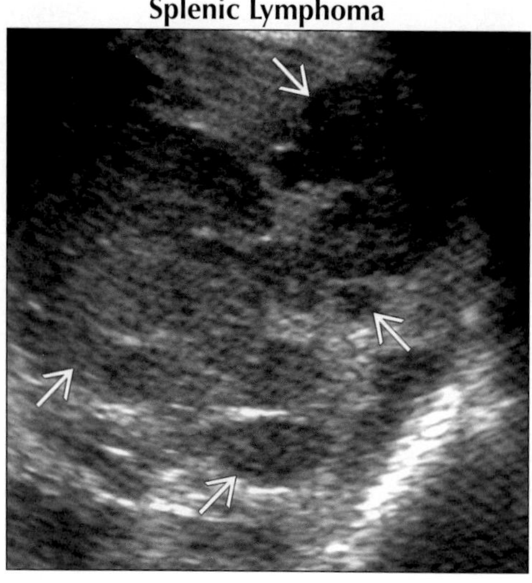

Splenic Lymphoma

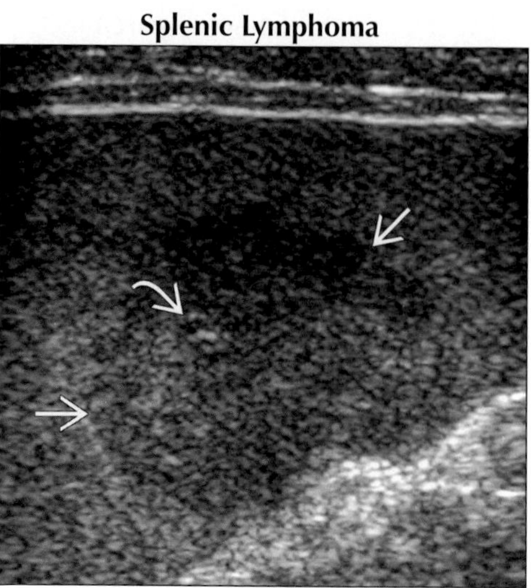

(Left) Transverse transabdominal ultrasound shows multiple, irregular, heterogeneous, hypoechoic, lymphomatous deposits ➡, some with a conglomerate geographic appearance. (Right) Longitudinal transabdominal ultrasound in another patient with splenic lymphoma shows a solitary hypoechoic mass ➡. The parenchymal architecture and internal vessels ➡ appear nondisplaced.

HYPOECHOIC SPLENIC LESION

Infection/Abscess

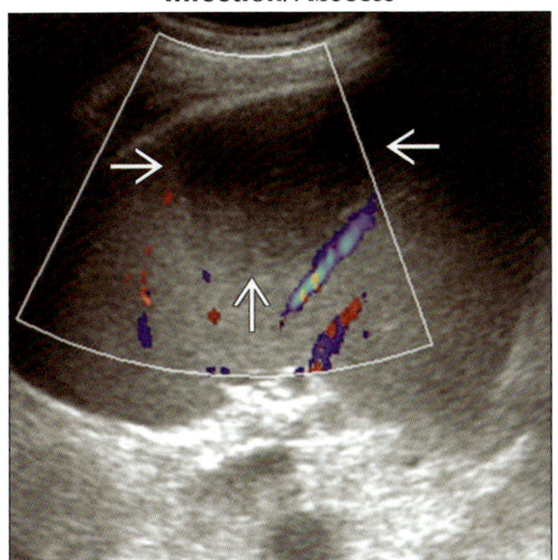

Infection/Abscess

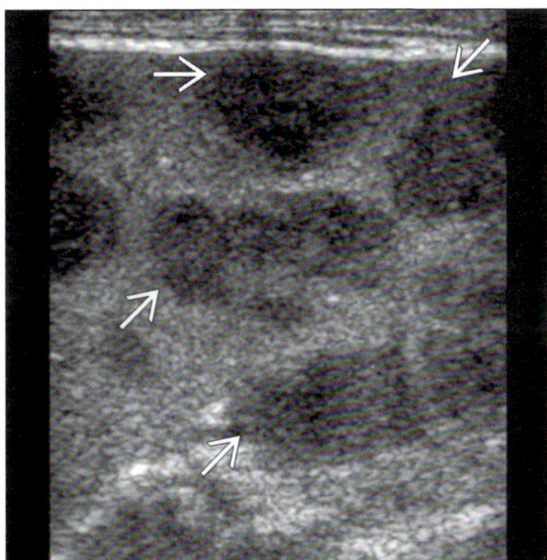

(Left) Oblique transabdominal ultrasound shows an ill-defined, hypoechoic, subcapsular, splenic lesion ➡. Mobile internal debris was seen, consistent with a liquefied abscess cavity in this septic patient. (Right) Oblique transabdominal ultrasound shows multiple, ill-defined, irregular, heterogeneous, hypoechoic masses ➡ in the spleen, representing tuberculomas in this immunocompromised patient with a disseminated TB infection.

Hemangioma

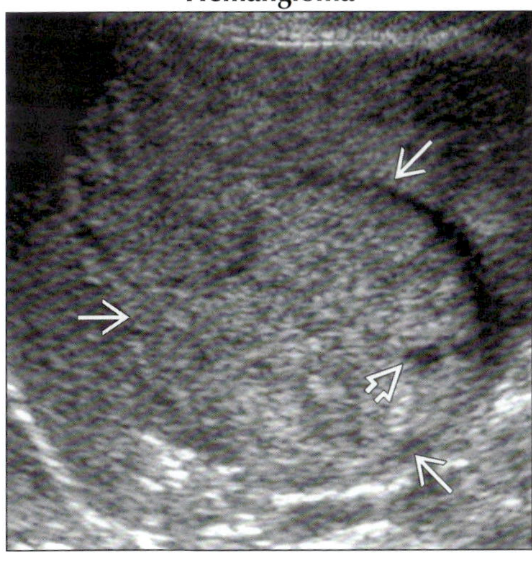

Hemangioma

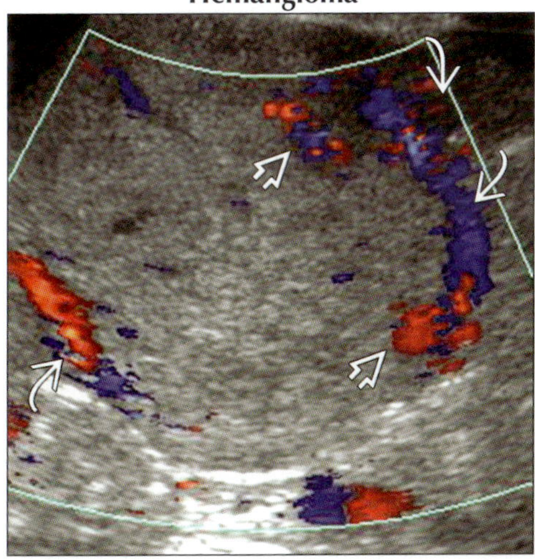

(Left) Oblique transabdominal ultrasound shows a large, round, well-circumscribed, isoechoic hemangioma ➡ with a small, peripheral, discrete, cystic area ➡. Hyperechoic or complex cystic splenic hemangiomas are more common. (Right) Oblique color Doppler ultrasound shows vascularity within the "cystic" area ➡, which represents a vascular lake, a common feature in splenic hemangiomata. Adjacent vessels ➡ are displaced by the tumor.

Lymphangioma

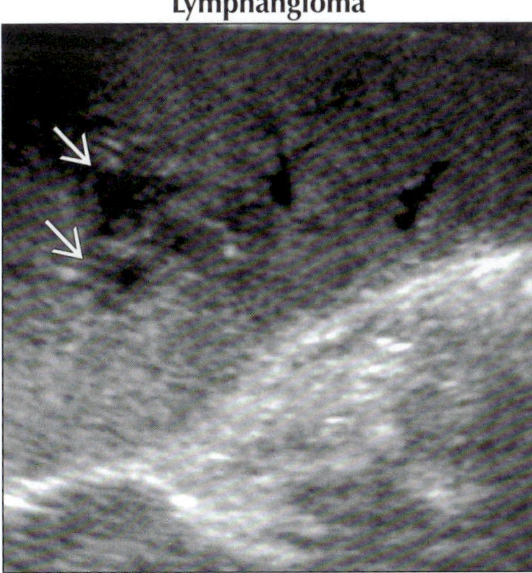

Angiosarcoma

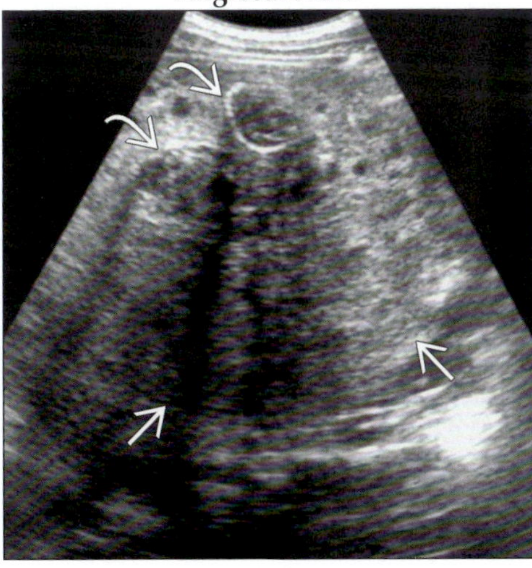

(Left) Longitudinal ultrasound of the spleen shows a well-defined, multiloculated cystic lesion ➡ representing a lymphangioma. Previous parenchymal injury with liquefaction may appear similarly, but there was no relevant history or sequential change. (Right) Transverse ultrasound of the spleen in an elderly man with LUQ pain shows a large, complex, heterogeneous, splenic tumor ➡ with calcific foci ➡. It was later confirmed as angiosarcoma.

DIFFERENTIAL DIAGNOSIS

Common
- Hematoma
- Splenic Calcification
  - Granuloma
  - Vascular Calcification
  - Gamna-Gandy Nodules
  - Calcification of Cyst Wall
- Hemangioma

Less Common
- Metastasis
- Lymphoma
- Invasion by Adjacent Mass (Mimic)

Rare but Important
- Hamartoma
- Primary Malignant Splenic Tumor
  - Angiosarcoma
- Metabolic Diseases
- Sarcoidosis

ESSENTIAL INFORMATION

Key Differential Diagnosis Issues
- Calcifications without associated soft tissue mass generally represent benign chronic calcification
  - Attention should be paid to curvilinear calcification for possible underlying aneurysm, pseudoaneurysm, or hydatid cyst
- Well-defined, homogeneously echogenic nodule: Hemangioma, hamartoma, metastasis (irregular contour, multiple, variable size, known malignancy)
- Heterogeneously hyperechoic mass can represent hemangioma > metastasis, lymphoma, primary splenic vascular tumor, or hamartoma
- Hematoma has history of trauma, ill-defined characteristics, amorphous appearance, surrounding edema, and avascular appearance on Doppler study

Helpful Clues for Common Diagnoses
- **Hematoma**
  - Spleen is most frequently injured intraperitoneal organ in blunt abdominal trauma
  - Intraparenchymal, subcapsular, or perisplenic

- Hyperacute/flowing blood appears hypoechoic
- Amorphous echogenic mass represents acute blood clot
- Check for integrity of major vascular pedicle and hemoperitoneum
- Sequential liquidation and regression
- **Splenic Calcification**
  - Look at pattern of calcification
    - Double-lined linear ± branching: Vascular
    - Curvilinear: Calcified cyst, hydatid cyst, pseudoaneurysm/aneurysm (rare), lymphangioma, or vascular tumor
    - Punctate, scattered: Gamna-Gandy nodules, granulomas, sarcoidosis
    - Amorphous, coarse calcification with acoustic shadow: Calcified granuloma, calcified hamartoma, chronic infarct, post-traumatic scarring, previous infection
  - **Granuloma**
    - Varies from punctate to larger, amorphous calcifications
    - Infectious etiologies include *Mycobacterium*, histoplasmosis, pneumocystic
  - **Vascular Calcification**
    - May see other signs of atherosclerosis
  - **Gamna-Gandy Nodules**
    - Foci of hemosiderin deposition with variable amount of fibrous tissue and calcium due to foci of intrasplenic hemorrhage
    - Causes: Portal hypertension, splenic vein thrombosis, hemolytic anemia, hemochromatosis, etc.
    - Punctate echogenic foci scattered in background of splenomegaly
    - MR more sensitive showing hypointense signal on all pulse sequences with blooming artifacts on gradient echo
- **Hemangioma**
  - Although uncommon, it is most common primary neoplasm of spleen (0.3-14% in autopsy series)
  - Usually small but can be as large as 17 cm
  - Appearance quite variable
    - Hyperechoic, heterogeneous, or hypoechoic solid mass

HYPERECHOIC SPLENIC LESION

- May see cystic areas or even be predominately cystic (rare)
- Appearance reflects relative proportion of capillary (solid, hyperechoic) and cavernous (cystic) component
- ○ Majority asymptomatic
  - Rarely, rupture can occur
- ○ May contain speckled calcification in solid component or curvilinear calcified in cystic component

Helpful Clues for Less Common Diagnoses
- **Metastasis**
  - ○ Variable size and echogenicity
  - ○ Hypo-, iso-, or hyperechoic
  - ○ Mucinous adenocarcinoma or melanoma metastases are echogenic
- **Lymphoma**
  - ○ Infiltrative, nodular/miliary or mass-like
  - ○ < 10% hyperechoic
  - ○ Majority are markedly hypoechoic; may mimic cystic lesion
- **Invasion of Adjacent Mass (Mimic)**
  - ○ Adjacent tumor invading/abutting spleen, e.g., pancreatic tail tumor, gastric fundal tumor

Helpful Clues for Rare Diagnoses
- **Hamartoma**
  - ○ Usually solitary
  - ○ Variable appearance
    - Well-defined hyperechoic solid to mixed, to purely cystic
  - ○ Solid lesions: Hyperechoic > iso- or hypoechoic with internal vascularity

- ○ Necrosis and calcification may occur in large lesion
- **Primary Malignant Splenic Tumor**
  - ○ **Angiosarcoma**
    - Most common primary malignant neoplasm of spleen
    - Appearance is nonspecific compared to other primary splenic tumors; could be solid, complex cystic to cystic appearance
    - Cystic component due to necrosis
    - Echogenic component: Solid portion or internal hemorrhage
    - Propensity to spontaneously rupture
- **Metabolic Diseases**
  - ○ Glycogen storage disease: Splenomegaly + multiple hypo-/hyperechoic nodules
  - ○ Amyloidosis: Discrete masses + 4-13% splenomegaly
- **Sarcoidosis**
  - ○ Usually seen as splenomegaly with hypoechoic nodules
  - ○ Diffuse punctate calcified granulomas in background of splenomegaly is sometimes seen
  - ○ Occasionally seen as necrotic mass with focal calcifications

Hematoma

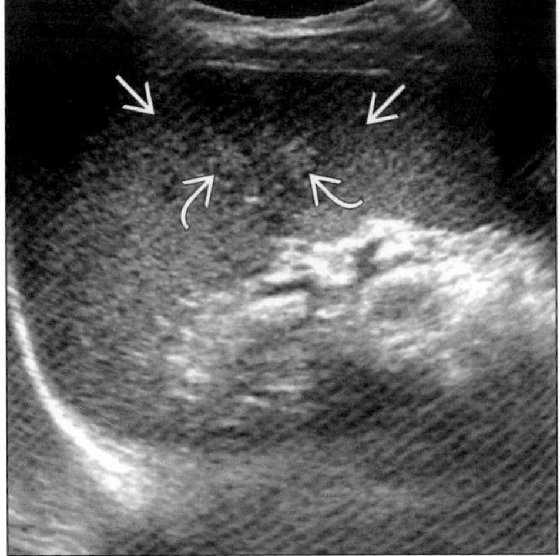

Oblique transabdominal ultrasound shows a splenic laceration ➡. Note that the hyperechoic blood clot ➡ stands out from the hypoechoic area of laceration.

Granuloma

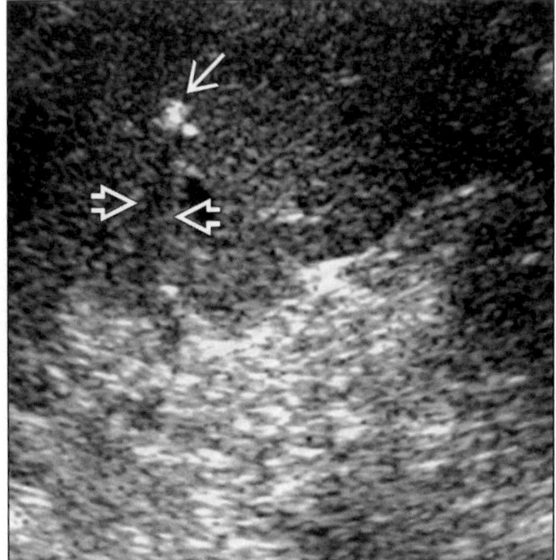

Longitudinal transabdominal ultrasound shows a small, irregular, markedly echogenic focus ➡ with acoustic shadowing ➡ in the spleen, representing a small focus of calcification in a splenic granuloma.

6

HYPERECHOIC SPLENIC LESION

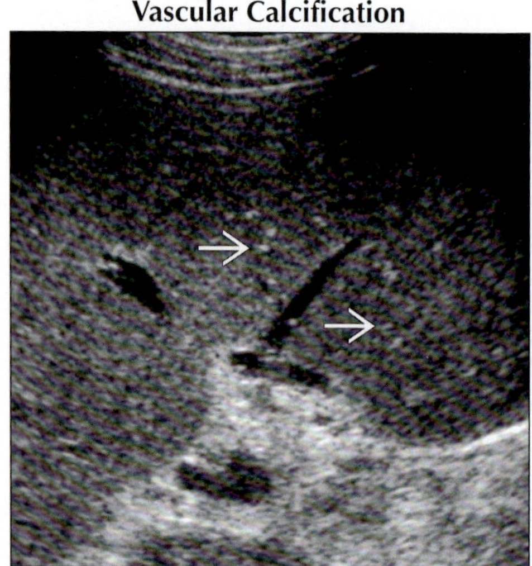

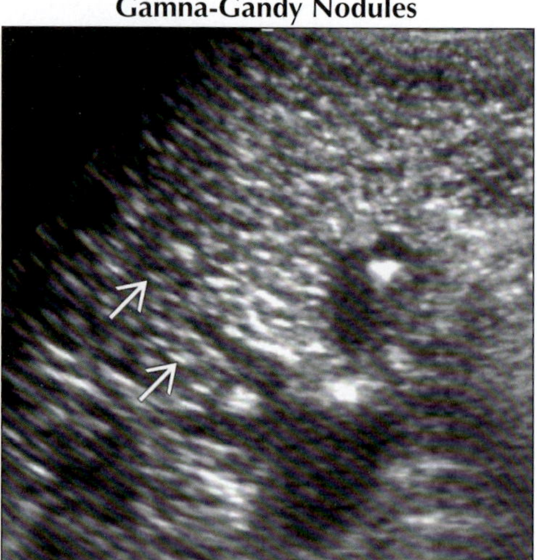

(Left) Oblique transabdominal ultrasound shows small calcified splenic arterial branches ➡. (Right) Oblique transabdominal ultrasound in this cirrhotic patient with portal hypertension and splenomegaly shows multiple tiny hyperechoic foci ➡, representing Gamna-Gandy bodies.

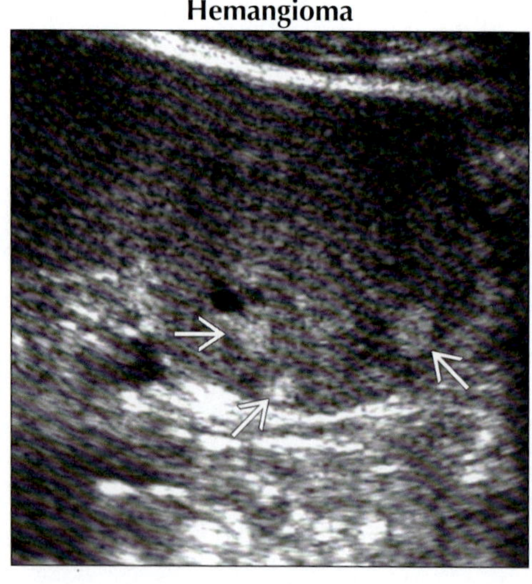

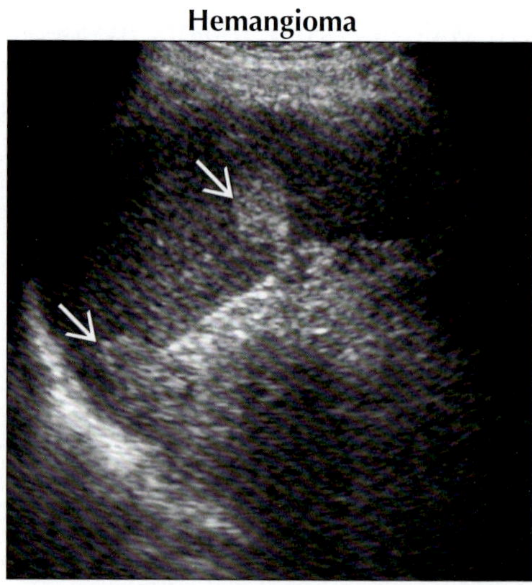

(Left) Longitudinal transabdominal ultrasound of the spleen shows multiple, well-defined, rounded, homogeneously hyperechoic lesions ➡, representing multiple hemangiomata. (Right) Oblique transabdominal ultrasound shows another case of splenic hemangiomata. Again they appear as well-defined, homogeneously hyperechoic masses ➡. This appearance is similar to that of hepatic hemangiomata.

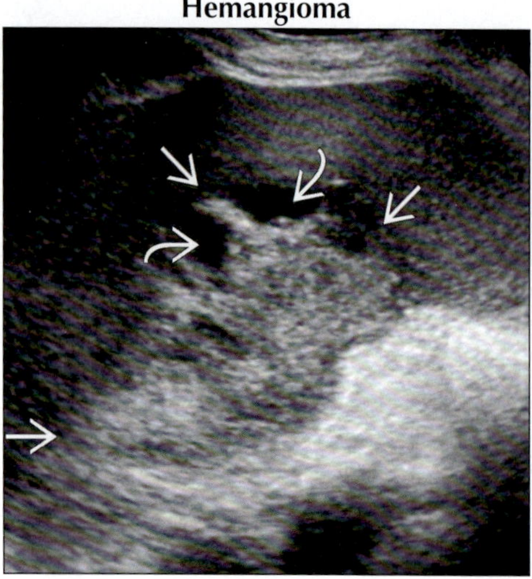

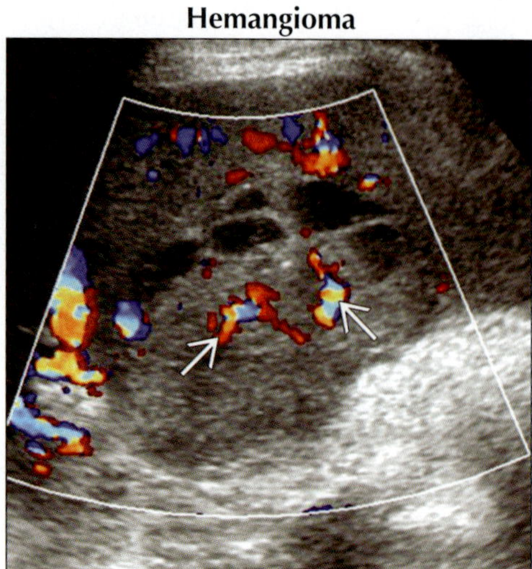

(Left) Longitudinal ultrasound shows a large splenic hemangioma ➡ in a patient with thrombocytopenia, a common association. Note the well-defined hyperechoic appearance with discrete cystic areas ➡. (Right) Color Doppler ultrasound shows internal vascularity ➡. Features are typical of splenic hemangioma. However, other malignant primary splenic tumors may appear similar. Biopsy or splenectomy is required for definitive diagnosis.

6

HYPERECHOIC SPLENIC LESION

Metastasis

Metastasis

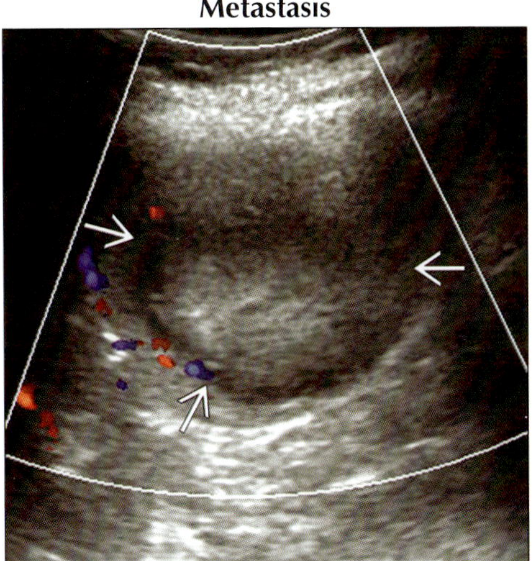

(Left) Longitudinal ultrasound shows multiple, irregular, echogenic nodules of varying sizes in the spleen, representing metastases ➡ from hepatocellular carcinoma. They were hypodense on CECT. The echogenic appearance may represent coagulative necrosis. (Right) Longitudinal color Doppler ultrasound of the spleen shows a heterogeneously hyperechoic mass ➡ representing a splenic metastasis from conjunctival melanoma.

Lymphoma

Lymphoma

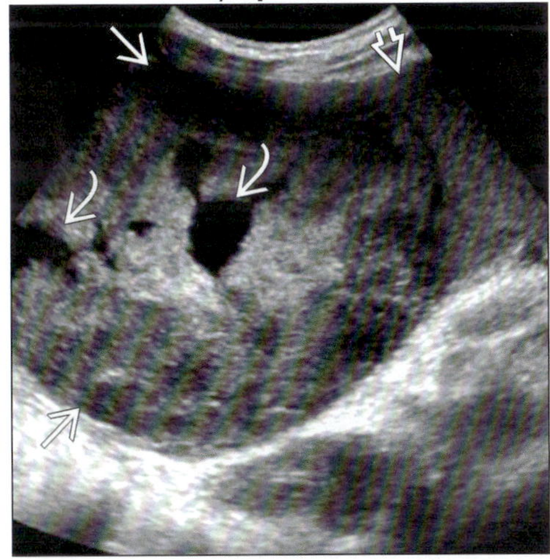

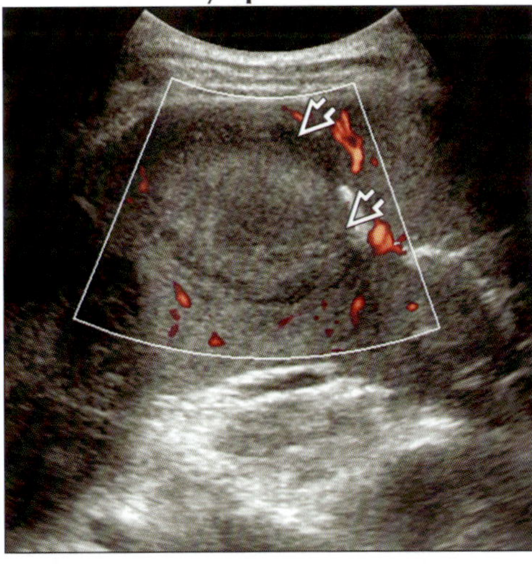

(Left) Longitudinal transabdominal ultrasound shows an exophytic gastric MALT lymphoma ➡ with direct invasion to the spleen ➡. Discrete irregular internal necrosis ➡ is present. (Right) Longitudinal power Doppler ultrasound of the spleen shows splenic metastasis from gastric MALT lymphoma ➡. Note the heterogeneously hyperechoic appearance. Most splenic lymphomas are hypoechoic and occasionally markedly hypoechoic to mimic cysts.

Hamartoma

Sarcoidosis

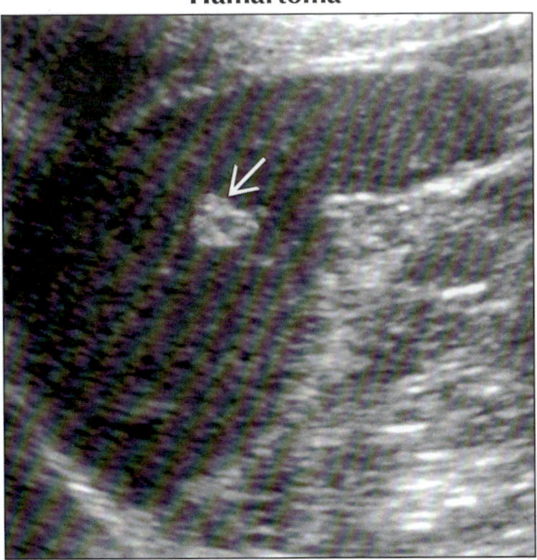

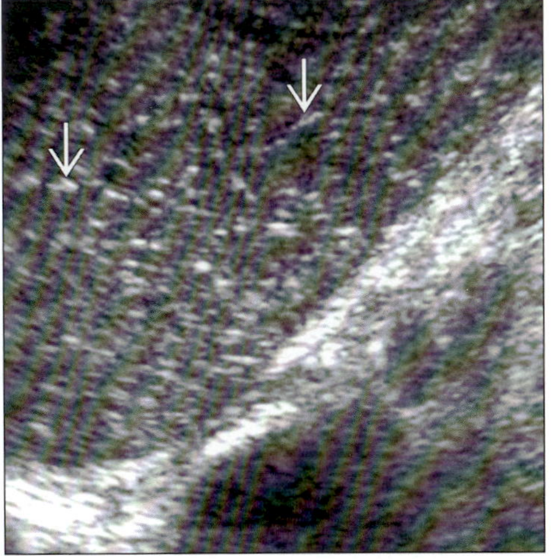

(Left) Longitudinal transabdominal ultrasound shows a calcified splenic hamartoma ➡. It is well defined and echogenic. The echogenicity is higher than that seen in a solid tumor, e.g., hemangioma, and is suggestive of a calcified lesion. (Right) Oblique transabdominal ultrasound shows splenomegaly and multiple punctate calcified granulomas ➡ due to splenic sarcoidosis.

6

SECTION 7
Adrenal Gland

BILATERAL ADRENAL ENLARGEMENT

DIFFERENTIAL DIAGNOSIS

Common
- Adenoma
- Metastases
- Hemorrhage and Infarction
- Diaphragmatic Crura (Mimic)

Less Common
- Bilateral Adrenal Hyperplasia (BAH)
  - Smooth Hyperplasia
  - Cortical Nodular Hyperplasia
- Pheochromocytoma
- Infection and Granulomatous Diseases

Rare but Important
- Lymphoma
- Primary Pigmented Nodular Adrenocortical Hyperplasia
- Myelolipoma
- Wolman Disease

ESSENTIAL INFORMATION

Key Differential Diagnosis Issues
- Thickened diaphragmatic crus may be mistaken for hyperplastic adrenal glands
- Smooth enlargement
  - Bilateral adrenal hyperplasia, adrenal infarction, infection or granulomatous disease, lymphoma, primary pigmented nodular adrenocortical hyperplasia, Wolman disease
- Macronodular enlargement
  - Cortical nodular hyperplasia in longstanding Cushing syndrome
- Bilateral adrenal masses
  - Hemorrhage: Hypoechoic when acute and sequential decrease in size
  - Other adrenal tumors, infections, or inflammatory conditions are generally nonspecific in appearance
  - Correlation with clinical symptoms; endocrine profile, urine catecholamine, MR, or CT is required for further evaluation

Helpful Clues for Common Diagnoses
- **Adenoma**
  - 2% prevalence, 10% bilateral
  - < 5 cm, average 2-2.5 cm
  - US nonspecific

  - Well defined, homogeneously hypoechoic, may calcify
  - CT
    - NECT: < 10 Hounsfield units (HU)
    - Delayed CECT: < 37 HU
    - Washout: > 50% after 10 minutes
  - MR: Marked hypointensity (compared to spleen) on opposed-phase GRE images
- **Metastases**
  - Adrenal gland common site of metastases, seen in 27% of epithelial malignancies
  - Sonographic appearances are nonspecific
  - More definite malignant features: > 3 cm, ill-defined heterogeneous masses ± necrosis ± local invasion
  - Smaller lesions are difficult to differentiate, especially < 3 cm
  - MR: Higher T2WI signal than adenoma, but appearances overlap in 20-30% cases
- **Hemorrhage and Infarction**
  - Bilateral involvement usually in setting of anticoagulation; may also be caused by stress-related hemorrhage
  - Traumatic hemorrhage and neonatal hemorrhage are usually unilateral (R > L); 10% bilateral
  - May be related to stasis and thrombosis of adrenal vein
  - Appearances
    - Well defined if spontaneous, more ill defined if traumatic cause
    - Echogenic in acute phase; organization and liquefaction in subacute to chronic phase, seen as hypoechoic to cystic areas
  - Suspect infarction when enlarged; hypoechoic adrenal glands are seen after severe hypotensive episode/stress
  - Risk of Addison crisis exists with bilateral adrenal hemorrhage &/or infarction

Helpful Clues for Less Common Diagnoses
- **Bilateral Adrenal Hyperplasia (BAH)**
  - **Smooth Hyperplasia**
    - Common
    - Normal-looking glands or diffuse uniform thickening
    - Most thickened and elongated glands seen in ectopic ACTH production, e.g., medullary carcinoma of thyroid, oat cell carcinoma of lung
  - **Cortical Nodular Hyperplasia**
    - Uncommon

- Macronodular hyperplasia: Thickened glands + nodules of varying size, up to 2.5 cm; seen in longstanding Cushing disease
- Micronodular hyperplasia: Normal or thickened glands ± micronodule; micronodule often too small to be appreciated on anatomical imaging
- **Pheochromocytoma**
  - Characteristic propensity of bilateral involvement
  - Multiplicity in 10% of nonfamilial adult cases, 32% of nonfamilial childhood cases, 65% of familial syndromes
  - Associated syndromes: MEN2A, 2B, neurofibromatosis, von Hippel-Lindau syndrome, familial pheochromocytomas
  - Markedly hypervascular on Doppler ultrasound
  - Spectrum of appearances
- **Infection and Granulomatous Diseases**
  - Tuberculosis, histoplasmosis, and granulomatous diseases
    - Usually bilateral and asymmetrical
    - Smooth enlargement, solid masses, cystic change
    - Calcification is common; reflects age of process and degree of necrosis
  - Diagnosis made by biopsy

Helpful Clues for Rare Diagnoses
- **Lymphoma**
  - Non-Hodgkin lymphoma > Hodgkin lymphoma, 50% bilateral
  - Often other sites of involvement, e.g., retroperitoneal lymphoma
  - Adrenal insufficiency is rare
  - Smooth enlargement (due to diffuse infiltration) or discrete or conglomerate hypoechoic masses
- **Primary Pigmented Nodular Adrenocortical Hyperplasia**
  - Seen in young adults and children
  - Cortisol secreted by pigmented nodules in cortex
  - Appearance similar to micronodular hyperplasia
  - Micronodules often too small to be seen on anatomical imaging
- **Myelolipoma**
  - Benign tumor composed of fat and hematopoietic elements
  - Very rarely bilateral
  - Homogeneous, echogenic masses
- **Wolman Disease**
  - Primary familial xanthomatosis
  - Rare autosomal recessive lipidosis that affects children
  - Accumulation of cholesterol esters and triglycerides in visceral foam cells + organs
  - Characteristic imaging features
    - Echogenic smooth enlargement of both adrenal glands + scattered calcification
    - Hepatosplenomegaly, fatty liver, thickened echogenic bowel wall (typically ileum and jejunum), enlarged echogenic lymph nodes

Metastases

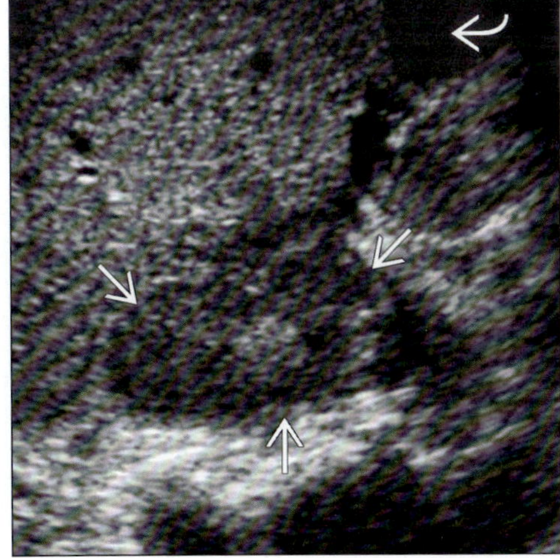

Longitudinal transabdominal ultrasound shows an irregular, heterogeneously hypoechoic mass ➔ in the right adrenal bed. Note the ascites ➔ in the subhepatic space.

Metastases

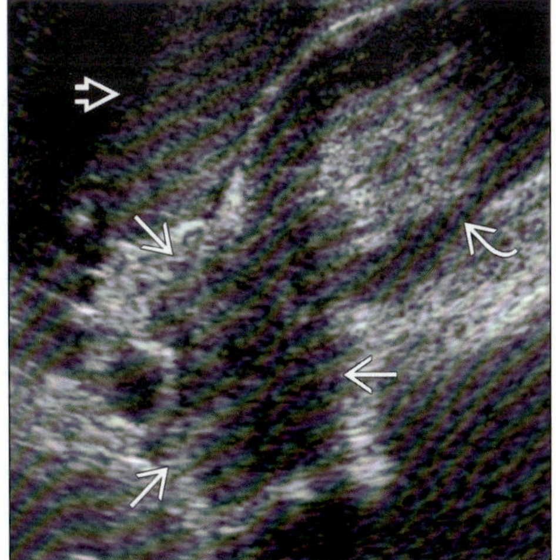

Longitudinal transabdominal ultrasound shows a left adrenal mass ➔ in the same patient, who had bilateral adrenal metastases from lung cancer. (Spleen ➔, left kidney ➔.)

BILATERAL ADRENAL ENLARGEMENT

Diaphragmatic Crura (Mimic)

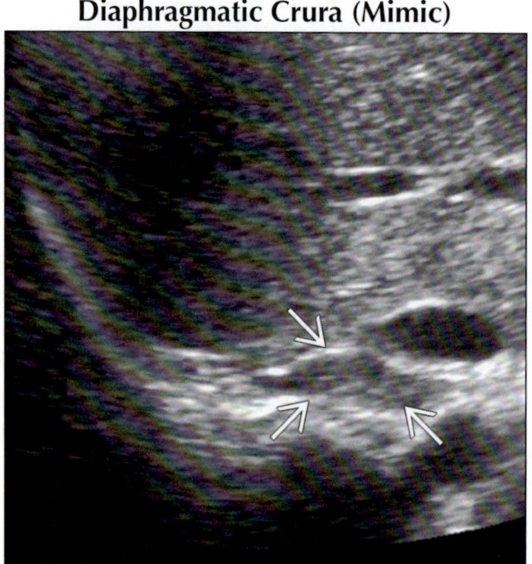

Diaphragmatic Crura (Mimic)

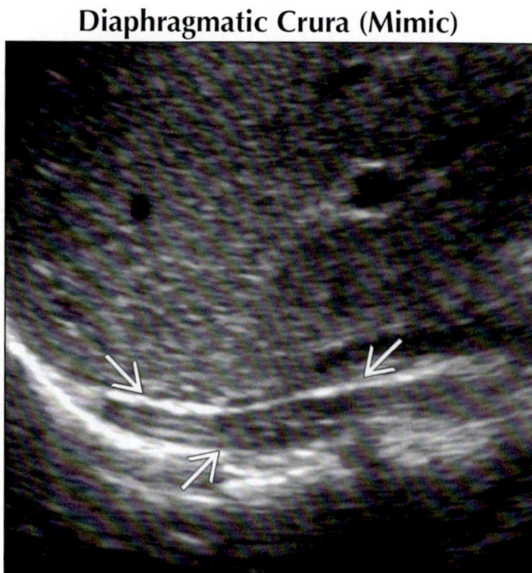

(Left) Transverse transabdominal ultrasound shows a prominent diaphragmatic crus ➡, which may mimic an enlarged adrenal gland. (Right) Longitudinal transabdominal ultrasound in the same patient shows the diaphragmatic crus ➡ once the transducer is turned 90°. Note the linear and tubular appearance.

Cortical Nodular Hyperplasia

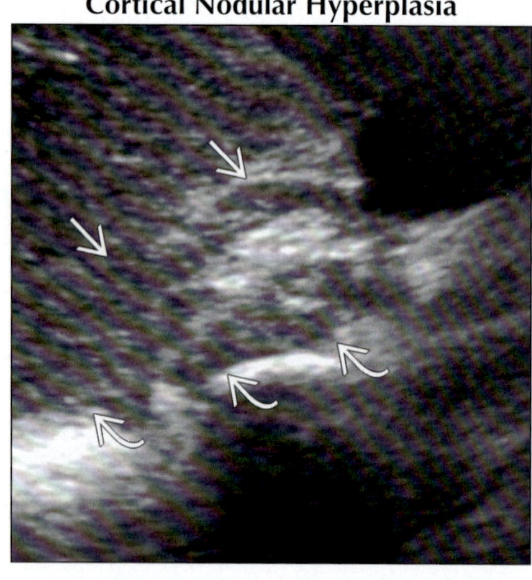

Cortical Nodular Hyperplasia

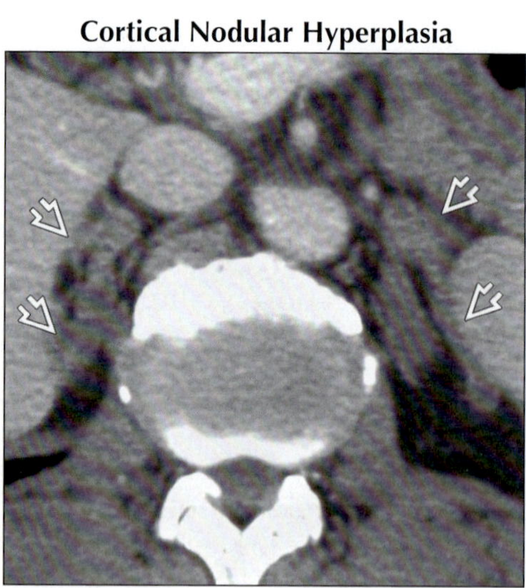

(Left) Transverse ultrasound shows marked enlargement of the right adrenal gland with thickened and elongated limbs, which have a macronodular appearance. Note the lateral ➡ and medial ➡ limbs. (Right) Correlative axial NECT shows the macronodular enlargement of both adrenal glands ➡. They are equally enlarged, but the left adrenal gland is more difficult to see on US due to the inherent limitation of an acoustic window for the left adrenal region.

Cortical Nodular Hyperplasia

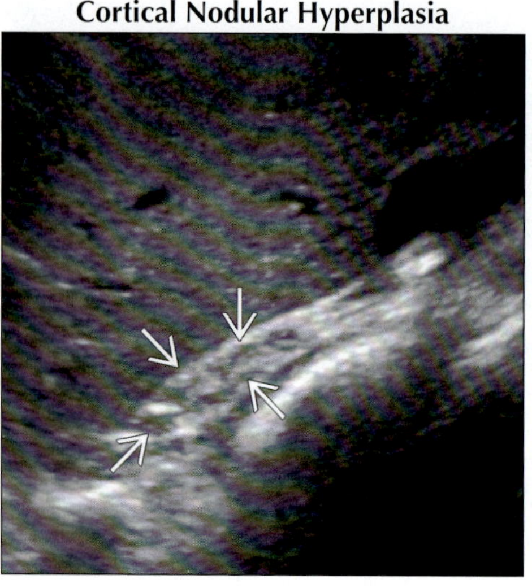

Cortical Nodular Hyperplasia

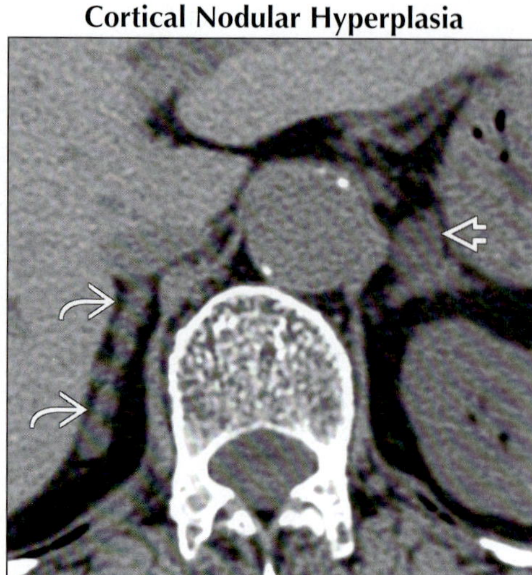

(Left) Transverse ultrasound shows elongated thickened limbs of the right adrenal ➡ with undulating contour, representing a micronodular change in a patient with bilateral adrenal hyperplasia. (Right) Correlative axial NECT shows the micronodular/early macronodular change of the right adrenal gland ➡. A coexisting adenoma ➡ is present in the left adrenal isthmus. The left adrenal limb, which also showed nodular change, did not fall into this scanning section.

BILATERAL ADRENAL ENLARGEMENT

Pheochromocytoma

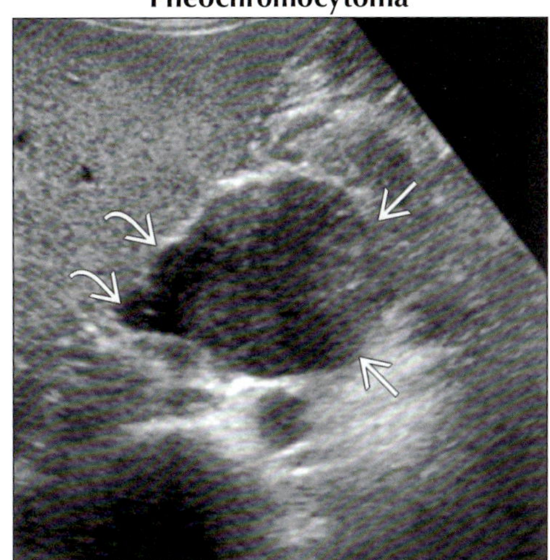

Pheochromocytoma

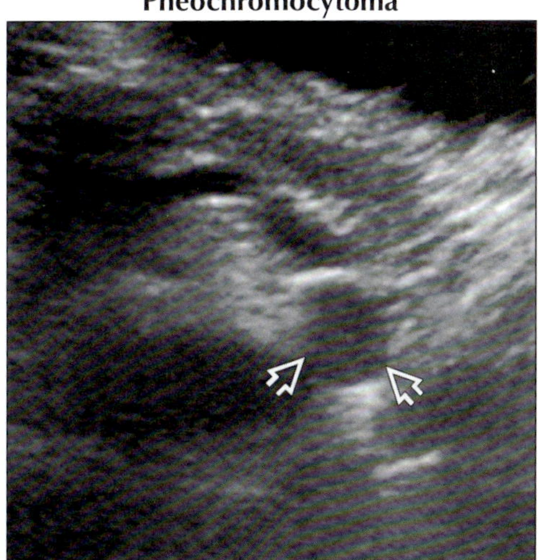

(Left) Oblique transabdominal ultrasound shows an irregular, heterogeneously hypoechoic, right adrenal mass ➡ with eccentric discrete areas of cystic change ➡. (Right) Transverse ultrasound shows a smaller, well-defined, hypoechoic nodule in the left adrenal bed ➡. This patient had a history of familial pheochromocytoma. The diagnosis of bilateral pheochromocytoma was confirmed by urinalysis and MIBG scan.

Infection and Granulomatous Diseases

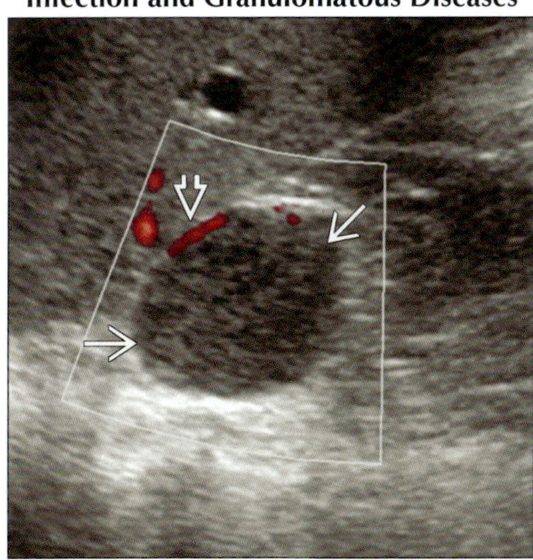

Infection and Granulomatous Diseases

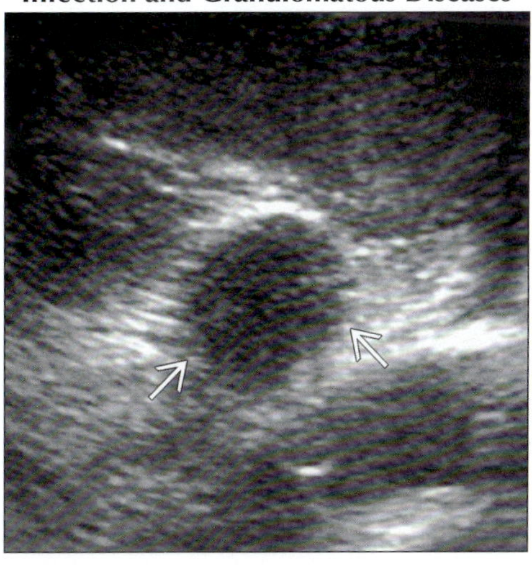

(Left) Longitudinal transabdominal color Doppler ultrasound of the right adrenal bed shows a well-defined, round, homogeneously hypoechoic nodule ➡ with mild peripheral vascularity ➡. (Right) Longitudinal scan of the left adrenal bed shows a similar but smaller nodule ➡. The appearances are nonspecific on US as well as on CT (not shown) in this asymptomatic patient. A subsequent biopsy specimen revealed granulomatous inflammation.

Myelolipoma

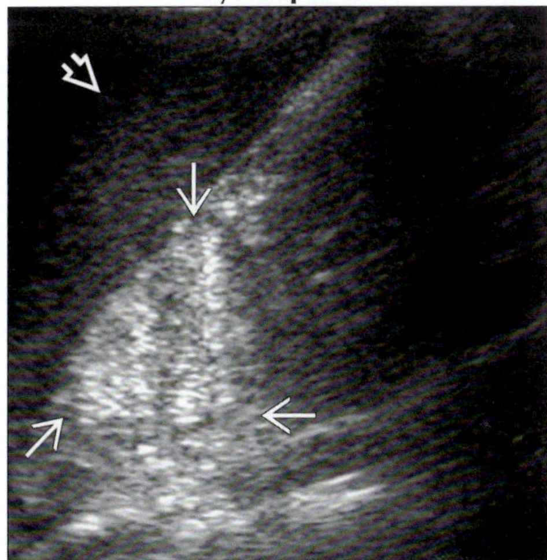

Myelolipoma

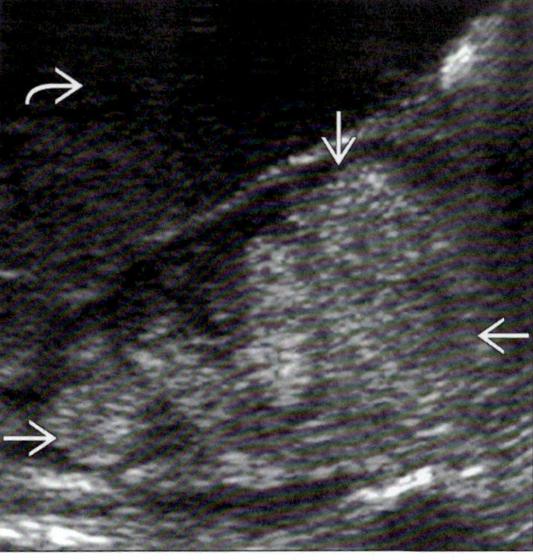

(Left) Oblique transabdominal ultrasound shows a diffusely hyperechoic mass in the right adrenal gland ➡ adjacent to the liver ➡ in a patient with bilateral adrenal myelolipomas. (Right) Longitudinal transabdominal ultrasound in the same patient shows a diffusely hyperechoic left adrenal mass ➡ with hypoechoic periphery adjacent to the spleen ➡.

CYSTIC ADRENAL MASS

DIFFERENTIAL DIAGNOSIS

Common
- Endothelial Cyst
- Pseudocyst
- Abscess
- Organizing Hematoma
- Mimics

Less Common
- Cystic Adenoma
- Cystic Neuroblastoma
- Cystic Pheochromocytoma
- Cystic Adrenocortical Carcinoma
- Cystic Adenomatoid Tumor

Rare but Important
- Cystic Metastases
- Epithelial Cysts, True Cyst
- Hydatid Cyst
- Cystic Schwannoma

ESSENTIAL INFORMATION

Key Differential Diagnosis Issues
- Differentiate adrenal cysts from cystic lesion of adjacent organs
- Always evaluate with color Doppler to confirm "cyst" is not aneurysm from adjacent artery
- Pseudocysts may be associated with benign or malignant adrenal tumors
  - Extensive pathologic sampling of macroscopically suspicious portion of resected tissue is essential to exclude tumor foci in cyst
- Many cystic tumors show overlapping appearances on US, MR, and needle biopsy
  - Surgical resection may be required for definitive diagnosis

Helpful Clues for Common Diagnoses
- **Endothelial Cyst**
  - 45-48% of all adrenal cysts
  - Not as commonly detected as pseudocyst since some endothelial cysts are small (1-15 mm)
  - Lymphangiomatous or angiomatous are most common types
  - Lymphangiomatous cysts (93%)
    - Multiloculated, septated; anechoic ± low-level mobile debris
  - Angiomatous cysts
    - Commonly unilocular with lobulated border and internal vascularity
    - Debris/pseudonodular appearance due to hemorrhage
- **Pseudocyst**
  - 39-42% of all adrenal cysts
  - Heterogeneous group of cysts
  - Most cysts believed to be due to organization of previous hematoma or infarction
  - Rarely associated with adrenal tumor, e.g., adrenal carcinoma, pheochromocytoma, or adenocarcinoma
  - Appearances
    - Unilocular, thin walled, or thick fibrous capsule ± septae
    - Anechoic or hypoechoic ± debris and fluid level
- **Abscess**
  - Pyogenic abscess due to hematological spread or superimposed infection of hematoma
  - Well-circumscribed, irregular, heterogeneously hypoechoic mass
  - Cystic areas develop as abscess liquefies
- **Organizing Hematoma**
  - In subacute to chronic phase of adrenal hematoma
  - Progressive liquefaction forms cystic spaces
  - Sequential reduction in size without treatment is diagnostic
- **Mimics**
  - Pedunculated cystic lesions, e.g., renal cyst, liver cyst, pancreatic pseudocyst
  - Splenic artery aneurysm

Helpful Clues for Less Common Diagnoses
- **Cystic Adenoma**
  - Larger than solid adenomas, typically between 5-20 cm
    - May reflect increased central ischemia with increasing tumor size
  - Almost entirely solid > focal cystic regions > completely cystic
  - Irregular wall ± soft tissue nodules protruding into cystic regions
  - Scattered, irregularly shaped calcifications or rim calcification in 1/3
- **Cystic Neuroblastoma**
  - Pediatric patients, peak age 2 years
  - Cystic area due to necrosis and hemorrhage, 85% calcified

CYSTIC ADRENAL MASS

- Characteristic endocrine abnormality and symptoms
- **Cystic Pheochromocytoma**
  - 16% of all pheochromocytomas
  - Cystic area due to hemorrhage/necrosis, but pure cystic appearance is rare
  - Characteristic symptoms, endocrine abnormalities, and scintigram with metaiodobenzylguanidine (MIBG)
- **Cystic Adrenocortical Carcinoma**
  - Typically large (5-50 cm reported)
  - Adult (40-70 years)
  - Endocrine dysfunction is common
  - Appearance overlap with cystic adenoma
    - Thick irregular wall; heterogeneous with hemorrhage, necrosis, or cystic degeneration
    - Entirely cystic appearance is rare
    - 30% calcified; rim calcification or irregular deposits
    - Metastases and invasion to inferior vena cava, liver, kidney, diaphragm
- **Cystic Adenomatoid Tumor**
  - Rare benign neoplasm usually confined to genital tract
  - Male predominance when adrenal gland involved
  - Small solid or large cystic appearance
  - Imaging features indistinguishable from other nonfunctioning adrenal tumors

Helpful Clues for Rare Diagnoses
- **Cystic Metastases**

- Extremely rare, e.g., from carcinoma of breast; calcification unlikely
- **Epithelial Cysts, True Cyst**
  - 9-10% of adrenal cysts
  - Glandular/retention cyst
  - Embryonal cyst
  - Mesothelial inclusion cyst
- **Hydatid Cyst**
  - Disseminated infection by *Echinococcus granulosus*
  - Asymptomatic or symptoms due to local visceral compression
  - Eosinophilia (25%), 90% sensitivity of serologic tests
  - Depends on stage of evolution of disease; most common classification by Gharbi
    - Type 1: Well defined, anechoic
    - Type 2: Separation of membrane; "water lily" sign due to undulating membrane
    - Type 3: Septa and intraluminal daughter cysts
    - Type 4: Nonspecific solid mass
    - Type 5: Solid mass with calcified capsule
- **Cystic Schwannoma**
  - Extremely rare but well recognized
  - Presents as asymptomatic, nonfunctioning adrenal tumor
  - Discrete cystic area is common, often surrounded by echogenic rim; purely cystic form has been reported

Pseudocyst

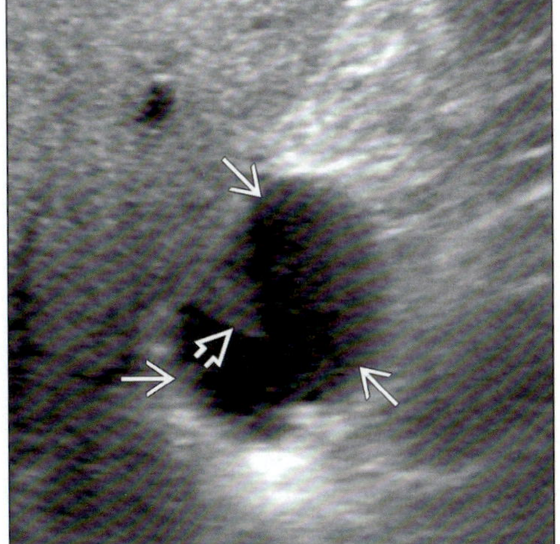

Oblique transabdominal ultrasound shows a thin-walled right adrenal cyst ➡ with a thin septation ➡. Note the anechoic content and posterior acoustic enhancement.

Pseudocyst

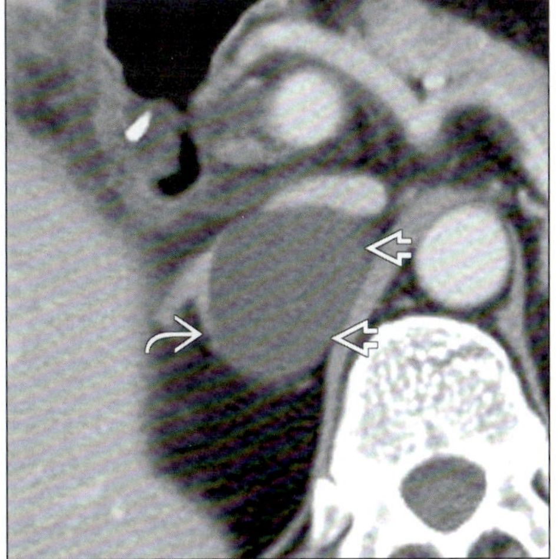

CECT in the same patient shows a cyst ➡ arising from the medial limb of the right adrenal ➡. The homogeneous fluid density and thin wall are consistent with sonographic findings of a simple cyst.

CYSTIC ADRENAL MASS

Pseudocyst

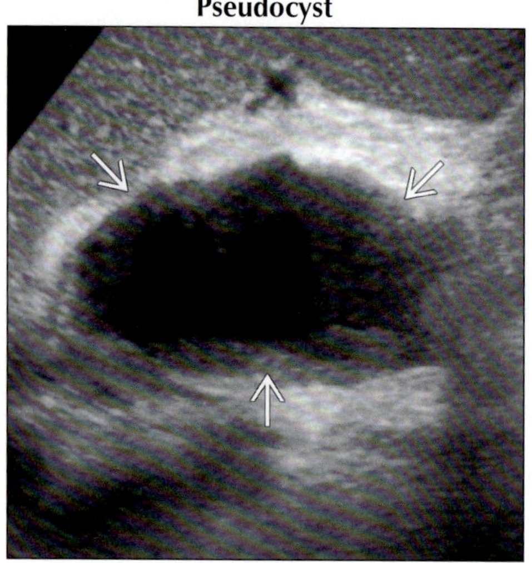

Pseudocyst

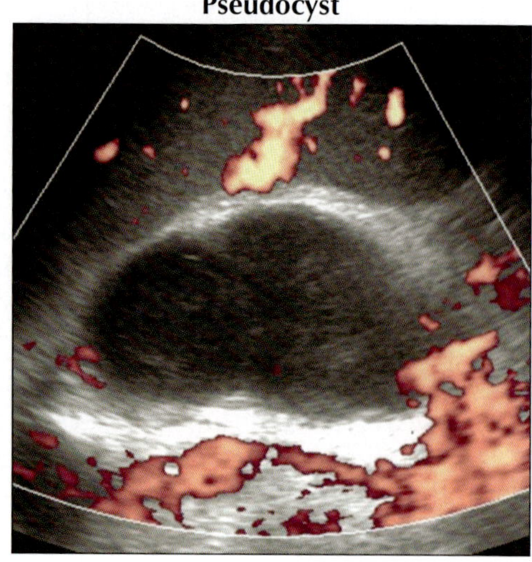

(Left) Longitudinal transabdominal ultrasound shows a left adrenal cyst ➡ with recent hemorrhage. The cyst wall is thickened and irregular. Echogenic foci within the cyst represent debris. *(Right)* Power Doppler ultrasound shows no internal vascularity. Note that the sonographic appearances of complicated cysts are nonspecific and indistinguishable from necrotic tumors or abscesses. The diagnosis of this patient was based on sequential regression on follow-up.

Abscess

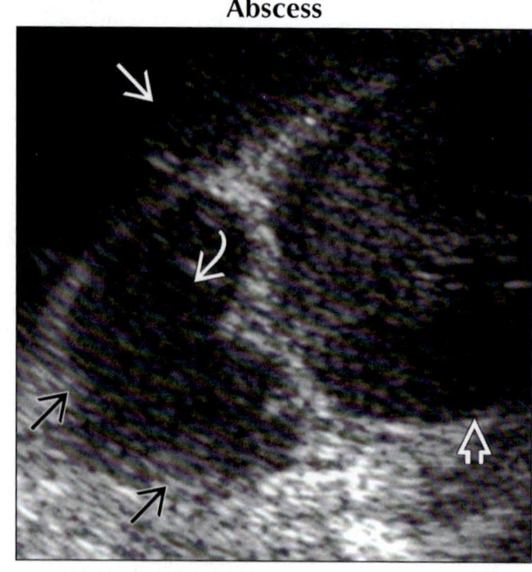

Abscess

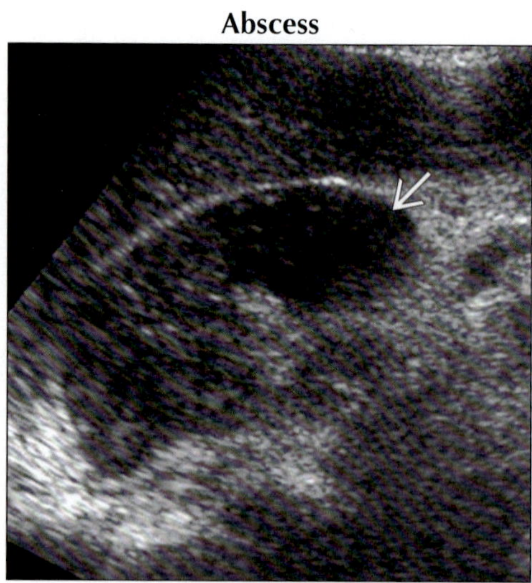

(Left) Longitudinal transabdominal ultrasound shows a right adrenal abscess ➡. It is well defined and lobulated in contour with low-level internal debris ➡. Note the liver ➡ and right kidney ➡. *(Right)* Longitudinal transabdominal ultrasound shows another adrenal abscess ➡ with more liquefied (hypoechoic) content.

Organizing Hematoma

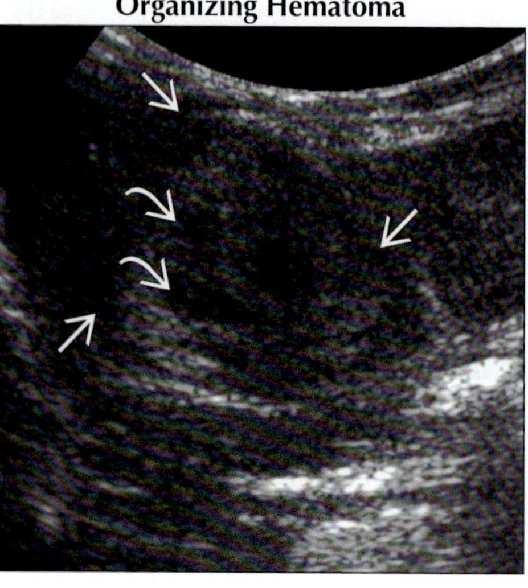

Organizing Hematoma

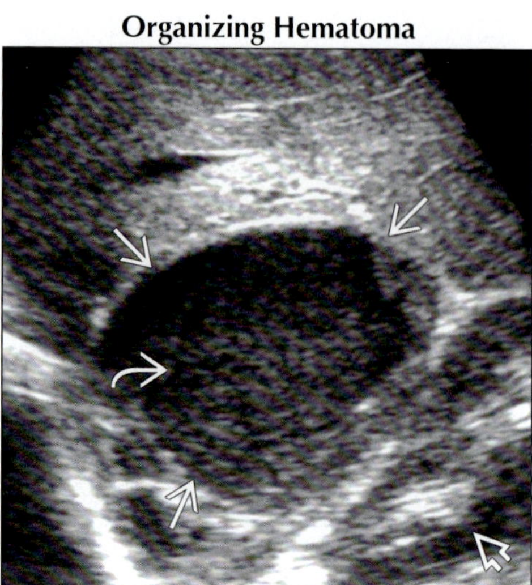

(Left) Oblique transabdominal ultrasound shows adrenal hematoma ➡ with early organization seen as small areas of cystic change ➡. Serial follow-up revealed progressive reduction in size. *(Right)* Longitudinal transabdominal ultrasound shows an organizing adrenal hematoma ➡. The internal content is nearly completely liquefied with dispersed low-level internal echoes, representing debris ➡. Note the right kidney ➡.

CYSTIC ADRENAL MASS

Mimics

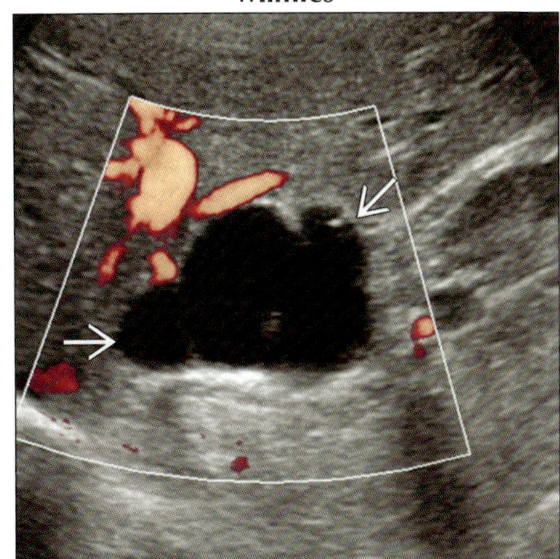

Mimics

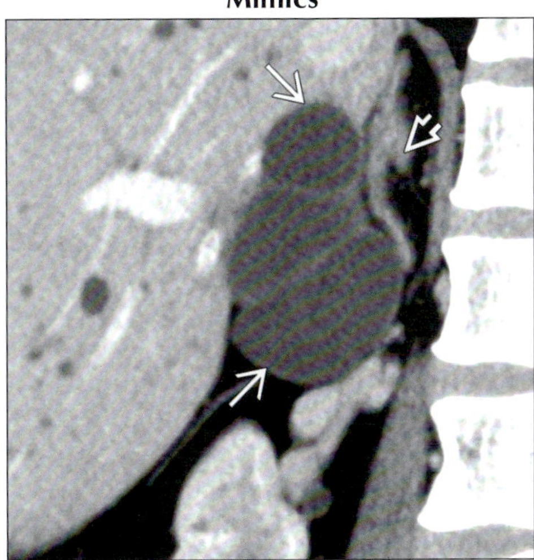

(Left) Longitudinal power Doppler ultrasound shows a multiloculated, thin-walled cyst ➡ in the right adrenal bed, mimicking a cystic adrenal lesion. No internal vascularity is detected on this power Doppler study. (Right) Oblique coronal reformatted CECT shows a tissue plane between the septated cyst ➡ and the right adrenal gland ➡. The cyst abuts the hepatic parenchyma, forming an acute angle, and represents a subcapsular pedunculated liver cyst.

Mimics

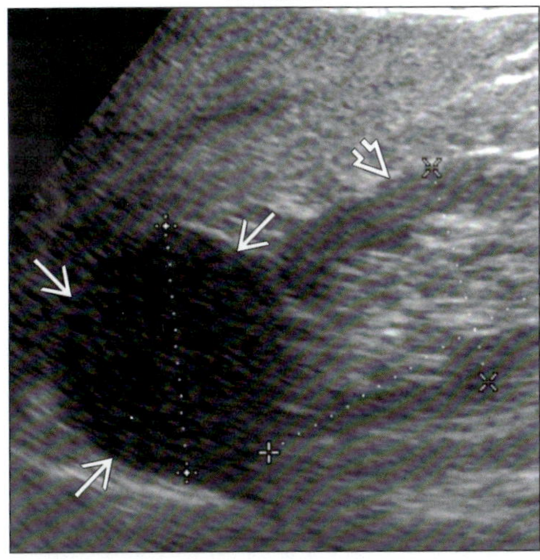

Mimics

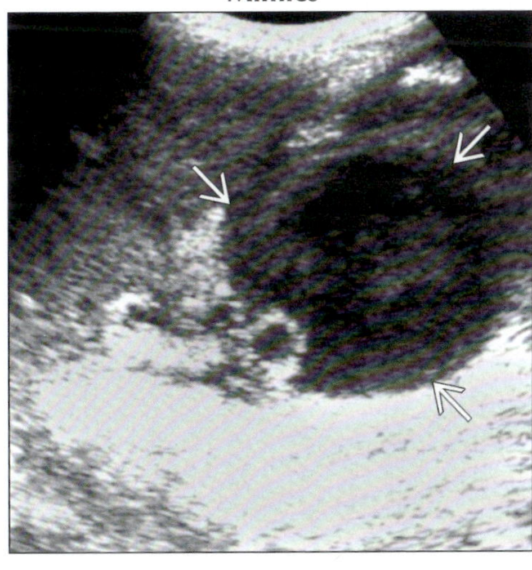

(Left) Longitudinal transabdominal ultrasound of the right kidney ➡ shows a pedunculated renal cyst ➡, which may occasionally mimic an adrenal cyst. (Right) Longitudinal transabdominal ultrasound shows a splenic artery pseudoaneurysm ➡ in the left adrenal bed. It is important to differentiate this mimic from an adrenal cyst so that a biopsy is not needlessly performed. Color Doppler (not shown) revealed internal turbulent flow.

Cystic Neuroblastoma

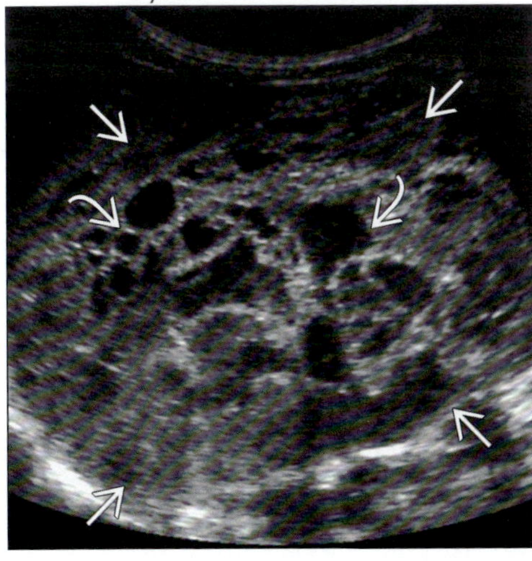

Cystic Pheochromocytoma

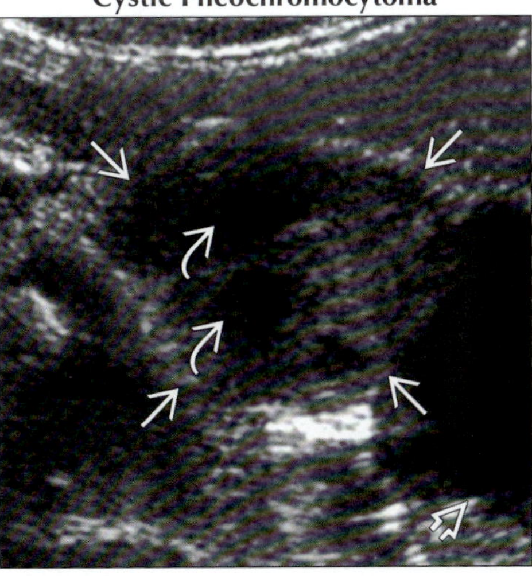

(Left) Oblique transabdominal ultrasound shows a huge neuroblastoma ➡ with a multicystic ➡ appearance. Cystic areas and calcification are common features of a neuroblastoma. (Right) Oblique transabdominal ultrasound shows a left adrenal pheochromocytoma ➡. Discrete cystic areas ➡ are a common feature in pheochromocytomas. Note the adjacent upper pole, renal cortical cyst ➡.

DIFFERENTIAL DIAGNOSIS

Common
- Adenoma
- Metastases
- Pseudotumors (Mimic)

Less Common
- Pheochromocytoma
- Adrenal Hemorrhage

Rare but Important
- Adrenal Cortical Carcinoma
- Lymphoma
- Infection or Inflammation

ESSENTIAL INFORMATION

Key Differential Diagnosis Issues
- Solid adrenal tumors generally lack specific diagnostic features on sonography
- Pheochromocytoma is identified by its characteristic clinical symptoms and endocrine profile
- Known diffuse metastatic disease or lymphoma helps in diagnosis
- Other tumors may require multiple examinations for definitive diagnosis
  - Statistically, smaller tumors (< 3 cm) with lack of growth over 6 months are more likely to be benign
  - NECT: ≤ 10 Hounsfield units (HU) is benign lipid-rich adenoma/cyst
    - Identifies 56% of adenomas
    - > 10 HU is indeterminate
  - CECT: Washout > 60% is lipid-poor adenoma
    - < 60% washout indeterminate
  - Chemical shift MR: Correctly classifies 90% of lesions indeterminate on CT
  - MIBG scintigraphy scan most specific for pheochromocytoma
  - Image-guided biopsy
    - For indeterminate lesions
    - 96-100% accuracy for malignancy
    - Caveat: Risk of precipitating hypertensive crisis in patient with pheochromocytoma

Helpful Clues for Common Diagnoses
- **Adenoma**
  - Prevalence higher with age, diabetes, and hypertension

- Hyperfunctioning (cortisol, aldosterone, androgen, or estrogen) or nonhyperfunctioning
- Appearances
  - Typically well defined, round, homogeneously hypoechoic, ± calcification
  - Central hemorrhage and necrosis may occur when large
  - Typical CT and MR appearances identify majority of benign adenomas
  - Large lesions indistinguishable from malignant adrenal tumor
- **Metastases**
  - Nonspecific imaging appearances
    - Similar to typical adenoma when small
    - Similar to any adrenal tumor with hemorrhage and necrosis when large
  - Widespread metastases in most patients
    - If adrenal is only suspected site of metastatic involvement, differentiation is critical to direct treatment
  - In patients with known primary malignancy, adrenal adenoma is still more common than adrenal metastasis
  - Features of malignant lesion
    - > 3 cm, poorly defined, local invasion, inhomogeneous, thick irregular wall
- **Pseudotumors (Mimic)**
  - Right side: Exophytic liver mass
  - Left side
    - Splenic lesion (accessory spleen, lobulated spleen)
    - Vascular lesion (thrombosed splenic vein or splenic artery aneurysm)
    - Pancreatic lesion (pancreatic tail tumor, pseudocyst)
    - Gastric diverticulum
  - Either side: Exophytic renal mass, retroperitoneal lymph node or masses

Helpful Clues for Less Common Diagnoses
- **Pheochromocytoma**
  - Characteristic clinical symptoms with elevated serum and urine catecholamines
    - Urine metanephrine or vanillylmandelic acid are elevated in > 90% with 24-hour urine collections
  - Multiplicity in 10% of nonfamilial cases and in 65% of those associated with familial syndromes
  - 10% malignant, 10% extraadrenal

HYPOECHOIC ADRENAL MASS

- Sonography
  - Round or irregular, well defined > ill defined
  - Hypoechoic, homogeneous, or heterogeneous
  - Heterogeneity is due to intratumoral hemorrhage/necrosis
  - Discrete cystic areas are often seen
  - Marked hypervascularity on Doppler
- Definitive diagnosis cannot be made on US
  - Urine catecholamine analysis
  - MIBG scan for confirmation/detection of bilateral, extraadrenal, or metastatic involvement
- **Adrenal Hemorrhage**
  - More common in neonates than in older children or adults
  - Majority unilateral, R > L
  - Sonography is particularly useful in neonates and children due to reduced retroperitoneal fat
  - Appearances
    - Round or oval mass centered in adrenal medulla
    - Evolution from acute to chronic stage, from hyperechoic to heterogeneous, hypoechoic, and cystic
    - Serial reduction in size

Helpful Clues for Rare Diagnoses
- **Adrenal Cortical Carcinoma**
  - All age groups, mean age 50 years
  - Functional tumor more common in females, L > R

- Appearances
  - Often nonspecific
  - Typically large, hypoechoic with central cystic area due to necrosis or old hemorrhage
  - May be heterogeneously hyperechoic if recent hemorrhage
  - Calcification in 30%
  - Hepatic or regional lymph node metastases
  - Extension to renal vein or inferior vena cava
  - Small tumors may be well defined and homogeneously hypoechoic; indistinguishable from benign adenomas
- **Lymphoma**
  - NHL (4%) > Hodgkin lymphoma
  - Bilateral in 50%
  - Appearances
    - Diffuse enlargement > nodular pattern
    - Well defined, homogeneously hypoechoic
    - Seldom isolated disease; most commonly retroperitoneal disease is associated
    - No pathognomic pattern; may be confused with granulomatous disease
- **Infection or Inflammation**
  - Pyogenic
    - Unilateral, enlarged hypoechoic adrenal
    - May see abscess formation
  - Granulomatous
    - Typically bilateral and symmetrical
    - Smooth enlargement/nonspecific hypoechoic nodules or masses ± Ca++

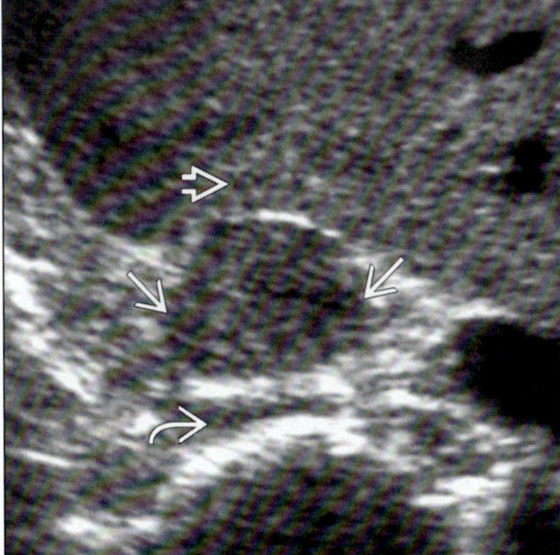

Adenoma

Transverse transabdominal ultrasound shows a nonfunctioning adrenal adenoma. It is well defined and homogeneously hypoechoic ➡. Note the liver ➡ anteriorly and right diaphragmatic crus ➡ posteriorly.

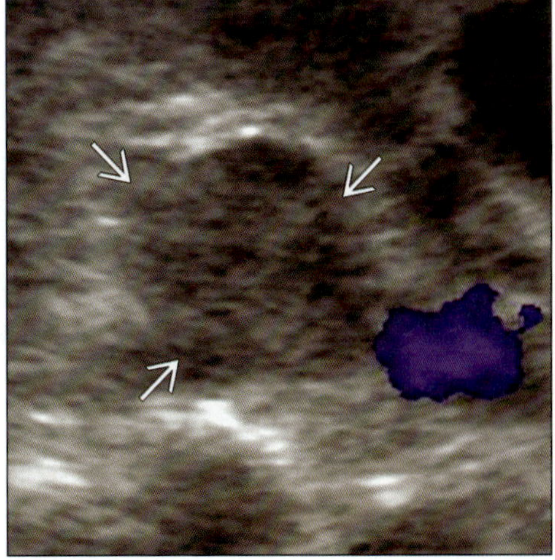

Adenoma

Longitudinal color Doppler ultrasound shows a round, hypoechoic, left adrenal incidentaloma ➡. Note that it is relatively avascular/hypovascular. Most small incidental lesions are nonfunctioning adenomas.

HYPOECHOIC ADRENAL MASS

Metastases

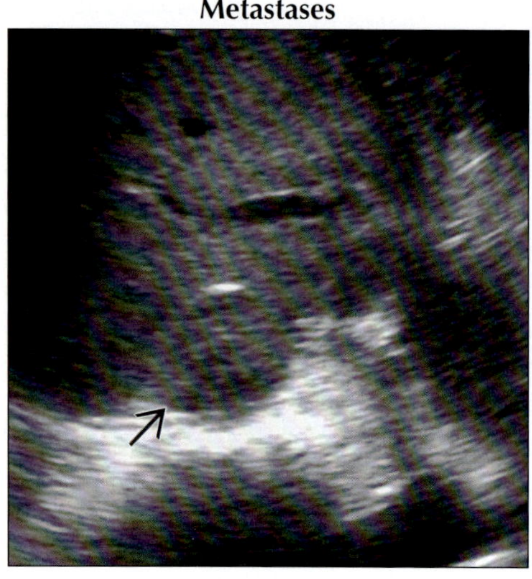

Metastases

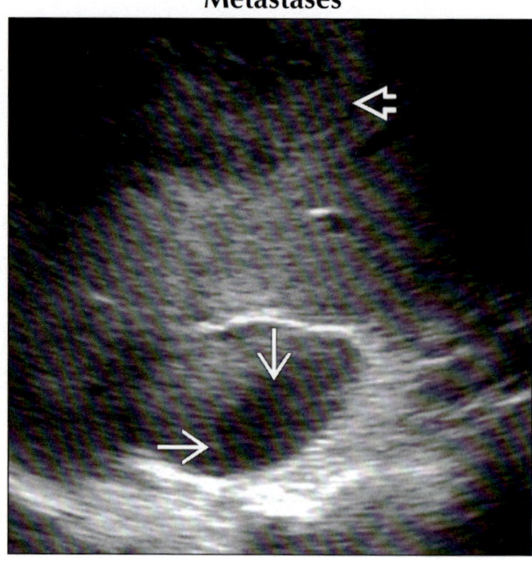

(Left) Transverse US shows a right adrenal metastasis ➡ from a leiomyosarcoma of the IVC. The round, well-defined, homogeneous appearance is indistinguishable from other small adrenal tumors, and a biopsy is required for diagnosis. *(Right)* Longitudinal US shows a right adrenal metastasis with necrosis ➡ from a small cell lung cancer. Necrosis is seldom seen in a small adenoma, making a metastasis more likely. Also note liver metastasis ➡.

Metastases

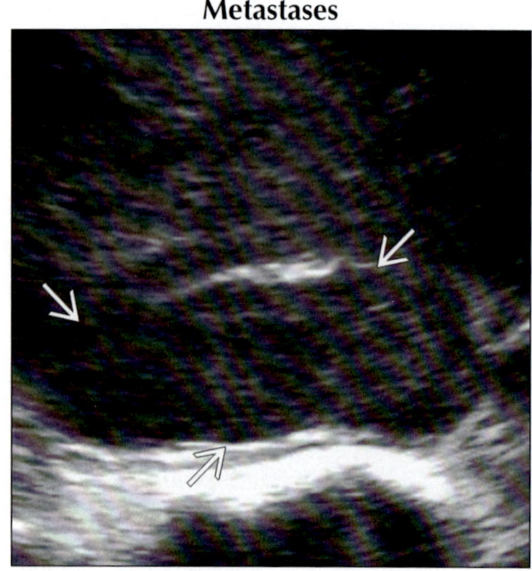

Metastases

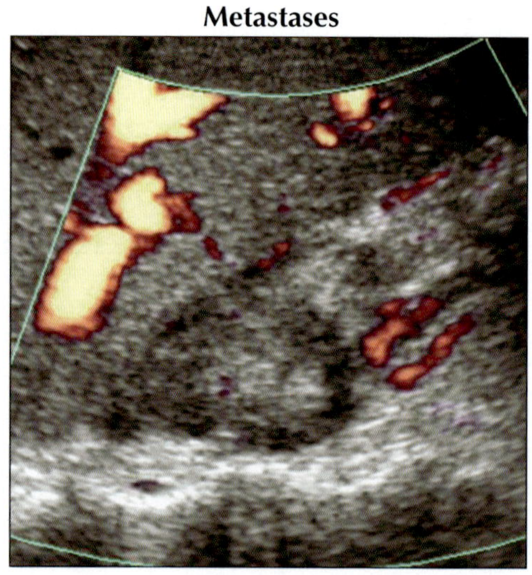

(Left) Transverse transabdominal ultrasound shows a right adrenal metastasis ➡ from small cell carcinoma of the lung. Note its irregular, heterogeneously hypoechoic appearance and large size (5 cm), suggestive of a malignant adrenal tumor. *(Right)* Longitudinal power Doppler ultrasound shows a right adrenal metastasis with an ill-defined border and heterogeneous echogenicity. The intratumoral vascularity is sparse in this case.

Pheochromocytoma

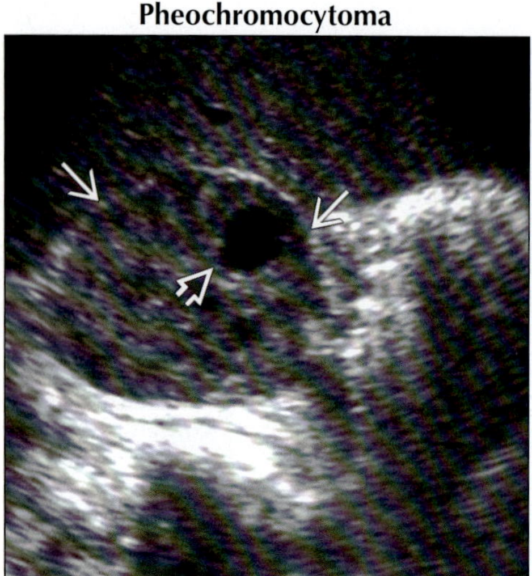

Pheochromocytoma

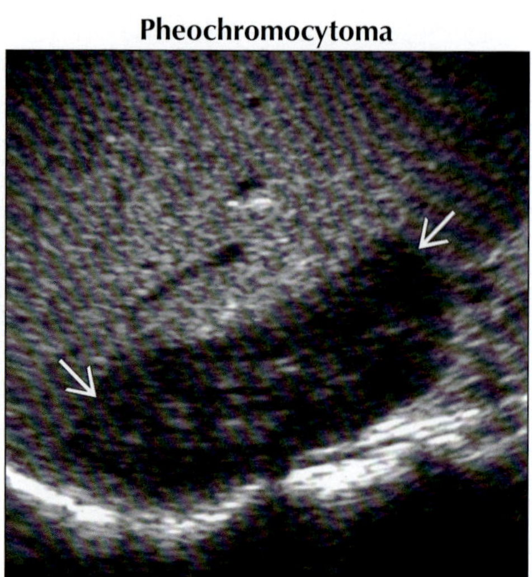

(Left) Transverse transabdominal ultrasound shows a round, hypoechoic, right adrenal pheochromocytoma ➡ in a patient with multiple paragangliomas. Note the internal cystic change ➡. *(Right)* Longitudinal ultrasound of the same pheochromocytoma ➡ reveals that it's appearance is markedly similar to that of a metastasis.

7

HYPOECHOIC ADRENAL MASS

Pheochromocytoma

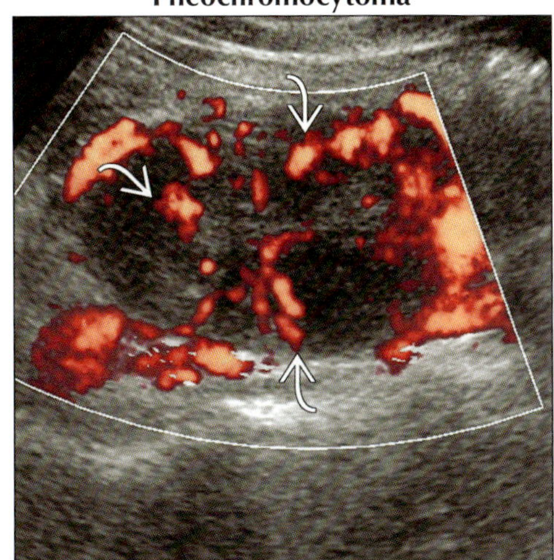

Pheochromocytoma

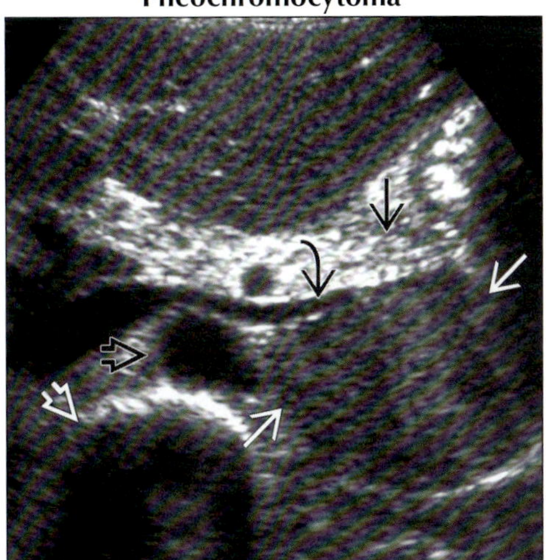

(Left) Longitudinal power Doppler US shows marked intrinsic vascularity ➡ of a pheochromocytoma, as seen in paragangliomas elsewhere in the body. (Right) Transverse ultrasound shows a large left pheochromocytoma ➡ that is well defined and homogeneously hypoechoic. Note the anatomic relation of the left adrenal bed to the adjacent structures. Anteriorly: Splenic vein ➡ and tail of pancreas ➡. Medially: Abdominal aorta ➡ and vertebral body ➡.

Adrenal Hemorrhage

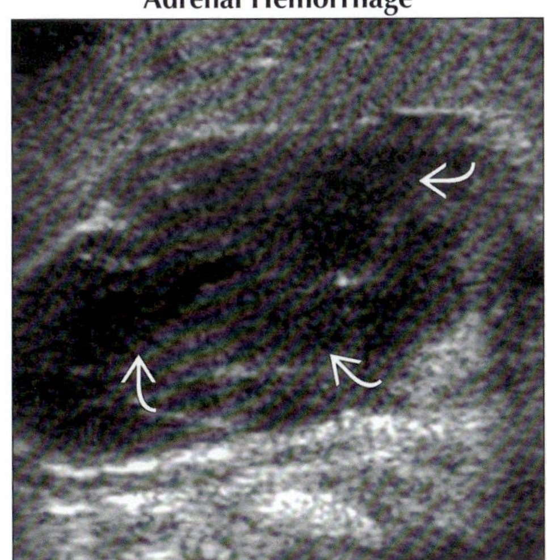

Adrenal Cortical Carcinoma

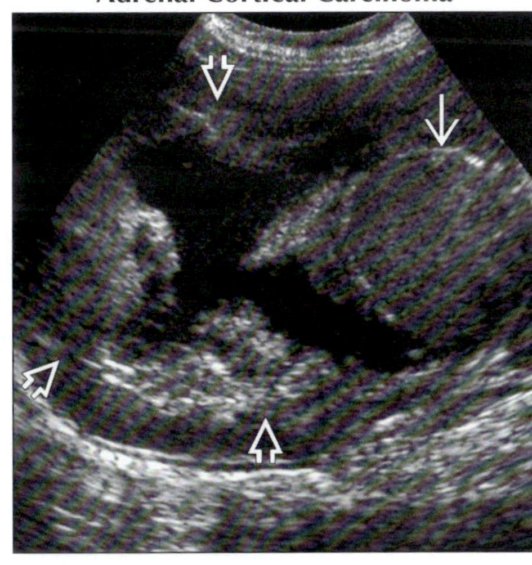

(Left) Longitudinal transabdominal ultrasound shows a hypoechoic subacute hemorrhage with organization and liquefaction seen as cystic change ➡. (Right) Longitudinal transabdominal ultrasound shows a well-defined, homogeneously hypoechoic, right adrenal cortical carcinoma ➡. The sonographic feature that suggests its possible malignant nature is not its size but the presence of an associated large, necrotic, liver metastasis ➡.

Infection or Inflammation

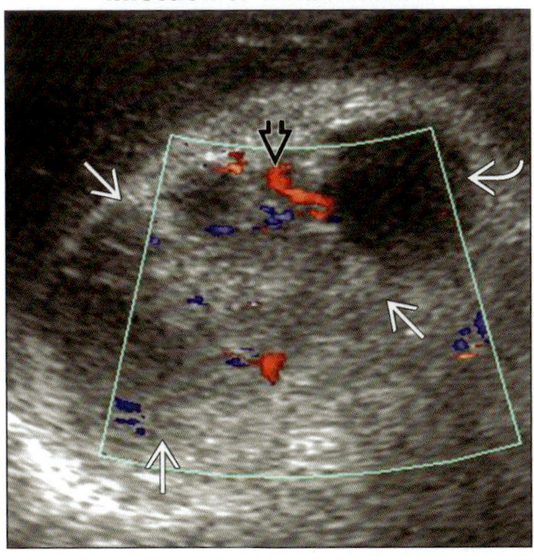

Infection or Inflammation

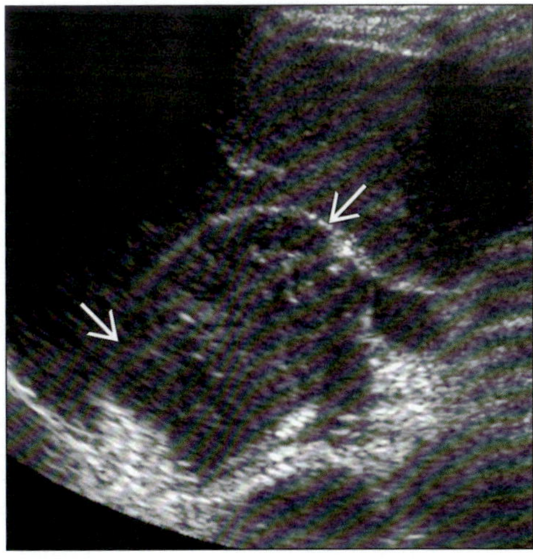

(Left) Longitudinal color Doppler ultrasound shows a right adrenal abscess ➡ with liquefaction ➡ and hypervascularity ➡, representing inflammatory phlegmon. (Right) Transverse transabdominal ultrasound shows adrenal involvement ➡ of disseminated intraperitoneal tuberculosis in a patient infected with HIV. The irregular, heterogeneous appearance overlaps with that of other malignant adrenal tumors and pheochromocytoma.

7

HYPERECHOIC ADRENAL MASS

DIFFERENTIAL DIAGNOSIS

Common
- Adrenal Hemorrhage
- Calcification

Less Common
- Myelolipoma
- Neuroblastoma
- Adrenocortical Carcinoma
- Pheochromocytoma
- Metastases

Rare but Important
- Hemangioma
- Hydatid Disease

ESSENTIAL INFORMATION

Key Differential Diagnosis Issues
- Adrenal hemorrhage and myelolipoma have characteristic ultrasound features
- Other adrenal tumors have significant overlap in appearance
  - Demonstration of local invasion and metastases is important to identify malignancy
  - Further differentiate by patient age group, clinical information, endocrine profile, and MR or scintigraphy in selected cases

Helpful Clues for Common Diagnoses
- **Adrenal Hemorrhage**
  - Most common abnormality of adrenal gland in neonates
    - Unilateral in 80%, majority are right-sided (up to 85%)
    - Most commonly present during 1st week of life
    - Birth trauma or neonatal stress, e.g., asphyxia, hypoxia, septicemia, bleeding diathesis, thrombus extending from renal vein
  - Trauma most common cause in adults
    - Unilateral (80%), R > L
  - Stress: Surgery, sepsis, hypotension, burns, pregnancy, exogenous steroids, and adrenocorticotrophic hormone, etc.
  - Anticoagulant therapy: Typically during 1st 3 weeks of treatment
    - Not due to excessive anticoagulation
    - Prothrombin level is within therapeutic range; no hemorrhage at other sites
    - May be due to stasis or thrombosis of adrenal veins leading to hemorrhage
  - Nontraumatic hemorrhage often bilateral
  - Ultrasound appearance
    - Well-circumscribed, rounded, or oval mass, centered in medulla
    - Hyperechoic when acute; echogenicity changes to heterogeneous, hypoechoic, and cystic with organization of clot
    - Regression on serial imaging without treatment is diagnostic
    - May eventually calcify
    - Traumatic hemorrhage is less well defined and may extend to surrounding peritoneal fat
- **Calcification**
  - Previous hemorrhage
  - Previous infection
    - Tuberculosis, histoplasmosis
  - Calcified neoplasm
    - Neuroblastoma (85%), myelolipoma (20%), pheochromocytoma (10%), adenoma (rare)
  - Addison disease
    - Small adrenal glands difficult to see except when calcified (in 25% of chronic disease patients)
  - Wolman disease
    - Diffuse, punctate calcifications in bilaterally enlarged glands

Helpful Clues for Less Common Diagnoses
- **Myelolipoma**
  - 0.08-0.4% prevalence on autopsy
  - 3% of all primary adrenal tumors
  - Composed of mature fat and myeloid tissue
  - Ultrasound appearance
    - Well-defined, diffusely echogenic mass
    - Variable hypoechoic areas due to myeloid component
    - Internal irregular echogenic/cystic areas may be seen with intratumoral hemorrhage (common) ± calcification
    - Apparent diaphragmatic disruption (propagation speed artifact): Decreased sound velocity through fatty mass (> 4 cm) creates apparent step defect in diaphragm
    - May be confused with retroperitoneal fat when small or retroperitoneal lipoma/liposarcoma when large

- CT to differentiate indeterminate lesion
- **Neuroblastoma**
  - 8-10% of all childhood cancer; 3rd most common malignant tumor in infancy
  - 97% < 10 years, peak age 2 years
  - Ultrasound appearances
    - Well or poorly circumscribed
    - Predominantly hyperechoic ± internal cystic areas due to hemorrhage or necrosis
    - Calcification (85%) with posterior acoustic shadowing
    - May be complex or cystic in infancy
    - Large tumor crosses midline ± vascular encasement and metastases
- **Adrenocortical Carcinoma**
  - Adults, 40-70 years
  - In pediatric age group, 3x more common than adenoma and pheochromocytoma
    - Patients present earlier, smaller tumor size, more hormonal dysfunction
  - Ultrasound appearance
    - Variable: Smaller lesions (< 3-4 cm) are well defined and fairly homogeneous; larger lesions are heterogeneous with cystic areas of necrosis and hemorrhage
    - Up to 30% predominantly echogenic
    - Calcification (20-30%) seen as small echogenic foci or denser clumps with posterior acoustic shadowing
    - Thick, echogenic capsule-like rim, may be seen partially or completely surrounding lesion
- **Pheochromocytoma**
  - 0.1% in autopsy series, 0.4-2% in hypertensive patients
  - Predominantly in adults, 5% in childhood
  - Characteristic clinical symptoms and endocrine dysfunction
  - Ultrasound appearance
    - 23% predominantly hyperechoic with heterogeneity and small hypoechoic areas, representing extensive macroscopic hemorrhage and small necrotic foci
    - May be homogeneously iso-/hypoechoic (small tumors), heterogeneous (large tumors), with large cystic areas
    - Cystic areas represent old hemorrhage or liquefactive necrosis
    - Markedly hypervascular on Doppler
- **Metastases**
  - Adrenal gland common site of metastatic involvement
  - Hypoechoic > echogenic

Helpful Clues for Rare Diagnoses
- **Hemangioma**
  - Benign vascular tumor
  - Rare in adrenal gland
- **Hydatid Disease**
  - Appearances similar to hydatid cyst involving other body regions
  - Initially "solid" looking with variable echogenicity

Adrenal Hemorrhage

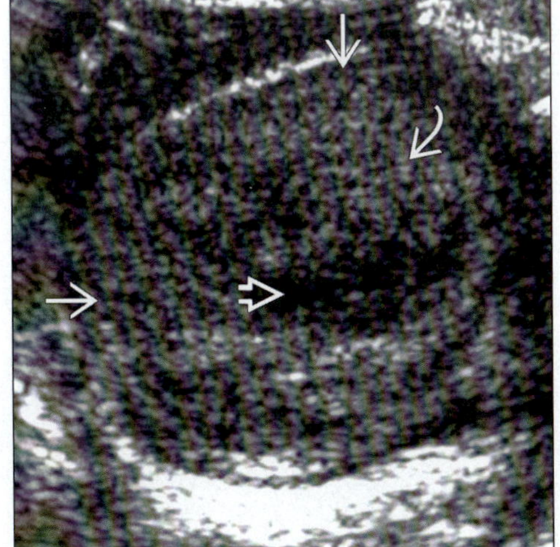

Longitudinal ultrasound shows a large acute adrenal hemorrhage ➡ that consists of both a hyperechoic component ➡ and small cystic areas ➡. Hemorrhage will become more hypoechoic and resolve over time.

Calcification

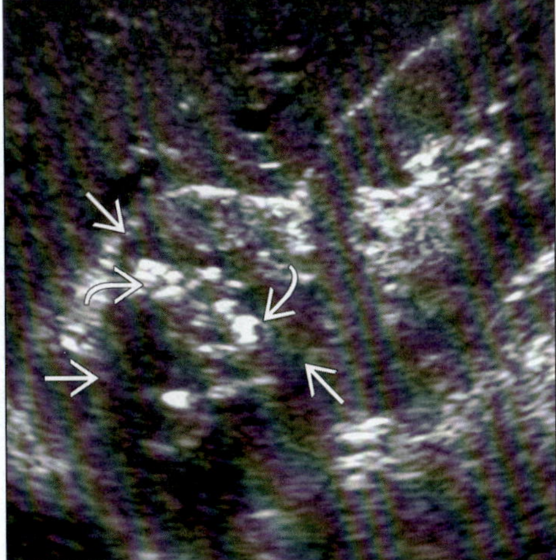

Longitudinal transabdominal ultrasound shows a well-defined adrenal adenoma ➡ with multiple foci of calcifications ➡.

HYPERECHOIC ADRENAL MASS

Myelolipoma

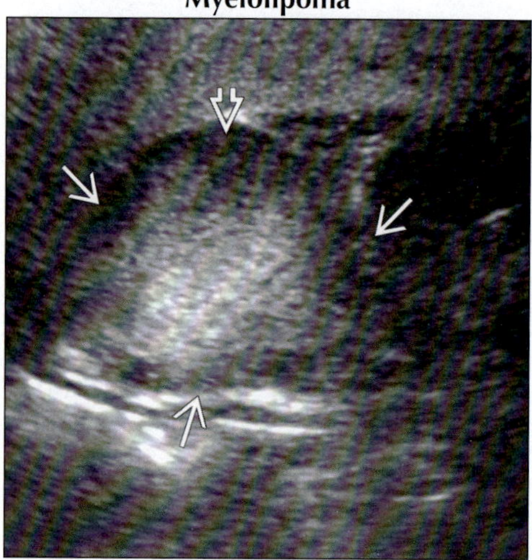

Myelolipoma

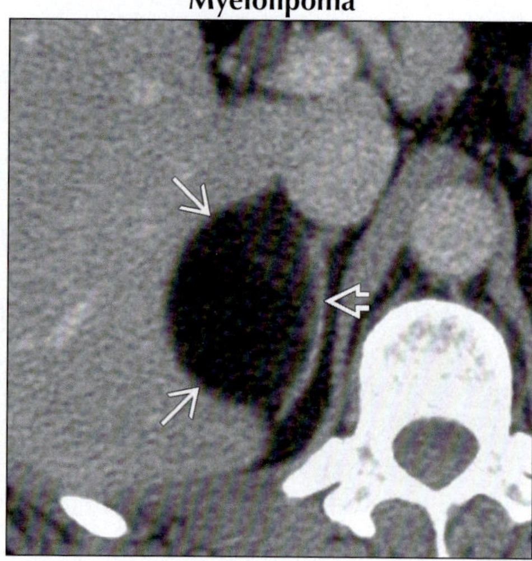

(Left) Longitudinal transabdominal ultrasound shows a predominantly hyperechoic right adrenal myelolipoma ➡ with a myeloid component ⇒ that appears hypoechoic. (Right) Axial CECT of the right adrenal myelolipoma ➡ in the same patient reveals slight enhancement ⇒ in the medial aspect of the periphery. This corresponds to the more hypoechoic, solid-looking area on ultrasound, representing a myeloid component.

Myelolipoma

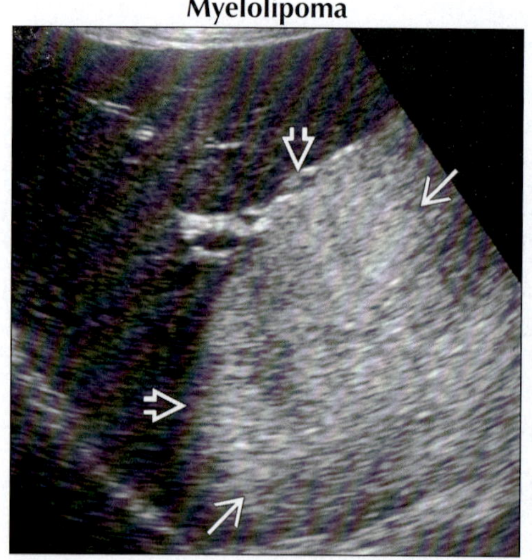

Neuroblastoma

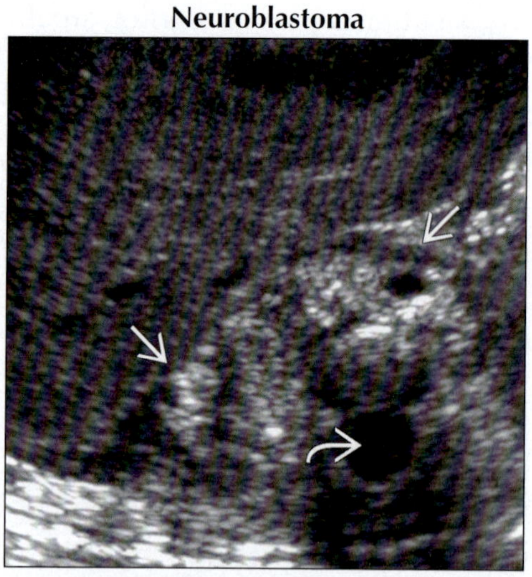

(Left) Longitudinal transabdominal ultrasound shows a large, homogeneously hyperechoic myelolipoma ➡ compressing the liver surface ⇒. (Right) Transverse transabdominal ultrasound shows a neuroblastoma ➡ in a neonate. There are hyperechoic foci throughout the mass with areas of cystic change ➡.

Neuroblastoma

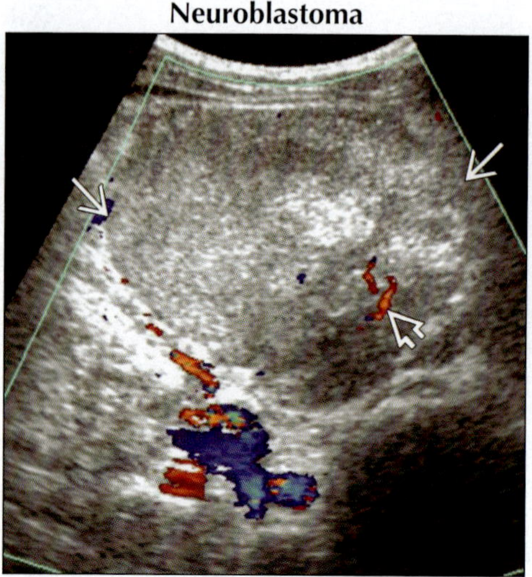

Neuroblastoma

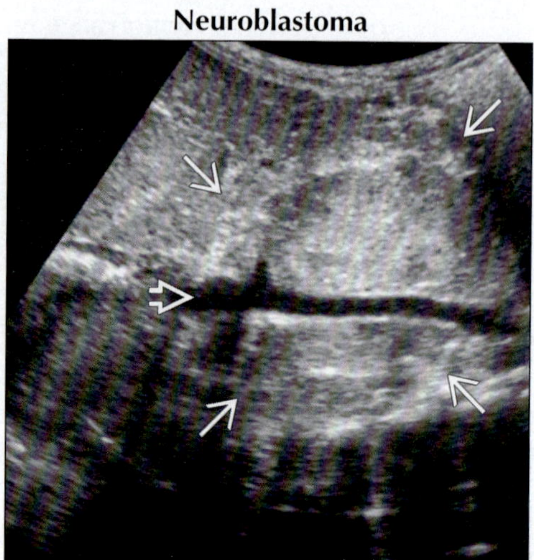

(Left) Longitudinal color Doppler ultrasound shows mild vascularity ⇒ in a large neuroblastoma ➡. (Right) Longitudinal transabdominal ultrasound shows the long axis of the neuroblastoma ➡ encasing and anteriorly displacing the abdominal aorta ⇒.

HYPERECHOIC ADRENAL MASS

Adrenocortical Carcinoma

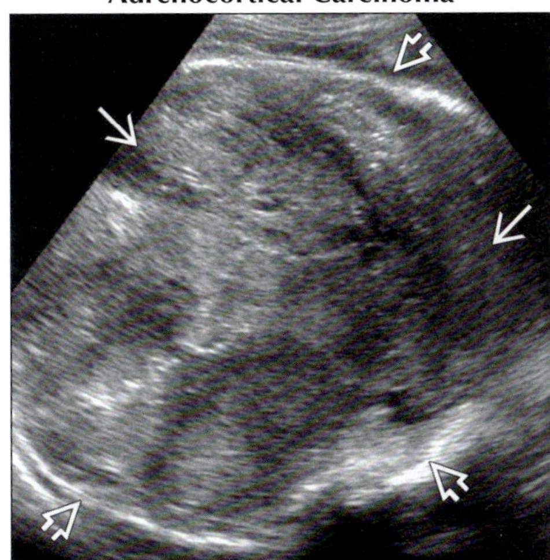

Adrenocortical Carcinoma

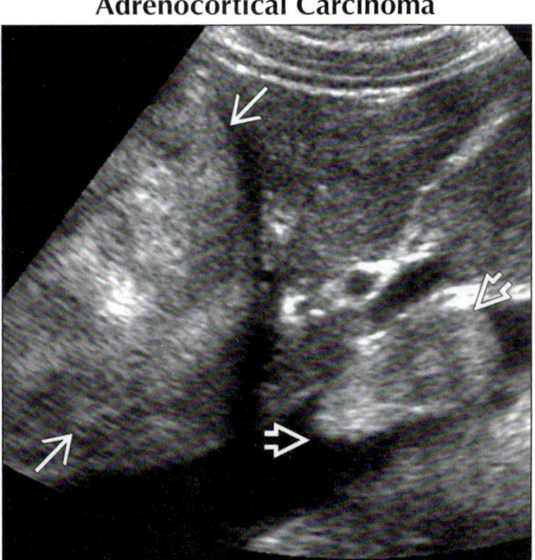

(Left) Transverse transabdominal ultrasound shows a large heterogeneous adrenocortical carcinoma ➡ surrounded by a thick echogenic capsule ➡. (Right) Longitudinal transabdominal ultrasound shows liver metastasis ➡ and inferior vena cava tumor thrombus ➡ from the adrenocortical carcinoma. The size of the tumor and metastatic involvement make a definitive diagnosis possible.

Adrenocortical Carcinoma

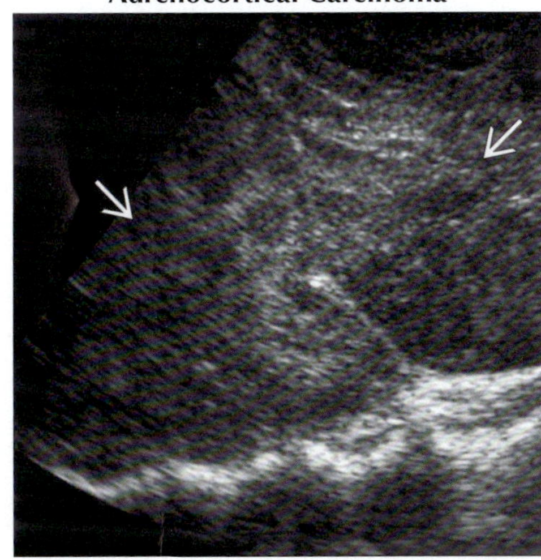

Pheochromocytoma

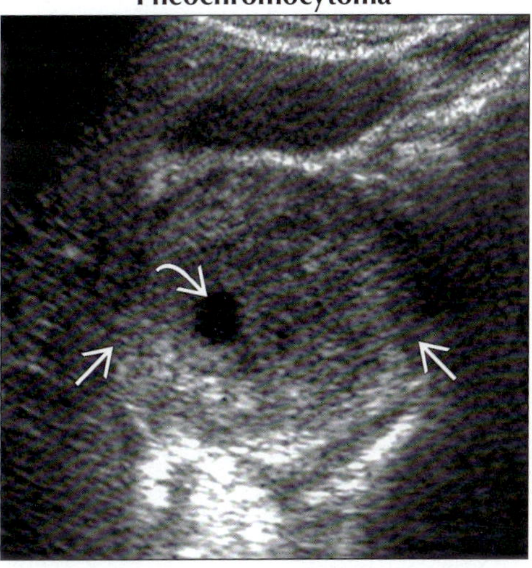

(Left) Longitudinal transabdominal ultrasound shows a large adrenocortical carcinoma ➡ with a heterogeneously hypoechoic echopattern. (Right) Oblique transabdominal ultrasound shows a slightly hyperechoic pheochromocytoma ➡ with a small hypoechoic/cystic area that represents macroscopic hemorrhage or necrosis ➡.

Pheochromocytoma

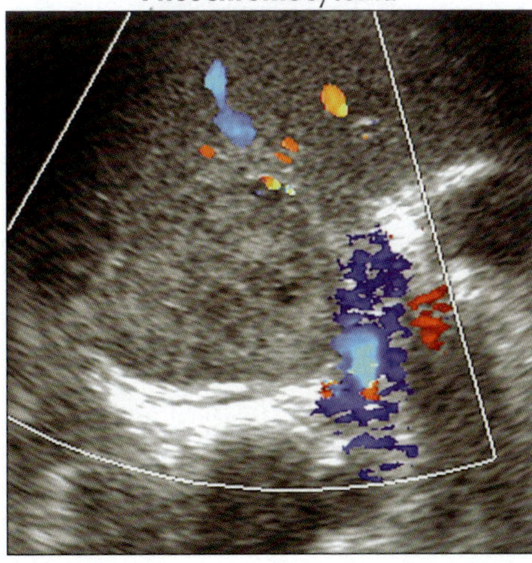

Hydatid Disease

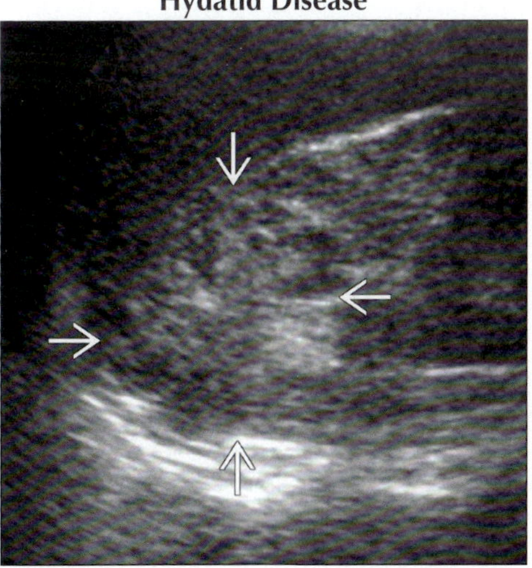

(Left) Transverse color Doppler ultrasound shows another slightly hyperechoic pheochromocytoma with sparse intratumoral vascularity. This is unusual, as most pheochromocytomas are hypervascular on Doppler. (Right) Longitudinal transabdominal ultrasound shows a solid left adrenal mass ➡, which was invasive hydatid disease. Hydatid disease may appear hyperechoic initially before evolving into its typical cystic appearance.

7

SECTION 8
Kidney

DIFFERENTIAL DIAGNOSIS

Common
- Autosomal Dominant Polycystic Kidney Disease (ADPKD)
- Hydronephrosis
- Acute Pyelonephritis
- Acute Glomerulonephritis (GN)
- Lupus Nephritis
- Compensatory Renal Hypertrophy
- Primary Renal Malignancy
- Diabetic Nephropathy
- Duplex Kidney

Less Common
- Multicystic Dysplastic Kidney (MDK)
- Renal Abscess
- Pyonephrosis
- Perinephric Fluid Collections
- Horseshoe Kidneys
- Acute Tubular Necrosis
- Acute Renal Vein Thrombosis

Rare but Important
- Autosomal Recessive Polycystic Kidney Disease (ARPKD)
- Acute Cortical Necrosis
- Exercise-Induced Nonmyoglobinuric Acute Renal Failure
- Leukemia
- Renal Lymphoma
- Xanthogranulomatous Pyelonephritis
- Acute Renal Infarction
- Renal Amyloidosis
- HIV Nephropathy
- Renal Parenchymal Malacoplakia

ESSENTIAL INFORMATION

Key Differential Diagnosis Issues
- Acute causes: Obstruction, infection, inflammation
- Chronic causes: Cellular hypertrophy, abnormal protein deposition, malignancies, infection, glomerular or microvascular proliferation
- Unilateral or bilateral
- Focal or diffuse

Helpful Clues for Common Diagnoses
- **Autosomal Dominant Polycystic Kidney Disease (ADPKD)**
  - Usually presents in adulthood
  - Bilateral large kidneys with innumerable cysts of varying sizes that distort normal renal architecture
- **Hydronephrosis**
  - Splitting of central renal echocomplex
  - Gross hydronephrosis may mimic multicystic dysplastic kidney, ovarian cyst, or ascites
- **Acute Pyelonephritis**
  - Renal size: Normal or enlarged
  - Echogenicity ↑/↓ ± wedge-shaped perfusion defect pointing to papilla
  - Cortical vascularity may ↓ due to cortical vasoconstriction and edema
- **Acute Glomerulonephritis (GN)**
  - Bilaterally enlarged kidneys with ↑ cortical echogenicity
- **Lupus Nephritis**
  - Histologically noted in most SLE patients
  - Acute: Normal or increased size bilaterally; cortical echogenicity variable
- **Compensatory Renal Hypertrophy**
  - Enlarged, otherwise unremarkable kidney
  - Occurs with contralateral renal disease, aplasia/dysplasia, or nephrectomy
- **Primary Renal Malignancy**
  - Renal cell carcinoma: Most common
  - Appears as exophytic echogenic renal mass when large
- **Diabetic Nephropathy**
  - Bilateral enlarged kidneys at early stage
- **Duplex Kidney**
  - Splitting of central, renal echocomplex into upper and lower pole moieties
  - 2 distinct ureters draining duplex kidney may be seen if obstructed distally

Helpful Clues for Less Common Diagnoses
- **Multicystic Dysplastic Kidney (MDK)**
  - Seen as large echogenic renal mass with multiple small cysts
  - Association with contralateral renal disease common
- **Renal Abscess**
  - Common in patients with diabetes mellitus, drug abuse, vesicoureteral reflux, renal calculi
  - Solitary or multiple heterogeneous intrarenal cystic lesions
- **Pyonephrosis**
  - Swollen kidney with debris or dependent echoes in collecting system

- **Perinephric Fluid Collections**
  - May be abscess, blood, urine, and lymph
  - May mimic large renal mass
- **Horseshoe Kidneys**
  - Lower poles joined by isthmus of functioning renal tissue or fibrous band
- **Acute Tubular Necrosis**
  - Normal or diffuse renal swelling
  - Prominent pyramids due to edema
- **Acute Renal Vein Thrombosis**
  - Nonneoplastic causes: Dehydration and fever in children; hypercoagulability and nephrotic syndrome in adults
  - Common in membranous GN
  - Renal enlargement with ↓ echogenicity

Helpful Clues for Rare Diagnoses

- **Autosomal Recessive Polycystic Kidney Disease (ARPKD)**
  - Detected in utero or in infancy
  - Bilaterally enlarged kidneys + ↑ reflectivity
- **Acute Cortical Necrosis**
  - Caused by abruptio placentae, postpartum hemorrhage, shock, sepsis, and toxins
  - Results from microvascular thrombosis with cortical ischemia
  - Enlarged echogenic kidney with hypoechoic subcapsular rim
- **Exercise-Induced Nonmyoglobinuric Acute Renal Failure**
  - Severe flank pain
  - Swollen kidney + ↓ cortical vascularity due to vasoconstriction
- **Leukemia**
  - Gross renal involvement uncommon
  - Lymphocytic > granulocytic
  - Symmetrically enlarged kidneys with distorted central sinus and ↓ corticomedullary differentiation
- **Renal Lymphoma**
  - Focal or diffuse renal enlargement
  - Infiltrative: Diffuse renal enlargement with disruption of internal architecture
  - Reactive: Bilaterally enlarged kidneys, otherwise unremarkable
- **Xanthogranulomatous Pyelonephritis**
  - 80% due to obstruction by stone, usually staghorn
  - Diffuse renal enlargement with calculi and thick debris in dilated calyces
  - Extensive perirenal inflammation with thickened renal fascia
  - Mimics renal tumor
- **Acute Renal Infarction**
  - Unilateral flank pain
  - Normal or enlarged kidney with wedge-shaped defect on color Doppler
- **Renal Amyloidosis**
  - Abnormal protein deposition in kidneys
  - Renal enlargement with ↓ echogenicity
- **HIV Nephropathy**
  - Normal or enlarged kidneys
  - About 50% with ↑ echogenicity
- **Renal Parenchymal Malacoplakia**
  - Focal (25%): Sharply demarcated renal mass ranging from 2-8 cm in size
  - Multifocal (75%): 1/2 are bilateral
  - Enlarged kidney + multiple small masses

Autosomal Dominant Polycystic Kidney Disease (ADPKD)

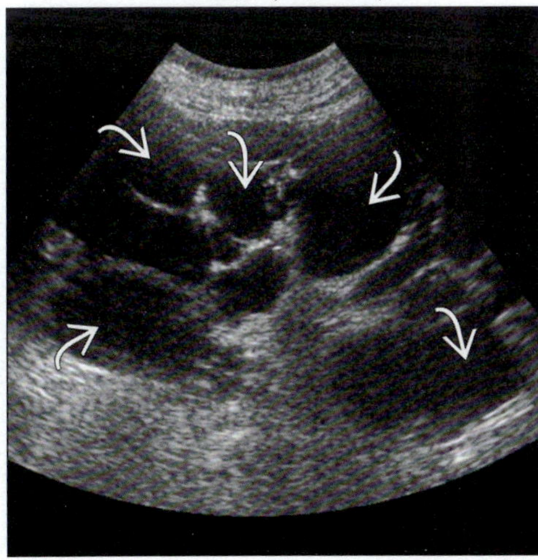

Longitudinal transabdominal ultrasound shows ADPKD. The kidney is grossly enlarged with numerous cysts ➔ of varying sizes. Classically, no normal renal parenchyma can be identified.

Hydronephrosis

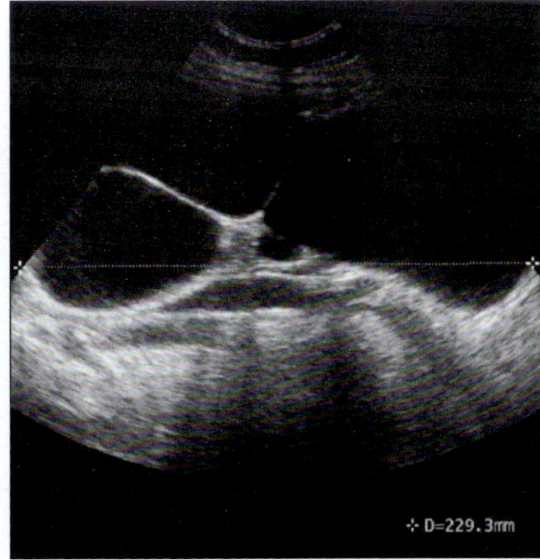

Longitudinal transabdominal ultrasound shows gross hydronephrosis with a "paper-thin" cortex mimicking MDK, ovarian cyst, or ascites. Communication between the cystic spaces is a clue to the diagnosis.

ENLARGED KIDNEY

(Left) Longitudinal transabdominal ultrasound shows acute pyelonephritis. The kidney is swollen and hypoechoic with decreased corticomedullary differentiation. (Right) Longitudinal transabdominal ultrasound shows membranous glomerulonephritis with renal enlargement but nonspecific parenchymal echogenicity.

Acute Pyelonephritis

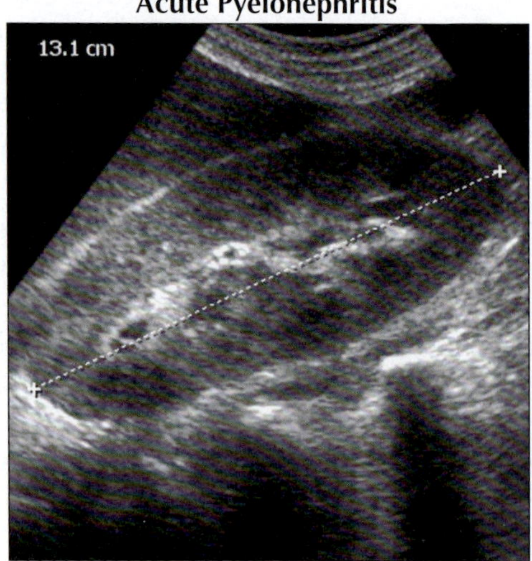

Acute Glomerulonephritis (GN)

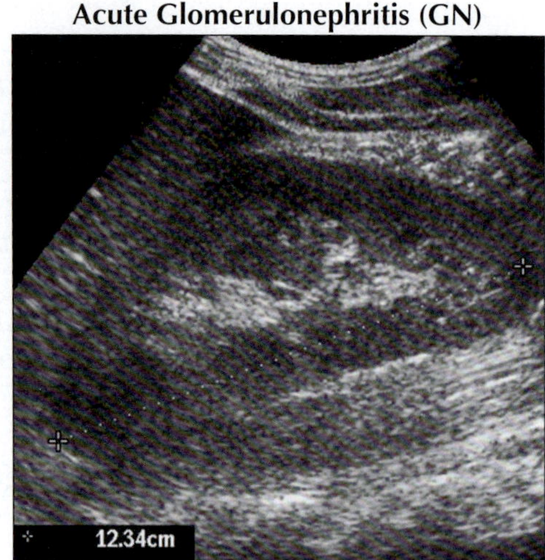

(Left) Longitudinal transabdominal ultrasound shows an enlarged but otherwise unremarkable kidney with histologically proven lupus nephritis. (Right) Longitudinal transabdominal ultrasound shows asymmetrical kidneys in a patient with a known history of TB kidney. The right kidney shows compensatory hypertrophy (upper) with a shrunken contralateral kidney (lower).

Lupus Nephritis

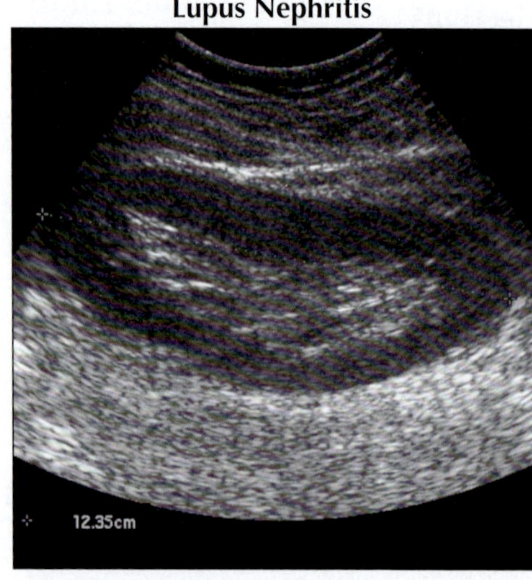

Compensatory Renal Hypertrophy

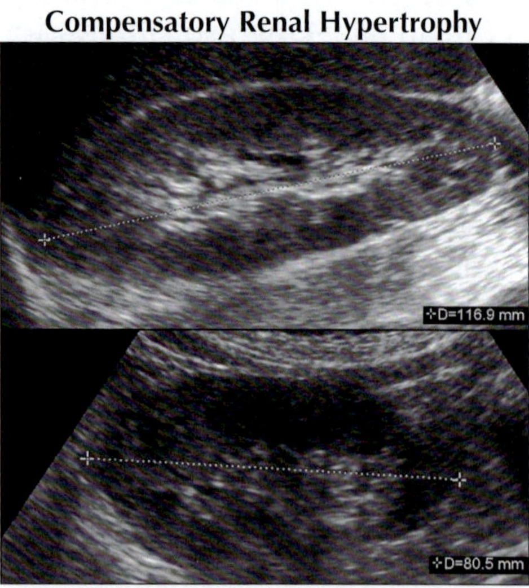

(Left) Longitudinal transabdominal ultrasound shows an enlarged kidney ➡ with its lower pole occupied by a large renal cell carcinoma ➡ with central necrosis. (Right) Longitudinal transabdominal ultrasound shows a nonobstructive duplex kidney with splitting of central sinus echoes by a hypoechoic band of tissue ➡. The duplex kidney is a normal variant that tends to be larger than a normal kidney with a single collecting system.

Primary Renal Malignancy

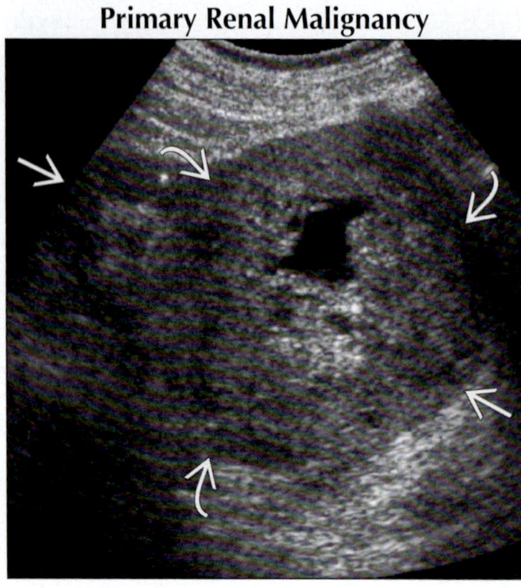

Duplex Kidney

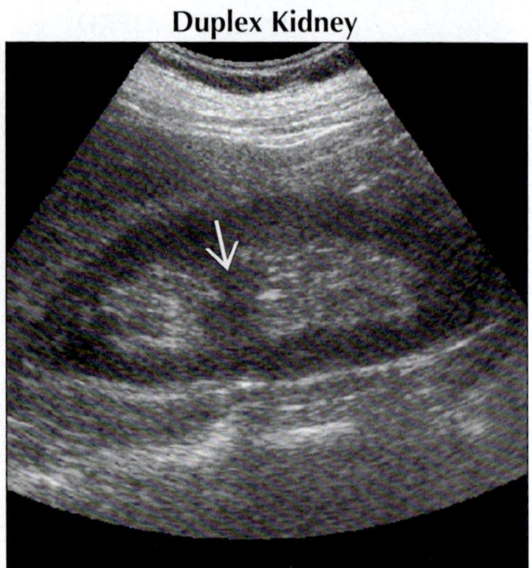

Pyonephrosis

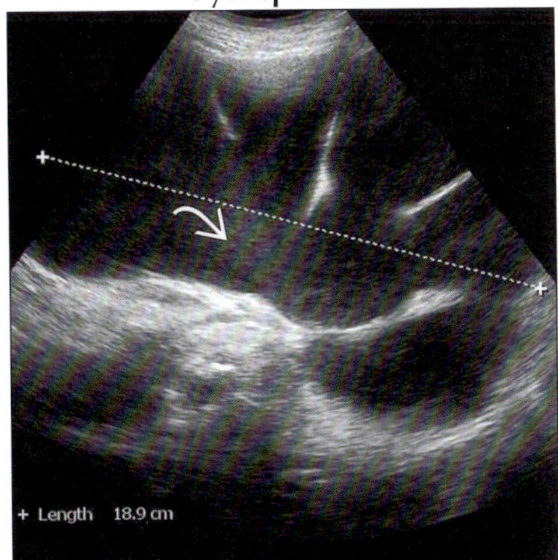

Perinephric Fluid Collections

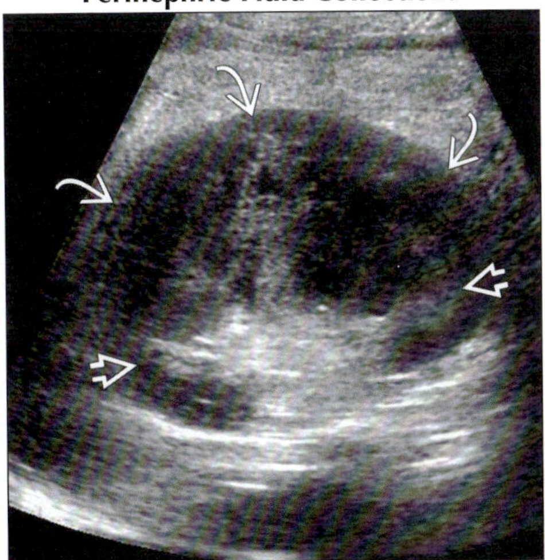

(Left) Longitudinal transabdominal ultrasound shows a grossly enlarged kidney with pyonephrosis. Purulent material ➔ is demonstrated in the dilated collecting system. *(Right)* Longitudinal transabdominal ultrasound shows a large perinephric hematoma ➔ encapsulating a normal-sized kidney ➔ due to renal biopsy. The appearance may mimic a swollen kidney.

Horseshoe Kidneys

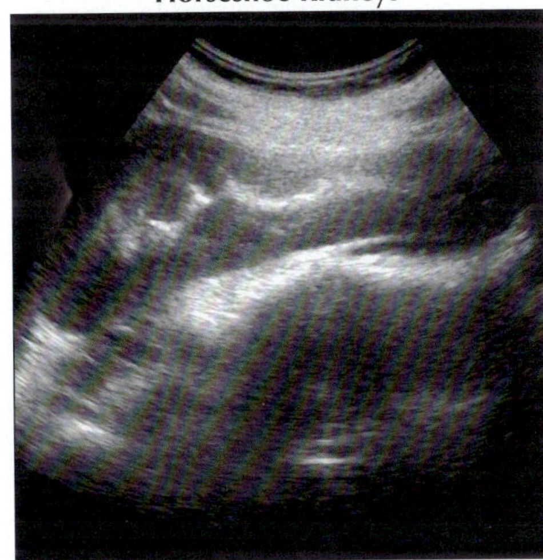

Horseshoe Kidneys

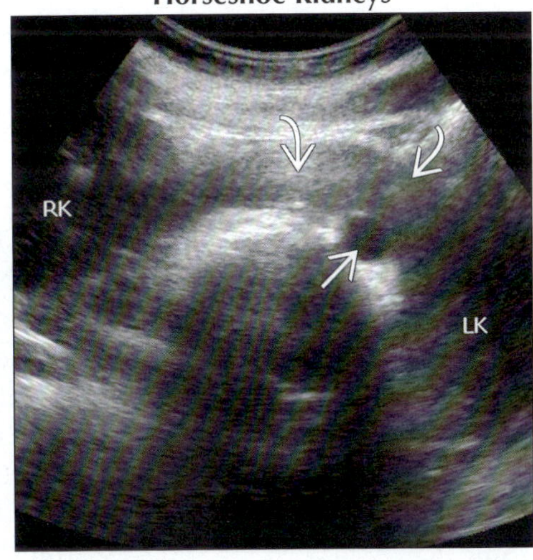

(Left) Longitudinal transabdominal ultrasound shows 1 limb of the horseshoe kidney, appearing as an exceptionally elongated kidney. *(Right)* Transverse transabdominal ultrasound shows the same horseshoe kidney. An isthmus of renal tissue ➔ is seen joining the 2 kidneys and bridging over the aorta ➔ anteriorly.

Acute Tubular Necrosis

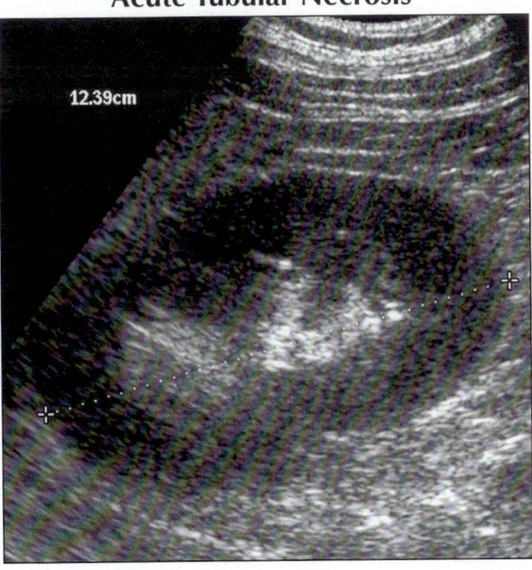

Xanthogranulomatous Pyelonephritis

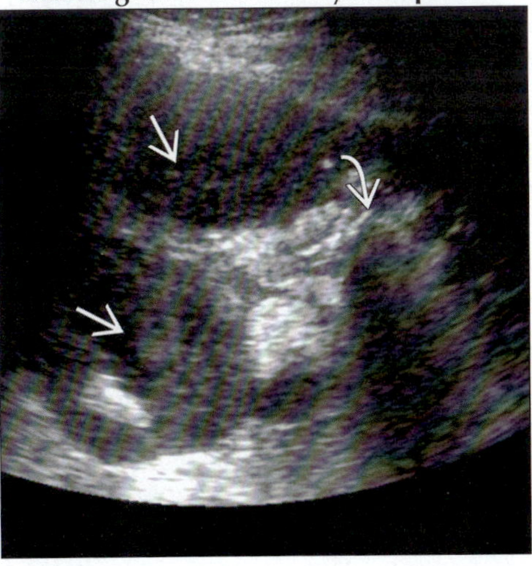

(Left) Longitudinal transabdominal ultrasound shows drug-induced acute interstitial nephritis with histological evidence of acute tubular necrosis. The affected kidney is swollen with an increase in both renal length and cortical thickness. *(Right)* Longitudinal transabdominal ultrasound shows xanthogranulomatous pyelonephritis. The kidney is grossly enlarged, simulating a renal mass with a central calculus ➔ and abscesses ➔ in the parenchyma.

DIFFERENTIAL DIAGNOSIS

Common
- Chronic Diabetic Nephropathy
- Chronic Glomerulonephritis (GN)
- Chronic Hypertensive (HT) Nephropathy
- Chronic Lupus Nephritis
- Chronic Reflux Nephropathy
- Chronic Pyelonephritis
- Postobstructive Atrophy

Less Common
- Partial Nephrectomy
- Renal Cystic Dysplasia
- Multicystic Dysplastic Kidney
- Chronic Renal Artery Stenosis (RAS)
- Chronic Renal Infarction
- Chronic Radiation Nephropathy
- Chronic Nephritis (Alport Syndrome)
- Chronic Renal Allograft Rejection

Rare but Important
- Tuberculous Autonephrectomy
- Post-Traumatic Renal Atrophy
- Renal Hypoplasia
- Supernumerary Kidney
- Chronic Lead Poisoning

ESSENTIAL INFORMATION

Key Differential Diagnosis Issues
- Causes of loss of renal substance
  - Hypoplasia, necrosis, atrophy, fibrosis, ischemia, surgical intervention
- Ultrasound findings are nonspecific and renal echogenicity variable
- Etiology of small kidneys usually depends on discerning clinical history

Helpful Clues for Common Diagnoses
- **Chronic Diabetic Nephropathy**
  - Small kidneys + ↑ cortical echogenicity
  - Corticomedullary differentiation (CMD) usually preserved, unless patient is in overt renal failure
- **Chronic Glomerulonephritis (GN)**
  - Small kidneys + smooth renal outline
  - Parenchyma remains echogenic
- **Chronic Hypertensive (HT) Nephropathy**
  - Due to progressive nephrosclerosis
  - Small kidneys + irregular cortical thinning
  - ↓ cortical vascularity due to arteriolar fibrosis and hyaline degeneration

- **Chronic Lupus Nephritis**
  - Small kidneys
  - Variable renal echogenicity and CMD
- **Chronic Reflux Nephropathy**
  - Unilateral or bilateral
  - May cause focal/diffuse renal scarring and atrophy
  - Small kidneys + irregular renal outline
- **Chronic Pyelonephritis**
  - Risk factors: Calculi, urinary tract obstruction, neurogenic bladder, and urinary diversion
  - Cortical scars are common in upper pole
  - Focal areas of compensatory hypertrophy seen adjacent to cortical scars
  - Small kidney + parenchymal scarring + focal cortical thinning + irregular outline
- **Postobstructive Atrophy**
  - Caused by longstanding uretropelvic junction (UPJ), ureteric, or bladder outlet obstruction
  - Results in progressive decrease in renal blood flow & glomerular filtration
  - Small kidney + cortical thinning + pyelocaliectasis

Helpful Clues for Less Common Diagnoses
- **Partial Nephrectomy**
  - Small residual kidney
  - Compensatory hypertrophy of contralateral kidney may be evident
- **Renal Cystic Dysplasia**
  - May be bilateral
  - Associated with posterior urethral valve, renal duplication, crossed-fused ectopia, horseshoe-shaped and pelvic kidney
  - Unilateral small kidney + ↑ echogenicity + small cortical cysts
- **Multicystic Dysplastic Kidney**
  - Unilateral enlarged kidney replaced by cysts of varying sizes
  - Usually undergoes partial or complete involution over 1st 2 years of life
  - May appear as small echogenic kidney in childhood
  - Contralateral diseases common such as vesicoureteric reflux, UPJ obstruction, and ureteric stenosis
- **Chronic Renal Artery Stenosis (RAS)**
  - Mostly atherosclerosis affects main, interlobar, or interlobular renal arteries or arterioles

SMALL KIDNEY

- ○ Progressive generalized reduction in kidney size caused by ischemia
- ○ Produces renal atrophy or collateralization
- **Chronic Renal Infarction**
  - ○ Renal atrophy after acute renal infarction caused by embolism or thrombosis
  - ○ Atrophy may be focal (segmental) or global
  - ○ Parenchymal loss depends on distribution of occluded artery
  - ○ Infarcted area may be contracted, producing renal scar
- **Chronic Radiation Nephropathy**
  - ○ Occurs after renal irradiation for bone marrow transplantation
  - ○ Begins months to years after irradiation
  - ○ Areas of diminished perfusion may be seen
  - ○ Small kidneys + ↑ renal echogenicity
- **Chronic Nephritis (Alport Syndrome)**
  - ○ Chronic hereditary nephritis
  - ○ Small kidneys + smooth renal outline
  - ○ ↑ cortical echogenicity due to cortical nephrocalcinosis
- **Chronic Renal Allograft Rejection**
  - ○ Irreversible cause of renal allograft dysfunction
  - ○ Small transplant kidney + cortical thinning + ↑ cortical echogenicity

Helpful Clues for Rare Diagnoses
- **Tuberculous Autonephrectomy**
  - ○ Caused by calcified caseous pyonephrosis with UPJ fibrosis
  - ○ Shrunken kidney + extensive calcification
- **Post-Traumatic Renal Atrophy**
  - ○ Caused by segmental renal infarction due to renal artery thrombosis after blunt renal trauma
  - ○ Contracted kidney + irregular outline
  - ○ Collateralization may be demonstrated
- **Renal Hypoplasia**
  - ○ At least 50% smaller than normal
  - ○ Has fewer calyces and papillae
  - ○ Renal function normal for its size
  - ○ Usually unilateral
    - ▪ Unipapillary kidney: Rare; usually associated with ipsilateral hypoplasia or contralateral kidney disease
    - ▪ Ask-Upmark kidney with few calyces and papillae: Segmental; usually affecting upper pole
    - ▪ Constitutional small kidney
  - ○ Differentiation from obstruction, chronic pyelonephritis, and ischemia difficult
- **Supernumerary Kidney**
  - ○ Extremely rare
  - ○ Hypoplastic
  - ○ Most are caudally placed
  - ○ Connected to dominant kidney either completely or by loose areolar connective tissue
- **Chronic Lead Poisoning**
  - ○ Bilateral small kidneys
  - ○ Indistinguishable sonographically from other causes of renal atrophy
  - ○ Blood test for lead concentration useful for diagnosis

Chronic Diabetic Nephropathy

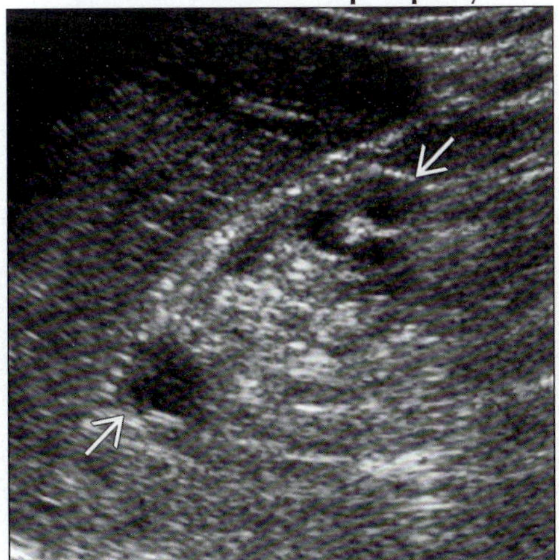

Longitudinal transabdominal ultrasound shows chronic diabetic nephropathy. The kidney ➡ is small with increased cortical echogenicity and preserved corticomedullary differentiation.

Chronic Hypertensive (HT) Nephropathy

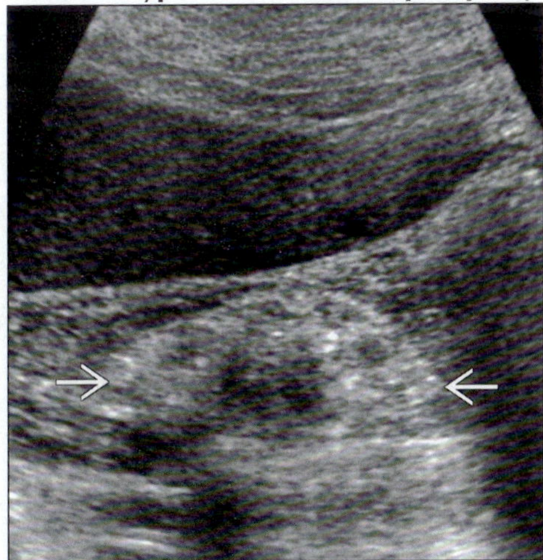

Longitudinal transabdominal ultrasound shows a small echogenic kidney ➡ due to chronic hypertensive nephropathy. The appearance is a nonspecific finding for chronic renal parenchymal disease.

SMALL KIDNEY

(Left) Longitudinal transabdominal ultrasound shows chronic GN (Immunoglobin A, IgA) with severe cortical thinning ➡. GN (IgA) is the most common type of GN that leads to chronic renal failure. *(Right)* Longitudinal transabdominal ultrasound shows chronic mesangiocapillary GN. The small kidney ➡ shows severe cortical thinning, loss of corticomedullary differentiation, and a renal cyst ➡.

Chronic Glomerulonephritis (GN)

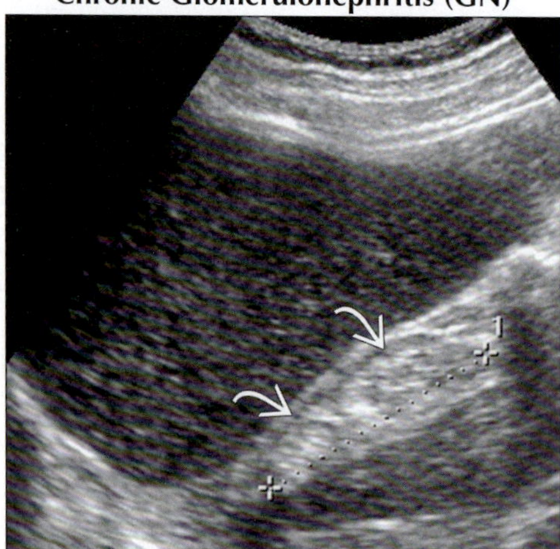

Chronic Glomerulonephritis (GN)

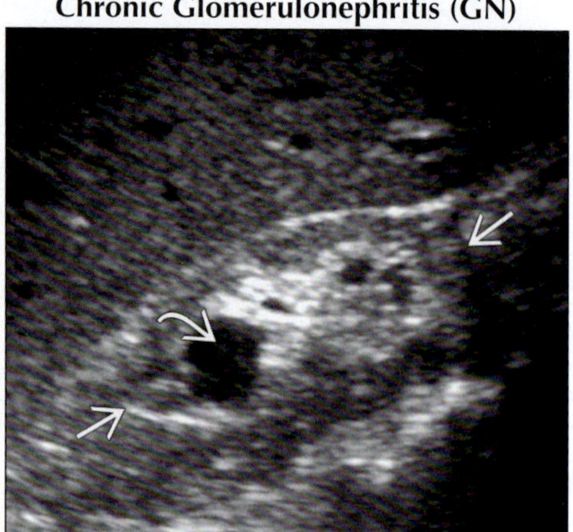

(Left) Longitudinal transabdominal ultrasound shows chronic lupus nephritis. The shrunken kidney ➡ is echogenic with absent corticomedullary differentiation. *(Right)* Longitudinal transabdominal ultrasound shows chronic reflux nephropathy. The kidney shows focal cortical thinning ➡ in the mid-pole with moderate hydronephrosis. Over time, the kidney may develop multiple scars and a gradual reduction in overall size.

Chronic Lupus Nephritis

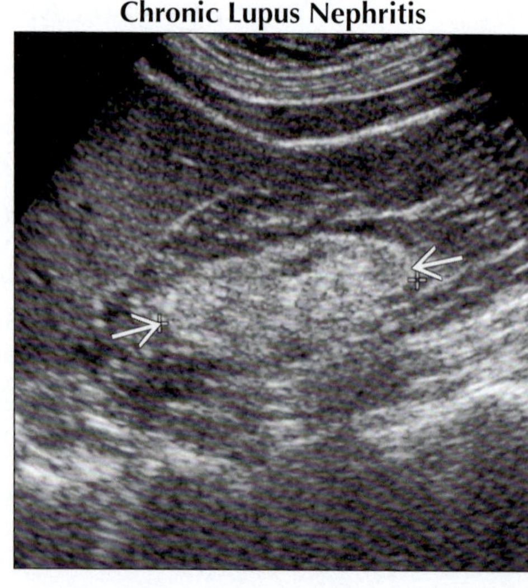

Chronic Reflux Nephropathy

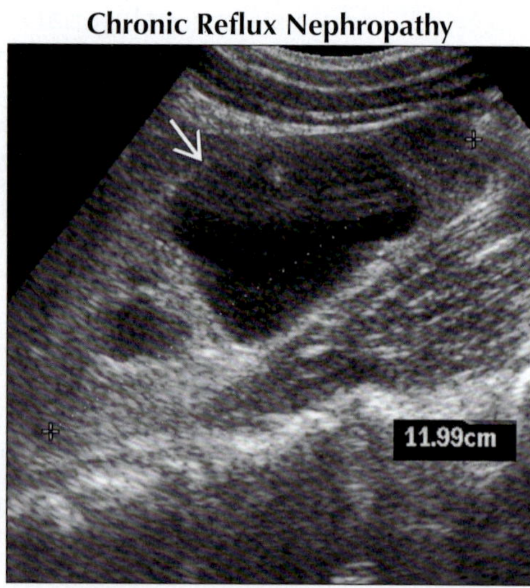

(Left) Longitudinal transabdominal ultrasound shows a small hydronephrotic kidney due to postobstructive atrophy. Note there is significant loss of renal parenchyma ➡. *(Right)* Longitudinal transabdominal ultrasound shows an atrophic duplex kidney due to chronic obstruction by a rectal tumor. Double dilated ureters ➡ are seen exiting the hydronephrotic duplex collecting systems ➡.

Postobstructive Atrophy

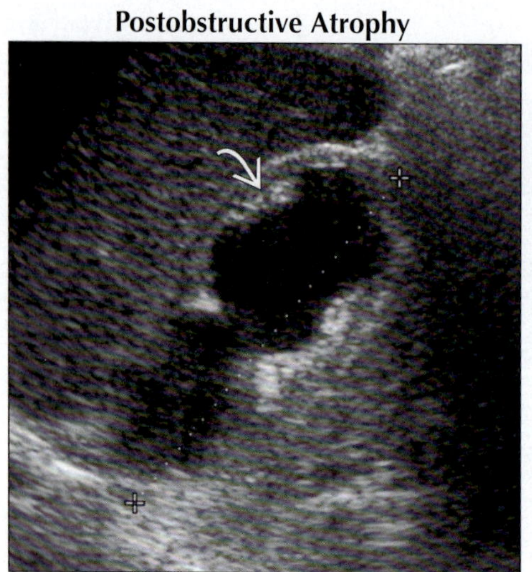

Postobstructive Atrophy

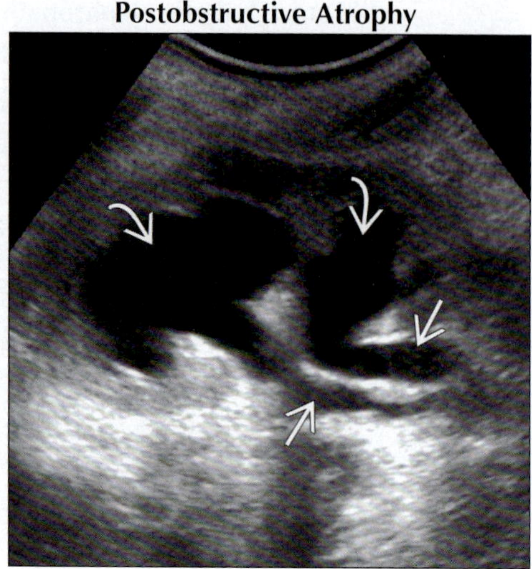

Multicystic Dysplastic Kidney

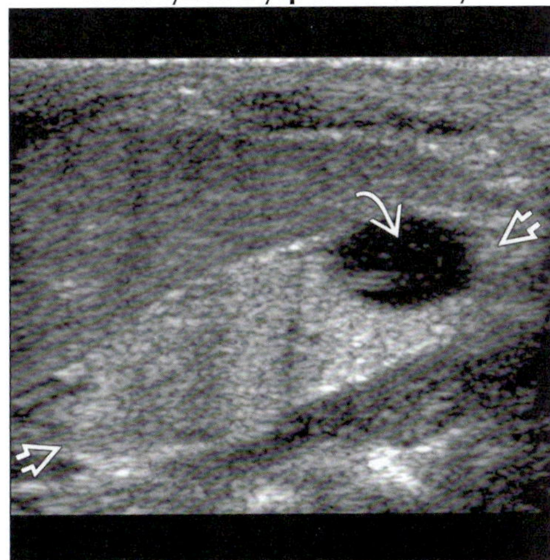

Chronic Renal Allograft Rejection

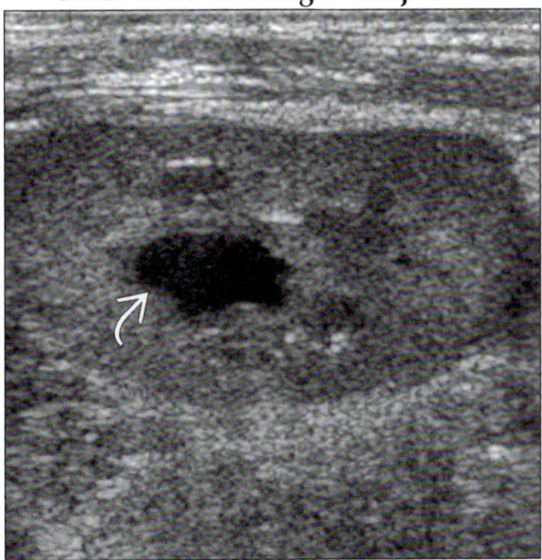

(Left) Longitudinal transabdominal ultrasound shows a small multicystic dysplastic kidney ⊞ with partial involution and a residual peripheral cyst ⊟. *(Right)* Longitudinal transabdominal ultrasound in a case of chronic renal allograft rejection. The transplanted kidney is atrophic and nonfunctioning with loss of corticomedullary differentiation and cystic change ⊞.

Chronic Renal Artery Stenosis (RAS)

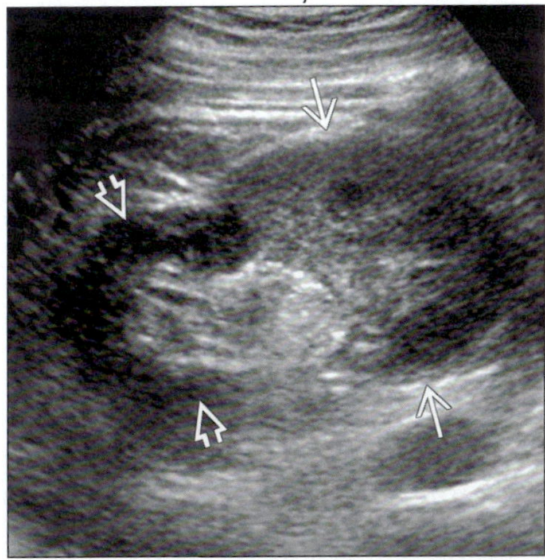

Chronic Renal Artery Stenosis (RAS)

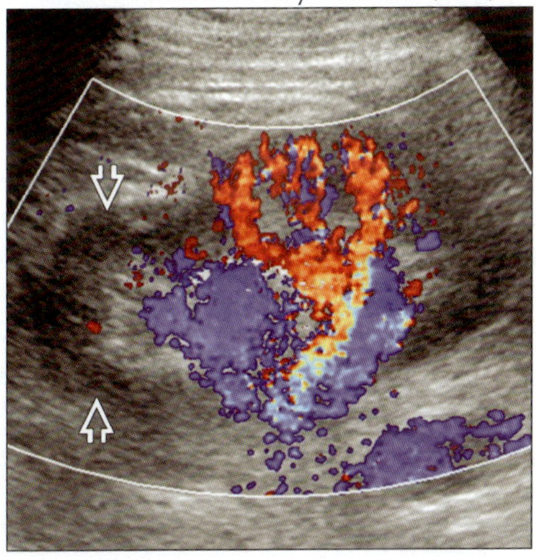

(Left) Longitudinal transabdominal ultrasound shows a difference in size and echotexture of the atrophic upper pole ⊞ and normal lower pole ⊟. *(Right)* Longitudinal color Doppler ultrasound in the same patient shows chronic segmental renal artery stenosis affecting the upper pole of the kidney, where there is an obvious perfusion defect ⊞ with absence of color signal and reduction in renal size.

Tuberculous Autonephrectomy

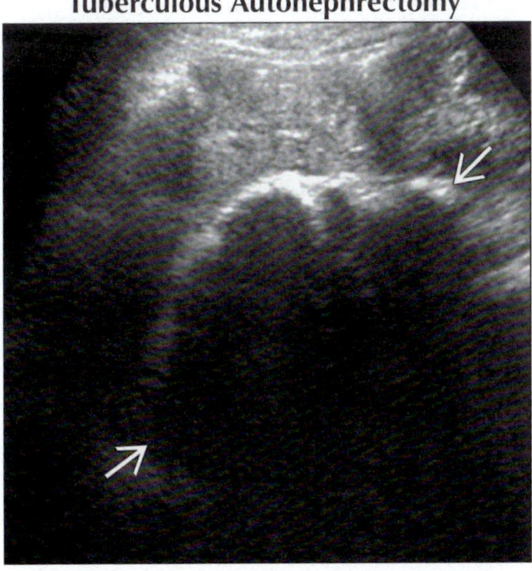

Tuberculous Autonephrectomy

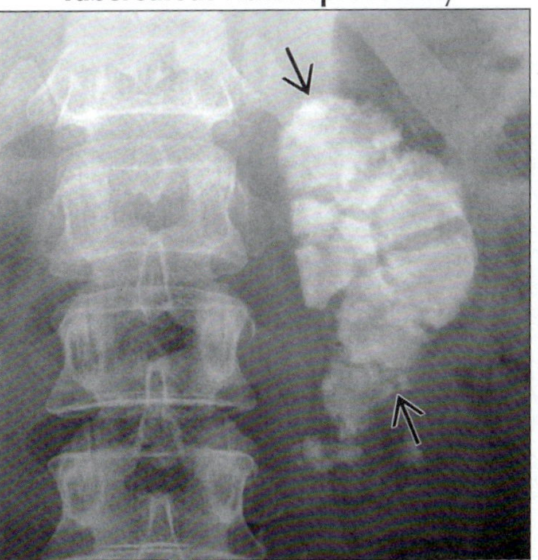

(Left) Longitudinal transabdominal ultrasound shows tuberculous autonephrectomy of the left kidney, which is densely calcified ⊞ and shrunken in size. *(Right)* Corresponding plain radiograph shows a radiopaque left kidney ⊟, consistent with tuberculous autonephrectomy.

DIFFERENTIAL DIAGNOSIS

Common
- Severe Fatty Liver (Mimic)
- Acute Pyelonephritis

Less Common
- Perinephric Hematoma
- Acute Renal Vein Thrombosis (RVT)
- Acute Renal Transplant Rejection

Rare but Important
- Xanthogranulomatous Pyelonephritis
- Acute Amyloidosis
- Acute RVT (Renal Transplant)
- Renal Artery Embolism
- Multiple Myeloma
- Renal Lymphoma

ESSENTIAL INFORMATION

Key Differential Diagnosis Issues
- Mostly related to benign conditions except in renal lymphoma and multiple myeloma

Helpful Clues for Common Diagnoses
- **Severe Fatty Liver (Mimic)**
  - Highly attenuating fatty liver resulting in appearance of hypoechoic kidney
- **Acute Pyelonephritis**
  - Diffusely hypoechoic renal parenchyma
  - On Doppler, ↓ cortical perfusion due to vasoconstriction
  - Ill-defined hypoechoic lesions ⇒ abscesses
  - ± urothelial wall thickening

Helpful Clues for Less Common Diagnoses
- **Perinephric Hematoma**
  - May occur spontaneously or after trauma
  - Hypoechoic reticular perirenal collection
  - Mimics enlarged hypoechoic renal mass
- **Acute Renal Vein Thrombosis (RVT)**
  - Enlarged and relatively hypoechoic kidney
  - Usually segmental or subsegmental RVT
  - Abnormally high resistivity index (RI)
- **Acute Renal Transplant Rejection**
  - Swollen and hypoechoic kidney ± urothelial thickening
  - RI > 0.9 highly specific for rejection

Helpful Clues for Rare Diagnoses
- **Xanthogranulomatous Pyelonephritis**
  - Diffuse (85%)
  - Large heterogeneous mass ± abscess, fibrosis, or chronic granuloma
  - Obstructive calculus in contracted pelvis
- **Acute Amyloidosis**
  - Enlarged hypoechoic kidney due to edema
- **Acute RVT (Renal Transplant)**
  - Swollen tender kidney + ↓ echogenicity
  - Doppler: Oscillating arterial flow
- **Renal Artery Embolism**
  - May affect main or segmental artery
  - Main renal artery embolism ⇒ swollen kidney and ↓ renal echogenicity
- **Multiple Myeloma**
  - Bilateral nephromegaly + ↓ echogenicity ± nephrocalcinosis or urate calculi
- **Renal Lymphoma**
  - Hypoechoic enlarged kidneys

Severe Fatty Liver (Mimic)

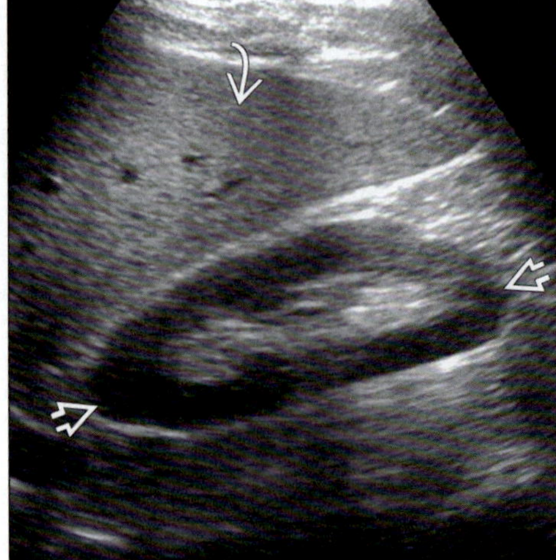

Longitudinal transabdominal ultrasound shows a normal kidney with an apparent decrease in renal echogenicity ⇉ due to the overlying attenuating fatty liver ⇗.

Acute Pyelonephritis

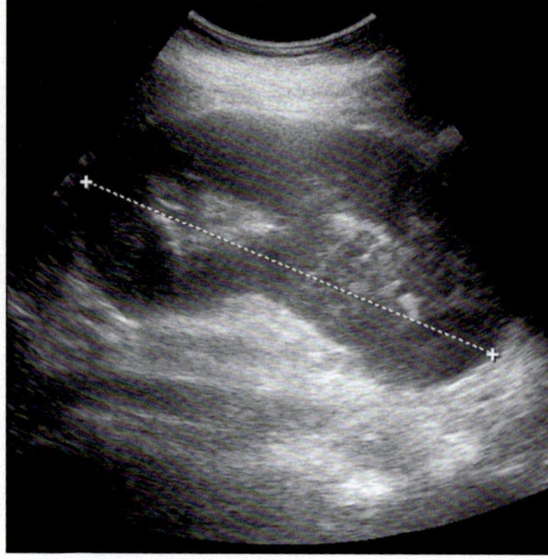

Longitudinal transabdominal ultrasound demonstrates a swollen hypoechoic kidney (calipers) due to uncomplicated acute pyelonephritis.

HYPOECHOIC KIDNEY

Perinephric Hematoma

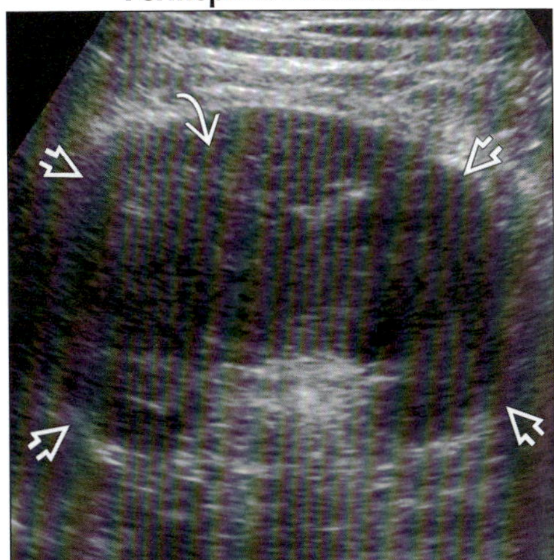

Perinephric Hematoma

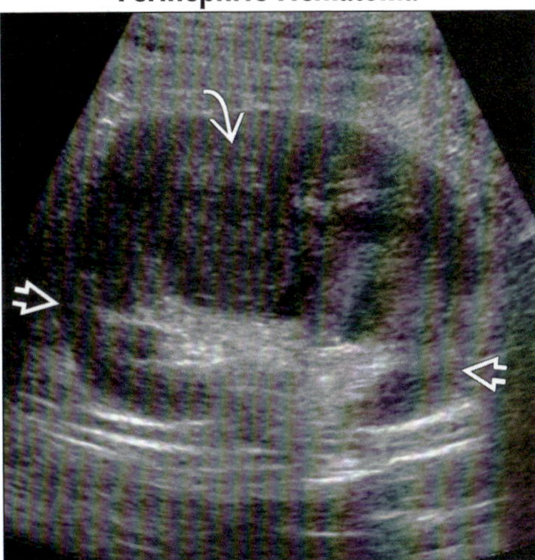

(Left) Longitudinal transabdominal ultrasound shows a large perinephric hematoma ➔ simulating a large hypoechoic renal mass ⇨ under a normal gain setting. *(Right)* Longitudinal transabdominal ultrasound shows the same perinephric hematoma ➔ after an increase in overall gain. Note that the kidney ⇨ embedded in the hematoma is better visualized at the higher gain setting.

Acute Renal Transplant Rejection

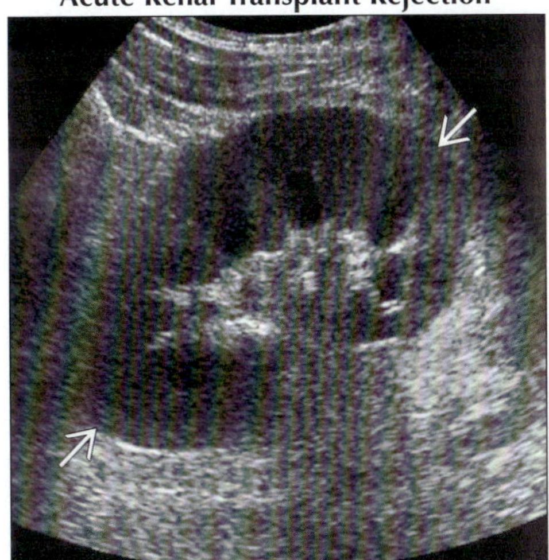

Acute Renal Transplant Rejection

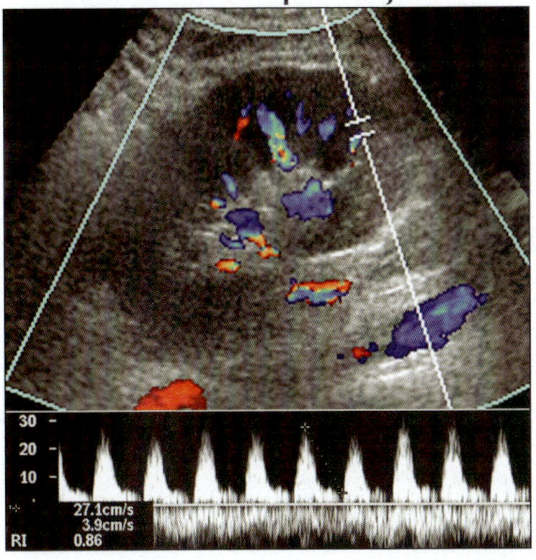

(Left) Longitudinal transabdominal ultrasound shows a hypoechoic renal transplant allograft ➔ with histologically proven acute rejection. Grayscale ultrasound appearances are nonspecific. *(Right)* Longitudinal color Doppler ultrasound shows the intrarenal flow of the acute rejection in the previous image. Note that RI is raised and approaching 0.9, which is suggestive of acute rejection.

Xanthogranulomatous Pyelonephritis

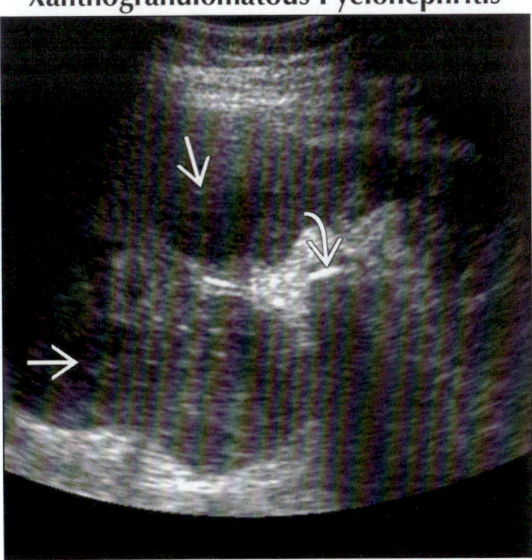

Multiple Myeloma

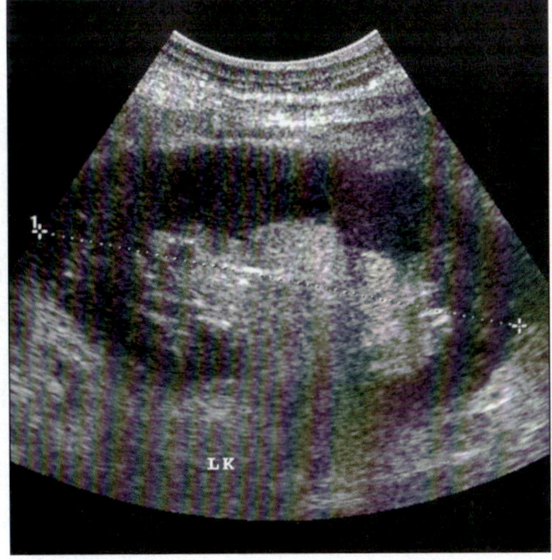

(Left) Longitudinal transabdominal ultrasound shows xanthogranulomatous pyelonephritis. The kidney is enlarged and hypoechoic with abscesses ➔. The pelvis is contracted, appearing as a central echogenic area with a shadowing calculus ➔. *(Right)* Longitudinal transabdominal ultrasound shows a diffusely enlarged and hypoechoic kidney (calipers) due to multiple myeloma. The contralateral kidney was also affected (not shown).

HYPERECHOIC KIDNEY

DIFFERENTIAL DIAGNOSIS

Common
- Diabetic Nephropathy
- Glomerulonephritis (GN)
- Medullary Nephrocalcinosis
- Hypertensive (HT) Nephrosclerosis
- Lupus Nephritis
- Acute Interstitial Nephritis
- Pediatric Acute Pyelonephritis

Less Common
- Renal Vein Thrombosis
- Cortical Nephrocalcinosis
- Multicystic Dysplastic Kidney (MCDK)
- Oxalosis
- Chronic Renal Transplant Rejection

Rare but Important
- HIV Nephropathy
- Renal Lymphoma
- Acute Cortical Necrosis
- Autosomal Recessive Polycystic Kidney Disease
- Renal Amyloidosis

ESSENTIAL INFORMATION

Key Differential Diagnosis Issues
- Increased renal echogenicity specific to abnormal kidneys but not any particular cause
- Echogenicity correlates well with interstitial disease but not with glomerular disease
- Degree of echogenicity correlates poorly with severity of renal impairment
- Renal biopsy indispensable in diagnosis of renal parenchymal disease

Helpful Clues for Common Diagnoses
- **Diabetic Nephropathy**
  - Single most important disease leading to renal failure in adults
  - Early: Normal or enlarged kidneys
  - ↑ resistivity index (RI) on Doppler studies with ↑ cortical echogenicity
  - Chronic: Small echogenic kidney with variable corticomedullary differentiation (CMD)
- **Glomerulonephritis (GN)**
  - Primary or secondary immunomediated renal disease
    - Proliferative: IgA disease, postinfective GN, mesangiocapillary GN, rapidly progressive GN
    - Nonproliferative: Minimal change GN, focal segmental glomerulosclerosis, membranous GN
    - Immunoglobulin A (IgA) disease (Berger nephropathy) most common type
  - Acute: Normal/enlarged kidney with ↑ renal echogenicity and CMD
  - Chronic: Small and hyperechoic kidney
- **Medullary Nephrocalcinosis**
  - Common causes: Hyperparathyroidism, renal tubular acidosis, medullary sponge kidney
  - ↑ echogenicity of renal medullae with reversed normal corticomedullary (CM) echogenicity
- **Hypertensive (HT) Nephrosclerosis**
  - Causes 25% of end-stage renal disease
  - Renal echogenicity depends on chronicity
  - ↑ RI with ↑ cortical echogenicity
- **Lupus Nephritis**
  - Acute: Renal echogenicity and size are nonspecific
  - Chronic: Small and echogenic kidney
- **Acute Interstitial Nephritis**
  - Common causes: Hypersensitivity reaction to drug or infective antigen
  - Mimics acute tubular necrosis clinically
  - Kidney size may be normal or enlarged
  - Cortical echogenicity may ↑ depending on severity of reaction
- **Pediatric Acute Pyelonephritis**
  - Normal/swollen kidney with ↑ echogenicity
  - Loss of normal CMD
  - Mild hydronephrosis due to urinary atony, reflux, or obstruction
  - Thickened urothelium
  - Focal hypoechoic areas or triangle-/wedge-shaped vascular defects

Helpful Clues for Less Common Diagnoses
- **Renal Vein Thrombosis**
  - Usually results from membranous GN, hypercoagulability, or tumor invasion
  - Dehydration is common cause in infants
  - Rare complication of kidney transplant
  - May involve main, segmental, or subsegmental veins
  - Doppler: ↓ or reversed diastolic flow, ↑ RI

HYPERECHOIC KIDNEY

- ○ Acute: Swollen kidney, ↓ renal echogenicity
- ○ Chronic: Contracted kidney, ↑ cortical echogenicity due to scarring and fibrosis
- **Cortical Nephrocalcinosis**
  - ○ Focal: Caused by trauma, infarction, or infection
  - ○ Diffuse: Due to renal cortical necrosis, kidney transplant rejection, chronic GN, Alport syndrome
  - ○ Characterized by peripheral parenchymal calcifications and ↑ cortical echogenicity
- **Multicystic Dysplastic Kidney (MCDK)**
  - ○ Appears as large unilateral renal mass
  - ○ Characterized by presence of multiple, randomly distributed, small cysts in hyperechoic dysplastic renal parenchyma
  - ○ Contralateral abnormalities common (30-50%), including MCDK, vesicoureteral reflux, and ureteropelvic obstruction
- **Oxalosis**
  - ○ Characterized by combined cortical and medullary nephrocalcinosis
  - ○ Early: ↑ cortical echogenicity
  - ○ Late: Hyperechoic kidneys; absent CMD
- **Chronic Renal Transplant Rejection**
  - ○ Mediated by humoral + cellular rejection
  - ○ Occurs months to years after transplantation
  - ○ Results in interstitial fibrosis
  - ○ Typically, kidney is echogenic with ↓ size

Helpful Clues for Rare Diagnoses
- **HIV Nephropathy**

- ○ Renal size may be normal or enlarged
- ○ > 50% show ↑ cortical echogenicity due to tubular changes
- ○ Common pathology: Focal segmental glomerulosclerosis
- **Renal Lymphoma**
  - ○ Homogeneously ↑ renal echogenicity (hepatization) when diffusely infiltrated
- **Acute Cortical Necrosis**
  - ○ Classically associated with abruptio placentae or postpartum hemorrhage
  - ○ May occur with shock, sepsis, snake bites, and exposure to toxins
  - ○ Due to microvascular thrombosis leading to cortical ischemia
  - ○ Diffuse ↑ parenchymal echogenicity
  - ○ Subcapsular area spared and seen as hypoechoic rim
- **Autosomal Recessive Polycystic Kidney Disease**
  - ○ May be detected prenatally by ultrasound
  - ○ Typical appearance: Symmetrically enlarged echogenic kidneys
  - ○ ↑ renal echogenicity due to multiple reflections from numerous small cyst walls
- **Renal Amyloidosis**
  - ○ Primary: Abnormal protein production with deposition in kidney
  - ○ Secondary: Dialysis related; due to failure to remove large protein molecules
  - ○ Acute: ↑ renal size, ↓ cortical echogenicity, preserved CMD
  - ○ Chronic: Same as other chronic renal diseases with ↓ renal size & ↑ echogenicity

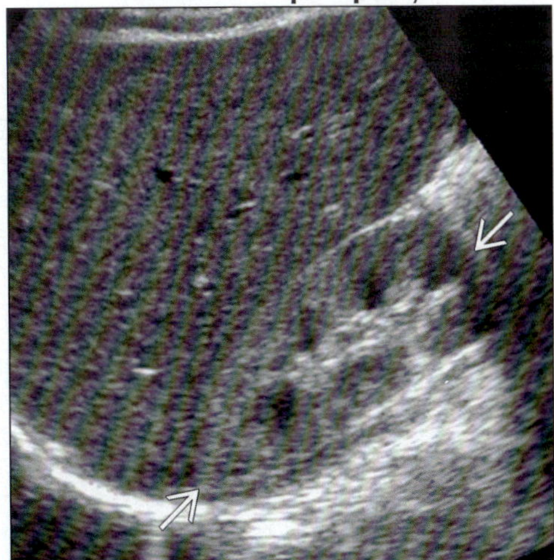

Diabetic Nephropathy

Longitudinal transabdominal US of the kidney ➡ shows a subtle ↑ in cortical echogenicity with preserved CMD. Renal echogenicity may be normal in early stages of disease, despite deranged renal function.

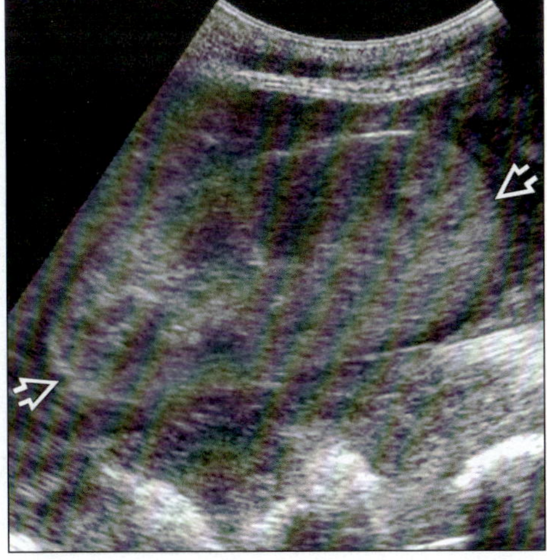

Diabetic Nephropathy

Longitudinal transabdominal ultrasound shows chronic diabetic nephropathy. The diseased kidney ⬵ is markedly echogenic and reduced in size.

HYPERECHOIC KIDNEY

(Left) Longitudinal transabdominal ultrasound shows mesangiocapillary GN ⮞ in a patient with POEMS syndrome, an extremely rare blood disorder affecting multiple systems with polyneuropathy, organomegaly, endocrinopathy, monoclonal gammopathy, and skin changes. (Right) Longitudinal transabdominal ultrasound in the same patient shows the contralateral kidney ⮞. Note that GN is a renal disease that affects both kidneys symmetrically.

Glomerulonephritis (GN)

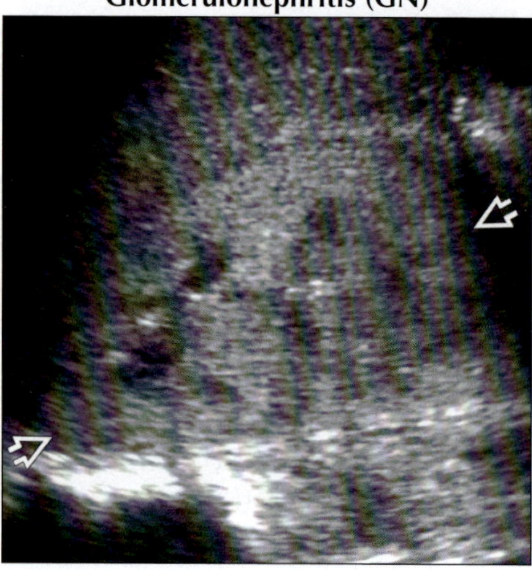

Glomerulonephritis (GN)

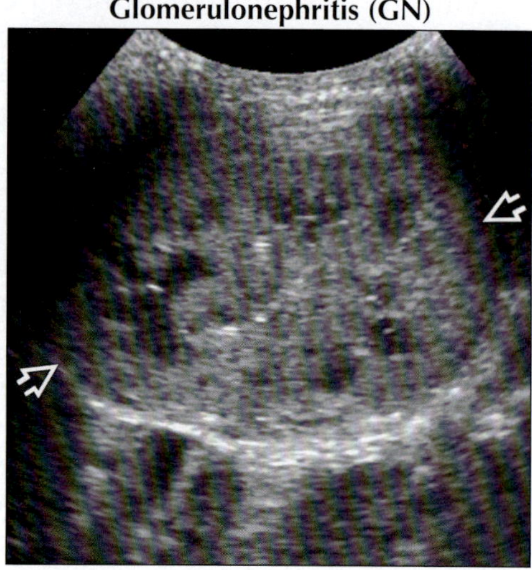

(Left) Longitudinal transabdominal ultrasound shows a normal-sized hyperechoic kidney ⮞ in a patient with macroscopic hematuria. Renal biopsy specimen showed IgA nephropathy with hyaline arteriosclerosis. (Right) Longitudinal color Doppler ultrasound in the same patient shows the intrarenal arterial flow resistance is within normal limits (RI = 0.57).

Glomerulonephritis (GN)

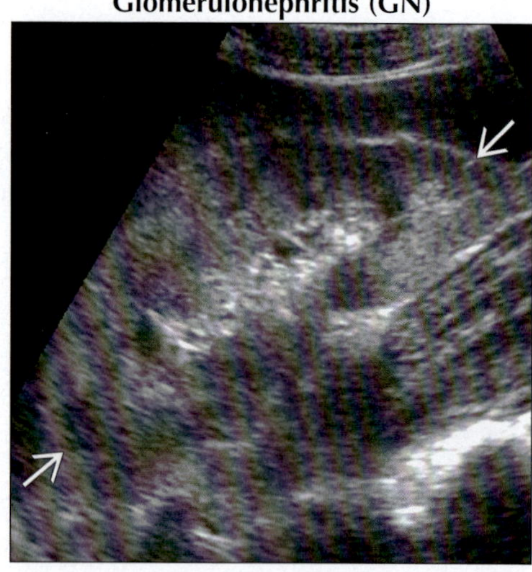

Glomerulonephritis (GN)

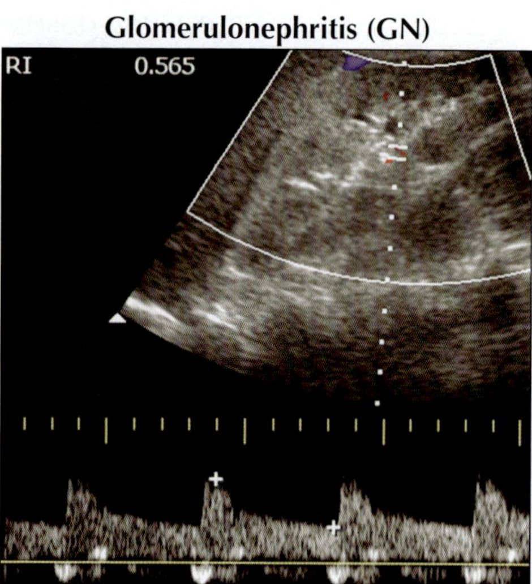

(Left) Longitudinal transabdominal US shows extensive medullary nephrocalcinosis. The deposition of calcium in the renal medullae increases the reflectivity of these areas ⮞ and reverses the normal corticomedullary echogenicity. (Right) Longitudinal transabdominal US shows a biopsy-proven, advanced, hypertensive, nephrosclerotic right kidney ⮞. Note that the echogenicity of the kidney is much higher than that of the liver ⮞.

Medullary Nephrocalcinosis

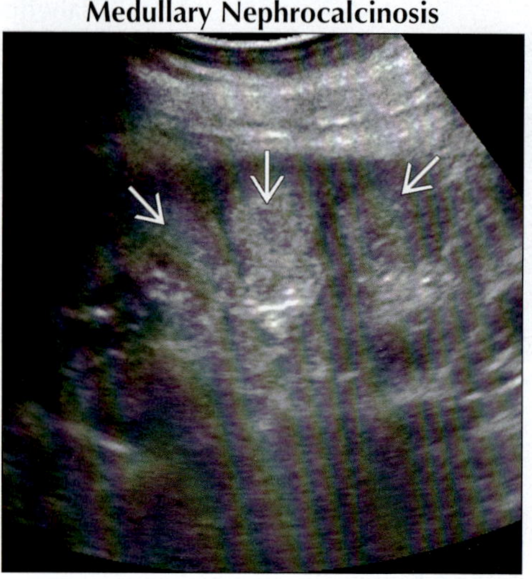

Hypertensive (HT) Nephrosclerosis

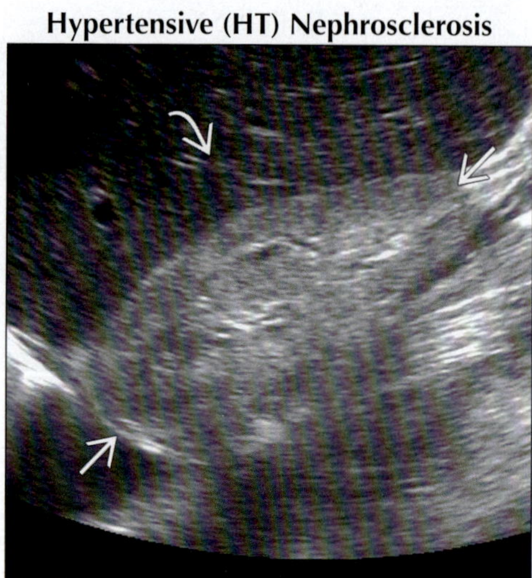

HYPERECHOIC KIDNEY

Hypertensive (HT) Nephrosclerosis

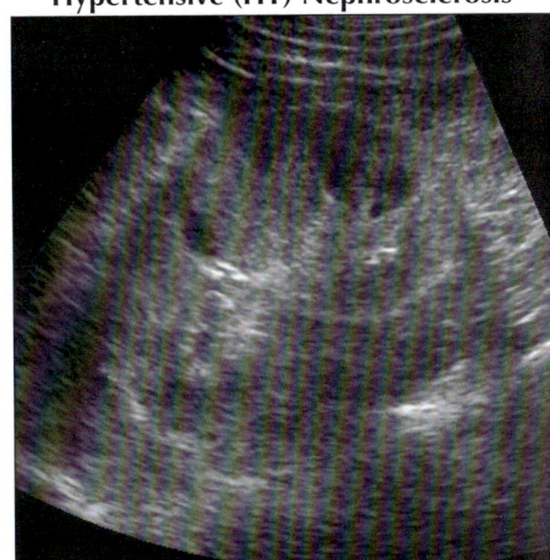

Hypertensive (HT) Nephrosclerosis

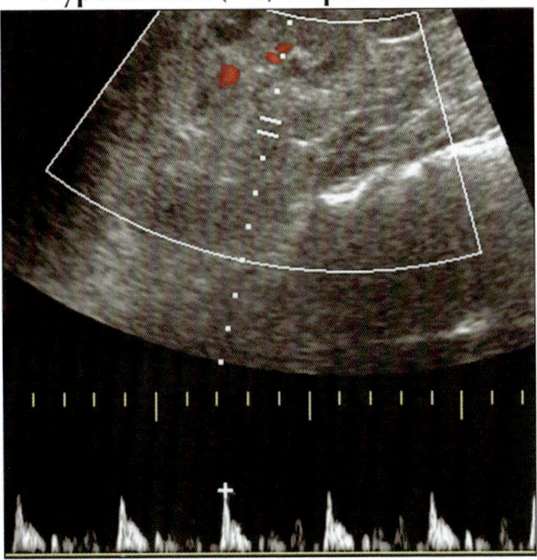

(Left) Longitudinal transabdominal ultrasound shows hypertensive nephrosclerosis. The diseased kidney is echogenic with reduced blood flow. *(Right)* Longitudinal color Doppler ultrasound shows intrarenal waveforms of the same kidney. It is evident that the intrarenal flow is reduced and is of high resistance.

Lupus Nephritis

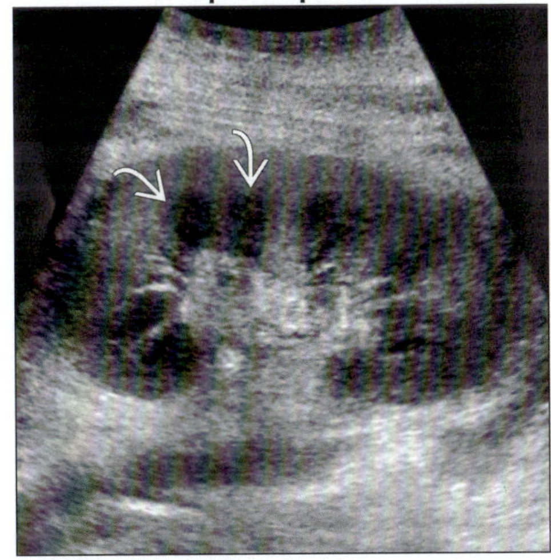

Lupus Nephritis

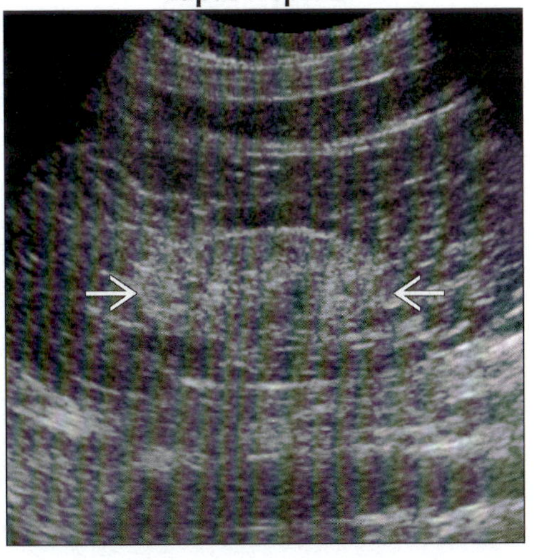

(Left) Longitudinal transabdominal ultrasound shows acute lupus nephritis in a patient with nephrotic syndrome. The kidney is mildly enlarged with increased cortical echogenicity and prominent CMD ➔. *(Right)* Longitudinal transabdominal ultrasound shows chronic lupus nephritis. The kidney is echogenic ➔ with a significant decrease in size. Differentiation of chronic lupus nephritis from other chronic renal disease is difficult.

Lupus Nephritis

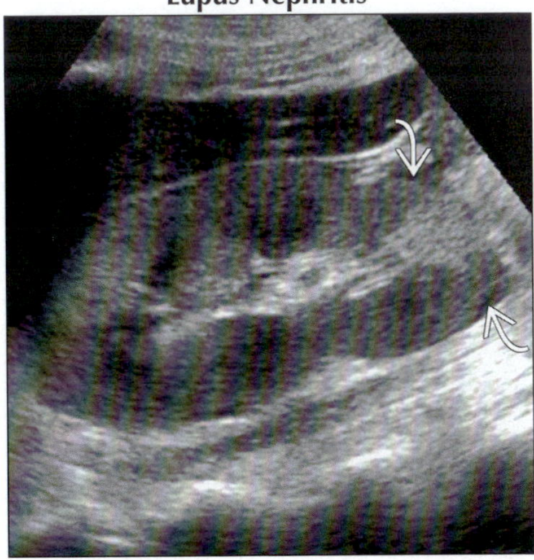

Pediatric Acute Pyelonephritis

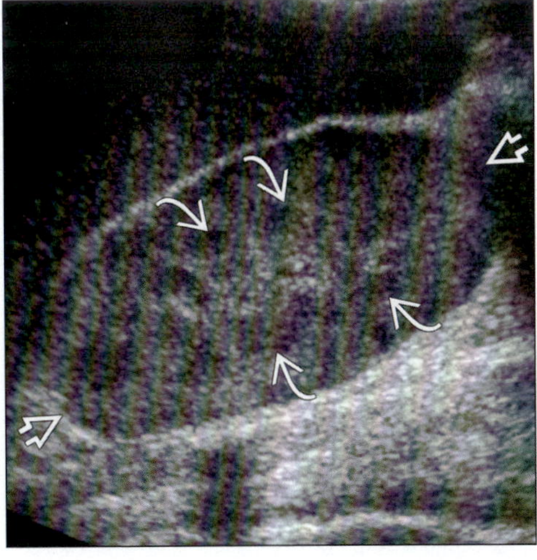

(Left) Longitudinal transabdominal ultrasound shows acute lupus nephritis. The kidney is swollen with increased cortical echogenicity. A thin film of perinephritic fluid ➔ is present in reaction to the inflammation. *(Right)* Longitudinal transabdominal ultrasound shows pediatric acute pyelonephritis. The infected kidney is swollen ➔ with a generalized increase in renal echogenicity and diminished corticomedullary differentiation ➔.

(Left) Longitudinal transabdominal ultrasound shows chronic renal vein thrombosis in a transplanted kidney. The renal cortical echogenicity ➡ is mildly increased. Note the thin film of perinephritic fluid ➡. (Right) Oblique color Doppler ultrasound in the same patient shows an oscillating flow in the renal artery of the allograft. This is characteristic of RVT in transplanted kidneys (but not in native kidneys) because of the absence of collaterals in transplants.

Renal Vein Thrombosis

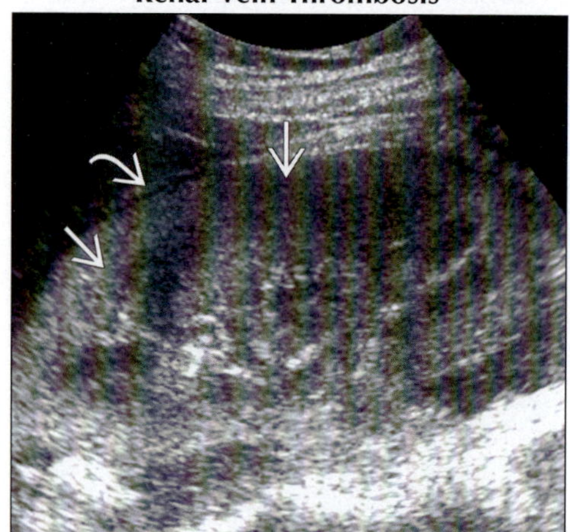

Renal Vein Thrombosis

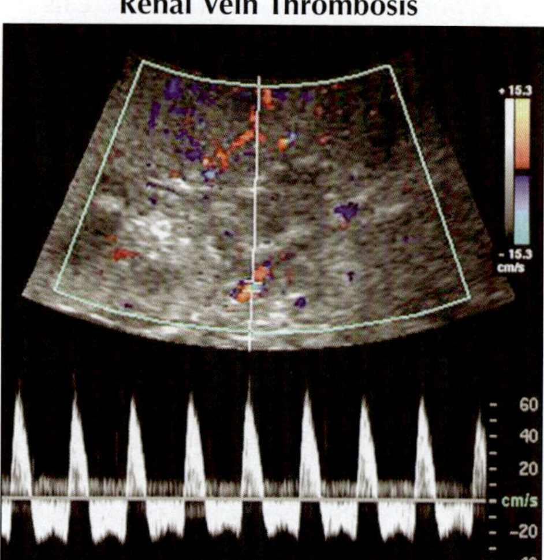

(Left) Longitudinal transabdominal ultrasound of a transplanted kidney shows diffusely increased in cortical echogenicity ➡ with prominent CMD. Renal biopsy revealed extensive cortical nephrocalcinosis due to rejection. (Right) Longitudinal transabdominal ultrasound shows a MCDK manifesting as a large renal mass with multiple small cysts randomly distributed in the echogenic dysplastic tissue ➡. Note that evaluation for contralateral renal disease is indicated.

Cortical Nephrocalcinosis

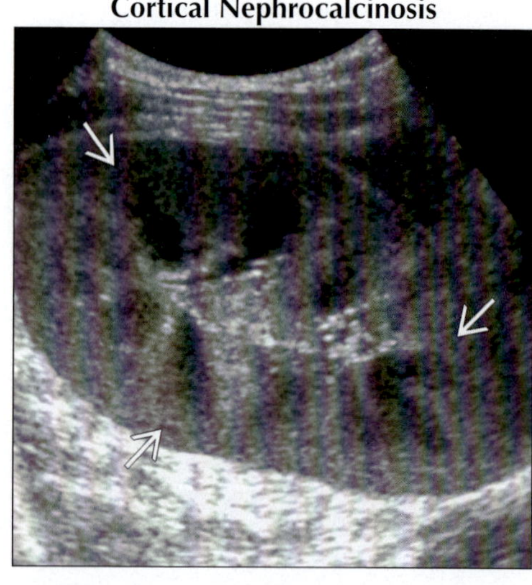

Multicystic Dysplastic Kidney (MCDK)

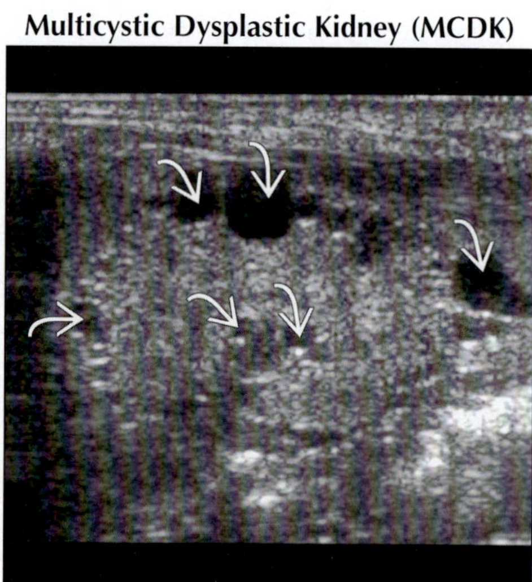

(Left) Longitudinal transabdominal ultrasound shows a nonfunctioning dysplastic kidney, which is small and echogenic ➡ with a dominant peripheral cyst ➡. (Right) Longitudinal transabdominal ultrasound in a 2-month-old infant shows a hyperechoic kidney ➡ caused by oxalosis with severe cortical and medullary nephrocalcinosis and absent corticomedullary differentiation.

Multicystic Dysplastic Kidney (MCDK)

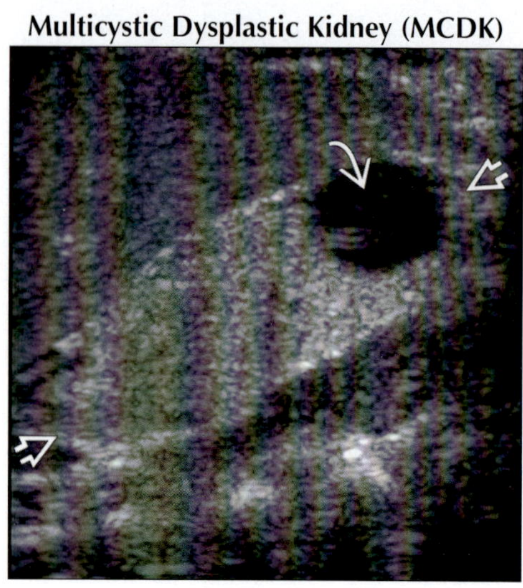

Oxalosis

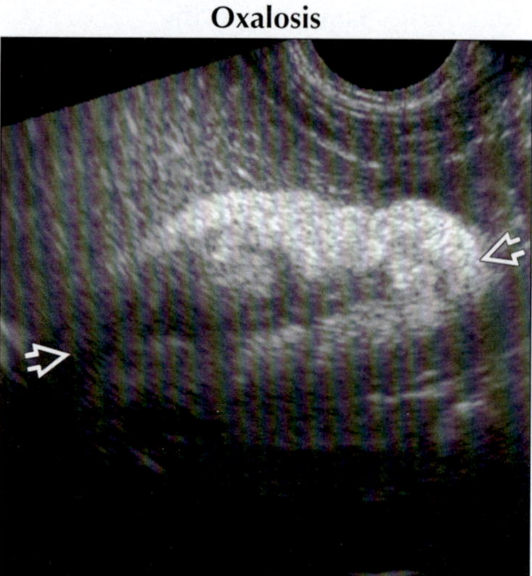

HYPERECHOIC KIDNEY

Chronic Renal Transplant Rejection

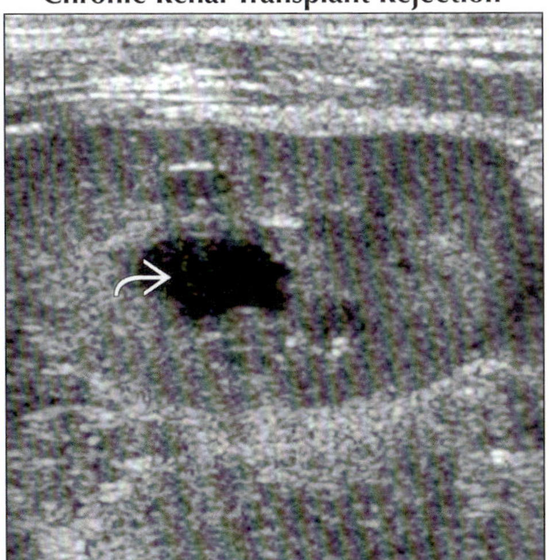

Renal Lymphoma

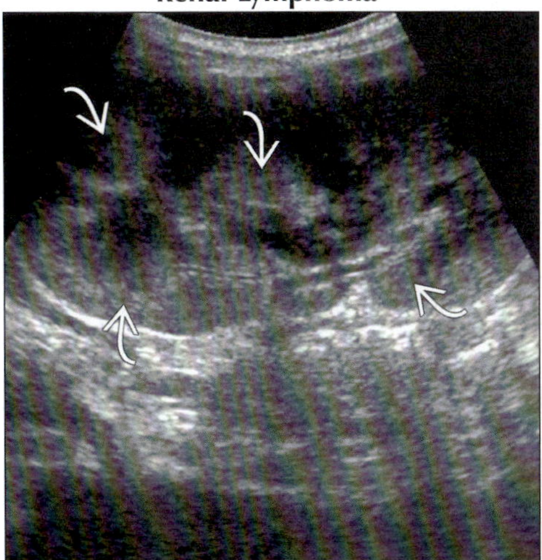

Acute Cortical Necrosis

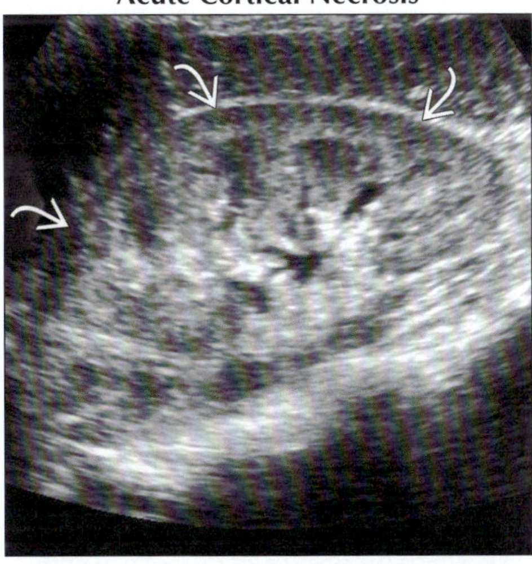

Autosomal Recessive Polycystic Kidney Disease

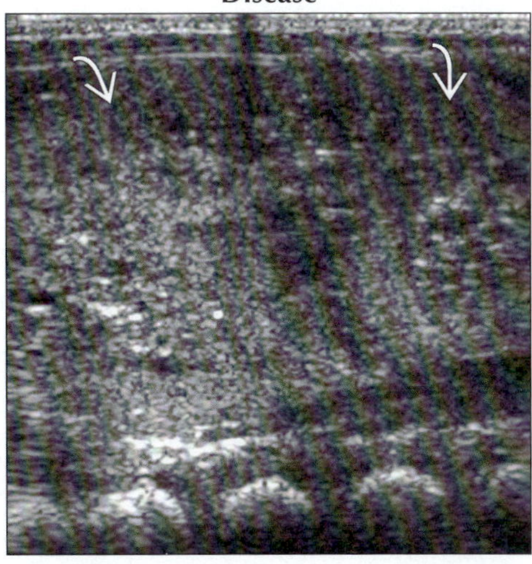

Autosomal Recessive Polycystic Kidney Disease

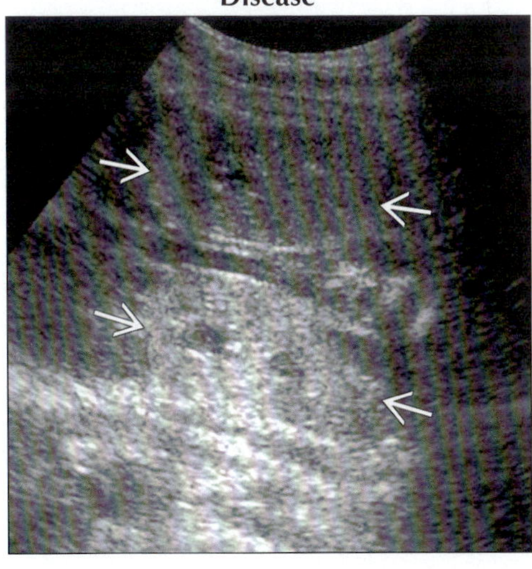

Autosomal Recessive Polycystic Kidney Disease

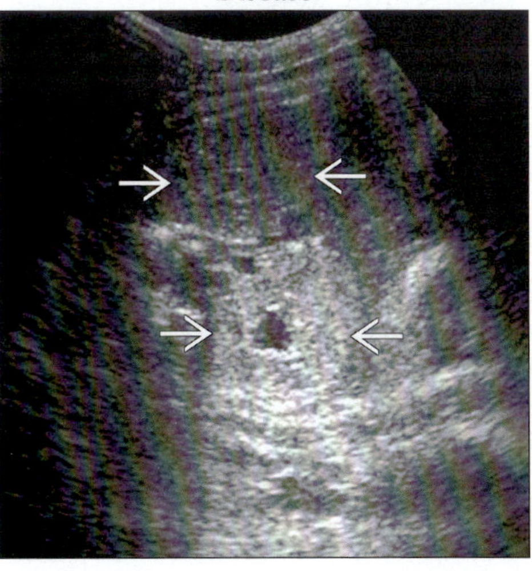

(Left) Longitudinal transabdominal ultrasound shows chronic renal transplant rejection. The kidney is overtly abnormal with decrease in size, increase in renal echogenicity, and loss of corticomedullary differentiation. A renal cyst ⊅ is also present. *(Right)* Longitudinal transabdominal ultrasound shows diffuse renal involvement by Burkitt lymphoma. Note the diffuse increase in size and parenchymal echogenicity ⊅. No discrete mass is seen.

(Left) Longitudinal transabdominal ultrasound shows acute cortical necrosis. There is an increase in parenchymal echogenicity with sparing of a thin rim of subcapsular cortical tissue ⊅, which is preserved by the capsular blood supply. *(Right)* Longitudinal transabdominal ultrasound shows infantile autosomal recessive polycystic kidney disease. The kidney is highly reflective ⊅ due to the presence of multiple acoustic interfaces from the tiny cyst walls.

(Left) Longitudinal ultrasound of the fetal abdomen shows autosomal recessive polycystic kidney disease detected in utero. Note that the fetal kidneys are symmetrically enlarged and bright ⊅. *(Right)* Transverse ultrasound of the kidney ⊅ in the same fetus. There is oligohydramnios surrounding the fetal abdomen, indicating that the kidneys are nonfunctioning.

DIFFERENTIAL DIAGNOSIS

Common
- Simple Renal Cyst
- Parapelvic Cyst
- Hydronephrosis
- Autosomal Dominant Polycystic Kidney Disease
- Cystic Disease of Dialysis
- Medullary Sponge Kidney

Less Common
- Multicystic Dysplastic Kidney
- Tuberous Sclerosis
- Congenital Megacalyces
- Perinephric Collection

ESSENTIAL INFORMATION

Key Differential Diagnosis Issues
- Beware of artifacts within anechoic cystic lesions caused by
  - Reverberation from skin-transducer interfaces superficial to cyst
  - Gain setting too high ⇒ acoustic interference
  - Echoes from adjacent tissue (partial volume effect)
- Posterior acoustic enhancement typically occurs with larger lesion, may not be seen if cyst is very small
- Occasionally cysts in upper pole of kidney may be difficult to differentiate from suprarenal, hepatic (right), or splenic (left) cysts
  - Try to delineate relationship on multiplanar real-time imaging
  - Important to ensure cyst is simple and echo free; conservative treatment is all that may be necessary

Helpful Clues for Common Diagnoses
- **Simple Renal Cyst**
  - Extremely common; frequency increases with age
  - Best diagnostic clue: Well-defined, round or oval, smooth, and thin walled
  - Entirely echo free, no septum or solid component
  - Posterior acoustic enhancement
  - ± displacement of central calyceal system
  - Location: Renal cortex, deep or superficial
  - Color Doppler: Lack of intracystic color signal
- **Parapelvic Cyst**
  - Lymphangiectasia of renal hilum
    - Develops from embryologic rests
  - Medially located cystic lesion with surrounding echogenic walls
  - Lies adjacent to renal pelvis at hilum
  - Rarely extends to corticomedullary junction or involves renal capsule (distinguished from cortical cyst)
  - Lack of communication with collecting system (distinguished from calyceal dilatation)
  - Most are asymptomatic; rarely associated with hematuria, hypertension
- **Hydronephrosis**
  - Dilated calyces coalesce centrally, appearing like fingers of a glove
  - Mild hydronephrosis
    - Normal bright sinus echoes and normal parenchymal thickness
  - Moderate hydronephrosis
    - Diminished sinus echoes, normal/thinned parenchymal thickness
  - Severe hydronephrosis
    - Loss of normal sinus echoes, cortical thinning
  - Pulsed Doppler
    - Obstructive hydronephrosis: RI > 0.7, or RI 0.1 higher than contralateral side without hydronephrosis
- **Autosomal Dominant Polycystic Kidney Disease**
  - Hereditary disorder (family history helps)
  - Multiple, bilateral, asymmetrical cysts of varying size
  - Well-defined round or oval cysts + thin imperceptible or calcified wall
  - Complicated cysts: Hemorrhage/infection, stone/dystrophic calcification
  - Massively enlarged, echogenic kidneys with lack of corticomedullary differentiation
  - Associated with cysts of other organs
    - Liver (75%),
    - Pancreas (10%)
    - Spleen (5%)
    - Other rare sites: Thyroid, ovary, endometrium, seminal vesicles, lung, brain, pituitary, breast, epididymis

- **Cystic Disease of Dialysis**
  - Clinical history of long-term renal dialysis, 70% incidence
  - 1 or more small cysts < 3 cm
  - Usually in small echogenic kidneys with loss of corticomedullary differentiation
  - Renal size may be enlarged due to acquired cysts
  - Cysts scattered in both renal cortex and medulla, especially at site of renal scars
  - May resemble polycystic kidney disease in advanced stage (distinguished by history)
- **Medullary Sponge Kidney**
  - Dilated, ectatic collecting tubes, unknown etiology
  - Medullary cysts, usually associated with multiple echogenic foci localized at renal medullary pyramids
  - Calculus occasionally seen if focus of calcification has eroded into collecting system

Helpful Clues for Less Common Diagnoses
- **Multicystic Dysplastic Kidney**
  - Caused by obstruction in first 10 weeks of intrauterine life
  - Also known as renal dysplasia/dysgenesis
  - Multiple cysts of varying size with no renal pelvis/ureter
  - Doppler study: No demonstrable renal blood flow or low velocity systolic peaks with absent diastolic flow
  - Usually unilateral involvement affecting entire kidney

- Bilateral, segmental, or focal involvement possible but rare
- May be associated with abnormality in contralateral kidney (up to 20%)
  - Vesicoureteric reflux or ureteropelvic junction obstruction
- **Tuberous Sclerosis**
  - Clinically characterized by adenoma sebaceum, mental retardation, and seizures
  - Multiple, bilateral, small cysts
  - Associated with small fat-containing angiomyolipomas (AML) and renal cell carcinoma (1-2%)
  - Bilateral renal cysts + multiple AMLs (confirmed by CT) ⇒ pathognomonic
- **Congenital Megacalyces**
  - Nonobstructive enlargement of calyces
  - Enlarged clubbed calyces, loss of papillary impression
  - Increased number of calyces, preserved cortical thickness
  - Usually unilateral
  - Nonprogressive, normal renal function, diagnosis by serial follow-up
  - May be associated with megaureter
- **Perinephric Collection**
  - Results from ruptured hydronephrosis or pyonephrosis
  - Occasionally direct extension of peritoneal or retroperitoneal infection
  - Cystic abnormality outside renal parenchyma
    - May cause indentation or distortion of renal contour

Simple Renal Cyst

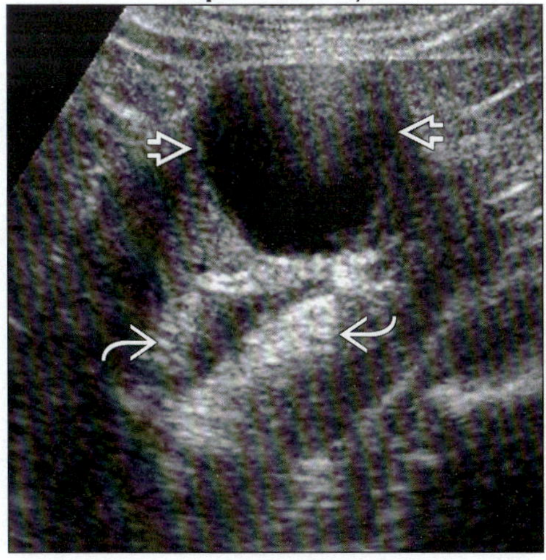

Oblique transabdominal ultrasound shows a simple renal cortical cyst ➡. The cyst is round, thin walled, and anechoic with posterior acoustic enhancement ➡.

Simple Renal Cyst

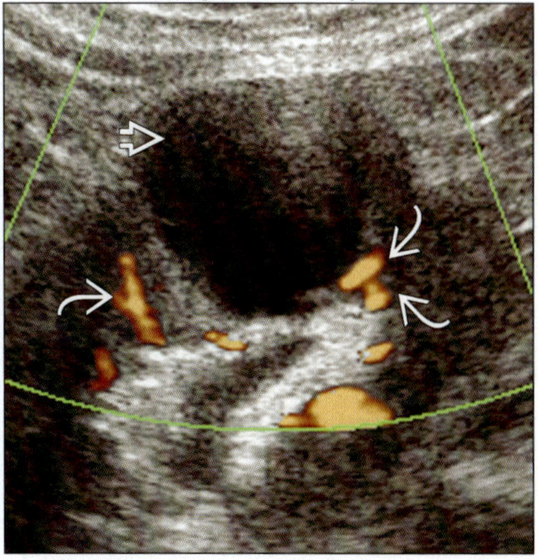

Oblique power Doppler ultrasound shows the same renal cyst ➡. Note the avascular nature of this lesion with splaying ➡ of the adjacent blood vessels.

ANECHOIC RENAL MASS

(Left) Longitudinal transabdominal ultrasound shows a typical anechoic renal cyst ⇨ within the renal parenchyma. Note the posterior acoustic enhancement ➡, which is typical of a simple cyst. (Right) Oblique transabdominal ultrasound shows a medially located cystic lesion ⇨ with surrounding echogenic wall ➡, representing lymphangiectasis of the renal hilum. It rarely extends to the corticomedullary junction.

Simple Renal Cyst

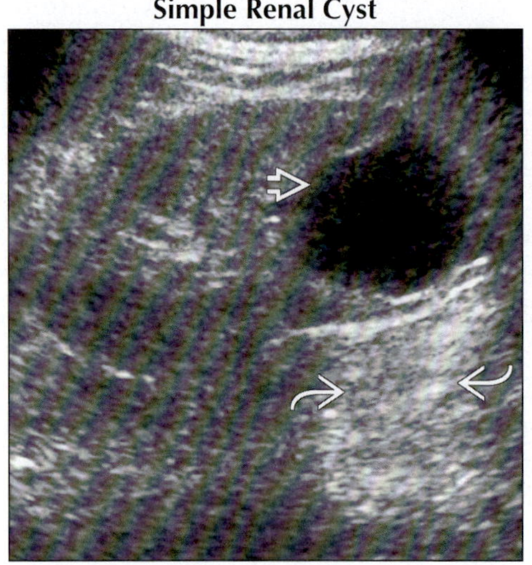

Parapelvic Cyst

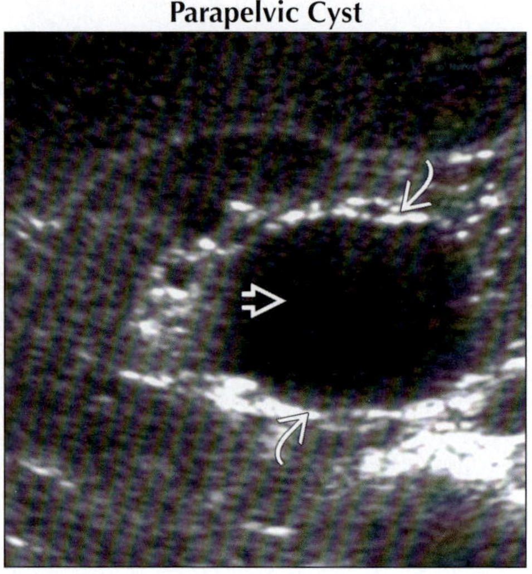

(Left) Oblique transabdominal ultrasound shows a dilated renal pelvis ➡ mimicking a renal cyst. Note the associated dilated calyces ⇨, which coalesce centrally with the renal pelvis. (Right) Longitudinal transabdominal ultrasound shows generalized caliectasis ➡ with cortical thinning ➡ in a patient with postobstructive uropathy.

Hydronephrosis

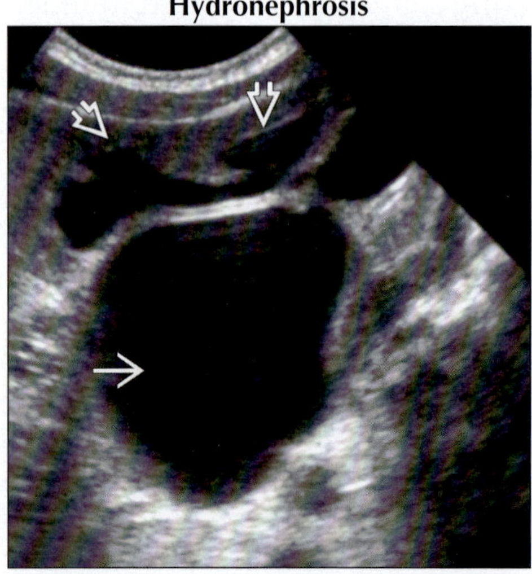

Hydronephrosis

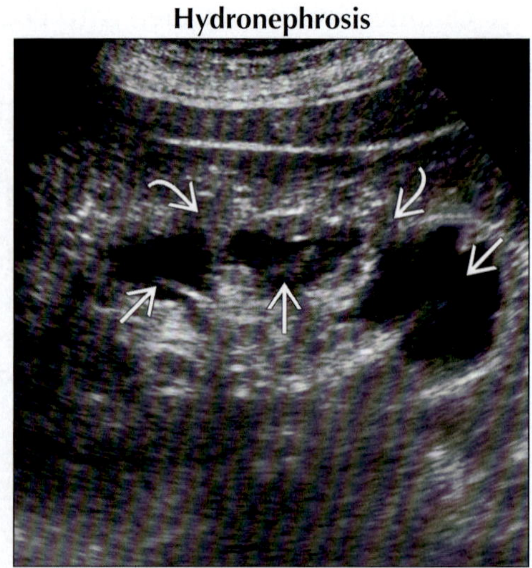

(Left) Longitudinal ultrasound shows an enlarged kidney with the renal parenchyma replaced by anechoic cysts ➡ of varying sizes. The corticomedullary differentiation is lost. The contralateral kidney had a similar appearance. (Right) Longitudinal transabdominal ultrasound shows a small echogenic kidney ➡ in a patient with renal failure on dialysis. Multiple cysts ➡ of varying size are randomly distributed throughout cortex and medulla.

Autosomal Dominant Polycystic Kidney Disease

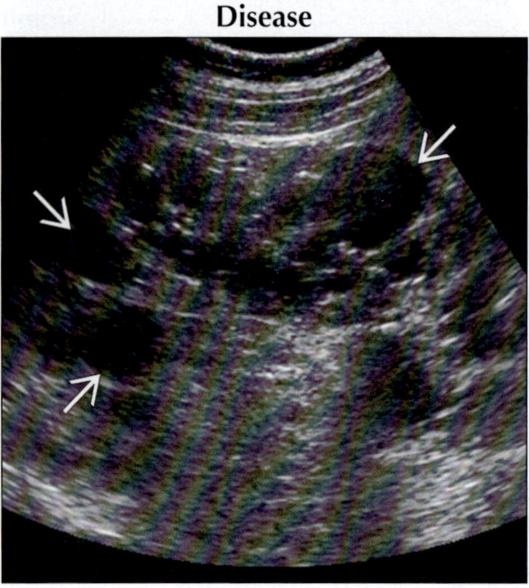

Cystic Disease of Dialysis

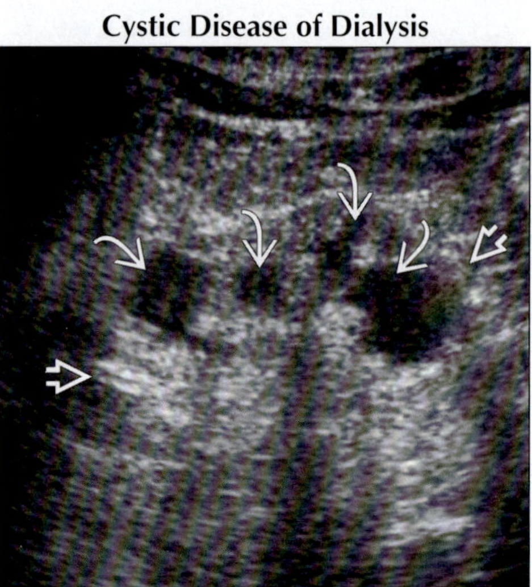

ANECHOIC RENAL MASS

Medullary Sponge Kidney

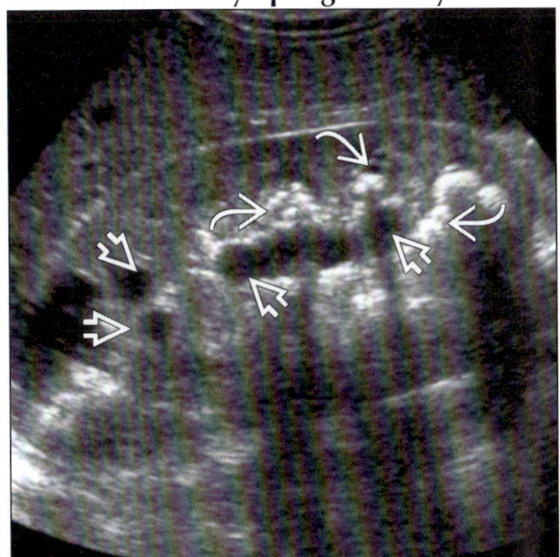

Multicystic Dysplastic Kidney

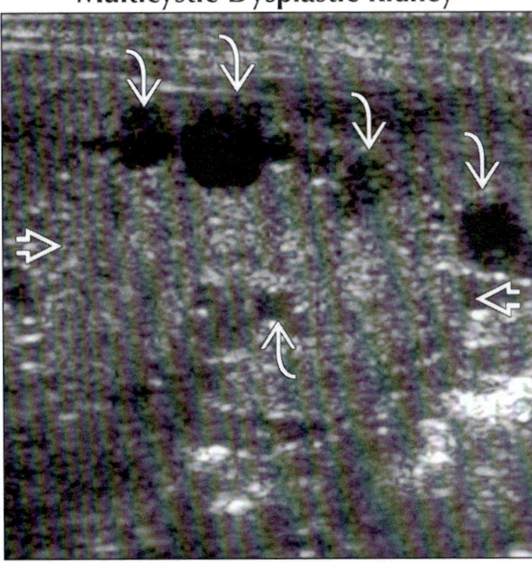

(Left) Longitudinal transabdominal ultrasound shows multiple cystic lesions representing dilated, ectatic collecting tubules ➡. The echogenic foci ➡, which represent calcifications, are localized to the medullary pyramids. *(Right)* Oblique transabdominal ultrasound shows a small echogenic kidney ➡ with multiple cysts ➡. Note the loss of corticomedullary differentiation. The contralateral kidney was normal.

Multicystic Dysplastic Kidney

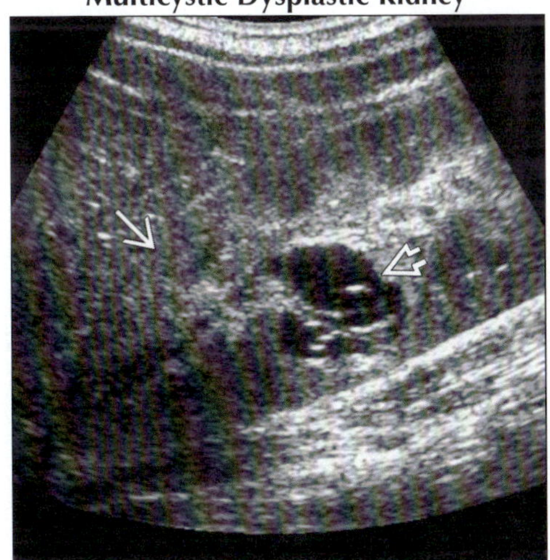

Tuberous Sclerosis

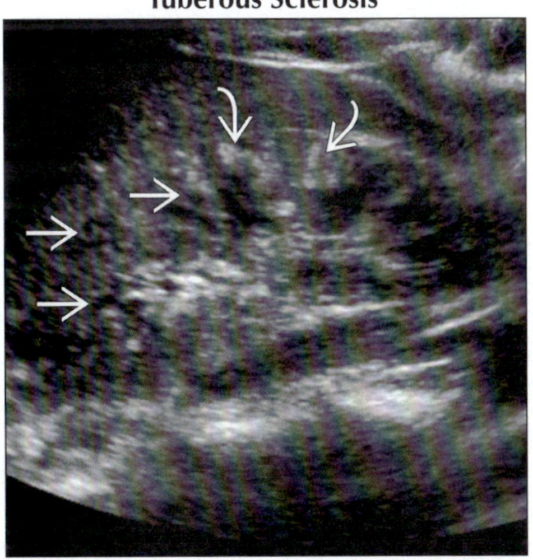

(Left) Oblique ultrasound shows a focal cystic area ➡ in an echogenic dysplastic kidney ➡ with reduced corticomedullary differentiation. This is a rare variant of multicystic dysplastic kidney. *(Right)* Longitudinal ultrasound shows multiple tiny renal cysts ➡ affecting the kidney in a patient with tuberous sclerosis. Tiny, echogenic, fat-containing, renal angiomyolipomas ➡ are also present. Similar changes were also seen in the contralateral kidney.

Congenital Megacalyces

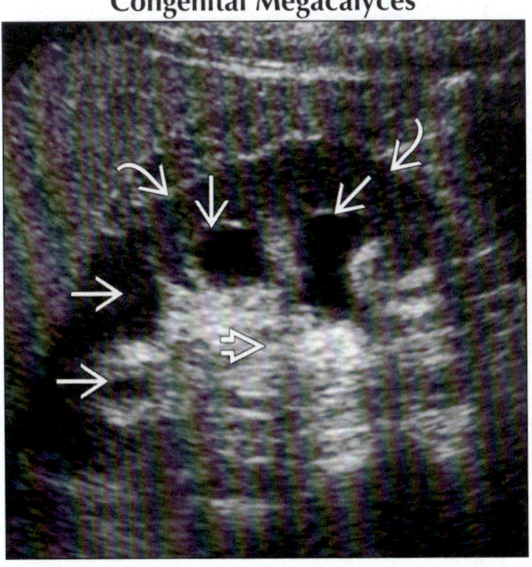

Perinephric Collection

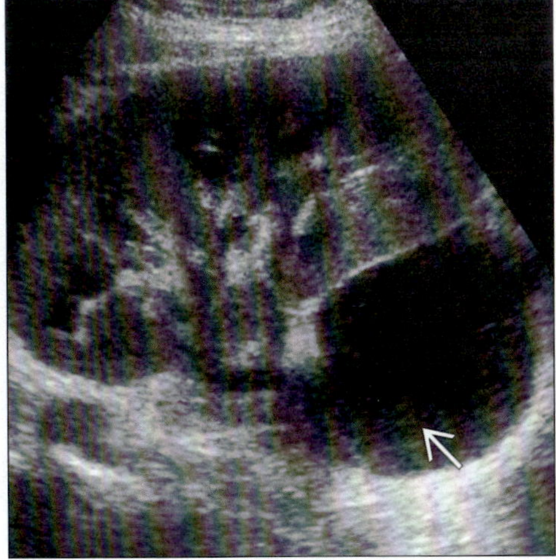

(Left) Oblique transabdominal ultrasound shows nonobstructive enlargement of calyces ➡. They have a polygonal shape differentiating them from cysts. The cortical thickness is normal ➡, and the renal pelvis ➡ is not dilated. *(Right)* Oblique transabdominal ultrasound shows an anechoic urinoma ➡ seen as a loculated perinephric fluid collection, indenting and causing distortion of the renal contour.

HYPO-/ISOECHOIC RENAL MASS

DIFFERENTIAL DIAGNOSIS

Common
- Renal Pseudotumor
  - Column of Bertin, Kidney
  - Dromedary Hump, Left Kidney
- Renal Cell Carcinoma
- Horseshoe Kidney
- Renal Metastases
- Wilms Tumor
- Renal Lymphoma
- Focal Bacterial Nephritis

Less Common
- Renal Tuberculosis
- Xanthogranulomatous Pyelonephritis
- Hematoma

ESSENTIAL INFORMATION

Key Differential Diagnosis Issues
- Do not mistake pseudotumor for true pathology
  - Pseudotumors are isoechoic to normal parenchyma and have normal kidney architecture
  - DMSA isotope scans aid diagnosis
    - Normal renal tissue takes up isotope, while renal tumor produces photo-deficient "cold" area
- Major role of US to identify solid renal tumor (excluding simple cortical cyst, which is most common renal mass)
- Look for signs of malignancy
  - Renal vein invasion, inferior vena cava (IVC) tumor thrombosis, regional lymphadenopathy, and liver metastasis
- Clinical history always helps
  - Consider infective causes in febrile patient; hematoma with trauma history

Helpful Clues for Common Diagnoses
- **Renal Pseudotumor**
  - **Column of Bertin, Kidney**
    - Hypertrophic medial bands of cortical tissue that separate pyramids of renal medulla
    - Best diagnostic clue: Isoechoic and continuous with renal cortex
    - Normal renal outline and normal vascularity on Doppler
  - **Dromedary Hump, Left Kidney**
    - Focal bulge in lateral border of left kidney midpole
    - Similar echopattern as rest of kidney
    - Best diagnostic clue: Calyces underlying hump extend into it
- **Renal Cell Carcinoma**
  - Most common primary renal malignancy
  - Variable grayscale US appearances: Solid or heterogeneous
  - Isoechoic (42%), hypoechoic (10%), hyperechoic (48%)
  - Large tumors tend to be hypoechoic, exophytic with anechoic necrotic areas
  - Color Doppler usually shows peripheral, intratumoral vascularity
  - Commonly associated with renal vein thrombosis (23%) and IVC tumor extension (7%)
- **Horseshoe Kidney**
  - Congenital anomaly of kidney where 2 kidneys are fused by isthmus at lower poles
  - Isthmus: Same echopattern as rest of kidney
    - Usually anterior to aorta and IVC at L4/5 level
  - Elongated kidneys, lower poles poorly defined with curved configuration
- **Renal Metastases**
  - Most common of primary cancers: Lung > breast > gastrointestinal tract
  - Usually small and round, occasionally wedge-shaped, mimics infarction
  - Usually intraparenchymal; rarely disrupts renal contour or capsule
  - Variable echogenicity, but majority are hypoechoic
  - Color Doppler: Mostly avascular or hypovascular
  - Look for other evidence of disseminated disease, e.g., liver, lymph node, lung involvement
- **Wilms Tumor**
  - Most common primary renal tumor in children > 1 year old, most presenting < 5 years of age
  - Well-circumscribed mass with hyper-/hypoechoic rim (pseudocapsule) compressing renal tissue
  - May contain areas of necrosis, hemorrhage, fat, and calcification

8

- ○ Tumor spread similar to renal cell carcinoma
  - ▪ Extension into renal vein, IVC, metastases to local lymph nodes, liver, or lung
- **Renal Lymphoma**
  - ○ Mainly by hematogenous spread (90%) or direct extension via retroperitoneal lymphatic channels
  - ○ Variable manifestations: Solitary, multiple, direct invasion, diffuse infiltration, or perirenal invasion
  - ○ Lesions are often hypoechoic or near anechoic (pseudocystic)
  - ○ Solitary: Focal hypoechoic mass indistinct from renal cell carcinoma
  - ○ Multiple: Usually bilateral, hypoechoic renal masses
  - ○ Infrequently associated with renal vein and IVC tumor thrombosis
- **Focal Bacterial Nephritis**
  - ○ Hypoechoic lesions due to liquefaction and abscess formation
  - ○ Usually wedge-shaped, poorly defined margin, ↓ focal vascularity on Doppler
  - ○ May have increased echogenicity due to hemorrhage
  - ○ Other associated features of renal inflammation: Renal enlargement, urothelial thickening of renal pelvis

Helpful Clues for Less Common Diagnoses
- **Renal Tuberculosis**
  - ○ Urinary tract infection by *Mycobacterium tuberculosis* via hematogenous spread from primary focus, usually lungs
  - ○ May be associated with ureteral and bladder disease
  - ○ Variable grayscale US appearance
    - ▪ Early stage: Multiple, hypoechoic, cortical lesions with poorly defined border ± calcifications
    - ▪ Progressive stage: Irregular hypoechoic mass, connecting to collecting system with distorted renal parenchyma
- **Xanthogranulomatous Pyelonephritis**
  - ○ Chronic renal inflammation associated with longstanding urinary calculus and obstruction (75%)
  - ○ Characterized by destruction and replacement of renal parenchyma by lipid-laden macrophages
  - ○ Anechoic/hypoechoic masses replacing normal parenchyma, ± abscesses
  - ○ Associated with highly reflective central echocomplex containing calculus
- **Hematoma**
  - ○ May be hypoechoic, hyperechoic, or heterogeneous depending on age of hematoma
  - ○ May be associated with perirenal fluid collection (subcapsular hematoma)
  - ○ History of blunt abdominal trauma or renal intervention suggests diagnosis, usually presents with acute flank pain

Renal Pseudotumor

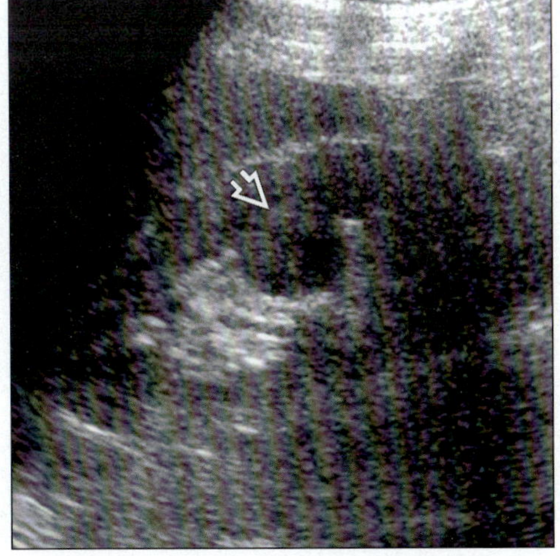

Longitudinal transabdominal ultrasound shows a column of Bertin ➡, which is isoechoic and continuous with the renal cortex. Note the smooth renal outline.

Renal Cell Carcinoma

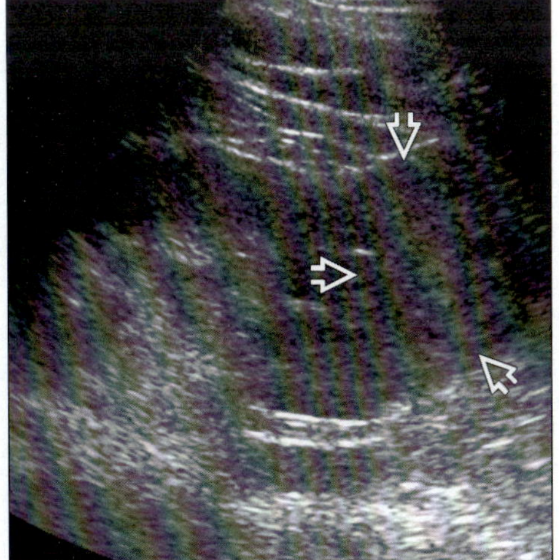

Oblique transabdominal ultrasound shows a fairly homogeneous isoechoic mass ➡ arising from the lower pole of the kidney. There is no intralesional cystic component or calcification.

HYPO-/ISOECHOIC RENAL MASS

(Left) Longitudinal transabdominal ultrasound shows a hypoechoic renal cell carcinoma ⮞. Note the disruption of the central sinus echo complex by the mass ⮞ but no associated hydronephrosis. (Right) Longitudinal power Doppler ultrasound shows an infiltrative, hypoechoic renal cell carcinoma ⮞ at the upper pole of kidney. There is a sparse intratumoral vascular signal ⮞. Residual normal renal parenchyma ➔ is noted at the lower pole.

Renal Cell Carcinoma

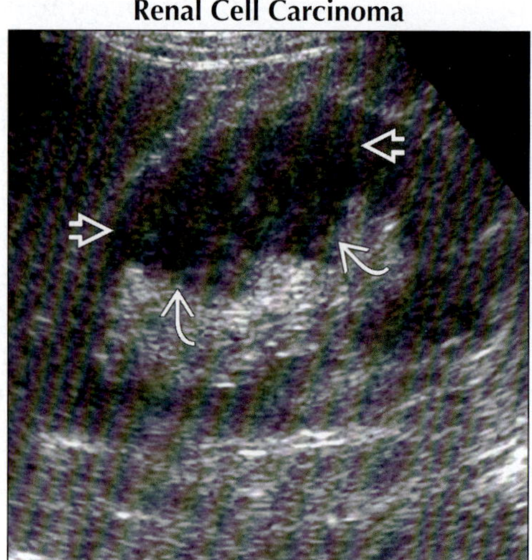

Renal Cell Carcinoma

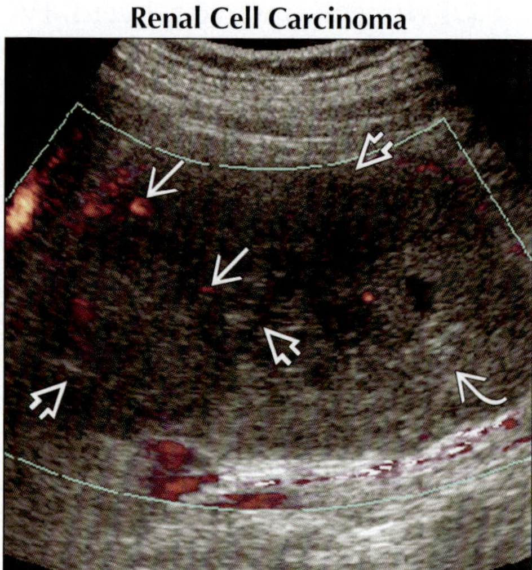

(Left) Longitudinal transabdominal ultrasound shows a low-lying right kidney with an elongated and poorly defined lower pole ⮞. (Right) Transverse color Doppler ultrasound shows the isthmus ➔ crossing the midline anterior to the inferior vena cava ⮞ and aorta ➔.

Horseshoe Kidney

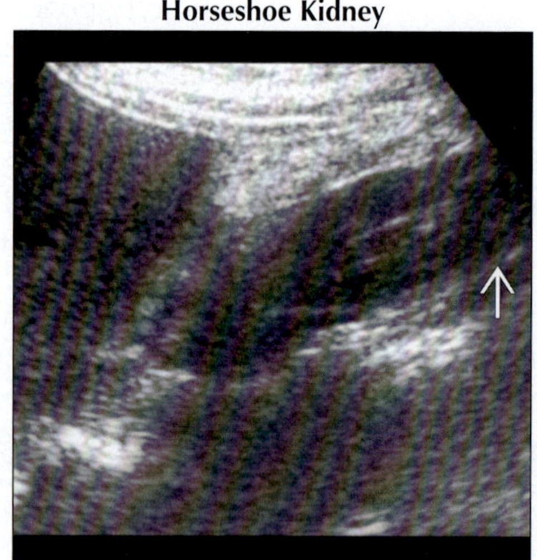

Horseshoe Kidney

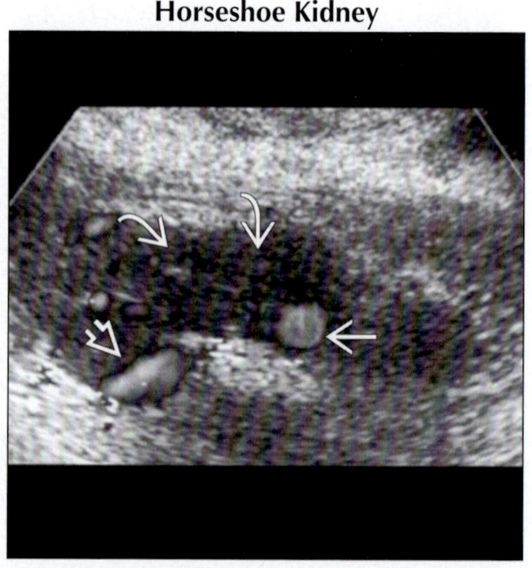

(Left) Transverse transabdominal ultrasound shows a well-defined hypoechoic mass ⮞ at the mid-pole of the kidney in this patient with lung carcinoma and disseminated metastases. (Right) Transverse color Doppler ultrasound shows the renal metastasis ⮞ in the same patient. The lesion is avascular and situated next to the normal vasculature ➔ without significant displacement.

Renal Metastases

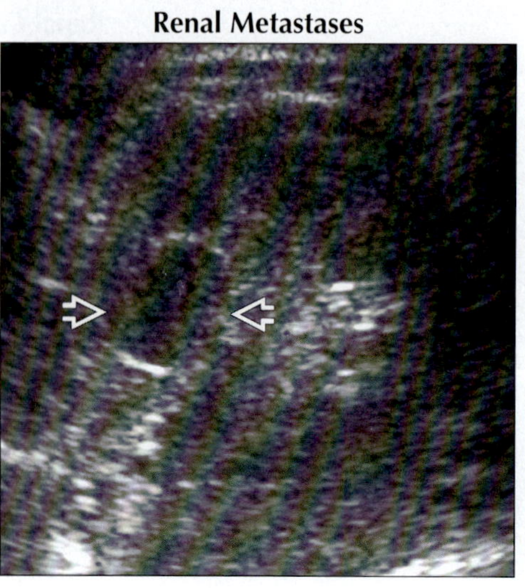

Renal Metastases

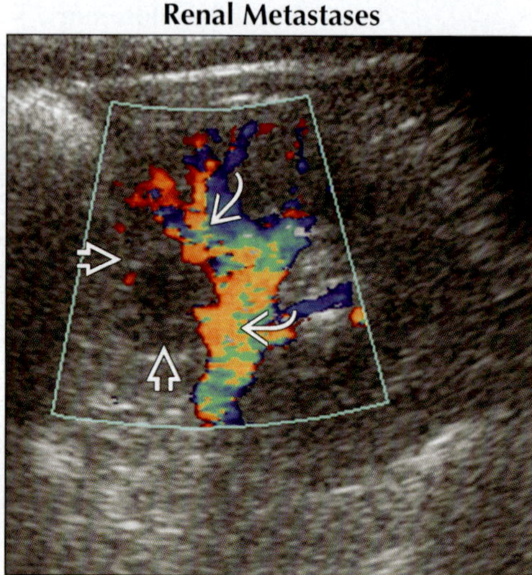

HYPO-/ISOECHOIC RENAL MASS

Wilms Tumor

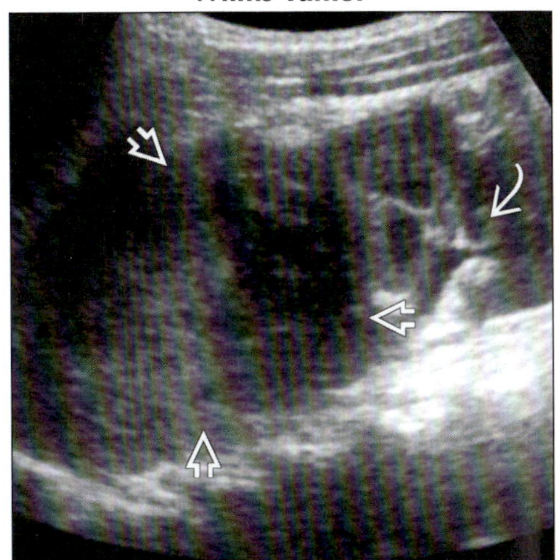

Renal Lymphoma

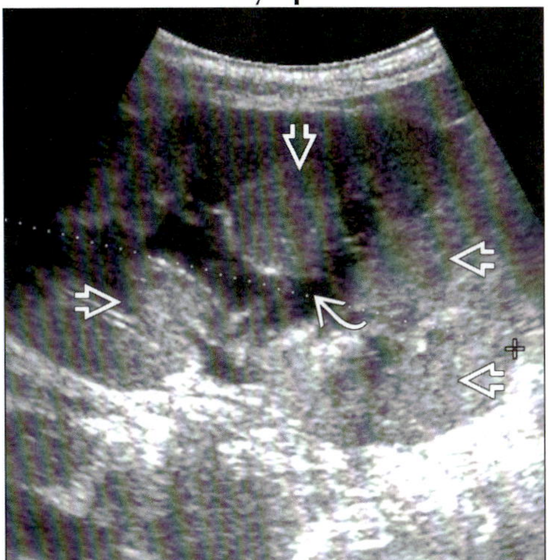

(Left) Longitudinal transabdominal ultrasound shows a large, heterogeneous, hypoechoic mass ⮞ arising from the upper kidney pole in a 4-year-old child. There is mild compressive hydronephrosis ➡. (Right) Longitudinal transabdominal ultrasound shows enlargement of the kidney with diffuse infiltration by hypo-/isoechoic masses ⮞. Note the loss of normal corticomedullary differentiation. The collecting system is mildly dilated ➡.

Focal Bacterial Nephritis

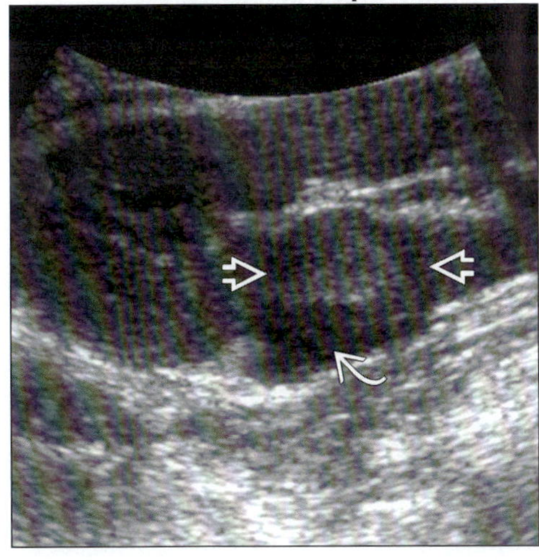

Focal Bacterial Nephritis

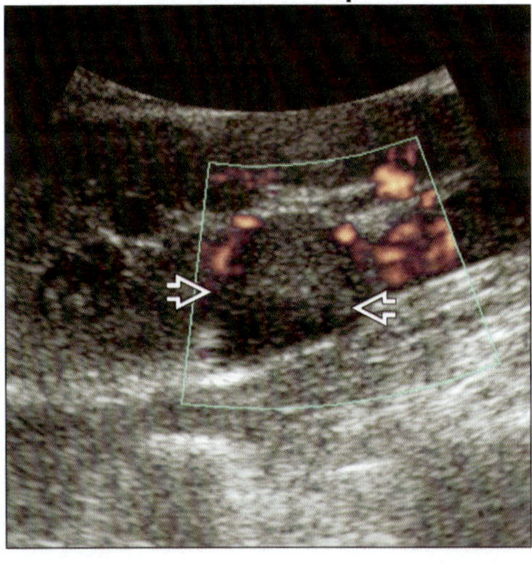

(Left) Longitudinal transabdominal ultrasound shows isoechoic to hypoechoic focal bacterial nephritis ⮞ in a febrile patient with flank pain. The hypoechoic component ➡ may represent liquefaction. (Right) Longitudinal power Doppler ultrasound shows a parenchymal vascular defect at the site of focal bacterial nephritis ⮞. In a proper clinical setting, sonographic findings are diagnostic of focal bacterial nephritis.

Renal Tuberculosis

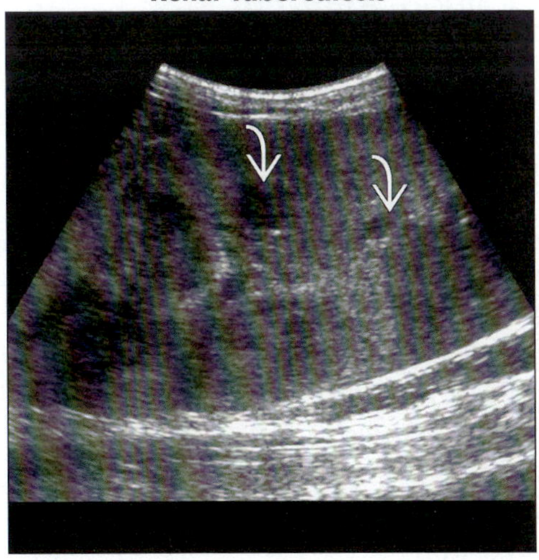

Xanthogranulomatous Pyelonephritis

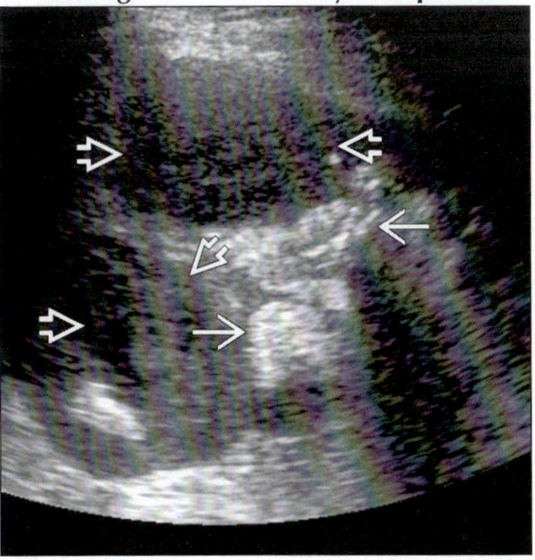

(Left) Longitudinal transabdominal ultrasound shows renal tuberculosis with distorted renal parenchyma. There are small, irregular, hypoechoic lesions ➡, which represent cavities connecting to the collecting system. (Right) Oblique transabdominal ultrasound shows diffuse xanthogranulomatous pyelonephritis. The kidney is enlarged, and the parenchyma is replaced by round hypoechoic masses ⮞. Calculi ➡ are seen obstructing the renal pelvis.

COMPLEX CYSTIC RENAL MASS

DIFFERENTIAL DIAGNOSIS

Common
- Hemorrhagic Cyst
- Septated Benign Cyst
- Milk of Calcium Cyst
- Calcified Cyst
- Infected Cyst
- Proteinaceous Cyst
- Renal Abscess
- Pyonephrosis

Less Common
- Cystic Renal Cell Carcinoma
- Transitional Cell Carcinoma
- Renal Papillary Necrosis
- Multilocular Cystic Nephroma
- Hematoma
- Renal Trauma
- Hydatid Cyst

ESSENTIAL INFORMATION

Key Differential Diagnosis Issues
- Either follow-up US or CT should be performed depending on level of suspicion
- Serial US follow-up probably sufficient if benign features present, such as
  - Low-amplitude internal echoes
  - Thin septation
  - Small amount of calcium
  - Milk of calcium
- CT ± surgical removal should be performed if features suspicious of malignancy present, such as
  - Thickened wall or mural nodularity
  - Septal irregularity and nodularity
  - Multiple complex septations
  - Solid mass at septal wall attachment
  - Extensive septal calcification
  - Thick, irregular, or amorphous calcification
  - Cyst wall/septum obscured by shadowing from calcifications
- Bosniak CT classification for renal cysts
  - Class I: Benign cysts (well defined, round, homogeneous, avascular, thin walled)
  - Class II: Minimally complicated cysts (mildly irregular, calcified, septae, avascular, hyperdense, ≤ 3 cm)
  - Class IIF: Likely benign (hyperdense, thick or nodular calcification in wall or septa, vaguely enhanced) but requires follow-up
  - Class III: Indeterminate
  - Class IV: Malignant lesions with large cystic or necrotic components (irregular wall thickening or enhancing mass)

Helpful Clues for Common Diagnoses
- **Hemorrhagic Cyst**
  - Appearance varies with age of blood
  - May appear as anechoic solid septate lesion or with fluid-debris level
  - Chronic lesion may be multiloculated ± thick calcified wall
- **Septated Benign Cyst**
  - Bosniak II and IIF
  - May be result of prior hemorrhage
- **Milk of Calcium Cyst**
  - "Comet tail" artifact
  - Calcification may layer creating fluid-debris level
- **Calcified Cyst**
  - Wall or septal calcification ± shadowing
- **Infected Cyst**
  - Infection in preexisting cyst
  - Thick wall with scattered internal echoes
  - ± debris-fluid level, representing pus
- **Proteinaceous Cyst**
  - May contain low-level echoes with bright reflectors or even layers of echoes
  - May simulate renal abscess or hemorrhagic cyst
- **Renal Abscess**
  - Develops from untreated or inadequately treated acute pyelonephritis
  - Characterized by parenchymal necrosis and hence abscess formation
  - Round, thick-walled, complex cystic mass with internal echoes, debris
  - Gas with irregular shadowing may present occasionally
  - Usually solitary; may spontaneously decompress into collecting system or perinephric space
  - Clinically febrile and septic patient
  - Risk factors include diabetes, urinary tract obstruction, infected renal stone, or immunocompromise
- **Pyonephrosis**
  - Purulent material within obstructed collecting system

COMPLEX CYSTIC RENAL MASS

- ○ Presence of mobile debris and layering of low-amplitude echoes in hydronephrotic kidney
- ○ Echogenic pus layering in dependent portion of collecting system
- ○ Gas and calculi may be present
- ○ Associated with thickening of urothelial lining of renal pelvis or ureter

Helpful Clues for Less Common Diagnoses
- **Cystic Renal Cell Carcinoma**
  - ○ Rare (< 5%) form of renal cell carcinoma
  - ○ Unilocular form
    - ▪ Hypoechoic mass with fluid-debris levels (hemorrhage and necrosis)
    - ▪ Thick and irregular wall
  - ○ Multilocular form
    - ▪ Multiple thick septations with nodules ± calcifications
  - ○ Solid tumor with extensive cystic necrosis
    - ▪ Debris-filled cystic spaces; appearance varies with degree of necrosis
- **Transitional Cell Carcinoma**
  - ○ May present as intraluminal soft tissue mass within dilated calyx, mimicking complex cystic mass
- **Renal Papillary Necrosis**
  - ○ Late stage: Multiple cystic cavities in medullary pyramids ± nonshadowing echogenic sloughed papillae
  - ○ Calcified sloughed papilla with strong acoustic shadowing simulates calculus; may cause obstructive hydronephrosis
- **Multilocular Cystic Nephroma**
  - ○ Nonhereditary benign cystic renal neoplasm
  - ○ Multiple noncommunicating anechoic cysts within well-defined mass
  - ○ Hyperechoic septa and fibrous capsule
    - ▪ Fine vessels may be seen within septae on Doppler
  - ○ No intracystic mural nodule
- **Hematoma**
  - ○ Variable appearance depending on time of injury
  - ○ Chronic form may simulate complex cyst with internal echoes ± calcification
- **Renal Trauma**
  - ○ Renal laceration appears as linear defect extending through kidney, associated with perirenal collection
  - ○ Subcapsular hematoma: Perirenal fluid collection flattens renal contour
  - ○ Shattered kidney: Multiple fragments of disorganized tissue within blood and urine collections
- **Hydatid Cyst**
  - ○ Simple or multiloculated with endocyst and membranes; calcified or solid (chronic)
  - ○ Mural nodularity suggests scolices
  - ○ Membrane of endocyst detaches and precipitates to form "hydatid sand"
  - ○ Calcification may resemble "eggshell" or reticular pattern
  - ○ Consider diagnosis in endemic region

Hemorrhagic Cyst

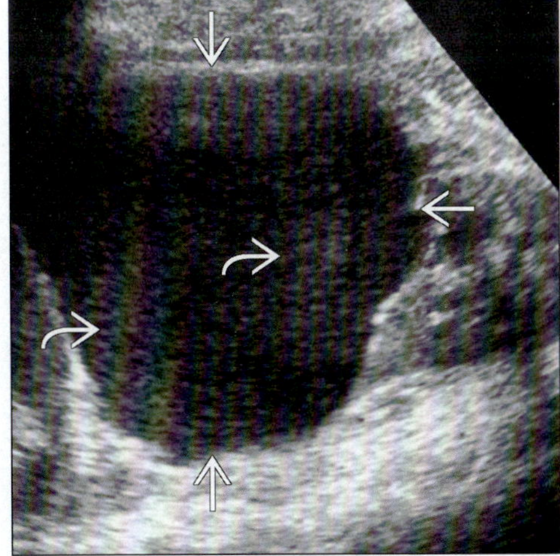

Oblique transabdominal ultrasound shows a large hemorrhagic cyst ➡ at the upper pole of the kidney with low-level echoes ➡ within the cyst.

Septated Benign Cyst

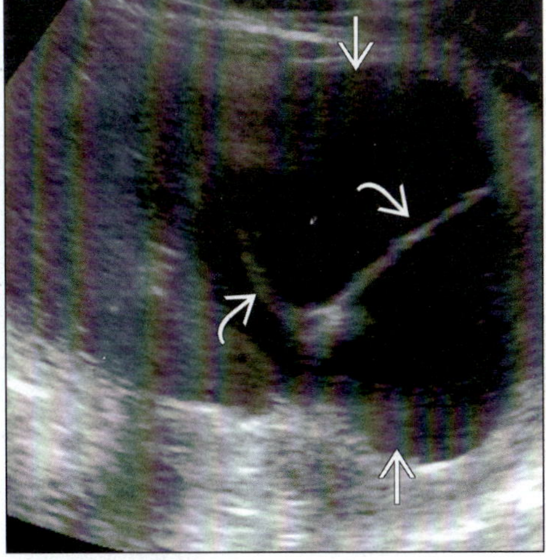

Oblique transabdominal ultrasound shows a large septated cyst ➡. Note that the septae ➡ are uniformly thin. There are no other solid components or echoes within the cystic compartments.

COMPLEX CYSTIC RENAL MASS

(Left) Transverse color Doppler ultrasound shows no color signal present within this cyst or along the septae, findings compatible with a benign cyst. *(Right)* Longitudinal transabdominal ultrasound shows a milk of calcium cyst ➡ at the upper pole of the kidney with characteristic "comet tail" artifacts ➡ posterior to the cyst. Another simple anechoic cyst ➡ is seen at the lower pole.

Septated Benign Cyst
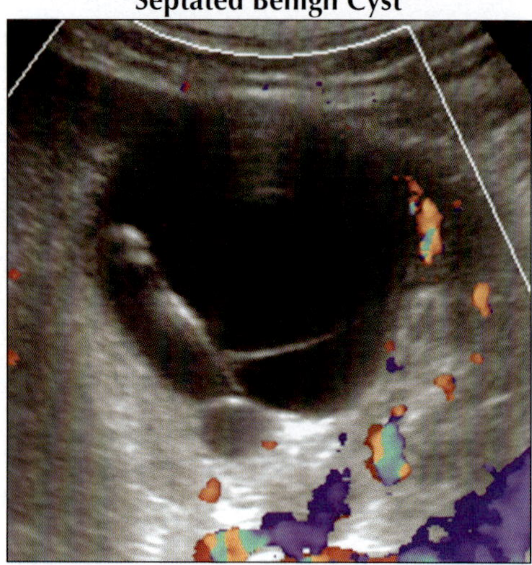

Milk of Calcium Cyst
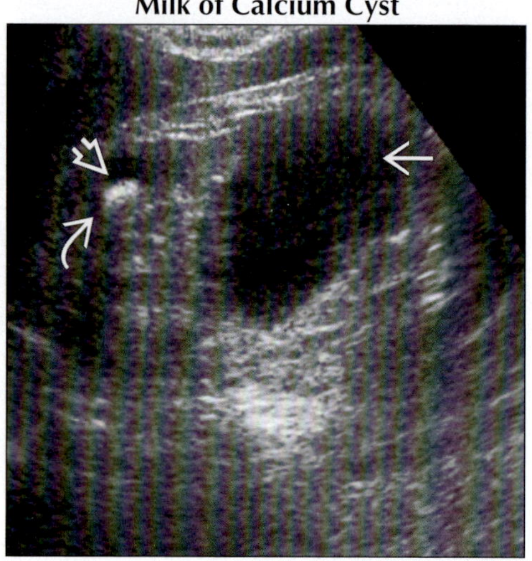

(Left) Longitudinal transabdominal ultrasound shows a milk of calcium cyst ➡ at the lower pole of the kidney with a characteristic "comet tail" artifact ➡ posterior to the cyst. *(Right)* Longitudinal transabdominal ultrasound shows a debris-fluid level ➡ representing pus in an infected cyst ➡ at the upper pole of the kidney.

Milk of Calcium Cyst
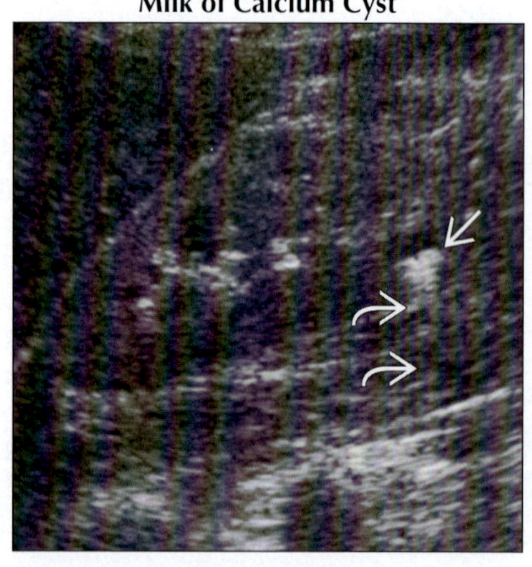

Infected Cyst
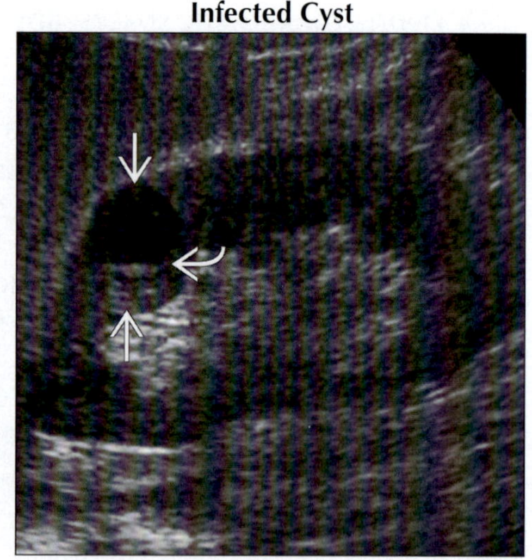

(Left) Transverse transabdominal ultrasound shows a well-defined cystic lesion ➡ with internal debris ➡. This patient presented with a high fever, suggesting an acute infective cause. *(Right)* Oblique transabdominal ultrasound shows a complex cystic mass with internal debris ➡ and septae ➡, compatible with a renal abscess, in a patient with a fever and elevated white blood cell count.

Renal Abscess
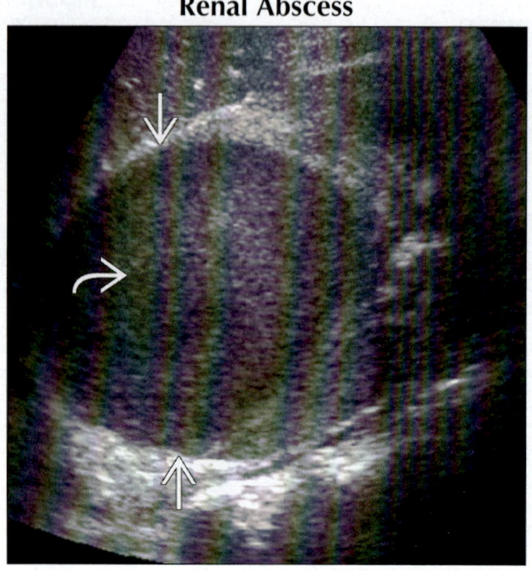

Renal Abscess
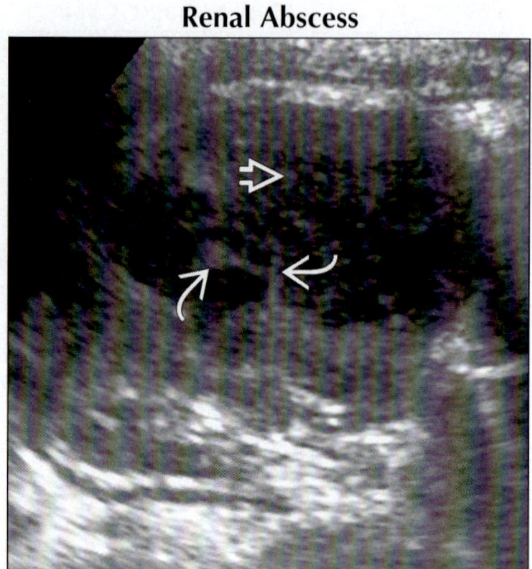

COMPLEX CYSTIC RENAL MASS

Pyonephrosis

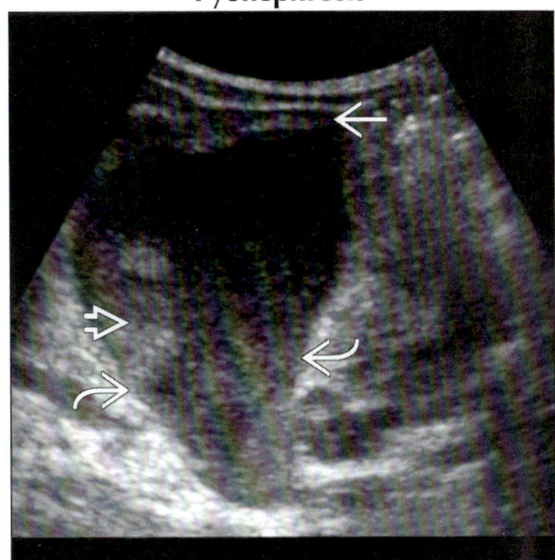

Pyonephrosis

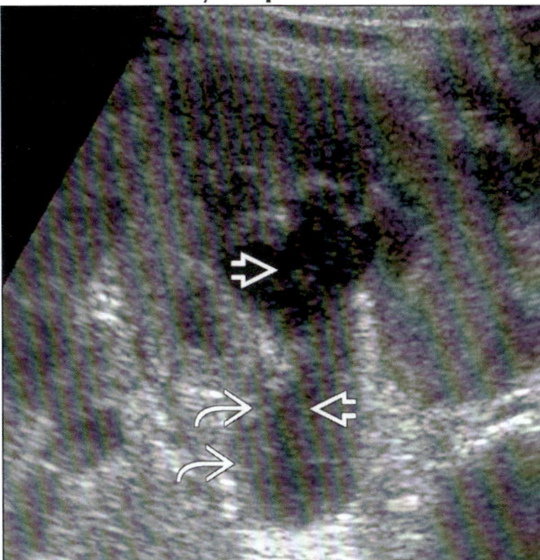

(Left) Transverse transabdominal ultrasound shows a chronically obstructed collecting system complicated by an infection. Echogenic pus ⮞ is present within the markedly dilated renal pelvis ➔. Note the marked thinning of the renal cortex ➔. (Right) Transverse transabdominal ultrasound shows echogenic pus ⮞ within the dilated calyceal system. There is urothelial thickening ➔ lining the renal pelvis.

Cystic Renal Cell Carcinoma

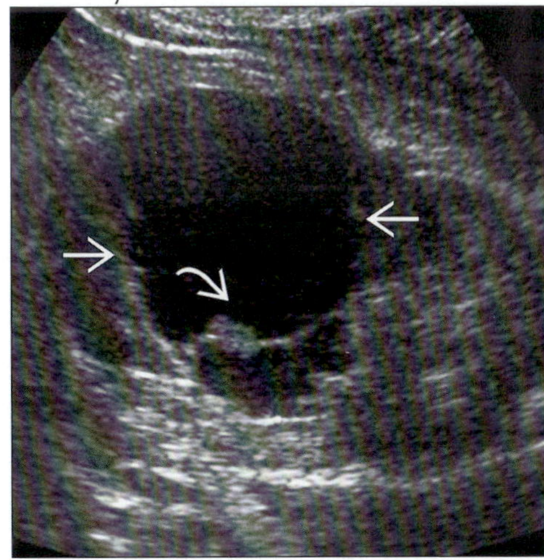

Cystic Renal Cell Carcinoma

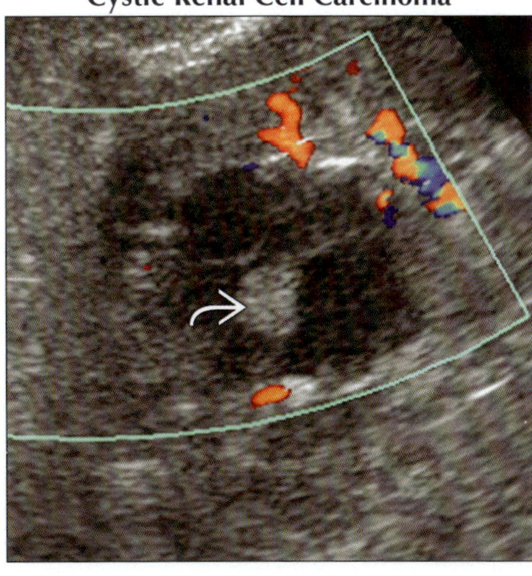

(Left) Longitudinal transabdominal ultrasound shows a mid-pole complex renal cyst ➔ with a nodule ➔ arising from the thick septum. Nodularity and thick septations are suspicious features for neoplasia. (Right) Transverse color Doppler ultrasound shows no demonstrable vascularity within the intracystic nodule ➔. However, contrast-enhanced CT is the recommended imaging modality to look for enhancement of the nodule.

Cystic Renal Cell Carcinoma

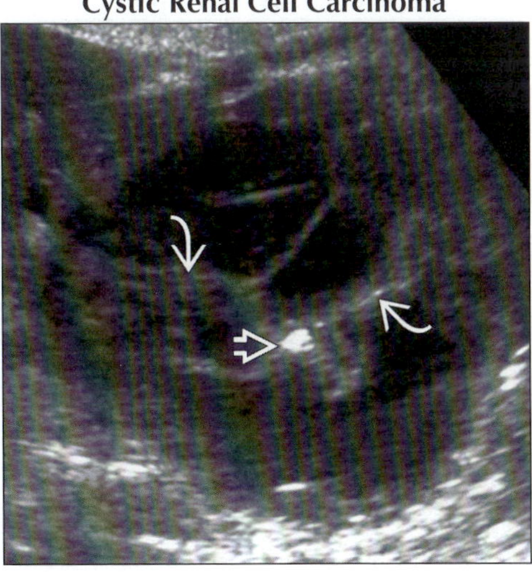

Cystic Renal Cell Carcinoma

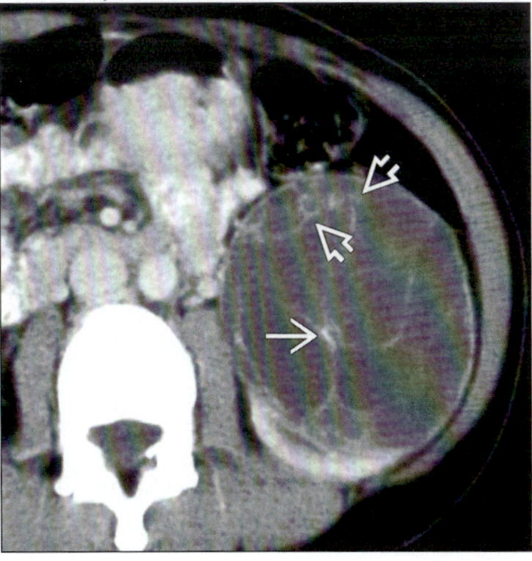

(Left) Oblique transabdominal ultrasound shows a large, multilocular, cystic renal cell carcinoma occupying the mid-lower pole of the left kidney. The tumor contains thick septations ➔ and septal calcification ⮞. (Right) CECT in the same patient shows the cystic renal cell carcinoma arising from the left kidney. Note the enhancing nodularity ⮞ and septal calcification ➔.

COMPLEX CYSTIC RENAL MASS

(Left) Longitudinal transabdominal ultrasound shows dilated calyces ➡, filled with echoes while the dilated renal pelvis contains a solid mass ➡. Histology confirmed transitional cell carcinoma arising from the renal pelvis. (Right) Longitudinal transabdominal ultrasound shows multiple cystic lesions ➡ representing dilated clubbed calyces. The necrotic papilla appears as an echogenic focus ➡ in the medullary pyramid surrounded by fluid.

Transitional Cell Carcinoma

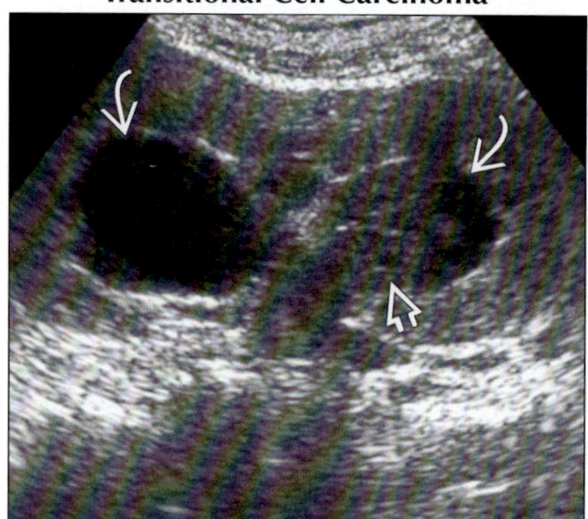

Renal Papillary Necrosis

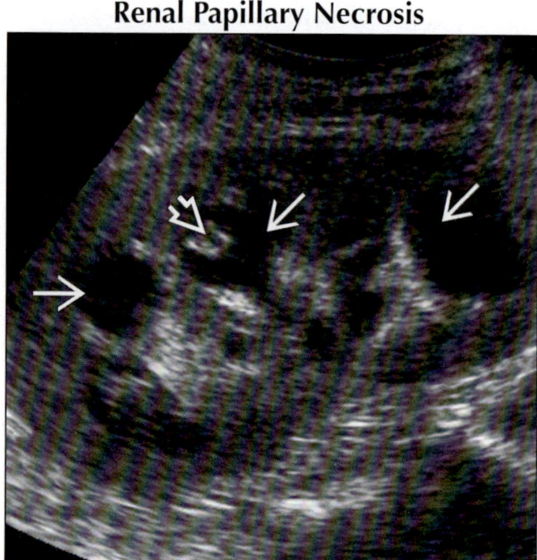

(Left) Longitudinal ultrasound shows multiple anechoic cysts separated by echogenic septae ➡. Portions of the lesion appear more solid ➡ due to multiple acoustic interfaces of numerous tiny cysts. (Right) Axial CECT shows a multiloculated, septated cystic mass occupying almost the entire left kidney with minimal, residual, functioning parenchymal tissue ➡. Note the enhancing septae ➡ and normal contralateral kidney.

Multilocular Cystic Nephroma

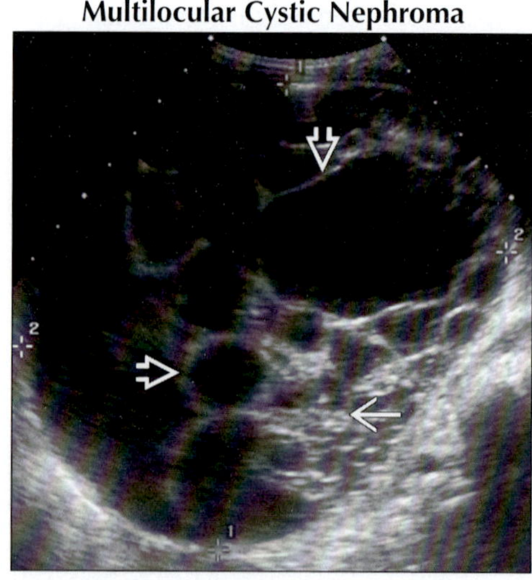

Multilocular Cystic Nephroma

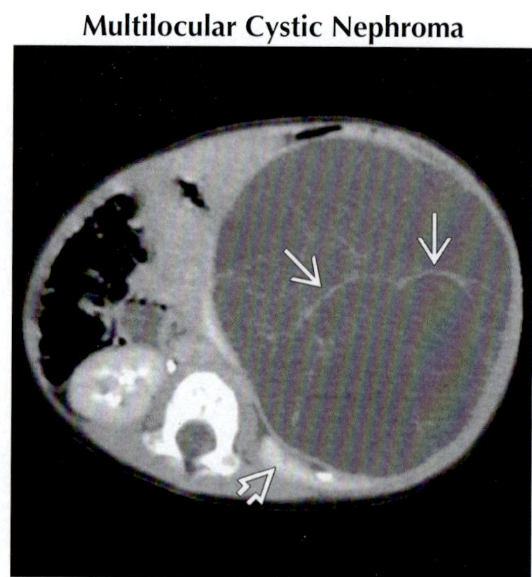

(Left) Oblique transabdominal ultrasound shows a variant of focal multilocular cystic nephroma. A septated cystic lesion ➡ occupies only the upper pole of the kidney. Otherwise the overall appearance is similar to the previous image. Such focal involvement of the kidney is rare. (Right) Oblique color Doppler ultrasound shows fine vessels ➡ within the echogenic septae.

Multilocular Cystic Nephroma

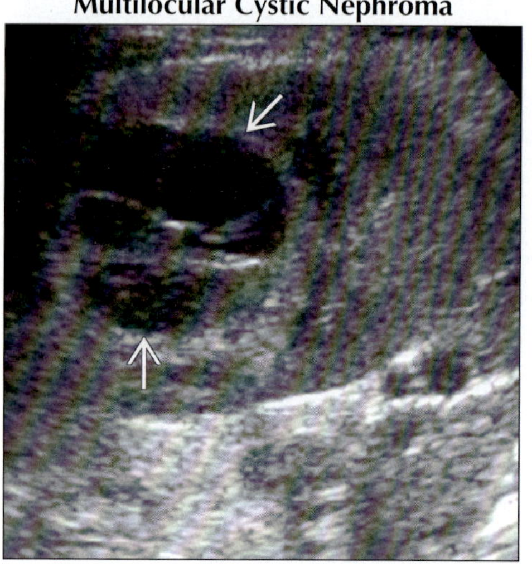

Multilocular Cystic Nephroma

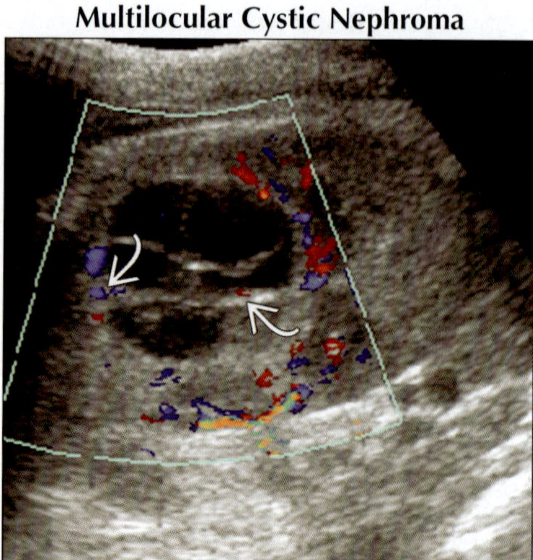

COMPLEX CYSTIC RENAL MASS

Hematoma

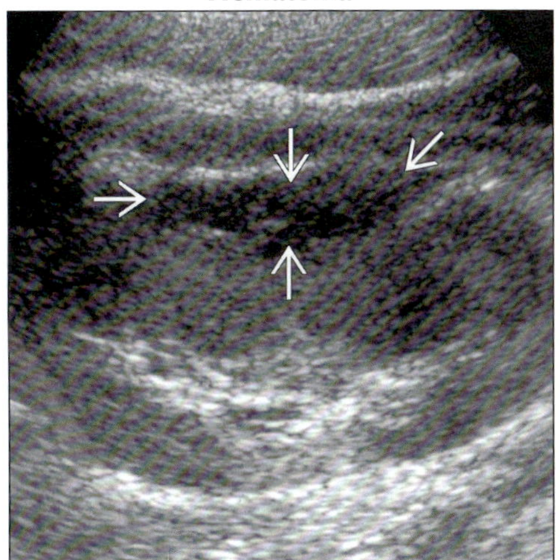

Hematoma

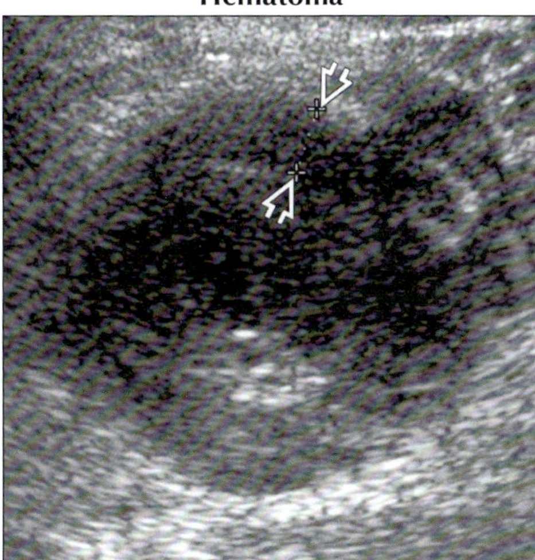

(Left) Longitudinal transabdominal ultrasound shows a perinephric cystic abnormality with internal echoes ➡ in a patient presenting with acute groin pain after a renal biopsy. (Right) Transverse transabdominal ultrasound shows the same crescentic collection ➡. In view of the recent biopsy, this is most likely a hematoma.

Renal Trauma

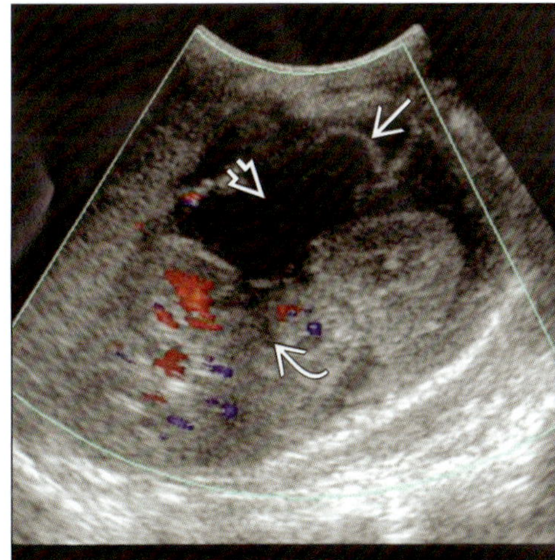

Renal Trauma

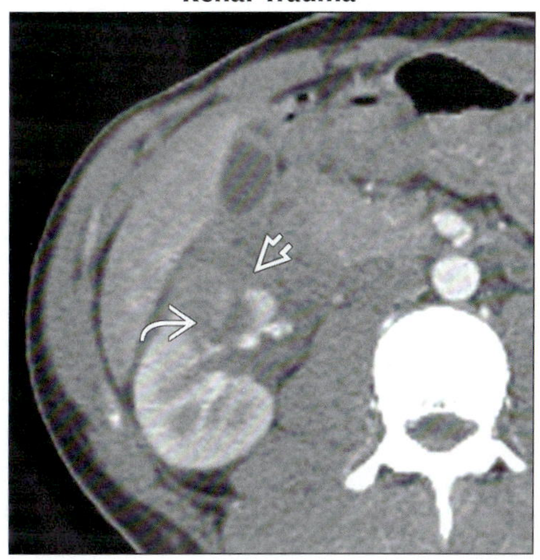

(Left) Longitudinal color Doppler ultrasound shows a cortical laceration ➡ extending into the calyceal system. The lower pole is distorted with fragments ➡ floating within a subcapsular hematoma ➡. (Right) Corresponding axial CECT shows the complete cortical laceration ➡ of the right kidney and adjacent subcapsular hematoma ➡.

Hydatid Cyst

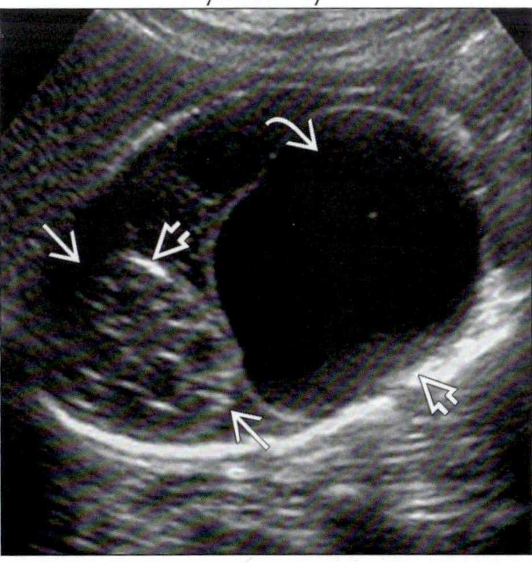

Hydatid Cyst

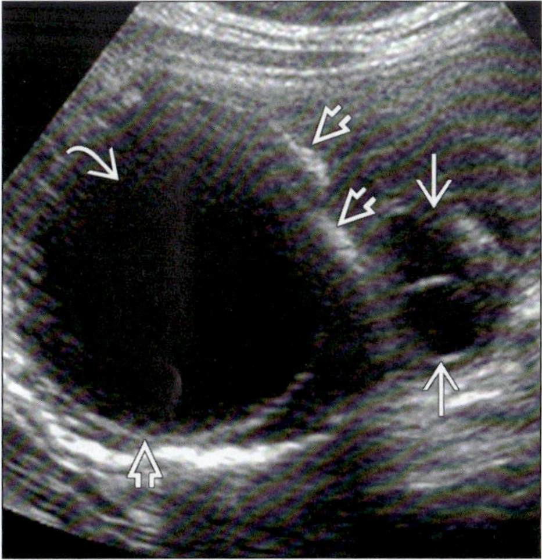

(Left) Longitudinal transabdominal ultrasound shows a renal hydatid cyst as a multiloculated cyst with an endocyst ➡ and daughter cysts ➡. "Eggshell" and cyst wall calcifications are also seen ➡. (Right) Oblique transabdominal ultrasound shows the same well-developed hydatid cyst, with an endocyst ➡ embedded in the calcified wall ➡ adjacent to the daughter cyst ➡.

DIFFERENTIAL DIAGNOSIS

Common
- Renal Angiomyolipoma (AML)
- Renal Cell Carcinoma (RCC)
- Wilms Tumor

Less Common
- Fat in Renal Scar
- Milk of Calcium Cyst
- Renal Junctional Line/Cortical Parenchymal Defect
- Renal Calculi
- Renal Papillary Necrosis
- Renal Abscess
- Emphysematous Pyelonephritis
- Renal Metastases

Rare but Important
- Focal Bacterial Nephritis
- Xanthogranulomatous Pyelonephritis
- Tuberculosis, Urinary Tract
- Renal Oncocytoma
- Renal Trauma

ESSENTIAL INFORMATION

Key Differential Diagnosis Issues
- Lesions that cause fat density (intensity) lesions on CT and MR usually produce echogenic lesions on US
  - However, echogenicity alone is not reliable indicator of fat content
  - Other sources of renal echogenicity include calcification and gas
  - Lesions with calcification: Milk of calcium cyst, RCC, Wilms tumor
  - Lesions with gas: Renal abscess, emphysematous pyelonephritis

Helpful Clues for Common Diagnoses
- **Renal Angiomyolipoma (AML)**
  - Well-defined hyperechoic mass, similar to renal sinus
  - Echogenicity created by high fat content and multiple vessel-tissue interfaces
  - May have posterior acoustic shadowing not typically seen with other masses
  - Small lesion: AML has much higher echogenicity than RCC
  - Larger tumors usually have prominent vascularity, visible on color Doppler
  - May have central necrosis simulating malignant lesion
  - US alone not reliable in diagnosing AML; requires NECT or CECT confirmation
- **Renal Cell Carcinoma (RCC)**
  - 30% of small RCCs appear as hyperechoic masses, mimic AML
    - Presence of necrosis in mass or anechoic rim favors RCC, but large overlap exists
  - Larger RCC may have foci of calcification (also echogenic), rarely fat
  - Mass with calcification and fat in adult = RCC, not AML
- **Wilms Tumor**
  - Highly variable morphology, including echogenic foci (fat &/or calcification)
  - Heterogeneous echopattern with areas of necrosis or hemorrhage
  - Consider Wilms for any renal mass in child (most present before age 5)

Helpful Clues for Less Common Diagnoses
- **Fat in Renal Scar**
  - Example: Following partial nephrectomy
    - Fat may be placed into cortical defect
- **Milk of Calcium Cyst**
  - Echogenic lesion associated with characteristic "comet tail"/ring-down artifact
  - Calcification may layer creating fluid-debris level
- **Renal Junctional Line/Cortical Parenchymal Defect**
  - Echogenic line at anterosuperior aspect, upper pole of right kidney, lower pole of left kidney
    - Infolding of renal capsule and fat creates hyperechoic line or "mass"
  - Can also see extension of renal sinus fat into same location
  - Less commonly appears as triangular focus known as parenchymal defect
- **Renal Calculi**
  - Usually hyperechoic with sharp shadowing
  - Calculi or milk of calcium may form within calyceal diverticulum, mimicking hyperechoic mass
  - Most stones show color and power Doppler "twinkling" artifacts
    - Useful ancillary finding in equivocal cases
- **Renal Papillary Necrosis**

- Early stage: Echogenic "ring" in medulla = necrotic papillae, surrounded by rim of fluid
- Late stage: Multiple cystic cavities in medullary pyramids ± nonshadowing echogenic sloughed papillae
- Calcified sloughed papilla with strong acoustic shadowing simulates stone, may cause obstructive hydronephrosis
- **Renal Abscess**
  - Gas-forming abscess is echogenic
- **Emphysematous Pyelonephritis**
  - Gas within infarcted, infected parenchyma is echogenic
    - Nondependent linear echos with posterior ring-down artifact and "dirty" shadowing
  - Extremely ill patient with fever, flank pain, and electrolyte imbalance
  - Different from emphysematous pyelitis where gas is limited to renal pelvis and calyces (less serious diagnosis)
- **Renal Metastases**
  - Variable echogenicity, typically hypoperfused masses
  - Look for metastases in other organs
  - Most common primary tumors include lung carcinoma, breast carcinoma, contralateral RCC

Helpful Clues for Rare Diagnoses
- **Focal Bacterial Nephritis**
  - Increased echogenicity is related to hemorrhage
- Usually wedge-shaped, poorly defined margin, ↓ focal vascularity on power Doppler
- Can be hypoechoic due to liquefaction and abscess formation
- Can be multiple lesions with patchy heterogeneous renal parenchyma
- Other associated features of renal inflammation: Renal enlargement, urothelial thickening of renal pelvis
- **Xanthogranulomatous Pyelonephritis**
  - Highly reflective central echo complex with strong shadowing corresponding to large stone
  - Echogenicity depends on amount of debris and necrosis within mass
- **Tuberculosis, Urinary Tract**
  - Active stage: Papillary destruction with echogenic masses near calyces
  - Late stage: Calcified granuloma or dense dystrophic calcification associated with shrunken kidneys
- **Renal Oncocytoma**
  - Cannot be differentiated from RCC on imaging
  - Variable in echogenicity; may contain central scar, central necrosis, or calcification
- **Renal Trauma**
  - Hematoma can be hyperechoic or heterogeneous during acute phase
  - Regional distortion of corticomedullary differentiation

Renal Angiomyolipoma (AML)

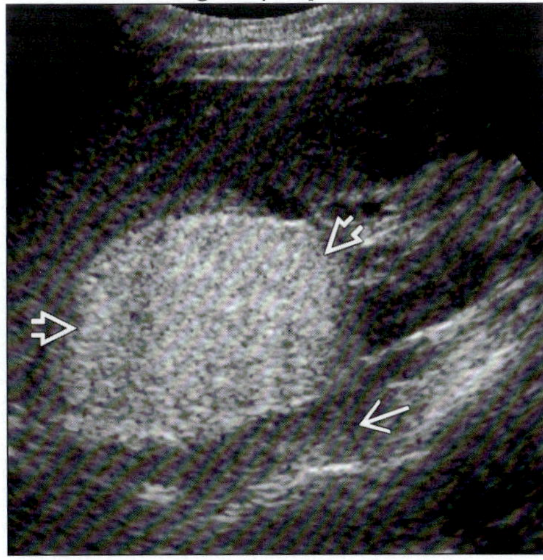

Longitudinal transabdominal ultrasound shows a typical large, homogeneous, hyperechoic mass ⊡ at the upper pole of the right kidney. Note the faint posterior acoustic shadowing ⊡.

Renal Angiomyolipoma (AML)

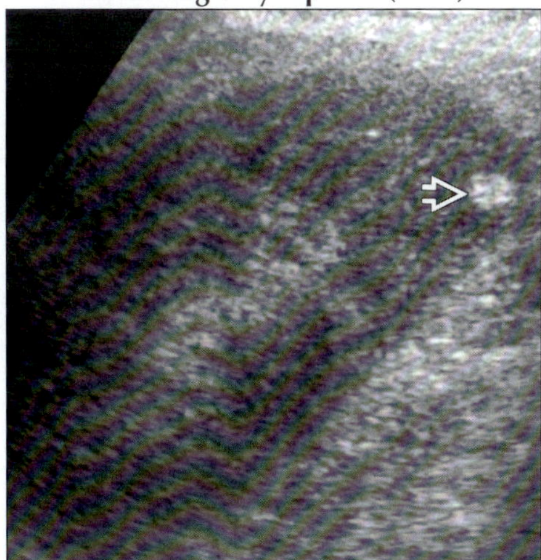

Oblique transabdominal ultrasound shows a typical small, homogeneous, echogenic lesion ⊡ at the lower pole of the kidney without alternation of renal contour. A small RCC is not typically this hyperechoic.

HYPERECHOIC RENAL MASS

(Left) Longitudinal transabdominal ultrasound shows 2, irregular, large, echogenic angiomyolipomas ⮕ in a patient with tuberous sclerosis. These lesions are heterogeneous in appearance and may mimic malignant lesions. *(Right)* Longitudinal transabdominal ultrasound shows a mildly echogenic lesion ⮕ in the upper pole of the right kidney that is not as echogenic as most small angiomyolipomas. A tiny intralesional cystic component ⮕ is present.

Renal Angiomyolipoma (AML)

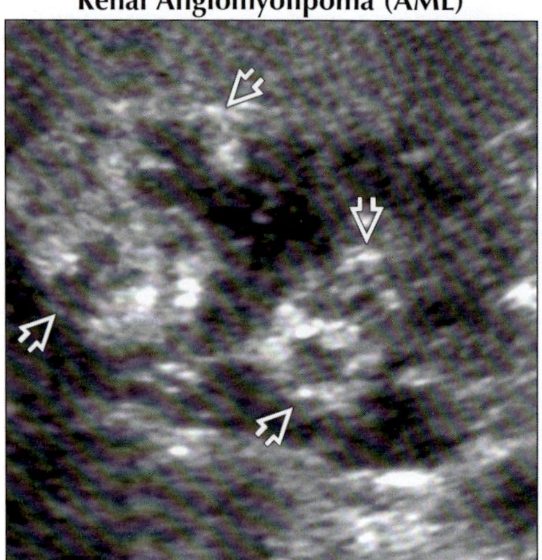

Renal Cell Carcinoma (RCC)

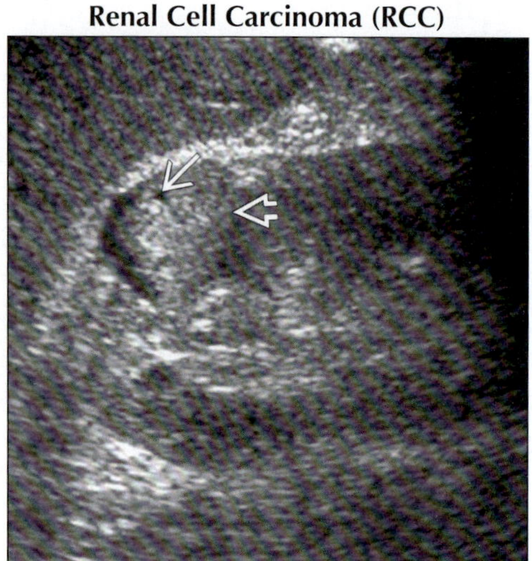

(Left) Longitudinal transabdominal ultrasound shows a large, exophytic, heterogeneous RCC that is mildly hyperechoic with tiny cystic ⮕ and calcific ⮕ foci. The tumor disrupts central sinus echoes ➔. *(Right)* Correlative longitudinal power Doppler ultrasound shows rich intratumoral vascularity. RCC is typically hypervascular, helping to differentiate it from hypovascular lesions such as renal metastasis, lymphoma, and transitional cell carcinoma.

Renal Cell Carcinoma (RCC)

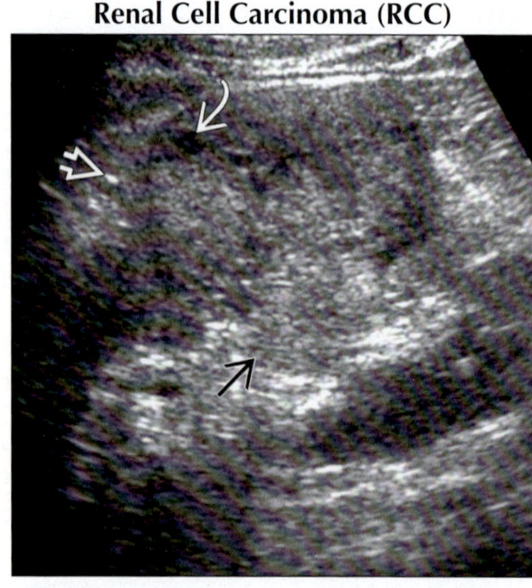

Renal Cell Carcinoma (RCC)

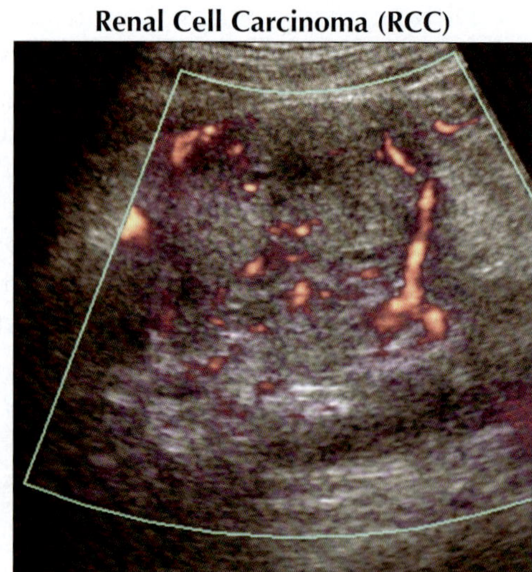

(Left) Longitudinal transabdominal ultrasound shows a large, slightly hyperechoic mass ⮕ at the upper pole of the right kidney in a 3-year-old boy. It is causing obstructive hydronephrosis ⮕. *(Right)* Oblique transabdominal ultrasound shows that the Wilms tumor ⮕ is heterogeneous and mildly hyperechoic compared to the normal renal parenchyma ⮕, which is displaced.

Wilms Tumor

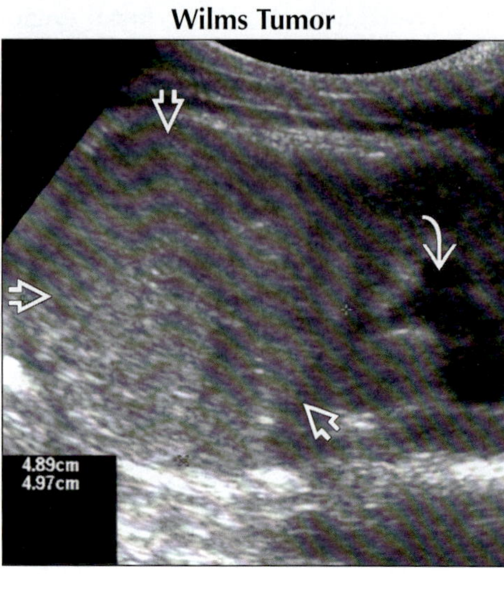

Wilms Tumor

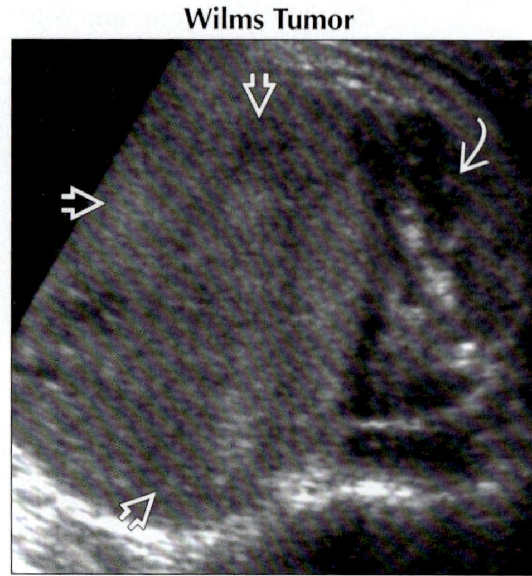

HYPERECHOIC RENAL MASS

Fat in Renal Scar

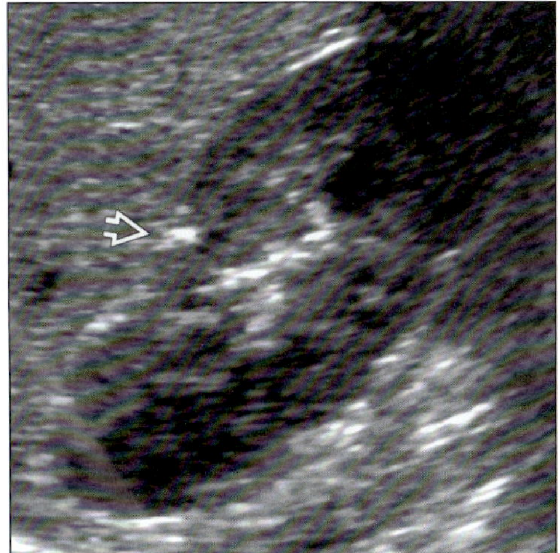

Milk of Calcium Cyst

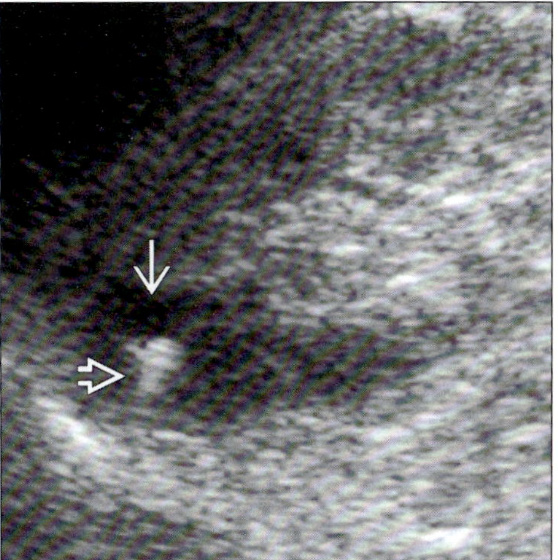

(Left) Oblique transabdominal ultrasound shows an echogenic focus with a focal contour depression ⇨ in the interpolar region of the right kidney, compatible with a focal renal scar. (Right) Oblique transabdominal ultrasound shows a bright echogenic focus with a ring-down artifact ⇨, compatible with calcium layering within a cyst ⇨.

Renal Junctional Line/Cortical Parenchymal Defect

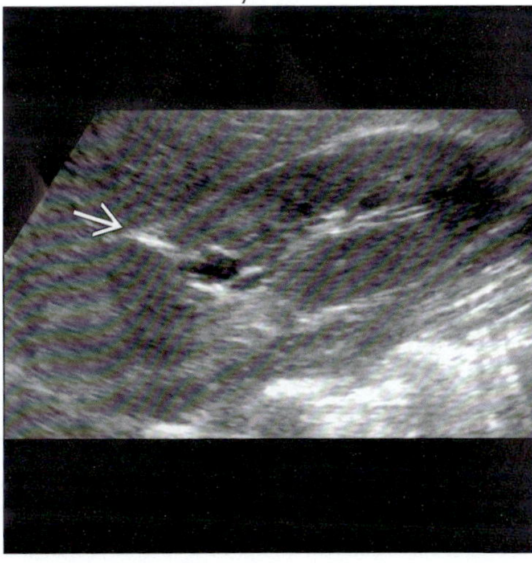

Renal Junctional Line/Cortical Parenchymal Defect

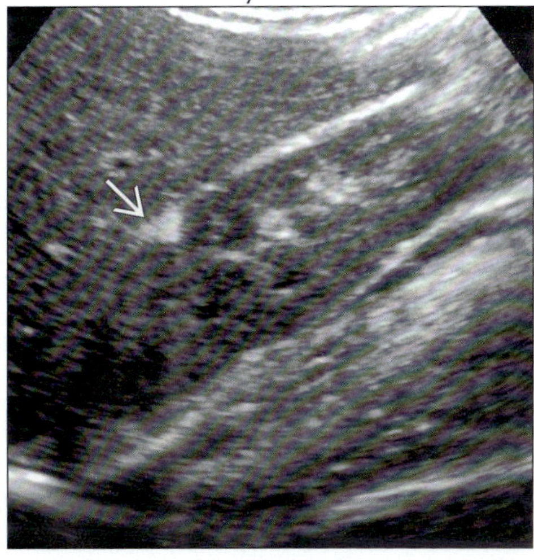

(Left) Longitudinal transabdominal ultrasound shows the typical appearance of a renal junction line ⇨ at the classic location of the anterosuperior aspect of the right kidney. (Right) Longitudinal transabdominal ultrasound shows a cortical parenchymal defect as a triangular echogenic focus ⇨ near the junction of the upper and middle 1/3 of the kidney.

Renal Calculi

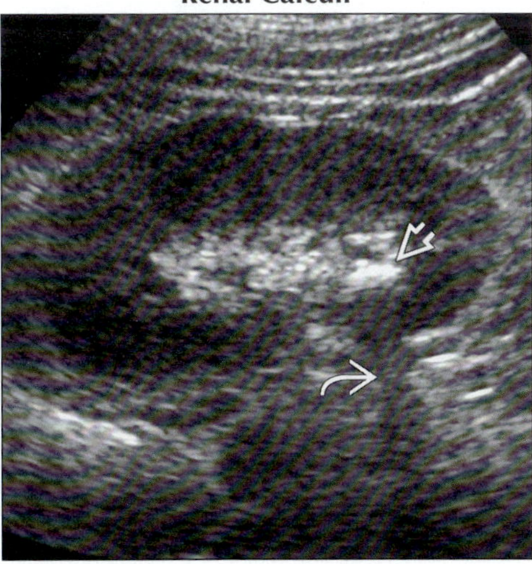

Renal Papillary Necrosis

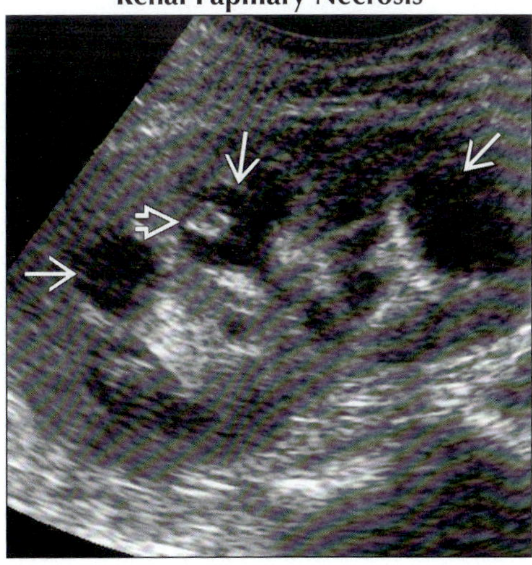

(Left) Longitudinal transabdominal ultrasound shows an echogenic stone ⇨ at the lower pole of the left kidney, associated with posterior acoustic shadowing ⇨. There is no associated obstructive calyceal dilatation. (Right) Longitudinal transabdominal ultrasound shows a necrotic papilla, appearing as an echogenic focus ⇨ with "ring" calcification in the medullary pyramid. It is surrounded by a rim of fluid in the dilated and clubbed calyces ⇨.

HYPERECHOIC RENAL MASS

(Left) Oblique transabdominal ultrasound shows multiple foci of echogenic gas ➡ around the renal pelvis and within the renal sinus. *(Right)* Transverse transabdominal ultrasound shows echogenic gas within the renal cortex ➡ and collecting system ⇨. Note the ring-down artifacts ➡, which are compatible with air bubbles trapped in fluid.

Emphysematous Pyelonephritis

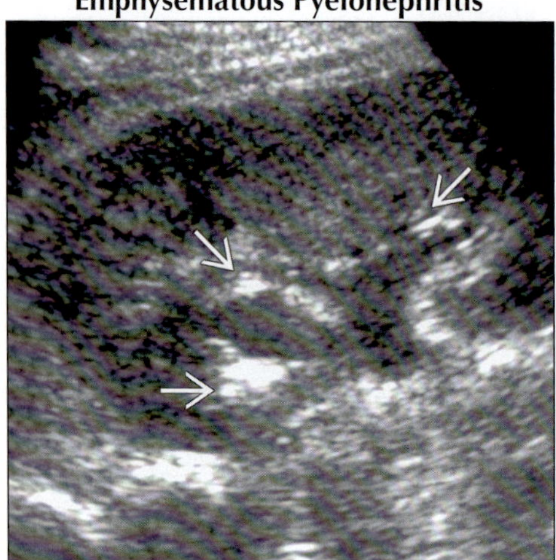

Emphysematous Pyelonephritis

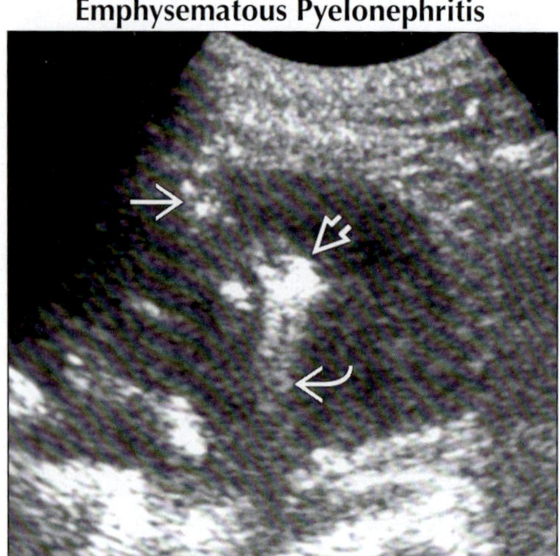

(Left) Longitudinal transabdominal ultrasound shows a large echogenic mass ⇨ at the interpolar region of the right kidney. Similar lesions were found in the contralateral kidney in this patient with known rhabdomyosarcoma. *(Right)* Transverse color Doppler ultrasound shows an echogenic mass ➡ at the mid-right kidney in a patient with carcinoma of the lung and multiple liver metastases. Note that the mass is hypovascular, which is typical of renal metastasis.

Renal Metastases

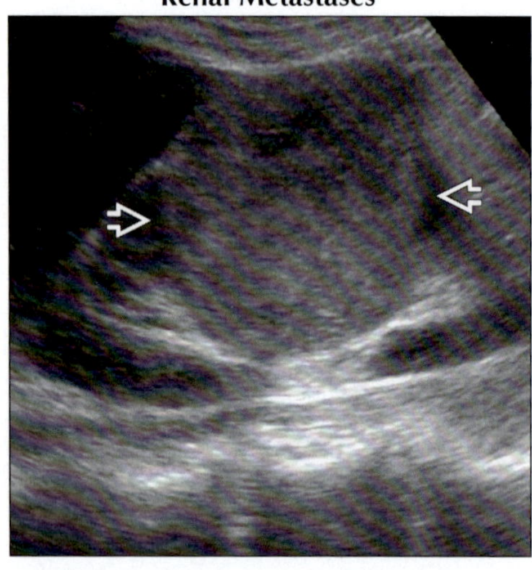

Renal Metastases

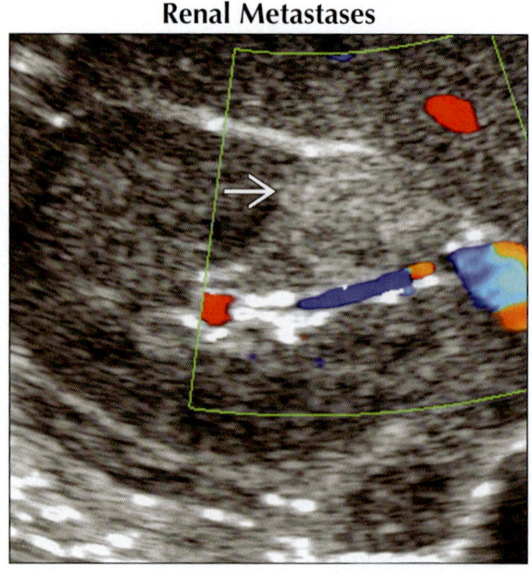

(Left) Longitudinal transabdominal ultrasound shows a wedge-shaped echogenic mass ⇨ in a febrile patient with flank pain. Increased echogenicity in focal bacterial nephritis is due to hemorrhage and may mimic a neoplastic lesion. Clinical correlation is important in the differentiation. *(Right)* Correlative longitudinal color Doppler ultrasound shows a parenchymal vascular defect ⇨ in the echogenic area of focal bacterial nephritis.

Focal Bacterial Nephritis

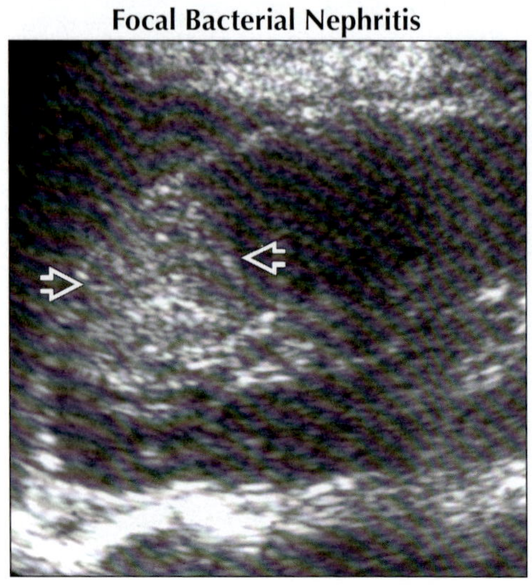

Focal Bacterial Nephritis

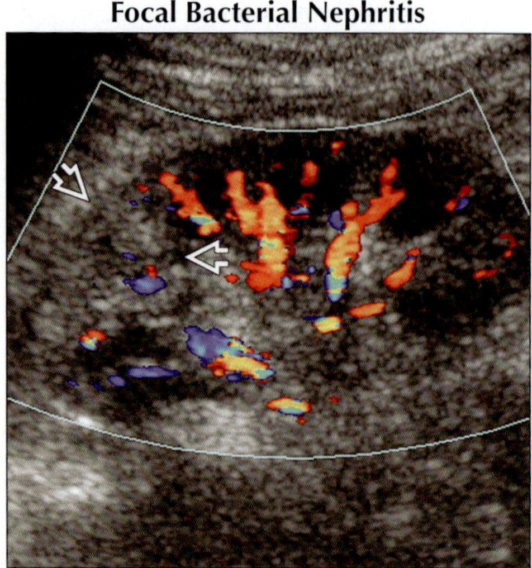

HYPERECHOIC RENAL MASS

Xanthogranulomatous Pyelonephritis

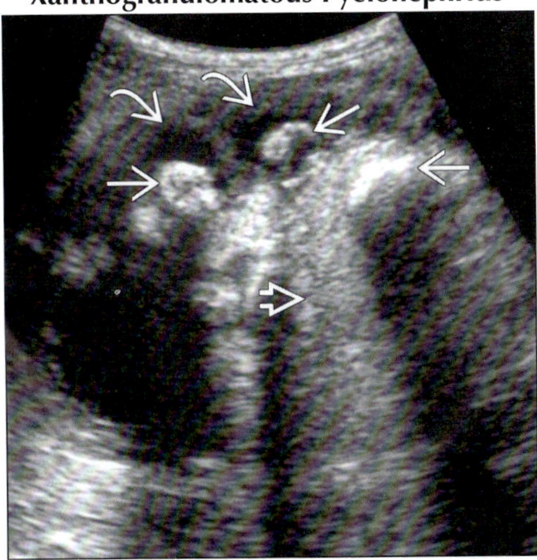

Xanthogranulomatous Pyelonephritis

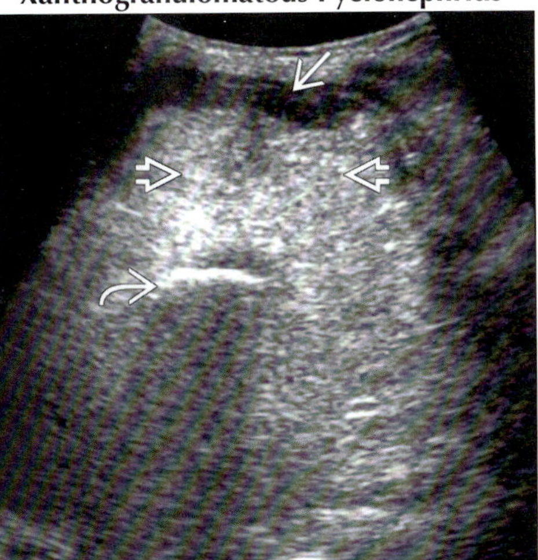

(Left) Longitudinal transabdominal ultrasound shows extensive peripelvic fat infiltration ➡ secondary to xanthogranulomatous pyelonephritis. Multiple echogenic calculi ➡ are present and associated with caliectasis ➡. *(Right)* Longitudinal transabdominal ultrasound shows renal parenchymal replacement by echogenic xanthogranulomatous tissue ➡ with generalized cortical thinning ➡. A large central calculus is present ➡.

Tuberculosis, Urinary Tract

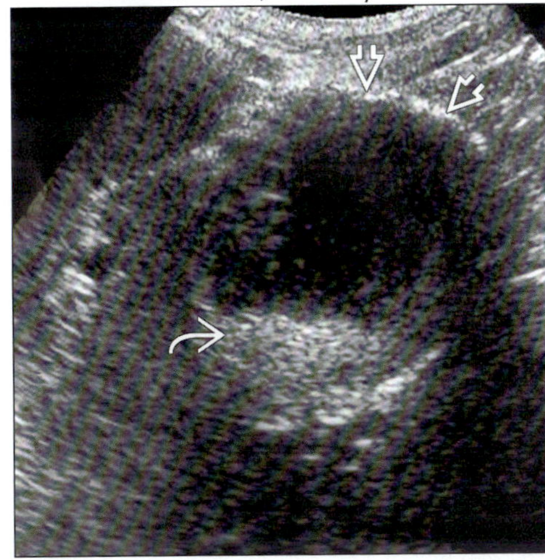

Renal Oncocytoma

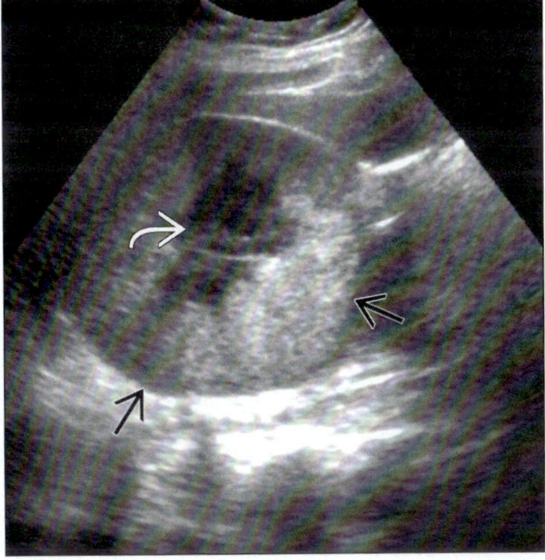

(Left) Transverse transabdominal ultrasound shows a renal TB abscess with internal echogenic debris ➡ & a calcified wall ➡. Abscess formation is secondary to stricture at the calyceal infundibulum. *(Right)* Longitudinal transabdominal ultrasound shows a large, mildly hyperechoic mass ➡ in the right kidney with a spiculated central hypoechoic scar ➡, suggestive of an onocytoma. As RCC cannot be excluded, excision is required.

Renal Trauma

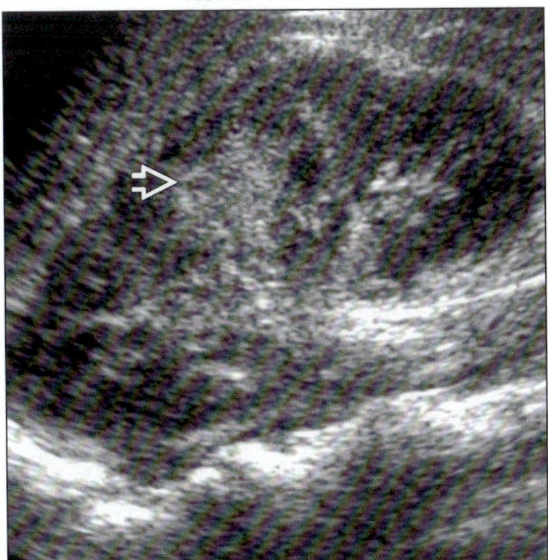

Renal Trauma

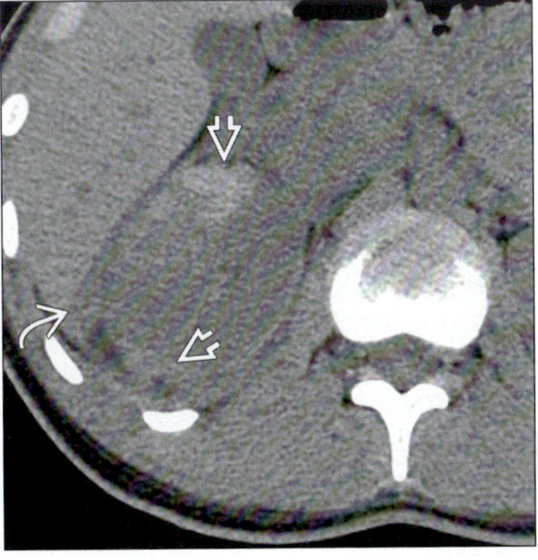

(Left) Longitudinal transabdominal ultrasound shows a focal poorly defined area of hyperechogenicity ➡ in the mid-pole of the right kidney, compatible with a contusion. Note that there is a loss of corticomedullary differentiation at the mid-pole when compared with the lower pole. *(Right)* Axial NECT in the same patient shows hyperdense hemorrhagic contusions ➡ in the right kidney. There is also a small perinephric hematoma ➡.

DIFFERENTIAL DIAGNOSIS

Common
- Urolithiasis
- Milk of Calcium
- Renal Junction Line, Junctional Parenchymal Defect
- Arcuate Arteries
- Medullary Sponge Kidney
- Nephrocalcinosis

Less Common
- Renal Papillary Necrosis
- Emphysematous Pyelonephritis

ESSENTIAL INFORMATION

Key Differential Diagnosis Issues
- Normal anatomical structures/variants (arcuate arteries and renal junction line) are recognized by their typical location
  - Should not be mistaken for renal calculus or cortical scar
- If posterior acoustic shadowing not seen in suspected urolithiasis; try color Doppler to look for "twinkling" artifact
  - Useful ancillary sign in equivocal cases
- Look for features associated with echogenic focus such as "comet tail" artifacts, medullary cysts

Helpful Clues for Common Diagnoses
- **Urolithiasis**
  - Most common types of stone: Calcium stones (75%-80%), calcium oxalate/calcium phosphate
  - Calculi seen as crescent-shaped echogenic foci with sharp posterior acoustic shadowing
  - Posterior border of stone usually obscured by strong posterior acoustic shadowing
  - May cause obstruction: Look for hydronephrosis/calyceal dilatation and cortical scars
  - Nonobstructive calculi may have similar echogenicity as central sinus echo, distinguished by acoustic shadowing
    - Acoustic shadowing varies according to size and composition of stone
    - Very small stones may not show obvious posterior acoustic shadowing
  - On color Doppler, most urinary tract stones show "twinkling" artifacts
    - Rapidly changing color posterior to stone with "comet tail"
  - Variable locations: Calyceal, renal pelvis, ureteropelvic junction, ureter, ureterovesicle junction
  - Calculi best visualized in kidney and at ureterovesicle junction
- **Milk of Calcium**
  - Calcium carbonate + calcium phosphate (carbonate apatite)
  - Common incidental finding in renal cortex
  - Associated with characteristic "comet tail"/ring-down artifacts
  - May be present within cortical cyst; calcification may layer, creating fluid-debris level
- **Renal Junction Line, Junctional Parenchymal Defect**
  - Pseudotumor: Line represents plane of embryologic fusion between fetal renal lobes
  - Best diagnostic clue: Echogenic line at anterosuperior aspect of kidney without disruption of renal contour
  - Most common location: Junction of upper and middle 1/3 of kidney
  - Uncommon location: Posteroinferior surface of kidney
  - Classical interrenuncular septum = echogenic line; connects perirenal space with renal sinus; occasionally may indent cortex
  - Some appear as triangular echogenic focus = junctional parenchymal defect
  - Size variable, depending on type of fusion defect
    - Small linear indentation or sulcus on renal surface
    - Deep fissure of varying depth
    - Hilar asymmetry as lateral wedge-shaped extension of anterosuperior recess of renal hilum
    - Complete cleft in continuity with lobar sulcus that opens into renal sinus
  - May be confused with cortical scar or tiny angiomyolipoma
- **Arcuate Arteries**
  - Normal vascular structures, commonly identified at corticomedullary junctions

ECHOGENIC RENAL FOCUS

- ○ May be mistaken for nephrocalcinosis or stone
- **Medullary Sponge Kidney**
  - ○ Dilated, ectatic collecting tubules; unknown etiology
  - ○ Anechoic medullary cysts representing ectatic collecting tubes
  - ○ Focal or diffuse
  - ○ Multiple echogenic foci localized at renal medullary pyramids
  - ○ Calculus occasionally seen if focus of calcification has eroded into collecting system
- **Nephrocalcinosis**
  - ○ Diffuse calcium deposition within renal substance
  - ○ Detected on screening of patients with known predisposing metabolic conditions such as renal tubular acidosis or hyperoxaluria
  - ○ Medullary type (95%) more common than cortical type (5%); coexisting medullary and cortical type is rare
  - ○ Best diagnostic clue: Calcification within renal parenchyma
  - ○ Acoustic shadowing may be absent with minimal or punctate calcification
  - ○ Medullary nephrocalcinosis
    - ▪ Earliest sign: Absence of normal hypoechoic papillary structures
    - ▪ Solitary focus of hyperechogenicity at tip of pyramid near fornix

- ▪ Hypoechoic rim at corticomedullary junction and along periphery of pyramids
- ▪ Advanced stage: Generalized increased echogenicity of renal pyramids ± shadowing
- ○ Cortical nephrocalcinosis
  - ▪ Homogeneously increased echogenicity of renal parenchyma
  - ▪ Kidney more echogenic than liver

Helpful Clues for Less Common Diagnoses
- **Renal Papillary Necrosis**
  - ○ Necrosis of renal papilla secondary to interstitial nephritis or ischemia
  - ○ Early stage: Echogenic "ring" in medulla = necrotic papillae, surrounded by rim of fluid
  - ○ Late stage: Multiple cystic cavities in medullary pyramids ± nonshadowing echogenic sloughed papillae
  - ○ Calcified sloughed papilla with strong acoustic shadowing simulates stone; may cause obstructive hydronephrosis
- **Emphysematous Pyelonephritis**
  - ○ Life-threatening, necrotizing upper urinary tract infection associated with gas within kidney
  - ○ Echogenic gas within infarcted, infected parenchyma
  - ○ Nondependent linear echogenic lines with strong posterior acoustic shadowing, ring-down artifact

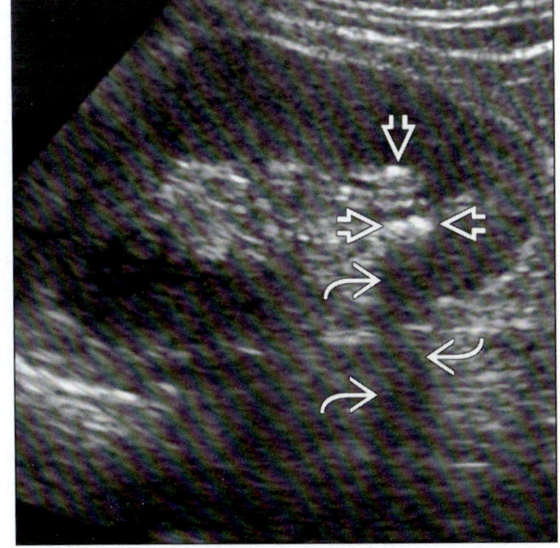

Urolithiasis

Longitudinal transabdominal ultrasound shows multiple echogenic calculi ▧ present at the lower pole of the kidney. These calculi are associated with characteristic posterior acoustic shadowing ▧.

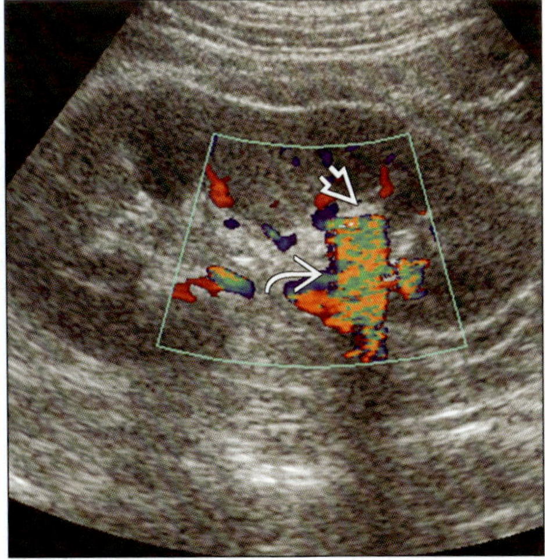

Urolithiasis

Longitudinal color Doppler ultrasound shows a "twinkling" artifact ▧ immediately behind an echogenic calculus ▧ in the lower pole of the kidney.

(Left) Longitudinal US shows a large echogenic stone 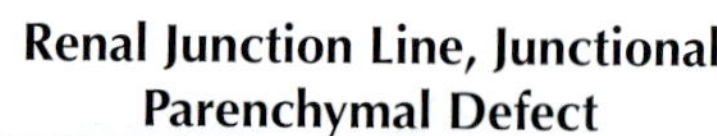 causing obstructive hydronephrosis ⇗ at the lower pole of the kidney. Note that the posterior surface of the stone is obscured by strong posterior acoustic shadowing ⇨. This is a typical feature of an oxalate stone. *(Right)* Oblique US shows an echogenic focus of milk of calcium ⇨ at the cortex of the upper pole of the kidney. Note that it is associated with a characteristic "comet tail" artifact ⇗.

Urolithiasis

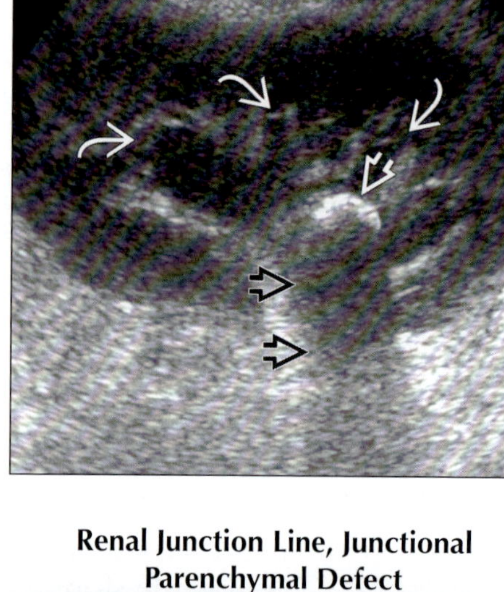

Milk of Calcium

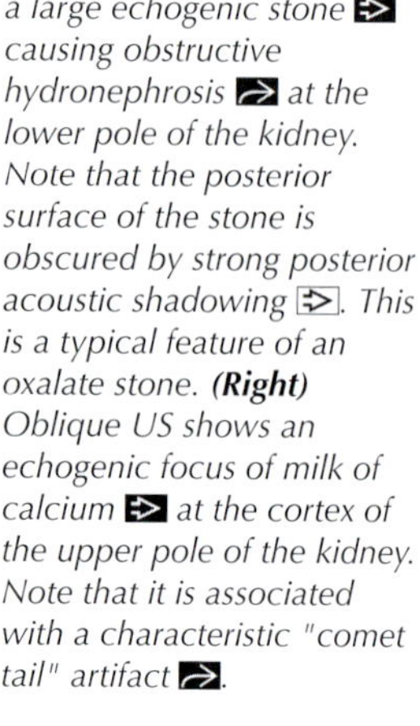

(Left) Longitudinal transabdominal ultrasound shows the typical location and appearance of a renal junction line ⇨ at the anterosuperior aspect of the right kidney. *(Right)* Longitudinal transabdominal ultrasound shows a junctional parenchymal defect as a triangular echogenic focus ⇨ near the junction of the upper and middle 1/3 of the kidney.

Renal Junction Line, Junctional Parenchymal Defect

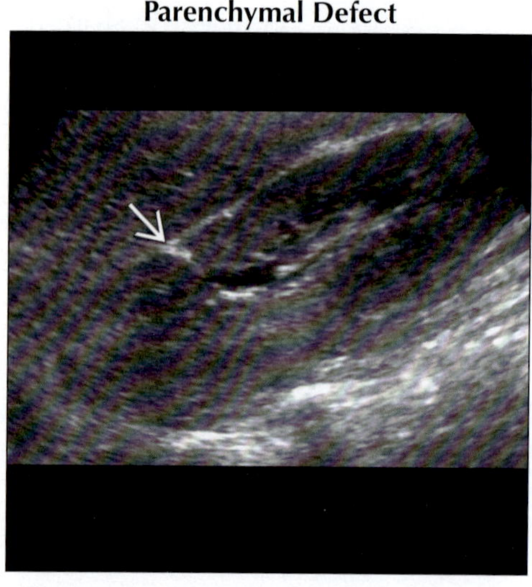

Renal Junction Line, Junctional Parenchymal Defect

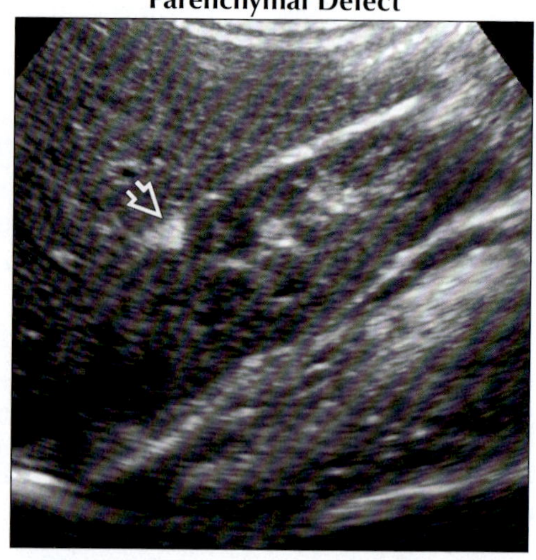

(Left) Longitudinal transabdominal ultrasound shows a discrete echogenic focus ⇨ at the corticomedullary junction, a typical site for arcuate arteries. A focus of milk of calcium ⇗ is present in the renal cortex. *(Right)* Longitudinal transabdominal ultrasound shows multiple echogenic foci representing calcification ⇨, localized to the medullary pyramids. Note the medullary cyst ⇗, which represents a dilated ectatic collecting tubule.

Arcuate Arteries

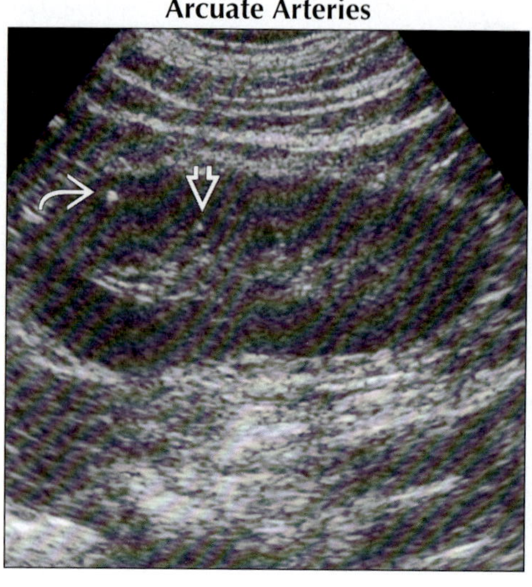

Medullary Sponge Kidney

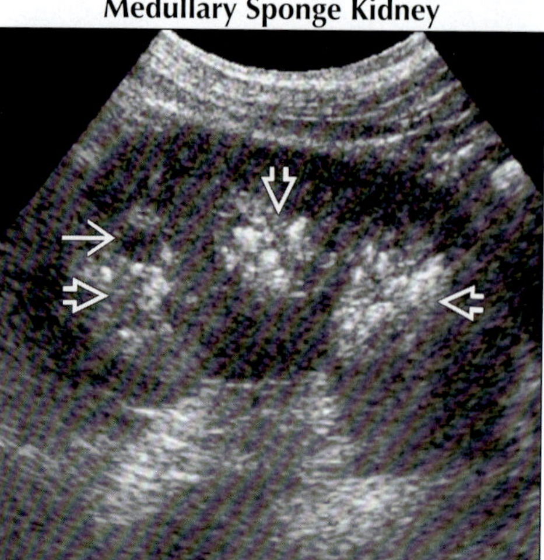

8

ECHOGENIC RENAL FOCUS

Nephrocalcinosis

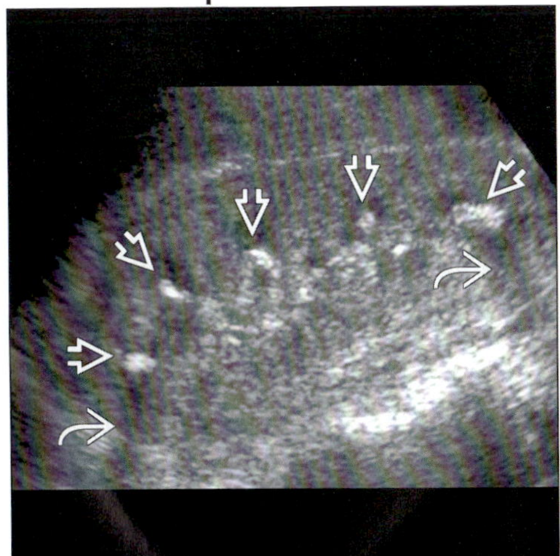

Nephrocalcinosis

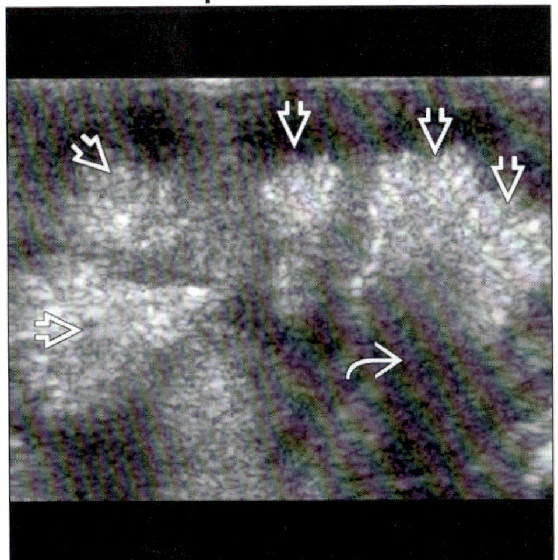

(Left) Longitudinal transabdominal ultrasound shows hyperechogenicity at the tip of the pyramids ⊳ associated with posterior acoustic shadowing ⇲. (Right) Longitudinal transabdominal ultrasound shows an advanced stage of nephrocalcinosis, with generalized increased echogenicity of the renal pyramids ⊳ and associated posterior acoustic shadowing ⇲.

Renal Papillary Necrosis

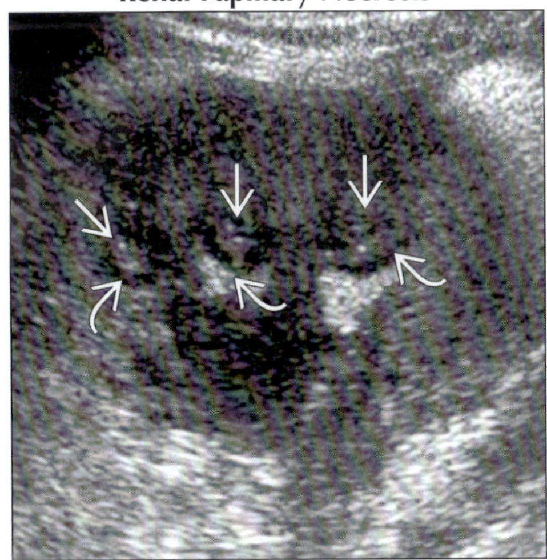

Renal Papillary Necrosis

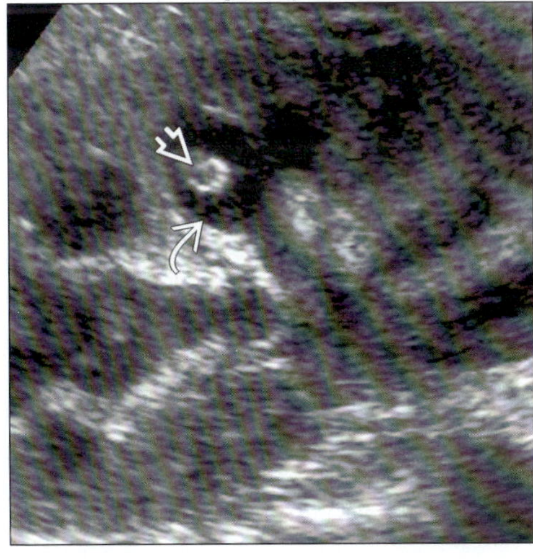

(Left) Longitudinal transabdominal ultrasound shows early papillary necrosis seen as echogenic medullary tips representing necrotic papillae ⇲, which are outlined by rims of fluid ⇲. (Right) Oblique transabdominal ultrasound shows a necrotic papilla seen as an echogenic focus ⊳ with "ring" calcification in the medullary pyramid surrounded by fluid ⇲. The surrounding fluid makes the necrotic papilla more conspicuous.

Emphysematous Pyelonephritis

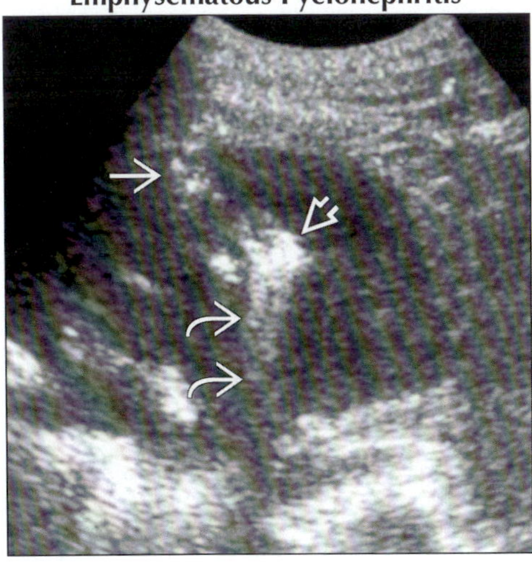

Emphysematous Pyelonephritis

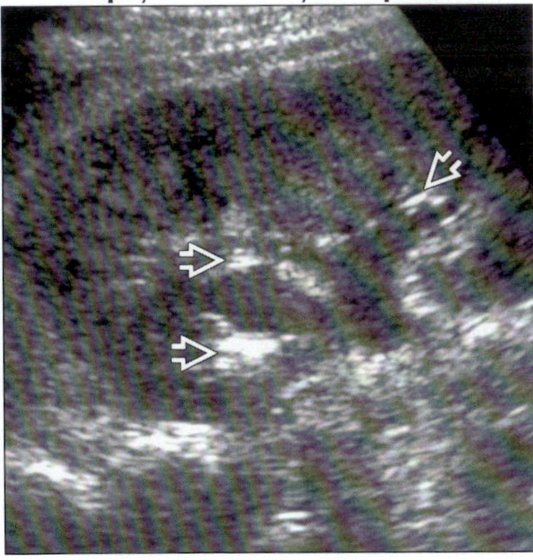

(Left) Transverse transabdominal ultrasound shows echogenic gas within the renal cortex ⇲ and deep parenchyma ⊳, with ring-down artifacts ⇲ also visible. (Right) Longitudinal transabdominal ultrasound shows multiple foci of echogenic gas ⊳ around the renal pelvis. Clinically, the patient was septic.

DIFFERENTIAL DIAGNOSIS

Common
- Column of Bertin
- Renal Junction Line, Junctional Parenchymal Defect
- Fetal Lobulation
- Dromedary Hump

ESSENTIAL INFORMATION

Key Differential Diagnosis Issues
- Be aware of typical locations of these pseudotumors
- Rarely cause focal mass effect or distortion of normal architecture of renal parenchyma

Helpful Clues for Common Diagnoses
- **Column of Bertin**
  - Hypertrophic medial bands of cortical tissue that separate pyramids of renal medulla
  - Best diagnostic clue: Isoechoic and continuous with renal cortex
  - Normal renal outline
  - No abnormal vascularity on color Doppler
  - Junction of upper and middle 1/3 of kidney most common site
  - Unilateral > bilateral (18% of cases)
  - May be confused with renal tumor
- **Renal Junction Line, Junctional Parenchymal Defect**
  - Line represents plane of embryologic fusion between fetal renal lobes
  - Best diagnostic clue: Echogenic line at anterosuperior aspect of kidney without disruption of renal contour
  - Junction of upper and middle 1/3 of kidney most common location
  - Posteroinferior surface of kidney uncommon location
  - Interrenuncular septum: Echogenic line, connects perirenal space with renal sinus, occasionally may indent cortex
  - Junctional parenchymal defect: Triangular echogenic focus in renal cortex
  - Variable size; ranges from small linear sulcus on renal surface to complete cleft in continuity with lobar sulcus opening into renal sinus
  - May be confused with scar or tiny angiomyolipoma
- **Fetal Lobulation**
  - Sign of fusion of fetal renal lobes
  - Indentations in renal outline, which lie between renal pyramids or calyces
  - Distinguished from scars that lie directly over calyces
- **Dromedary Hump**
  - a.k.a "splenic hump", only occurs in left kidney
  - Focal bulge in lateral border of mid-pole of left kidney with similar echopattern as rest of kidney
  - Diagnostic clue: Calyces underlying hump extend laterally into hump
  - May be confused with renal tumor

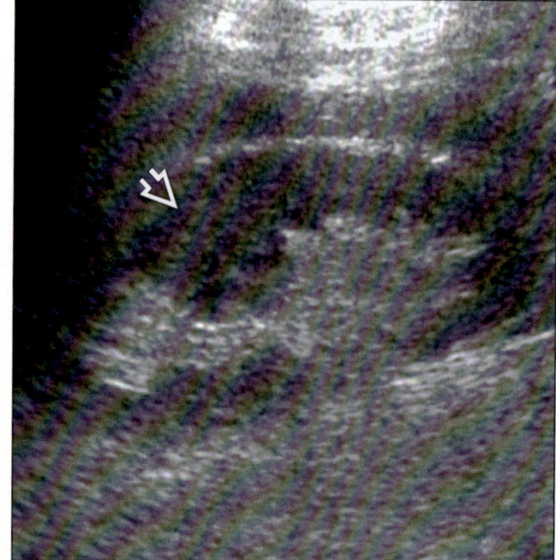

Column of Bertin

Longitudinal transabdominal ultrasound shows a column of Bertin ▷, which is isoechoic and continuous with the renal cortex. Note the smooth renal outline.

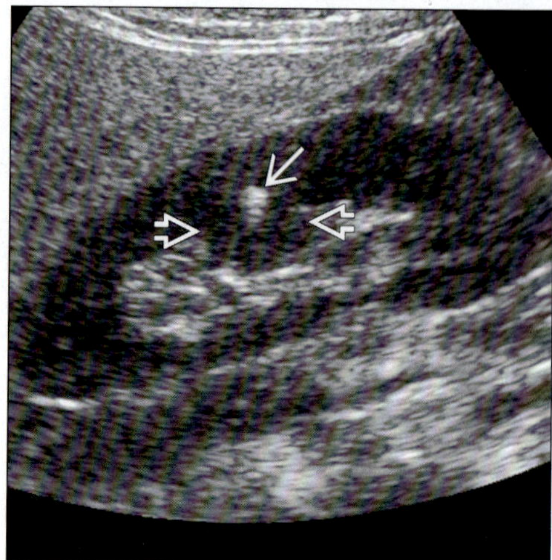

Column of Bertin

Longitudinal transabdominal ultrasound shows a classic column of Bertin ▷, with a focus of milk of calcium ▷ in the overlying cortex. Both features are commonly seen as benign entities on ultrasound.

RENAL PSEUDOTUMOR

Column of Bertin

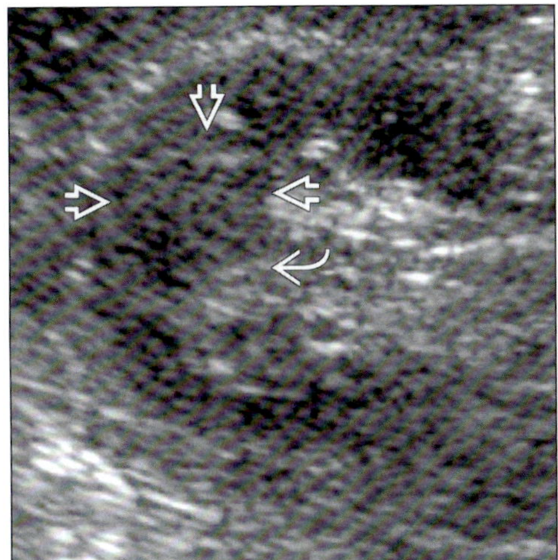

Renal Junction Line, Junctional Parenchymal Defect

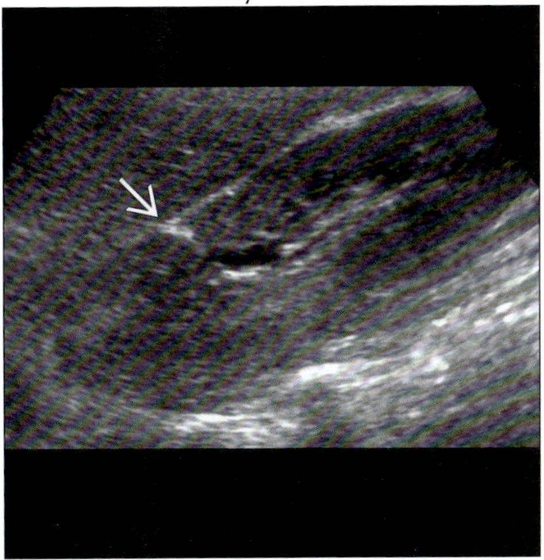

(Left) Transverse transabdominal ultrasound shows a column of Bertin ⇨, which is isoechoic and continuous with the adjacent cortex, indenting the central renal sinus ⇨. *(Right)* Longitudinal transabdominal ultrasound shows the typical appearance of an echogenic renal junctional line ⇨ at the anterosuperior aspect of right kidney. Note its location at the junction of the upper and middle 1/3 of the kidney.

Renal Junction Line, Junctional Parenchymal Defect

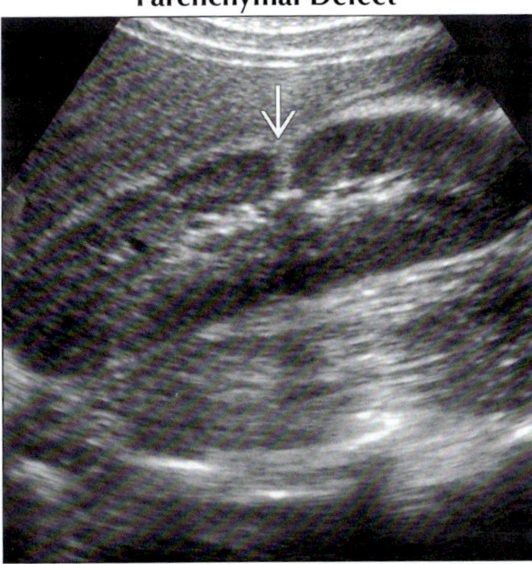

Renal Junction Line, Junctional Parenchymal Defect

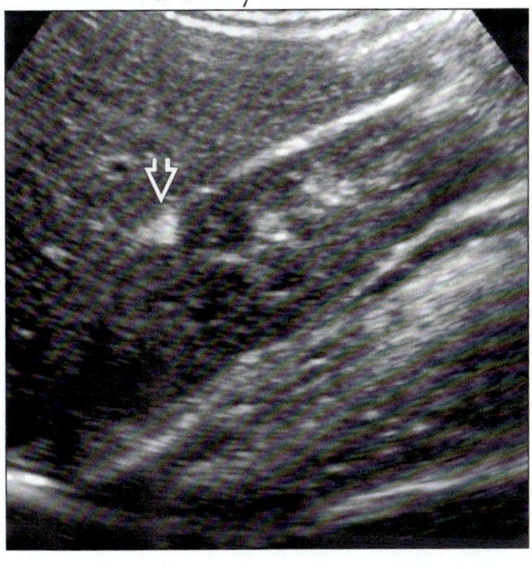

(Left) Longitudinal transabdominal ultrasound shows an echogenic line ⇨ at the middle 1/3 of the right kidney. This location of the renal junction line is less common than the one at the anterosuperior aspect. *(Right)* Longitudinal transabdominal ultrasound shows a junctional parenchymal defect as a triangular echogenic focus ⇨ at junction of upper and middle 1/3 of the kidney. This is a typical site for both junction line and junctional parenchymal defect.

Fetal Lobulation

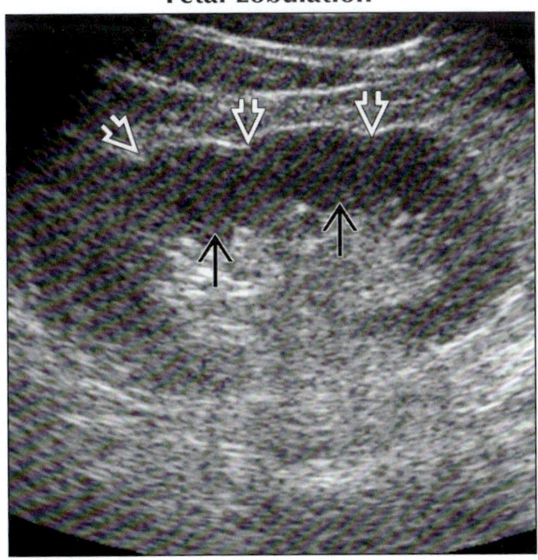

Dromedary Hump

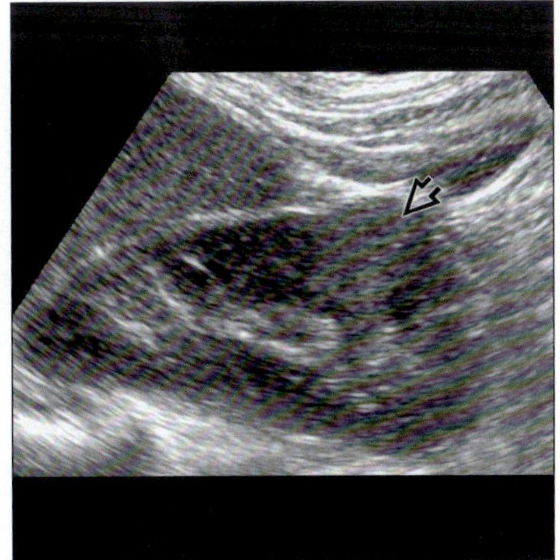

(Left) Longitudinal transabdominal ultrasound shows regular indentations ⇨ in the renal outline. They lie between the renal pyramids ⇨ or calyces, distinguishing fetal lobulations from a renal scar. *(Right)* Longitudinal transabdominal ultrasound shows a bulge ⇨ in the lateral border of the mid-pole of the left kidney. The echopattern of this hump is similar to the rest of the kidney.

DIFFERENTIAL DIAGNOSIS

Common
- Simple Renal Cyst
- Renal Angiomyolipoma
  - Tuberous Sclerosis
- Cystic Disease of Dialysis

Less Common
- AD Polycystic Kidney Disease
- Multicystic Dysplastic Kidney
- Renal Metastases
- von Hippel-Lindau Disease
- Acute Pyelonephritis
- Xanthogranulomatous Pyelonephritis

ESSENTIAL INFORMATION

Key Differential Diagnosis Issues
- Note pattern of distribution, size, and echogenicity of underlying kidneys
- Correlate with clinical history and associated syndromes, if any

Helpful Clues for Common Diagnoses
- **Simple Renal Cyst**
  - Frequently multiple in elderly
  - Well defined, smooth, thin walled, anechoic with posterior enhancement
- **Renal Angiomyolipoma**
  - Well-defined hyperechoic mass, similar to renal sinus echogenicity
  - May require CT confirmation to look for presence of fat within these lesions
  - When multiple, consider tuberous sclerosis

- **Cystic Disease of Dialysis**
  - Bilateral; in patients with chronic renal disease and long-term dialysis
  - Early stage: Small cysts < 3 cm seen in small echogenic kidneys
  - Advanced stage: Large kidneys + multiple small cysts

Helpful Clues for Less Common Diagnoses
- **AD Polycystic Kidney Disease**
  - Autosomal dominant disorder (family history helps)
  - Multiple, bilateral, asymmetrical cysts of varying size, ± liver, pancreas involvement
  - Massively enlarged, echogenic kidneys
- **Multicystic Dysplastic Kidney**
  - Multiple cysts of varying size with no renal pelvis/ureter
  - Usually affecting entire kidney, unilateral involvement
- **Renal Metastases**
  - Variable echogenicity, hypoperfused masses, ± evidence of disseminated disease
  - Common primary tumors: Lung, breast
- **von Hippel-Lindau Disease**
  - Bilateral cysts and renal cell carcinomas
- **Acute Pyelonephritis**
  - Swollen kidneys with microabscesses or focal areas of necrosis
  - ↓ vascularity on power Doppler
- **Xanthogranulomatous Pyelonephritis**
  - Hypoechoic masses replacing normal parenchyma
  - + calculus, ± focal abscesses

Renal Angiomyolipoma

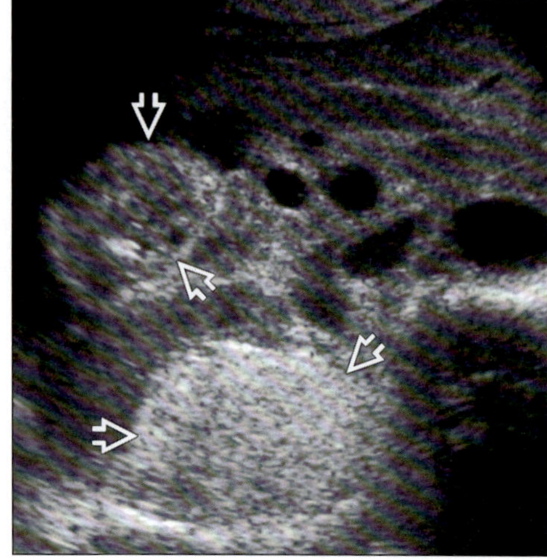

Oblique transabdominal ultrasound of the kidney shows multiple, well-defined, hyperechoic masses ➡.

Tuberous Sclerosis

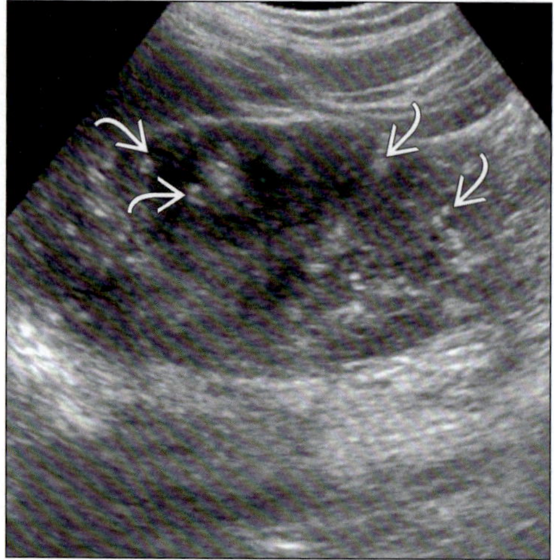

Longitudinal US in a patient with tuberous sclerosis shows numerous, small, echogenic lesions ➡ in both kidneys. The echogenic lesions were shown to be fat-containing angiomyolipomas on CT.

MULTIFOCAL RENAL MASS

Cystic Disease of Dialysis

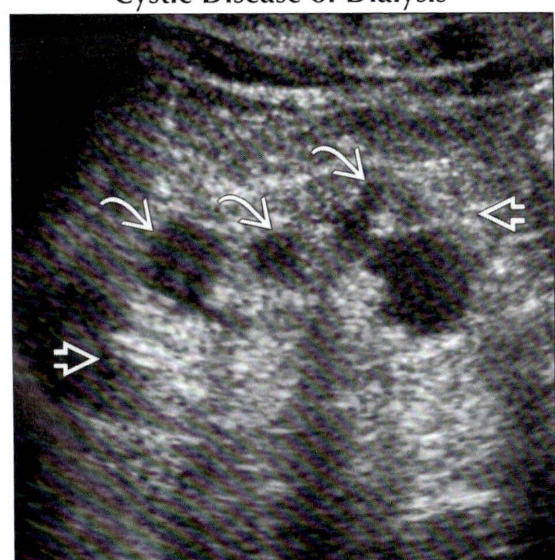

AD Polycystic Kidney Disease

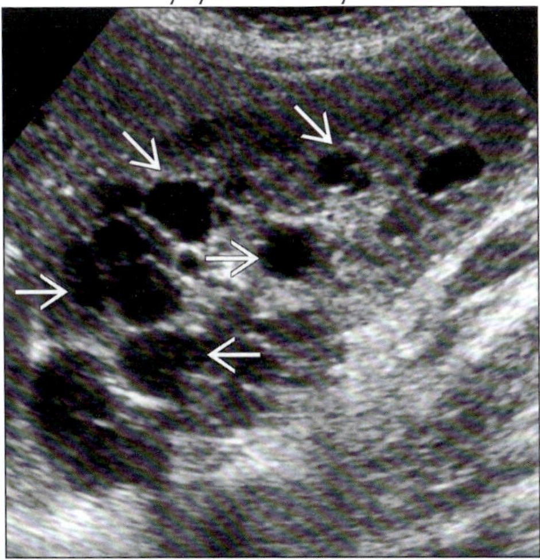

(Left) Longitudinal transabdominal ultrasound shows a small echogenic kidney ➡. Multiple cysts ➡ are present throughout the cortex and medulla; the opposite kidney had a similar appearance. This patient had a history of long-term dialysis. (Right) Longitudinal transabdominal ultrasound shows multiple cysts ➡ of varying size, which were present in both kidneys. The kidneys are enlarged and echogenic with a loss of corticomedullary differentiation.

Multicystic Dysplastic Kidney

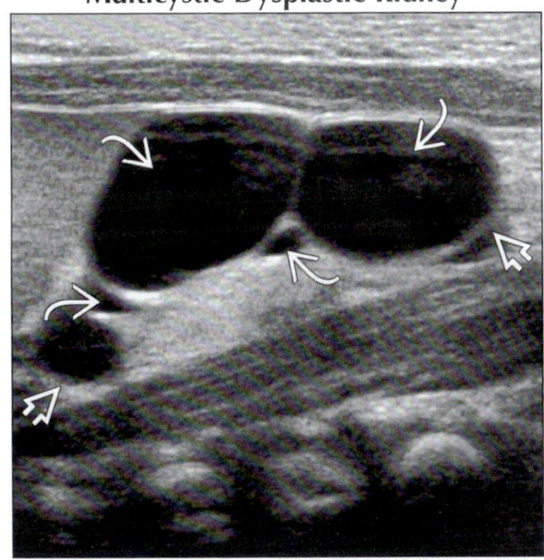

Renal Metastases

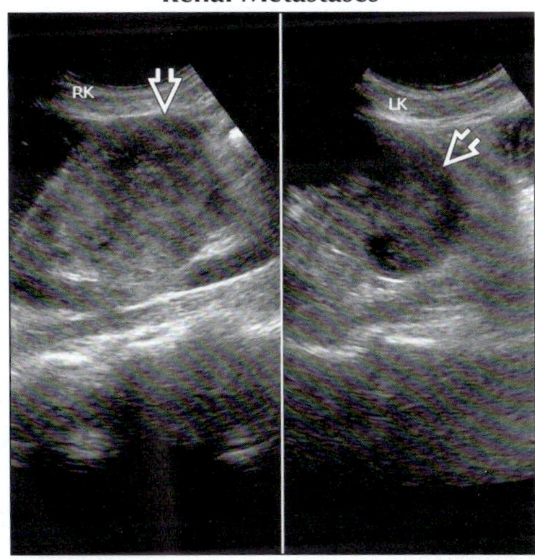

(Left) Longitudinal ultrasound shows a small echogenic kidney ➡ without corticomedullary differentiation in a young child. Multiple cysts of varying size ➡ are present with no normal parenchyma or renal pelvis. (Right) Longitudinal ultrasound shows large heterogeneous hypoechoic masses ➡ in both right and left kidneys in a patient with a known history of lung carcinoma. There was other evidence of disseminated disease.

Acute Pyelonephritis

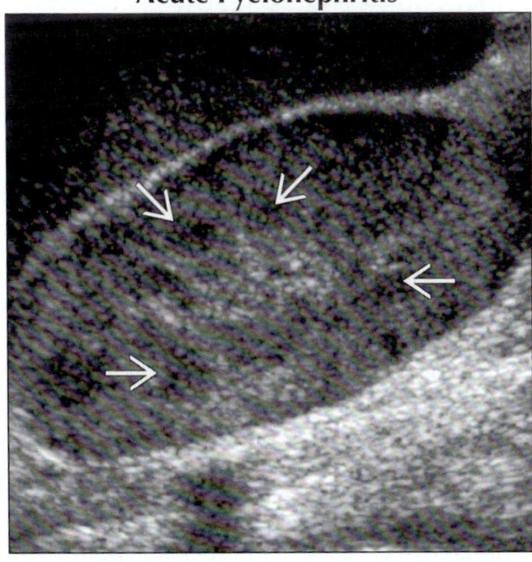

Xanthogranulomatous Pyelonephritis

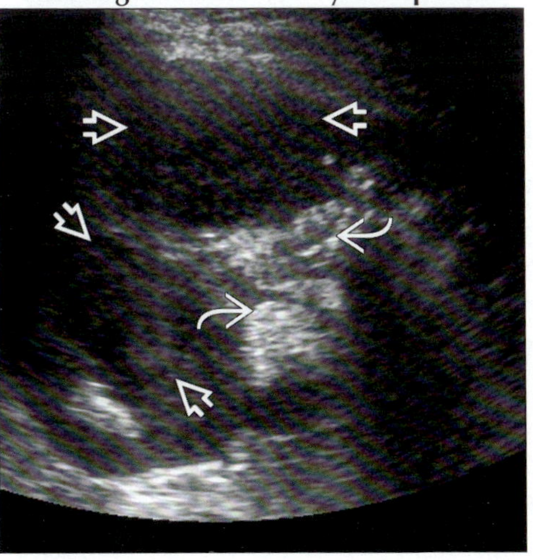

(Left) Longitudinal transabdominal ultrasound shows a swollen kidney with multiple, small, hypoechoic lesions ➡ representing small abscesses. This infected kidney has lost its corticomedullary differentiation and normal sinus echoes. (Right) Oblique transabdominal ultrasound shows an enlarged kidney with multiple, round, hypoechoic masses ➡. Calculi ➡ are seen obstructing the renal pelvis.

DILATED RENAL PELVIS

DIFFERENTIAL DIAGNOSIS

Common
- Normal Distended Renal Pelvis
- Obstructed Renal Pelvis
- Refluxing Renal Pelvis
- Extrarenal Pelvis
- Parapelvic Cyst
- Prominent Renal Vein
- Transitional Cell Carcinoma

Less Common
- Pyonephrosis
- Hemonephrosis
- Renal Sinus Hemorrhage
- Pararenal Fluid Collections
- Peripelvic Cyst
- Atypical Renal Cyst
- Intrarenal Abscess
- Pancreatic Pseudocyst
- Calyceal Diverticulum
- Renal Artery Aneurysm
- Acute Renal Vein Thrombosis

Rare but Important
- Pyelogenic Cyst
- Arteriovenous Malformation (AVM)
- Intrarenal Varices
- Lucent Sinus Lipomatosis
- Renal Lymphoma
- Renal Lymphangiomatosis
- Circumcaval (Retrocaval) Ureter

ESSENTIAL INFORMATION

Key Differential Diagnosis Issues
- Important to differentiate between obstructive and nonobstructive dilatation
- Mimicking lesions may be
  - Extrarenal or intrarenal
  - Vascular or avascular
  - Neoplastic or normal structure

Helpful Clues for Common Diagnoses
- **Normal Distended Renal Pelvis**
  - Commonly associated with full bladder and pregnancy
- **Obstructed Renal Pelvis**
  - Isolated dilatation of renal pelvis is uncommon
  - Depending on level of obstruction, caliectasis ± hydroureter may be seen
- **Refluxing Renal Pelvis**
  - Mild: Transient dilatation of ureter and renal pelvis
  - Severe: Pelvicalyceal dilatation ± hydroureter
  - May be indistinguishable from obstructive renal pelvis
- **Extrarenal Pelvis**
  - Common finding in neonates
  - Appearance may simulate early obstruction
  - Not commonly associated with pelvicalyceal dilatation
- **Parapelvic Cyst**
  - Lymphocyst/embryological remnant
  - Parenchymal in origin; usually solitary
  - May cause extrinsic compression of collecting system
  - May mimic dilated renal pelvis or extrarenal pelvis
- **Prominent Renal Vein**
  - May mimic mild hydronephrosis
  - Color Doppler useful in differentiation
- **Transitional Cell Carcinoma**
  - Hypoechoic mass in dilated pelvis
  - Mimics blood clot or pus
  - Intratumoral vascularity on color Doppler is helpful clue

Helpful Clues for Less Common Diagnoses
- **Pyonephrosis**
  - Pus in dilated pelvicalyceal system
  - Debris-fluid level may be seen
- **Hemonephrosis**
  - Blood in dilated pelvicalyceal system
  - Internal echoes of variable echogenicity
- **Renal Sinus Hemorrhage**
  - May occur in renal sinus or in wall or lumen of renal pelvis
  - 2° to renal tumor, AVM, arteritis, aneurysm, trauma, coagulation disorders
  - Cystic lesion of variable echogenicity disrupting central echocomplex
  - May narrow renal pelvis, major infundibula, or proximal ureter
- **Pararenal Fluid Collections**
  - Secondary to obstruction, infection, biopsy, or trauma of pelvicalyceal system and post-renal transplantation
  - Include urinoma, hematoma, abscess, and lymphocele near renal hilum
- **Peripelvic Cyst**
  - Thought to arise from lymphatic ectasia
  - Usually multiple and septated; bilateral

- **Atypical Renal Cyst**
  - May result from infection, hemorrhage, ischemia, and malignancy
- **Intrarenal Abscess**
  - Acute: Solitary or multiple hypoechoic lesions with low-level echoes
  - Chronic: Complex intrarenal mass
  - May extend into perinephric space
- **Pancreatic Pseudocyst**
  - Prevalent location: Lesser sac (abdomen)
  - Anterior pararenal space involvement: Left > right
- **Calyceal Diverticulum**
  - Location: Fornix > renal pelvis
  - Appears as simple cyst or hydrocalyx
  - May contain calculi
  - If large, causes infundibular/calyceal compression and displacement
  - Contrast CT with delayed excretion phase images shows filling of diverticulum
- **Renal Artery Aneurysm**
  - Aneurysm near hilum may be confused with dilated pelvis
  - May reach up to 10 cm in size
  - Prone to rupture in pregnancy, polyarteritis nodosa, and when lacking aneurysmal calcification
- **Acute Renal Vein Thrombosis**
  - Dilated vein with hypoechoic thrombus
  - Absent venous signal and increased renal vascular resistance

Helpful Clues for Rare Diagnoses
- **Pyelogenic Cyst**
  - Intraparenchymal renal cavity lined with transitional epithelium
  - Communicates with pelvicalyceal system at fornix through neck
  - Small in size (< 2 cm)
  - May contain calculi or milk of calcium
- **Arterivenous Malformation (AVM)**
  - Appearance identical to simple cyst
  - Large AVM near pelvicalyceal system may compress renal pelvis
  - Color Doppler ideal for diagnosis: Mixed color flow with high velocities
- **Intrarenal Varices**
  - May present as cystic renal mass
  - May mimic hydronephrosis
- **Lucent Sinus Lipomatosis**
  - Sinus fat: Echogenic (typical), lucent (rare)
  - Common in patients with Cushing syndrome, obesity, & chronic urolithiasis
- **Renal Lymphoma**
  - Due to direct invasion from paracaval or paraaortic lymphomatous disease
  - May mimic dilated renal pelvis
- **Renal Lymphangiomatosis**
  - Multiple cystic lesions in both parapelvic and perirenal areas
  - Related to lymphatic obstruction
- **Circumcaval (Retrocaval) Ureter**
  - May present as "7" or reversed "J" configuration
  - Typically causes partial obstruction of right ureter
  - Dilatation of proximal ureter and pelvicalyceal system

Obstructed Renal Pelvis

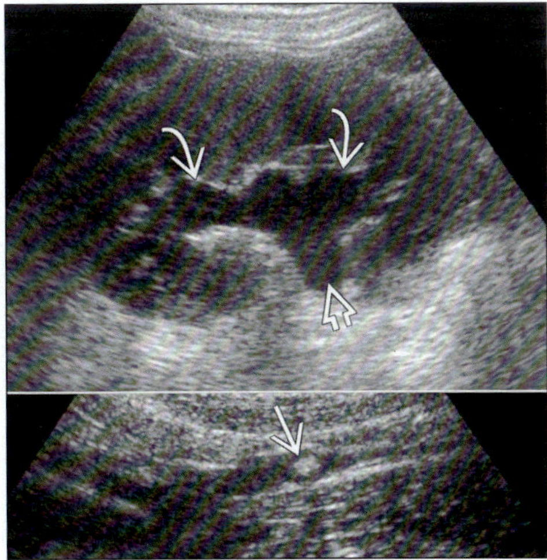

Longitudinal transabdominal ultrasound shows a dilated renal pelvis ⇢ with associated dilatation of the calyceal system ⇢ (upper), which is obstructed by a ureteric calculus ⇢ (lower).

Extrarenal Pelvis

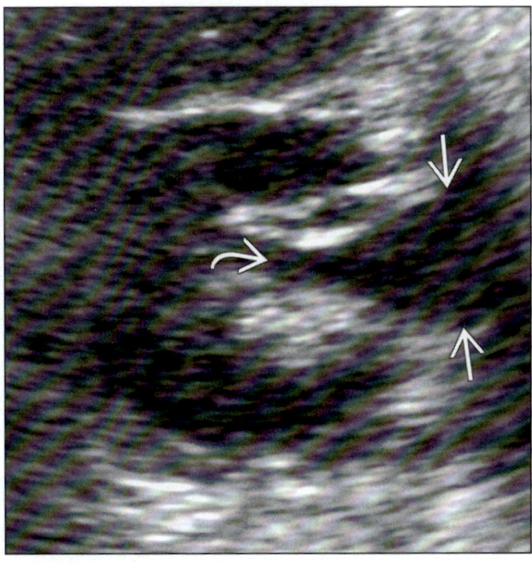

Transverse transabdominal ultrasound shows an extrarenal pelvis. Note that the dilated renal pelvis ⇢ is outside the confines of the kidney, and there is no associated calyceal dilatation ⇢.

DILATED RENAL PELVIS

(Left) Transverse transabdominal ultrasound shows a tubular hypoechoic structure ➡, which could represent either a dilated renal pelvis and hydroureter or a prominent renal vein. **(Right)** Transverse color Doppler ultrasound confirms a renal vein ➡. Color Doppler is very useful for differentiating between dilated renal pelvis and prominent renal vein in equivocal cases.

Prominent Renal Vein

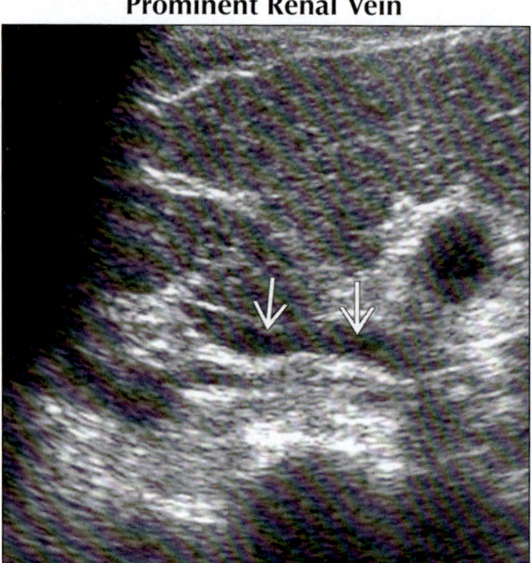

Prominent Renal Vein

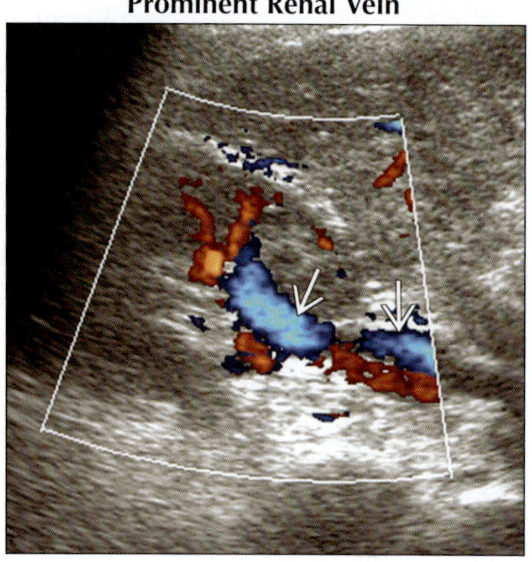

(Left) Transverse transabdominal ultrasound shows a parapelvic cyst ➡ at the renal hilum causing extrinsic compression of the calyceal system ➡. **(Right)** Transverse transabdominal ultrasound shows pyonephrosis with debris ➡ in the obstructed pelvicalyceal system of an infected kidney. Pyonephrosis cannot be distinguished from hemonephrosis on ultrasound alone.

Parapelvic Cyst

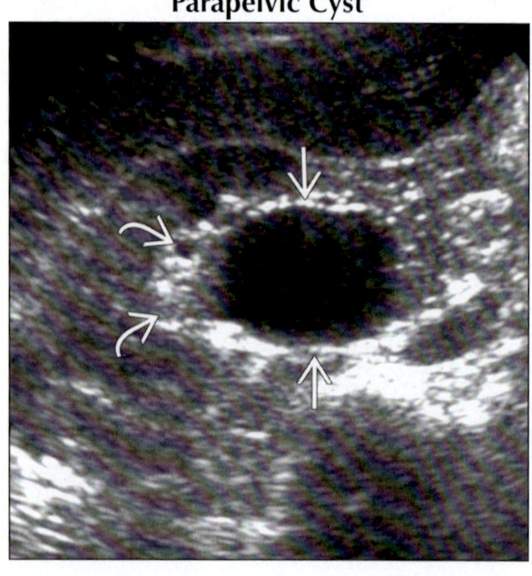

Pyonephrosis

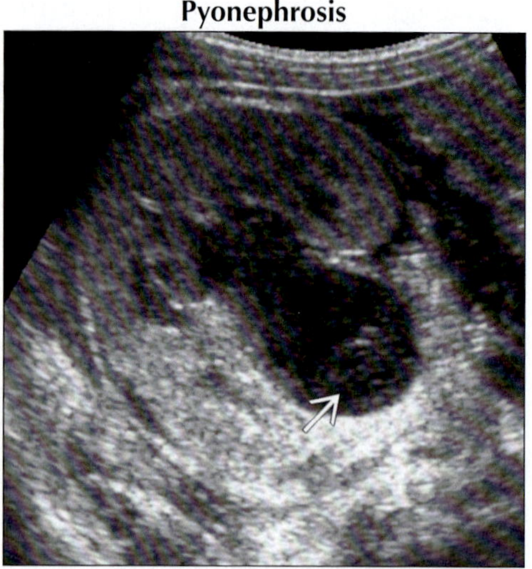

(Left) Transverse transabdominal ultrasound shows hemonephrosis with mid-level echoes in the dilated renal pelvis ➡. Note the echogenicity of blood may vary depending on blood products. **(Right)** Longitudinal color Doppler ultrasound shows a renal sinus hemorrhage ➡ in an atrophic kidney. Note that the hemorrhagic lesion is well defined and avascular, replacing most of the central echocomplex.

Hemonephrosis

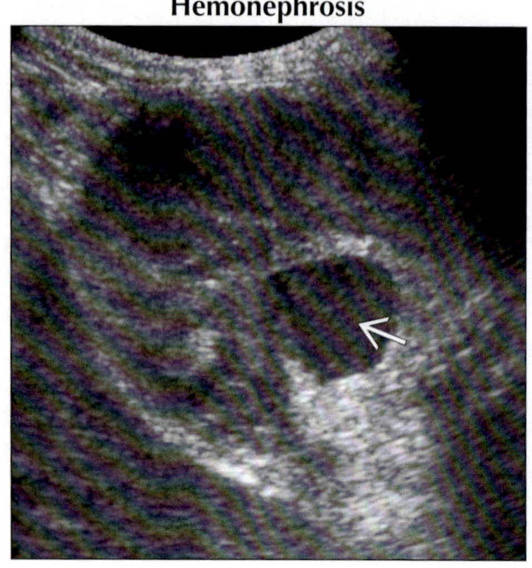

Renal Sinus Hemorrhage

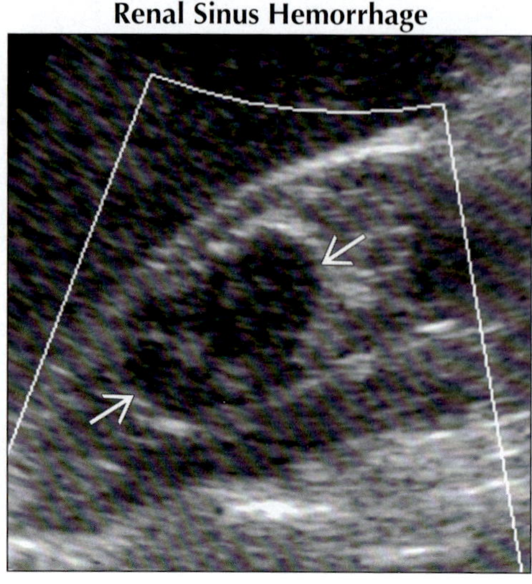

DILATED RENAL PELVIS

Renal Sinus Hemorrhage

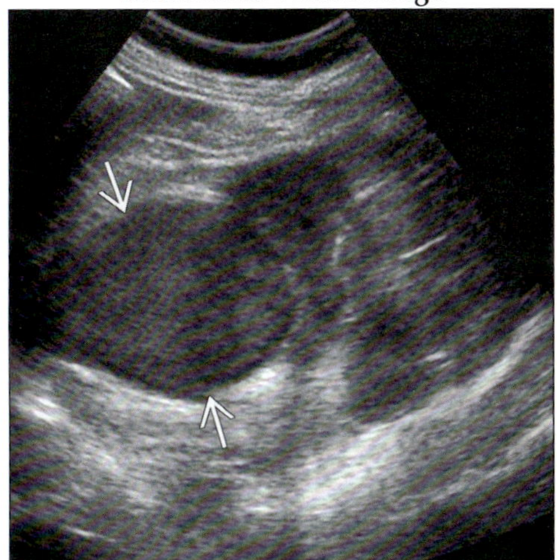

Renal Sinus Hemorrhage

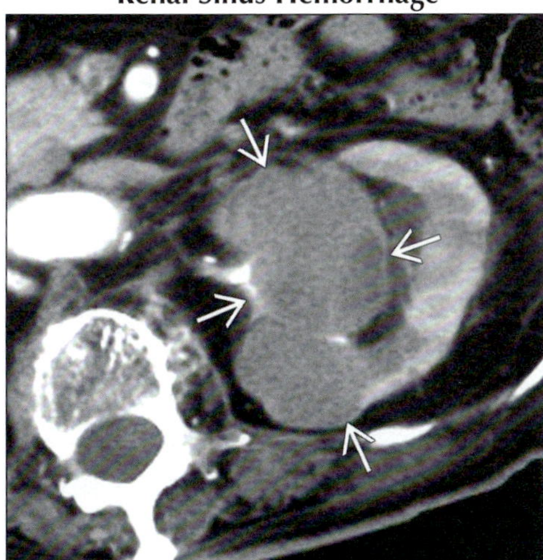

(Left) Transverse transabdominal ultrasound shows a renal sinus hemorrhage due to a hemorrhagic renal tumor at the hilum. The tumor appears as a large cyst ➡ with echogenic internal echoes representing blood. *(Right)* Corresponding axial CECT shows a large, heterogeneously enhancing mass ➡ in the left renal hilum and posterior cortex, representing the hemorrhagic renal tumor.

Pararenal Fluid Collections

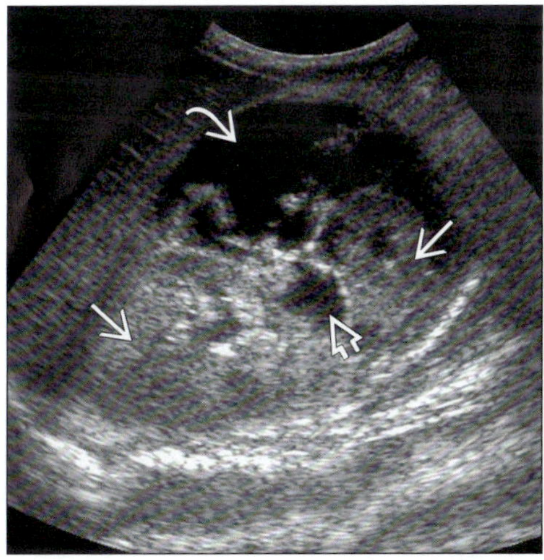

Acute Renal Vein Thrombosis

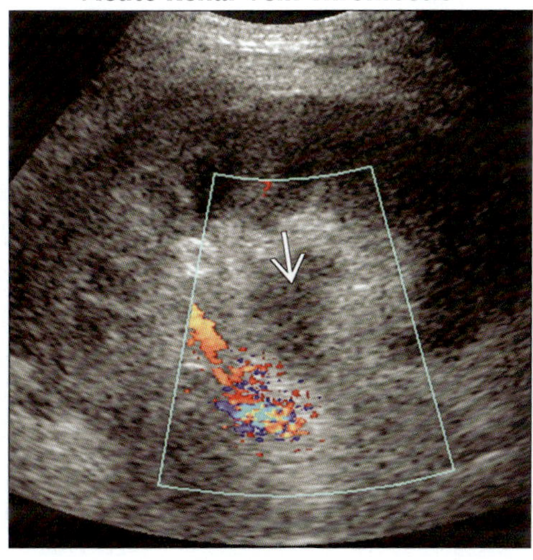

(Left) Longitudinal transabdominal US shows a fractured kidney ➡ surrounded by a large subcapsular hematoma ➡. The blood fills the deep laceration ➡, mimicking a dilated renal pelvis. *(Right)* Longitudinal color Doppler US shows acute renal vein thrombosis (RVT) ➡ in which the vein is filled with hypoechoic thrombus and devoid of color flow. On grayscale imaging, RVT is indistinguishable from a dilated renal pelvis filled with blood, pus, or tumor.

Peripelvic Cyst

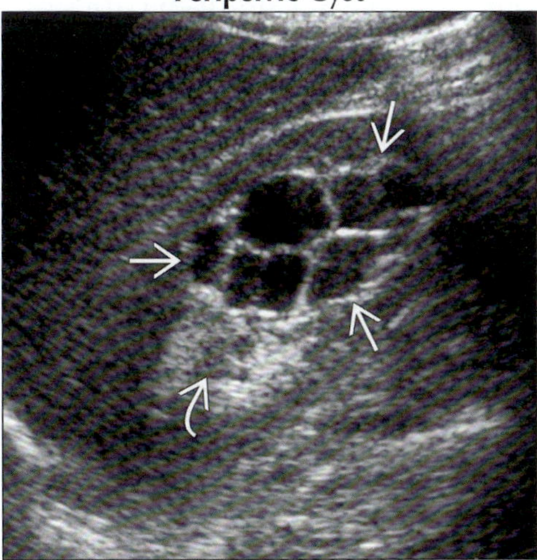

Peripelvic Cyst

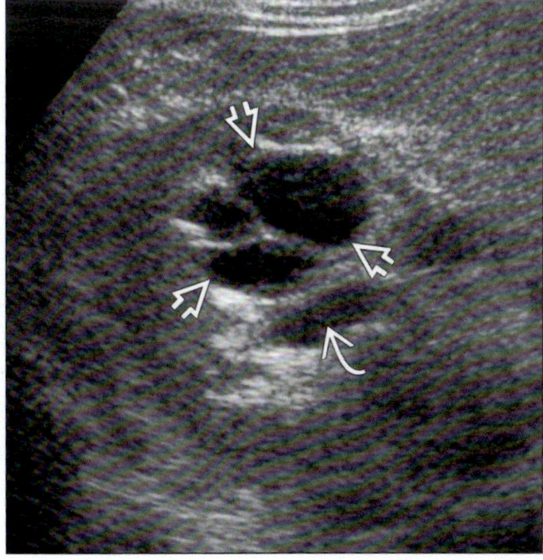

(Left) Longitudinal transabdominal ultrasound shows a peripelvic cyst ➡. The cyst is multiseptated, arising from the renal sinus ➡ of the mid-lower pole and is thought to represent lymphatic ectasia. *(Right)* Transverse transabdominal ultrasound shows the previous peripelvic cyst ➡ at the level of the renal pelvis ➡. The appearance resembles a dilated renal pelvis with associated hydrocalyces.

DIFFERENTIAL DIAGNOSIS

Common
- Fresh Blood Clot
- Benign Urothelial Thickening
- Prominent Renal Papilla

Less Common
- Transitional Cell Carcinoma (TCC)
- Renal Cell Carcinoma (RCC) Invasion
- Renal Lymphoma
- Renal Pelvic Metastasis

Rare but Important
- Suburothelial Hematoma
- Ectopic Renal Papilla
- Hydatid Cyst
- Papilloma
- Leiomyoma
- Neurofibroma
- Mucinous Cystadenoma
- Pyelitis Cystica

ESSENTIAL INFORMATION

Key Differential Diagnosis Issues
- Hypoechoic lesions in renal pelvis should be considered potentially malignant unless proven otherwise
- Blood clot is common entity that may be confused with renal pelvic malignancies
- Further investigation may be warranted to exclude malignancy as underlying cause of bleeding

Helpful Clues for Common Diagnoses
- **Fresh Blood Clot**
  - Hypoechoic
    - Echogenicity of blood clot varies over time
  - Occurs in urinary tract infection, calculus disease, renal neoplasm, and trauma
  - May be confused with TCC
- **Benign Urothelial Thickening**
  - Appears as circumferential wall thickening
  - Echogenicity similar to that of renal parenchyma
  - May be seen in urinary tract infection, chronic urinary reflux, and acute rejection in renal allograft
- **Prominent Renal Papilla**
  - May protrude into renal pelvis, mimicking soft tissue lesion
  - Useful to scan lesion in 2 orthogonal planes to demonstrate continuation of papilla with medullary pyramid

Helpful Clues for Less Common Diagnoses
- **Transitional Cell Carcinoma (TCC)**
  - Appearance depends on whether tumor is sessile, papillary, or obstructive
  - If obstructive, hydronephrosis ± blood in pelvicalyceal (PC) system is present
  - Discrete, single or multiple, hypoechoic solid masses in renal pelvis
  - Synchronous lesions may be found in bladder
  - Reniform shape of kidney usually preserved
- **Renal Cell Carcinoma (RCC) Invasion**
  - Cortical renal tumor; typically exophytic
  - Usually heterogeneous but may be hypoechoic
  - Typically hypervascular
  - May be intrarenal or infiltrative, extending into renal pelvis
  - May simulate TCC
  - PC system may be disrupted
- **Renal Lymphoma**
  - Non-Hodgkin disease > Hodgkin disease
  - Presentations: Multiple cortical masses > diffuse infiltration > single mass > direct extension from extrarenal disease
  - Direct invasion to renal pelvis from retroperitoneal lymphomatous disease is rare
  - Typically hypoechoic and hypovascular
- **Renal Pelvic Metastasis**
  - Common primaries are lung, breast, colon, and melanoma
  - Rarely from esophageal carcinoma and sarcoma
  - RCC metastasis to contralateral renal pelvis or ureter extremely rare
  - Invariably causes urinary obstruction

Helpful Clues for Rare Diagnoses
- **Suburothelial Hematoma**
  - Also called Antopol-Goldman lesions
  - Either forms in perirenal area or in renal pelvis
  - Mild: Appears as pelvic or ureteral wall thickening
  - Severe: Hypoechoic mass in renal pelvis compressing PC system
  - Associated with coagulation disorders

- **Ectopic Renal Papilla**
  - May be intrainfundibular or in intrarenal portion of renal pelvis
  - May appear as small, hypoechoic, ovoid or round lesion with smooth outline
  - Careful scanning may show extrinsic origin of papilla
- **Hydatid Cyst**
  - Location: Renal parenchyma > renal pelvis
  - May appear as unilocular cyst simulating simple renal cyst
  - Debris or small cysts ("bunch of grapes" sign) may be seen within renal pelvis
  - Cyst may rupture into PC system (10-20%) causing hydatiduria
- **Papilloma**
  - Benign transitional epithelial tumor
  - Location: Ureter and bladder > upper urinary tract
  - With polypoid lesion, however, ultrasound unable to demonstrate stalk
  - Appears as hypoechoic lesion mimicking renal pelvic tumor
  - Inverted papilloma with central core composed of transitional epithelium extremely rare
- **Leiomyoma**
  - Rare mesenchymal tumor in kidney
  - Size ranges from 1 cm to > 10 cm
  - Location: Subcapsular region > renal cortex > renal pelvis
  - Appears as well-defined, hypoechoic lesion
  - NECT: Hyperdense to renal cortex
  - CECT: Hypodense to renal cortex

- Imaging techniques cannot readily differentiate it from other renal malignancies
- **Neurofibroma**
  - Rare nerve tumor involving kidney
  - Renal pelvic lesions have echogenicity similar to renal cortex
  - Parapelvic lesions may cause extrinsic compression on renal pelvis
  - > 60% show cystic changes
- **Mucinous Cystadenoma**
  - Cystic tumor that may undergo malignant transformation to cystadenocarcinoma
  - Large size at presentation
  - Mucinous nephrosis due to mucin production by tumor
- **Pyelitis Cystica**
  - Multiple, small, subepithelial cysts arising from pelvic wall
  - May be unilateral or bilateral
  - Excretory urogram shows multiple, small, smooth, round filling defects in renal pelvis
  - Caused by degeneration of basal layer of urothelium due to chronic urinary tract infection

Fresh Blood Clot

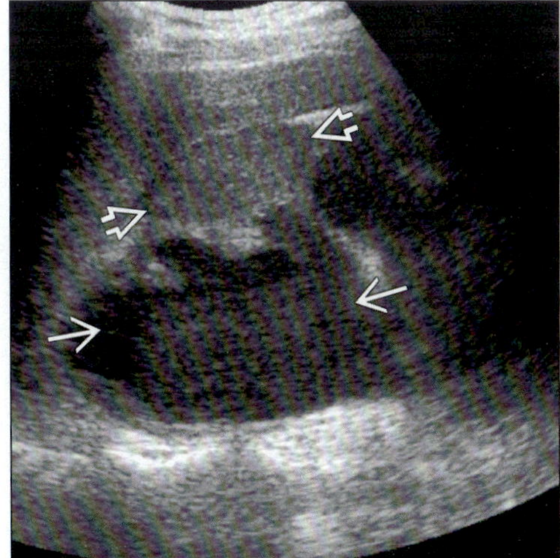

Longitudinal transabdominal ultrasound shows a fresh blood clot ➡ in the dilated PC system of a patient with gross hematuria. A cortical tumor ▶ is also noted, suspicious of renal malignancy.

Benign Urothelial Thickening

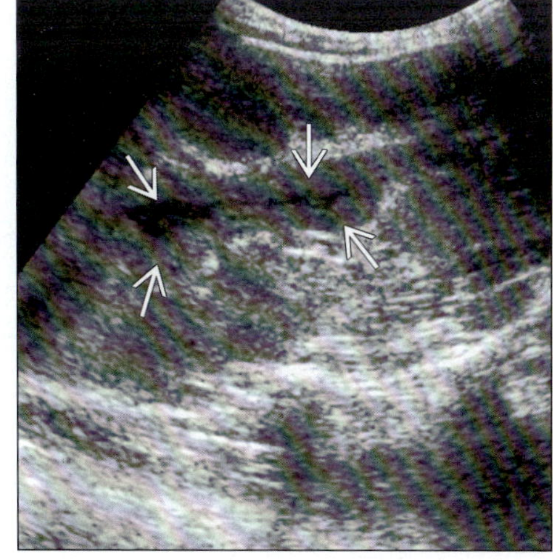

Longitudinal transabdominal ultrasound shows a grossly thickened urothelium ➡ in the renal pelvis of a patient with confirmed renal tuberculosis.

HYPOECHOIC RENAL PELVIC LESION

(Left) Oblique transabdominal ultrasound shows a round lesion ➡ in the renal pelvis, suspicious of a small soft tissue mass. *(Right)* Transverse transabdominal ultrasound shows the same renal pelvic lesion to be a renal papilla ➡ protruding into the mildly distended renal pelvis ➡. The contrast offered by fluid in the distended pelvis makes the renal papilla more conspicuous.

Prominent Renal Papilla

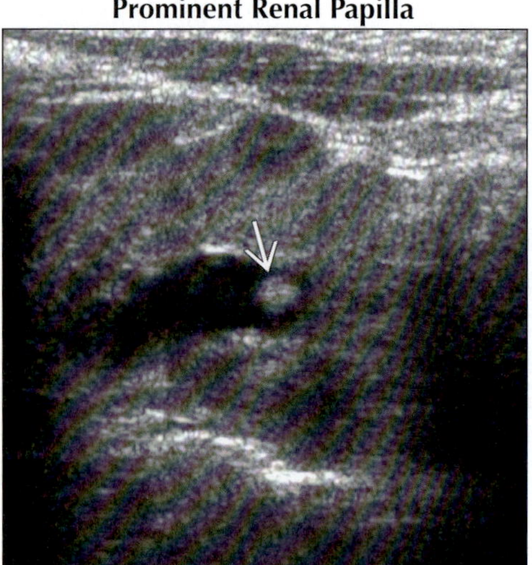

Prominent Renal Papilla

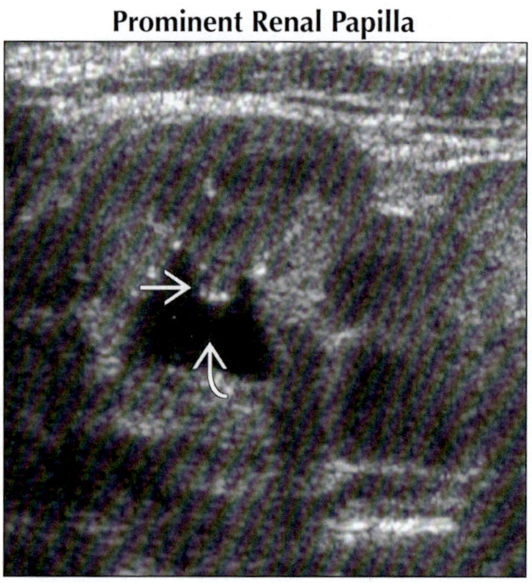

(Left) Longitudinal transabdominal ultrasound shows a multifocal transitional cell carcinoma in a hydronephrotic kidney. Note multiple hypoechoic lesions ➡, which appear similar to organized blood or debris. *(Right)* Transverse transabdominal ultrasound in the same patient shows multifocal transitional cell carcinoma with the renal pelvis obstructed by hypoechoic material ➡.

Transitional Cell Carcinoma (TCC)

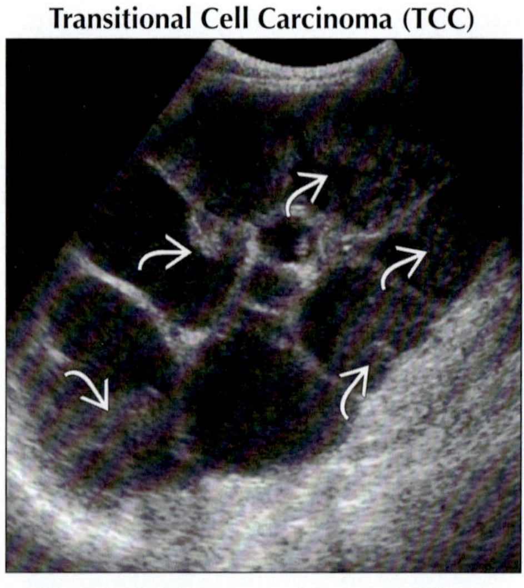

Transitional Cell Carcinoma (TCC)

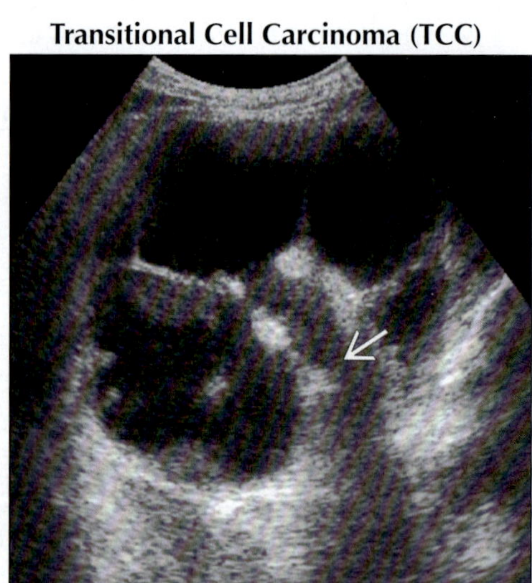

(Left) Longitudinal transabdominal ultrasound shows a TCC ➡ obstructing the renal pelvis with associated hemonephrosis. Note that the low-level echoes ➡ within the collecting system likely represent urine mixed with debris and red blood cells. *(Right)* Corresponding longitudinal color Doppler ultrasound shows vascularity ➡ in the TCC. On grayscale imaging, differentiation between blood clot and tumor may be difficult.

Transitional Cell Carcinoma (TCC)

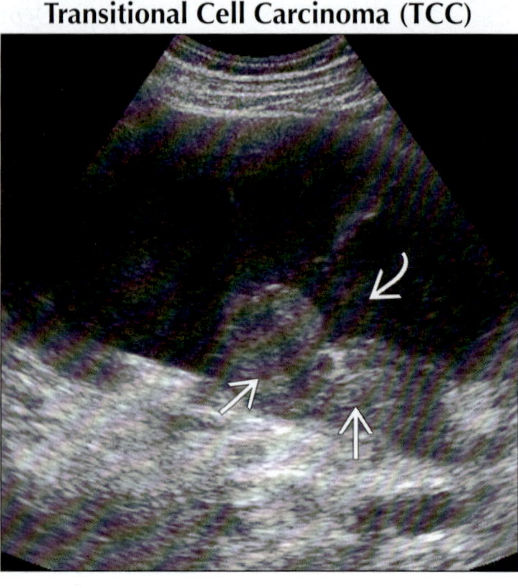

Transitional Cell Carcinoma (TCC)

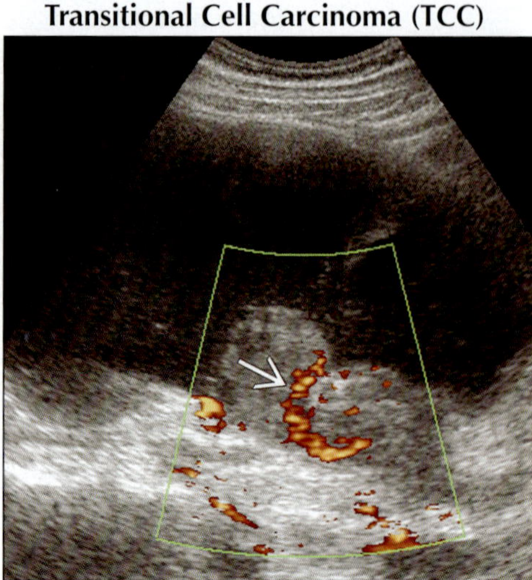

HYPOECHOIC RENAL PELVIC LESION

Transitional Cell Carcinoma (TCC)

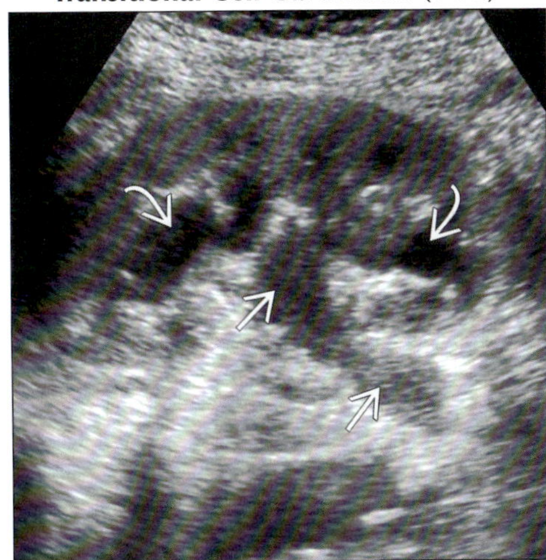

Transitional Cell Carcinoma (TCC)

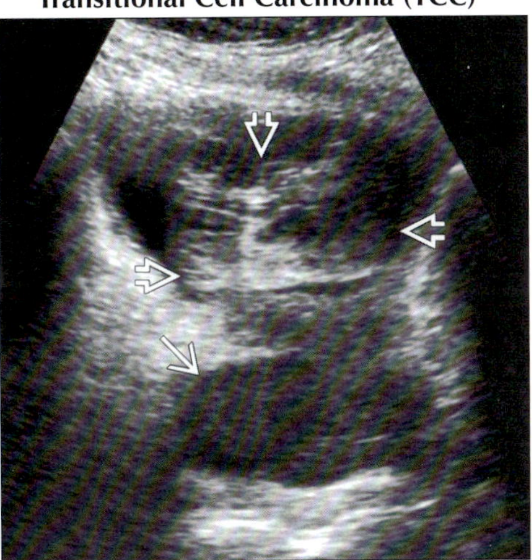

(Left) Longitudinal transabdominal ultrasound of the renal pelvis in a patient with bladder TCC. The tumor is hypoechoic, filling the upper ureter and renal pelvis ➡, causing hydronephrosis ➡. Synchronous TCC is common. (Right) Longitudinal transabdominal ultrasound of the pelvis in the same patient shows a large heterogeneous mass ➡ in the bladder with posterior extension to the vaginal stump ➡.

Renal Cell Carcinoma (RCC) Invasion

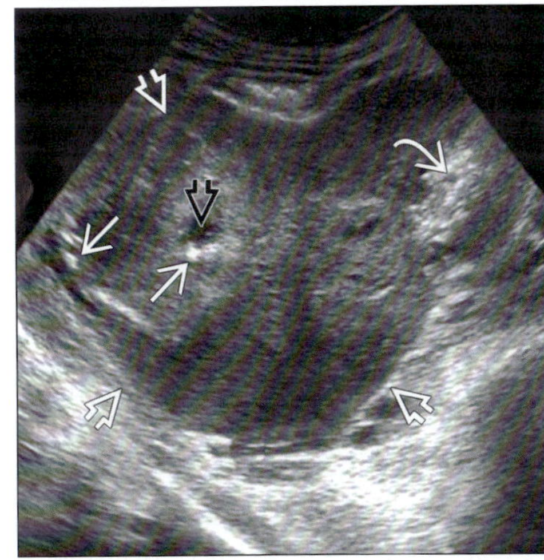

Renal Cell Carcinoma (RCC) Invasion

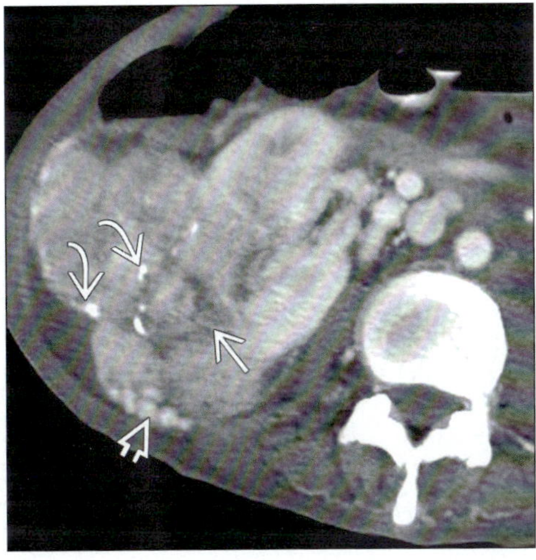

(Left) Transverse transabdominal ultrasound shows a large, lobulated renal cell carcinoma ➡ extending into the PC system ➡ of the kidney. The tumor is hypoechoic with central necrosis ➡ and intraparenchymal and rim calcifications ➡. (Right) Corresponding axial CECT shows PC system involvement by the renal cell carcinoma. The tumor is heterogeneously enhanced with small cystic areas ➡, calcifications ➡, and peritumoral vascularity ➡.

Renal Lymphoma

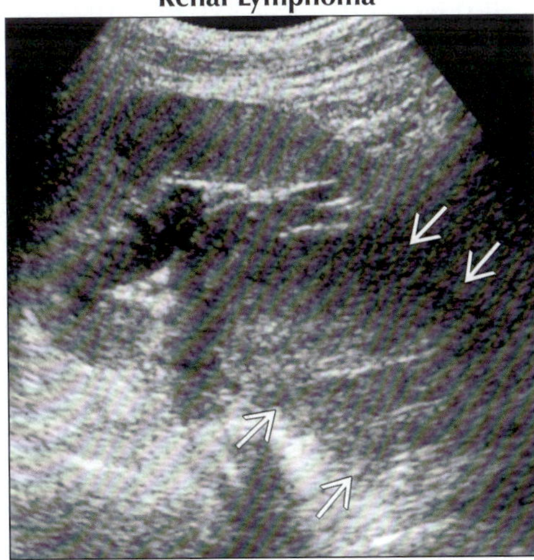

Papilloma

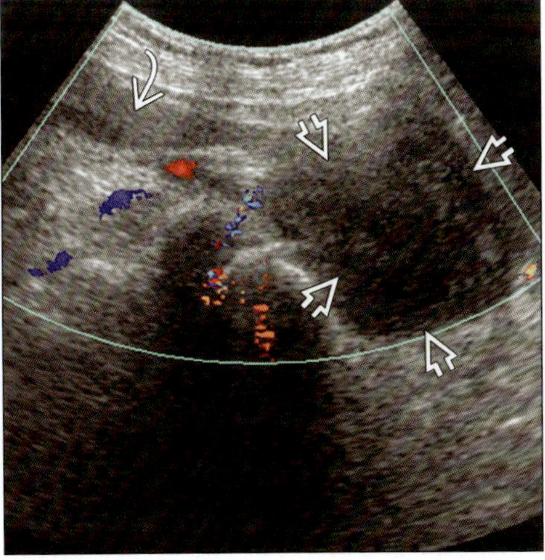

(Left) Transverse transabdominal ultrasound shows a retroperitoneal lymphomatous mass ➡ extending into the renal hilum. The appearance simulates a large mass in the dilated renal pelvis. (Right) Oblique color Doppler ultrasound shows a large papilloma ➡ in the distal ureter ➡ causing urinary obstruction. The tumor is hypoechoic and avascular. In the renal pelvis, papillomas may mimic a transitional cell carcinoma.

DIFFERENTIAL DIAGNOSIS

Common
- Calcium Stone
- Nephrocalcinosis
- Surgical Stent or Drainage Catheter
- Adjacent Calcified Renal Artery
- Adjacent Milk of Calcium Cyst
- Adjacent Renal Angiomyolipoma
- Urinary Sludge
- Blood Clot
- Transitional Cell Carcinoma (TCC)

Less Common
- Sloughed Papilla
- Struvite (Infection) Stone
- Urate Calculus
- Gas in Pelvicalyceal (PC) System
- Squamous Cell Carcinoma (SCCa)

Rare but Important
- Fungal Ball (Mycetoma)
- Hemangioma
- Leukoplakia or Cholesteatoma
- Hydatid Cyst
- Renal Replacement Lipomatosis (RRL)
- Medullary Carcinoma
- Adenocarcinoma
- Melamine Stone

ESSENTIAL INFORMATION

Key Differential Diagnosis Issues
- Calcium stone most common
- Echogenic malignant lesions rare in renal pelvis

Helpful Clues for Common Diagnoses
- **Calcium Stone**
  - Accounts for ~ 70% of renal stones
  - Echogenic renal focus with posterior acoustic shadowing
- **Nephrocalcinosis**
  - Commonly caused by medullary sponge kidney or hypercalcemia due to primary hyperparathyroidism or renal tubular acidosis
  - Hyperechoic foci ± shadowing or diffuse hyperechogenicity in renal pyramids
- **Surgical Stent or Drainage Catheter**
  - Echogenic parallel lines in renal pelvis; history of intervention
- **Adjacent Calcified Renal Artery**
  - Calcified plaque in renal arterial wall
  - Mimics small renal pelvic calculus
- **Adjacent Milk of Calcium Cyst**
  - Collection of calcific granules in urine
  - Frequently seen in calyceal diverticulum, simple cyst, or polycystic kidneys
  - Produces "comet tail" artifacts
- **Adjacent Renal Angiomyolipoma**
  - Highly echogenic renal mass depending on fat content
  - May grow to 20 cm in size
  - Large exophytic lesion may distort pelvicalyceal system and cause obstruction
  - May mimic renal cell carcinoma with renal pelvic invasion
- **Urinary Sludge**
  - Urinary precipitate of calcium crystals, infective or hemorrhagic material
  - Appearance varies with change in patient's position
- **Blood Clot**
  - Echogenicity varies with time
  - ↑ echogenicity in chronic blood clot
- **Transitional Cell Carcinoma (TCC)**
  - High-grade TCC may be densely echogenic due to formation of keratin "pearls"
  - Do not produce posterior acoustic shadowing

Helpful Clues for Less Common Diagnoses
- **Sloughed Papilla**
  - Sequelae of renal papillary necrosis
  - May appear as soft tissue lesion with ring-shaped peripheral calcification or echogenic lesion mimicking calculi
- **Struvite (Infection) Stone**
  - Commonly occurs in urinary tract infection due to gram-negative enteric organisms
  - Accounts for 70% of staghorn stones
- **Urate Calculus**
  - Nonradiopaque stone that may produce posterior acoustic shadowing
  - Occurs in patients with gout, neoplastic disease on chemotherapy or radiation therapy, and Lesch-Nyhan syndrome
- **Gas in Pelvicalyceal (PC) System**
  - Iatrogenic causes: Vesicoureteric reflux of air during introduction of Foley catheter or ureterocystoscopy

HYPERECHOIC RENAL PELVIC LESION

- ○ Infective causes: Emphysematous pyelonephritis, pyonephrosis, or pyelitis due to gas-producing organisms
- ○ Hyperechoic focus with "dirty" shadowing
- **Squamous Cell Carcinoma (SCCa)**
  - ○ Echogenic, solid, renal pelvic tumor
  - ○ Associated with retroperitoneal lymphadenopathy
  - ○ Usually presents with advanced disease at diagnosis
  - ○ Frequently associated with stones or chronic irritation

Helpful Clues for Rare Diagnoses
- **Fungal Ball (Mycetoma)**
  - ○ Appears as echogenic nonshadowing mass in collecting system
  - ○ Secondary to renal infection in isolated or disseminated fungal infection
  - ○ Common in immunocompromised and diabetic patients
- **Hemangioma**
  - ○ Usually solitary and unilateral
  - ○ Echogenic or hyperechoic ± anechoic center corresponding to blood-filled spaces
  - ○ Echogenicity ≈ renal sinus
  - ○ Mostly located in renal pelvis or at medullary junction
  - ○ May mimic renal cell carcinoma or TCC
- **Leukoplakia or Cholesteatoma**
  - ○ Associated with chronic infection &/or calculus disease
  - ○ Location: Renal pelvis > proximal ureter
  - ○ Bilateral in 10% of cases

- ○ Leukoplakia: Flat mass or focal urothelial wall thickening
- ○ Cholesteatoma: Keratinized soft tissue mass simulating renal pelvic calculus
- **Hydatid Cyst**
  - ○ With wall calcification ⇒ densely echogenic shadowing mass
- **Renal Replacement Lipomatosis (RRL)**
  - ○ Result of chronic inflammation; associated with calculus disease
  - ○ Renal parenchyma destroyed and replaced by echogenic fibrofatty tissue
  - ○ Involves renal sinus, renal hilum, and perirenal space
  - ○ May coexist with xanthogranulomatous pyelonephritis
- **Medullary Carcinoma**
  - ○ Afflicts young men with sickle cell trait
  - ○ Centrally located infiltrating mass with ↑ echogenicity and sinus fat invasion
  - ○ Associated with retroperitoneal adenopathy and caliectasis
  - ○ Venous invasion often present
- **Adenocarcinoma**
  - ○ Echogenic mass in renal pelvis
  - ○ Dystrophic tumoral calcification relatively common
  - ○ Frequently associated with calculi or chronic irritation
- **Melamine Stone**
  - ○ Due to consumption of melamine-tainted milk or products
  - ○ Echogenic ± weak posterior shadowing

Calcium Stone

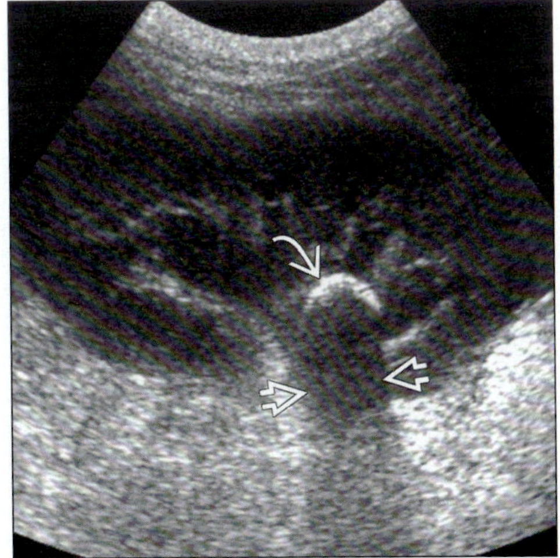

Longitudinal transabdominal ultrasound shows an echogenic calculus ➡ *with dense posterior acoustic shadowing* ➡ *in the renal pelvis. This appearance most likely represents a calcium stone.*

Surgical Stent or Drainage Catheter

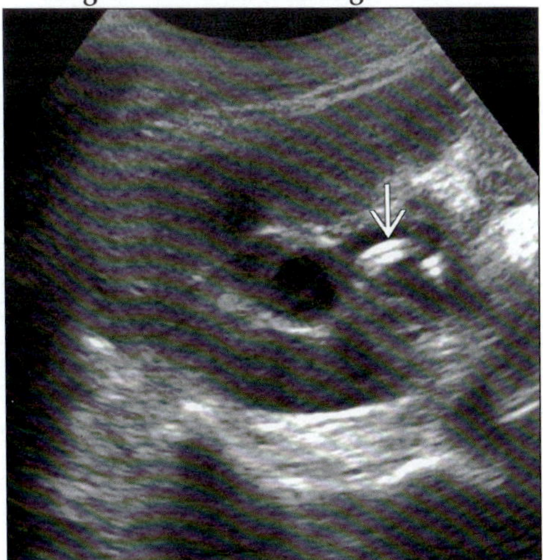

Transverse ultrasound of the kidney shows a "pigtail" drainage catheter ➡ *as hyperechoic parallel lines in a dilated renal pelvis. Differentiation of the stent from other echogenic renal pelvic lesions is straightforward.*

HYPERECHOIC RENAL PELVIC LESION

(Left) Transverse transabdominal ultrasound shows a small milk of calcium cyst ➡ adjacent to the renal pelvis with a characteristic "comet tail" artifact. (Right) Longitudinal transabdominal ultrasound shows a large exophytic renal angiomyolipoma ➡. Note that the pelivcalyceal system is obliterated with only the central sinus of the lower pole preserved ➡. A hydrocalyx ➡ is also visible.

Adjacent Milk of Calcium Cyst

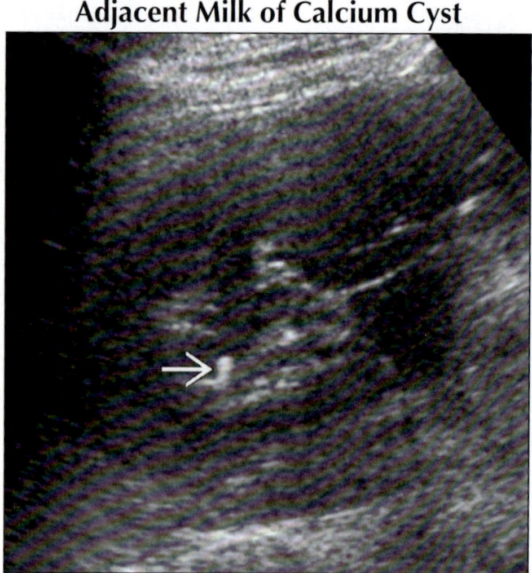

Adjacent Renal Angiomyolipoma

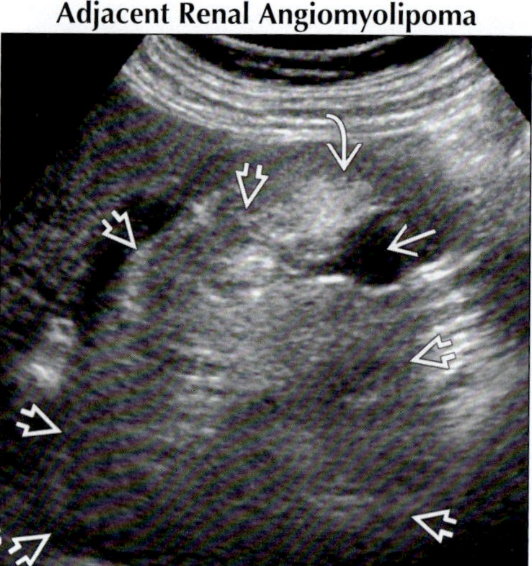

(Left) Longitudinal transabdominal ultrasound shows echogenic sludge or pus ➡ in a pyonephrotic kidney. A staghorn calculus ➡ with shadowing is seen in the lower pole. (Right) Longitudinal transabdominal ultrasound shows an echogenic blood clot ➡ in the renal pelvis confirmed by ureteroscopy. Note the sonographic resemblance of the blood clot and the sludge. The appearance may also mimic urothelial malignancies.

Urinary Sludge

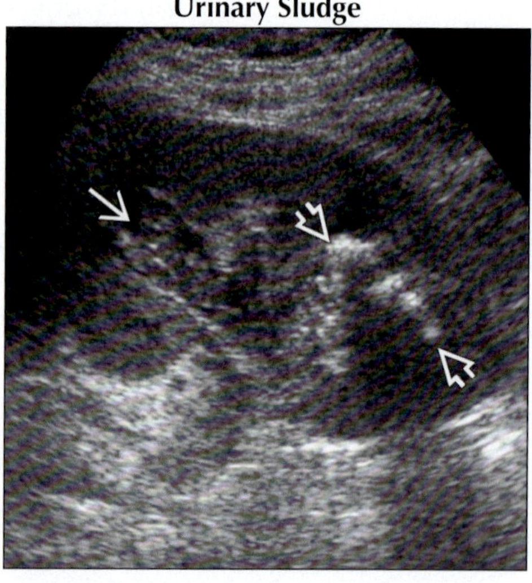

Blood Clot

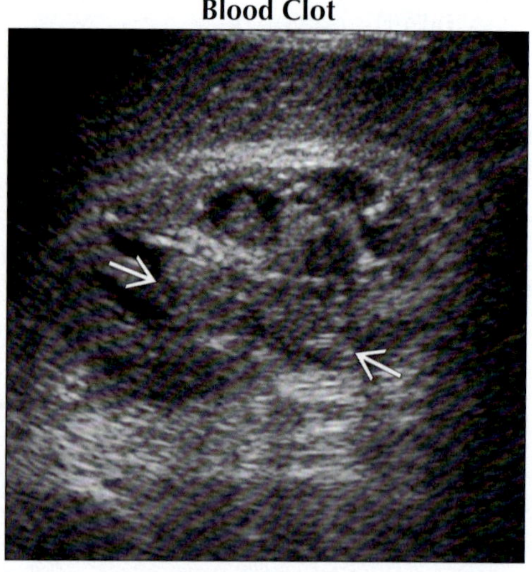

(Left) Transverse transabdominal ultrasound shows a high-grade TCC ➡ causing hemonephrosis with echogenic blood ➡. The tumor shows an increase in echogenicity due to keratinization. (Right) Longitudinal transabdominal ultrasound shows an echogenic lesion ➡ in a fluid-filled medullary cavity, which is continuous with the calyx ➡. Note that the lesion has ring-shaped peripheral calcification, typical of a sloughed papilla.

Transitional Cell Carcinoma (TCC)

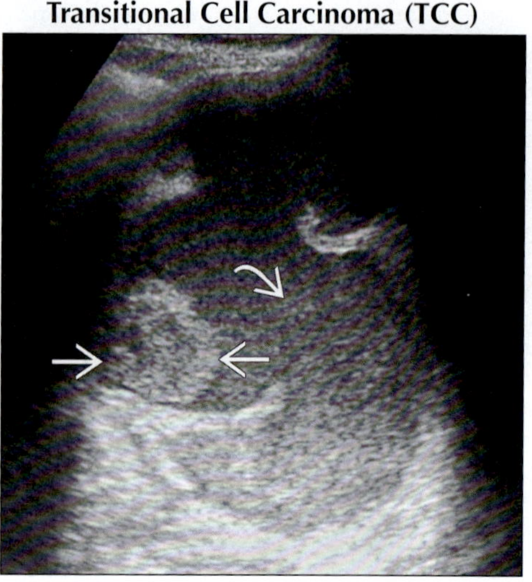

Sloughed Papilla

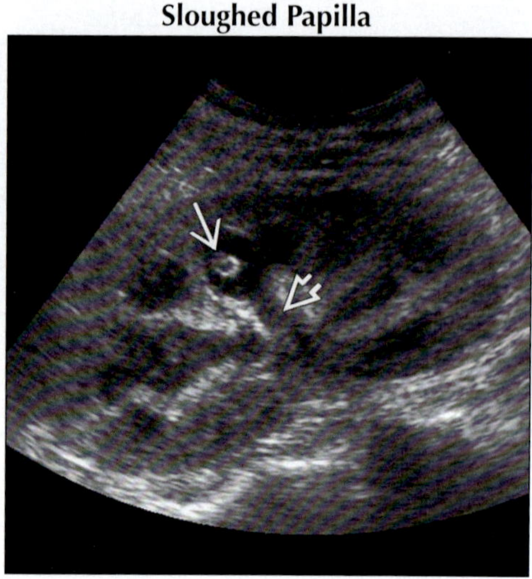

8

HYPERECHOIC RENAL PELVIC LESION

Struvite (Infection) Stone

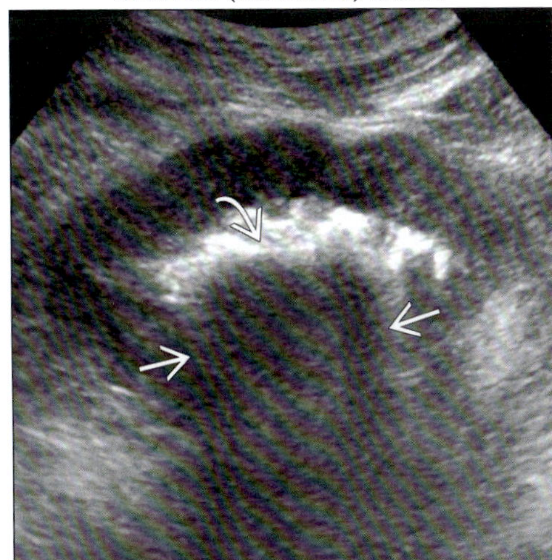

Gas in Pelvicalyceal (PC) System

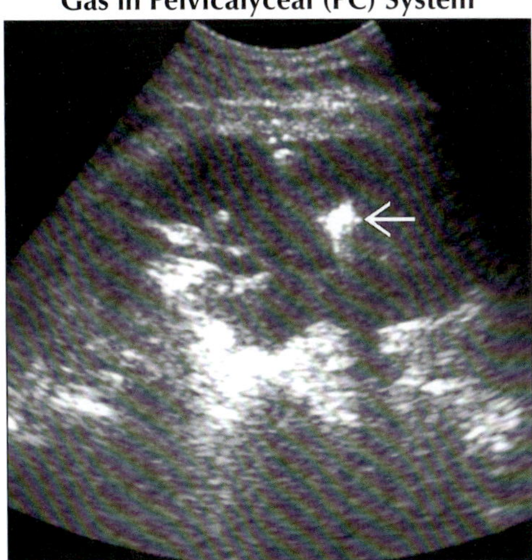

(Left) Longitudinal transabdominal ultrasound shows a large staghorn calculus ➡ with posterior acoustic shadowing ➡ in the pelvicalyceal system. This calculus probably represents a struvite stone caused by a urinary tract infection. *(Right)* Longitudinal transabdominal ultrasound shows emphysematous pyelonephritis with gas ➡ in the renal parenchyma, mimicking gas or calculus in the renal pelvis.

Squamous Cell Carcinoma (SCCa)

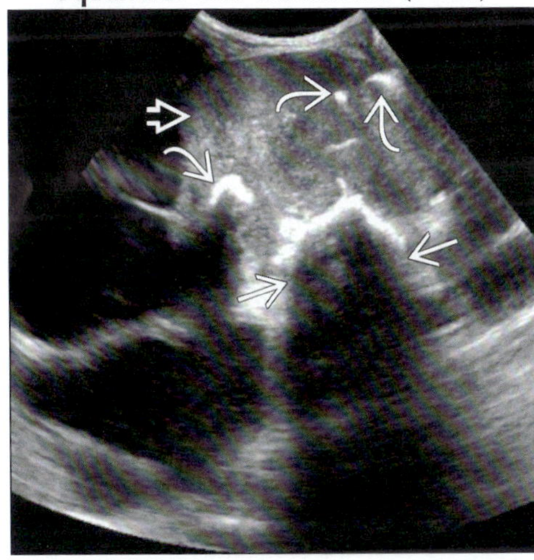

Squamous Cell Carcinoma (SCCa)

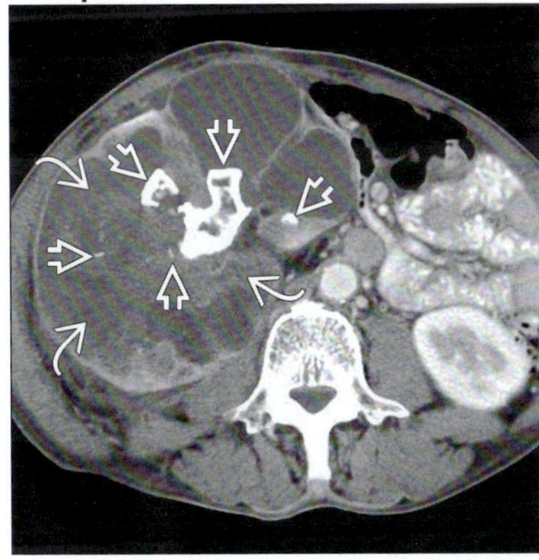

(Left) Longitudinal transabdominal ultrasound shows renal squamous cell carcinoma ➡ in a grossly hydronephrotic kidney. The tumor is echogenic with internal calcifications ➡ occupying the lower half of the PC system, which is obstructed by a large staghorn stone ➡ in the renal pelvis. *(Right)* Corresponding axial CECT shows the SCCa ➡ in the grossly enlarged kidney. The staghorn stone and small calcifications ➡ are clearly shown within the tumor.

Fungal Ball (Mycetoma)

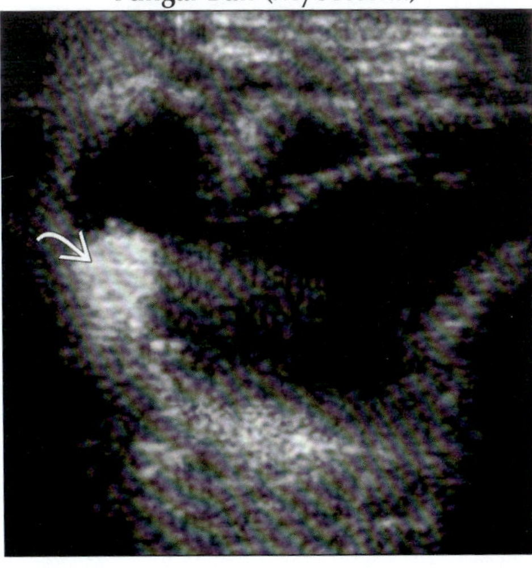

Renal Replacement Lipomatosis (RRL)

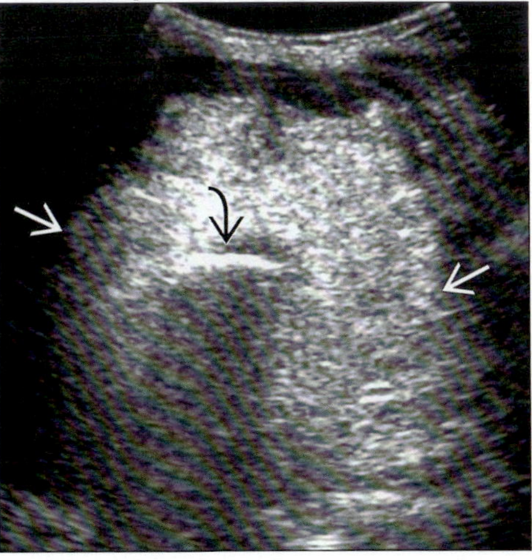

(Left) Longitudinal transabdominal ultrasound in an immunocompromised patient shows a fungal ball ➡, which is echogenic and nonshadowing in the dilated PC system due to a Candida infection. *(Right)* Transverse transabdominal ultrasound shows RRL in xanthogranulomatous pyelonephritis with marked hyperechoic fat ➡ replacing the normal renal parenchyma, resulting in an enlarged renal sinus with an obstructing calculus ➡.

SECTION 9
Abdominal Wall/Peritoneal Cavity

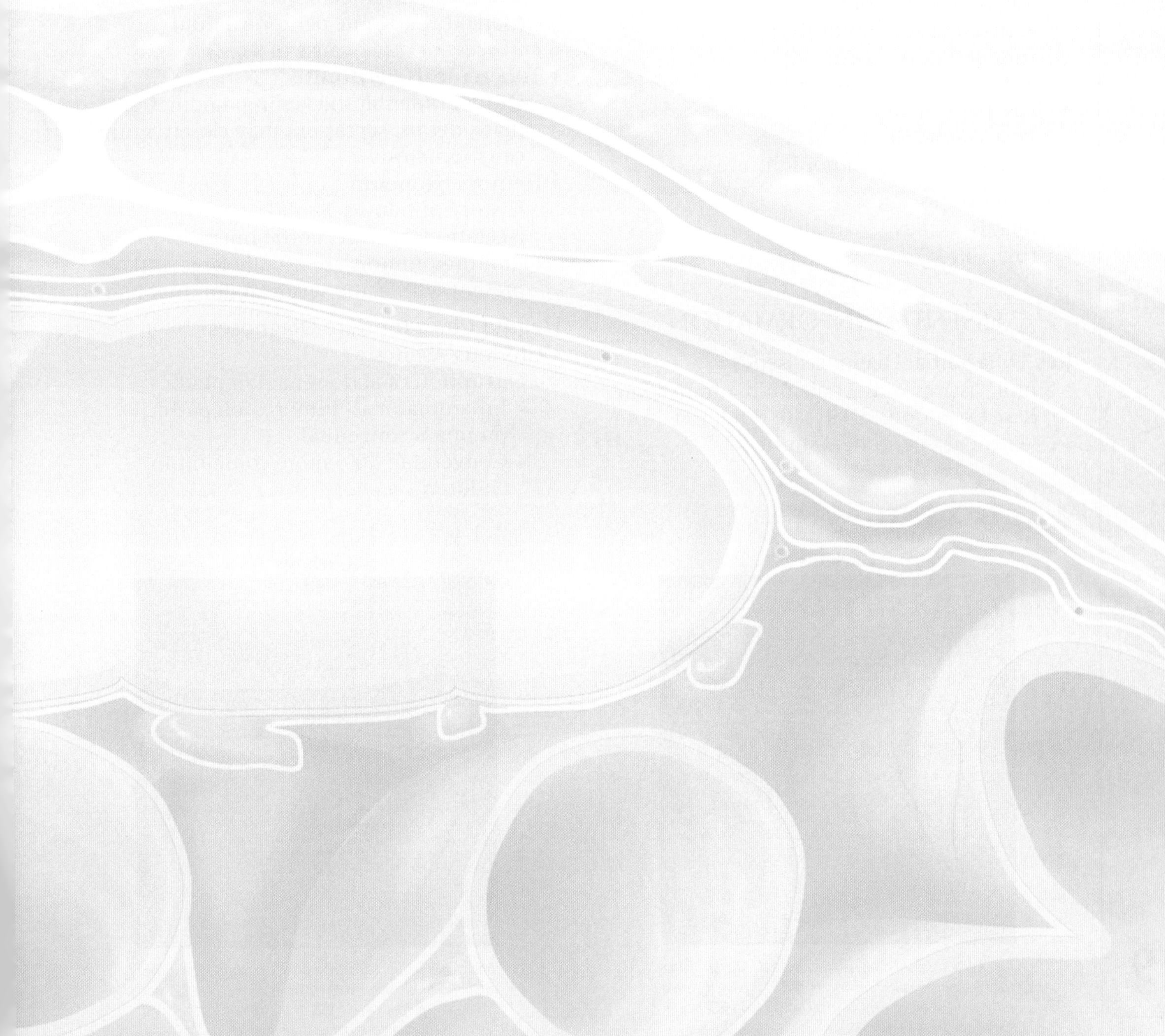

DIFFUSE PERITONEAL FLUID

DIFFERENTIAL DIAGNOSIS

Common
- Transudate
  - Portal Hypertension
    - Cirrhosis
    - Portal Vein Thrombosis
    - Budd-Chiari Syndrome
  - Poor Cardiac Output
  - Fluid Overload
    - Chronic Renal Failure

Less Common
- Exudate
  - Carcinomatosis
  - Peritonitis
    - Pyogenic Peritonitis
    - Tuberculosis Peritonitis
  - Inflammatory Cause
    - Pancreatitis, Polyserositis
- Hemoperitoneum
  - Post-Traumatic
  - Intraabdominal Tumor Rupture

Rare but Important
- Chylous Ascites
- Urine, Bile, CSF

ESSENTIAL INFORMATION

Key Differential Diagnosis Issues
- Simple ascites = anechoic fluid = transudate
  - Rare exceptions: Dialysate fluid, CSF from ventriculo-peritoneal shunt
- Complicated ascites = echogenic fluid, debris, septae = exudate, hemorrhagic, or chylous
  - Septae suggest subacute to chronic nature

Helpful Clues for Common Diagnoses
- **Transudate**
  - Look for cause: Cirrhotic liver, engorged hepatic veins in heart failure, chronic renal parenchymal disease

Helpful Clues for Less Common Diagnoses
- **Carcinomatosis**
  - Peritoneal deposits, omental cake, other evidence of metastases or primary
- **Pyogenic Peritonitis**
  - Dilated, fluid-filled bowel with ↓ peristalsis
  - Marked echogenic peritoneal fluid
  - Abscess or other cause of sepsis
- **Tuberculosis Peritonitis**
  - Diffuse omental thickening, nodules or mass, debris, septation; may closely mimic carcinomatosis
- **Hemoperitoneum**
  - History of trauma ± solid organ laceration/fracture, aortic injury
  - Ruptured tumors are usually large and present with acute severe abdominal pain

Helpful Clues for Rare Diagnoses
- **Chylous Ascites**
  - Disruption of abdominal lymphatics
    - Inflammatory > tumor > idiopathic > trauma > congenital
    - Congenital: 40% more common in children

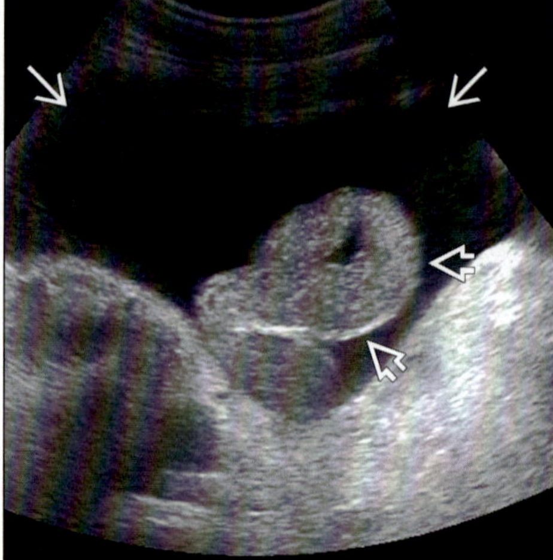

Cirrhosis

Transverse transabdominal ultrasound shows large volume, diffuse, anechoic ascites ➡ in a patient with a cirrhotic liver. A segment of small bowel loop ➡ is seen floating in the ascitic fluid.

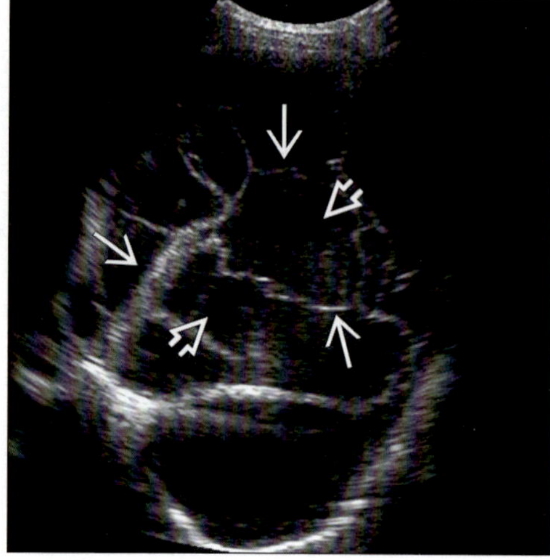

Cirrhosis

Transverse transabdominal ultrasound shows multiloculated ascites with multiple thick septae ➡ and low-level internal debris ➡ in a cirrhotic patient with previous spontaneous bacterial peritonitis.

DIFFUSE PERITONEAL FLUID

Carcinomatosis

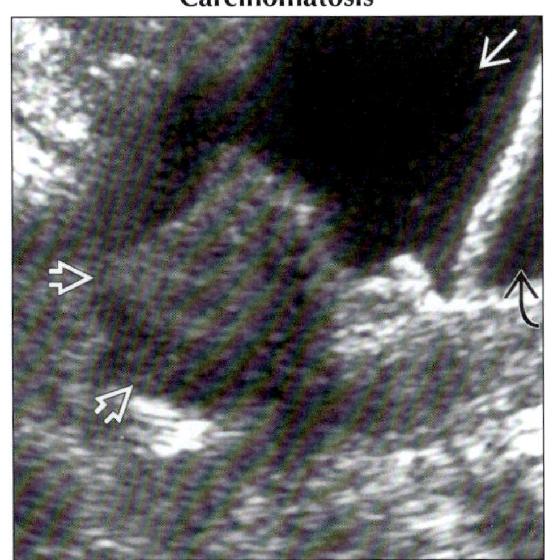

Carcinomatosis

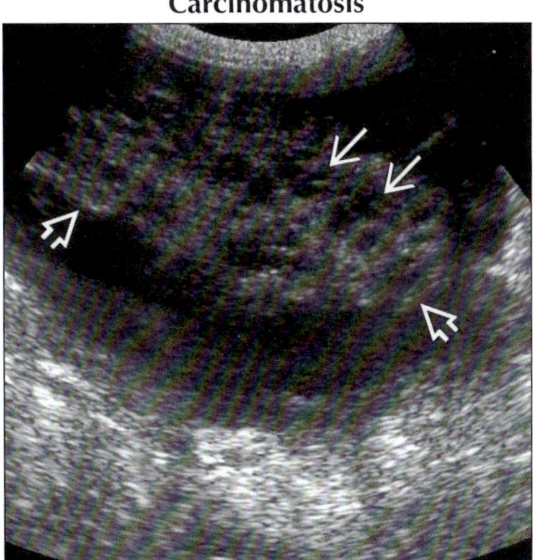

(Left) Longitudinal transabdominal US shows anechoic ascites ➡ associated with multiple, irregular, hypoechoic soft tissue nodules ⇉, representing metastatic deposits with malignant ascites. Note the urinary bladder ➔. *(Right)* Transverse transabdominal US shows pseudomyxoma peritonei with ascites. Note that the pseudomyxoma peritonei is seen as an irregular, soft tissue mass ⇉ with numerous internal cystic spaces ⇉.

Peritonitis

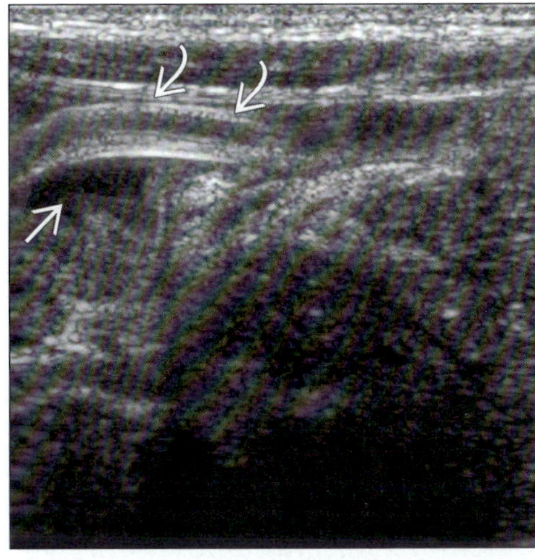

Pyogenic Peritonitis

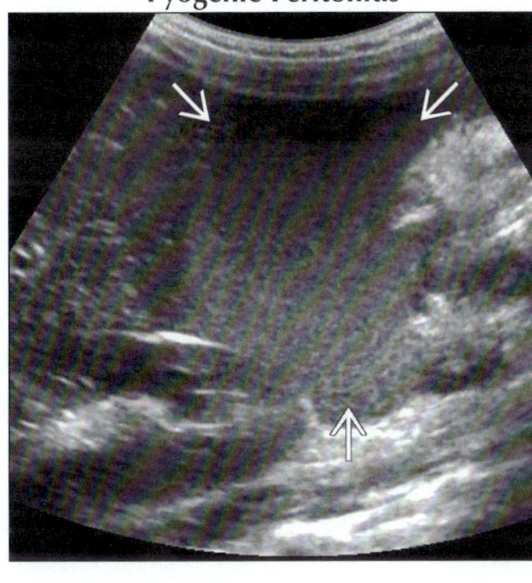

(Left) Longitudinal transabdominal US in RLQ shows a small amount of ascites ➡ in this patient with a mobile tubular structure, representing round worm infestation ➡ with peritonitis. *(Right)* Longitudinal US in RLQ shows markedly echogenic peritoneal fluid ➡ with no loculation or septae, suggesting acute, complicated ascites (pus or blood). This was peritonitis with frank pus in this patient with a ruptured acute appendicitis.

Tuberculosis Peritonitis

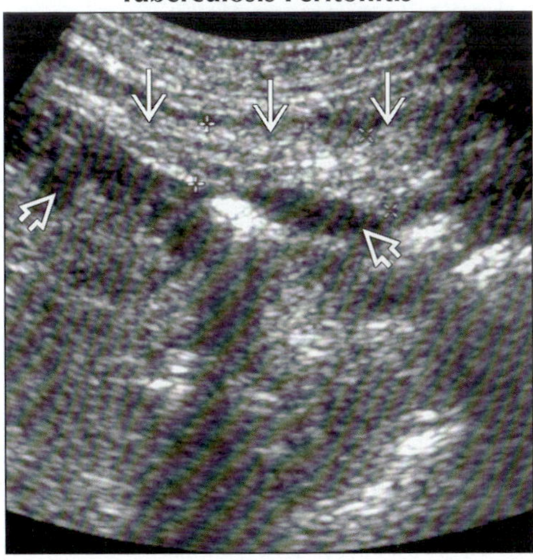

Intraabdominal Tumor Rupture

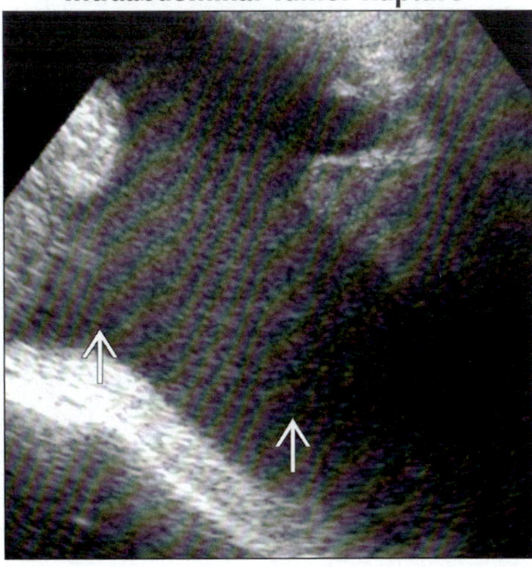

(Left) Transverse transabdominal ultrasound shows a small amount of ascites ⇉ with peritoneal thickening ➡ in a patient with tuberculous peritonitis. *(Right)* Longitudinal ultrasound shows complicated ascites filled with low-level echoes ➡ in this case of hemoperitoneum due to ruptured hepatocellular carcinoma.

DIFFERENTIAL DIAGNOSIS

Common
- Abscess
- Organizing Hematoma
- Complicated Ascites
- Pancreatic Pseudocyst
- Cystic Ovarian Masses

Less Common
- Localized Collections
  - Biloma, Urinoma, CSF Pseudocyst
- Pedunculated Cyst/Diverticula
- Peritoneal Inclusion Cyst
- Cystic Malignant Neoplasm
  - Cystic Metastasis
  - Pseudomyxoma Peritonei
  - Pedunculated Cystic Tumor
    - Gastrointestinal Stromal Tumor (GIST)
    - Cystic Leiomyosarcoma
    - Pancreatic Mucinous Cystadenoma/Cystadenocarcinoma
  - Cystic Mesenchymal Tumor
    - Malignant Fibrous Histiocytoma
    - Synovial Sarcoma
- Cystic Benign Neoplasm
  - Mesenteric Teratoma
  - Multicystic Mesothelioma
- Cystic Lymph Nodes

Rare but Important
- Mesenteric/Omental Cyst
  - Lymphangioma
  - Nonpancreatic Pseudocyst
  - Enteric Duplication Cyst
  - Enteric Cyst
  - Mesothelial Cyst
- Urachal Cyst/Abscess
- Infarcted Accessory Spleen

ESSENTIAL INFORMATION

Key Differential Diagnosis Issues
- Lesions with relevant history
  - Abscess, organizing hematoma
- Lesions with characteristic appearances
  - Peritoneal inclusion cyst, pseudomyxoma peritonei, mature teratoma (dermoid), enteric duplication cyst
- Lesions with thin-walled cystic appearance unless complicated
  - Mesenteric/omental cysts
  - Pedunculated cyst from adjacent organs
- Lesions with complicated appearance
  - Any cystic neoplasm mentioned above or cystic lesion with complication (infection/hemorrhage)
  - Bowel wall origin suggests GIST
  - Other lesions nonspecific, need clinical info to narrow DDx, biopsy to confirm

Helpful Clues for Common Diagnoses
- **Abscess**
  - Pyogenic
    - Unilocular/multiloculated; thin/thick walled plus debris-fluid level
    - Echogenic foci with "comet tail" artifacts/"dirty" shadow = gas locule = gas forming abscess/bowel perforation
  - Tuberculous
    - With features of TB peritonitis or GI/renal/mesenteric lymph node involvement
  - Parasitic
    - Hydatid disease: 12% affects peritoneum
    - Variable appearance: Heterogeneous solid-looking mass to complex cystic mass
- **Organizing Hematoma**
  - History of trauma, coagulopathy, or anticoagulant therapy
  - Organization with liquefaction in subacute to chronic stage
  - Localized collection with multiple thick septae horizontally aligned ± layering debris
- **Complicated Ascites**
  - Infection, hemorrhage, inflammation
  - Septations and loculation ↑ with time
    - Multiple, thick, irregular septae in chronic cases
- **Cystic Ovarian Masses**
  - Mucinous and serous cystadenoma and cystadenocarcinoma

Helpful Clues for Less Common Diagnoses
- **Localized Collections**
  - Perforation of gallbladder or urinary bladder wall due to infection, trauma, or postoperative complication
  - CSF pseudocyst associated with ventriculoperitoneal shunt, due to inflammation or infection
    - Cysts are close to shunt tip
- **Pedunculated Cyst/Diverticula**
  - Hepatic, renal cyst, GI diverticula

CYSTIC PERITONEAL MASS

- ○ Origin may be difficult to trace
- ○ May cause abdominal pain and palpable mass if hemorrhagic or infected
- **Peritoneal Inclusion Cyst**
  - ○ Normal ipsilateral ovary; surrounding loculated fluid conforms to space
  - ○ Characteristic "spider in web" appearance
  - ○ May appear complicated if containing debris/hemorrhage
  - ○ Low-resistance flow sometimes present in septae from vessels in mesothelial lining
- **Cystic Malignant Neoplasm**
  - ○ **Cystic Metastasis**
    - ▪ Most common: GIST, ovarian carcinoma
    - ▪ Thick irregular wall to thin walled (especially after imatimib treatment)
  - ○ **Pseudomyxoma Peritonei**
    - ▪ Characteristic appearance of voluminous, loculated pseudoascites
    - ▪ Irregular soft tissue mass with cystic spaces
    - ▪ Typically from cystadenocarcinoma of ovary or appendix; also associated with several other tumors
  - ○ **Pedunculated Cystic Tumor**
    - ▪ Look for organ of orgin
    - ▪ Cystic leiomyosarcoma: 66% extrinsic, about 1/2 from ileum; usually large (> 6 cm), connection with bowel wall seen, ± dystrophic calcification
    - ▪ GIST, cystic pancreatic neoplasm
  - ○ **Cystic Mesenchymal Tumor**
    - ▪ Rare, but malignant fibrous histiocytoma is most common histologic type
- ▪ Varies from thick irregular wall (with central necrosis) to completely cystic ± mural nodule plus debris/hemorrhage
- **Cystic Benign Neoplasm**
  - ○ **Mesenteric Teratoma**
    - ▪ Purely cystic (10-15%), complex cystic (66%), predominantly solid (10-13%)
    - ▪ Fat-fluid level is characteristic, but chylous pseudocyst may look similar
    - ▪ Tooth (calcification) and hair are specific
- **Cystic Lymph Nodes**
  - ○ Tuberculosis, metastatic (cervix, ovary), inflammatory (celiac disease)

Helpful Clues for Rare Diagnoses
- **Mesenteric/Omental Cyst**
  - ○ **Lymphangioma**
    - ▪ Pediatric patients; thin walled, usually with multiple thin septae; anechoic > hypoechoic
  - ○ **Nonpancreatic Pseudocyst**
    - ▪ Lined by fibrous capsule; sequelae of previous infection, inflammation, or hemorrhage
  - ○ **Enteric Duplication Cyst**
    - ▪ Double-layered wall (mucosa and muscularis) ± peristalsis
  - ○ **Enteric Cyst**
    - ▪ Single layer (no muscle layer)
- **Urachal Cyst/Abscess**
  - ○ Anywhere from anteroventral aspect of urinary bladder to umbilical level
  - ○ Complicated appearance of abscess may mimic urachal carcinoma

Abscess

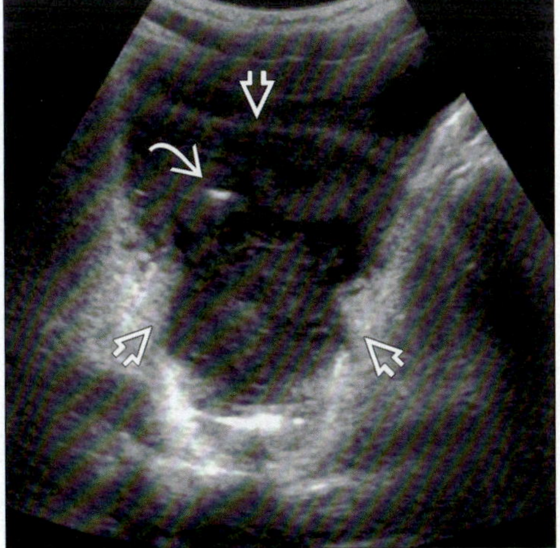

Longitudinal transabdominal ultrasound of RLQ shows a loculated abscess ➡ with internal debris. The echogenic foci with "comet tail" artifact ➡ represent gas from a gas-forming organism or perforated bowel.

Organizing Hematoma

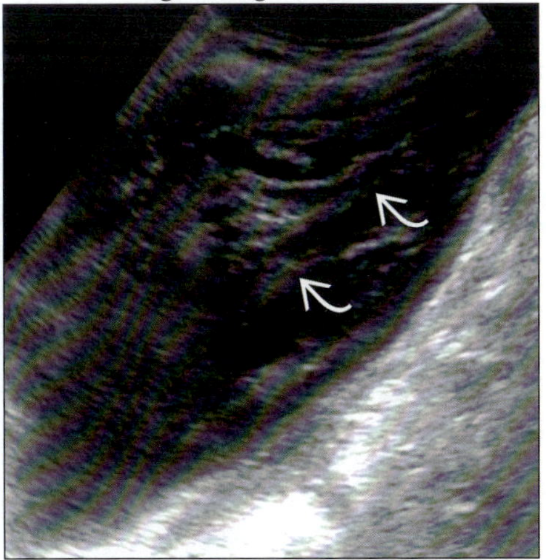

Longitudinal transabdominal ultrasound shows an irregular collection with multiple thick, irregular, horizontal, internal septae ➡, findings typical of an organizing hematoma.

CYSTIC PERITONEAL MASS

(Left) Transverse US shows a multiloculated cystic lesion in the left paracolic gutter. Note the thick wall, insinuating border ➡, and multiple thick, irregular internal septae ➡, consistent with chronic complicated ascites, here due to Crohn disease. *(Right)* Transverse US shows a large, unilocular, thin-walled cyst ➡ with debris in the central abdomen, initially mistaken for a mesenteric cyst. Diagnosis of hemorrhagic liver cyst was made on CECT (not shown).

Complicated Ascites

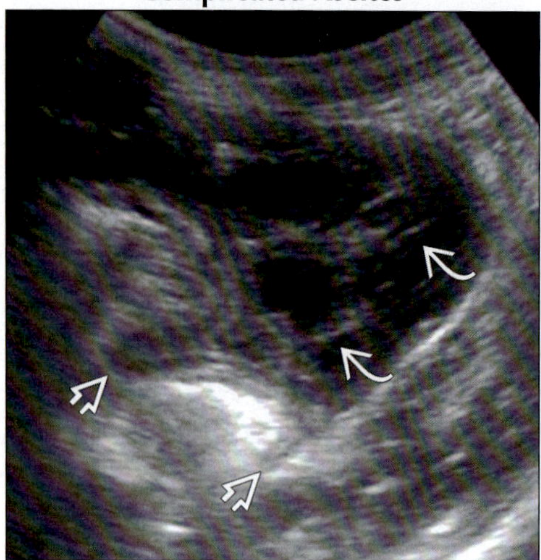

Pedunculated Cyst/Diverticula

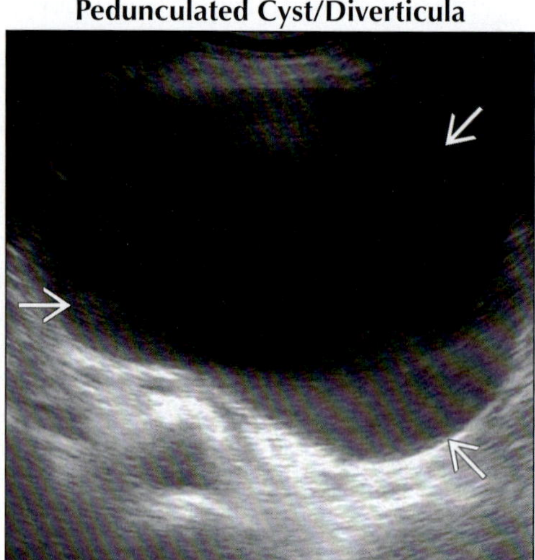

(Left) Longitudinal transvaginal US of the right adnexa shows a multiloculated, thin-walled, cystic lesion ➡ conforming to the peritoneal space. The right ovary ➡ is located eccentrically and tethered by peritoneal adhesions ➡, creating a "spider in web" appearance. *(Right)* Transverse transabdominal US shows a malignant leiomyosarcoma of GI tract. Note its typical round/ovoid, well-defined, hypoechoic appearance with central cystic areas/necrosis ➡.

Peritoneal Inclusion Cyst

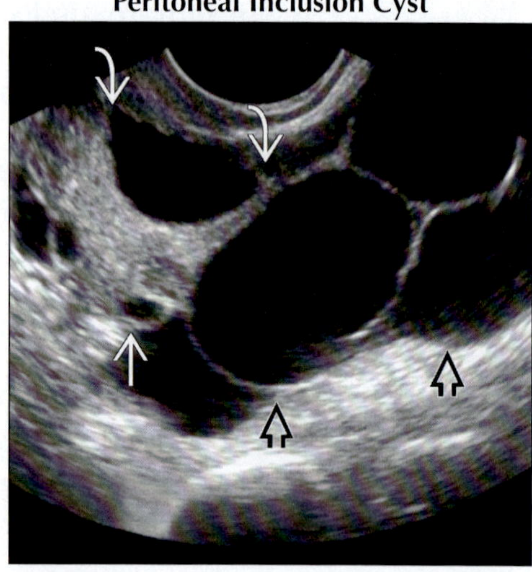

Cystic Leiomyosarcoma

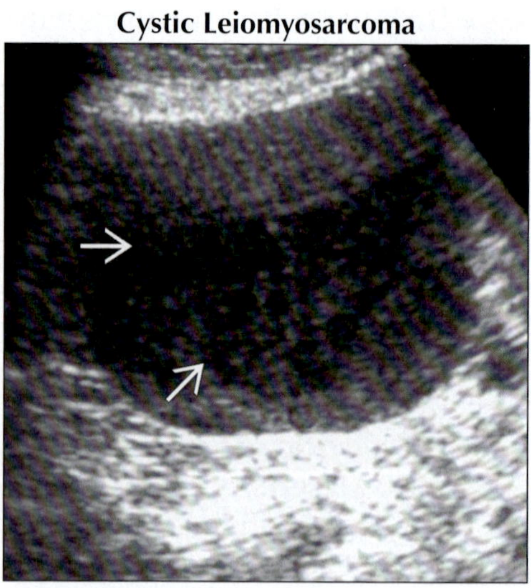

(Left) Transverse transabdominal ultrasound shows a large metastatic deposit in the right paramedian region of the central abdomen. Note the large irregular necrotic component ➡. *(Right)* Longitudinal US shows an irregular, heterogeneously hypoechoic, soft tissue deposit on the greater omentum with a central cystic/necrotic area ➡ (metastasis from an ovarian primary). Note the small amount of ascitic fluid ➡.

Cystic Metastasis

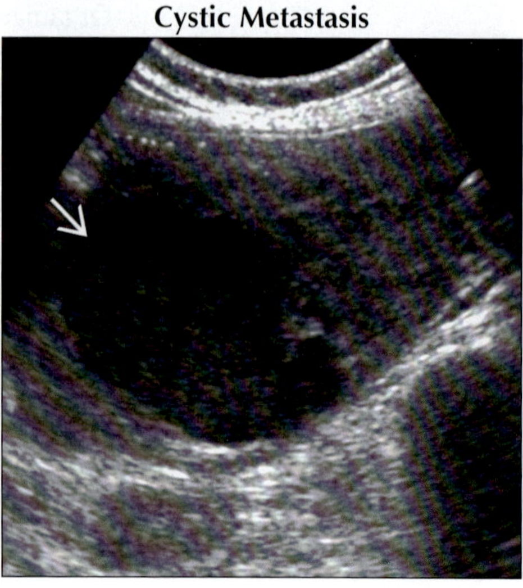

Cystic Metastasis

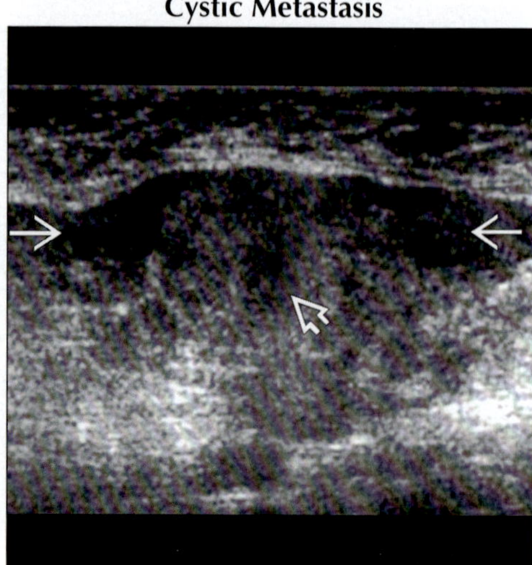

9

CYSTIC PERITONEAL MASS

Pseudomyxoma Peritonei

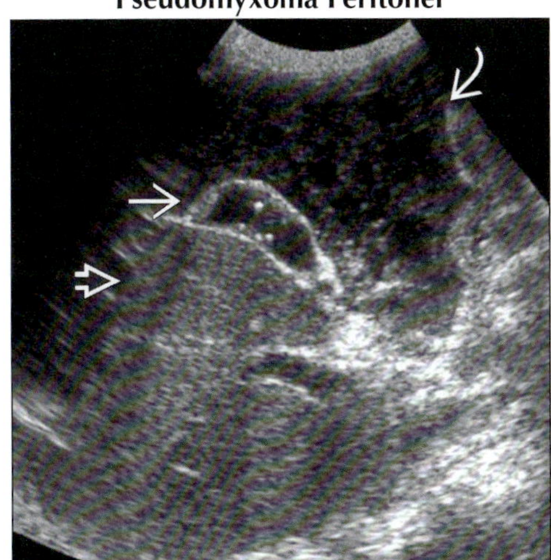

Pseudomyxoma Peritonei

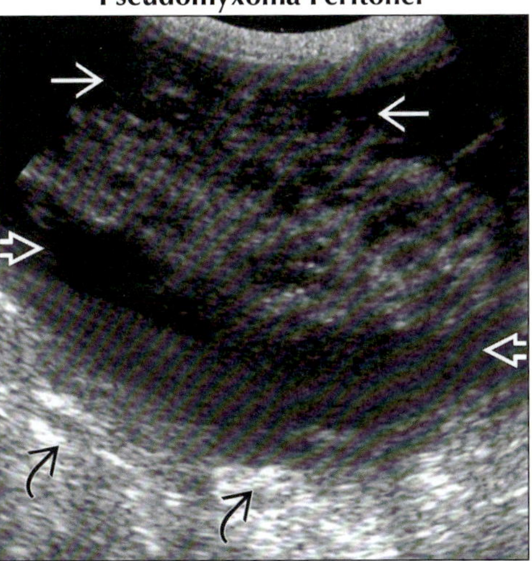

(Left) Transverse US demonstrates the typical appearance of pseudomyxoma peritonei, seen as a voluminous multiseptated pseudoascites ➡ with mass effect displacing the liver ➡ and gallbladder ➡ from the anterior peritoneal wall. (Right) Longitudinal transabdominal ultrasound shows the broad peritoneal base ➡ of the cystic mass, standing out from the surrounding true ascitic fluid ➡. Note the gas within the bowel loops ➡.

Mesenteric Teratoma

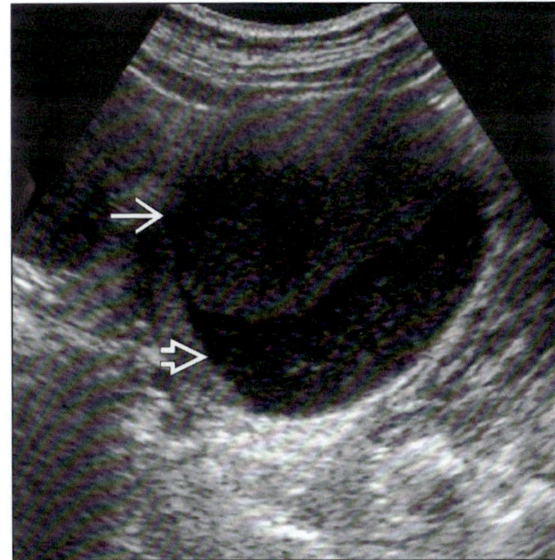

Mesenteric Teratoma

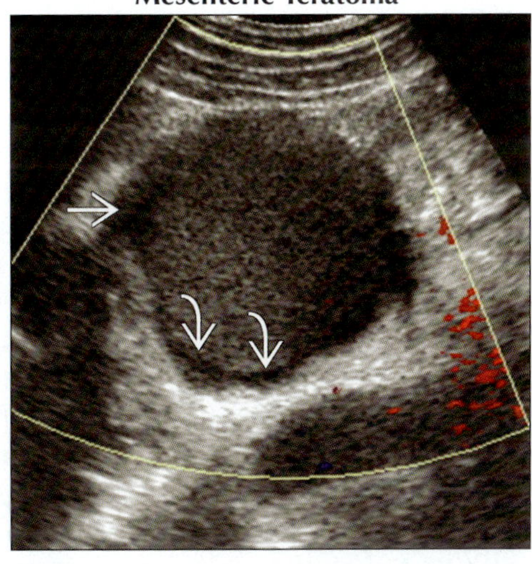

(Left) Longitudinal transabdominal ultrasound shows a mesenteric teratoma with a classic fat-fluid level. Note the layer of echogenic superficial fat ➡ and the layer of hypoechoic, dependent fluid ➡. (Right) Transverse power Doppler ultrasound of the epigastric region shows a mesenteric teratoma ➡ with a well-defined border and dispersed homogeneous internal echoes and a fat-fluid level ➡.

Lymphangioma

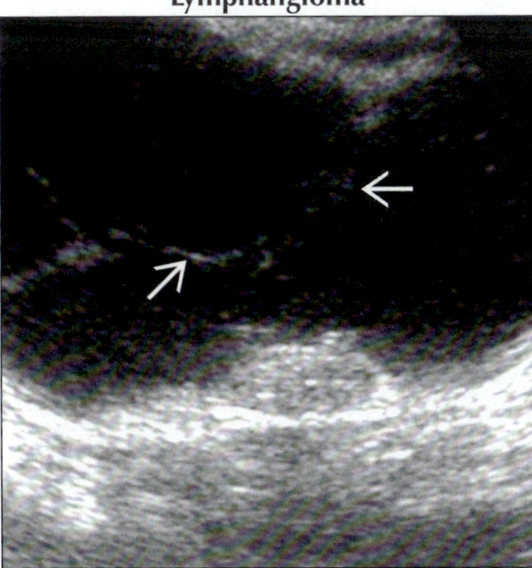

Enteric Cyst

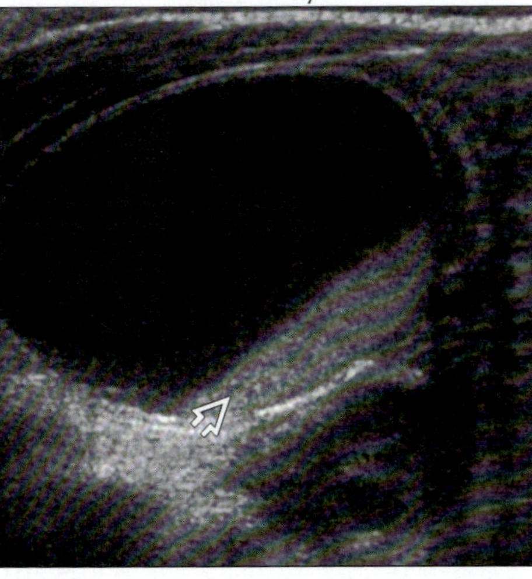

(Left) Transverse transabdominal ultrasound shows a mesenteric lymphangioma with characteristic multiple thin septations ➡ and anechoic content. (Right) Longitudinal transabdominal ultrasound shows a thin-walled, single-layered, unilocular enteric cyst with fluid-debris level ➡. Note the single-layered wall vs. the double-layered wall that would be seen in an enteric duplication cyst.

9

SOLID PERITONEAL MASS

DIFFERENTIAL DIAGNOSIS

Common
- Lymphadenopathy
- Peritoneal Carcinomatosis
- Peritoneal Lymphomatosis
- Secondary Inflammatory Changes
- Mesenteric Hematoma
- Mimics
  - Pedunculated Mass from Abdominal Organs
  - Bowel Mass

Less Common
- Peritoneal Tuberculosis
- Malignant Peritoneal Mesothelioma
- Malignant Mesenchymal Tumors
  - Malignant Fibrous Histiocytoma

Rare but Important
- Primary Malignant Peritoneal Tumors
  - Papillary Serous Carcinoma
  - Desmoplastic Small Round Cell Tumor
- Carcinoid
- Benign Mesenchymal Tumor
- Tumor-like Conditions
  - Desmoid Tumor
  - Castleman Disease
- Systemic Diseases
  - Extramedullary Hematopoiesis
  - Systemic Amyloidosis

ESSENTIAL INFORMATION

Key Differential Diagnosis Issues
- Peritoneal tumors generally lack specific features for definitive diagnosis
- Secondary peritoneal tumor much more common than primary peritoneal or mesenchymal tumor
  - However, primary peritoneal tumors are generally more aggressive
- Image-guided biopsy for histological type

Helpful Clues for Common Diagnoses
- **Lymphadenopathy**
  - Solid nodules along lymphatic distribution
  - Metastasis, lymphoma, leukemia > sarcoidosis, tuberculosis, mastocytosis, Crohn disease, Whipple disease, and nontropical sprue
- **Peritoneal Carcinomatosis**
  - Metastatic tumoral seeding of peritoneal surface, peritoneal ligaments, omentum, and mesentery
  - Common sites of orgin: Ovary, stomach, and colon
  - 3 morphological forms
    - Peritoneal deposits: Multiple hypoechoic nodules or plaques on peritoneal surface; commonly involve pouch of Douglas, Morrison pouch, right subphrenic space
    - Omental cake: Large conglomerate soft tissue mass on peritoneum/omentum
    - Mesenteric infiltration: Infiltration of mesenteric leaves with thickening; may give "sunburst" appearance
- **Peritoneal Lymphomatosis**
  - Common in non-Hodgkin lymphoma but unusual if only site of involvement at presentation
    - Appearances indistinguishable from peritoneal carcinomatosis, except lymphadenopathy and solid deposits may be more bulky
- **Secondary Inflammatory Changes**
  - Local peritoneal inflammation secondary to adjacent inflammatory process, e.g., appendicitis or pancreatitis
  - May form ill-defined echogenic/hypoechoic mass due to inflamed mesentry with adhesion
  - Identification of underlying cause important
- **Mesenteric Hematoma**
  - Traumatic or spontaneous hemorrhage in patients with clotting derangement
  - Ill-defined border
  - Echogenicity depends on age of hematoma, from echogenic to heterogeneously hypoechoic over time
  - ± hemoperitoneum or ascites

Helpful Clues for Less Common Diagnoses
- **Peritoneal Tuberculosis**
  - Up to 38% of patients with pulmonary tuberculosis (~ 50% show no typical findings of thoracic involvement)
  - Appearances closely mimic peritoneal carcinomatosis
  - Necrotic mesenteric lymphadenopathy ± calcification
  - Consider *Mycobacterium avium-intracellulare* in AIDS patients

SOLID PERITONEAL MASS

- **Malignant Peritoneal Mesothelioma**
  - Asbestos exposure is risk factor, but < 1/2 patients have significant asbestos exposure
  - Any age group, adult predominance
  - Rapid fatal course, median survival 6-12 months
  - Appearance is again similar to peritoneal carcinomatosis
  - Biopsy with immunohistochemical markers useful for diagnosis
- **Malignant Mesenchymal Tumors**
  - Derived from lymphatic, vascular, neuromuscular, or fatty tissues
  - Generally lacks distinguishing features (ill-defined soft tissue masses ± local invasion)
  - **Malignant Fibrous Histiocytoma**
    - Single most common peritoneal sarcoma
    - Solid hypoechoic ± central necrosis, which may appear cystic with thick septations
    - 7-20% show calcification due to osteoid and chondroid metaplasia

Helpful Clues for Rare Diagnoses
- **Primary Malignant Peritoneal Tumors**
  - **Papillary Serous Carcinoma**
    - Imaging appearance and histology closely mimic metastatic papillary serous ovarian carcinoma, but with much worse prognosis
    - Extensive calcification is common
  - **Desmoplastic Small Round Cell Tumor**
    - Highly aggressive, affects adolescents and young adults
    - Multiple hypoechoic, round peritoneal masses ± internal necrosis ± ascites
    - Omentum and paravesicular regions more frequently involved
- **Carcinoid**
  - Arises within bowel wall; strong fibrotic reaction of mesentry causing radiating appearance of mesenteric vessels on color Doppler study
- **Benign Mesenchymal Tumor**
  - Mesenteric plexiform neurofibroma in NF1 is most common manifestation
  - Leiomyomatosis peritonealis disseminata primarily affects reproductive-age females
- **Tumor-like Conditions**
  - **Desmoid Tumor**: Benign, locally aggressive proliferative process with tendency to recur locally; irregular hypoechoic mass, 1/3 mesenteric infiltration
  - **Castleman Disease**: Hypertrophic lymphadenopathy ± hypervascular soft tissue masses; foci of coarse calcification (5-10%); hepatosplenomegaly
- **Systemic Diseases**
  - **Extramedullary Hematopoiesis**: May involve mesentery as soft tissue masses; other sites of extramedullary hematopoiesis present
  - **Systemic Amyloidosis**: Rarely multifocal or diffuse mesenteric infiltration, dystrophic Ca++ important clue

Lymphadenopathy

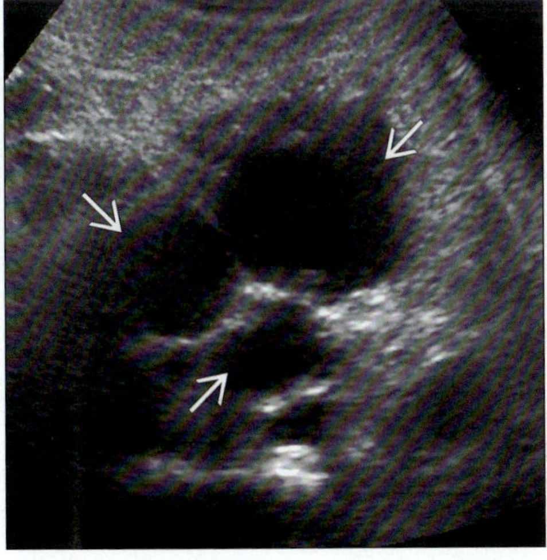

Transverse transabdominal ultrasound shows a cluster of malignant celiac lymph nodes ➡ in a patient with carcinoma of the colon.

Peritoneal Carcinomatosis

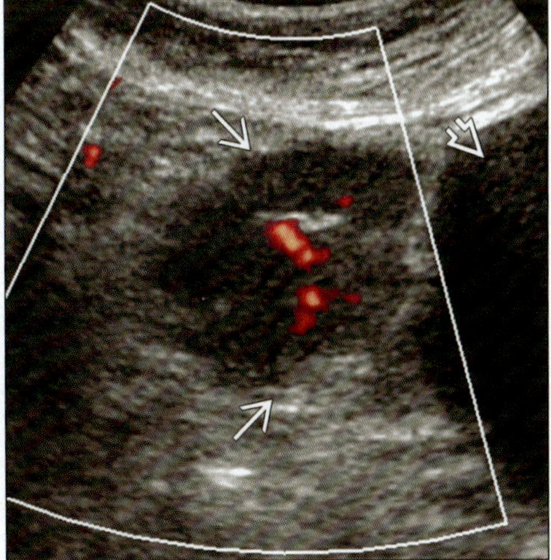

Longitudinal transabdominal ultrasound shows a well-defined hypoechoic peritoneal deposit ➡ just superior to the dome of the urinary bladder ➡.

SOLID PERITONEAL MASS
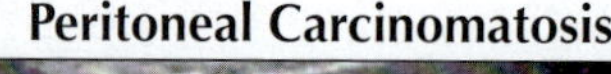

(Left) Oblique transabdominal ultrasound shows a hyperechoic peritoneal deposit ➡ with ascites ➡ in Morrison pouch between the right lobe of the liver ➡ and the kidney ➡. *(Right)* Transverse transabdominal ultrasound shows ascites filled with internal echoes ➡ and echogenic debris ➡ in a patient with peritoneal carcinomatosis.

Peritoneal Carcinomatosis
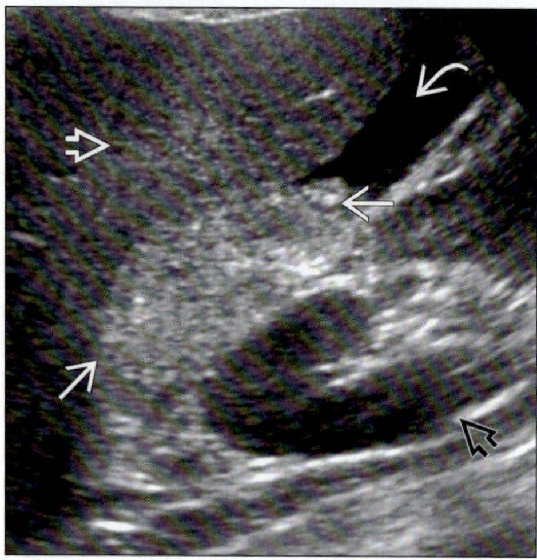

Peritoneal Carcinomatosis
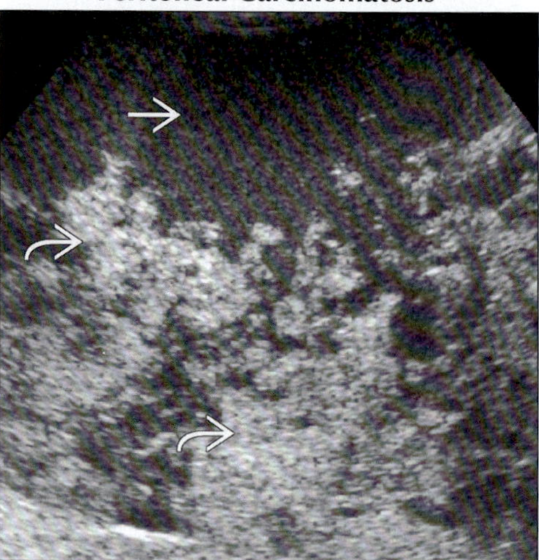

(Left) Transverse ultrasound shows a large omental cake ➡. The diagnosis is either primary peritoneal carcinoma or metastasis from a primary ovarian tumor. *(Right)* Correlative axial CECT of the pelvis shows diffuse peritoneal carcinomatosis ➡ with multiple scattered specks of calcification ➡, typically seen in ovarian or primary peritoneal malignancy. A biopsy will differentiate between the 2 entities. Note the urinary bladder ➡.

Peritoneal Carcinomatosis
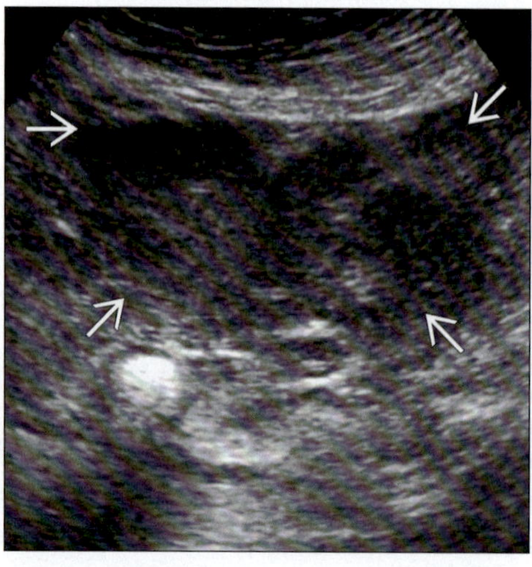

Peritoneal Carcinomatosis
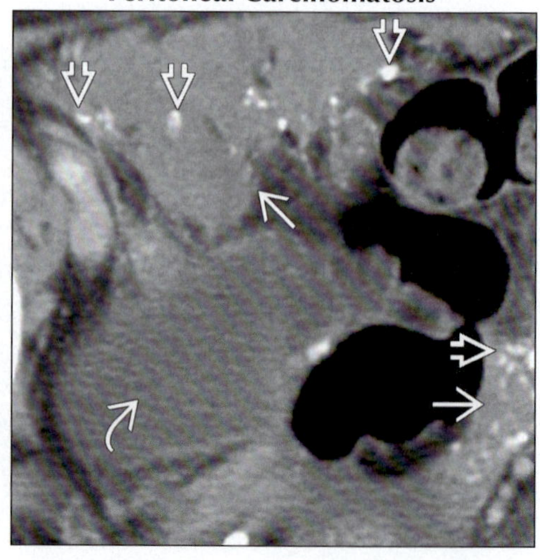

(Left) Transverse transabdominal ultrasound shows markedly thickened and echogenic mesenteric leaves ➡ with the classic "sunburst" appearance ➡. *(Right)* Transverse color Doppler ultrasound of the RLQ shows an inflammatory mass due to a ruptured appendicitis. The inflamed mesentry wraps around the ruptured appendix to form a mass ➡ with peripheral vascularity ➡.

Peritoneal Carcinomatosis
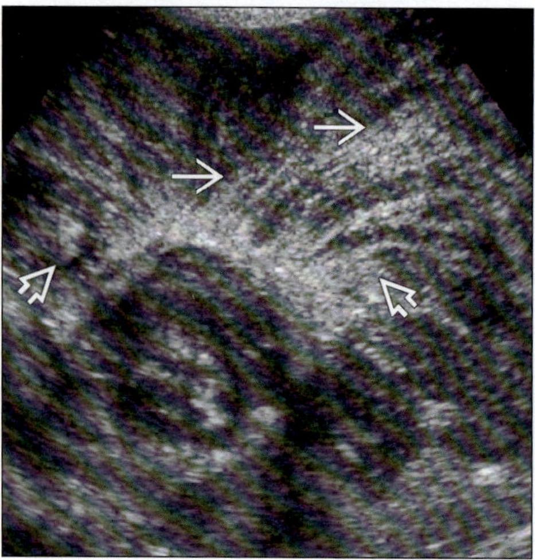

Secondary Inflammatory Changes
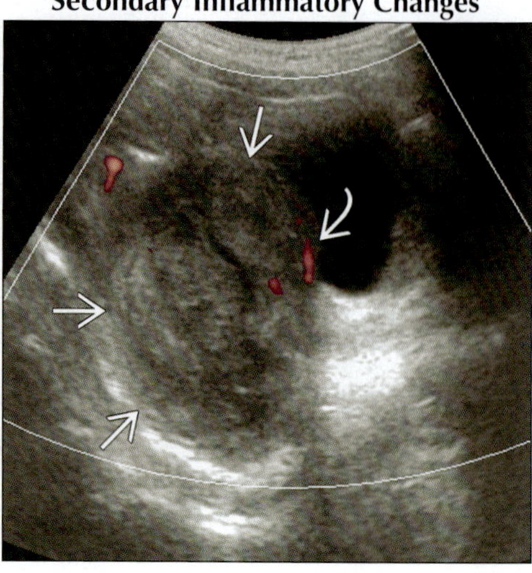

SOLID PERITONEAL MASS

Peritoneal Lymphomatosis

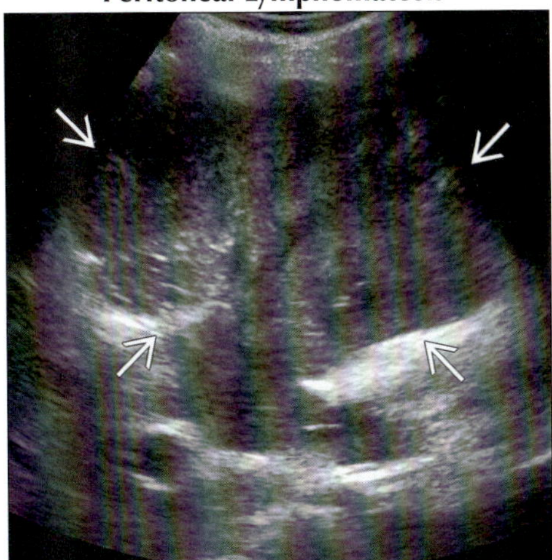

Peritoneal Lymphomatosis

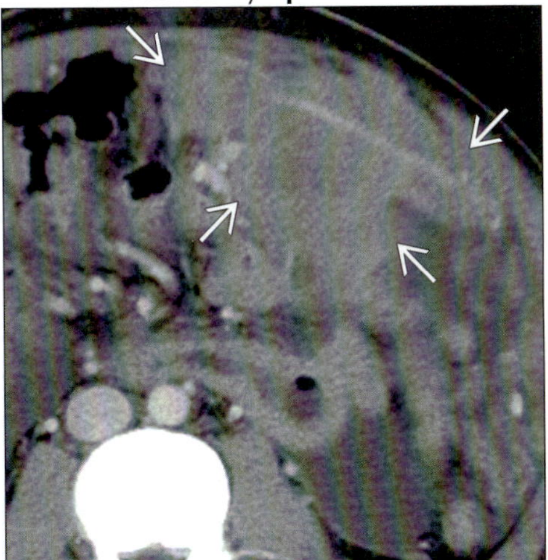

(Left) Transverse transabdominal ultrasound shows a large hypoechoic peritoneal infiltrate with a lobulated contour ➡ in a patient with Burkitt lymphoma. (Right) Correlative axial CECT shows the large lymphomatous peritoneal infiltrate ➡ with heterogeneous contrast enhancement. The stomach wall (not shown) was diffusely thickened, consistent with lymphomatous involvement.

Mimics

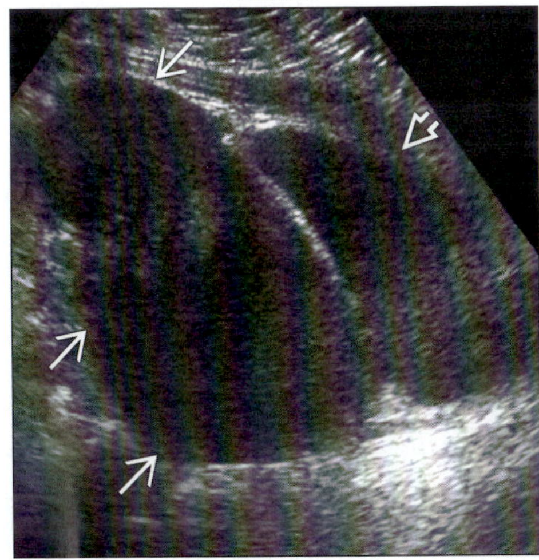

Mimics

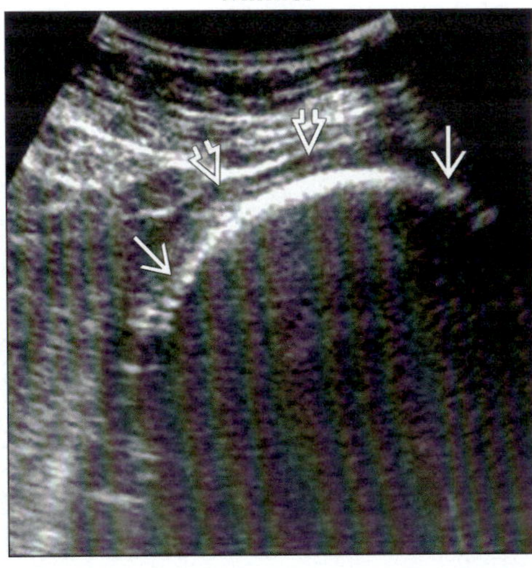

(Left) Oblique transabdominal ultrasound shows 2 well-defined, homogeneously hypoechoic, pedunculated subserosal fibroids ➡, mimicking peritoneal masses. Note the urinary bladder ➡. (Right) Transverse transabdominal ultrasound of the epigastric region shows a curvilinear echogenic interface ➡ with dense posterior acoustic shadowing. This represents the superficial surface of a heavily calcified bezoar in the stomach ➡, mimicking a calcified peritoneal mass.

Peritoneal Tuberculosis

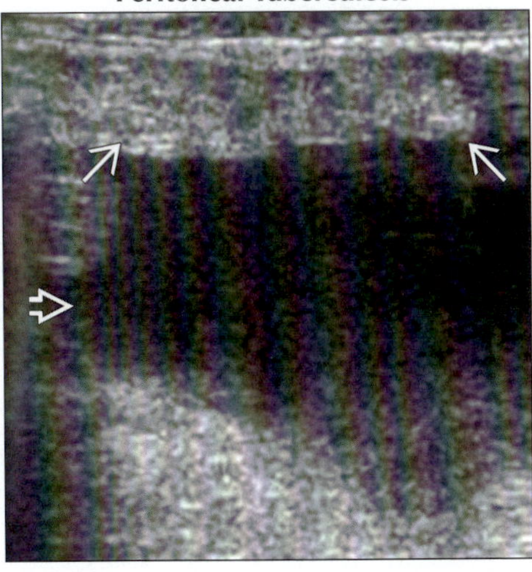

Malignant Mesenchymal Tumors

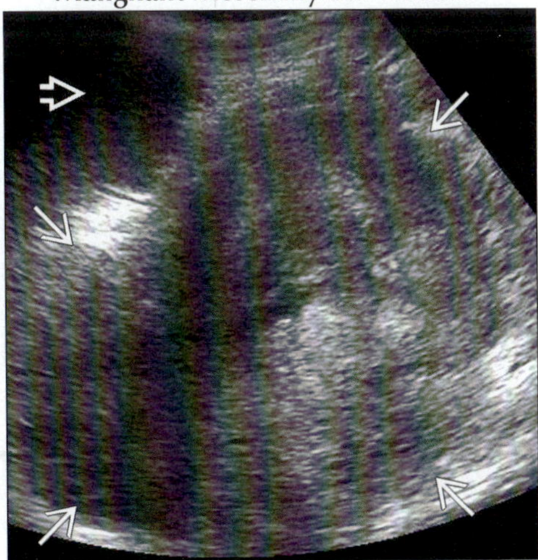

(Left) Transverse transabdominal ultrasound shows omental thickening ➡ in a patient with peritoneal tuberculosis. Note that the omental thickening is outlined by the ascitic fluid ➡. (Right) Longitudinal transabdominal ultrasound shows a large peritoneal sarcoma ➡ in the left upper quadrant, inferior to the spleen ➡. The margin is ill defined and inseparable from adjacent structures, suggesting of its aggressive nature.

DIFFERENTIAL DIAGNOSIS

Common
- Acute Appendicitis
- Gynecological Abnormalities
- Intussusception

Less Common
- Terminal Ileitis
- Abscess
- Colitis
- Colonic Tumor
  - Colon Carcinoma
  - Lymphoma
- Lymphadenopathy
- Musculoskeletal Abnormalities
  - Psoas Abscess
  - Iliac Lesion

Rare but Important
- Vascular Conditions
- Peritoneal/Retroperitoneal Abnormalities

ESSENTIAL INFORMATION

Key Differential Diagnosis Issues
- Appendicitis is most common condition
  - Ultrasound makes definitive diagnosis
  - Finding normal appendix may prevent unnecessary surgical intervention
- Ileal/cecal thickening is another common nonspecific finding
  - Causes include secondary inflammation due to acute appendicitis, diverticulitis, local perforation, infection, inflammatory bowel disease, malignancy

Helpful Clues for Common Diagnoses
- **Acute Appendicitis**
  - Noncompressible appendix > 6 mm has sensitivity of 100% but specificity of only 64%
  - Noncompressible appendix > 7 mm has sensitivity of 94% and specificity of 88%
  - Laminated wall thickening due to edema and inflammation, wall thickness > 2 mm
    - "Target" appearance in transverse plane
  - Increased flow within wall of appendix on Doppler
  - Loss of layer differentiation plus decreased/absent vascularity suggest gangrene
  - Appendix tip is most frequently involved
  - Increased echogenicity in surrounding peritoneal fat due to inflammation
  - Periappendiceal fluid, enlarged mesenteric nodes
  - Presence of appendicolith in acute appendicitis suggests high chance of perforation/gangrene
  - Many potential pitfalls so care must be taken in scanning
  - Normal terminal ileum mistaken as thickened appendix
    - Terminal ileum is peristaltic and much thicker
    - Demonstrating both terminal ileum and appendix will prevent confusion
  - May miss focal appendicitis of appendiceal tip; easy to miss, particularly if ruptured
    - Decompression makes appendix less thick than expected
    - Demonstration of intact appendix tip is essential
- **Gynecological Abnormalities**
  - Acute gynecological conditions generally seen as complex cystic lesions associated with relevant history and signs
    - DDx includes ectopic pregnancy, tubo-ovarian abscess, ovarian torsion, hemorrhagic or ruptured ovarian cyst
- **Intussusception**
  - Telescoping of proximal segment of bowel into lumen of distal segment
  - Classic "target" sign on transverse scan and "pseudokidney" sign on longitudinal scan
  - Presence of flow in intussusceptum is good predictor of reducibility
  - Absence decreases mural vascularity of intussusceptum suggests ischemia/infarction → risk of perforation
  - Typically ileocolic in pediatric idiopathic cases
  - Look for underlying tumor/mass if not ileocolic or in adult
  - Treatment by pneumatic reduction, which can be done under ultrasound guidance with normal saline
  - 4-10% recurrent intussusception

Helpful Clues for Less Common Diagnoses
- **Terminal Ileitis**
  - Thickened cecum, terminal ileum (diffuse or segmental), and ileocecal valve

RIGHT LOWER QUADRANT PAIN/MASS

- ○ Causes: Inflammatory bowel disease (Crohn disease), tuberculosis, typhilitis (neutropenic colitis), other infections (amebiasis, typhlitis)
- ○ Occasionally, appendix may be secondarily involved; differentiation depends on relative involvement/epicenter of abnormality
- ○ Colonoscopy plus biopsy for further evaluation
- **Abscess**
  - ○ Due to acute appendicitis, diverticulitis, colitis, bowel perforation, etc.
  - ○ Unilocular or multilocular
  - ○ Mobile internal echogenic foci due to pus ± gas (echogenic foci with "comet tail" artifacts or "dirty" shadow)
    - ▪ Due to anaerobes ± expelled appendicolith (curvilinear echogenic interface with dense posterior acoustic shadowing)
  - ○ Extension to pelvis is common
- **Colitis**
  - ○ Pseudomembranous colitis: Rectum > right + transverse colon > pancolitis
  - ○ Ischemic colitis: Segmental involvement of any part of colon
    - ▪ Most commonly splenic flexure and rectosigmoid junction, 11% pancolitis
  - ○ Infective colitis
    - ▪ Pancolitis: Cytomegalovirus, *E. coli*
    - ▪ Right colon: *Shigella*, *Salmonella*
- **Colonic Tumor**
  - ○ **Colon Carcinoma**
    - ▪ Concentric/eccentric thickening of cecum with loss of mural layer differentiation due to tumor invasion
    - ▪ Disorganized vascularity on Doppler
    - ▪ ± local invasion or regional lymph node, liver metastases
  - ○ **Lymphoma**
    - ▪ Occasionally infiltrates ileocecal junction causing diffuse mural thickening
- **Lymphadenopathy**
  - ○ Lymphomatous, metastatic, infective, reactive
- **Musculoskeletal Abnormalities**
  - ○ **Psoas Abscess**
    - ▪ Thickened, hypoechoic, heterogeneous, and hypervascular psoas muscle compared to normal side
    - ▪ Cystic areas with liquefaction
  - ○ **Iliac Lesion**
    - ▪ Any breach or irregularity of ventral cortex of right ilium should raise suspicion of underlying bony lesion, e.g., metastasis or primary bone neoplasm
    - ▪ Radiograph, CT, or MR is then required to further evaluate

Helpful Clues for Rare Diagnoses

- **Vascular Conditions**
  - ○ Aneurysm, pseudoaneurysm of external iliac or femoral artery
- **Peritoneal/Retroperitoneal Abnormalities**
  - ○ Sarcoma, carcinoid, retroperitoneal lymphadenopathy

Acute Appendicitis

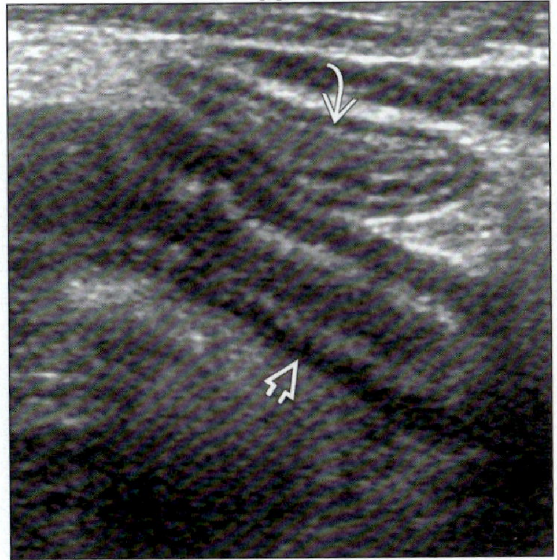

Oblique transabdominal ultrasound shows typical acute appendicitis. Note the thickened, noncompressible appendix ➡ and adjacent normal-looking terminal ileum ➡ with usual peristaltic activity on real-time scan.

Acute Appendicitis

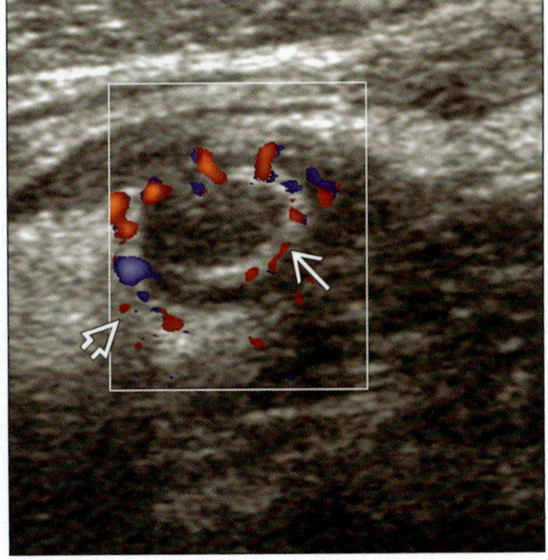

Transverse color Doppler ultrasound shows increased vascularity in the appendiceal wall ➡ and mesoappendix ➡. The absence of wall vascularity should raise the concern of gangrene.

Intussusception

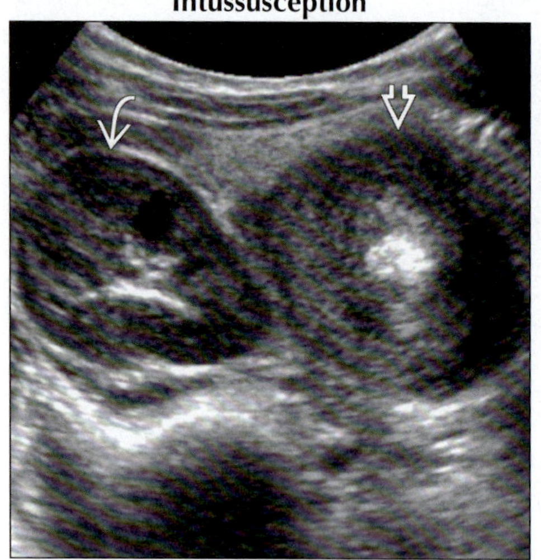

Intussusception

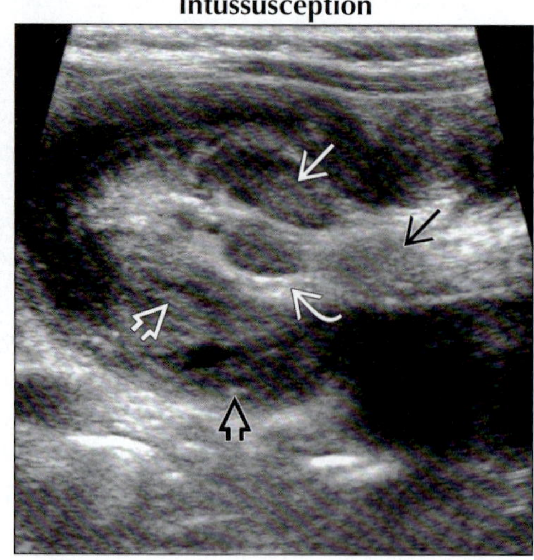

(Left) Transverse ultrasound shows an ileocolic intussusception. The intussusceptum ➡ with a "target" appearance is visible medial to the right kidney ➡. *(Right)* Longitudinal ultrasound shows an enlarged mesenteric lymph node ➡ acting as a lead point for an intussusception. From outer to inner there is the intussuscipiens ➡, returning limb ➡, mesentery ➡, entering limb of intussusceptum ➡.

Terminal Ileitis

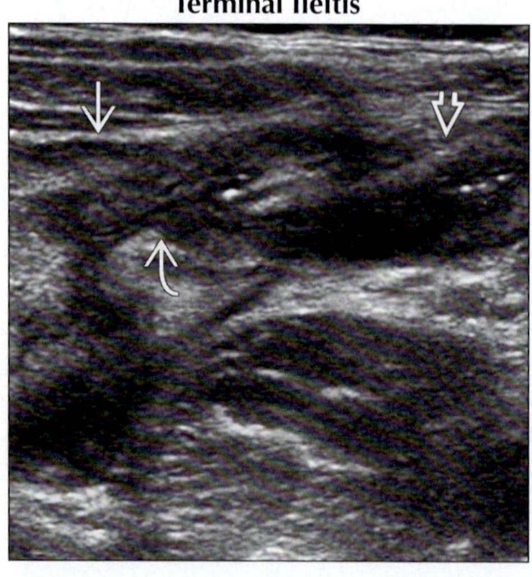

Terminal Ileitis

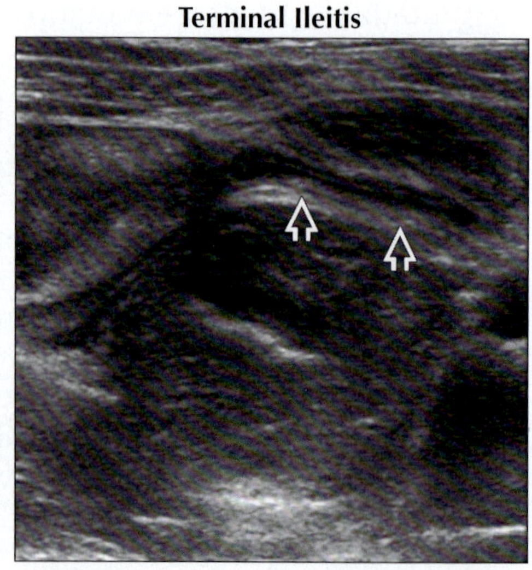

(Left) Transverse transabdominal ultrasound shows the ileocecal junction with thickened bowel wall. Mild inflammatory change is evident in the surrounding peritoneal fat as increased echogenicity. Note the cecum ➡, terminal ileum ➡, and ileocecal valve ➡. *(Right)* Transverse transabdominal ultrasound in the same patient shows a normal appendix ➡, excluding appendicitis as the cause of inflammatory ileocecal change.

Abscess

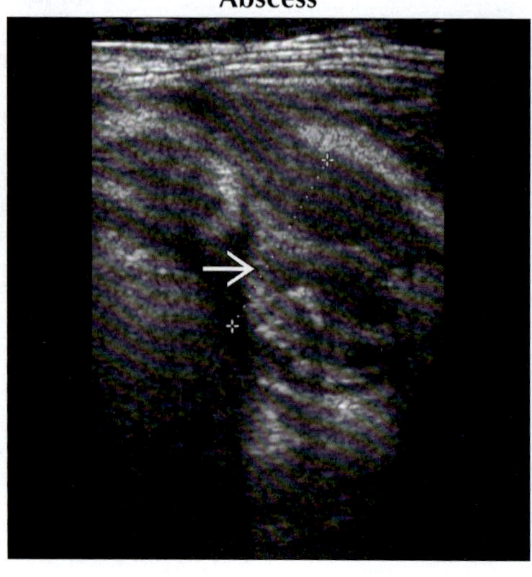

Colitis

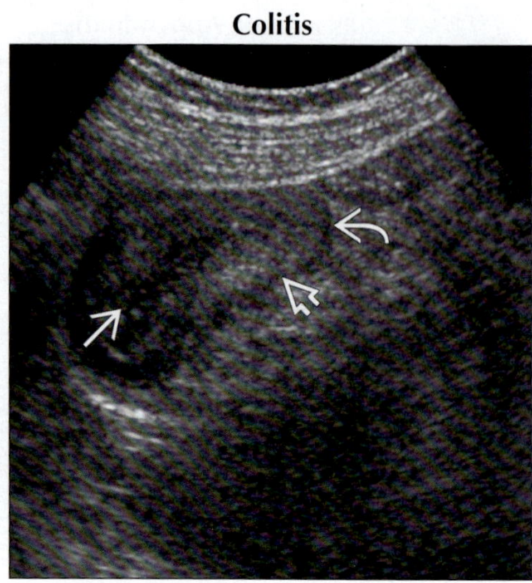

(Left) Oblique transabdominal ultrasound shows an appendiceal abscess ➡ in the right lower quadrant due to a ruptured appendix. An expelled appendicolith may be seen within the abscess. *(Right)* Transverse transabdominal ultrasound shows an inflamed cecum with transmural thickening. Note that the layers of bowel wall are maintained. Serosa ➡, muscularis ➡, and lumen ➡ are clearly visible.

9

RIGHT LOWER QUADRANT PAIN/MASS

Colitis

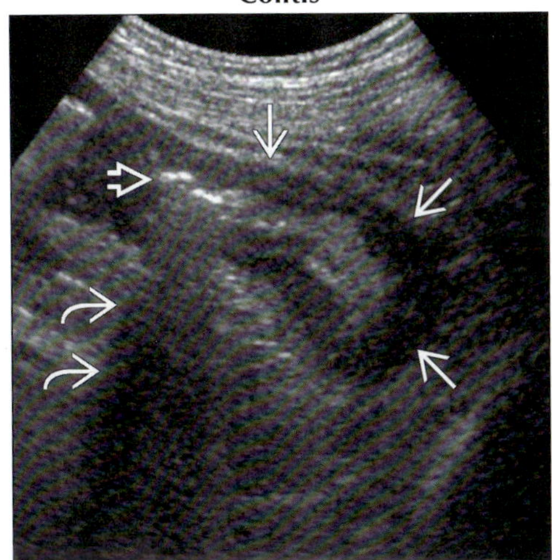

Colon Carcinoma

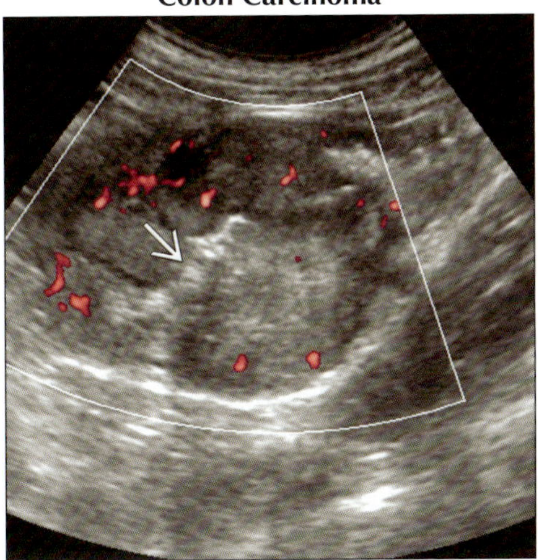

(Left) Oblique ultrasound in a patient with pseudomembranous colitis shows a thickened descending colon 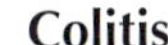 (echogenic bowel gas with "dirty" shadow). On real-time US, the entire colon was involved. *(Right)* Oblique power Doppler ultrasound of the RLQ shows a carcinoma of the cecum. Note the marked, transmural thickening, irregular contour, loss of layer differentiation, and scattered peripheral vascularity. Note the residual stenotic bowel lumen.

Lymphadenopathy

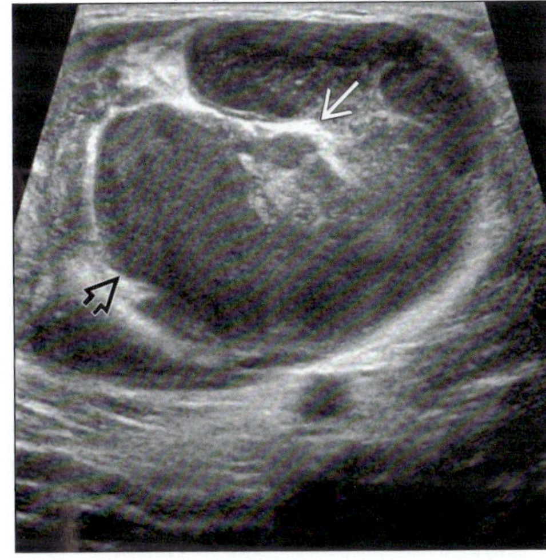

Lymphadenopathy

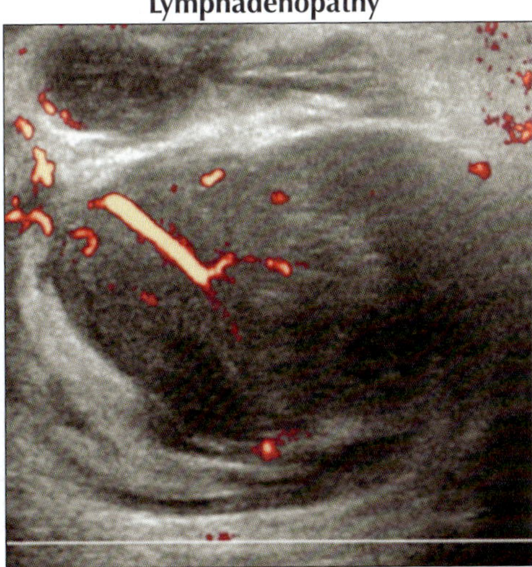

(Left) Transverse ultrasound of the RLQ shows a large, rounded, heterogeneously hypoechoic, soft tissue mass with an eccentric, echogenic linear center, representing an abnormal external iliac lymph node with cortical hypertrophy and preserved hilar architecture. *(Right)* Transverse color Doppler ultrasound shows central hilar vascularity. The features suggest a malignant lymph node, most likely due to lymphoma. Excisional biopsy confirmed the diagnosis.

Psoas Abscess

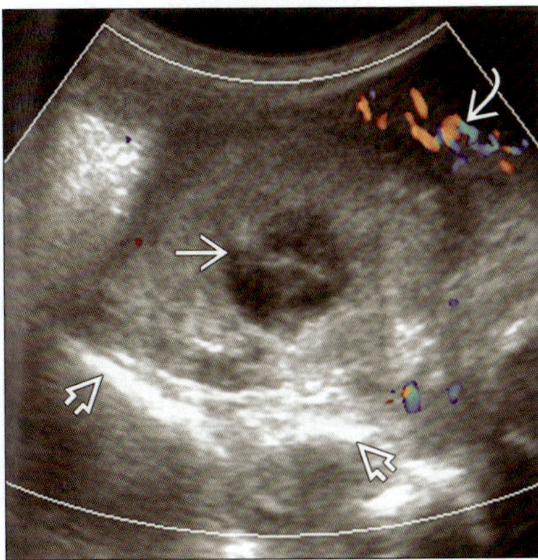

Psoas Abscess

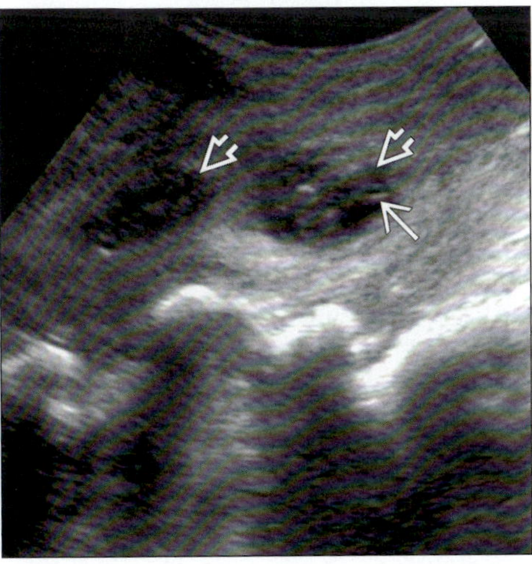

(Left) Transverse color Doppler ultrasound of the RLQ shows a soft tissue mass with central cystic necrosis and increased perilesional vascularity. The echogenic interface with posterior shadowing represents the inner cortex of the right ilium. *(Right)* Longitudinal transabdominal ultrasound reveals multiloculated collections within the edematous right psoas muscle, consistent with a psoas abscess. Note the internal debris.

SECTION 10
Bladder

DIFFERENTIAL DIAGNOSIS

Common
- Bladder Calculi, Cystolithiasis
- Bladder Sludge
- Foley Catheter
- Blood Clot
- Bladder Carcinoma
- Ureterocele

Less Common
- Deflux Injection
- Fungus Ball

ESSENTIAL INFORMATION

Key Differential Diagnosis Issues
- Distinguish intraluminal bladder mass mobility or nonmobility by scanning patient in different positions
- Look for posterior acoustic shadowing, which is characteristic feature of calculi
- Immobile bladder mass suspicious for fungating tumor arising from bladder wall

Helpful Clues for Common Diagnoses
- **Bladder Calculi, Cystolithiasis**
  - Best diagnostic clue: Mobile echogenic focus within bladder with posterior acoustic shadowing
  - Usually located in midline with patient in supine position
  - Eccentric location if within bladder augmentation or diverticulum
- **Bladder Sludge**
  - Less discrete, sand-like, mobile, echogenic debris within bladder
  - No posterior acoustic shadowing
- **Foley Catheter**
  - Characteristic round shape ± midline echogenic tubular structure
- **Blood Clot**
  - Medium-level, slightly speckled echoes without posterior acoustic shadowing
  - Diagnosis suggested if history of hematuria
- **Bladder Carcinoma**
  - Polypoid tumor may mimic intraluminal mass, nonmobile
  - Color Doppler: Increased intratumoral vascularity
- **Ureterocele**
  - Thin-walled, cystic, intravesical mass near ipsilateral ureter
  - Fluctuates in size with ureteric peristalsis
  - Orthotopic ureterocele: Normal insertion at trigone and otherwise normal ureter
  - Ectopic ureterocele: Inserts below trigone, duplicated collecting systems in 80%

Helpful Clues for Less Common Diagnoses
- **Deflux Injection**
  - Pseudoureterocele: Focal mucosal bulging after deflux injection in treatment of vesicoureteric reflux
- **Fungus Ball**
  - Occurs in diabetic or immunocompromised patients
  - Medium-level echoes; nonshadowing, round mobile lesion in bladder

Bladder Calculi, Cystolithiasis

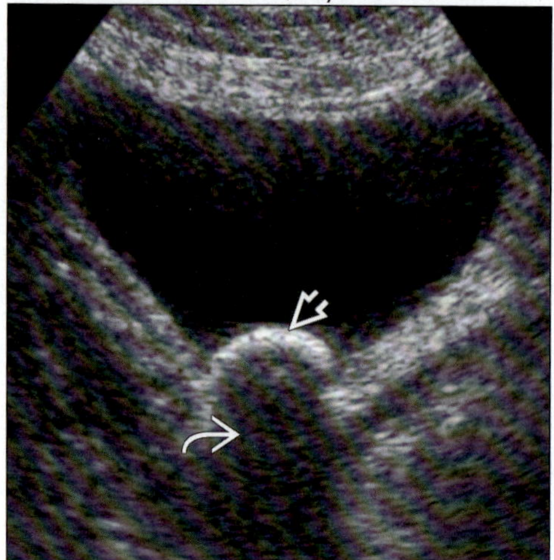

Transverse transabdominal ultrasound shows a large echogenic bladder calculus ➡ associated with strong posterior acoustic shadowing ➡. The calculus was mobile on real-time ultrasound.

Bladder Sludge

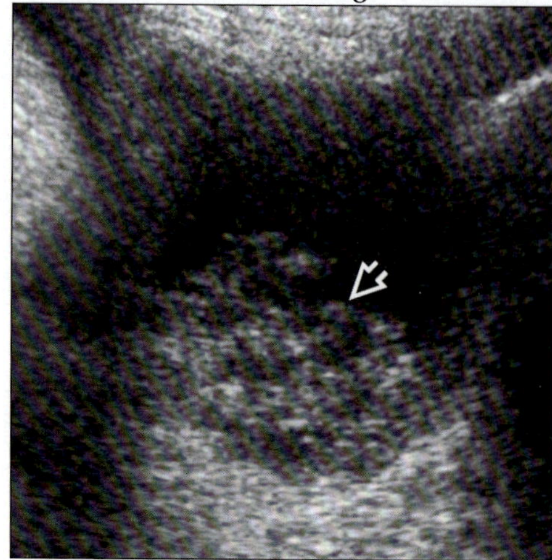

Transverse transabdominal ultrasound shows mobile, nonshadowing, echogenic sludge ➡ within the urinary bladder. The sludge is less discrete and less echogenic than a bladder calculus.

INTRALUMINAL BLADDER MASS

Foley Catheter

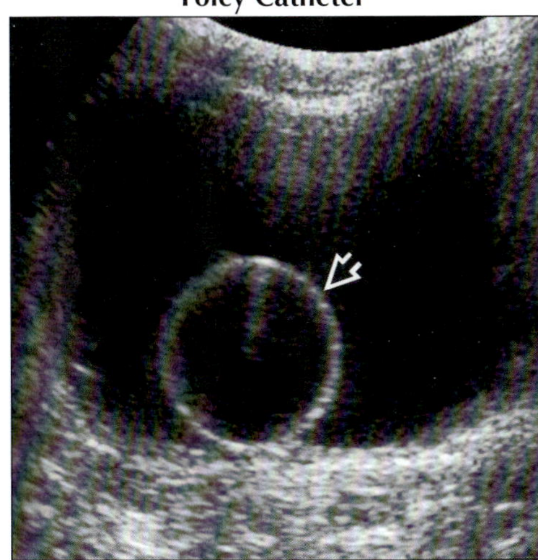

Blood Clot

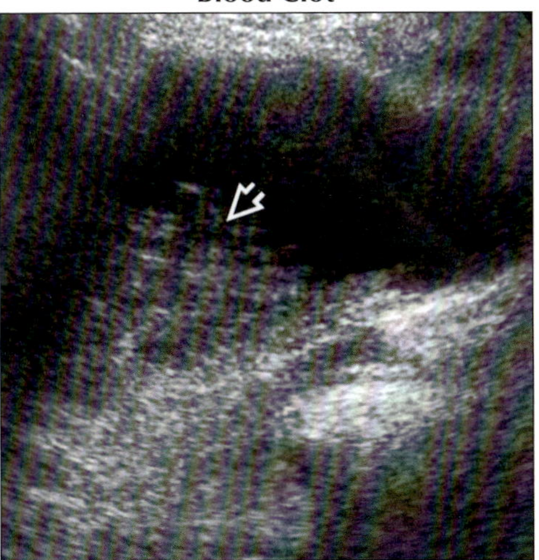

(Left) Transverse transabdominal ultrasound shows the round configuration of the inflated balloon ⮞ of a Foley catheter. The balloon is characteristic in appearance and should not be mistaken for an organic lesion. *(Right)* Oblique transabdominal ultrasound shows an echogenic blood clot ⮞ within the urinary bladder of a patient with gross hematuria. The blood clot can be mobile or adhere to the bladder wall.

Bladder Carcinoma

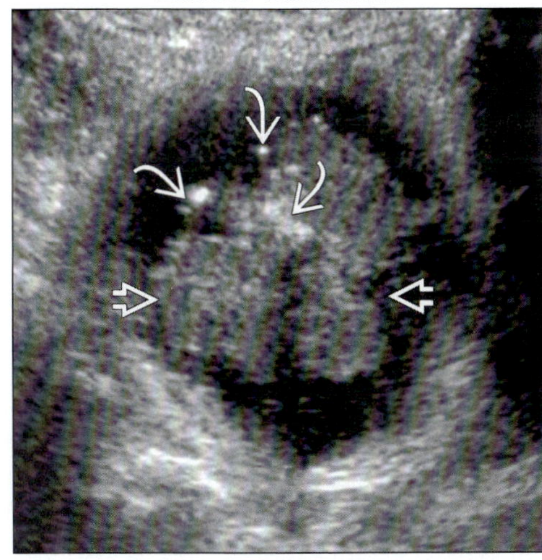

Ureterocele

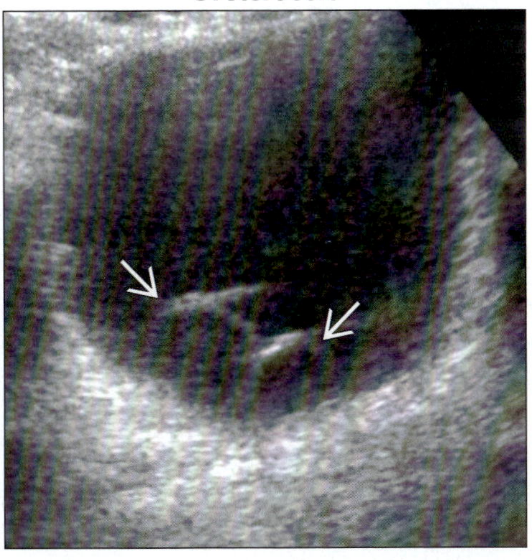

(Left) Transverse transabdominal ultrasound shows an irregular, intravesicular, polypoid mass ⮞ resembling a "cauliflower" arising from the right lateral bladder wall. Punctate calcifications ➤ are present within the tumor, which was not mobile. *(Right)* Transverse transabdominal ultrasound shows bilateral ureteroceles ➤ present in the bladder trigone, adjacent to the vesicoureteric junctions. There is no evidence of obstructive hydronephrosis.

Deflux Injection

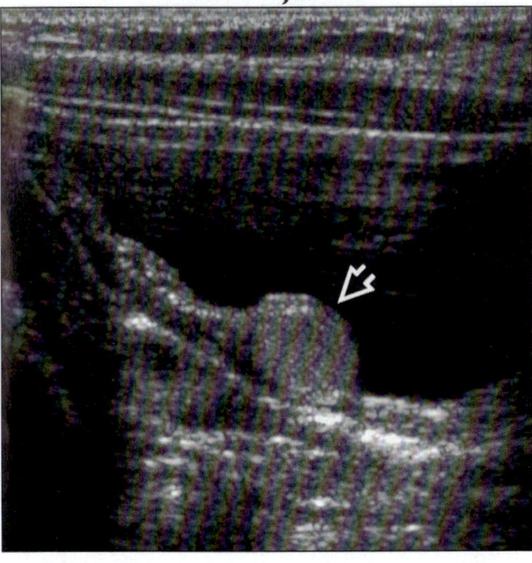

Fungus Ball

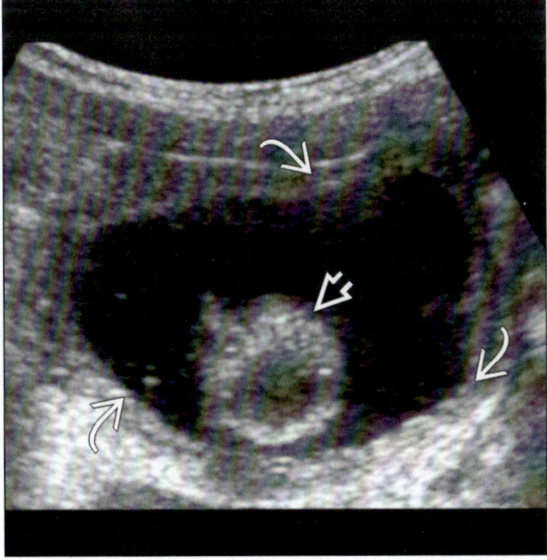

(Left) Transverse transabdominal ultrasound shows a pseudoureterocele ⮞ resulting from focal mucosal bulging after deflux injection for treatment of vesicoureteric reflux. Correlation with treatment history helps to derive a correct diagnosis. *(Right)* Transverse transabdominal ultrasound shows a mobile fungus ball ⮞ in a patient with fungal cystitis. Note the diffuse bladder wall thickening ➤.

BLADDER WALL THICKENING

DIFFERENTIAL DIAGNOSIS

Common
- Underfilling of Bladder
- Normal Trigone
- Bacterial Cystitis
- Neurogenic Bladder
- Chronic Bladder Outlet Obstruction
- Bladder Carcinoma
- Invasion by Pelvic Neoplasm

Less Common
- Fungal Cystitis
- Tuberculous Cystitis
- Bladder Schistosomiasis
- Emphysematous Cystitis
- Invasion by Pelvic Inflammatory Disease

ESSENTIAL INFORMATION

Key Differential Diagnosis Issues
- Check status of bladder distension before commenting on bladder wall thickness
- Be aware of sites of normal thickening near trigone
- Classify bladder wall thickening as focal or diffuse pattern
- Color Doppler helps to identify intralesional vascularity in malignant conditions
- Check kidneys and ureters for other clues of infectious causes, such as TB and schistosomiasis

Helpful Clues for Common Diagnoses
- **Underfilling of Bladder**
  - Bladder wall thickness returns to normal when bladder distends
- **Normal Trigone**
  - Normal finding of focal thickening between ureteral orifices (interureteric ridge)
- **Bacterial Cystitis**
  - Risk factors
    - Transurethral invasion of bladder by perineal flora in sexually active women
    - Bladder outlet obstruction and urinary stasis in men
  - Usually smooth diffuse bladder wall thickening
  - Recurrent bacterial infection: Malakoplakia
    - Associated with *E. coli* infection
    - Granulomatous inflammatory process
    - Caused by deficient function of lysosomes in macrophages
  - Chronic cystitis associated with decreased bladder capacity and vesicoureteric reflux
  - Other complications associated with chronic cystitis
    - Hyperplastic uroepithelial cell clusters (Brunn nests) form in bladder submucosa
    - Fluid accumulation → pseudocysts = cystitis cystica, potentially malignant
    - Transformation into gland: Cystitis glandularis
- **Neurogenic Bladder**
  - Diffuse bladder thickening
  - Typical "Christmas tree"-shaped bladder
  - Detrusor hyper-reflexia: Gross trabeculation and abnormal shape
- **Chronic Bladder Outlet Obstruction**
  - Trabeculated bladder
  - Usually diffuse bladder wall thickening
  - Muscular hypertrophy leading to irregular outline of inner bladder wall (trabeculation)
  - ± focal pseudopolyps, which are indistinguishable from tumor
  - Most common cause: Benign prostatic hypertrophy in males
- **Bladder Carcinoma**
  - Commonly appears as focal bladder wall thickening
    - Polypoidal or broad-based most common
    - May see frond-like projections
  - Best diagnostic clue: Focal nonmobile mass in bladder, of mixed echogenicity, absent posterior acoustic shadowing
  - Color Doppler shows increased vascularity in most large tumors
  - Reported sensitivity for bladder tumor detection by US range from 50-95%
  - US most useful for detection of tumor arising in bladder diverticulum, inaccessible by cystoscopy due to narrow neck of diverticulum
  - Diverticular tumor appears as moderately echogenic, nonshadowing mass
  - Tumor near bladder base in male may be confused with prostatic enlargement
    - Transrectal US differentiates bladder tumors from prostatic lesions

- Bladder tumors and prostatic enlargement often coexist; bladder tumors may invade prostate
  - Recent advances: 3D rendering may help to discriminate between superficial stage, pT1, and muscle invasive carcinoma > pT1
- **Invasion by Pelvic Neoplasm**
  - Common tumors
    - Male: Rectal, prostate carcinoma
    - Female: Cervical, ovarian, or vaginal carcinoma
  - Color Doppler: Vascularity of tumor outside bladder cavity may be demonstrated

Helpful Clues for Less Common Diagnoses
- **Fungal Cystitis**
  - *Candida* is most common organism
  - May be associated with fungal ball within bladder
- **Tuberculous Cystitis**
  - Infection by *Mycobacterium tuberculous* via hematogenous spread from primary focus, usually lungs
  - Secondary to renal involvement ± ureteric involvement
  - Earliest form of bladder TB starts around ureteral orifice
  - Small, fibrotic, thick-walled bladder
  - Echogenic foci or calcification (granulomas) in bladder wall near ureteric orifice
  - Associated with localized or generalized pyonephrosis

- Look for clues in kidneys and ureters
  - Papillary destruction with echogenic masses near calyces
  - Distorted renal parenchyma
  - Irregular hypoechoic masses connected to collecting system ± renal pelvic dilatation
  - Mucosal thickening in ureter ± stricture
  - Late stage: Small shrunken kidney, paper-thin cortex, & dense dystrophic calcification in collecting system
- **Bladder Schistosomiasis**
  - Infection of urinary system by parasite *Schistosoma hematobium*
  - Thick-walled fibrotic bladder
  - Echogenic calcification within bladder wall
  - Small capacity bladder with inability to completely empty
  - ± hydronephrosis and hydroureter due to distal ureteric stricture
  - Late complication: Squamous cell carcinoma of bladder
- **Emphysematous Cystitis**
  - Infection by gas-forming organism
  - Echogenic foci within area of bladder wall thickening with ring-down artifact
- **Invasion by Pelvic Inflammatory Disease**
  - Crohn disease: Inflamed bowel or fistula formation
  - Endometriosis
  - Color Doppler: Vascularity demonstrated within inflammatory tissue outside bladder cavity

Underfilling of Bladder

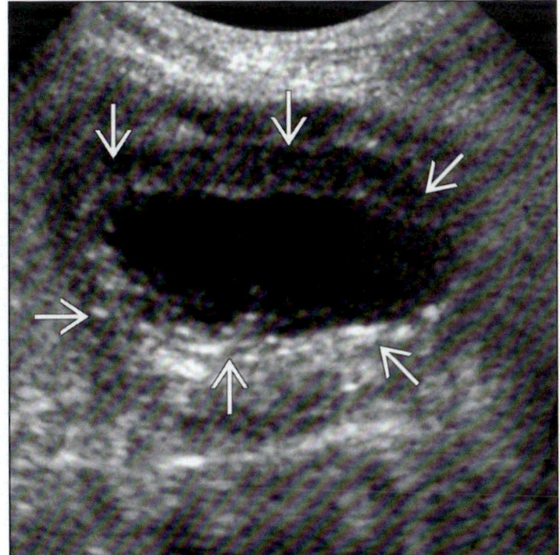

Transverse transabdominal ultrasound shows an apparent uniformly thickened bladder wall ➡ in a small volume urinary bladder. It was normal after filling.

Normal Trigone

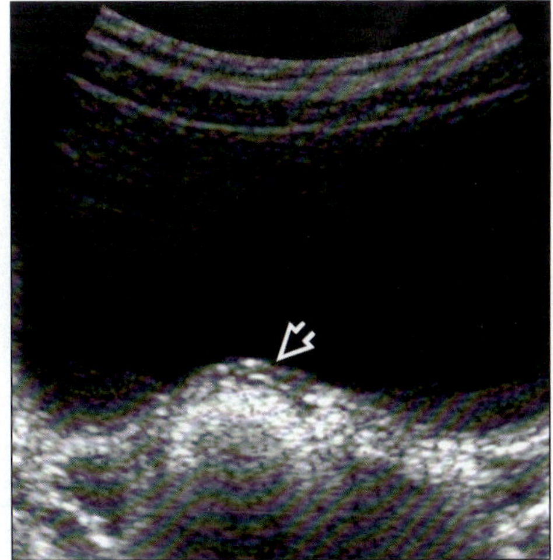

Transverse transabdominal ultrasound shows a focal thickening ➡ at the interureteric ridge. This is a normal finding.

BLADDER WALL THICKENING

(Left) Transverse transabdominal ultrasound shows smooth bladder wall thickening ➡ in a patient with a urinary tract infection, with positive bacterial growth on urine culture. (Right) Transverse transabdominal ultrasound shows wall thickening and an irregular inner bladder surface (trabeculations) ➡ in a neurogenic bladder. Note the long anteroposterior dimension of the bladder.

Bacterial Cystitis

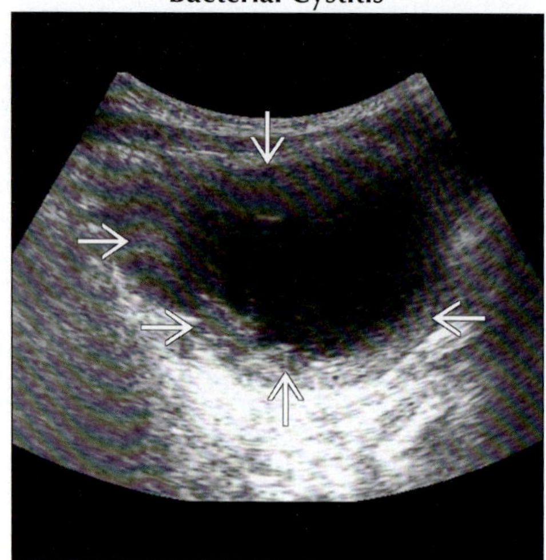

Neurogenic Bladder

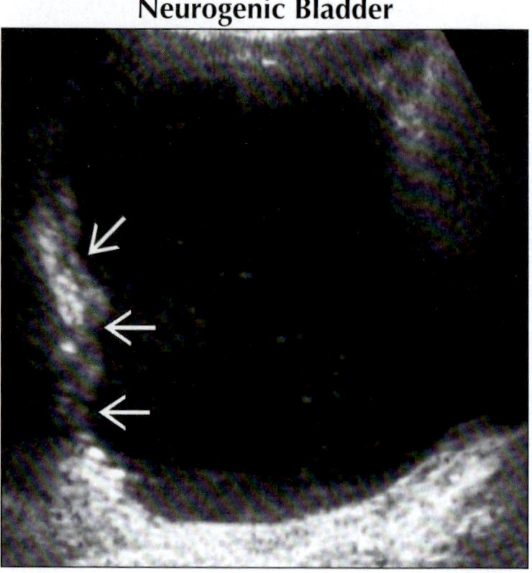

(Left) Transverse transabdominal ultrasound shows an irregular inner bladder outline, compatible with trabeculations ➡, in a patient with chronic outflow obstruction. (Right) Longitudinal transabdominal ultrasound shows benign prostatic hypertrophy ➡ with a lobulated contour, indenting the bladder base. This is a common cause of chronic bladder outlet obstruction in elderly male patients.

Chronic Bladder Outlet Obstruction

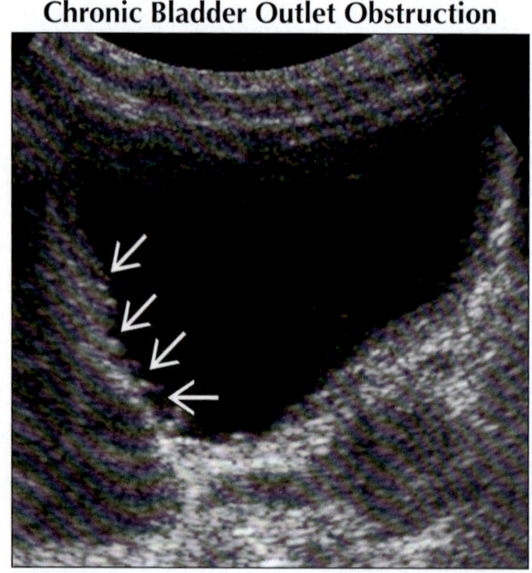

Chronic Bladder Outlet Obstruction

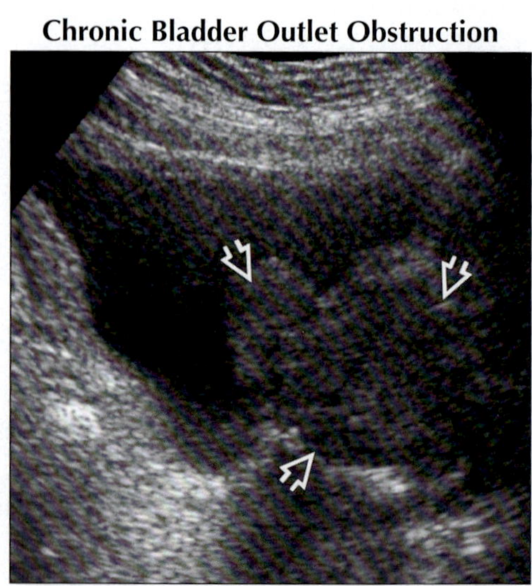

(Left) Oblique color Doppler ultrasound shows increased vascularity ➡ within a bladder carcinoma ➡ at the base of the urinary bladder. The rest of the bladder wall ➡ is not thickened. (Right) Transverse transabdominal ultrasound shows a fungating tumor ➡ occupying almost the entire lumen of the urinary bladder. There is generalized bladder wall thickening with poor distensibility of the bladder, indicating the infiltrative nature of this tumor.

Bladder Carcinoma

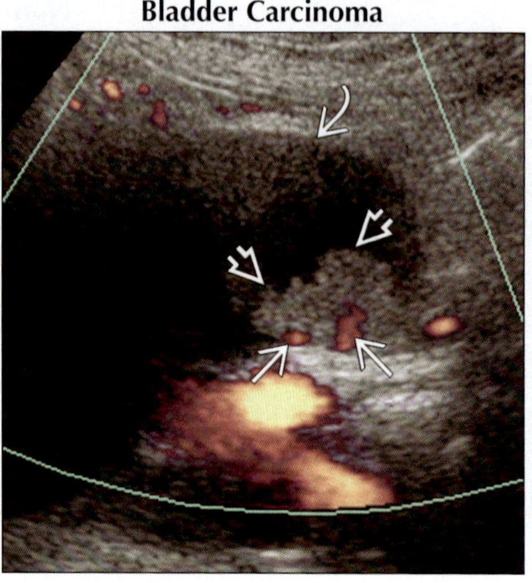

Bladder Carcinoma

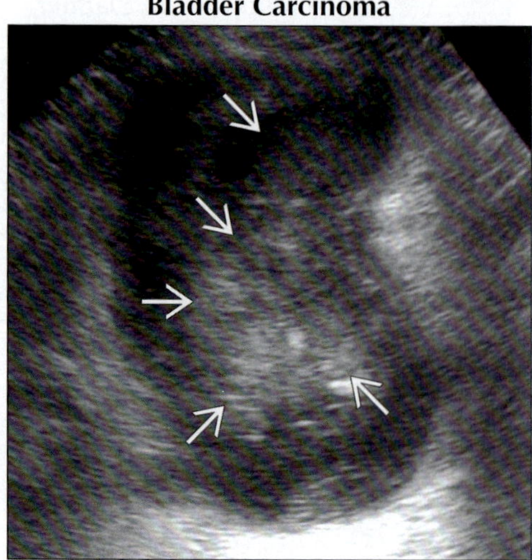

BLADDER WALL THICKENING

Invasion by Pelvic Neoplasm

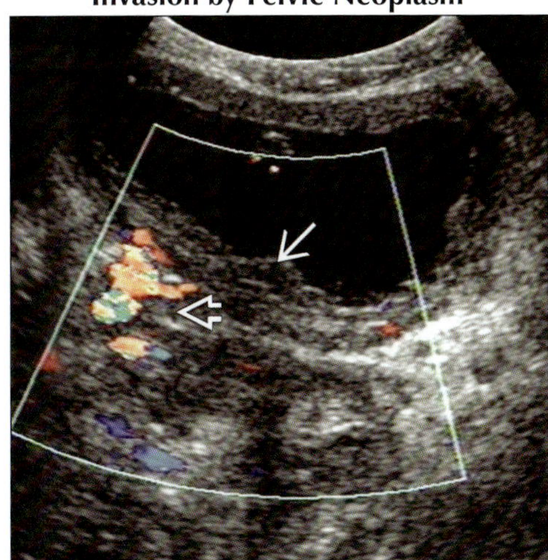

Fungal Cystitis

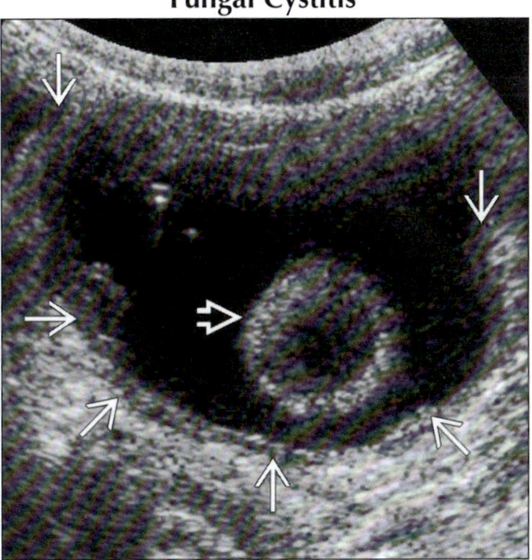

(Left) Longitudinal color Doppler ultrasound shows bladder wall thickening ➡ due to local invasion by uterine cancer. Increased vascularity is present in the tumor tissue ⬊. (Right) Transverse transabdominal ultrasound shows diffuse bladder wall thickening ➡ and a fungal ball ⬊ in the bladder of a patient with fungal cystitis.

Tuberculous Cystitis

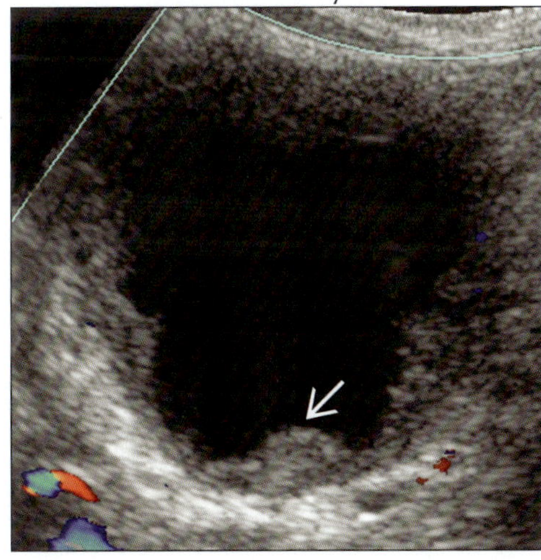

Tuberculous Cystitis

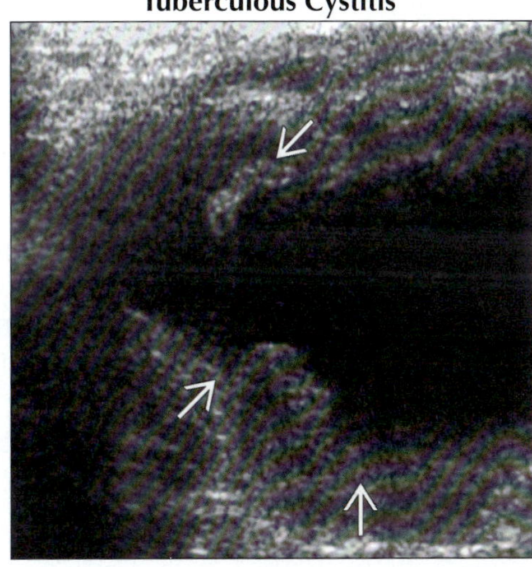

(Left) Longitudinal color Doppler ultrasound shows a urinary bladder infected by tuberculosis. There is irregular mucosal thickening ➡ without significant vascularity near the ureteric orifice, which is the earliest site for the onset of tuberculous cystitis. (Right) Transverse transabdominal ultrasound shows a bladder infected by TB with an irregularly thickened bladder wall ➡. Tuberculous cystitis may be indistinguishable from other forms of bacterial cystitis.

Bladder Schistosomiasis

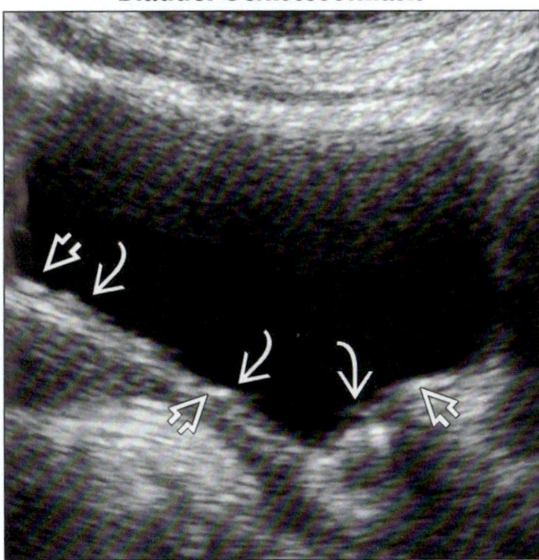

Emphysematous Cystitis

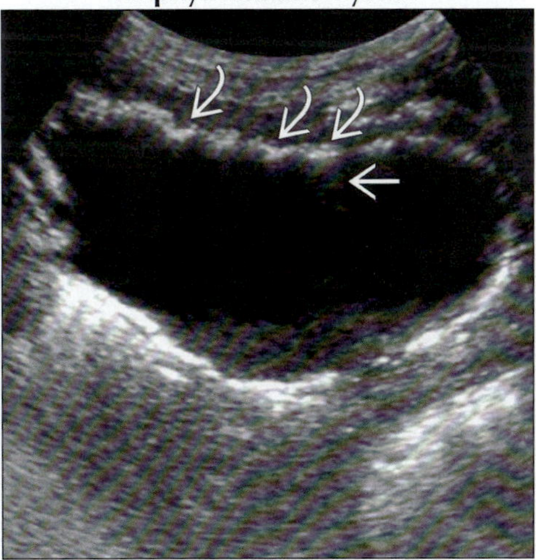

(Left) Longitudinal transabdominal ultrasound shows multiple echogenic foci of calcifications ⬊ and mucosal irregularity ➡ of the posterior bladder wall. The bladder volume is reduced. (Right) Transverse transabdominal ultrasound shows intramural gas as echogenic foci ➡ with ring-down artifact ➡. Also note the markedly thickened bladder wall.

IRREGULAR BLADDER CONTOUR

DIFFERENTIAL DIAGNOSIS

Common
- Bladder Trabeculation
- Bladder Diverticulum/Diverticula
- Ureterocele
- Urachal Remnant
- Extrinsic Compression by Pelvic Mass

Less Common
- Extrinsic Compression by Inflammatory Conditions

ESSENTIAL INFORMATION

Key Differential Diagnosis Issues
- Differentiate between focal and diffuse irregular bladder contour
  - Diffuse irregular bladder contour suggests trabeculations
  - Cystic nature of bladder irregularities suggests benign lesions
- Color Doppler helps to demonstrate vascularity in neoplasm and inflammatory conditions causing extrinsic compression

Helpful Clues for Common Diagnoses
- **Bladder Trabeculation**
  - Irregular outline of inner bladder wall due to muscular hypertrophy
  - Associated with chronic bladder outlet obstruction and neurogenic bladder
- **Bladder Diverticulum/Diverticula**
  - Best diagnostic clue: Perivesical cystic mass connected to bladder lumen
  - Sac formed by herniation of bladder mucosa and submucosa through muscular wall
- **Ureterocele**
  - Best diagnostic clues
    - Orthotopic: Thin-walled, sac-like structure, continuous with distal ureter at trigone
    - Ectopic: Continuous with hydroureter and hydronephrotic obstructive moiety
    - Everted ureterocele: Resume intravesicle appearance following partial bladder emptying
- **Urachal Remnant**
  - Cord-like embryonic remnant that connects bladder apex with umbilicus
  - Midline in position
- **Extrinsic Compression by Pelvic Mass**
  - Benign prostate hypertrophy is most common cause of extrinsic compression in males
  - May be caused by other pelvic neoplasms
    - Cancer arising from prostate, rectum, ovary, uterus, or cervix

Helpful Clues for Less Common Diagnoses
- **Extrinsic Compression by Inflammatory Conditions**
  - Endometriosis: Heterogeneous adnexal cyst with diffuse low-level echoes
  - Crohn disease: Inflamed bowel, fistula formation, fluid collections

Bladder Trabeculation

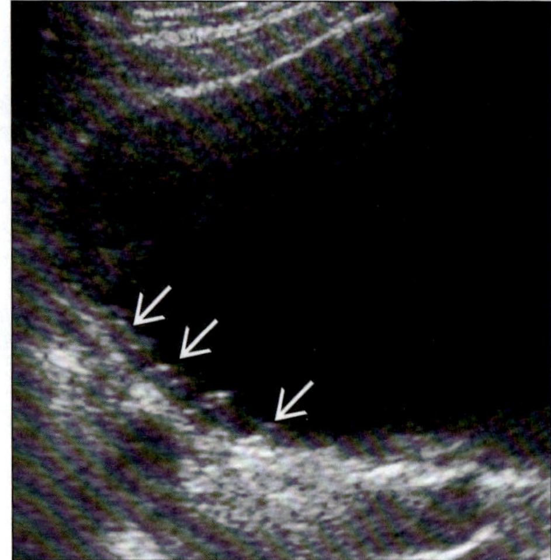

Oblique transabdominal ultrasound in a patient with a neurogenic bladder shows an irregular inner bladder outline ➡, compatible with trabeculations.

Bladder Diverticulum/Diverticula

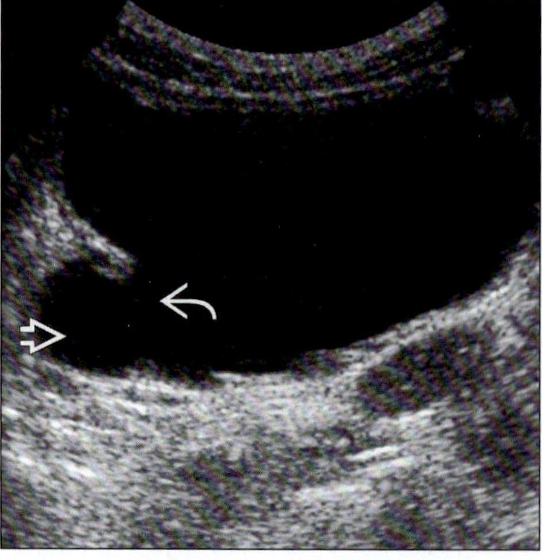

Transverse transabdominal ultrasound shows a typical diverticulum ➡ arising from the posterolateral wall of the urinary bladder. Note the wide neck ➡.

IRREGULAR BLADDER CONTOUR

Bladder Diverticulum/Diverticula

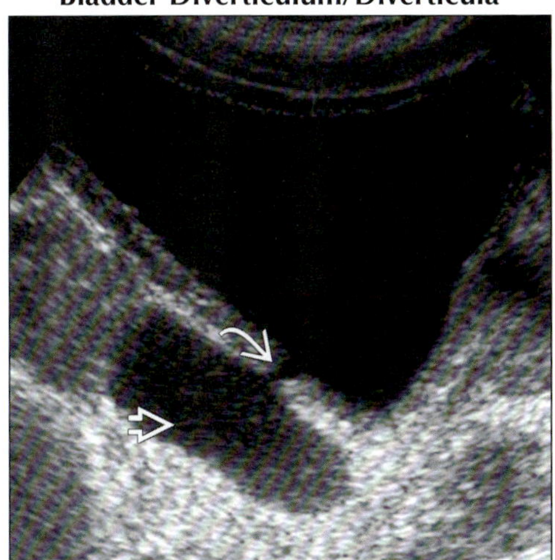

Bladder Diverticulum/Diverticula

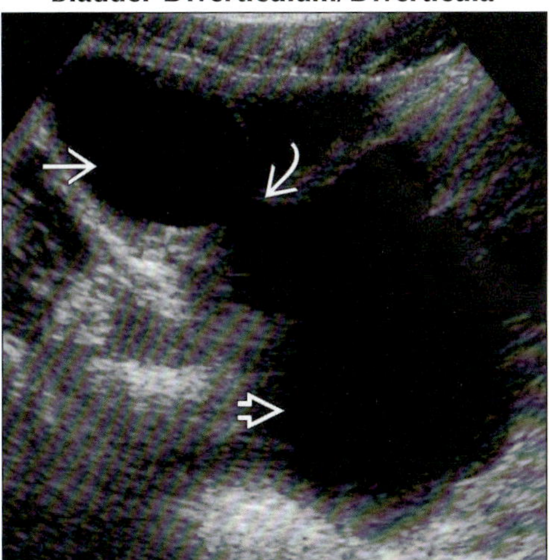

(Left) Longitudinal transabdominal ultrasound shows a Hutch diverticulum ➡, with a narrow neck ➡ arising from the posterolateral wall. *(Right)* Transverse transabdominal ultrasound shows a large diverticulum ➡ with a wide neck ➡ arising from the urinary bladder ➡. Note that the diverticulum is larger than the urinary bladder.

Ureterocele

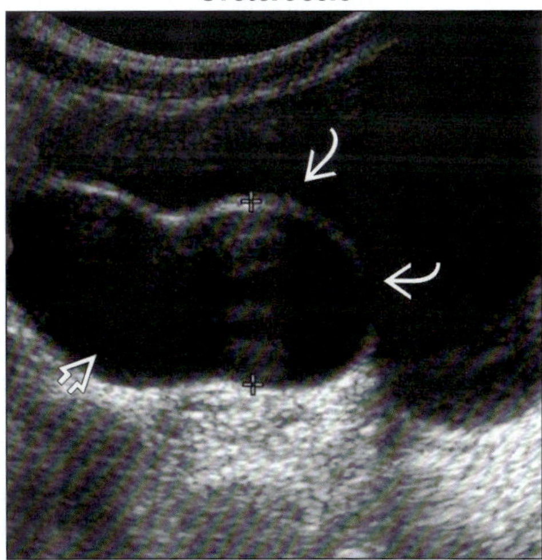

Urachal Remnant

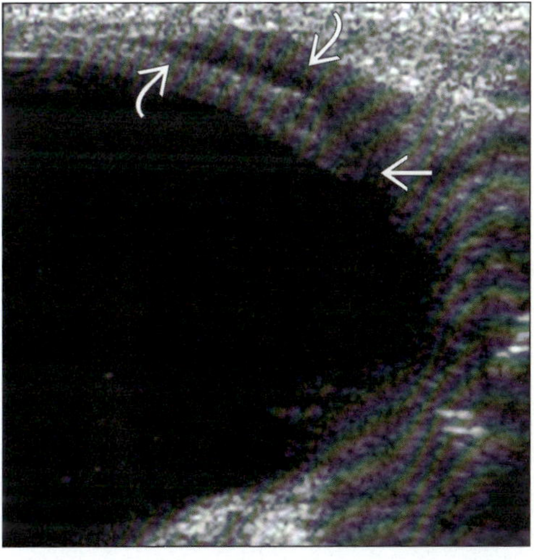

(Left) Transverse transabdominal ultrasound shows an everted ureterocele ➡, which indents the inferoposterior wall of the urinary bladder ➡. The ureterocele assumes the more usual; intravesicular appearance on partial bladder emptying. *(Right)* Longitudinal transabdominal ultrasound shows a thin, fluid-filled, cord-like structure ➡ extending from the bladder apex ➡ to umbilicus, consistent with patent urachus.

Extrinsic Compression by Pelvic Mass

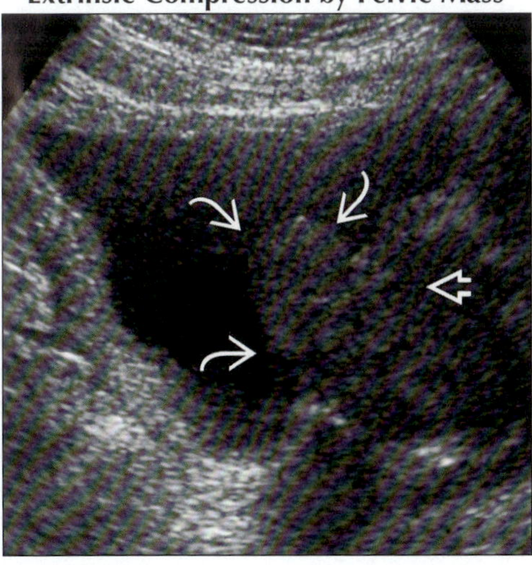

Extrinsic Compression by Pelvic Mass

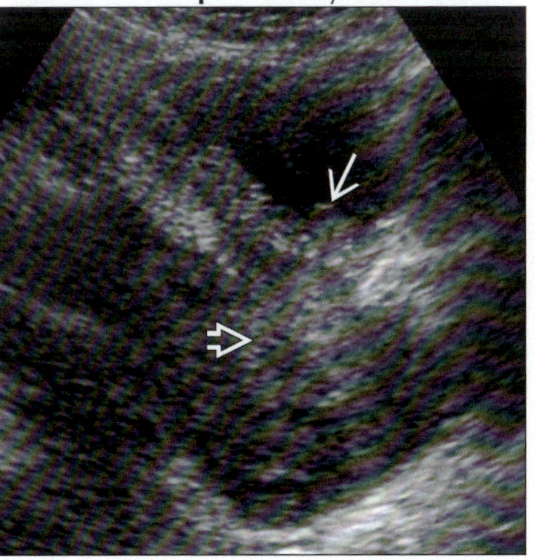

(Left) Longitudinal transabdominal ultrasound shows indentation of the bladder base ➡ by an enlarged prostate ➡. This patient with benign prostatic hypertrophy presented with dysuria. *(Right)* Longitudinal transabdominal ultrasound shows a large uterine tumor ➡ indenting the base of the urinary bladder ➡.

SECTION 11
Prostate

DIFFERENTIAL DIAGNOSIS

Common
- Benign Prostatic Hypertrophy
- Prostatic Cyst
- Prostatic Carcinoma

Less Common
- Acute Prostatitis
- Prostatic Abscess
- Bladder Cancer with Local Invasion

Rare but Important
- Tuberculosis Prostatitis
- Giant Multilocular Prostatic Cystadenoma
- Prostatic Phyllodes Tumor

ESSENTIAL INFORMATION

Key Differential Diagnosis Issues
- Age may help in assessing differentials
  - < 50 years: Bacterial prostatitis common
  - 50-80 years: Prostatic hypertrophy (50%)
  - > 80 years: Prostatic carcinoma (80%)
- Biopsy may be required for diagnosis

Helpful Clues for Common Diagnoses
- **Benign Prostatic Hypertrophy**
  - Diffusely enlarged transitional zone abutting bladder base
  - Heterogeneous nodular echotexture
- **Prostatic Cyst**
  - Large Müllerian duct cyst and ejaculatory duct cyst often extend above prostatic base
- **Prostatic Carcinoma**
  - Advanced infiltrative disease seen as irregularly enlarged prostate

Helpful Clues for Less Common Diagnoses
- **Acute Prostatitis**
  - Normal or enlarged prostate
  - Shows subtle periurethral and periglandular hypoechogenicity
  - ↑ glandular or periprostatic vascularity
  - Often coexists with urinary tract infection
  - Abscess formation uncommon
- **Prostatic Abscess**
  - More common in elderly, diabetic, or immunocompromised patients
- **Bladder Cancer with Local Invasion**
  - May mimic enlarged central gland in prostatic hypertrophy

Helpful Clues for Rare Diagnoses
- **Tuberculosis Prostatitis**
  - Acute: Diffusely enlarged gland + multiple abscesses ⇒ prostatic/periurethral cavities
  - Chronic: Extensive prostatic calcifications
- **Giant Multilocular Prostatic Cystadenoma**
  - May appear as large prostatic multiloculated cyst or as distinct extraprostatic lesion with retroperitoneal spread
- **Prostatic Phyllodes Tumor**
  - Prostatic stromal proliferation of uncertain malignancy potential
  - Huge retroperitoneal tumor, which may compress or invade bladder or rectum
  - May recur; associated with sarcomas with local invasion or distant metastasis

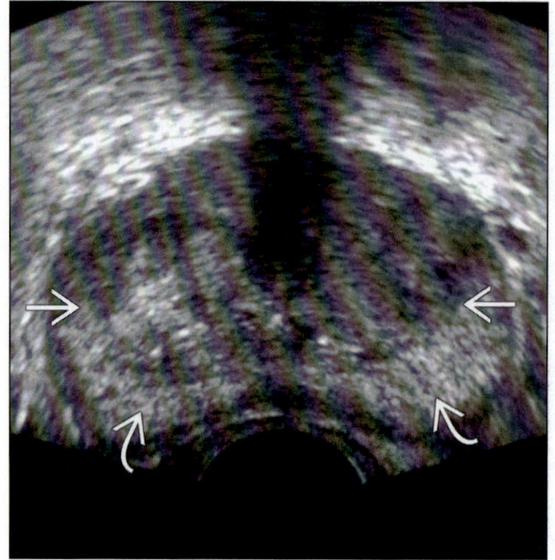

Benign Prostatic Hypertrophy

Transverse transrectal ultrasound shows prostatic hypertrophy with a symmetrically enlarged transitional zone ➡. The enlarged central gland causes thinning and outward displacement of the peripheral zone ➡.

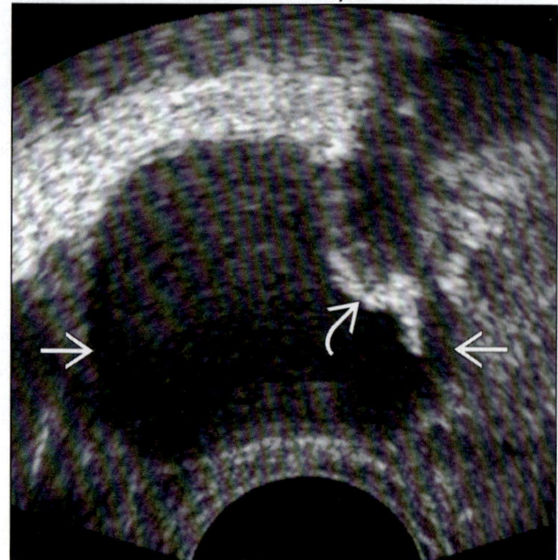

Prostatic Cyst

Transverse transrectal ultrasound (TRUS) shows a large prostatic ejaculatory duct cyst ➡ that contains calcification ➡.

ENLARGED PROSTATE

Prostatic Carcinoma

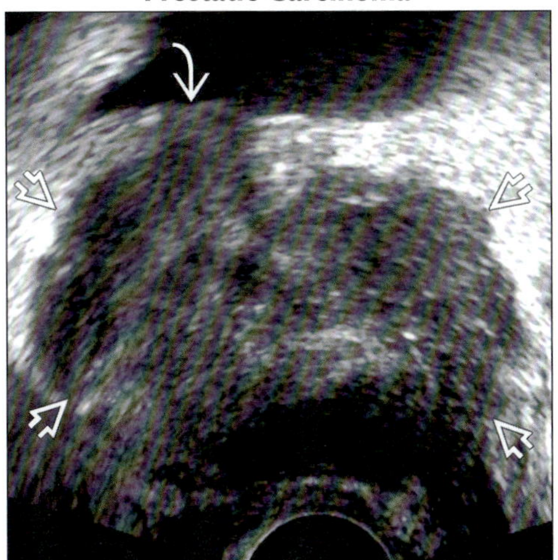

Acute Prostatitis

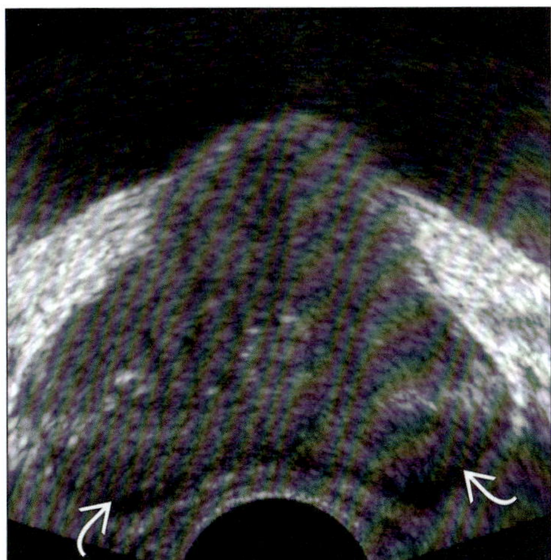

(Left) Transverse TRUS shows advanced prostatic carcinoma appearing as an enlarged gland with an irregular outline ➡. Note the gland is heterogeneous with extracapsular extension ➡ into the bladder base. (Right) Transverse TRUS shows uncomplicated acute prostatitis. Note that the gland is swollen and hypoechoic with a thin periglandular hypoechoic rim ➡.

Prostatic Abscess

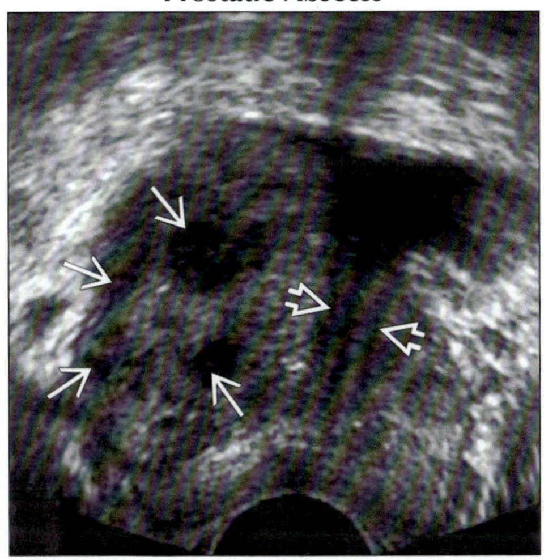

Prostatic Abscess

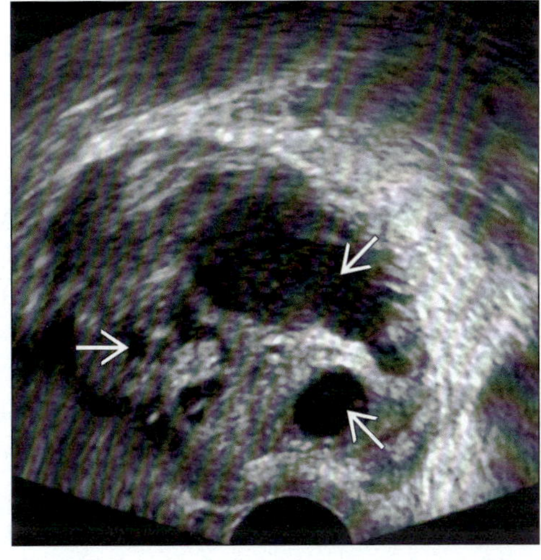

(Left) Transverse TRUS shows acute prostatitis complicated by multiple, small abscesses ➡, predominantly in the right lobe. Note that there is marked periurethral edema ➡. (Right) Oblique TRUS in the same patient shows acute prostatitis with multiple abscesses ➡ in the right lobe of the gland.

Bladder Cancer with Local Invasion

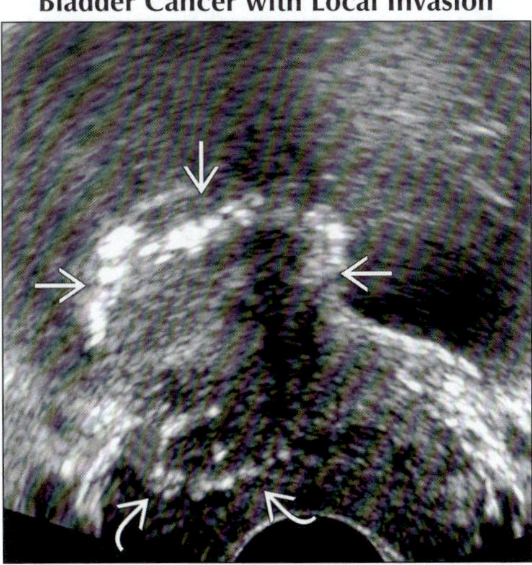

Tuberculosis Prostatitis

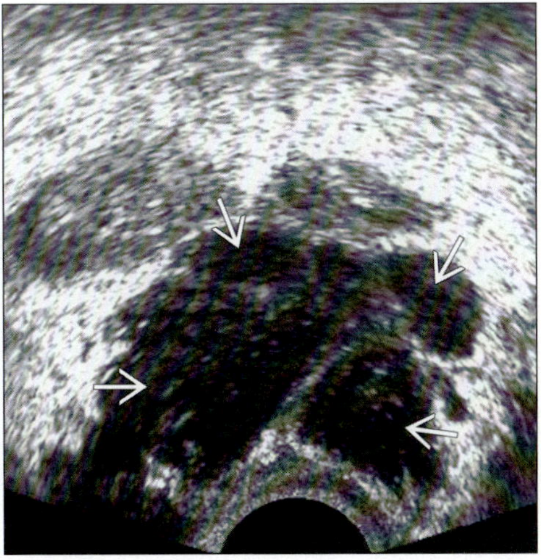

(Left) Transverse TRUS shows a large bladder cancer ➡ near the bladder base with posterior extension into the prostate gland ➡. (Right) Transverse TRUS shows cavitating tuberculosis prostatitis. The gland shows multiple, well-circumscribed, hypoechoic areas representing multiple abscesses ➡. Such multiple abscesses are typical of tuberculosis prostatitis.

DIFFERENTIAL DIAGNOSIS

Common
- Benign Prostatic Hyperplasia (BPH), Hyperplastic Nodules
- BPH, Cystic Degeneration
- Prostatic Calcification
- Prostatic Carcinoma
- Retention Cyst
- Utricle Cyst
- Müllerian Duct Cyst

Less Common
- Focal Prostatitis
- Prostatic Abscess
- Metastases and Lymphoma of Prostate
- Ejaculatory Duct Cyst (EDC) or Diverticulum
- Seminal Vesicle Cyst or Ductal Ectasia
- Vas Deferens Cyst

Rare but Important
- Cystic Prostatic Carcinoma
- Multilocular Prostatic Cystadenoma
- Hydatid Cyst
- Prostatic Urethral Diverticulum

ESSENTIAL INFORMATION

Key Differential Diagnosis Issues
- Focal lesion may be discovered by palpation (digital rectal exam) as incidental finding or part of screening
  - Or in patient with symptoms, signs, or abnormal laboratory evaluation
    - Fever, pain, dysuria, hemospermia, painful ejaculation
    - ↑ prostate specific antigen
- Location of cystic lesion helps in diagnosis
  - EDC and utricle cysts normally communicate with urethra; Müllerian duct cysts rarely do

Helpful Clues for Common Diagnoses
- **Benign Prostatic Hyperplasia (BPH), Hyperplastic Nodules**
  - Hyperechoic nodules in enlarged gland
  - Located in transitional and periurethral zones
  - May be confused with prostatic carcinoma
  - May undergo cystic degeneration
- **BPH, Cystic Degeneration**
  - Arises within hyperplastic nodules
  - Typically located in transitional zone

- **Prostatic Calcification**
  - Common feature of chronic prostatitis
  - Caused by calcium precipitation inside acini, with ducts obstructed by inflammation
  - Intraglandular or periurethral
  - In young patients, calcifications are usually periurethral
- **Prostatic Carcinoma**
  - > 90% are hypoechoic (less commonly iso- or hyperechoic)
  - ~ 70% occur in peripheral zone
  - 30% of tumors not evident on ultrasound
    - Indistinguishable from hyperplastic nodules in transitional zone
  - Extracapsular extension common in advanced disease
- **Retention Cyst**
  - Results from obstructed glandular acinus
  - Unilocular with smooth walls
  - Location variable; size ~ 1-2 cm
  - May be indistinguishable from BPH
- **Utricle Cyst**
  - Cystic dilatation of prostatic utricle, acquired or congenital
    - Congenital results from abnormality in regression of Müllerian duct system
  - Intraprostatic; midline, arises from verumontanum
  - Usually small; tubular or pear shaped
  - Normally communicates with urethra
  - Associated with hypospadias, undescended testes, and unilateral renal agenesis
- **Müllerian Duct Cyst**
  - Originates from remnant of Müllerian duct
  - Extraprostatic; midline
  - Usually large; extends above prostatic base
  - Oval/teardrop-shaped; rarely communicates with urethra
  - May contain calculi (rare)
  - Differentiation from utricle cyst is difficult

Helpful Clues for Less Common Diagnoses
- **Focal Prostatitis**
  - Clinical: Tender and warm to palpation
  - Acute: Size may be normal but often enlarged; ill-defined margin; hypoechoic areas with ↑ vascularity
  - Chronic: Normal-sized gland; heterogeneous echo pattern ± Ca++
- **Prostatic Abscess**
  - As complication of prostatitis

11

FOCAL LESION IN PROSTATE

- ○ 1 or multiple prostatic cystic lesions with internal debris ± septae ± gas
- **Metastases and Lymphoma of Prostate**
  - ○ Metastases most frequent from direct extension from carcinoma of rectum, bladder, seminal vesicle
  - ○ Lymphoma: Usually part of disseminated disease
- **Ejaculatory Duct Cyst (EDC) or Diverticulum**
  - ○ Intraprostatic, along ejaculatory duct
  - ○ Paramedian at base, midline at verumontanum
  - ○ Normally communicates with urethra
  - ○ Intracystic calculi common
  - ○ Ejaculatory duct diverticulum is rare
- **Seminal Vesicle Cyst or Ductal Ectasia**
  - ○ Variable in size; rarely bilateral
  - ○ Unilocular or multilocular
  - ○ Associated with renal agenesis/dysgenesis
  - ○ Ductal ectasia caused by ejaculatory duct or vas deferens obstruction
- **Vas Deferens Cyst**
  - ○ Extraprostatic, superior to gland
  - ○ Associated with ectopic vas deferens with abnormal vas ureteral communications

Helpful Clues for Rare Diagnoses
- **Cystic Prostatic Carcinoma**
  - ○ Complex cyst with solid components
  - ○ Predominantly peripheral in location
  - ○ Extracapsular extension is specific for malignancy, differentiating it from other cystic lesions

- **Multilocular Prostatic Cystadenoma**
  - ○ Rare, benign, prostatic tumor
  - ○ Can enlarge, causing urinary obstruction
- **Hydatid Cyst**
  - ○ Simple or multiloculated with endocysts
  - ○ "Eggshell" cyst/wall calcification common
- **Prostatic Urethral Diverticulum**
  - ○ Anterior: Commonly due to instrumentation trauma or infection
  - ○ Posterior: Commonly related to rupture of prostatic abscess
  - ○ May be single or multiple
  - ○ Wide or narrowed neck with smooth or ragged walls

Alternative Differential Approaches
- Cystic lesion
  - ○ Midline: Utricle cyst, Müllerian duct cyst, prostatic urethral diverticulum, EDC or diverticulum
  - ○ Paramedian: Vas deferens cyst, EDC or diverticulum
  - ○ Lateral: Seminal vesicle cyst, BPH cystic degeneration (transitional zone)
  - ○ Variable: Retention cyst, abscess, hydatid cyst, cystic prostatic carcinoma (Ca)
- Solid lesion
  - ○ Central: BPH hyperplastic nodules (transitional zone)
  - ○ Peripheral: Prostatic Ca (70%)
  - ○ Variable: Calcifications, focal prostatitis, metastasis or lymphoma, multilocular cystadenoma, prostatic Ca (30%)

Benign Prostatic Hyperplasia (BPH), Hyperplastic Nodules

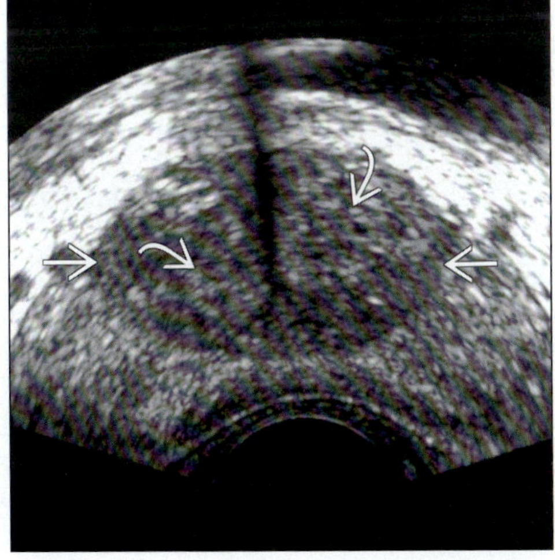

Coronal transrectal ultrasound (TRUS) of the prostate shows BPH with hyperechoic nodules ⇗ and enlargement of the transitional zone ⇥. These lesions, though typical of BPH, may mimic prostatic carcinoma.

BPH, Cystic Degeneration

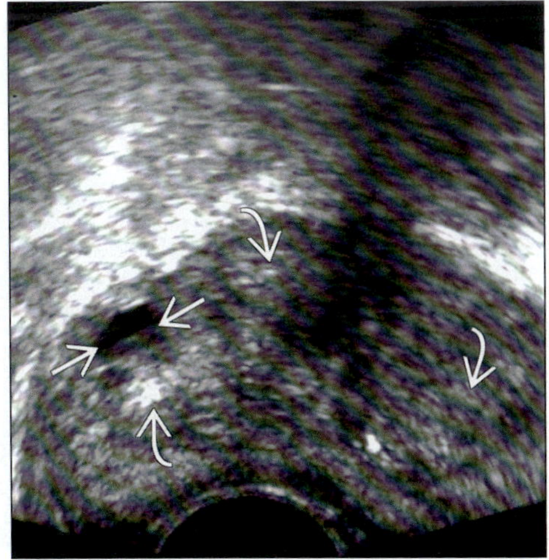

Coronal TRUS of the prostate shows BPH with multiple hyperplastic nodules ⇥ in the transitional zone. Note the small degenerative cyst ⇥ in 1 of the nodules.

(Left) Coronal TRUS of the prostate shows dense periurethral calcification ➡ with posterior acoustic shadowing ➡. This feature is common in young patients with chronic prostatitis due to calcium precipitation in obstructed acini. *(Right)* Longitudinal TRUS of the prostate shows an irregular hypoechoic nodule ➡ in the peripheral zone, suspicious for prostatic carcinoma. Over 90% of prostatic carcinomas are hypoechoic, and about 70% are in the peripheral zone.

Prostatic Calcification

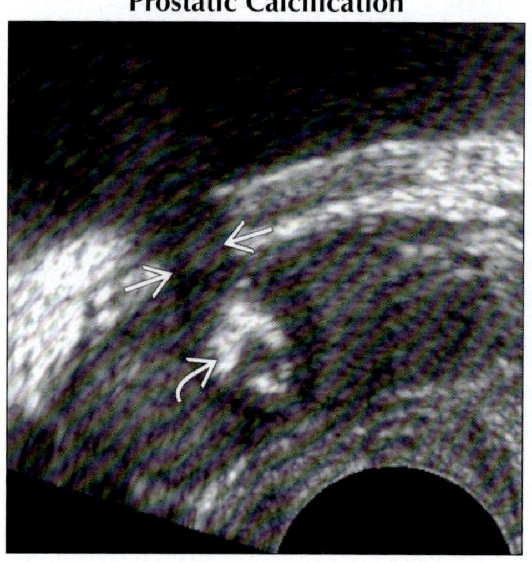

Prostatic Carcinoma

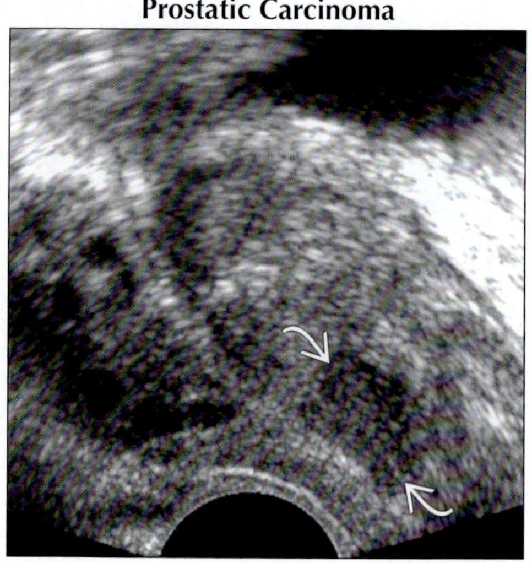

(Left) Coronal TRUS of the prostate shows a midline cyst ➡. To distinguish among ejaculatory duct cyst (EDC), utricle cyst, or Müllerian duct cyst, examine the relationship of the cyst to the urethra. *(Right)* Longitudinal TRUS in the same patient shows the cyst ➡ cephalic to, and separate from, the ejaculatory duct ➡ and communicating with the urethra ➡. The features favor an utricle cyst.

Utricle Cyst

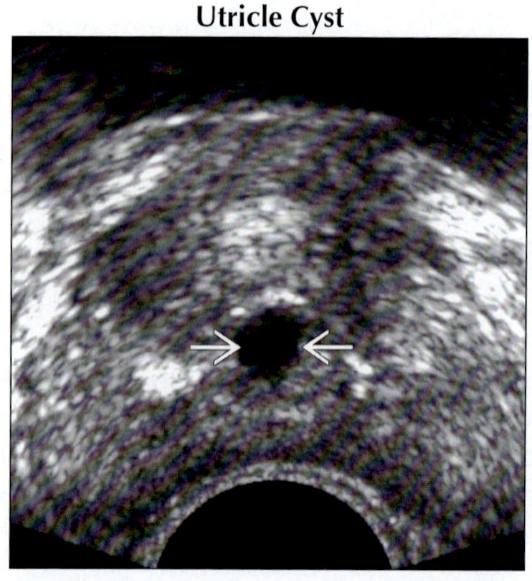

Utricle Cyst

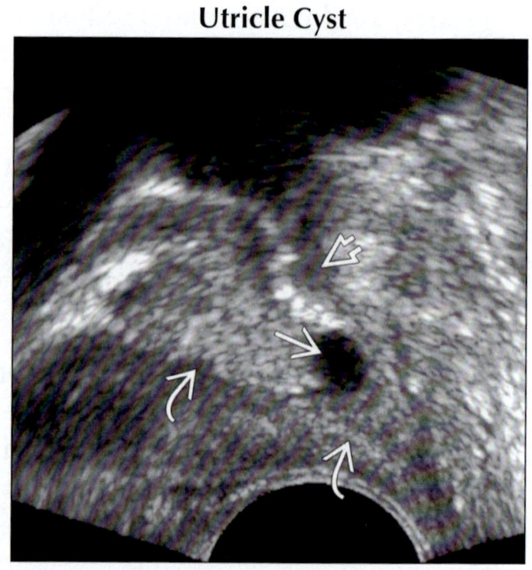

(Left) Coronal TRUS of the prostate shows a midline cyst at the level of the prostatic base, suggestive of a Müllerian duct cyst ➡. An EDC is less likely, because at this level, an EDC should be paramedian instead of median. *(Right)* Longitudinal TRUS in the same case shows the cyst ➡ with no obvious communication with the urethra ➡. Note that a Müllerian duct cyst is usually larger than a utricle cyst and rarely communicates with the urethra.

Müllerian Duct Cyst

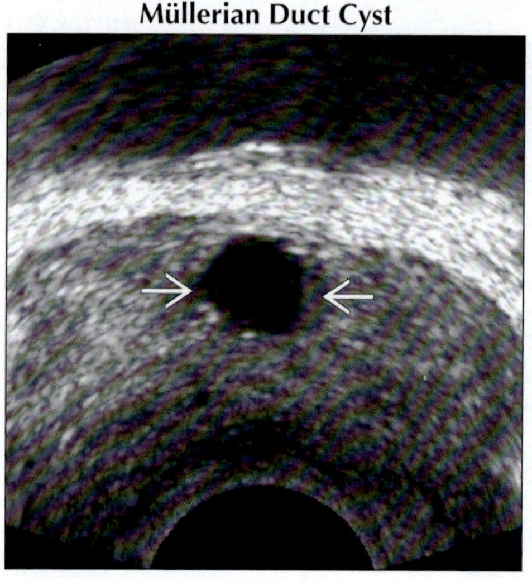

Müllerian Duct Cyst

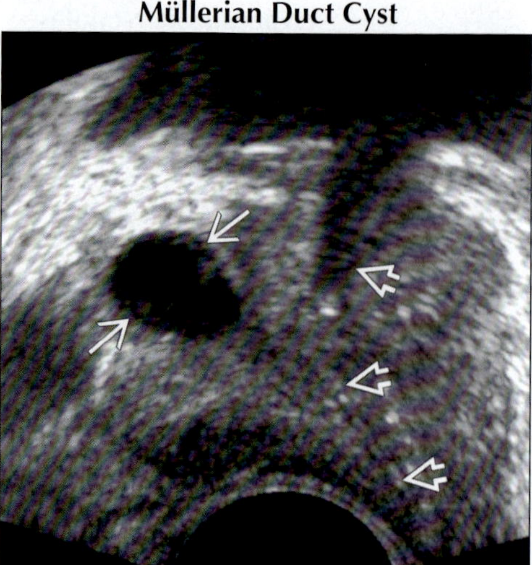

FOCAL LESION IN PROSTATE

Müllerian Duct Cyst

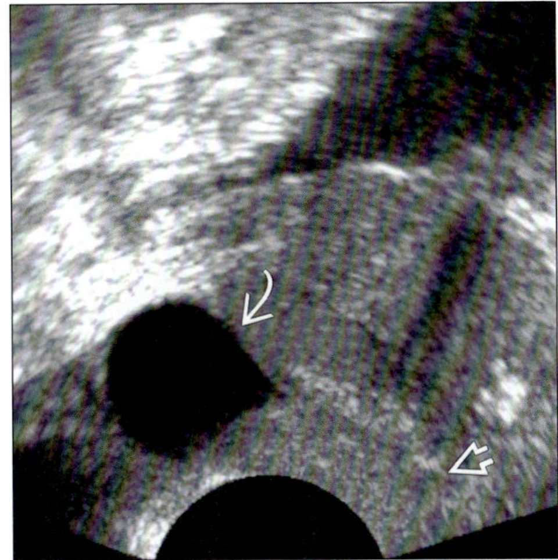

Prostatic Abscess

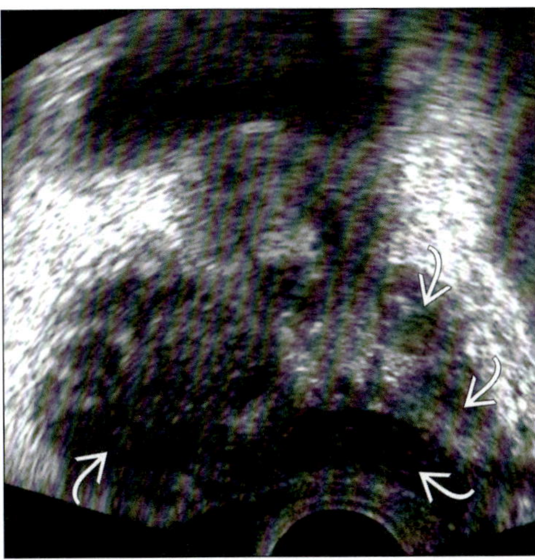

(Left) Longitudinal TRUS of the prostate shows a teardrop-shaped cystic lesion ➾, typical of a Müllerian duct cyst, lying posterior to the verumontanum ➾. When large, such cysts may extend cephalad above the prostatic base. (Right) Coronal TRUS shows an enlarged prostate deformed by multiple cystic lesions ➾ in a patient with acute prostatitis. Note that the cysts contain internal debris. These findings are suggestive of abscess formation.

Ejaculatory Duct Cyst (EDC) or Diverticulum

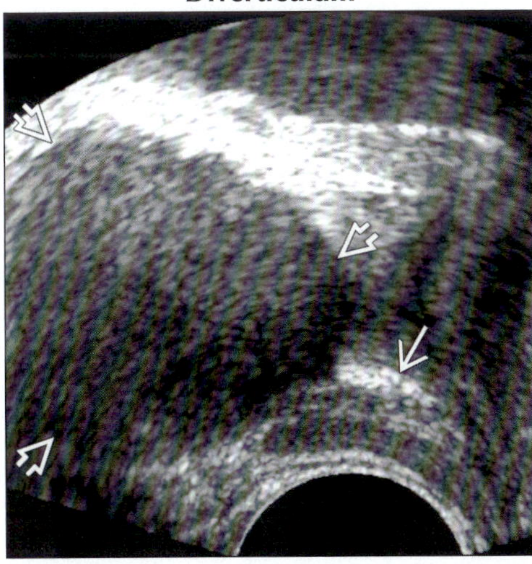

Ejaculatory Duct Cyst (EDC) or Diverticulum

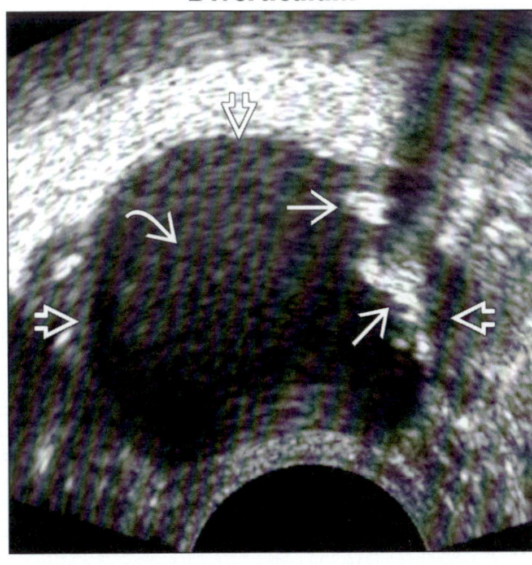

(Left) Longitudinal TRUS of the prostate shows a large cyst ➾ in a patient with hemospermia. The cyst arises from the ejaculatory duct ➾ and extends beyond the prostatic base. The aspirate contained spermatozoa, confirming it to be an EDC. (Right) Coronal TRUS of the prostate in the same patient shows internal echoes within the cyst ➾, which represent hemorrhage ➾ and calcification ➾, common findings in an EDC.

Seminal Vesicle Cyst or Ductal Ectasia

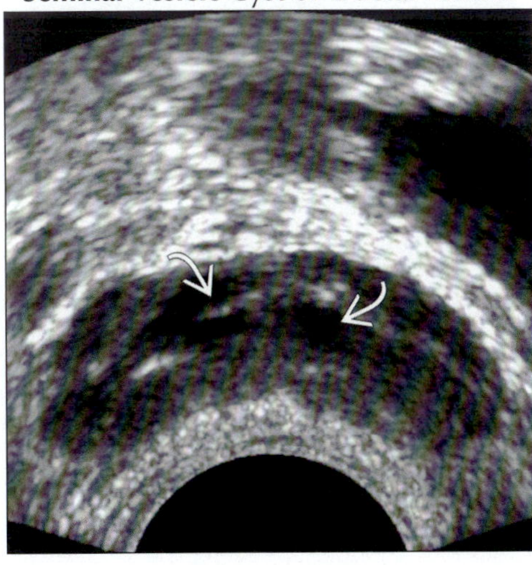

Cystic Prostatic Carcinoma

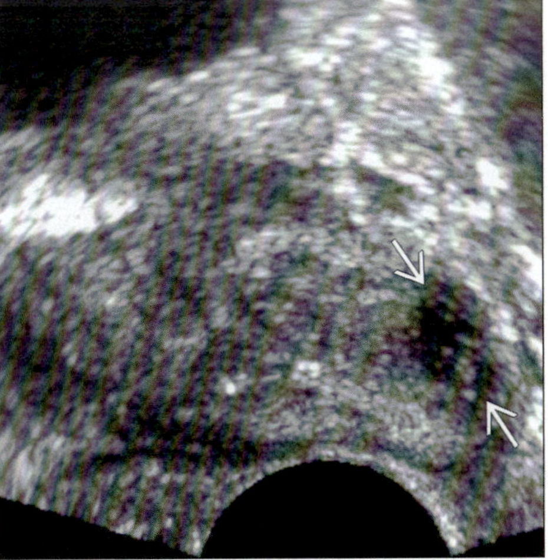

(Left) Coronal TRUS of the seminal vesicles shows ductal ectasia ➾, which may be caused by ejaculatory duct obstruction due to calculi, large midline cysts, and congenital causes, such as agenesis of the ejaculatory duct or vas deferens. (Right) Longitudinal TRUS of the prostate shows a histologically proven cystic prostatic Ca ➾. Note that the mass has an irregular wall and internal echoes mimicking an abscess.

11

SECTION 12
Scrotum

DIFFUSE TESTICULAR ENLARGEMENT

DIFFERENTIAL DIAGNOSIS

Common
- Orchitis
- Testicular Torsion/Infarction
- Testicular Carcinoma
- Scrotal Trauma

Less Common
- Testicular Lymphoma
- Testicular Metastases
- Testicular Cyst

ESSENTIAL INFORMATION

Key Differential Diagnosis Issues
- Diagnosis depends not on sonographic appearances alone, but on combination of clinical and ultrasound features

Helpful Clues for Common Diagnoses
- **Orchitis**
  - Characterized by edema of testes contained within rigid tunica albuginea
  - Heterogeneous parenchymal echogenicity and septal accentuation, seen as hypoechoic bands
  - Diffuse increase in testicular parenchymal vascularity on color Doppler ultrasound
- **Testicular Torsion/Infarction**
  - Acute infarction: Diffusely enlarged hypoechoic testis
  - Chronic infarction: Small, shrunken, heterogeneous testis
  - "Whirlpool" or "torsion knot" at level of spermatic cord; dampened or absent vascularity in testis
- **Testicular Carcinoma**
  - Discrete hypoechoic or mixed echogenic testicular mass, ± vascularity
  - Although seminomas are usually discrete hypoechoic lesions, they may cause diffuse enlargement of involved testis
  - Tumors < 1.5 cm commonly hypovascular; tumors > 1.6 cm more often hypervascular on color Doppler
- **Scrotal Trauma**
  - History of scrotal trauma
  - Focal hypoechoic area, discrete linear/irregular fracture plane within testis
  - Abnormal testicular parenchymal echogenicity, avascular mass; echogenicity of hematoma depends on its age

Helpful Clues for Less Common Diagnoses
- **Testicular Lymphoma and Metastases**
  - Multiple lesions; 50% of cases bilateral
  - Metastases are rare; most common sites include prostate, lung, and GI tract
  - Often large in size at time of diagnosis; associated with disseminated disease
    - Ill-defined, mostly hypoechoic lesions
- **Testicular Cyst**
  - Intratesticular cysts are usually simple cysts located near mediastinum testis
  - Need to differentiate them from cystic neoplasms
    - Search carefully for solid components

Orchitis

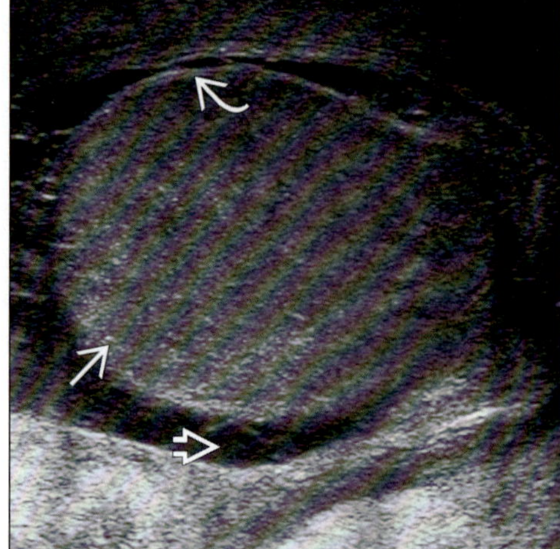

Longitudinal ultrasound shows an enlarged, diffusely hypoechoic testis ➦, suggesting acute orchitis. Note the globular shape of the testis, relative prominence of tunica albuginea ➦, and mild reactive hydrocele ➦.

Orchitis

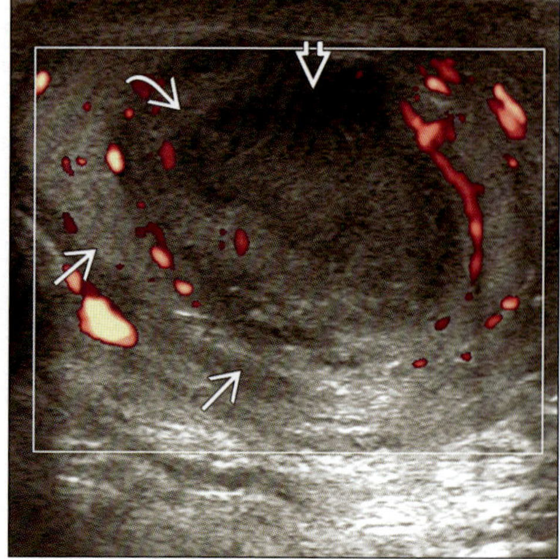

Longitudinal power Doppler ultrasound shows diffusely enlarged testis ➦ with a large, thick-walled ➦, hypoechoic, intratesticular abscess. Note avascularity at center ➦ of this lesion due to liquefactive necrosis.

DIFFUSE TESTICULAR ENLARGEMENT

Testicular Torsion/Infarction

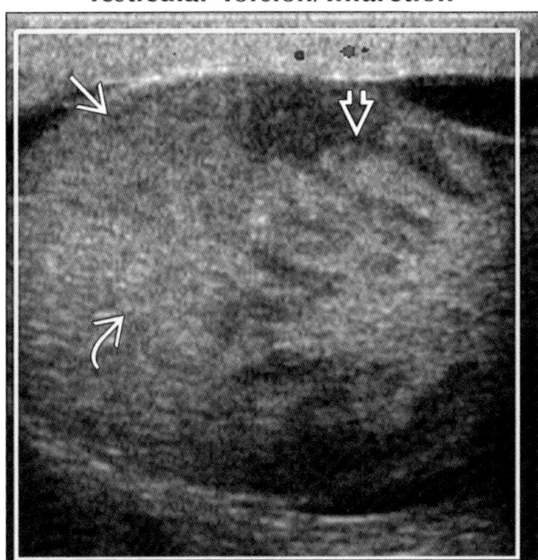

Testicular Carcinoma

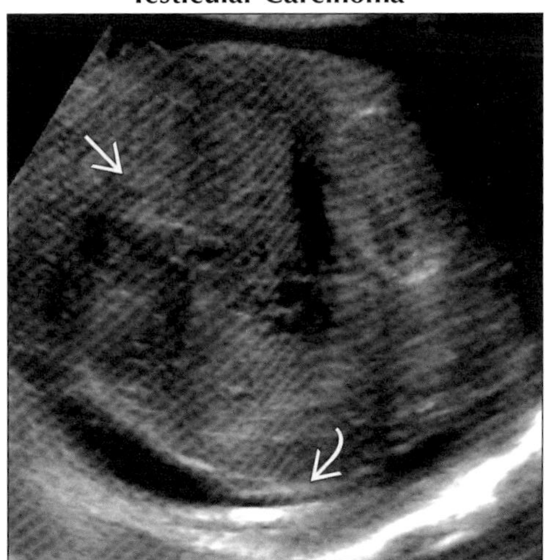

(Left) Longitudinal color Doppler ultrasound shows diffuse enlargement of the testis ➡ due to ischemia caused by torsion of spermatic cord. Note the absence of intrinsic testicular vascularity ➡ and internal heterogeneity ➡ due to developing infarcts. *(Right)* Longitudinal ultrasound shows a large, indistinct, heterogeneous, intratesticular seminoma ➡ diffusely enlarging and distorting the testis, without invading the tunica albuginea ➡.

Scrotal Trauma

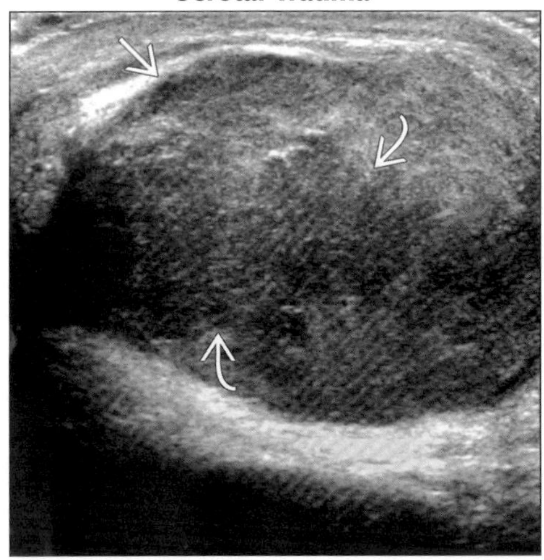

Testicular Lymphoma

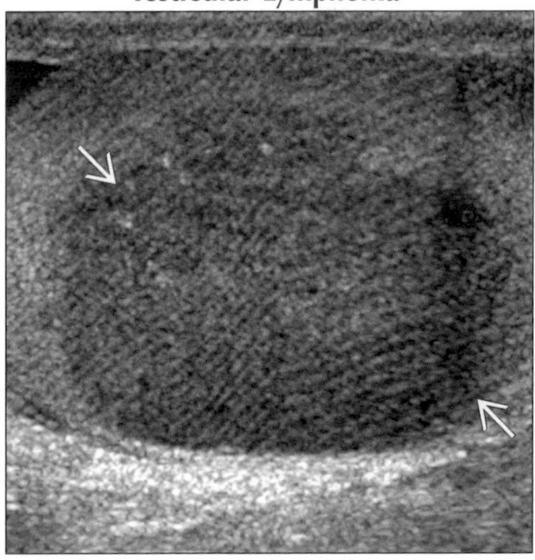

(Left) Longitudinal ultrasound shows a diffusely enlarged testis ➡ in a patient with scrotal trauma. Note the ill-defined hypoechoic hematoma ➡ distorting the testicular echopattern. *(Right)* Longitudinal ultrasound shows a large, focal, hypoechoic ➡ mass, diffusely enlarging the testis. The final diagnosis was testicular lymphoma. Without clinical correlation, it is difficult to differentiate other primary testicular tumors from lymphoma.

Testicular Metastases

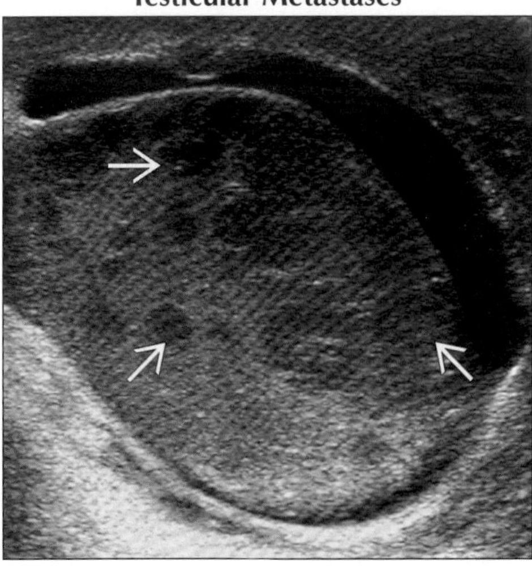

Testicular Cyst

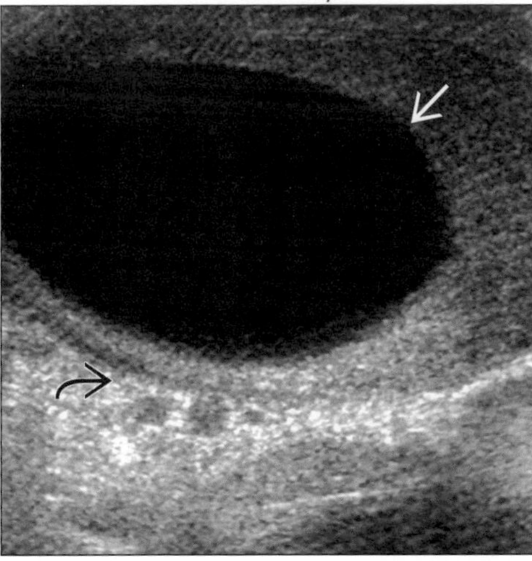

(Left) Longitudinal ultrasound shows multiple, small, hypoechoic, intratesticular masses ➡ of varying size in a patient with known rhabdomyosarcoma. The final diagnosis was testicular metastases. *(Right)* Longitudinal ultrasound shows a well-defined, intratesticular, anechoic cyst ➡ with an imperceptible wall, posterior acoustic enhancement ➡, and diffusely enlarging testis, all features of a simple testicular cyst.

12

DECREASED TESTICULAR SIZE

DIFFERENTIAL DIAGNOSIS

Common
- Testicular Infarction
- Scrotal Trauma
- Chronic Mass Effect
- Undescended Testis

Rare but Important
- Hypogonadism
- Polyorchidism

ESSENTIAL INFORMATION

Key Differential Diagnosis Issues
- Consider testicular atrophy if combined axis measurements of testes differ by 10 mm or more, or if testicular size < 4 x 2 cm
- Reduction in size considered significant if volume of affected testis reduced to 50% of unaffected testis
- Critical to identify viability of testis to determine whether orchiopexy or orchiectomy is needed

Helpful Clues for Common Diagnoses
- **Testicular Infarction**
  - Ischemic orchitis is known complication of inguinal hernia surgery
  - Epididymo-orchitis may result from severe inflammation/induration of cord
  - Missed torsion: In utero cord torsion (45%)
  - Uniformly hypoechoic or focal mixed echogenicity of testis are features of diffuse or focal infarction, respectively
  - Reduced echogenicity is sensitive marker of poor outcome compared to clinical parameters
- **Scrotal Trauma**
  - Acute testicular hematoma may lead to ischemia/infarction of viable parenchyma due to raised intratesticular pressure
    - Resorption of nonviable testicular tissue leads to atrophy or scarring
- **Chronic Mass Effect**
  - Longstanding scrotal mass may compromise blood flow and result in atrophy
- **Undescended Testis**
  - Exhibits different degrees of atrophy with altered parenchymal echogenicity
    - Less echogenic and smaller than normally descended testis
  - Testes < 1 cm often not detected by US

Helpful Clues for Rare Diagnoses
- **Hypogonadism**
  - Pituitary neoplasm, Kallmann syndrome, hypogonadotrophic hypogonadism
  - Diffuse heterogeneous echopattern
- **Polyorchidism**
  - Supernumerary or duplicated testis
    - Tunica albuginea surrounds and separates bifid testis
    - Epididymis may also duplicate
    - Homogeneously echogenic oval structure with echopattern identical to that of normal testis, but smaller in size

Testicular Infarction

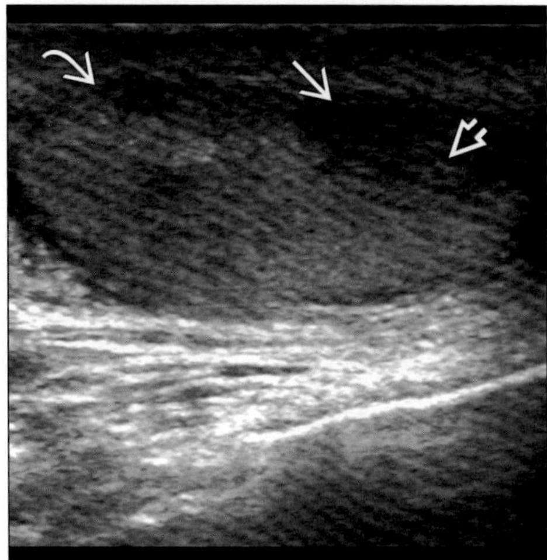

Oblique ultrasound shows a moderately shrunken heterogeneous testis ➡ in a patient with recurrent epididymo-orchitis. Note the patchy hypoechoic areas ➡ due to inflammation and ill-defined infarcts ➡.

Testicular Infarction

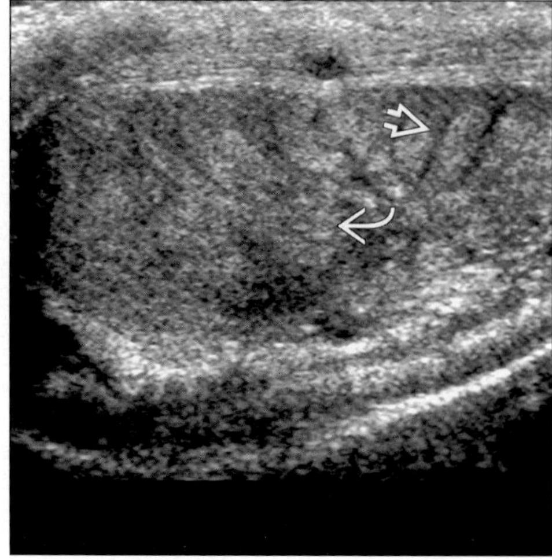

Longitudinal ultrasound shows a small, shrunken, intrascrotal testis in a 14-year-old boy with a history of recurrent torsion. Note the heterogeneous internal echopattern ➡ with multiple hypoechoic bands ➡.

DECREASED TESTICULAR SIZE

Scrotal Trauma

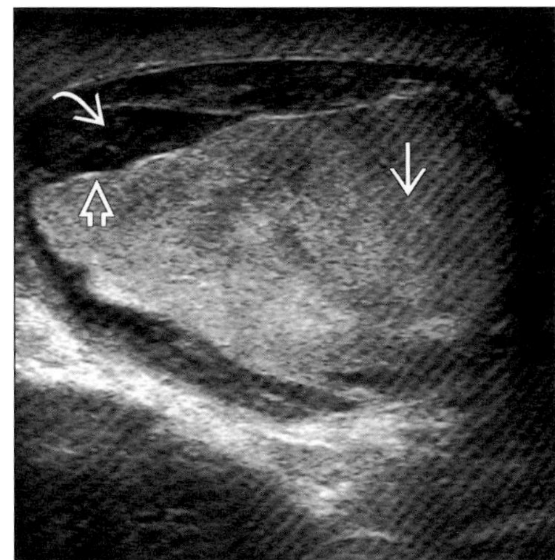

Chronic Mass Effect

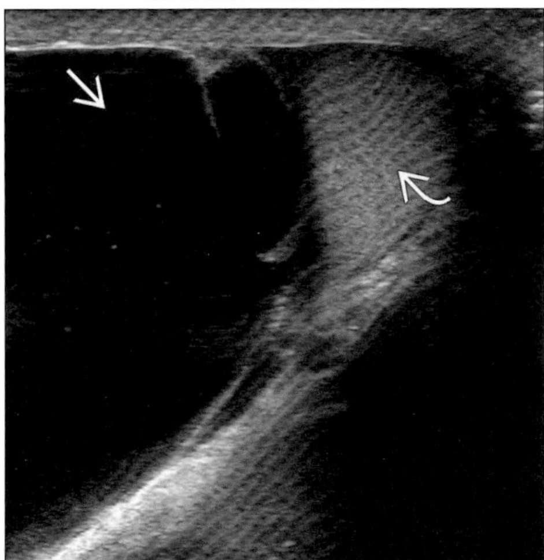

(Left) Longitudinal ultrasound shows a distorted testicular contour ⇒ due to chronic extrinsic pressure from a hematocele following trauma. Note heterogeneous echopattern ➡ and small amount of residual hematocele ➡. *(Right)* Oblique ultrasound shows a large septated spermatocele ➡ in the head of the epididymis, which displaces the testis outward and laterally. Note also the compressed and moderately atrophied testis ⇒ due to mass effect.

Chronic Mass Effect

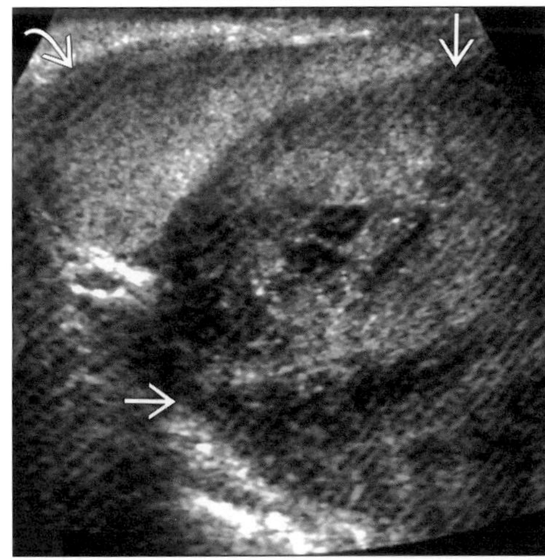

Undescended Testis

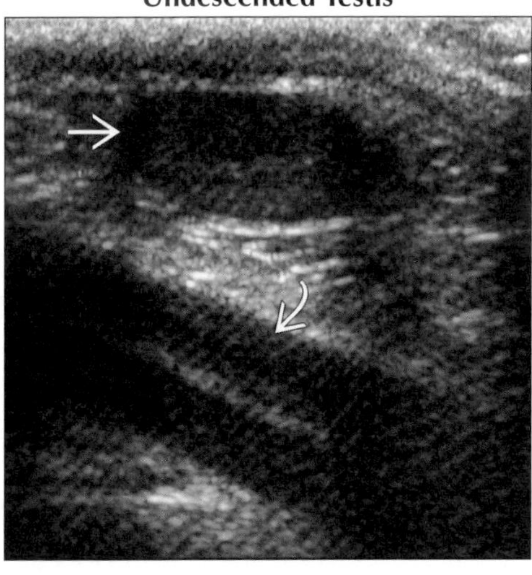

(Left) Oblique ultrasound shows a large, hypoechoic, paratesticular rhabdomyosarcoma ➡. Note the displaced, moderately atrophied testis ➡ due to chronic mass effect. *(Right)* Oblique ultrasound shows a well-defined, small, hypoechoic structure ➡ located in the inguinal canal, consistent with an undescended testis. Note the adjacent external iliac vessels ➡.

Hypogonadism

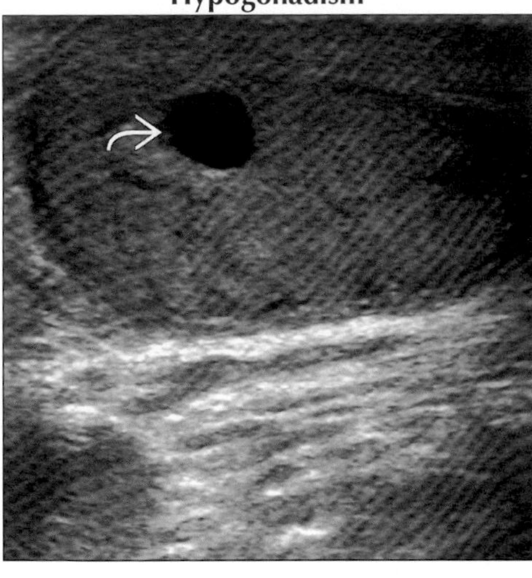

Polyorchidism

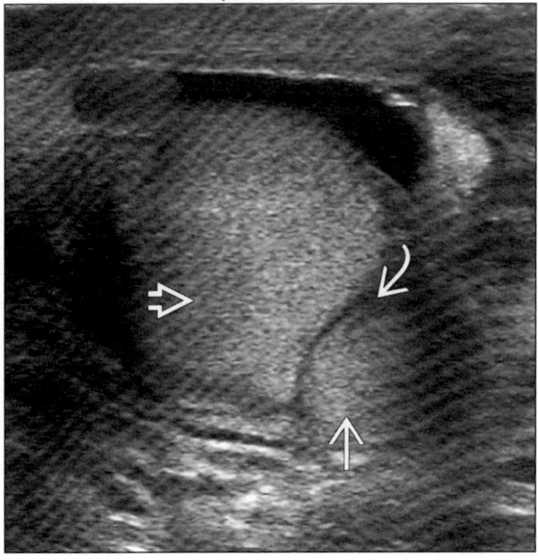

(Left) Longitudinal ultrasound shows a moderately shrunken, heterogeneous testis in a 17-year-old boy with hypogonadotrophic hypogonadism. Note the incidental simple intratesticular cyst ➡. *(Right)* Oblique US shows a small homogeneous globular structure ➡, isoechoic to the adjacent testis ➡. These features suggest a duplicated or supernumerary testis. Note the hypoechoic tunica albuginea ➡ separating the duplicated testes.

FOCAL TESTICULAR LESION

DIFFERENTIAL DIAGNOSIS

Common
- Epididymo-orchitis
- Testicular Germ Cell Tumor
  - Testicular Seminoma
  - Testicular Teratoma
  - Testicular Embryonal Cell Carcinoma
  - Choriocarcinoma
- Testicular Torsion/Infarction
- Testicular Microlithiasis
- Testicular Hematoma
- Tubular Ectasia of Rete Testis
- Testicular Lymphoma

Less Common
- Testicular Abscess
- Gonadal Stromal Tumor
  - Sertoli Cell Tumor
  - Leydig Cell Tumor
- Testicular Metastases
- Testicular Cyst
- Testicular Epidermoid Cyst
- Testicular Lipomatosis/Hamartoma

Rare but Important
- Testicular Adrenal Rest Tumors

ESSENTIAL INFORMATION

Key Differential Diagnosis Issues
- Age and clinical presentation help make diagnosis
- Sonographic findings are key but overlap among various tumors

Helpful Clues for Common Diagnoses
- **Epididymo-orchitis**
  - Primarily involves epididymis
    - Orchitis is usually secondary, occurring in 20-40% of cases with epididymitis due to contiguous spread of infection
    - Primary orchitis is typically viral (mumps) and bilateral
  - Orchitis characterized by inflammation, edema, and swelling of testis
    - Diffuse orchitis: Testis diffusely enlarged with heterogeneous echopattern
    - Focal orchitis: Hypoechoic focal area, usually adjacent to inflamed epididymis
  - Increase in vascularity on color Doppler without any displacement of vessels
- **Testicular Germ Cell Tumor**
  - Best diagnostic clue: Discrete, hypoechoic or mixed echogenic, testicular mass; ± vascularity
    - Tumor ≤1.5 cm, commonly hypovascular
    - Tumor > 1.5 cm, often hypervascular
  - **Testicular Seminoma**
    - Most common neoplasm in males 15-39 years old
    - Well-defined, lobulated, hypoechoic, solid lesion without calcification or tunica invasion
  - **Testicular Teratoma**
    - Complex solid-cystic mass
    - Heterogeneous internal echogenicity due to calcification (cartilage, immature bone) ± fibrosis
    - May be mature or immature
  - **Testicular Embryonal Cell Carcinoma**
    - Heterogeneous, predominantly solid, mixed echogenicity mass
    - Poorly marginated; 1/3 have necrosis
    - Invasion of tunica albuginea with distortion of testicular contour
  - **Choriocarcinoma**
    - Mixed echogenicity, heterogeneous mass
    - Calcification common; hemorrhage with focal necrosis typical feature
    - Invasion of tunica albuginea
    - Proclivity for early hematogenous spread, especially to brain
- **Testicular Torsion/Infarction**
  - Trauma, torsion, or diffuse inflammation are common causes of infarction
    - Hypercoagulable states or advanced atherosclerosis (e.g., diabetes) are other etiological factors
  - May be focal or involve entire testis
  - Focal or diffuse hypoechoic, avascular, intratesticular area
  - Linear appearance of focal infarctions not uncommon
  - Chronic infarcts may appear as ill-defined hyperechoic areas (hemorrhage/fibrosis)
  - Diffusely hypoechoic, small testis in late complete infarction
- **Testicular Hematoma**
  - History of scrotal trauma
    - Focal hypoechoic area or discrete linear or irregular fracture plane within testis

FOCAL TESTICULAR LESION

- Avascular mass, distorted intratesticular vascularity with interruption of vessels in area of hematoma or injury
- Echogenicity depends on age of hematoma; acute → hypoechoic, whereas chronic lesions are heterogeneous ± calcification
- **Tubular Ectasia of Rete Testis**
  - Normal variant of dilated seminiferous tubules in mediastinum of testis
  - Multiple small, branching, anechoic cystic lesions; no flow on color Doppler
  - May be associated with spermatocele
- **Testicular Lymphoma and Metastases**
  - Lymphoma
    - Most common testicular tumor in men older than 60 years; 50% of cases bilateral
    - Often large at time of diagnosis; commonly occurs in association with disseminated disease
    - Multiple ill-defined, predominantly hypoechoic lesions with significant intrinsic vascularity on color Doppler
    - Epididymis and spermatic cord commonly involved
    - Hemorrhage or necrosis rare
  - Metastases
    - Rare, most commonly from prostate, lung, and GI tract
    - Multiple poorly or well-defined, hypoechoic lesions
    - Testis frequent site of relapse in male patients with acute leukemia

Helpful Clues for Less Common Diagnoses
- **Testicular Abscess**
  - Epididymal abscess (6%), testicular abscess (6%)
  - Microabscess formation usually seen in low-grade infections, i.e., tuberculosis
    - Also seen in immunocompromised hosts
  - Well-defined, discrete, round, hypoechoic lesion(s) in testicular parenchyma
  - Necrotic center shows no vascularity on color Doppler studies
- **Gonadal Stromal Tumor**
  - Bilateral in 3%; < 3 cm usually benign, > 5 cm usually malignant
  - Indistinguishable from germ cell tumors on imaging
  - **Sertoli Cell Tumor**
    - Small, hypoechoic, solid-cystic masses
    - ± punctate calcification, large calcified mass in calcifying Sertoli cell tumor
    - Hemorrhage may lead to heterogeneity
  - **Leydig Cell Tumor**
    - Small, solid, hypoechoic, testicular mass
    - In larger tumor, hemorrhage or necrosis leads to heterogeneous echopattern

Helpful Clues for Rare Diagnoses
- **Testicular Adrenal Rest Tumors**
  - Identified in patients with congenital adrenal hyperplasia
  - On ultrasound, ill-defined, hypoechoic, intratesticular masses
  - Indistinguishable from other testicular tumors, especially Leydig cell tumors

Epididymo-orchitis

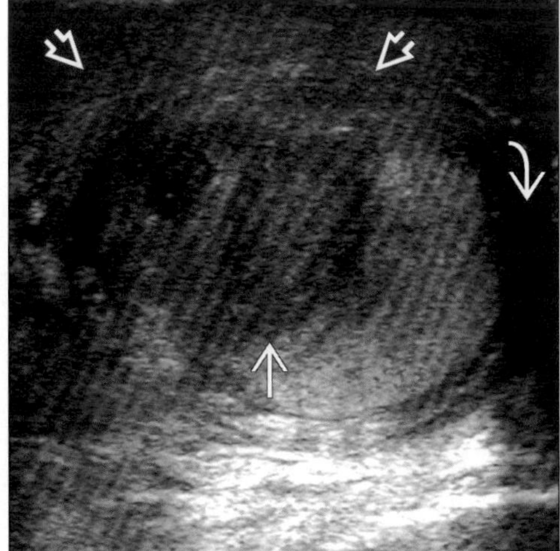

Longitudinal US shows an ill-defined, hypoechoic, intratesticular lesion ➡ *from focal orchitis. Note reactive thickening of the tunica albuginea, layers of the scrotal wall* ▱ *, and a small reactive hydrocele* ▱ *.*

Epididymo-orchitis

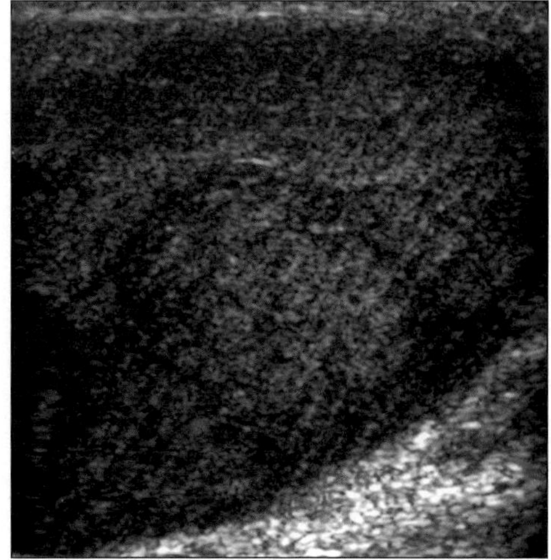

Transverse grayscale ultrasound shows an enlarged, lobulated testis with a heterogeneous internal echopattern in this patient with tuberculous orchitis.

12

FOCAL TESTICULAR LESION

(Left) Oblique ultrasound shows a large, ill-defined, mixed echogenicity mass ➡ completely distorting the testicular architecture in this patient with a mixed germ cell tumor. Note the invasion of the tunica albuginea ➡. *(Right)* Transverse US shows a well-circumscribed, hypoechoic, intratesticular mass ➡. Note a few similar smaller lesions ➡. The final diagnosis was mixed germ cell tumor. Invasion of tunica albuginea ➡ is common in nonseminomatous germ cell tumors.

Testicular Germ Cell Tumor

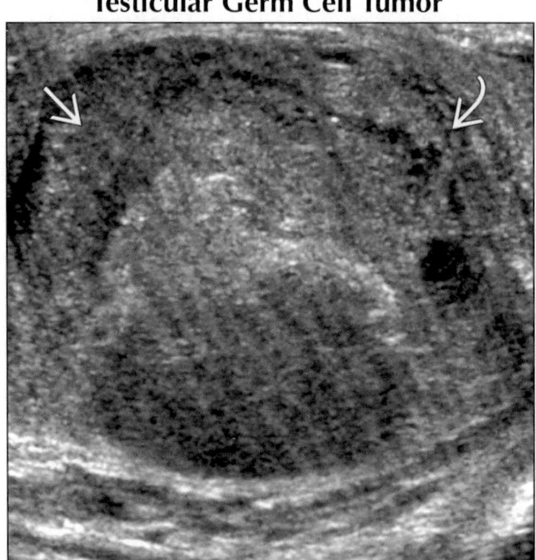

Testicular Germ Cell Tumor

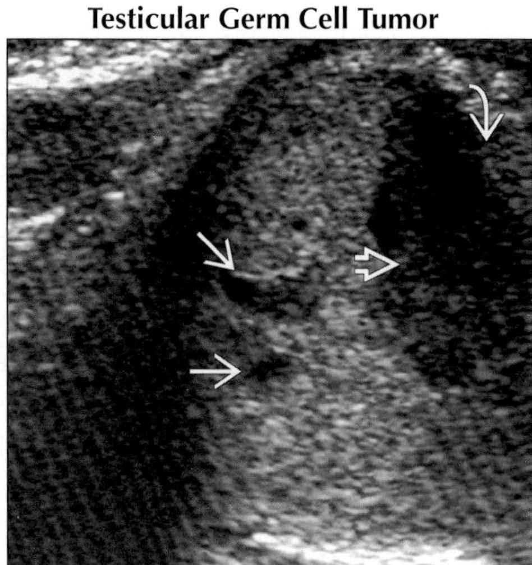

(Left) Longitudinal ultrasound shows a large, lobulated, hypoechoic, intratesticular mass ➡ without internal calcification or any focal area of necrosis, features suggestive of seminoma. Note the intact tunica albuginea ➡. *(Right)* Longitudinal ultrasound shows a well-circumscribed, hyperechoic mass ➡ with hypoechoic areas ➡ within, representing small cystic spaces. The final diagnosis was immature testicular teratoma.

Testicular Seminoma

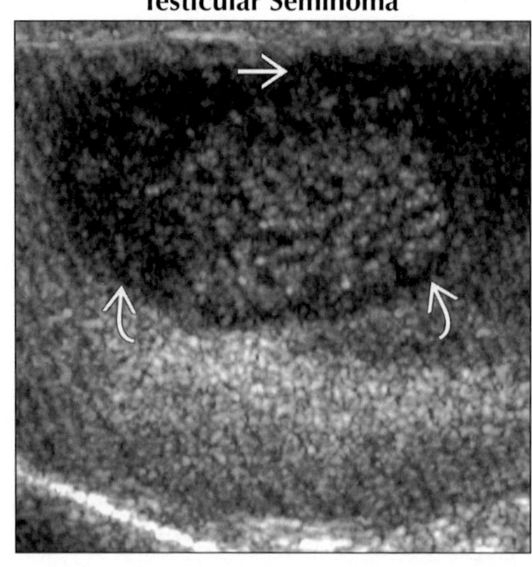

Testicular Teratoma

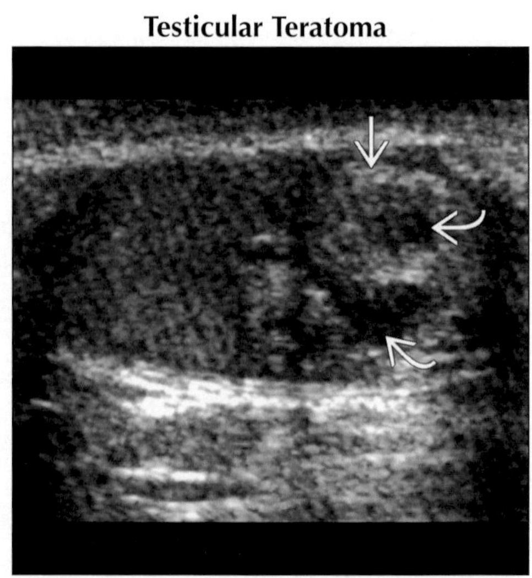

(Left) Transverse ultrasound shows cystic areas ➡ within a large, heterogeneous, intratesticular, mature teratoma. Note the few small echogenic foci of calcification ➡, causing posterior acoustic shadowing ➡. *(Right)* Longitudinal ultrasound shows a small, ill-defined, hypoechoic, intratesticular mass ➡ invading the tunica albuginea ➡. The final diagnosis was embryonal cell carcinoma.

Testicular Teratoma

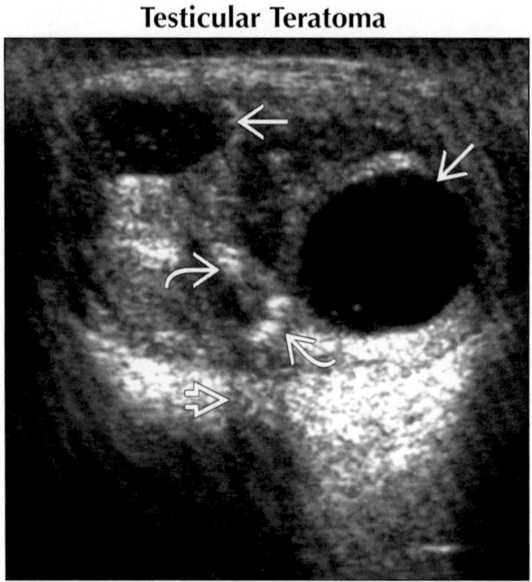

Testicular Embryonal Cell Carcinoma

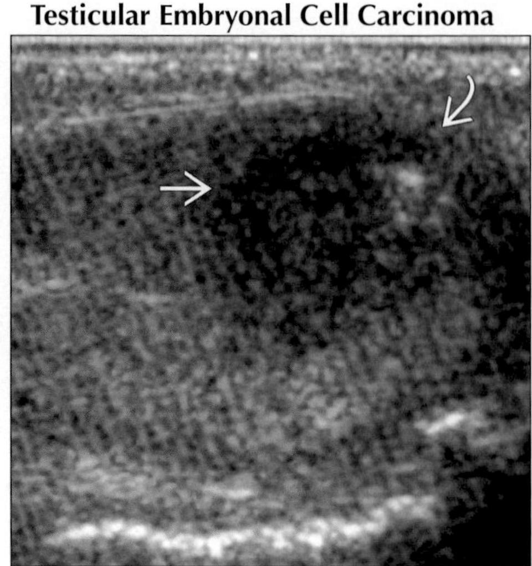

12

FOCAL TESTICULAR LESION

Testicular Embryonal Cell Carcinoma

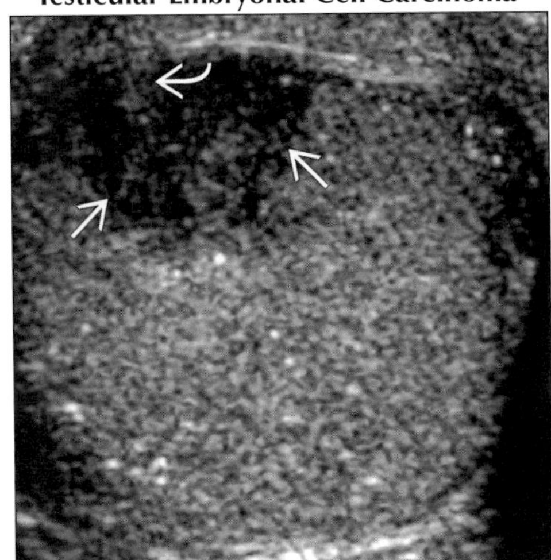

Testicular Microlithiasis

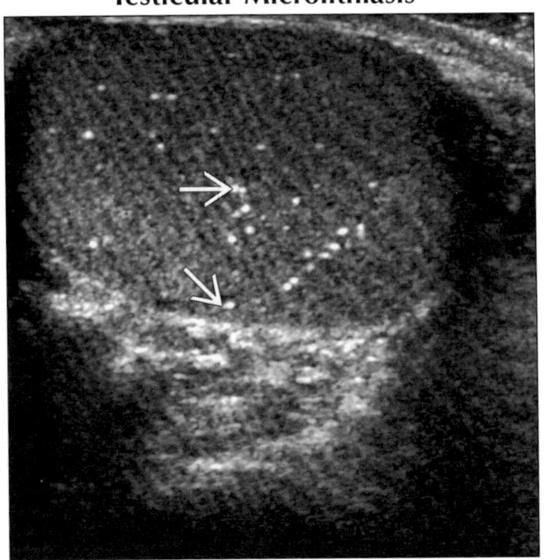

(Left) Transverse ultrasound shows an ill-defined, hypoechoic, intratesticular mass ➡. Note the tumor invasion ➡ of the tunica albuginea. The final diagnosis was embryonal cell carcinoma. *(Right)* Oblique ultrasound shows multiple small, hyperechoic nonshadowing, intratesticular foci ➡, features suggestive of testicular microlithiasis. It is very important to search for any focal neoplasm in such testes.

Testicular Hematoma

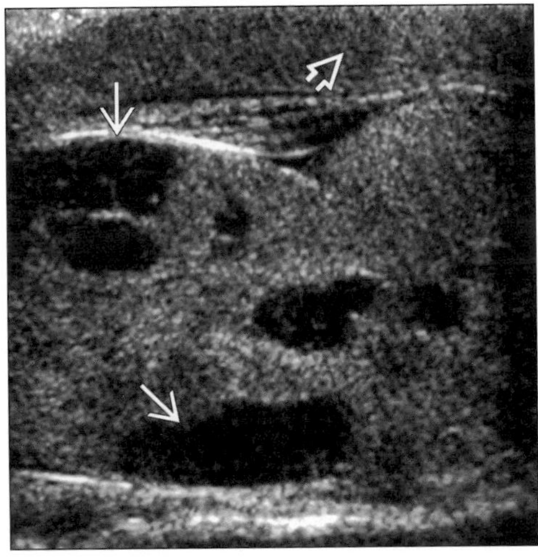

Tubular Ectasia of Rete Testis

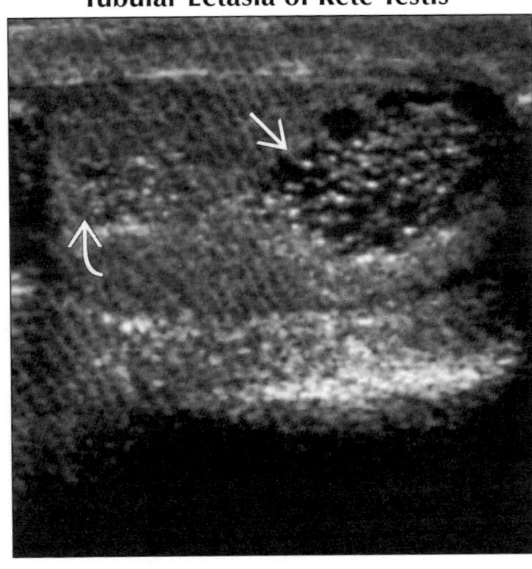

(Left) Oblique US shows multiple small, hypoechoic, intratesticular foci ➡ in a patient with recent scrotal trauma, features suggesting multiple hematomas. Note swollen scrotal wall ➡. *(Right)* Longitudinal ultrasound shows multiple small, branching, anechoic, circular masses ➡ of varying size converging at the mediastinum testis ➡, representing tubular ectasia of the rete testis.

Testicular Lymphoma

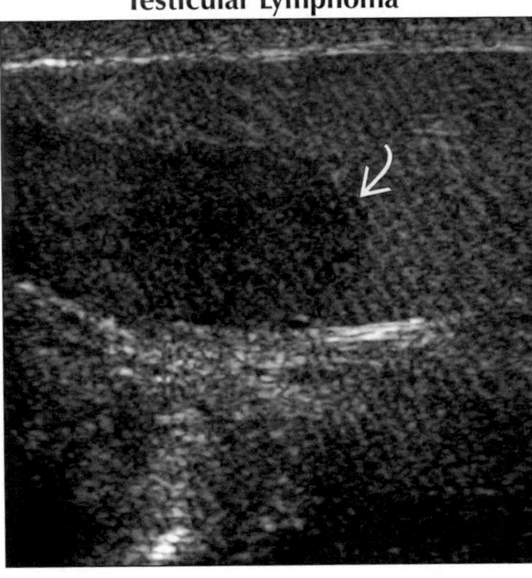

Testicular Abscess

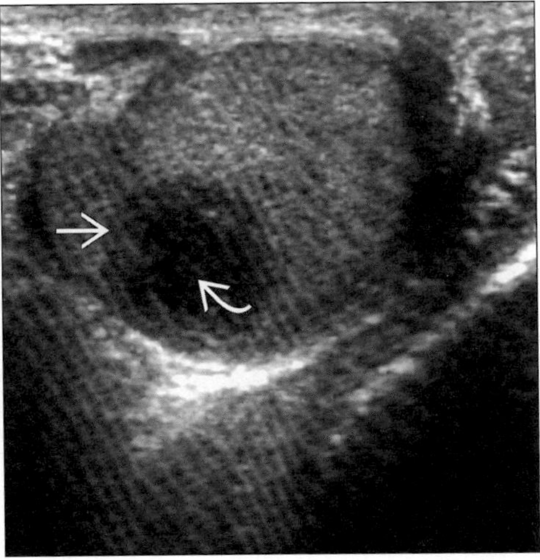

(Left) Longitudinal US shows a well-defined, homogeneous, hypoechoic, intratesticular mass ➡. The final diagnosis was testicular lymphoma, 50% of which is bilateral and often multifocal. *(Right)* Oblique US shows a well-defined, hypoechoic, intratesticular lesion ➡ in a patient with previous epididymo-orchitis, features suggestive of an early testicular abscess. Note relatively more hypoechoic center ➡ due to early liquefactive change.

FOCAL TESTICULAR LESION

(Left) Longitudinal color Doppler ultrasound shows a well-developed, thick-walled, intratesticular abscess ➡. Note the adjacent hypoechoic parenchyma ➡ due to orchitis. *(Right)* Longitudinal US shows a well-defined, homogeneously hypoechoic, intratesticular mass ➡. The final diagnosis was gonadal stromal tumors. Sonographically, gonadal stromal tumors cannot be differentiated from other testicular tumors.

Testicular Abscess

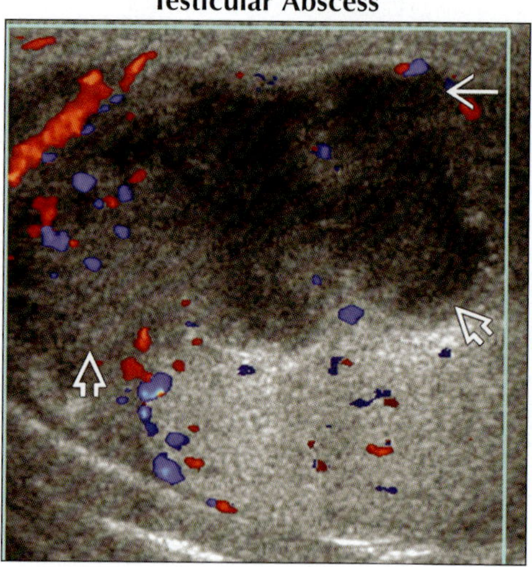

Gonadal Stromal Tumor

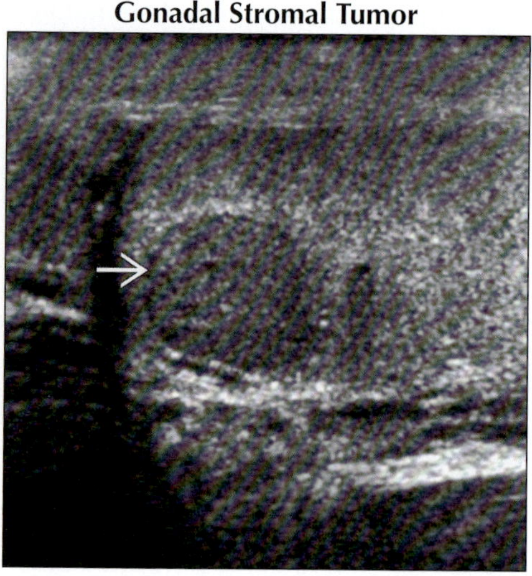

(Left) Longitudinal ultrasound shows a well-circumscribed, hypoechoic, solid mass ➡ in an 8-year-old boy. Note the areas of shadowing ➡ due to rim calcification. The final diagnosis was gonadal stromal tumor. *(Right)* Transverse color Doppler ultrasound shows an ill-defined, heterogeneous, mixed echogenicity, intratesticular mass ➡ in a 6-year-old boy. Note the peripheral vascularity ➡ in this patient with a Sertoli cell tumor.

Gonadal Stromal Tumor

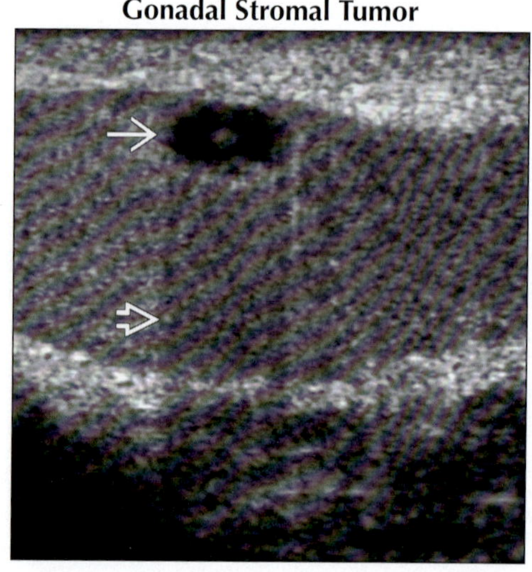

Sertoli Cell Tumor

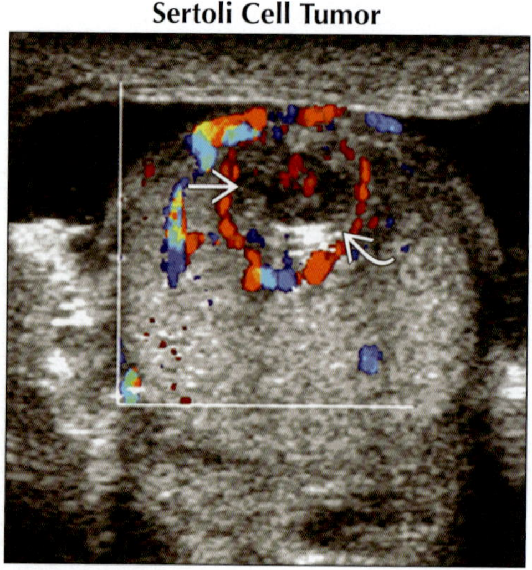

(Left) Transverse ultrasound shows a well-defined, lobulated, isoechoic, intratesticular mass ➡ in this patient with a Leydig cell tumor. *(Right)* Oblique ultrasound shows multiple large, well-defined, hypoechoic masses ➡, features suggestive of testicular metastases. Note the characteristic "punched out" margins ➡ of these masses.

Leydig Cell Tumor

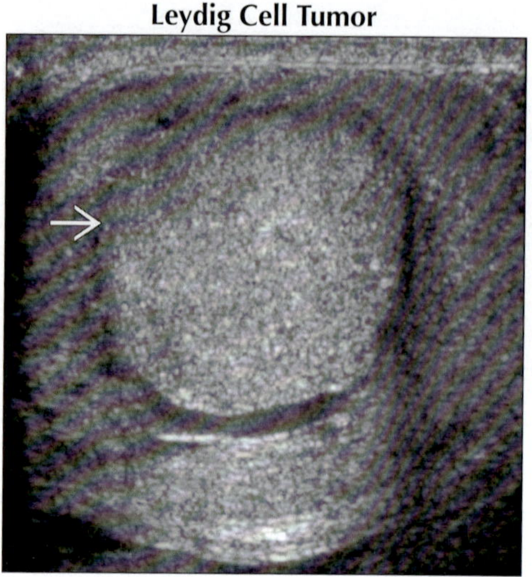

Testicular Metastases

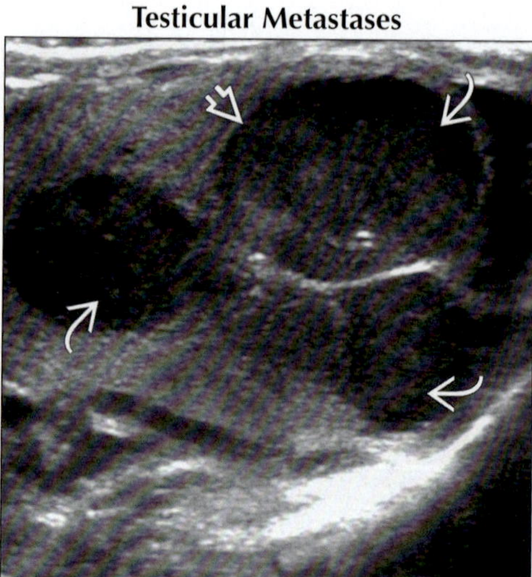

FOCAL TESTICULAR LESION

Testicular Cyst

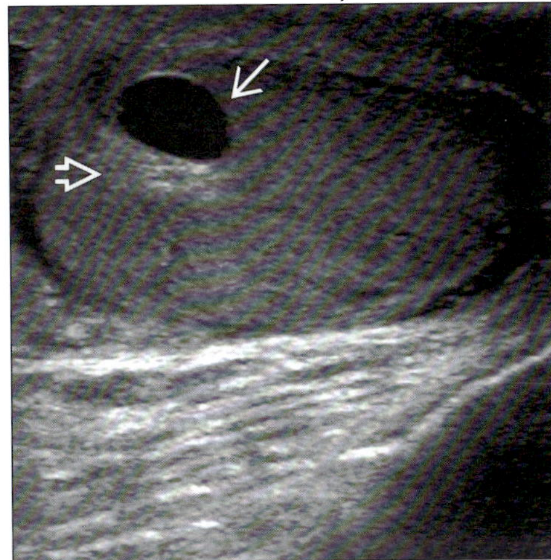

Testicular Epidermoid Cyst

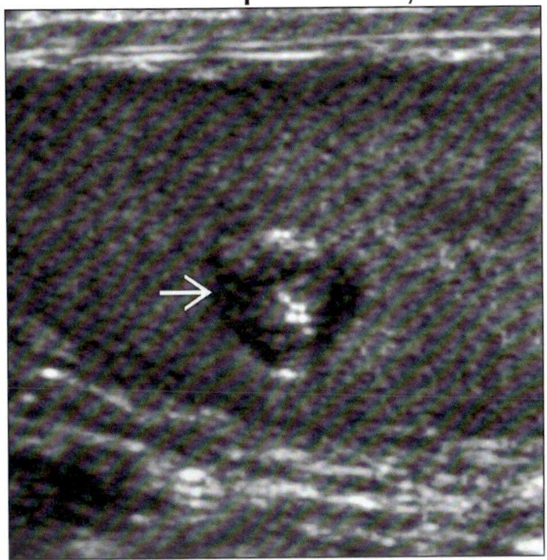

(Left) Oblique US shows a well-defined anechoic cyst ➡ in the superficial aspect of the testis. Note the posterior acoustic enhancement ➡. Testicular cysts are incidentally detected on sonography in 8-10% of population. *(Right)* Oblique US shows a well-circumscribed, mixed echogenicity, intratesticular mass ➡. Note the characteristic lamellated appearance due to increased intrinsic keratin content, features suggestive of an epidermoid cyst.

Testicular Epidermoid Cyst

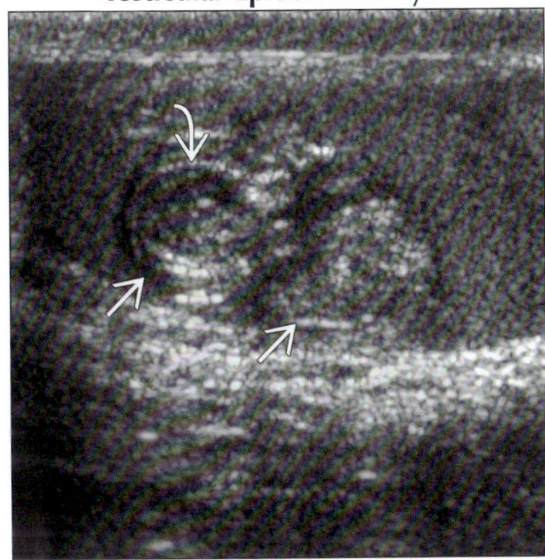

Testicular Lipomatosis/Hamartoma

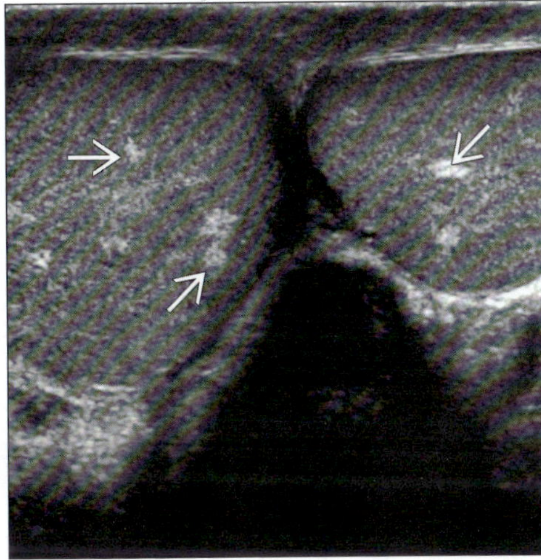

(Left) Longitudinal ultrasound shows a large, lobulated, hyperechoic, intratesticular mass ➡ with a lamellated appearance ➡ in this patient with an epidermoid cyst. *(Right)* Transverse ultrasound shows multiple small, nonconfluent, hyperechoic foci ➡ in both testes, features suggestive of testicular lipomatosis (or testicular hamartomas). These findings have a strong association with Cowden disease.

Testicular Adrenal Rest Tumors

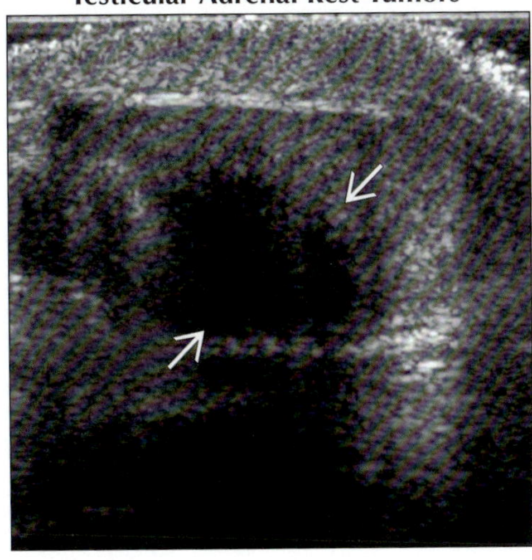

Testicular Adrenal Rest Tumors

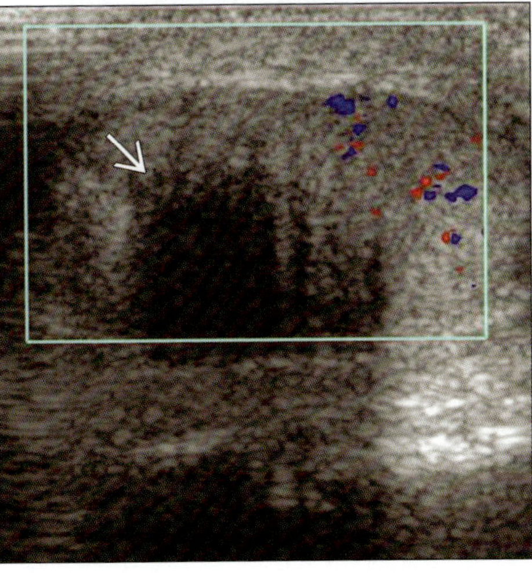

(Left) Longitudinal ultrasound shows an ill-defined, hypoechoic, intratesticular mass ➡ in a patient with bilateral adrenal hyperplasia. These ill-defined, hypoechoic masses represent adrenal rest tumors. *(Right)* Longitudinal color Doppler ultrasound in the same patient shows adrenal rest tumors ➡ with no significant intrinsic vascularity. Adrenal rest tumors are treated with steroid therapy rather than orchiectomy.

SOLID-APPEARING TESTICULAR MASS

DIFFERENTIAL DIAGNOSIS

Common
- Epididymitis/Orchitis
- Testicular Carcinoma
- Testicular Torsion/Infarction
- Testicular Hematoma

Less Common
- Testicular Abscess
- Testicular Lymphoma and Metastases
- Gonadal Stromal Tumor
- Testicular Epidermoid Cyst

ESSENTIAL INFORMATION

Key Differential Diagnosis Issues
- Correlate ultrasound with age and clinical features
- Sonographic findings are key but overlap among various tumors
- Histopathological correlation needed

Helpful Clues for Common Diagnoses
- **Epididymitis/Orchitis**
  - Primarily involves epididymis
    - Orchitis is usually secondary, occurring in 20-40% of cases with epididymitis due to contiguous spread of infection
    - Primary orchitis is typically viral (mumps) and bilateral
  - Orchitis is characterized by inflammation, edema, and swelling of testis
    - Diffuse orchitis: Testis is diffusely enlarged with heterogeneous echopattern
    - Focal orchitis: Hypoechoic focal area, usually adjacent to inflamed epididymis
  - Increase in vascularity on color Doppler without displacement of vessels
- **Testicular Carcinoma**
  - Best diagnostic clue: Discrete hypoechoic or mixed echogenicity testicular mass, ± vascularity
    - Tumor ≤ 1.5 cm is commonly hypovascular
    - Tumor > 1.5 cm is more often hypervascular
    - Discrete mass on grayscale ultrasound with abnormal intrinsic vascularity on color Doppler should raise suspicion of testicular carcinoma
  - Seminoma
    - Most common neoplasm in males 15-39 years old
    - Well-defined, lobulated, hypoechoic, solid lesion without calcification or tunica invasion
    - May undergo necrosis and appear partly cystic
  - Teratoma/teratocarcinoma
    - Heterogeneous, complex, solid-cystic mass
    - Calcification (cartilage, immature bone) ± fibrosis characterizes teratoma/teratocarcinoma
  - Embryonal cell carcinoma
    - Heterogeneous, predominantly solid, mixed echogenicity mass
    - Poorly marginated; 1/3 have cystic necrosis
    - May invade tunica albuginea and distort testicular contour
  - Choriocarcinoma
    - Mixed echogenicity, heterogeneous mass
    - Cystic areas and calcification common
    - Hemorrhage with focal necrosis is typical feature of choriocarcinoma
    - May invade tunica albuginea
    - Proclivity for early hematogenous spread, especially to brain
- **Testicular Torsion/Infarction**
  - Findings of torsion vary with duration and degree of cord rotations
    - Grayscale appearance in early torsion may be normal
    - Decreased or absent flow on color Doppler (always compare to contralateral normal side)
    - Diffusely hypoechoic small testis/focal mass in infarcted testis
    - Hyperechoic regions (hemorrhage, fibrosis)
  - Segmental infarction may be sequela of inflammatory process (orchitis) or surgical complication (hernia repair)
    - Focal infarctions may have linear appearance
  - Infarction may occur in patients with hypercoagulable states or advanced atherosclerosis, such as diabetes
- **Testicular Hematoma**
  - History of scrotal trauma

SOLID-APPEARING TESTICULAR MASS

- o Abnormal testicular parenchymal echogenicity
  - ▪ Echogenicity depends on age of hematoma
- o Discrete linear or irregular fracture plane within testis
- o Color Doppler
  - ▪ Hematoma forms avascular mass within testis
  - ▪ Distorted intratesticular vascularity with interruption of vessels in area of hematoma or injury

Helpful Clues for Less Common Diagnoses
- **Testicular Abscess**
  - o Epididymal abscess (6%)
  - o Testicular abscess (6%)
  - o Microabscess formation is usually seen in low-grade infections (e.g., tuberculosis)
    - ▪ Also seen in immunocompromised hosts
  - o Well-defined, discrete, round, hypoechoic lesion(s) in testicular parenchyma
  - o Necrotic center shows no vascularity on color Doppler studies
- **Testicular Lymphoma and Metastases**
  - o Lymphoma
    - ▪ Most common testicular tumor in men older than 60 years; multiple lesions; 50% of cases bilateral
    - ▪ Often large at time of diagnosis
    - ▪ Commonly occurs in association with disseminated disease
    - ▪ Ill-defined, predominantly hypoechoic lesions

- ▪ High vascularity on color Doppler
- ▪ Involvement of epididymis and spermatic cord is common
- ▪ Hemorrhage or necrosis is rare
- o Metastases are rare
  - ▪ Most common primaries include prostate, lung, and GI tract
- o Testis is frequent site of recurrence in male patients with lymphoma and acute leukemia
- **Gonadal Stromal Tumor**
  - o Bilateral in 3%
    - ▪ < 3 cm usually benign
    - ▪ > 5 cm usually malignant
  - o Leydig cell tumor
    - ▪ Small solid hypoechoic testicular mass
    - ▪ In larger tumor, hemorrhage or necrosis leads to heterogeneous echopattern
  - o Sertoli cell tumor
    - ▪ Small hypoechoic mass
    - ▪ Solid and cystic components
    - ▪ Punctate calcification may be present; large calcified mass in calcifying Sertoli cell tumor
    - ▪ Hemorrhage may lead to heterogeneity
  - o Indistinguishable from other testicular tumors by ultrasound findings
- **Testicular Epidermoid Cyst**
  - o Cystic cavity lined by stratified squamous epithelium
  - o "Onion skin" appearance on ultrasound due to alternating layers of keratin and desquamated squamous cells
  - o May have peripheral calcified rim

Epididymitis/Orchitis

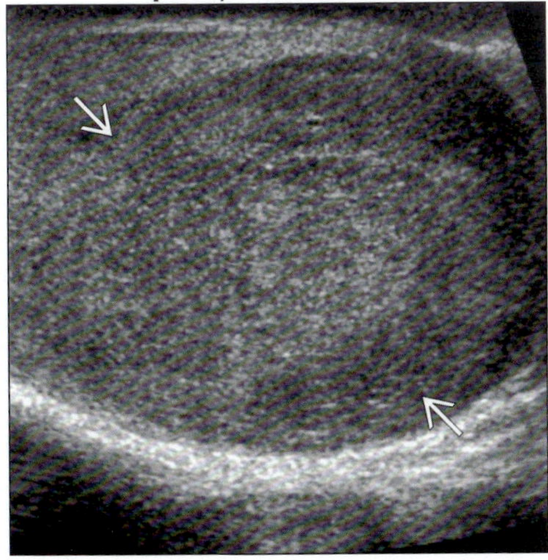

Oblique ultrasound shows an enlarged, diffusely hypoechoic testis ➡. A history of acute onset scrotal pain, combined with these sonographic findings, suggests acute orchitis.

Epididymitis/Orchitis

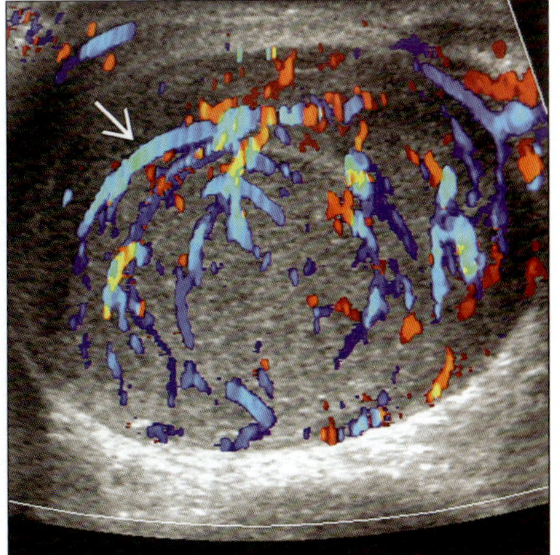

Correlative oblique color Doppler ultrasound shows marked testicular hypervascularity. Note the undisplaced course of the intratesticular vessels ➡.

SOLID-APPEARING TESTICULAR MASS

(Left) Oblique ultrasound shows a heterogeneous, hypoechoic, solid, testicular seminoma ➡. Note the typical lobulated appearance of the tumor without any calcification or necrosis. *(Right)* Longitudinal ultrasound shows a large, heterogeneous, solid, intratesticular mass ➡. Foci of intrinsic calcification cause posterior acoustic shadowing ➡. Note the ill-defined areas of necrosis within this mass ➡. The final diagnosis was immature teratoma.

Testicular Carcinoma

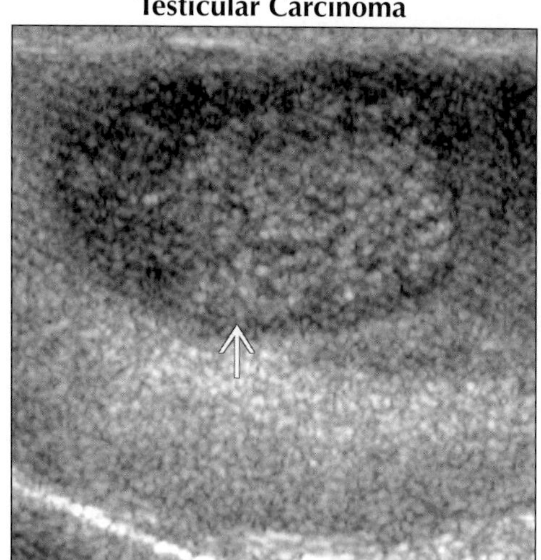

Testicular Carcinoma

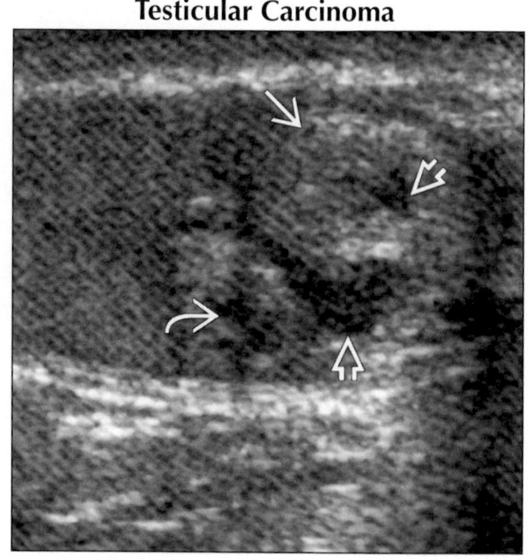

(Left) Transverse ultrasound shows a well-defined, hypoechoic, intratesticular mass ➡ with neither intrinsic calcification nor central necrosis. The features are nonspecific and suggest testicular carcinoma in this patient with mixed germ cell tumor. *(Right)* Longitudinal ultrasound shows an ill-defined, hypoechoic, heterogeneous, intratesticular mass ➡. Note the proximity of this mass to tunica albuginea ➡. Final diagnosis was embryonal cell carcinoma.

Testicular Carcinoma

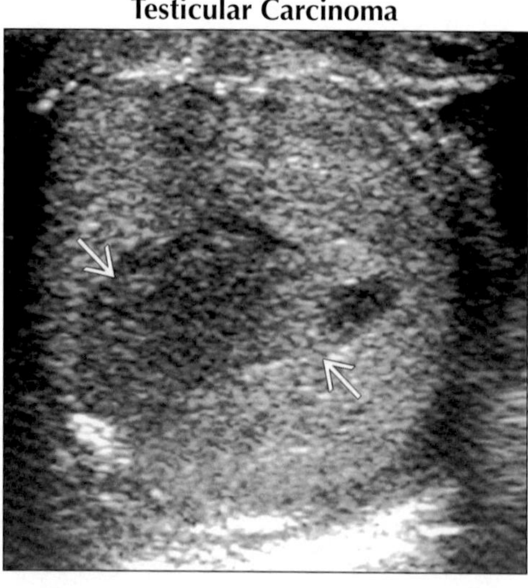

Testicular Carcinoma

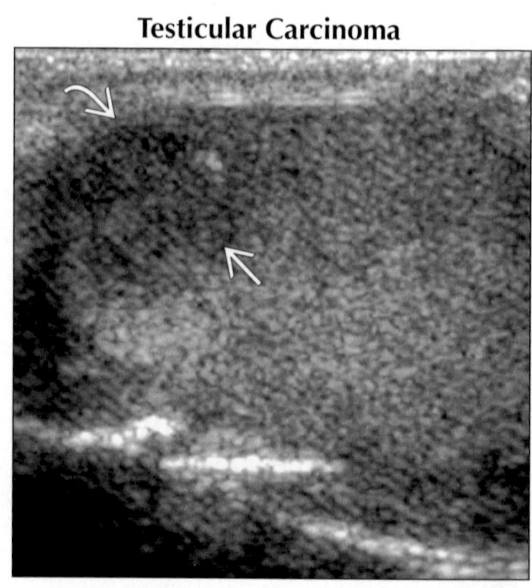

(Left) Oblique color Doppler ultrasound shows a diffusely enlarged, hypoechoic testis ➡ with nearly absent blood flow ➡, suggesting an acute infarction due to torsion. *(Right)* Oblique ultrasound shows a heterogeneous testicular echopattern ➡ with a few poorly defined hypoechoic areas ➡ within. These sonographic features suggest testicular hematoma in this patient with scrotal trauma.

Testicular Torsion/Infarction

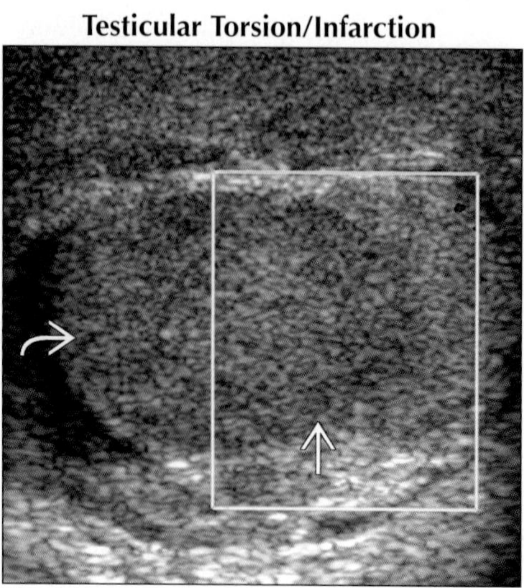

Testicular Hematoma

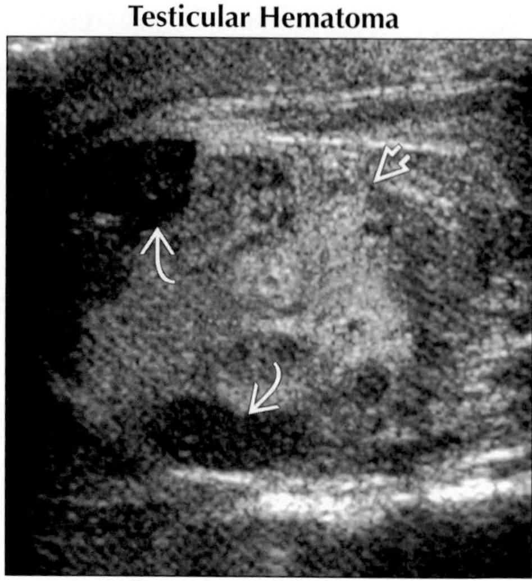

SOLID-APPEARING TESTICULAR MASS

Testicular Abscess

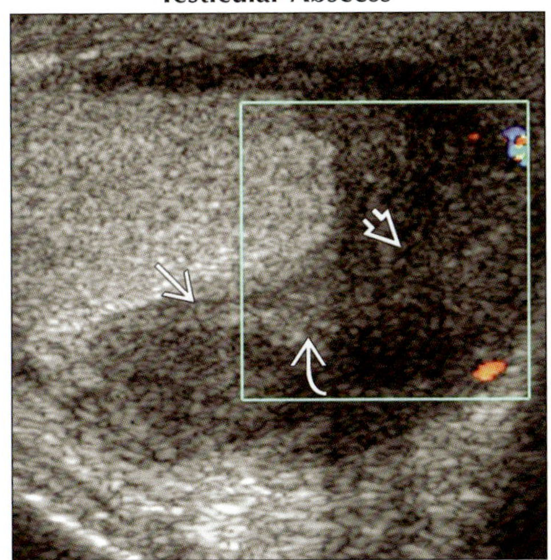

Testicular Lymphoma and Metastases

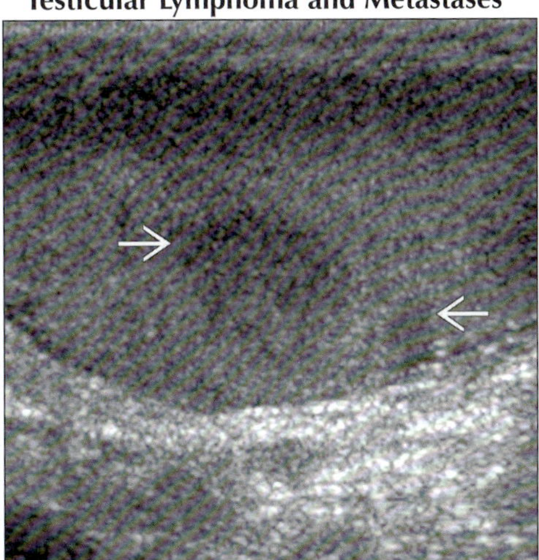

(Left) Oblique color Doppler ultrasound shows an ill-defined hypoechoic area ➡ in the testis with irregular thick walls ➡. Note the lack of vascularity ➡ within this lesion. These features suggest a testicular abscess. *(Right)* Longitudinal ultrasound shows ill-defined hypoechoic lesions ➡ within the testis in this patient with testicular lymphoma. In more than 50% of patients, lymphomatous lesions are multiple and involve both testes.

Testicular Lymphoma and Metastases

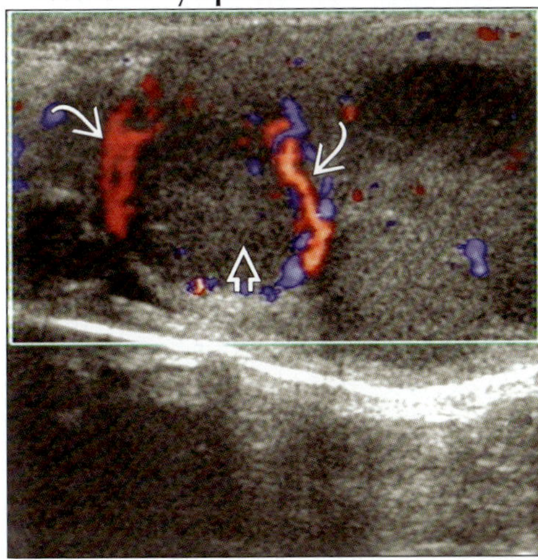

Gonadal Stromal Tumor

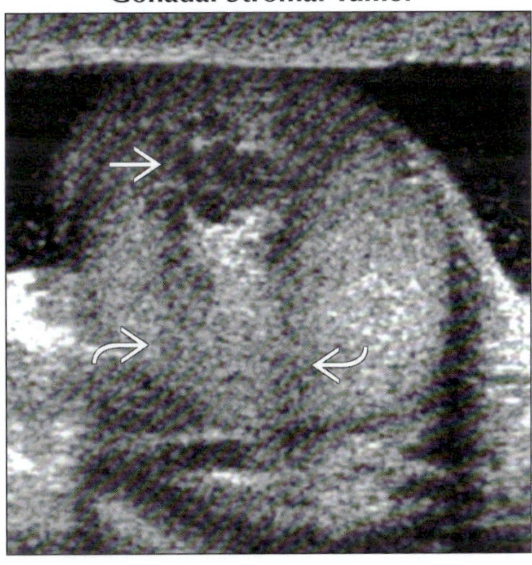

(Left) Oblique color Doppler ultrasound shows multiple large, well-defined, hypoechoic, intratesticular masses. Note the intratumoral hypovascularity ➡ and the displacement of the adjacent vessels ➡. *(Right)* Oblique ultrasound shows a heterogeneous, solid, testicular mass ➡ in a 6-year-old boy. Note the areas of acoustic shadowing ➡ due to rim calcification. Final diagnosis was Sertoli cell tumor.

Gonadal Stromal Tumor

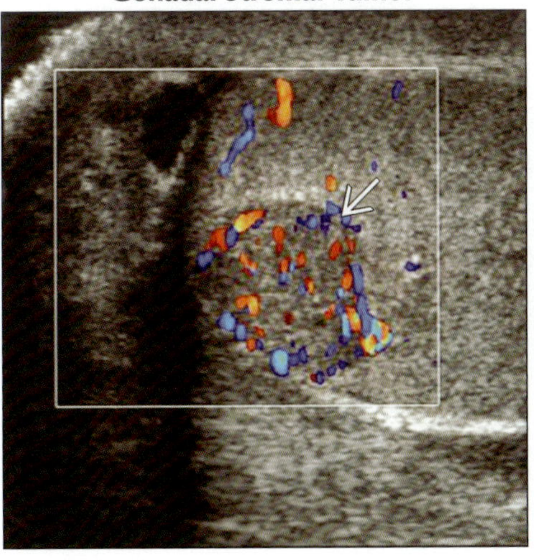

Testicular Epidermoid Cyst

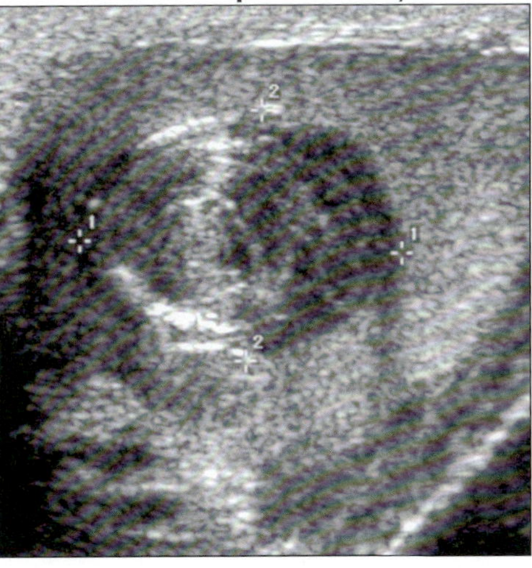

(Left) Longitudinal color Doppler ultrasound shows a well-defined, hypoechoic, vascular, intratesticular mass ➡ in this patient with a gonadal stromal tumor. *(Right)* Transverse ultrasound shows a hypoechoic mass within the testis with a characteristic lamellated or "onion skin" appearance. Because an epidermoid cyst is filled with keratin rather than fluid, the cysts often have a solid appearance on ultrasound ("pseudosolid" lesion).

CYSTIC TESTICULAR LESION

DIFFERENTIAL DIAGNOSIS

Common
- Nonseminomatous Germ Cell Tumor
- Intratesticular Cyst
- Tubular Ectasia of Rete Testis
- Tunica Albuginea Cyst
- Testicular Abscess

Less Common
- Tunica Vaginalis Cyst
- Necrosis or Hemorrhage in Tumor
- Epidermoid Cyst

ESSENTIAL INFORMATION

Key Differential Diagnosis Issues
- Testicular cysts are common (8-10% of men)
- Most cystic neoplasms have "complex" features
  - Mural nodularity, hemorrhage, or necrosis
  - Flow on color Doppler imaging

Helpful Clues for Common Diagnoses
- **Nonseminomatous Germ Cell Tumor**
  - Teratoma or teratomatous components in mixed germ cell tumor
    - Cysts are common feature, ± anechoic or complex, depending on cyst contents
  - Cystic necrosis of tumor not uncommon in other nonseminomatous testicular carcinomas
- **Intratesticular Cyst**
  - Simple cyst, 2-18 mm diameter
  - Near mediastinum testis

- **Tubular Ectasia of Rete Testis**
  - Variable-sized cystic lesions near mediastinum testis
    - On turning transducer, these elongate into tubular channels
  - No flow on color Doppler
  - May be bilateral, asymmetrical
  - Often with associated spermatocele
- **Tunica Albuginea Cyst**
  - Within tunica surrounding testis
  - Usually solitary, 2-3 mm diameter; can be septate
- **Testicular Abscess**
  - Usually complication of epididymo-orchitis
  - Enlarged testis with hypoechoic or mixed echopattern
  - Imaging alone cannot distinguish it from tumor

Helpful Clues for Less Common Diagnoses
- **Tunica Vaginalis Cyst**
  - Rare; arises from visceral or parietal layer of tunica vaginalis
  - Usually anechoic; may have septations or internal echoes due to hemorrhage
- **Epidermoid Cyst**
  - Contents are "cheesy" keratin
  - Occasionally anechoic, but layered keratin often creates lamellated "onion skin" appearance
  - May have calcified capsule
  - Presents as painless nodule in young man

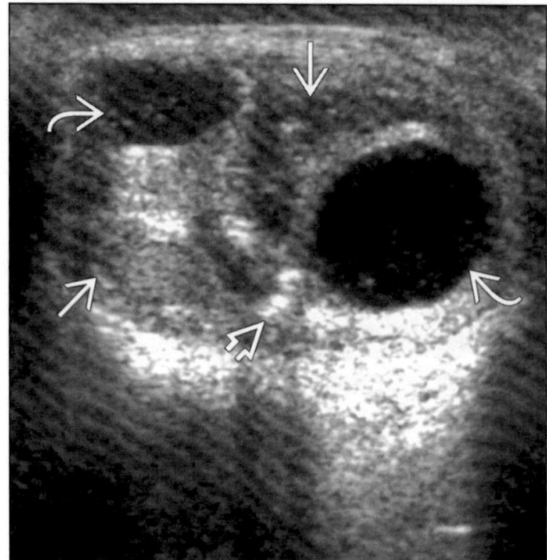

Nonseminomatous Germ Cell Tumor

Transverse ultrasound shows a large, heterogeneous, intratesticular mass ➡ with internal calcification ⬇ and intervening cysts ➡. This was a mature teratoma.

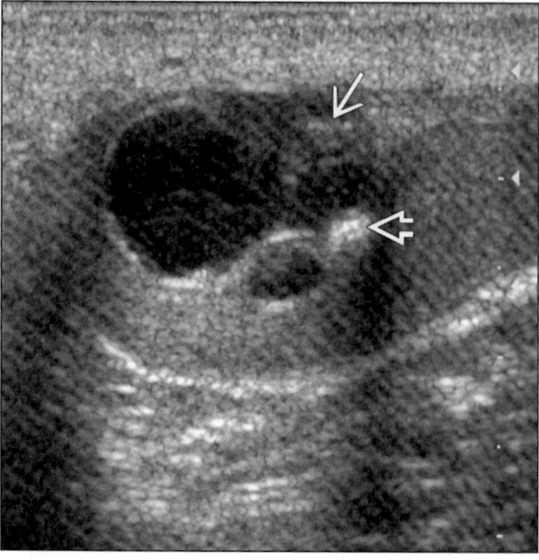

Nonseminomatous Germ Cell Tumor

Longitudinal ultrasound shows a cystic mass within the testis. The mass is heterogeneous with solid areas ➡ and calcification ⬇. The presence of cystic areas suggests that this tumor has teratomatous components.

CYSTIC TESTICULAR LESION

Intratesticular Cyst

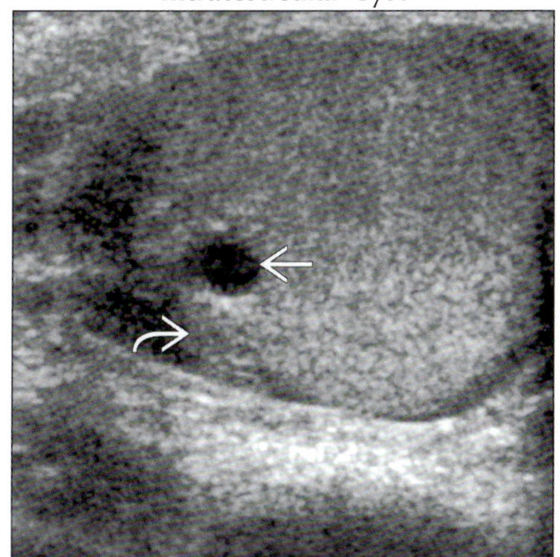

Tubular Ectasia of Rete Testis

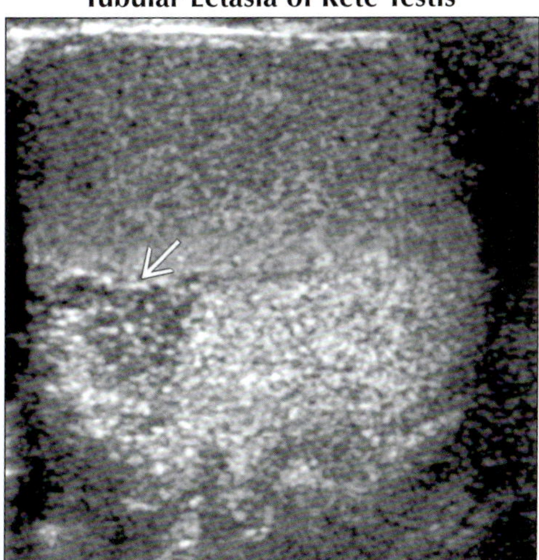

(Left) Oblique ultrasound shows a well-defined, intratesticular, anechoic cyst ➡ with an imperceptible wall and posterior acoustic enhancement ➘, features of a simple testicular cyst. *(Right)* Oblique ultrasound shows multiple small, branching, tubular, anechoic structures ➡ adjacent to the mediastinum testis, findings suggestive of mild to moderate tubular ectasia.

Tunica Albuginea Cyst

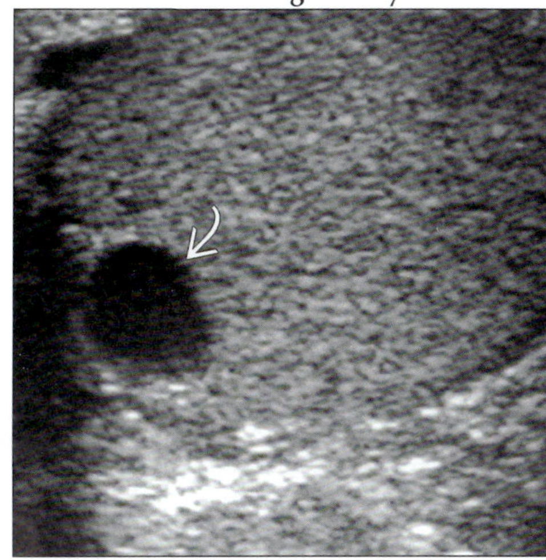

Testicular Abscess

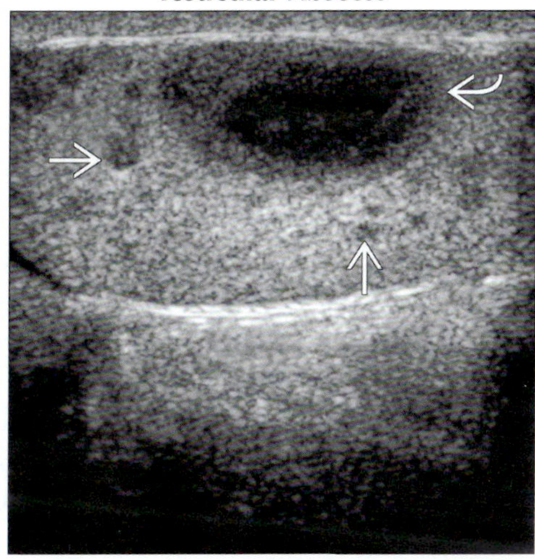

(Left) Oblique ultrasound shows a small, well-defined, anechoic cyst ➡ in the anterior aspect of the testis. Tunica albuginea cysts form within the layers of the tunica albuginea and may appear as either intra- or extratesticular cysts. *(Right)* Oblique ultrasound in a patient with epididymo-orchitis shows an ill-defined hypoechoic area ➡ with an irregular thick wall, suggesting a testicular abscess. Note several small abscesses/granulomas ➡ elsewhere in the testis.

Necrosis or Hemorrhage in Tumor

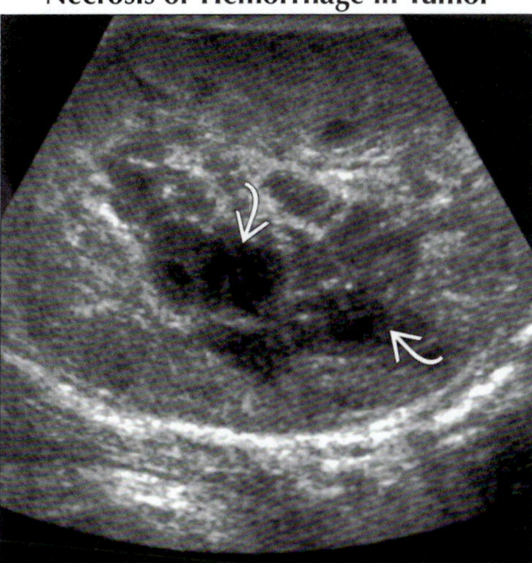

Epidermoid Cyst

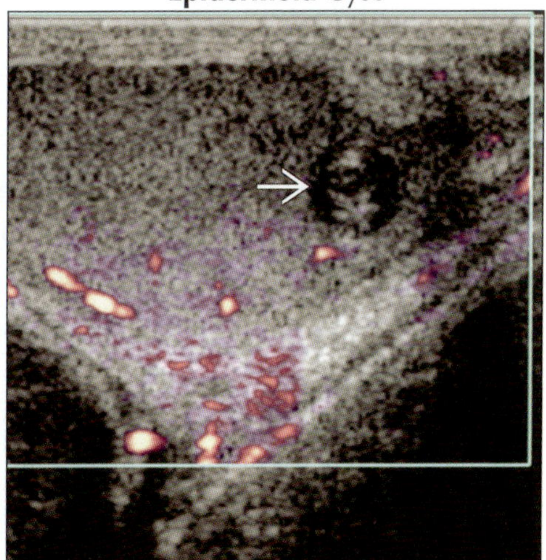

(Left) Oblique ultrasound shows an ill-defined, variegated, intratesticular mass with irregular areas of central necrosis ➘. The final diagnosis was teratoma with necrosis. *(Right)* Longitudinal power Doppler ultrasound shows a well-circumscribed, avascular, hypoechoic "mass" ➡ with a concentric lamellar pattern often referred to as an "onion skin" appearance. This is characteristic of epidermoid cysts.

12

EPIDIDYMAL/SPERMATIC CORD LESION

DIFFERENTIAL DIAGNOSIS

Common
- Epididymitis
- Spermatocele
- Epididymal Cyst
- Varicocele
- Spermatic Cord Torsion

Less Common
- Papillary Cystadenoma
- Fatty Deposition
- Lipoma
- Adenomatoid Tumor
- Hematoma
- Fibrous Pseudotumor
- Encysted Hydrocele of Cord
- Leiomyoma
- Epididymal/Scrotal Wall Abscess
- Inguinal Hernia
- Tuberculous Epididymitis

Rare but Important
- Sarcoidosis
- Metastases
- Rare Tumors
  - Sclerosing Lipogranuloma
  - Liposarcoma
  - Leiomyosarcoma
  - Malignant Schwannoma
  - Epididymal Rhabdomyosarcoma

ESSENTIAL INFORMATION

Key Differential Diagnosis Issues
- Diagnosis based on combination of clinical and sonographic features
- Acute pain: Epididymitis, hematoma, torsion, strangulated inguinoscrotal hernia
- Chronic pain: Varicocele, tumors
- Incidental finding: Epididymal cyst, spermatocele

Helpful Clues for Common Diagnoses
- **Epididymitis**
  - Most common cause of acutely painful scrotum
  - Acute epididymitis
    - *N. gonorrhoeae, C. trachomatis* most common pathogens
    - Enlarged, heterogeneous, predominantly hypoechoic epididymis
    - Reactive thickening of scrotal wall ± hydrocele
  - Chronic epididymitis
    - Granulomatous infection caused by tuberculosis, brucellosis, syphilis, and fungal infection
    - Usually bilateral involvement
    - Enlarged epididymis with heterogeneous appearance, ranging from hypoechoic to hyperechoic, ± calcification
  - Internal echogenicity depends on stage of disease
  - Hyperemic epididymis &/or testis on color Doppler ultrasound
    - Compare with contralateral side
- **Spermatocele**
  - Size: 1-2 cm, may be very large
  - Retention cyst of tubules connecting rete testis to head of epididymis
    - Obstruction and dilatation of efferent ductal system
    - Usually seen in individuals with previous vasectomy
  - Appearance similar to epididymal cyst: Anechoic, cystic with low-level echoes
    - Rarely spermatoceles may be hyperechoic
    - Large spermatoceles may have internal septations
- **Epididymal Cyst**
  - Usually ≤ 1 cm
  - Well-defined anechoic lesion with posterior acoustic enhancement
  - Large cysts (true cysts or spermatocele) may have septation and may be confused with hydroceles
    - Cysts displace testis, while hydrocele envelop it
- **Varicocele**
  - Dilatation of veins of pampiniform plexus > 2-3 mm in diameter due to retrograde flow in internal spermatic vein
  - Best imaging tool: Color Doppler US
    - Dilated serpiginous veins behind superior pole of testis
    - Veins enlarge with Valsalva maneuver

Helpful Clues for Less Common Diagnoses
- **Papillary Cystadenoma**
  - 1-4 cm solid mass, identified in men with von Hippel-Lindau disease (50-70%)
  - On US, variable appearance: Large, solid tumors, echogenic, ± cystic spaces

12

EPIDIDYMAL/SPERMATIC CORD LESION

- **Lipoma**
  - 1 of most common extratesticular neoplasms, usually involves spermatic cord
  - Homogeneous, well-circumscribed, variable-sized, hyperechoic, solid mass
- **Adenomatoid Tumor**
  - Most common tumor of epididymis; 1/3 of all paratesticular neoplasms
    - 3-50 mm, most common in men older than 20 years
    - Usually unilateral, common on left side
  - Variable US appearance
    - Typically seen as well-circumscribed, round to oval, homogeneous mass, isoechoic to normal epididymis
- **Hematoma**
  - Associated with trauma, torsion
  - Complex echogenic fluid with layering debris ± internal septation
  - Acute or chronic
    - Relatively cystic if acute; solid mass with internal septation if chronic
  - Identification of intact testicular vascularity very important, as enlarging hematoma may compress testicular vessels
- **Fibrous Pseudotumor**
  - Reactive fibrous proliferation in epididymis
    - Tunica albuginea may be another site for such fibrous proliferation
    - Lesions may be as large as 8 cm
  - Generally hypoechoic ± posterior acoustic shadowing
- **Encysted Hydrocele of Cord**
  - Patent processus vaginalis seen in infants; associated ascites may also be seen
  - Elongated fluid collection within layers of spermatic cord located above level of testis and epididymis
- **Leiomyoma**
  - 2nd most common epididymal neoplasm
  - Slow growing, hence delayed presentation (generally 5th decade)
  - Solid or cystic, variable US appearance, ± calcifications
- **Inguinal Hernia**
  - Herniation of abdominal contents into scrotum
  - Accentuated by Valsalva maneuver
  - Solid, irreducible mass if obstruction/strangulation
  - Ill-defined echogenic structure representing mesentery ± bowel in herniated sac
    - Obstruction at neck of hernia sac leads to strangulation of herniated contents

Helpful Clues for Rare Diagnoses
- **Metastases**
  - 25% of solid tumors of epididymis are malignant; majority of these are metastases
  - On ultrasound, most metastatic lesions are hypoechoic, but no other specific feature differentiates them from other epididymal neoplasms
- **Sclerosing Lipogranuloma**
  - Rare, hypoechoic paratesticular mass, histopathological correlation

Epididymitis

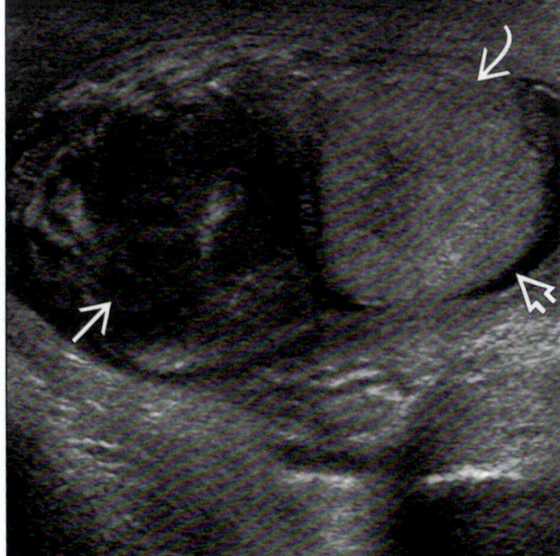

Transverse ultrasound shows a markedly thickened, predominantly hypoechoic head of epididymis ➡, features suggestive of acute epididymitis. Note the normal testis ➡ and minimal reactive hydrocele ➡.

Epididymitis

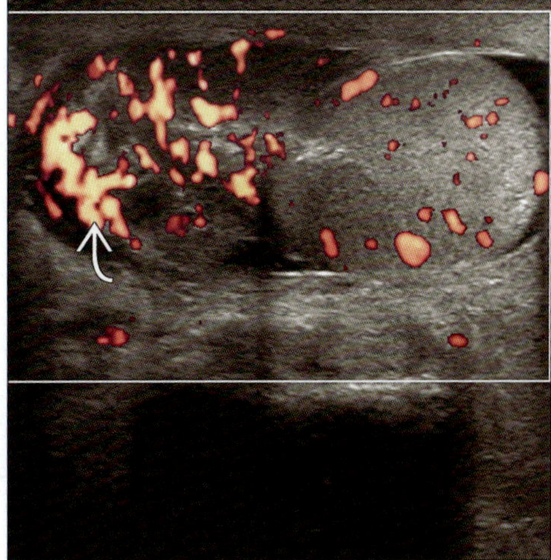

Oblique power Doppler ultrasound in the same patient shows marked increase in intrinsic vascularity ➡ of inflamed epididymis. Note the undisplaced pattern of vessels, helping differentiate this from a neoplasm.

EPIDIDYMAL/SPERMATIC CORD LESION

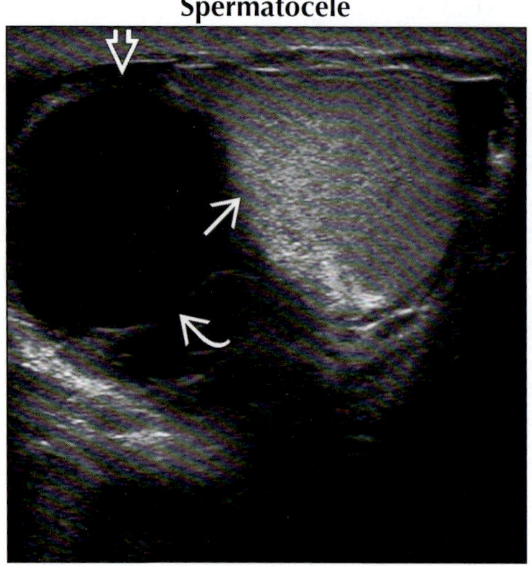

Spermatocele

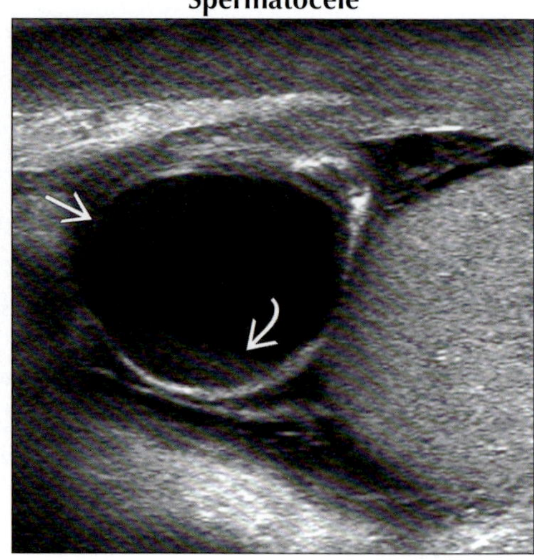

Spermatocele

(Left) Oblique US shows a large, septate ➜, anechoic cyst in the head of the epididymis, displacing the testis ➔ anteriorly. Features suggest a large spermatocele. Note the compressed epididymal head ➔. Larger spermatoceles may show low-level internal echoes due to spermatozoa. (Right) Longitudinal ultrasound shows a well-circumscribed cystic lesion ➔ in the head of the epididymis. Note layering of internal echoes ➔ due to spermatozoa within the spermatocele.

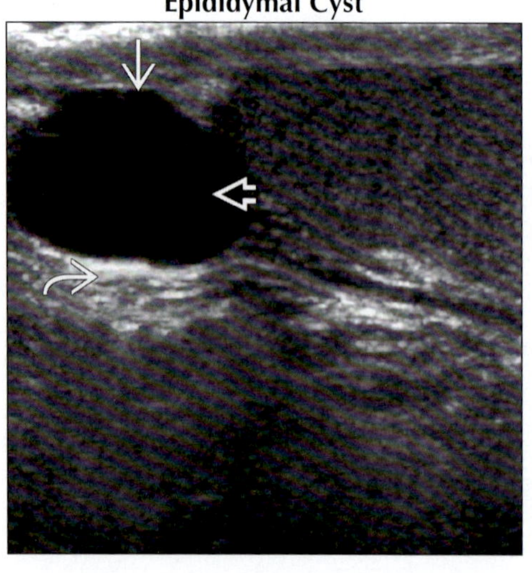

Epididymal Cyst

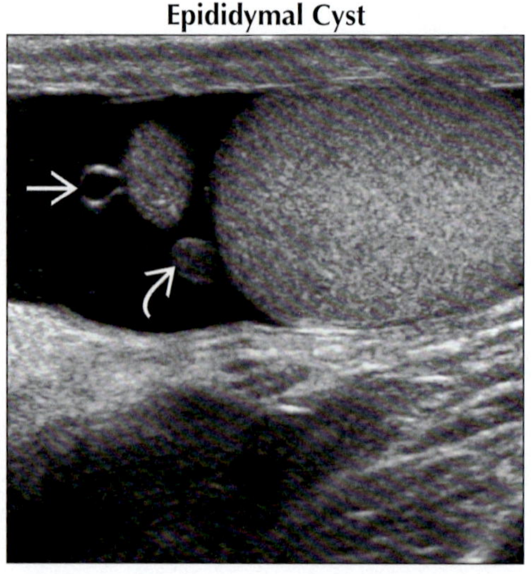

Epididymal Cyst

(Left) Oblique ultrasound shows a well-circumscribed anechoic lesion ➔ in the head of the epididymis, features suggestive of a simple epididymal cyst. Note the anechoic internal contents ➔ and posterior acoustic enhancement ➔. (Right) Oblique ultrasound shows a small, well-defined, pedunculated, anechoic, cystic lesion ➔ arising from the epididymal head. The features suggest a simple cyst of the epididymal appendix. Note the testicular appendix ➔.

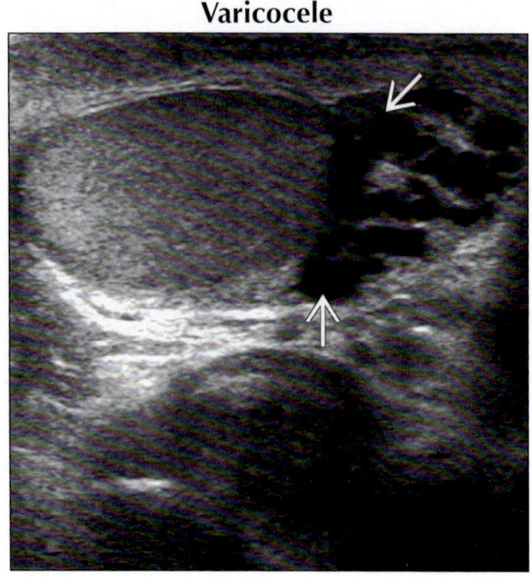

Varicocele

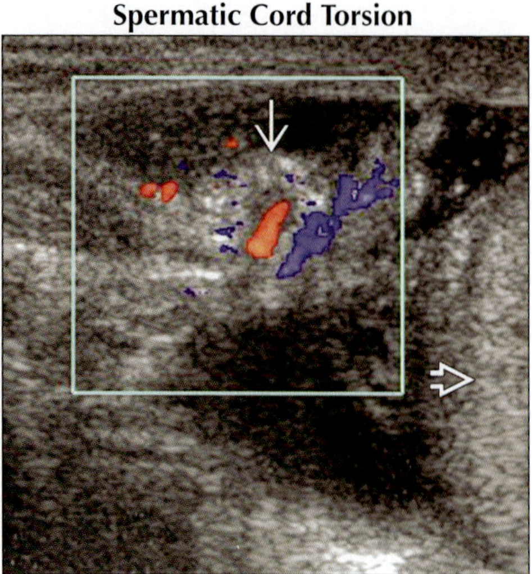

Spermatic Cord Torsion

(Left) Oblique ultrasound shows dilated, tortuous varicose veins of the pampiniform plexus ➔ in the spermatic cord, along the posterosuperior aspect of the testis, features of a varicocele. (Right) Oblique color Doppler ultrasound shows a "torsion knot" ➔ or "whirlpool" pattern of spermatic cord just immediately cranial to the testis ➔, features suggesting an acute torsion of spermatic cord. The testis is prone to infarct due to compromised vascularity.

12

EPIDIDYMAL/SPERMATIC CORD LESION

Papillary Cystadenoma

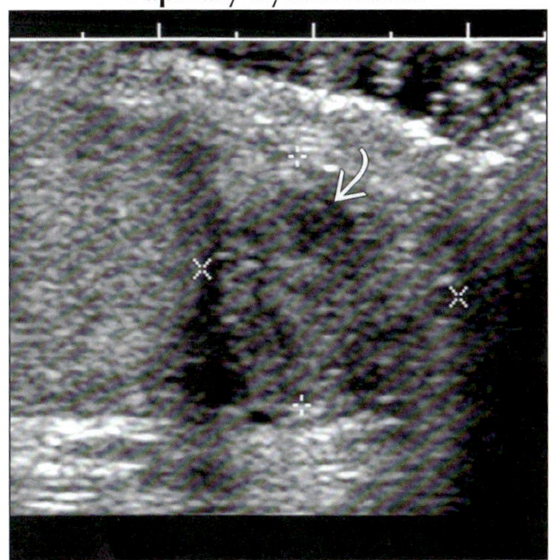

Fatty Deposition

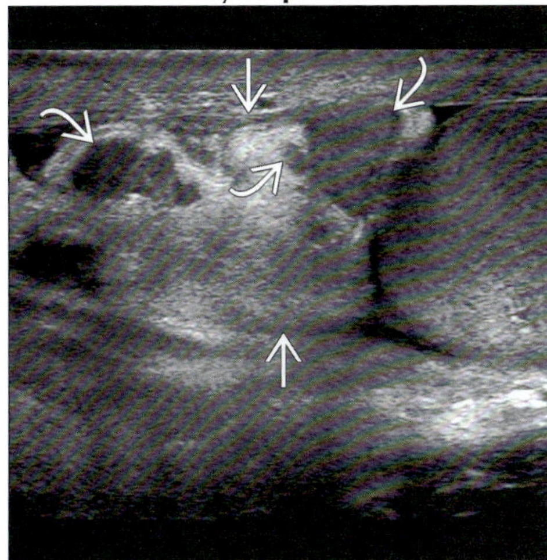

(Left) Longitudinal US shows an ill-defined heterogeneous mass (calipers) in the tail of the epididymis with scattered small cysts ➡ within. The final diagnosis was papillary cystadenoma. (Right) Longitudinal ultrasound shows an ill-defined hyperechoic structure ➡ surrounding the epididymis. No discrete mass is identifiable. This "pseudomass" is due to the deposition of fat, and parts of the epididymis are seen as small hypoechoic areas ➡ within it.

Lipoma

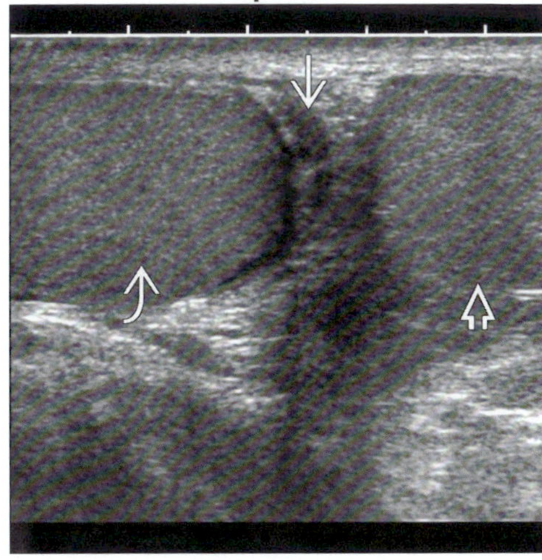

Lipoma

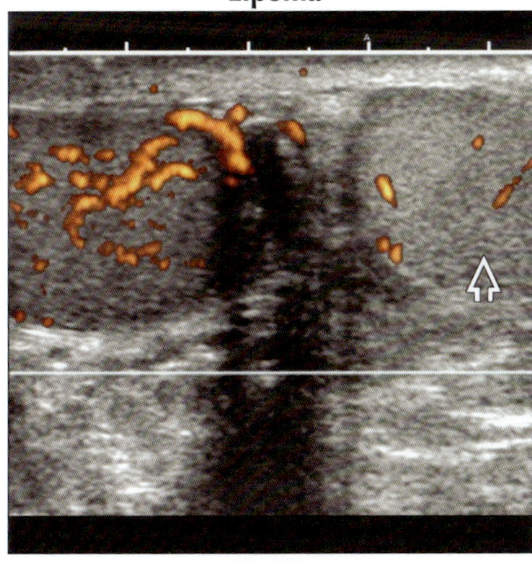

(Left) Longitudinal ultrasound shows a well-defined homogeneous mass ➡, slightly hyperechoic to the adjacent testis ➡, arising from the spermatic cord. These features are suggestive of a lipoma. Note the compressed portion of the normal epididymis ➡ between the mass and normal testis. (Right) Longitudinal power Doppler ultrasound in the same patient shows relative hypovascularity ➡ within the epididymal lipoma.

Adenomatoid Tumor

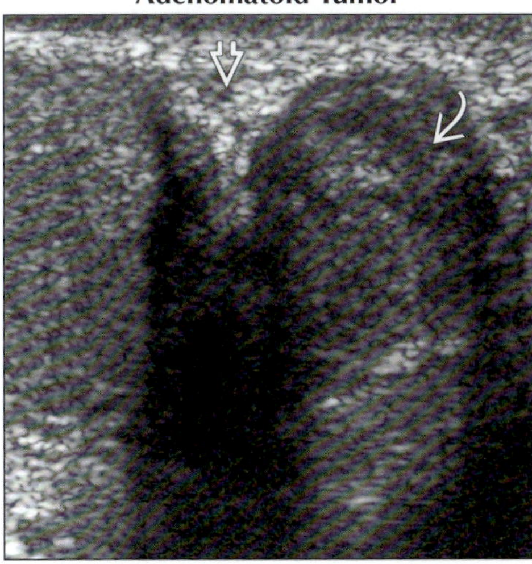

Adenomatoid Tumor

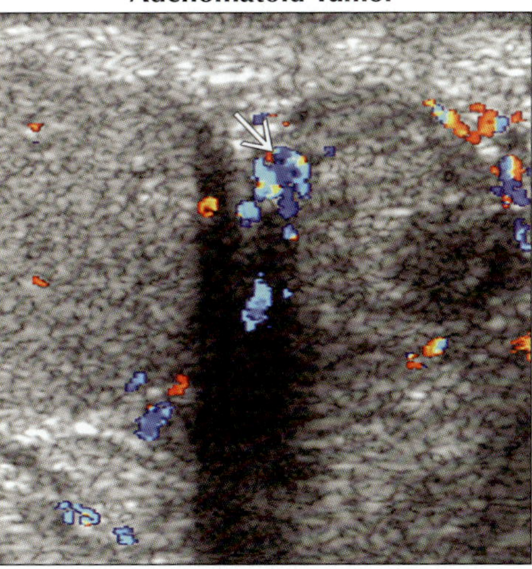

(Left) Longitudinal ultrasound shows a well-circumscribed, hypoechoic, solid mass ➡ adjacent to the head of the epididymis ➡ in this patient with an adenomatoid tumor. The majority of adenomatoid tumors are isoechoic relative to the adjacent normal epididymis. (Right) Longitudinal color Doppler ultrasound in the same patient shows peripheral vascularity ➡ in the adenomatoid tumor.

EPIDIDYMAL/SPERMATIC CORD LESION

(Left) Oblique ultrasound shows a large, complex, extratesticular mass ➡. Note the compressed head of the epididymis ➡ and testis ➡. (Right) Longitudinal ultrasound shows an elongated anechoic fluid collection ➡ within layers of the distal spermatic cord in the inguinoscrotal region. Note the splayed layers ➡ of the proximal spermatic cord, features suggestive of an encysted hydrocele of the spermatic cord.

Hematoma

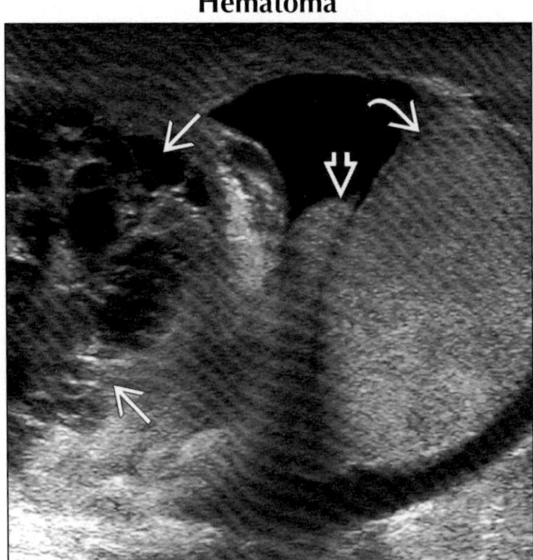

Encysted Hydrocele of Cord

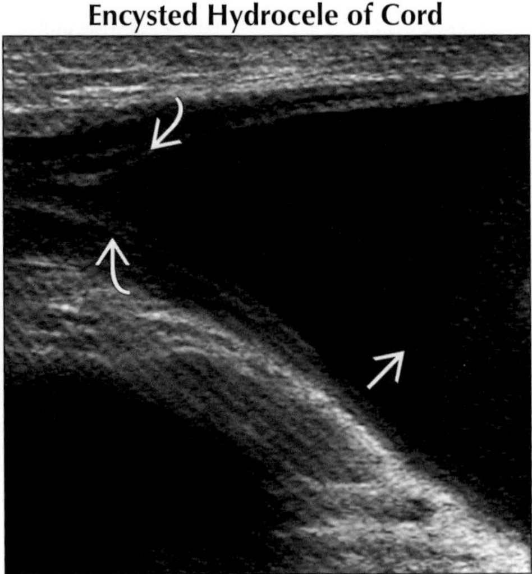

(Left) Transverse ultrasound shows a chronic, septated fluid ➡ collection ➡ in the inguinoscrotal region representing an encysted hydrocele of the spermatic cord. (Right) Oblique ultrasound shows a poorly defined, hypoechoic abscess ➡ within the layers of the scrotum, due to the spread of infection from the adjacent inflamed epididymis ➡. Note the track ➡ along which the infection has reached the scrotal wall.

Encysted Hydrocele of Cord

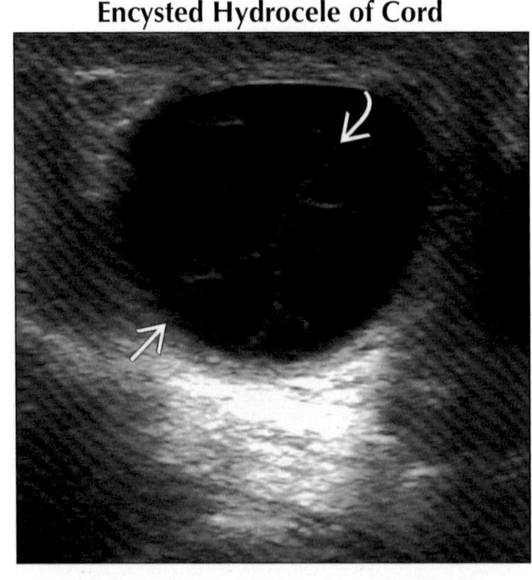

Epididymal/Scrotal Wall Abscess

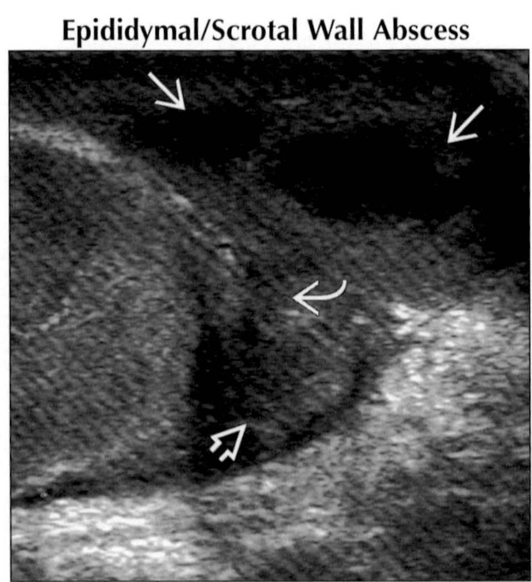

(Left) Oblique ultrasound shows a markedly enlarged epididymis ➡ with central liquefactive necrosis ➡ indicating abscess formation. (Right) Oblique ultrasound shows an inguinoscrotal hernia, containing small bowel loops ➡, and mesentery ➡. Note the bowel wall ("gut signature"), which distinguishes this from a cord or epididymal mass. Note the fluid in the hernia sac ➡.

Epididymal/Scrotal Wall Abscess

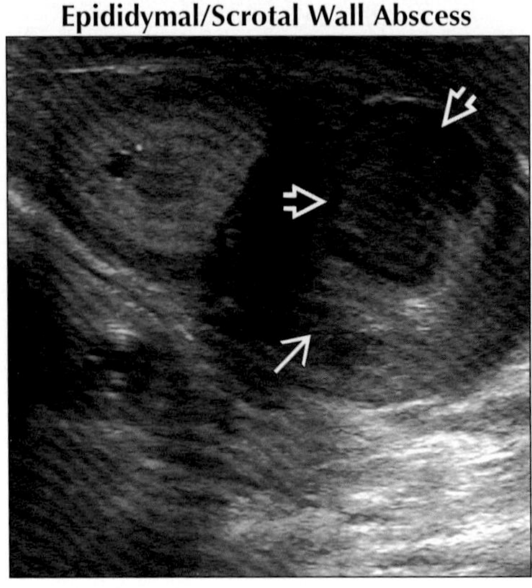

Inguinal Hernia

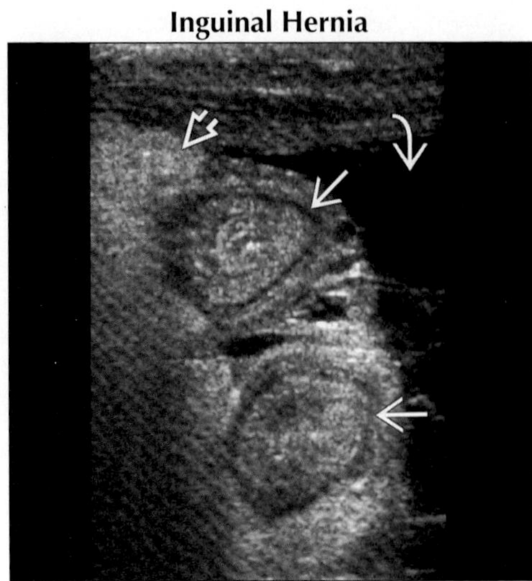

EPIDIDYMAL/SPERMATIC CORD LESION

Inguinal Hernia

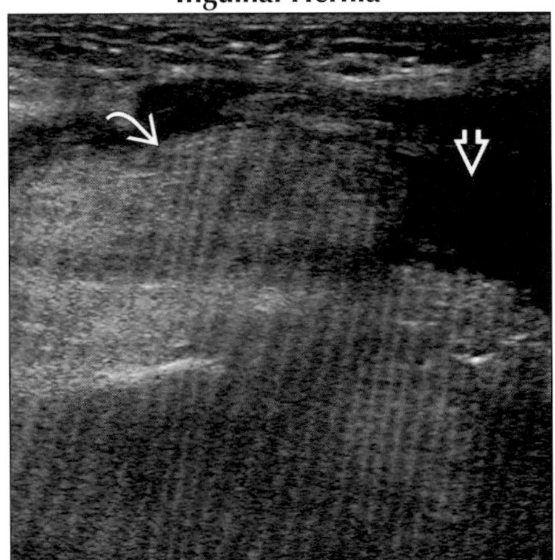

Sarcoidosis

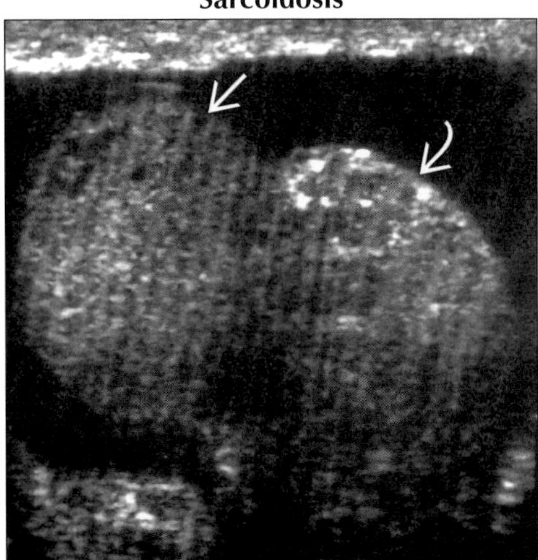

(Left) Longitudinal ultrasound shows an ill-defined, lobulated, echogenic ➡ structure herniating into the scrotum ➡, features suggestive of an omentocele. (Right) Oblique ultrasound shows a markedly enlarged, heterogeneous, predominantly hypoechoic ➡ epididymis, suggesting granulomatous disease in this patient with sarcoidosis. Note the normal testis ➡.

Tuberculous Epididymitis

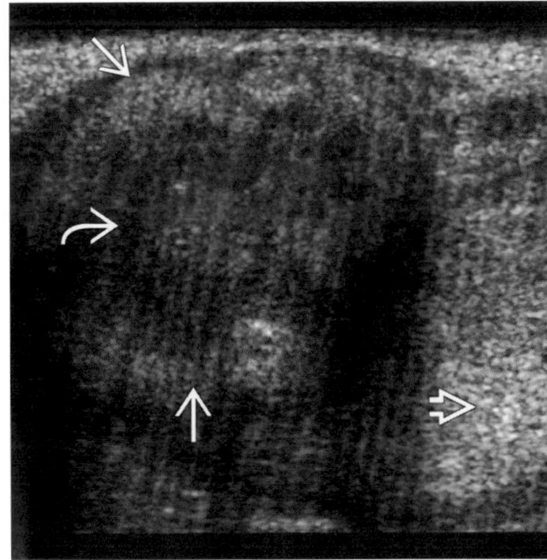

Tuberculous Epididymitis

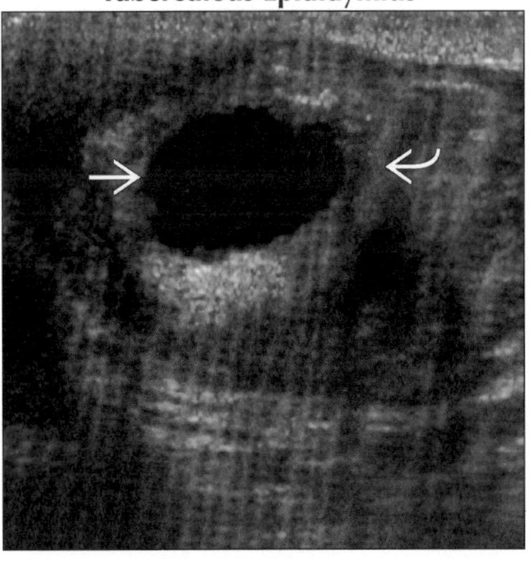

(Left) Transverse ultrasound shows an enlarged, lobulated, epididymal head ➡. Note the heterogeneous intrinsic echopattern ➡, features suggestive of a chronic granulomatous inflammatory mass in this patient with tuberculous epididymitis. Note the normal testis ➡. (Right) Oblique ultrasound follow-up performed 2 years later in the same patient shows a well-developed area of necrosis ➡ within the chronically inflamed epididymal head ➡.

Metastases

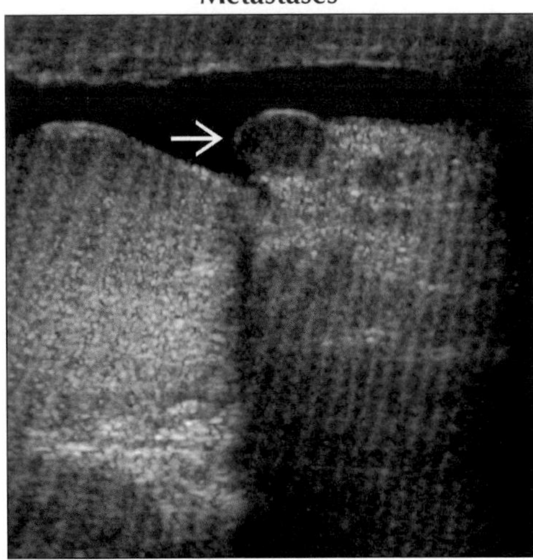

Epididymal Rhabdomyosarcoma

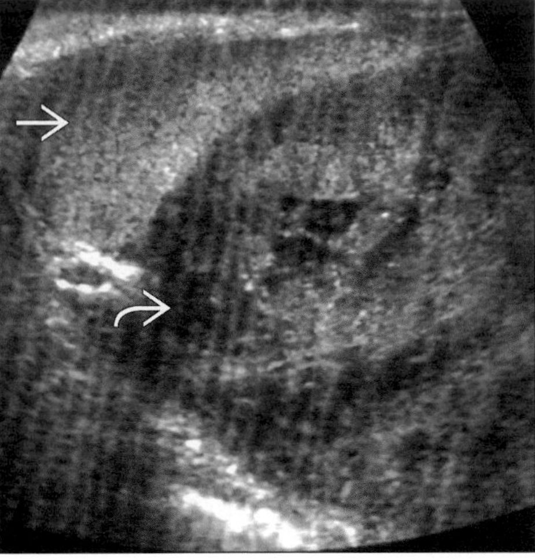

(Left) Oblique ultrasound shows a small, well-defined, hypoechoic lesion ➡ within the head of the epididymis in this patient with known disseminated malignancy. The final diagnosis was epididymal metastases. (Right) Longitudinal ultrasound shows a large, heterogeneous, paratesticular mass ➡ compressing the testis ➡. The epididymis could not be seen separately in this patient with epididymal rhabdomyosarcoma.

EXTRATESTICULAR CYSTIC MASS

DIFFERENTIAL DIAGNOSIS

Common
- Hydrocele
- Varicocele
- Spermatocele
- Epididymal Cyst

Less Common
- Tunica Albuginea Cyst
- Acute Hematocele
- Pyocele

ESSENTIAL INFORMATION

Helpful Clues for Common Diagnoses
- **Hydrocele**
  - Congenital or acquired
  - Fluid collection in tunica vaginalis
  - Envelops testis except for "bare area" where tunica vaginalis is deficient
- **Varicocele**
  - Dilation of veins of pampiniform plexus greater than 2-3 mm in diameter, due to retrograde flow in internal spermatic vein
  - Dilated serpiginous veins behind superior pole of testis on color Doppler US (best imaging tool)
  - Enlarges with Valsalva maneuver
  - Left (78%), right (6%), bilateral (16%)
- **Spermatocele**
  - Retention cyst of tubules connecting rete testis to head of epididymis
  - Located in head of epididymis; contains spermatozoa
  - Large spermatoceles have low-level echoes and septations within lesion
  - Often associated with tubular ectasia of rete testis
    - Normal variant of dilated seminiferous tubules in mediastinum of testis
    - Intratesticular; but if with spermatocele, gives appearance of complex intra-/extratesticular mass
    - No flow on color Doppler
- **Epididymal Cyst**
  - Located in epididymal head, body, tail
  - Anechoic, does not contain spermatozoa
    - Shows all features of simple cyst

Helpful Clues for Less Common Diagnoses
- **Tunica Albuginea Cyst**
  - Located within layers of tunica albuginea
    - May appear as intra-/extratesticular cyst
  - Usually solitary but can be multiple
    - 2-3 mm diameter
  - Asymptomatic
- **Acute Hematocele**
  - Associated with trauma, torsion, and infarction
  - Varies in appearance with evolution of blood products
  - Look for associated testicular injury
- **Pyocele**
  - Sequela of scrotal infections
  - Septate fluid with low-level internal echoes
  - Chronicity may lead to thickening of tunica and scrotal wall

Hydrocele

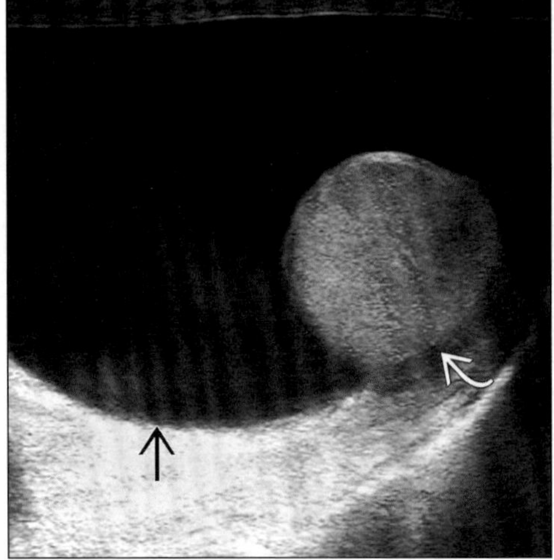

Longitudinal ultrasound of scrotum shows anechoic fluid ➜ within the tunica vaginalis, indicative of a simple hydrocele. Fluid in the tunica vaginalis envelops the testis except posteriorly ➜, where it is deficient.

Varicocele

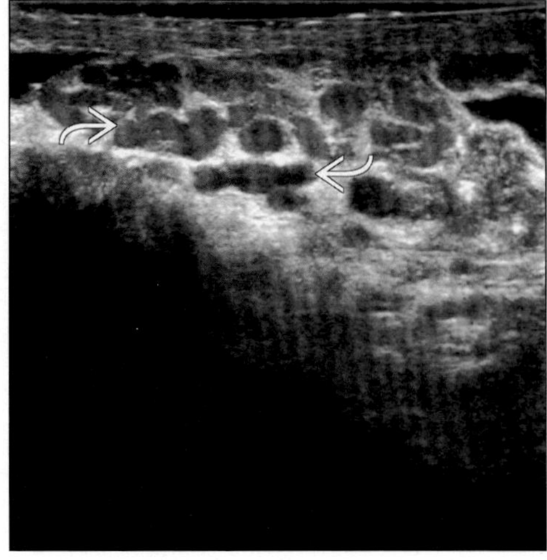

Oblique ultrasound of scrotum shows multiple serpiginous dilated veins ➜ in pampiniform plexus of the cord, along the posterosuperior aspect of the testis. Marked flow was seen on color Doppler.

EXTRATESTICULAR CYSTIC MASS

Spermatocele

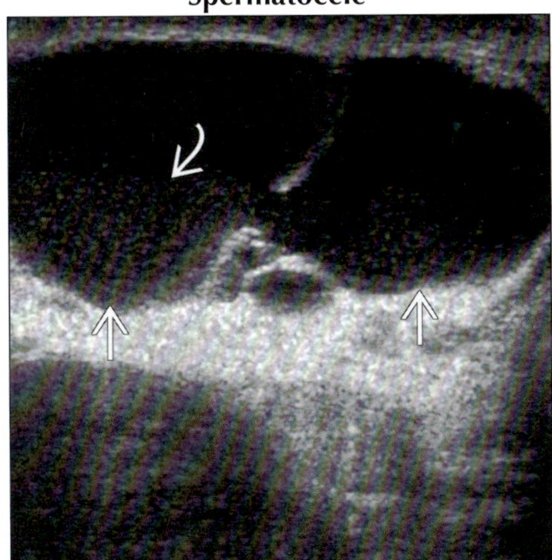

Spermatocele

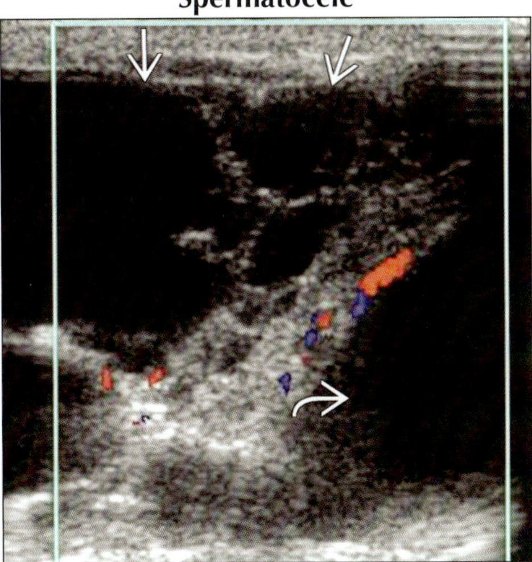

(Left) Longitudinal US shows a large septated cyst ➡ in the epididymal head. Note the floating internal echoes ➡ representing spermatozoa. *(Right)* Transverse color Doppler US shows multiple avascular, circular structures of varying size ➡ in the testis, representing tubular ectasia (cystic transformation) of the rete testis. A spermatocele ➡ is also seen, giving the appearance of a complex intra-/extratesticular mass.

Epididymal Cyst

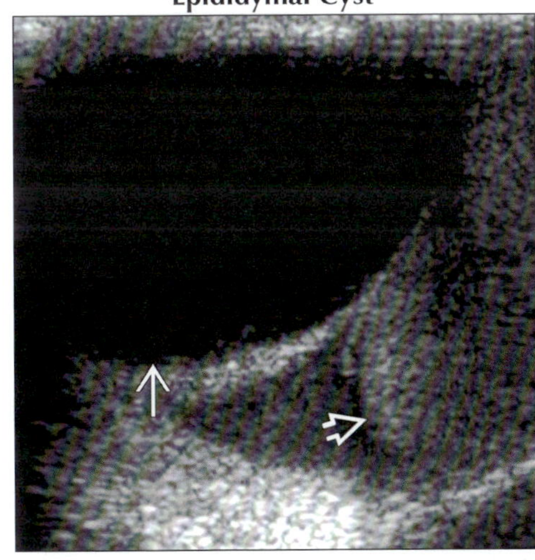

Tunica Albuginea Cyst

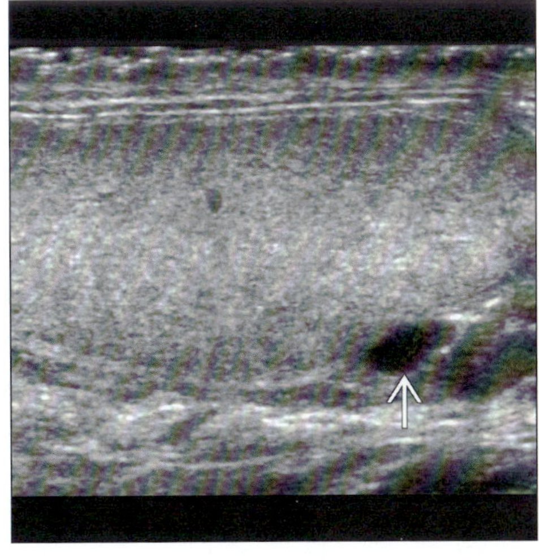

(Left) Oblique ultrasound shows a well-defined cyst ➡ in the head of the epididymis (testis ➡). Note the anechoic nature of the cyst, a feature helping to differentiate it from a spermatocele. Aspiration of fluid to rule out spermatozoa is diagnostic but seldom necessary, as both lesions are benign. *(Right)* Longitudinal ultrasound shows a small, well-defined, anechoic cyst ➡ along the periphery of the testis, a classic appearance of a tunica albuginea cyst.

Acute Hematocele

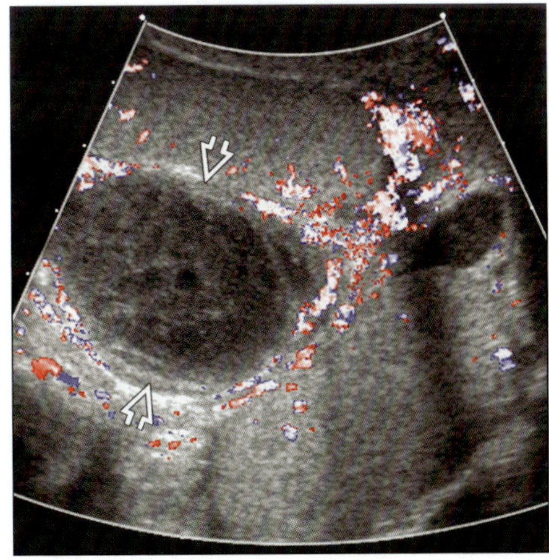

Pyocele

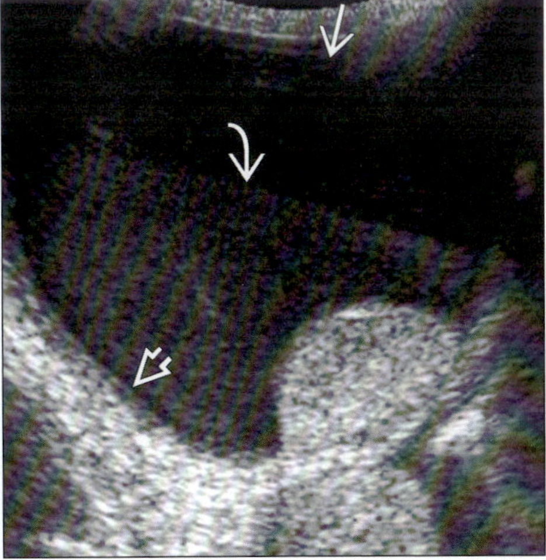

(Left) Color Doppler ultrasound of the scrotum shows an avascular, complex, extratesticular fluid collection ➡ in a man who recently had a vasectomy. The hematoma resolved on follow-up studies. *(Right)* Longitudinal ultrasound shows a moderate-sized fluid collection ➡ within the tunica vaginalis with layering of low-level echoes and debris ➡. There is also associated thickening of the scrotal wall ➡, all features of a pyocele.

EXTRATESTICULAR SOLID MASS

DIFFERENTIAL DIAGNOSIS

Common
- Epididymitis
- Chronic Hematocele
- Inguinal Hernia
- Scrotal Pearl
- Adenomatoid Tumor
- Fibrous Pseudotumor

Less Common
- Mesenchymal Tumors, Scrotum
- Papillary Cystadenoma, Epididymis

ESSENTIAL INFORMATION

Key Differential Diagnosis Issues
- Clinical presentation & US findings are key

Helpful Clues for Common Diagnoses
- **Epididymitis**
  - Variable echogenicity depending on whether acute or chronic stage
  - Enlarged hyperemic epididymis &/or testis on color Doppler US
  - Compare with contralateral side
- **Chronic Hematocele**
  - Associated with trauma, torsion, infarct
  - Complex echogenic fluid
    - May be chronic and fibrotic, appearing as solid mass
  - No intrinsic vascularity seen
  - Ipsilateral testis should be separately identified to exclude injury
- **Inguinal Hernia**
  - Inguinoscrotal hernia; indirect type
  - Bowel or echogenic omental fat seen within scrotum
    - Important to identify vascularity of bowel to exclude strangulation
- **Scrotal Pearl**
  - Detached and calcified testicular appendages; post-inflammation or secondary to prior torsion
- **Adenomatoid Tumor**
  - Most common epididymal tumor
    - 30% of all extratesticular neoplasms
  - Well-defined, solid, hypoechoic mass
  - Peripheral vascularity on color Doppler
- **Fibrous Pseudotumor**
  - Reactive fibrous proliferation, usually associated with tunica albuginea
  - Generally hypoechoic with strong posterior acoustic shadowing
  - May be as large as 8 cm in diameter

Helpful Clues for Less Common Diagnoses
- **Mesenchymal Tumors, Scrotum**
  - Lipoma most common benign neoplasm
    - Often appears hypoechoic
  - Most common malignant tumors include rhabdomyosarcoma and liposarcoma
    - Large, irregular, heterogeneous masses
- **Papillary Cystadenoma, Epididymis**
  - Epididymal component of von Hippel-Lindau (VHL) syndrome
    - Seen in 65% of patients with VHL
  - Often bilateral; found in young adults
  - Ill-defined solid mass with scattered cysts

Epididymitis

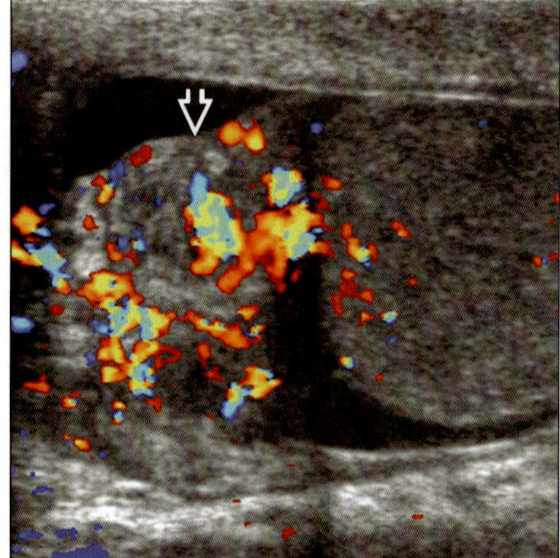

Longitudinal color Doppler ultrasound shows an enlarged and hyperemic epididymis ➡ in a man with 2 days of scrotal pain and swelling.

Chronic Hematocele

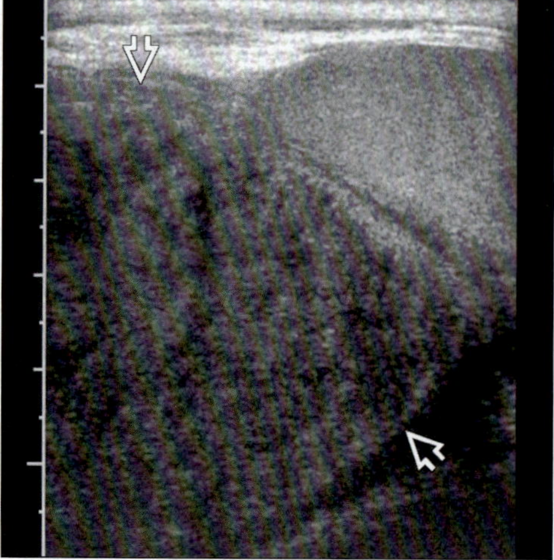

Longitudinal ultrasound shows a large, solid-appearing, extratesticular mass ➡. The patient reported that it had not changed in years. It was excised, and pathology showed a chronic fibrosed hematoma.

EXTRATESTICULAR SOLID MASS

Inguinal Hernia

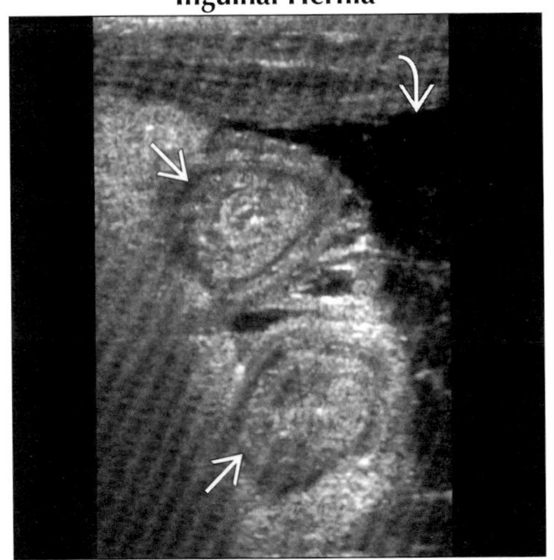

Scrotal Pearl

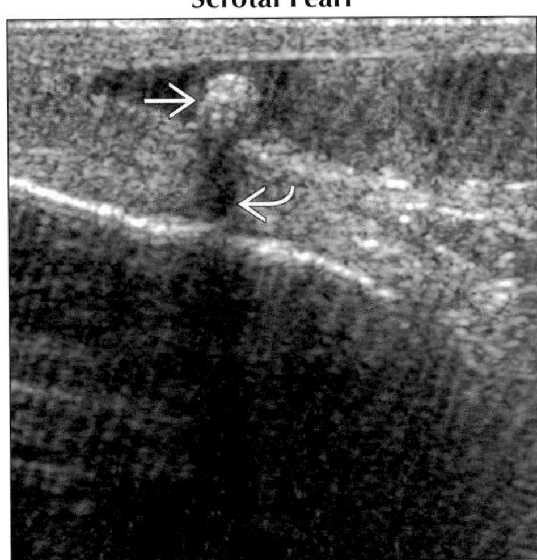

(Left) Oblique ultrasound shows herniated bowel loops ➡ in the scrotum in this patient with a inguinoscrotal hernia. Note the moderately sized hydrocele ➡. Vascularity of the herniated omentum and bowel wall should be assessed to exclude strangulation. (Right) Oblique ultrasound shows a small intrascrotal (extratesticular) calcified body ➡ with posterior acoustic shadowing ➡. This is typical of a scrotal pearl (scrotolith).

Adenomatoid Tumor

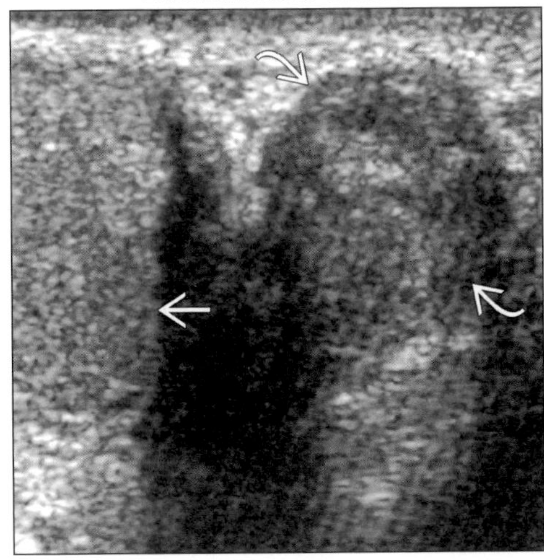

Fibrous Pseudotumor

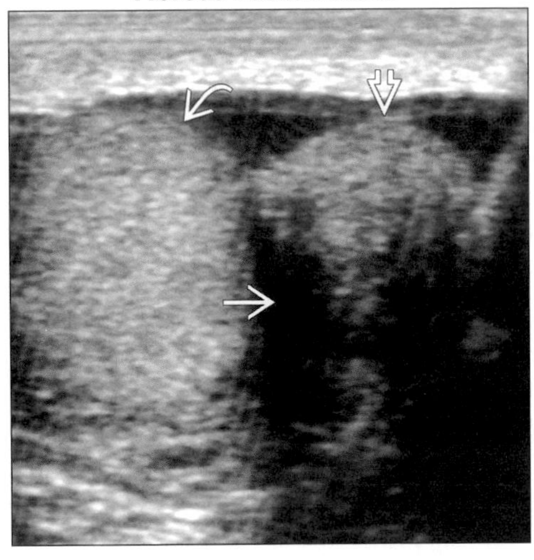

(Left) Transverse ultrasound shows a well-defined, hypoechoic, solid mass ➡ in the head of the epididymis. This lesion showed peripheral vascularity on color Doppler. Note the normal testis ➡. (Right) Transverse ultrasound shows a well-defined, hypoechoic, extratesticular mass ➡ adjacent to the testis ➡. Note the marked posterior acoustic shadowing ➡, which is often seen with these fibrous masses.

Mesenchymal Tumors, Scrotum

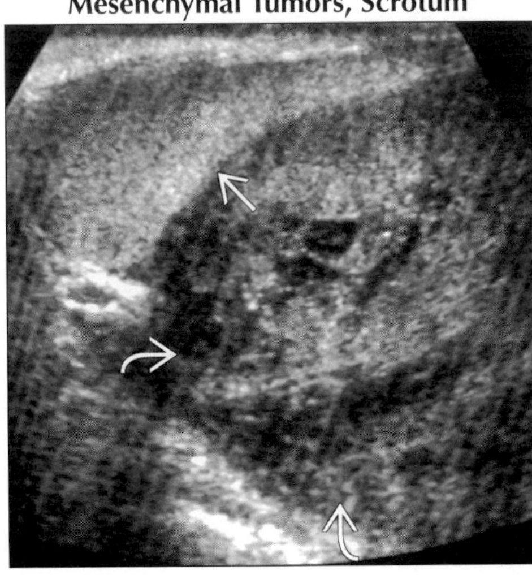

Papillary Cystadenoma, Epididymis

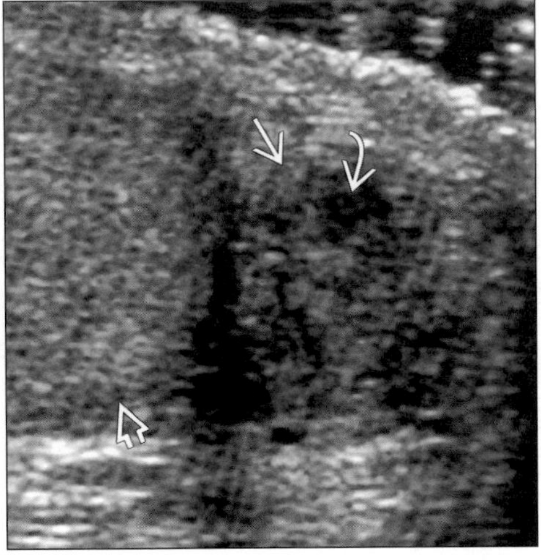

(Left) Oblique ultrasound shows a large, heterogeneous, paratesticular mass ➡ compressing the testis ➡. The epididymis could not be seen separately on real-time scanning in this patient with epididymal rhabdomyosarcoma. (Right) Longitudinal ultrasound shows an ill-defined, solid, heterogeneous mass ➡ with scattered small cysts ➡ in the epididymal tail. The testis is normal ➡.

SCROTAL CALCIFICATION

DIFFERENTIAL DIAGNOSIS

Common
- Testicular Microlithiasis
- Nonseminomatous Germ Cell Tumor
- Sertoli Cell Tumor

Less Common
- Scrotal Trauma
- Scrotal Pearl
- Epidermoid Cyst
- Scrotal Abscess

ESSENTIAL INFORMATION

Key Differential Diagnosis Issues
- Correlation between clinical and sonographic features essential
  - Incidental finding: Testicular microlithiasis, scrotal pearl
  - History of pain: Abscess, chronic infections, tumors
  - Mass with intrinsic calcification: Testicular tumors, epidermoid cyst
  - Associated with trauma: Testicular hematoma, hematocele

Helpful Clues for Common Diagnoses
- **Testicular Microlithiasis**
  - Multiple, discrete, small, nonshadowing, 2-3 mm, echogenic, intratesticular foci
  - Unilateral or bilateral involvement
  - Concurrent germ cell tumor in up to 40%
- **Nonseminomatous Germ Cell Tumor**
  - Complex solid-cystic testicular mass
  - Heterogeneous echogenic foci due to calcification ± fibrosis
  - Calcifications more common in tumors that contain teratomatous components
- **Sertoli Cell Tumor**
  - Small, hypoechoic, solid-cystic mass
  - Punctate calcification may be present
  - Occasionally, tumoral calcification may form large calcified mass, known as large calcifying Sertoli cell tumor

Helpful Clues for Less Common Diagnoses
- **Scrotal Trauma**
  - Chronic hematocele
    - Associated with trauma
    - Complex echogenic fluid
    - If chronic, appears as heterogeneous echogenic mass, ± calcification
    - No intrinsic vascularity on Doppler
    - ± ipsilateral testicular trauma
- **Scrotal Pearl**
  - Calcification of detached testicular epididymal appendages due to previous inflammation or torsion of appendages
  - Solitary, discrete, echogenic focus in tunica vaginalis
- **Epidermoid Cyst**
  - Lamellated appearance on ultrasound
  - May have peripheral calcified rim
- **Scrotal Abscess**
  - Tuberculous infections may produce intrascrotal calcifications, scrotal sinuses
  - Granulomas appear as small echogenic foci, ± calcification

Testicular Microlithiasis

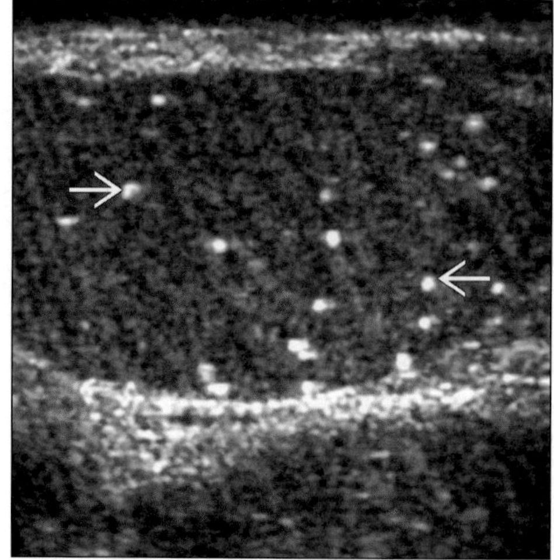

Oblique ultrasound shows multiple tiny, nonshadowing, echogenic foci ➡ representing diffuse testicular microlithiasis. For diffuse variety, more than 5 echogenic foci should be identified in any scan plane.

Nonseminomatous Germ Cell Tumor

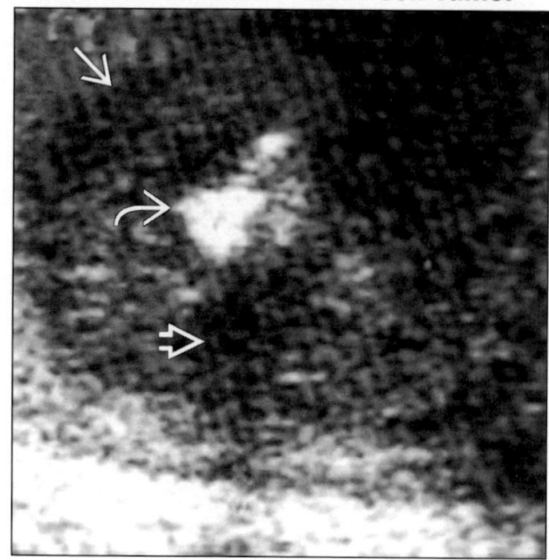

Oblique ultrasound shows an ill-defined, hypoechoic, intratesticular mass ➡ with coarse internal calcifications ➡. Note the posterior acoustic shadowing ➡. The final diagnosis was embryonal cell carcinoma.

SCROTAL CALCIFICATION

Nonseminomatous Germ Cell Tumor

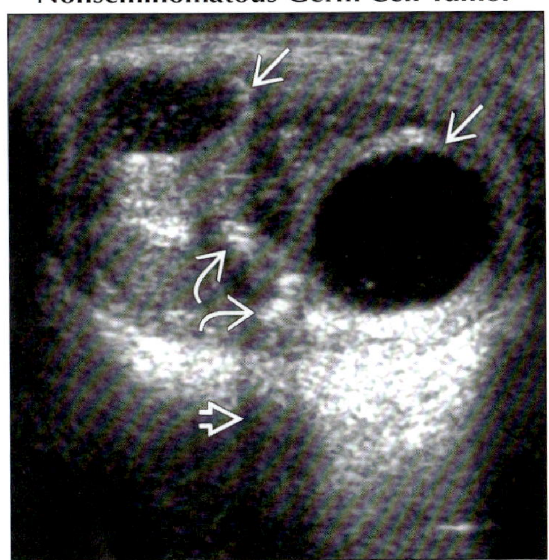

Sertoli Cell Tumor

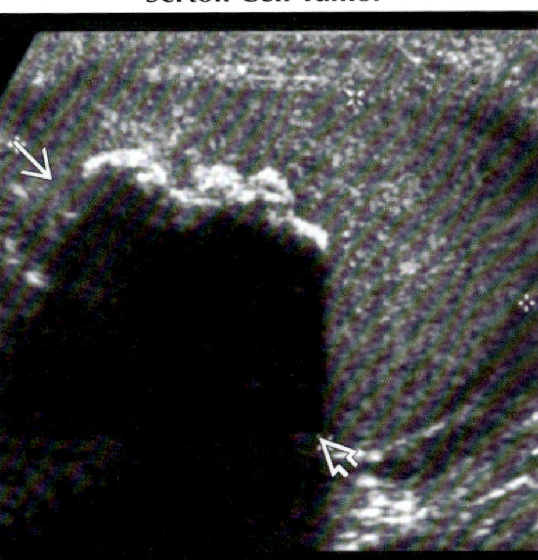

(Left) Transverse ultrasound shows a large, heterogeneous, intratesticular mature teratoma ➡. Note the few small echogenic foci ➡ of calcification that cause posterior acoustic shadowing ➡. (Right) Oblique ultrasound shows an intratesticular, ill-defined, dense focus of calcification ➡ with strong posterior acoustic shadowing ➡. The final diagnosis was a large calcified Sertoli cell tumor.

Scrotal Trauma

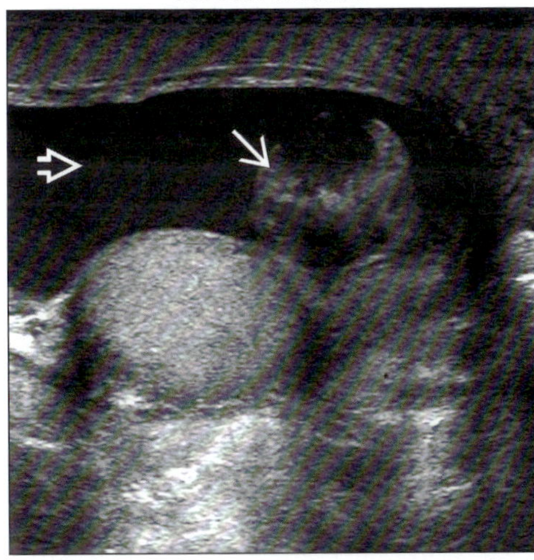

Scrotal Pearl

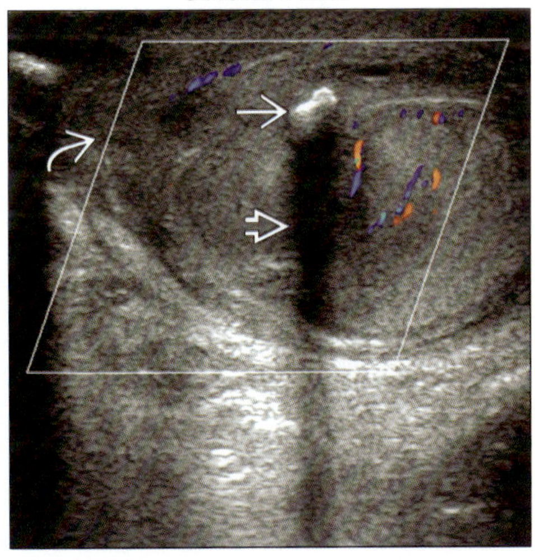

(Left) Oblique US shows an irregular heterogeneous lesion ➡ within the tunica vaginalis in a patient with scrotal trauma. Features suggest organized hematoma. Note the surrounding hematocele with internal echoes ➡. (Right) Oblique color Doppler US shows a small, intrascrotal, echogenic focus ➡ with strong posterior shadowing ➡, features of a scrotal pearl. This was an incidental finding in a patient with epididymo-orchitis. Note the enlarged epididymis ➡.

Scrotal Pearl

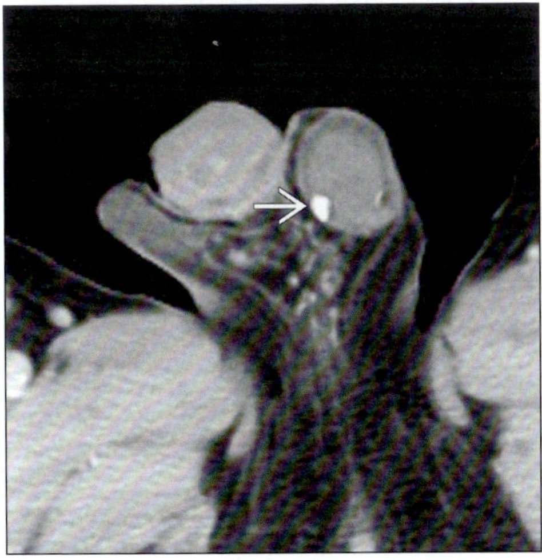

Epidermoid Cyst

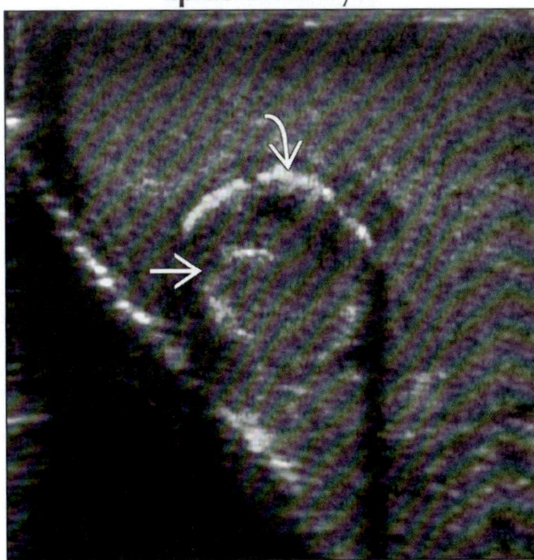

(Left) Axial CECT shows a well-defined calcific focus ➡ within the tunica vaginalis, representing a scrotal pearl (scrotolith). (Right) Oblique ultrasound shows a well-circumscribed, predominantly hypoechoic, intratesticular mass ➡ with a calcified rim ➡, features of an epidermoid cyst.

SECTION 13
Female Pelvis

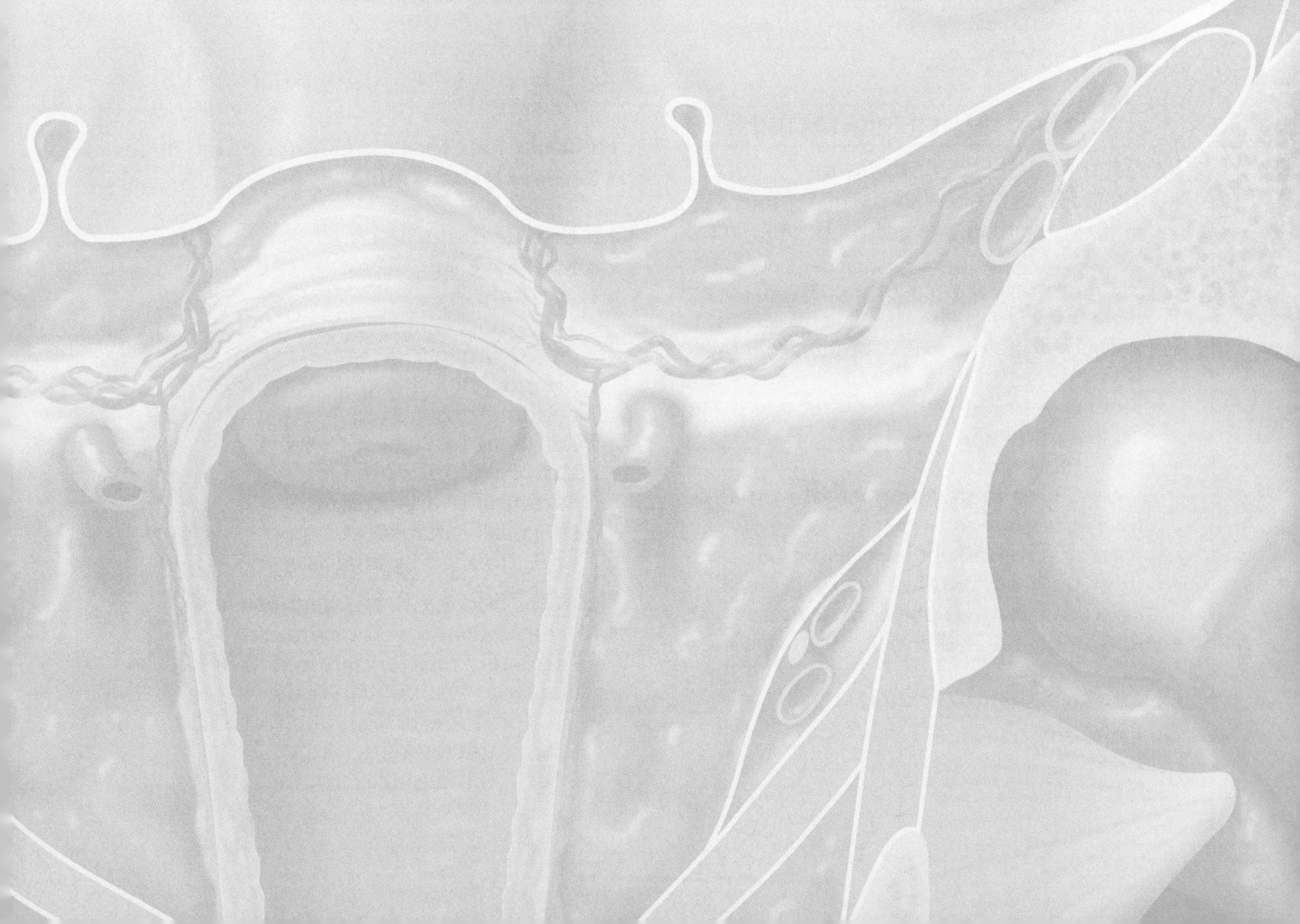

ANECHOIC CYSTIC ADNEXAL MASS

DIFFERENTIAL DIAGNOSIS

Common
- Physiologic Cysts
  - Follicular Cyst
  - Corpus Luteal Cyst
- Paraovarian Cyst
- Paratubal Cysts
- Postmenopausal Adnexal Cyst
- Inclusion Cyst, Ovary

Less Common
- Serous Cystadenoma
- Hydrosalpinx
- Peritoneal Inclusion Cysts

Rare but Important
- Dermoid (Mature Teratoma)
- Serous Cystadenocarcinoma
- Anechoic Adnexal Cyst (Mimic)
  - Loop of Bowel
  - Bladder Diverticulum
  - Tarlov Cyst
  - Gut Duplication Cyst
  - Complex Cyst (Mimic)
  - Solid Lesion (Mimic)
  - Nabothian Cyst
- Adnexal Torsion

ESSENTIAL INFORMATION

Key Differential Diagnosis Issues
- Thin-walled anechoic cysts are benign
  - Solid elements increase risk of malignancy
- Rule of 1-2-3
  - 1 cm cyst in 1st week of menstrual cycle is follicle
  - 2 cm cyst in 2nd week of menstrual cycle is dominant follicle
  - 3 cm cyst in 3rd week of menstrual cycle is corpus luteum
- Size is important
  - Cyst < 3 cm in premenopausal woman is likely physiologic
  - Cyst > 6 cm is likely neoplastic
- Follow-up sonogram in 6 weeks typically shows resolution of physiologic cysts
- Pain can be due to size of cyst or torsion of cyst
- Is cyst separate from ovary?
  - Paraovarian cyst
  - Paratubal cysts
  - Hydrosalpinx
  - Loop of bowel

Helpful Clues for Common Diagnoses
- **Physiologic Cysts**
  - Resolve over time
  - Scan 6 weeks later so patient is in different phase of menstrual cycle
  - Birth control pills can decrease formation of new cysts while current cyst resolves
- **Paraovarian and Paratubal Cysts**
  - Separate from ovary
  - Thin walled, anechoic
  - Tend to not change in size over time
- **Postmenopausal Adnexal Cyst**
  - Cysts may be present in postmenopausal women
  - If thin walled and anechoic, cyst likely benign
  - May change in size over time
  - Use of tamoxifen associated with adnexal cysts
- **Inclusion Cyst, Ovary**
  - Invagination of ovarian cortical surface epithelium with lost connection to surface
  - Typically small caliber (1-13 mm) but may be up to 10 cm
  - Thin, smooth wall
  - Typically within 1-2 mm of outer surface of ovary

Helpful Clues for Less Common Diagnoses
- **Serous Cystadenoma**
  - Thin-walled cyst
  - Usually unilocular
  - May have thin septation
- **Hydrosalpinx**
  - Tube-shaped mass
  - Cysts connect
  - Prior pelvic inflammatory disease or endometriosis
- **Peritoneal Inclusion Cysts**
  - History of prior surgery
  - Surround ovarian tissue
  - Irregularly shaped with poorly defined walls (formed by adjacent organs)

Helpful Clues for Rare Diagnoses
- **Dermoid (Mature Teratoma)**
  - Extremely rare for dermoid to present as anechoic cyst but can occur
  - Calcifications in wall or echogenic nodule raise suspicion of dermoid
- **Serous Cystadenocarcinoma**

ANECHOIC CYSTIC ADNEXAL MASS

- ○ Extremely rare for serous cystadenocarcinoma to present as anechoic cyst
- ○ If cyst is large, small solid element could be missed at imaging
- **Anechoic Adnexal Cyst (Mimic)**
  - ○ Use transvaginal scanning to assess for internal echotexture to exclude solid elements or septations
  - ○ At real-time scanning assess for peristalsis
  - ○ Ensure that gain is set appropriately to detect solid elements
  - ○ Assess for flow within presumed cyst to ensure it is not homogeneous, hypoechoic, solid lesion
  - ○ Ensure that lesion is in adnexa and not related to bowel or spine
  - ○ **Complex Cyst (Mimic)**
    - ▪ May appear anechoic due to transabdominal technique or gain set too low
  - ○ **Solid Lesion (Mimic)**
    - ▪ May appear as anechoic cyst if gain set too low and color Doppler not used
  - ○ **Nabothian Cyst**
    - ▪ Can be confused for adnexal cyst if location in cervix is not noted
- **Adnexal Torsion**
  - ○ Rare for adnexal torsion to present as anechoic cyst
  - ○ Cyst 5-10 cm in size can act as lead point for torsion
  - ○ Ipsilateral pain out of proportion to size of cyst suggests torsion

- ○ Blood flow analysis typically not helpful, because anechoic cysts do not demonstrate flow

Alternative Differential Approaches
- Multiple cysts
  - ○ Multiple physiologic cysts
  - ○ Hydrosalpinx folded on itself
  - ○ Peritoneal inclusion cyst
  - ○ Inclusion cysts
  - ○ Theca lutein cysts
  - ○ Hyperstimulated ovaries
  - ○ Hyperreactio luteinalis
- Bilateral cysts
  - ○ Peritoneal inclusion cyst
  - ○ Theca lutein cysts
  - ○ Hyperstimulated ovaries
  - ○ Hyperreactio luteinalis
  - ○ Hydrosalpinx
  - ○ Cystadenoma
- Pregnant patient
  - ○ Corpus luteum
  - ○ Serous cystadenoma
  - ○ Theca lutein cyst
  - ○ Hyperstimulated ovaries
  - ○ Hyperreactio luteinalis

Physiologic Cysts

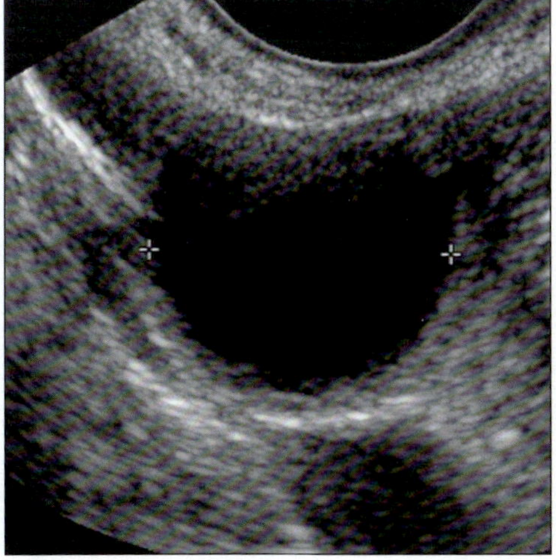

Longitudinal transvaginal ultrasound shows a 2.5 cm anechoic cyst (calipers). This cyst is in the physiologic range and does not require follow-up in a woman of menstrual age.

Paraovarian Cyst

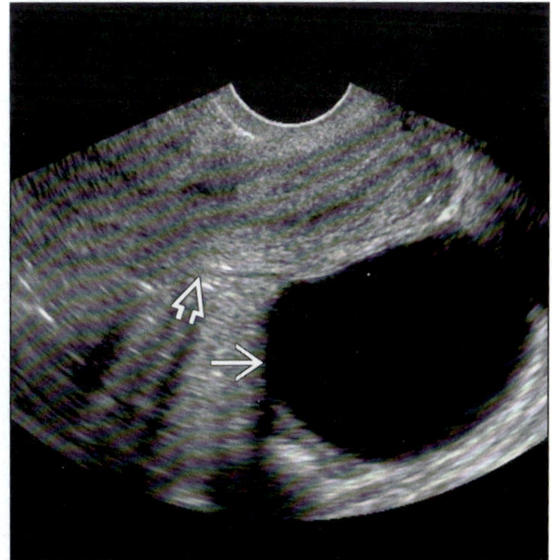

Longitudinal transvaginal US shows a thin-walled anechoic cyst ➡ posterior to the uterus ⊟ and separate from the ovary. A follow-up study 6 wks later showed no change in size or appearance of the cyst.

13

ANECHOIC CYSTIC ADNEXAL MASS

(Left) Longitudinal transabdominal ultrasound shows a 6 cm thin-walled anechoic pelvic cyst (calipers) anterior to the uterus ⮞ and the bladder ⮡. *(Right)* Transverse transvaginal ultrasound shows a 3 cm cyst (calipers) in the left adnexa. Because the cyst increased in size over time, it was removed. Histologic diagnosis was a cortical inclusion cyst.

Paratubal Cysts

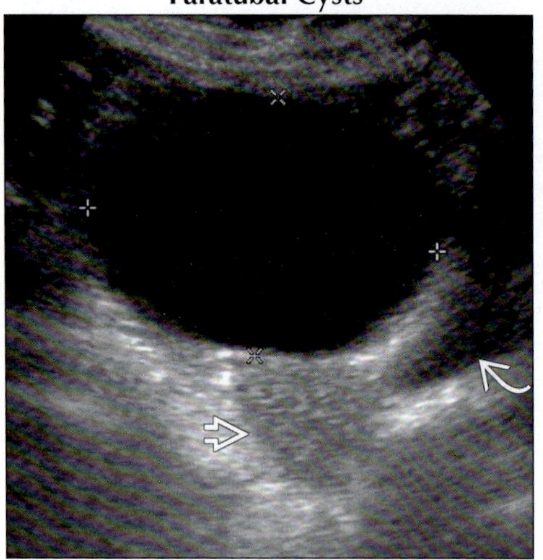

Inclusion Cyst, Ovary

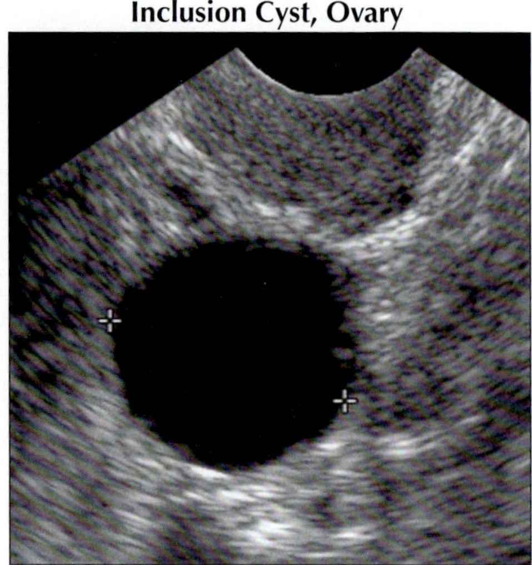

(Left) Oblique transvaginal ultrasound shows a 3.5 cm anechoic right adnexal cyst with a "claw" sign showing that the cyst is exophytic from the ovary ⮞. Note the adjacent free fluid ⮡. *(Right)* Longitudinal transabdominal ultrasound shows a 20 cm anechoic cyst (calipers) rising out of the pelvis. Note the lack of echoes and the thin wall of the cyst. Despite its size, this was a benign serous cystadenoma.

Serous Cystadenoma

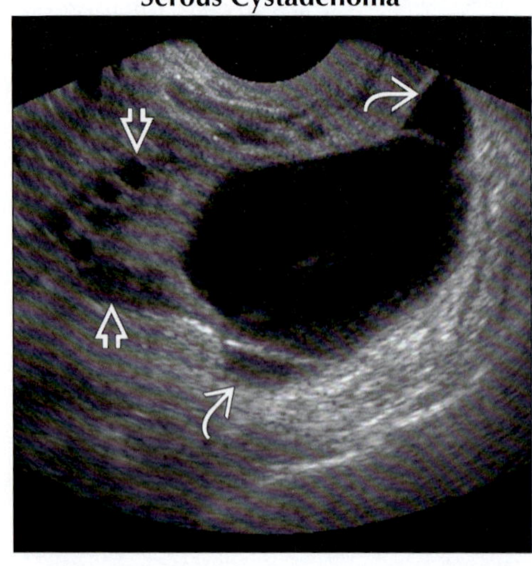

Serous Cystadenoma

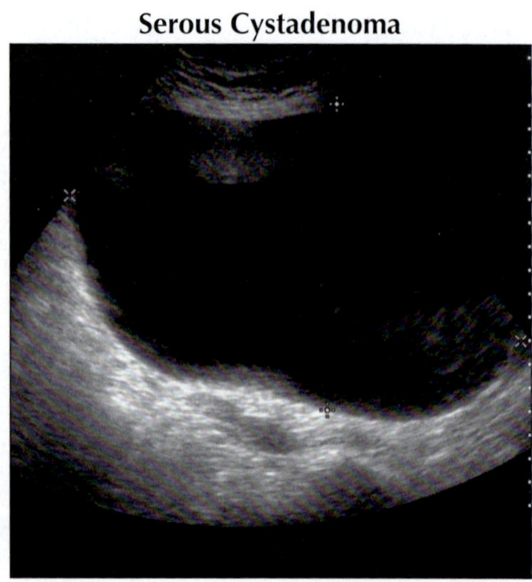

(Left) Transverse transvaginal ultrasound shows what appears to be a septated cyst ⮞ or 2 adjacent cysts. *(Right)* Oblique transvaginal ultrasound in the same patient shows the oblong nature of the "cyst" (calipers). Imaging may be needed in multiple planes in order to demonstrate that shapes appearing to be cysts actually communicate as a tube.

Hydrosalpinx

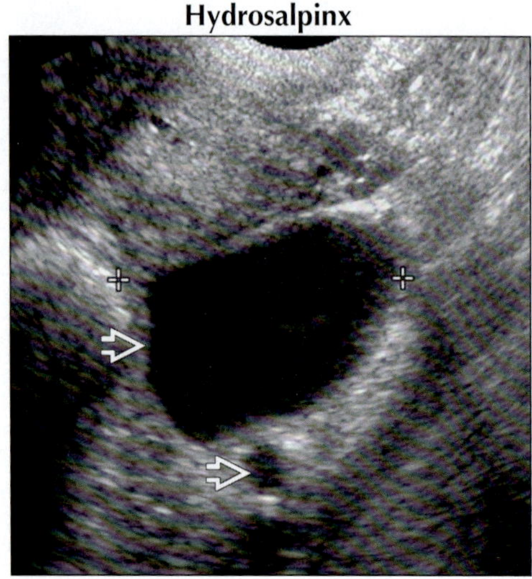

Hydrosalpinx

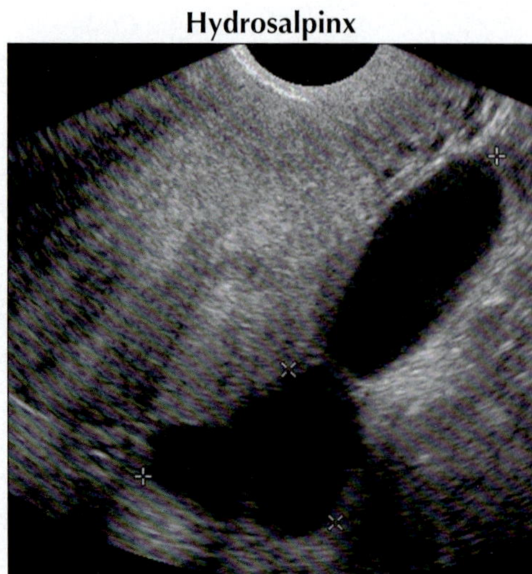

ANECHOIC CYSTIC ADNEXAL MASS

Loop of Bowel

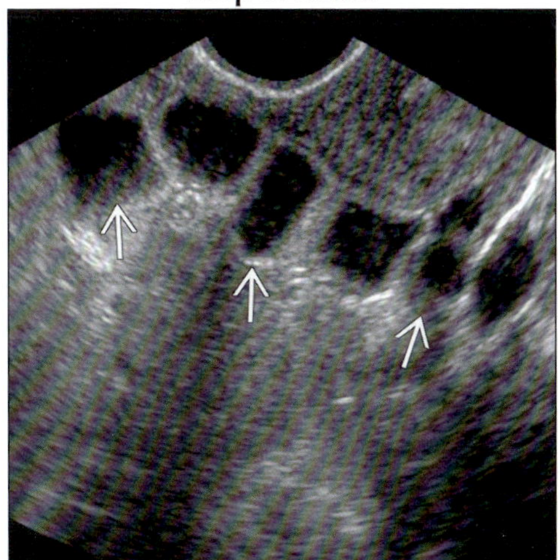

Bladder Diverticulum

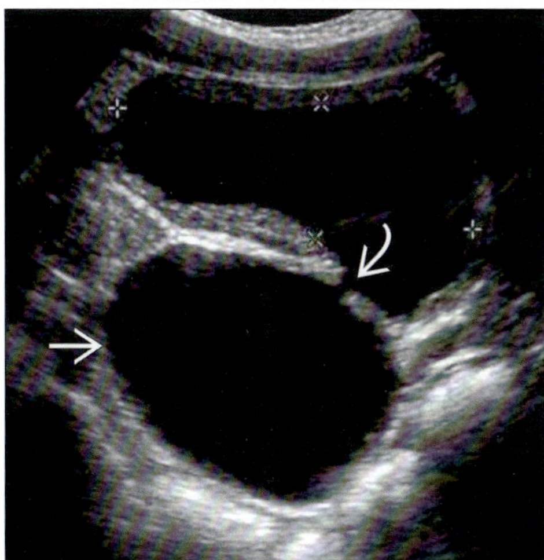

(Left) Oblique transvaginal ultrasound shows fluid-filled loops of bowel ➡. Loops of bowel are typically obvious due to peristalsis. However, they can be mistaken for adnexal cysts. (Right) Oblique transabdominal ultrasound shows a large bladder diverticulum ➡ posterior to the thick-walled bladder (calipers). Note the communication ➡ between the diverticulum and the bladder.

Complex Cyst (Mimic)

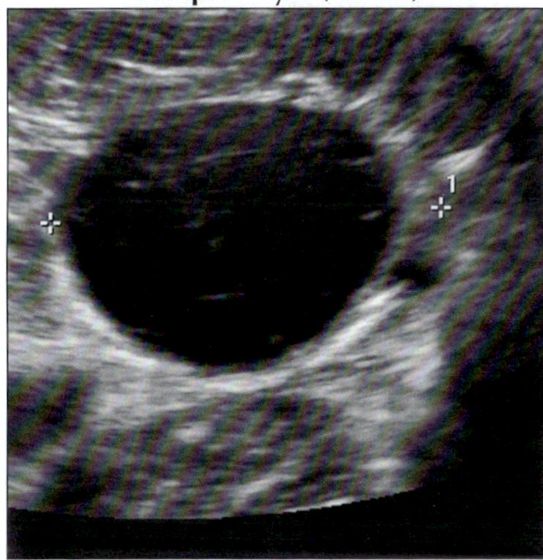

Complex Cyst (Mimic)

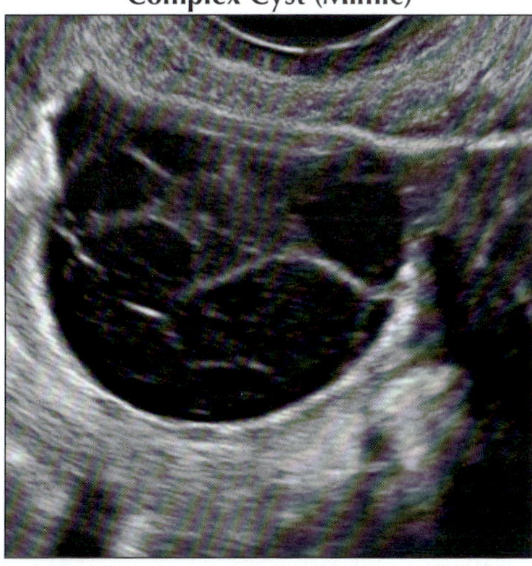

(Left) Transverse transabdominal ultrasound shows a 4 cm right adnexal cyst. On a transabdominal scan, it is difficult to characterize internal echotexture, and this could be mistaken for an anechoic cyst if the gain was set too low. (Right) Longitudinal transvaginal ultrasound in the same patient shows a classic "cobweb" appearance of the clot in this woman with a hemorrhagic corpus luteal cyst.

Nabothian Cyst

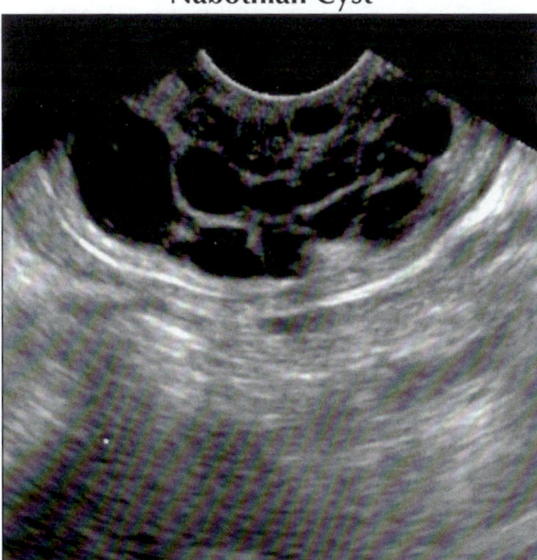

Adnexal Torsion

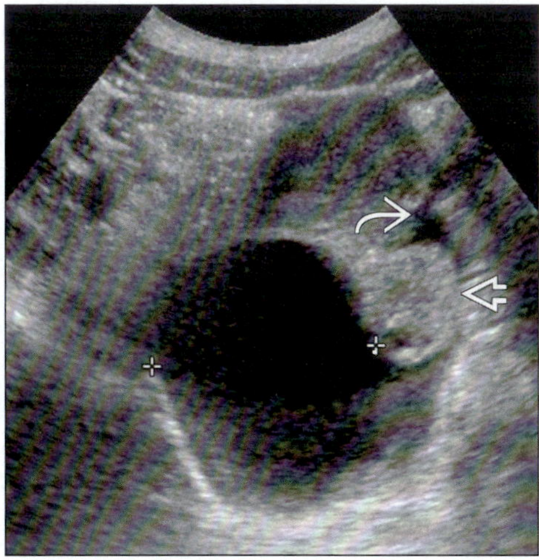

(Left) Transverse transvaginal ultrasound shows multiple cysts in the cervix. These can be confused for adnexal cysts if attention is not paid to their location. (Right) Transverse transabdominal ultrasound shows a 5 cm cyst (calipers) posterior to the uterus. The left ovary ➡ is enlarged and edematous with adjacent free fluid ➡. This was a paraovarian cyst that acted as a lead point for adnexal torsion.

COMPLEX CYSTIC ADNEXAL MASS

DIFFERENTIAL DIAGNOSIS

Common
- Hemorrhagic Cysts, Ovary
- Dermoid (Mature Teratoma)
- Endometrioma

Less Common
- Cystadenoma
  - Serous Cystadenoma
  - Mucinous Cystadenoma
- Cystadenocarcinoma
  - Serous Cystadenocarcinoma
  - Mucinous Cystadenocarcinoma
- Granulosa Cell Tumor
- Cystadenofibroma
- Endometrioid Carcinoma, Ovary
- Hydrosalpinx
- Tubo-Ovarian Abscess
- Peritoneal Inclusion Cysts
- Adnexal Torsion

Rare but Important
- Theca Lutein Cysts
- Ovarian Hyperstimulation Syndrome
- Hyperreactio Luteinalis

ESSENTIAL INFORMATION

Key Differential Diagnosis Issues
- Endovaginal examination essential to depict internal echotexture
- Evaluate for change in appearance over time
  - 6-week follow-up of hemorrhagic cysts will show change in appearance of internal echoes
- Pain when scanning over region
  - Hemorrhagic cysts, ovary
  - Adnexal torsion
  - Tubo-ovarian abscess
- Findings that increase likelihood of malignancy
  - Thick irregular septations
  - Solid elements
  - Thick wall
  - Blood flow in solid elements
  - Elevated CA-125
  - Older age of patient
  - Ascites
  - Metastatic disease
- Cysts in pregnancy
  - Corpus luteal cyst
  - Theca lutein cysts

- Ovarian hyperstimulation syndrome
- Hyperreactio luteinalis
- Benign and malignant ovarian neoplasms

Helpful Clues for Common Diagnoses
- **Hemorrhagic Cysts, Ovary**
  - Variety of appearances depending on age of hemorrhage
    - Echogenic when acute
    - Clot retracts from wall of cyst
    - Acute angles
    - Thick irregular wall
    - May have prominent flow in wall of cyst
    - Strands of internal echogenicity
    - Rapid change in appearance of cyst over time
    - No flow in solid-appearing components
- **Dermoid (Mature Teratoma)**
  - Variety of appearances depending on type of tissue
    - Echogenic mass
    - Cyst with linear bright echoes
    - Echogenic nodule with shadowing
    - Fluid-fluid level
    - Can be mistaken for bowel
  - Most common ovarian neoplasm; 20% of ovarian tumors
  - 10-20% bilateral
  - 80% of patients of childbearing age
- **Endometrioma**
  - "Chocolate" cyst with diffuse homogeneous low-level internal echoes
  - May have punctate calcifications in wall of cyst
  - May have septations with blood flow

Helpful Clues for Less Common Diagnoses
- **Serous Cystadenoma**
  - Thin-walled cyst
  - Usually unilocular
  - May have thin septations
- **Mucinous Cystadenoma**
  - Thin-walled cyst
  - Usually multilocular
  - Components of cyst have differing echogenicity
- **Cystadenocarcinoma**
  - Thick irregular wall
  - Thick irregular septations
  - Solid elements with flow suggest malignancy
    - Doppler useful to prove solid-appearing areas are not blood clot

13

COMPLEX CYSTIC ADNEXAL MASS

- Resistive index tends to be low in malignancy (< 0.4)
  - Resistive index is neither sensitive nor specific for malignancy
- Bilateral lesions increase likelihood of malignancy
- Risk of malignancy increases with patient age
- Signs of metastatic disease
  - Ascites
  - Omental thickening
  - Serosal metastases on liver &/or spleen
- **Granulosa Cell Tumor**
  - Due to estrogen secretion, associated with postmenopausal bleed and precocious puberty, depending on patient age
- **Endometrioid Carcinoma, Ovary**
  - 30% are bilateral
  - Associated with endometriosis in 15-20%
- **Hydrosalpinx**
  - Cystic components connect
  - Tubular structure
- **Tubo-Ovarian Abscess**
  - Complex hypoechoic mass
  - Irregular margins
  - Free fluid
  - Clinical findings of infection
    - Vaginal discharge
    - Cervical motion tenderness
    - Pain
    - Fever
    - Elevated white blood cell count
- **Peritoneal Inclusion Cysts**
  - History of prior surgery

- Cysts surround ovarian tissue
- Septations with blood flow can simulate malignancy
- **Adnexal Torsion**
  - Complex cyst presenting with torsion usually due to underlying adnexal pathology
  - Unilateral lesion in patient with severe ipsilateral pain
  - Pain out of proportion to appearance of cyst suggests torsion
  - Blood flow may be absent on affected side
  - Not all cases of torsion have abnormal blood flow

Helpful Clues for Rare Diagnoses
- **Theca Lutein Cysts**
  - Increased HCG levels
    - Fertility drugs
    - Gestational trophoblastic disease
  - Bilateral, multiple

Alternative Differential Approaches
- Patient age/menstrual status aids in differential diagnosis
  - Prepubertal girls
    - Granulosa cell tumor
    - Immature teratoma, ovary
  - Postmenopausal women
    - Cystadenoma
    - Cystadenocarcinoma
    - Undifferentiated carcinoma
    - Endometrioid carcinoma
    - Granulosa cell tumor

Hemorrhagic Cysts, Ovary

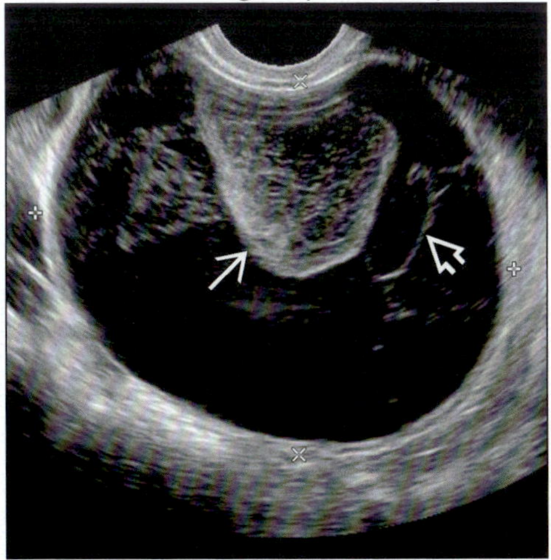

Longitudinal transvaginal ultrasound shows an 8 cm cyst (calipers) with a retractile clot ➔*. Note the adjacent cobweb appearance* ➔*.*

Dermoid (Mature Teratoma)

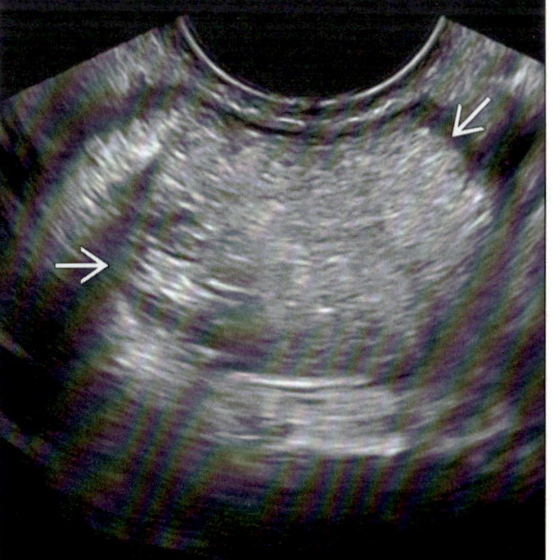

Longitudinal oblique transvaginal ultrasound shows a diffusely echogenic mass ➔ *with linear bright echoes. Note that the cyst mimics a loop of bowel.*

13

COMPLEX CYSTIC ADNEXAL MASS

(Left) Transverse transvaginal ultrasound shows a cyst with diffuse, homogeneous, low-level internal echoes. Note the punctate echogenicity in the cyst ➡ and a septation ➡. There is also a fluid-fluid layer in the dependent portion of the cyst ➡. (Right) Longitudinal transvaginal ultrasound shows a 5 cm complex right adnexal cyst (calipers) with septations and solid elements.

Endometrioma

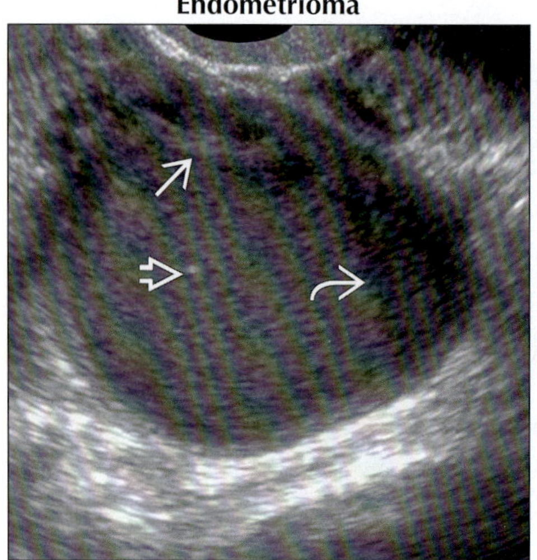

Serous Cystadenoma

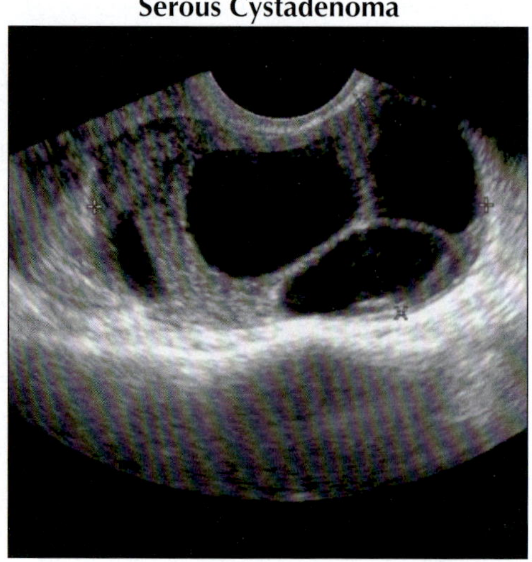

(Left) Longitudinal power Doppler ultrasound shows a 17 cm cyst with septations with blood flow. Note the low-level echoes in the cyst contents. (Right) Transverse transabdominal ultrasound shows a 10 cm cyst with a mural nodule (calipers). This is a borderline serous cystadenocarcinoma.

Mucinous Cystadenoma

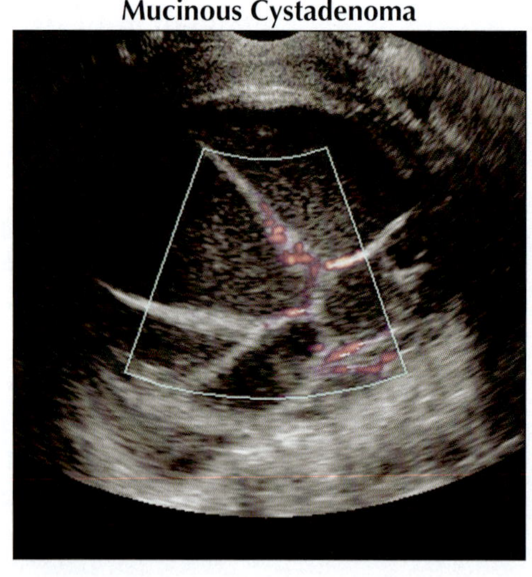

Cystadenocarcinoma

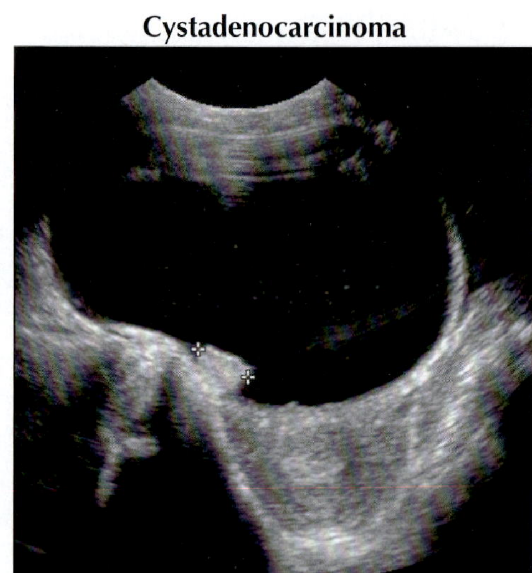

(Left) Longitudinal transvaginal ultrasound shows an 11 cm right complex cyst with a solid portion ➡ that has multiple septations. Note the layering debris ➡. (Right) Longitudinal transvaginal ultrasound in a 68 year old shows a cystic and solid adnexal mass (calipers). The solid portion has areas of increased echogenicity ➡, consistent with calcifications. The complex nature of this mass in a postmenopausal woman suggests an ovarian neoplasm.

Cystadenocarcinoma

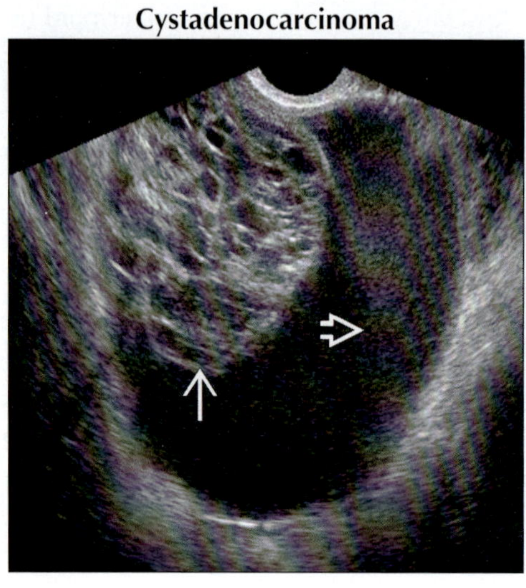

Cystadenofibroma

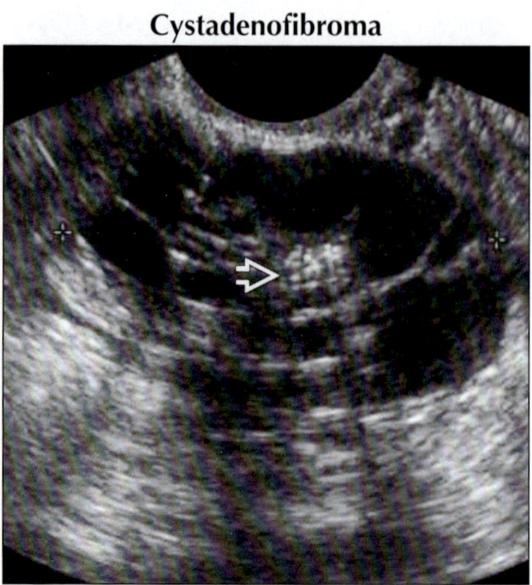

COMPLEX CYSTIC ADNEXAL MASS

Hydrosalpinx

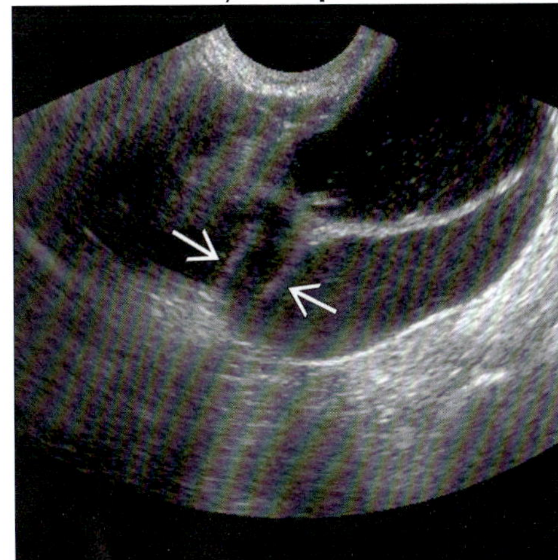

Tubo-Ovarian Abscess

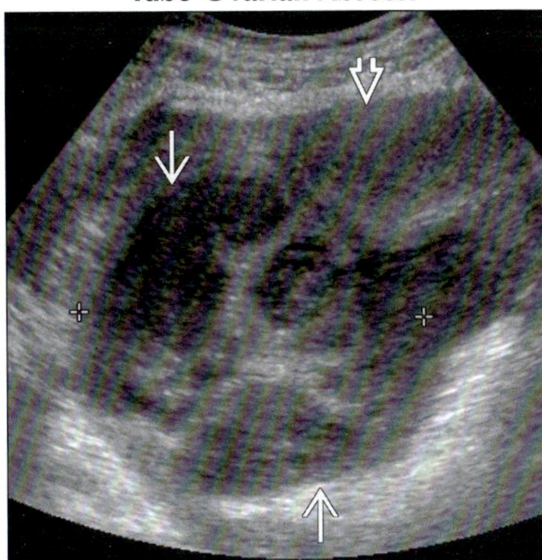

(Left) Oblique transvaginal ultrasound shows an oblong cyst folded on itself. Note that the "septations" ➡ do not extend from 1 wall to the other and that fluid can be seen to communicate throughout the "cyst." *(Right)* Transverse transabdominal ultrasound shows a large complex fluid collection ➡ located posterior to the uterus ➡.

Peritoneal Inclusion Cysts

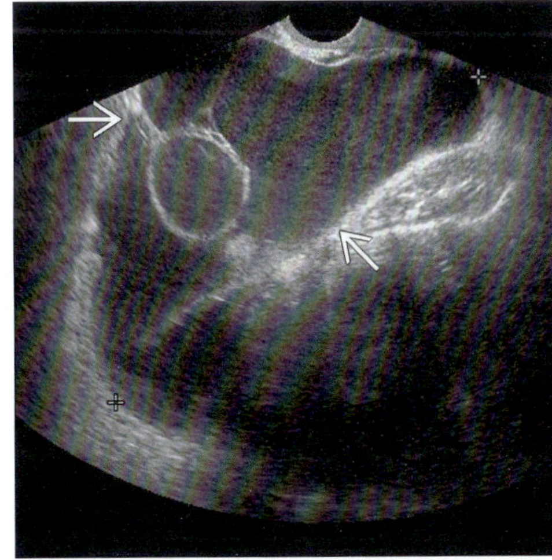

Peritoneal Inclusion Cysts

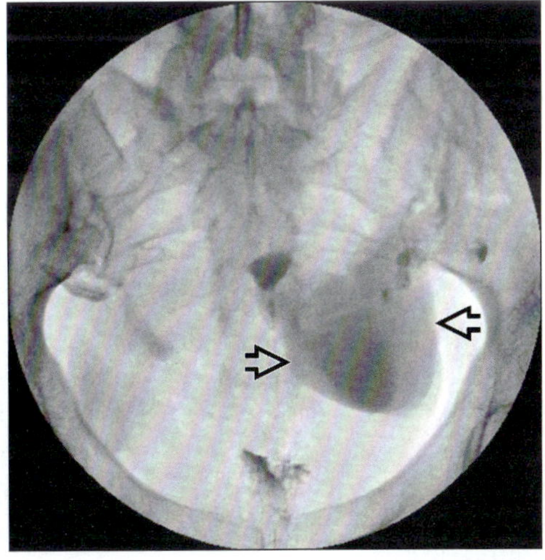

(Left) Longitudinal transvaginal ultrasound shows an oblong, septated cyst (calipers and ➡) with debris within the cyst. Peritoneal inclusion cysts typically form around the ovaries, but at times the ovaries are not visualized. *(Right)* Anteroposterior hysterosalpingogram in the same patient shows a loculated spill ➡ due to adhesions.

Ovarian Hyperstimulation Syndrome

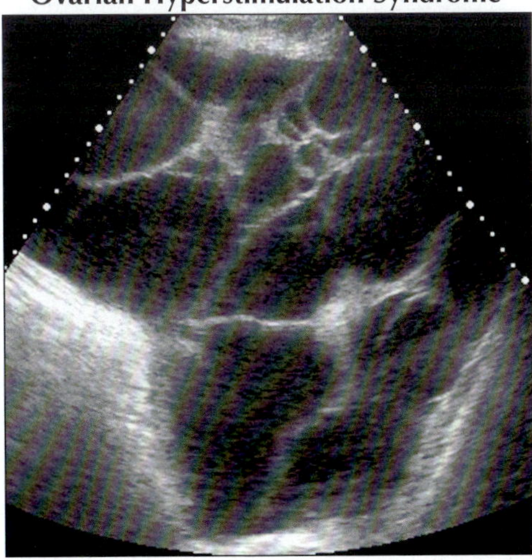

Hyperreactio Luteinalis

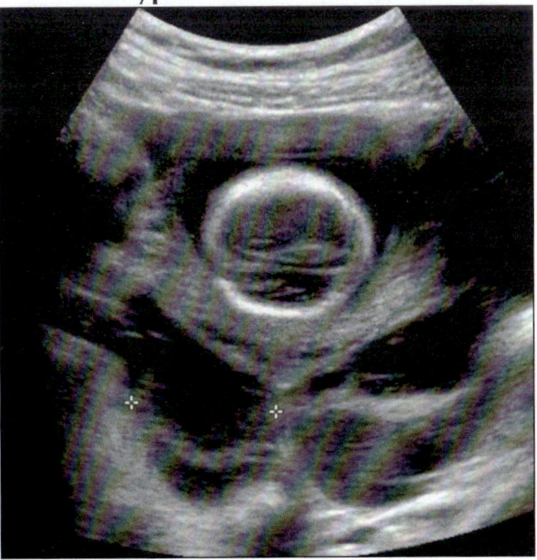

(Left) Transverse transabdominal ultrasound shows massive enlargement of the ovary (31 cm) due to hyperstimulation in a patient who underwent in vitro fertilization and presented with pleural effusion and shortness of breath. *(Right)* Transverse transabdominal ultrasound shows enlarged ovaries with multiple cysts in a pregnant patient. The cysts resolved postpartum.

13

SOLID ADNEXAL MASS

DIFFERENTIAL DIAGNOSIS

Common
- Leiomyoma

Less Common
- Adnexal Torsion
- Metastases, Ovary
- Primary Ovarian Malignancy
  - Mucinous Cystadenocarcinoma
  - Serous Cystadenocarcinoma
  - Endometrioid Carcinoma
- Fibrothecoma
- Solid Adnexal Mass (Mimics)
  - Hemorrhagic Ovarian Cyst
  - Obstructed Uterine Duplication
  - Pelvic Kidney
  - Rectosigmoid Carcinoma

Rare but Important
- Ovarian Lymphoma
- Tubo-Ovarian Abscess
- Tubal Carcinoma
- Luteoma of Pregnancy
- Adenofibroma
- Granulosa Cell Tumor
- Brenner Tumor
- Germ Cell Tumor
  - Dermoid (Mature Teratoma)
  - Immature Teratoma
  - Dysgerminoma
  - Choriocarcinoma

ESSENTIAL INFORMATION

Key Differential Diagnosis Issues
- Ovaries visualized separate from mass suggests nonovarian etiology
- If mass appears fibrotic with shadowing, tends to be benign fibrous lesions
  - Leiomyoma
  - Fibrothecoma
  - Adenofibroma
- Bilateral lesions
  - Primary ovarian malignancy
  - Lymphoma
  - Metastases
  - Endometrioid carcinoma
- Hormonally active lesion
  - Thecoma
  - Granulosa cell tumor

Helpful Clues for Common Diagnoses
- **Leiomyoma**
  - May be subserosal, exophytic, pedunculated
  - Ovaries are seen separate from mass
  - Fibrous appearance with shadowing
  - Blood flow is seen connecting mass to uterus
  - MR helpful in establishing etiology (leiomyoma vs. primary ovarian tumor)
  - Can grow during pregnancy due to hormonal stimulation
    - Causes pain
    - Appears as growing, solid adnexal mass

Helpful Clues for Less Common Diagnoses
- **Adnexal Torsion**
  - Unilateral lesion in patient with severe ipsilateral pain
  - Enlarged ovary
  - Multiple, small, peripheral follicles or mass acting as lead point
  - Blood flow may be absent on affected side, but not all cases of torsion have abnormal blood flow
- **Metastases, Ovary**
  - Patient with known primary carcinoma, most commonly from colon, gastric, breast, lung, or contralateral ovary
  - Krukenberg tumors are metastatic ovarian tumors that contain mucin-secreting signet-ring cells, usually of GI origin
- **Primary Ovarian Malignancy**
  - May have other signs of malignancy such as ascites, omental thickening, serosal metastases on liver &/or spleen
  - **Endometrioid Carcinoma**
    - 30% are bilateral
    - Typical mixed cystic and solid adnexal mass but may appear solid
    - Associated with endometriosis in 15-20%
- **Fibrothecoma**
  - Typically seen in women age 40-60
  - May be associated with hirsutism and amenorrhea if it secretes androgen
  - May be associated with endometrial thickening if it secretes estrogen
- **Solid Adnexal Mass (Mimics)**
  - **Hemorrhagic Ovarian Cyst**
    - May masquerade as solid lesion when acute

13

- Clues to diagnosis are increased through transmission and lack of blood flow within lesion
- Short-term follow-up will show rapid change in appearance of blood products
○ **Obstructed Uterine Duplication**
  - Look for deviation of uterus/endometrial stripe away from side of obstructed horn
  - Look for duplication of cervix
○ **Pelvic Kidney**
  - Look for reniform shape, collecting system, and ipsilateral empty renal fossa

Helpful Clues for Rare Diagnoses
- **Ovarian Lymphoma**
  ○ Most cases of ovarian involvement are in patients with systemic disease
  ○ Primary ovarian lymphoma is rare
  ○ Homogeneous, bilateral, solid masses with lack of ascites
- **Tubo-Ovarian Abscess**
  ○ Patient with pelvic pain, vaginal discharge, elevated white blood cell count
- **Tubal Carcinoma**
  ○ May be associated with hydrosalpinx
  ○ Seen between uterus and ovary
  ○ Tube may be enlarged with tubular-shaped, solid mass
- **Luteoma of Pregnancy**
  ○ Solid, ovarian, nonneoplastic mass that occurs during pregnancy
  ○ Elevated androgen levels
  ○ May cause virilization
  ○ Regresses postpartum

- **Adenofibroma**
  ○ Fibrous lesion with shadowing
  ○ Benign epithelial tumor
  ○ Bilateral in 10-20% of cases
- **Granulosa Cell Tumor**
  ○ Due to estrogen secretion, associated with postmenopausal bleeding and precocious puberty, depending on patient age
- **Brenner Tumor**
  ○ Almost always benign
  ○ May have calcifications

Alternative Differential Approaches
- Patient age/menstrual status aids in differential diagnosis
  ○ Prepubertal girls
    - Granulosa cell tumor
    - Germ cell tumor
    - Immature teratoma, ovary
  ○ Reproductive age
    - Leiomyoma, subserosal
    - Dermoid (mature teratoma)
    - Primary ovarian malignancy
    - Fibrothecoma, ovary
  ○ Postmenopausal
    - Fibrothecoma, ovary
    - Primary ovarian malignancy
    - Metastases, ovary
    - Leiomyoma
  ○ Pregnant patient
    - Luteoma of pregnancy
    - Leiomyoma, subserosal, exophytic, pedunculated, within broad ligament

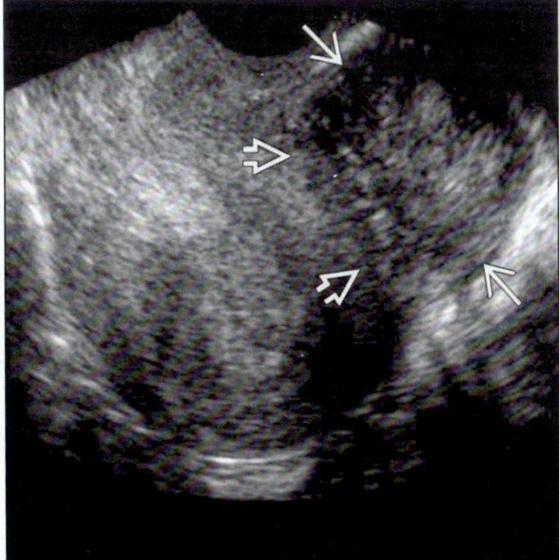

Leiomyoma

Longitudinal transvaginal ultrasound shows a mass ➡ exophytic off the uterus, with a broad base of attachment ➡.

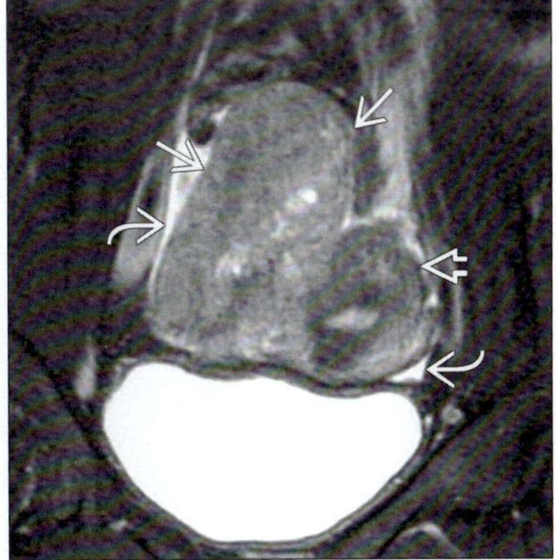

Leiomyoma

Coronal T2WI FS MR in the same patient shows the mass ➡ to the right of the uterus ➡. Note the small amount of ascites ➡.

SOLID ADNEXAL MASS

(Left) Longitudinal transvaginal ultrasound shows a mobile solid mass ➡ posterior to the uterus ⮕. (Right) Transverse transabdominal ultrasound in a woman with severe right lower quadrant pain shows a large right-sided mass (calipers). Note the edematous appearance of the ovary.

Leiomyoma

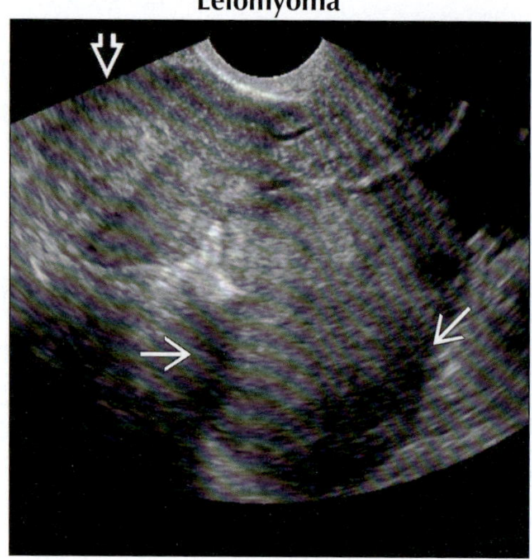

Adnexal Torsion

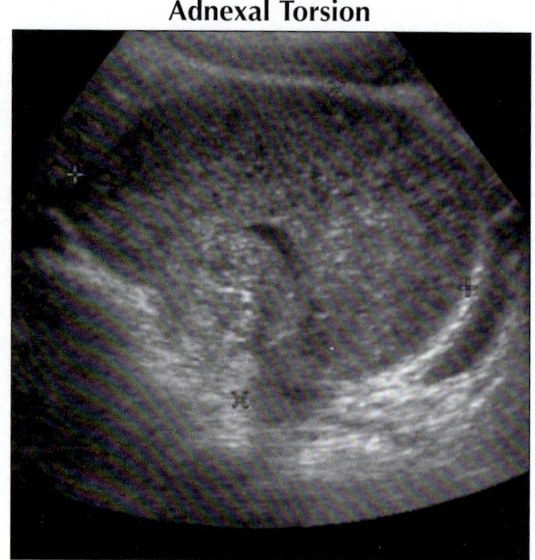

(Left) Longitudinal color Doppler ultrasound shows a bilobed solid adnexal mass ⮕ with blood flow centrally. (Right) Transverse transabdominal ultrasound shows multiple lobulated solid masses ⮕.

Metastases, Ovary

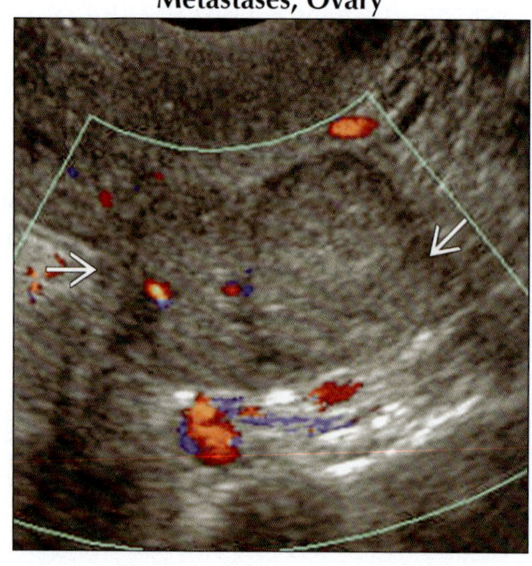

Metastases, Ovary

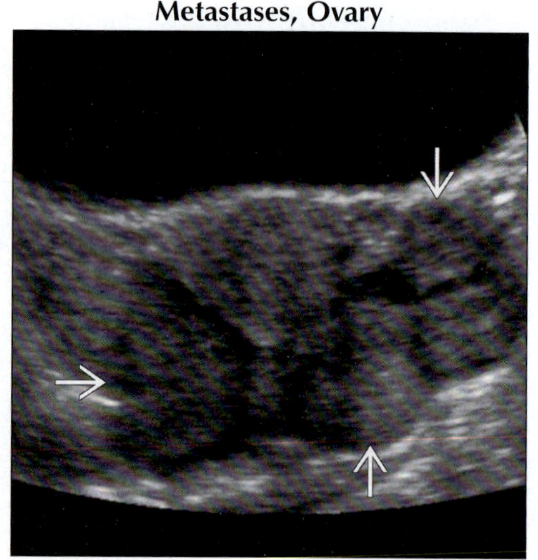

(Left) Oblique transabdominal ultrasound shows a solid-appearing mass (calipers) with increased through transmission ⮕. (Right) Oblique color Doppler ultrasound shows pronounced blood flow with tortuous vessels centrally.

Mucinous Cystadenocarcinoma

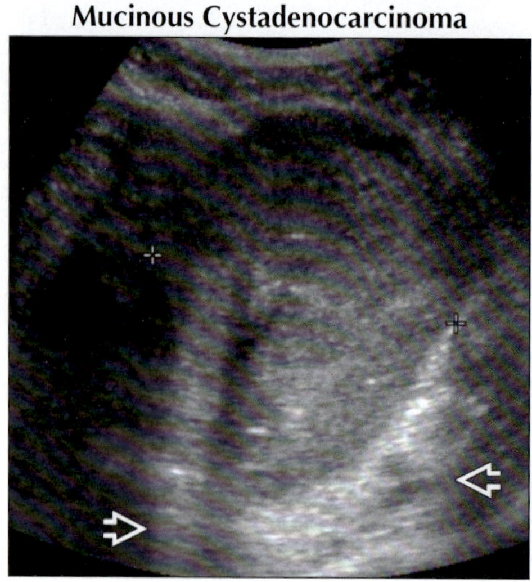

Mucinous Cystadenocarcinoma

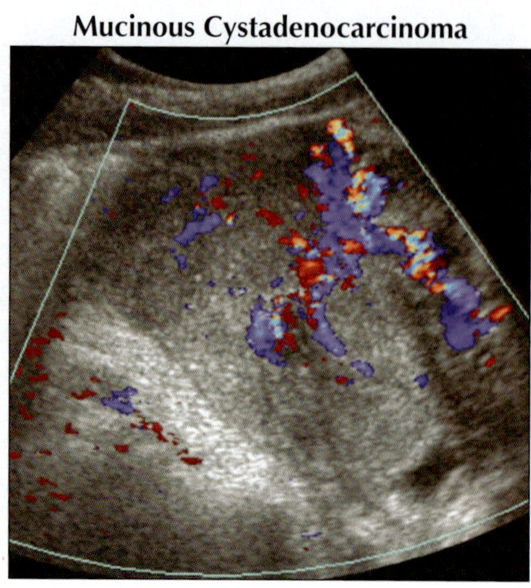

13

SOLID ADNEXAL MASS

Fibrothecoma

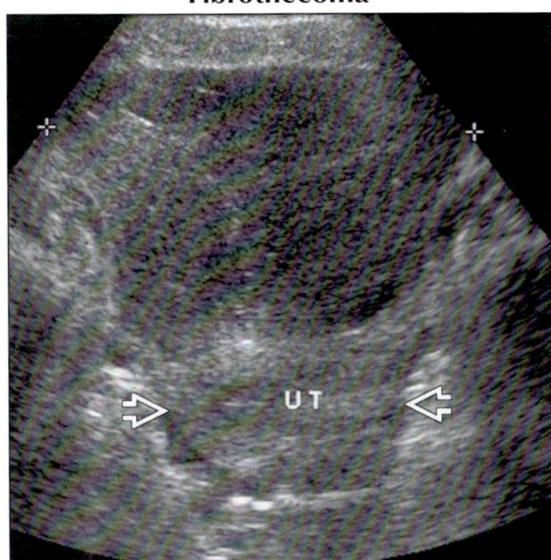

Fibrothecoma

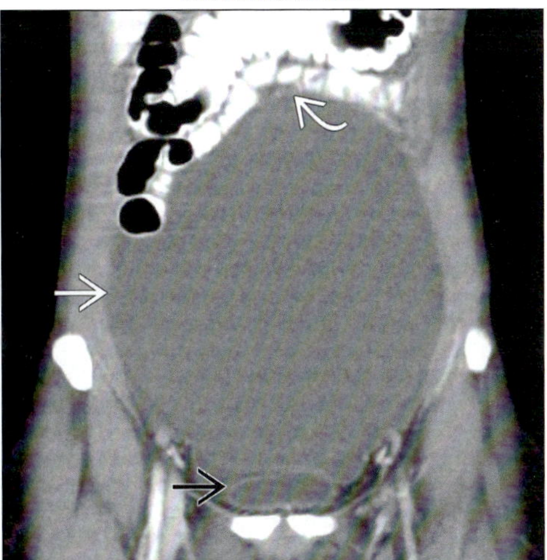

(Left) Transverse transabdominal ultrasound shows a solid pelvic mass (calipers) located anterior to the uterus (UT, ➡). *(Right)* Coronal CECT in the same patient shows the large solid mass ➡ deviating the bowel loops superiorly ➡. Note the bladder ➡ inferior to the mass.

Fibrothecoma

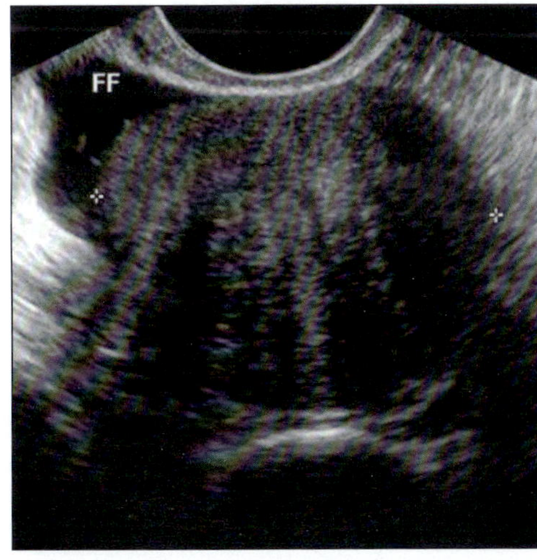

Hemorrhagic Ovarian Cyst

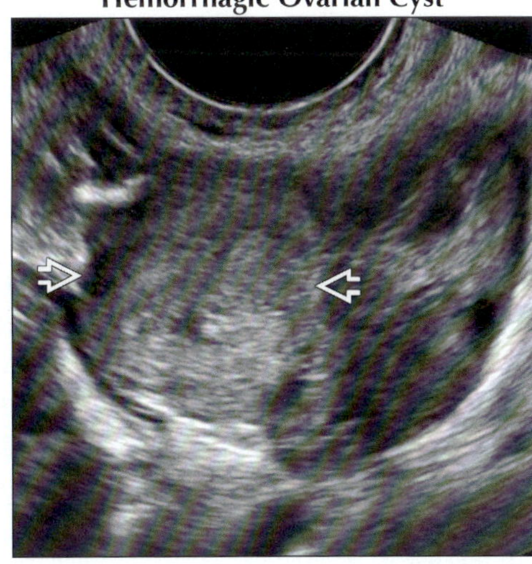

(Left) Longitudinal transvaginal ultrasound shows a 5 cm solid mass (calipers) with a small amount of ascites (FF). Note the alternating rays of shadowing, suggesting a fibrous etiology to the mass. *(Right)* Oblique transvaginal ultrasound shows an exophytic, echogenic mass ➡ off the ovary with through transmission, consistent with an acutely hemorrhagic cyst. This can mimic a solid lesion but the appearance changes on short-term follow-up.

Ovarian Lymphoma

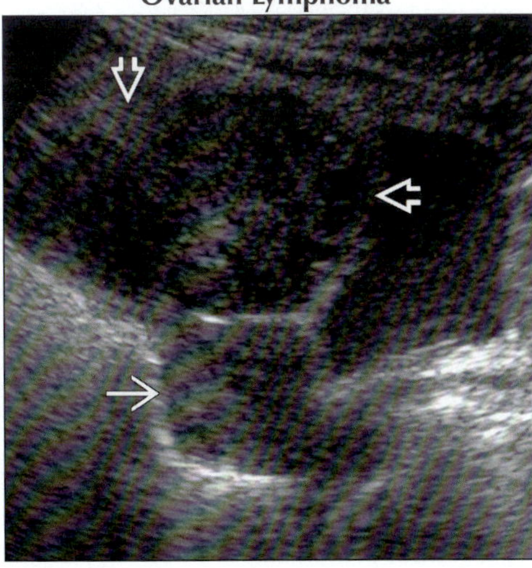

Ovarian Lymphoma

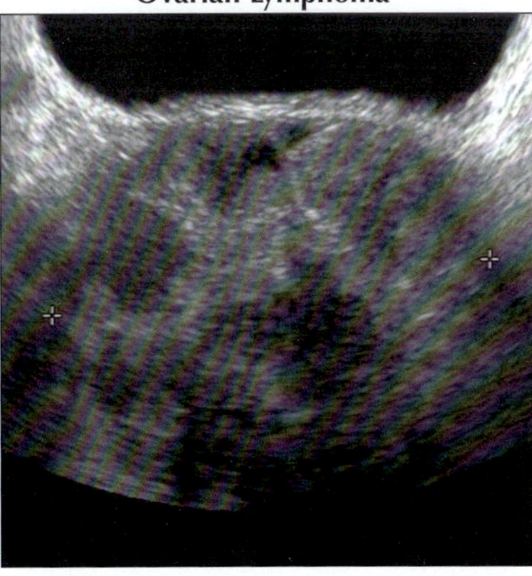

(Left) Longitudinal transabdominal ultrasound shows a large solid mass ➡ above the uterus ➡. *(Right)* Transverse transvaginal ultrasound in the same patient shows the mass (calipers) to be heterogeneous. This was confirmed to be lymphoma.

13

EXTRA-OVARIAN ADNEXAL MASS

DIFFERENTIAL DIAGNOSIS

Common
- Tubal Ectopic Pregnancy
- Endometrioma
- Subserosal Leiomyoma
- Paraovarian Cyst
- Paratubal Cyst
- Exophytic Ovarian Mass

Less Common
- Fallopian Tube Leiomyoma
- Hydrosalpinx
- Tubo-Ovarian Abscess
- Peritoneal Inclusion Cysts
- Lymphocele
- Nongynecologic Mass in Adnexal Region
  - Bowel Loop
  - Pelvic Varices
  - Appendicitis
  - Diverticulitis
  - Hydroureter
  - Bladder Diverticulum
  - Renal Ectopia (Pelvic Kidney)
  - Duplication Cyst
  - Tarlov Cyst

Rare but Important
- Hematosalpinx
- Tubal Torsion
- Heterotopic Pregnancy
- Tubal Carcinoma

ESSENTIAL INFORMATION

Key Differential Diagnosis Issues
- Is mass separate from ovary?
  - If adherent to ovary, may be exophytic ovarian mass
  - Tubal lesions may compress ovary and appear to arise from ovary
- Is mass separate from uterus?
  - Leiomyomas may show broad base of attachment to uterus
  - Leiomyomas may show blood flow from uterus
- Does blood flow connect mass to uterus or ovary?
- Is patient pregnant?
  - Ectopic pregnancy, tubal
  - Ectopic pregnancy, heterotopic
- Is patient febrile with elevated white blood cell count?

- Hydrosalpinx
- Tubo-ovarian abscess
- Appendicitis
- Diverticulitis

Helpful Clues for Common Diagnoses
- **Tubal Ectopic Pregnancy**
  - Pain &/or bleeding in 1st trimester
  - Echogenic ring-like mass separate from ovary
  - May see yolk sac or embryo
  - Free fluid with debris is blood
- **Endometrioma**
  - "Chocolate" cyst with diffuse homogeneous low-level internal echoes
  - ± layering debris
  - Thick wall
  - May have punctate calcifications in wall of cyst
  - May have septations with blood flow
  - Cyclic pelvic pain
- **Subserosal Leiomyoma**
  - Fibrous appearance with shadowing
  - Connection to uterus may be visualized
  - Blood flow from uterus may be present
  - MR helpful in establishing etiology (leiomyoma vs. primary ovarian tumor)
- **Paraovarian and Paratubal Cysts**
  - Separate from ovary
  - Thin walled
  - Anechoic
  - Tend not to change in size over time

Helpful Clues for Less Common Diagnoses
- **Hydrosalpinx**
  - Tubular mass
  - Cysts connect
  - Real-time scanning helpful to visualize connecting cysts
  - Prior pelvic inflammatory disease or endometriosis
- **Tubo-Ovarian Abscess**
  - Complex hypoechoic mass
  - Irregular margins
  - Free fluid
  - Clinical findings of infection
    - Pain
    - Fever
    - Elevated white blood cell count
  - Vaginal discharge
  - Cervical motion tenderness
- **Peritoneal Inclusion Cysts**
  - History of prior surgery

13

EXTRA-OVARIAN ADNEXAL MASS

- ○ Surround ovarian tissue
- ○ Irregular shape with poorly defined walls (formed by adjacent organs)
- ○ Septations with blood flow can simulate malignancy
- **Bowel Loop**
  - ○ Assess for peristalsis
  - ○ Change in appearance over time
- **Appendicitis**
  - ○ Rebound tenderness to scanning in right lower quadrant
  - ○ Dilated tubular blind-ending structure in region of patient's pain
  - ○ Tubular structure noncompressible
  - ○ ± adjacent fluid or appendicolith
  - ○ Clinical signs of infection
    - Pain
    - Fever
    - Elevated white blood cell count
- **Renal Ectopia (Pelvic Kidney)**
  - ○ Reniform shape of mass
  - ○ Collecting system
  - ○ Absent kidney in ipsilateral renal fossa

Helpful Clues for Rare Diagnoses
- **Hematosalpinx**
  - ○ Associated with tubal ectopic pregnancy or endometriosis
  - ○ Distended fallopian tube with fluid with debris
- **Tubal Torsion**
  - ○ Acute, colicky pain
  - ○ Associated with tubal mass or paraovarian cyst

- ○ Elongated cystic mass that tapers near cornua
- **Heterotopic Pregnancy**
  - ○ Intra- and extrauterine pregnancy
  - ○ Common in patients undergoing assisted fertilization
  - ○ Check for ovary separate from mass
- **Tubal Carcinoma**
  - ○ May be associated with hydrosalpinx
  - ○ Seen between uterus and ovary
  - ○ Tube may be enlarged with tubular solid mass

Alternative Differential Approaches
- Tubular mass
  - ○ Hydrosalpinx
    - Thin walled, anechoic
  - ○ Pyosalpinx
    - Thick walled, internal debris, patient with signs of infection
  - ○ Hematosalpinx
    - Filled with internal debris in patient with symptoms of ectopic pregnancy or endometriosis
- Bowel etiology of mass
  - ○ Peristalsis of normal bowel
  - ○ Abscess or cyst associated with bowel
  - ○ Appendicitis in right lower quadrant
  - ○ Diverticulitis in left lower quadrant

Tubal Ectopic Pregnancy

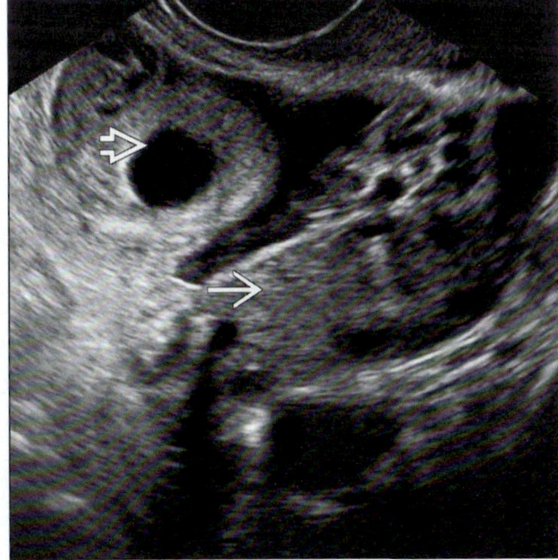

Oblique transvaginal ultrasound shows an echogenic ring-like mass ➡ separate from the left ovary ➡. There is adjacent free fluid with debris, consistent with blood.

Endometrioma

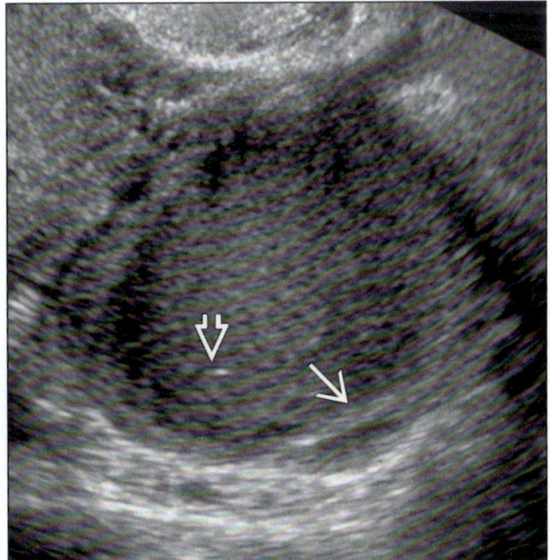

Longitudinal transvaginal ultrasound shows a cyst with diffuse, homogeneous, low-level, internal echoes. Note a punctate echogenicity in the cyst ➡ and a septation ➡.

13

EXTRA-OVARIAN ADNEXAL MASS

(Left) Longitudinal transvaginal ultrasound shows a mass ➡ exophytic off the uterus ➡ with a broad base of attachment to the uterus. (Right) Oblique transvaginal ultrasound shows 2 cysts in the right adnexa. There is a thick-walled cyst ➡, consistent with a corpus luteum. Adjacent to the ovary is an anechoic, thin-walled, paraovarian cyst (calipers).

Subserosal Leiomyoma

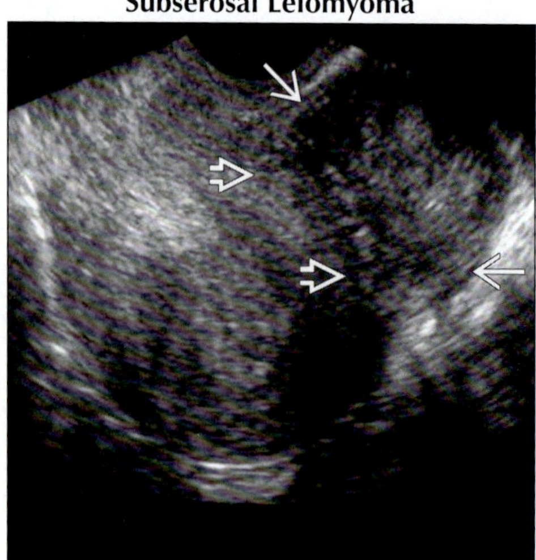

Paraovarian Cyst

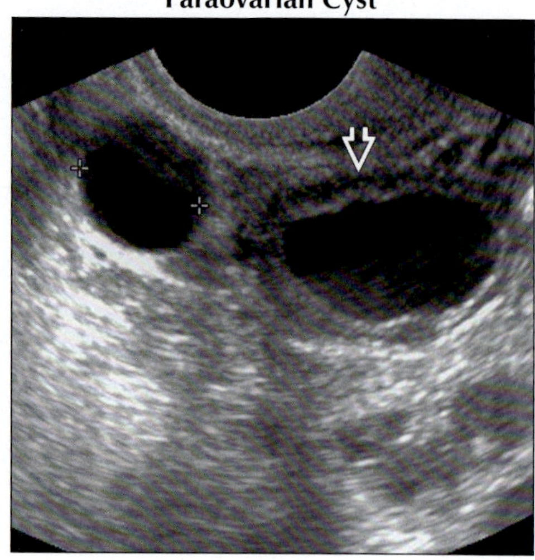

(Left) Longitudinal transabdominal ultrasound shows a 6 cm anechoic cyst ➡ anterior to the uterus (calipers). (Right) Transverse transvaginal ultrasound shows 2 cysts in the left adnexal region ➡. The ovaries are not seen separate from the cysts. This appearance could be due to 2 adjacent cysts or a hydrosalpinx folded on itself. At surgery, paratubal cysts were found.

Paratubal Cyst

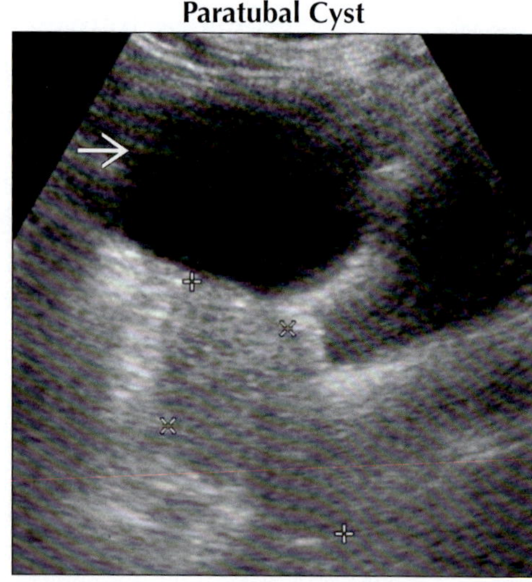

Paratubal Cyst

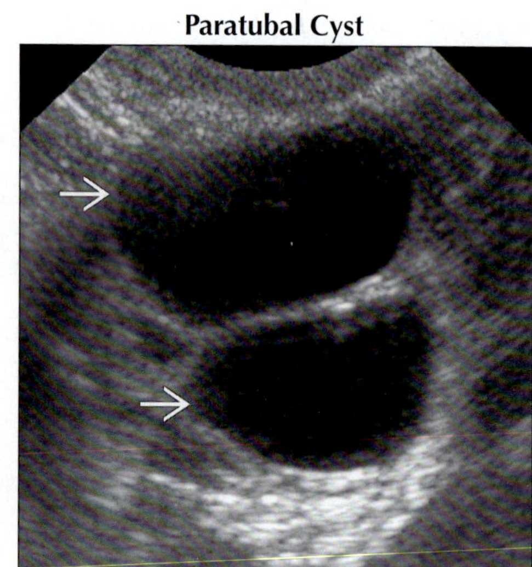

(Left) Oblique transvaginal ultrasound shows a 4 cm, complex, echogenic, thick-walled cyst ➡ exophytic off the right ovary ➡, which resolved on follow-up. On occasion, hemorrhagic cysts can be exophytic off the ovary and masquerade as an ectopic pregnancy. (Right) Transverse transvaginal ultrasound shows a serpiginous cystic structure ➡ in the right adnexa.

Exophytic Ovarian Mass

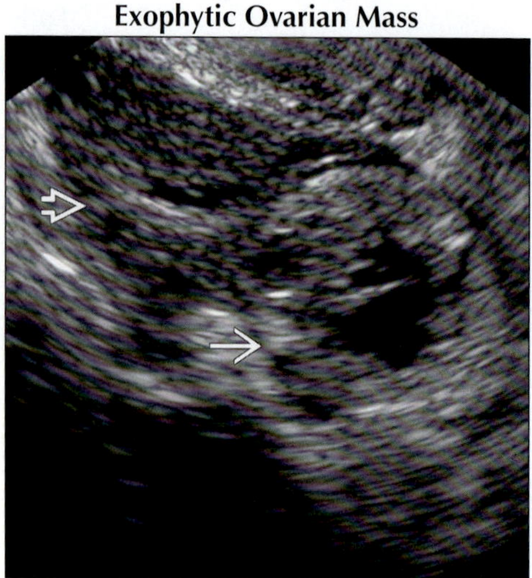

Hydrosalpinx

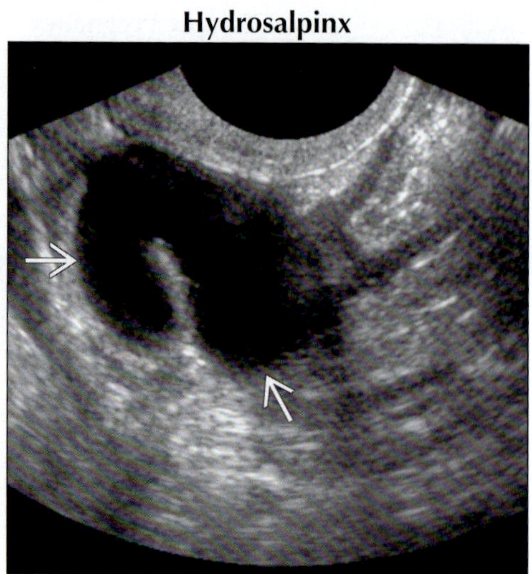

EXTRA-OVARIAN ADNEXAL MASS

Hydrosalpinx

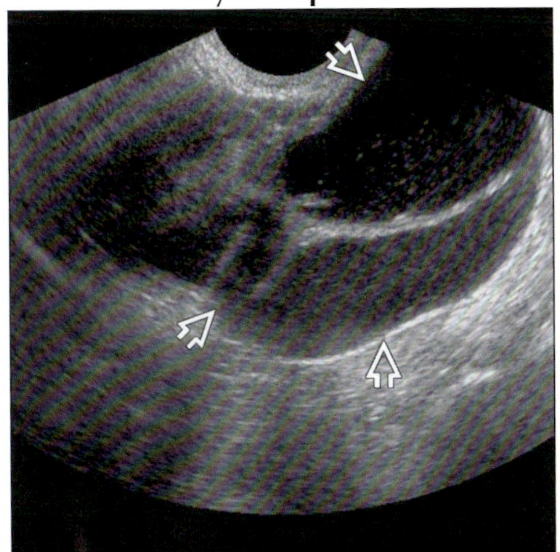

Tubo-Ovarian Abscess

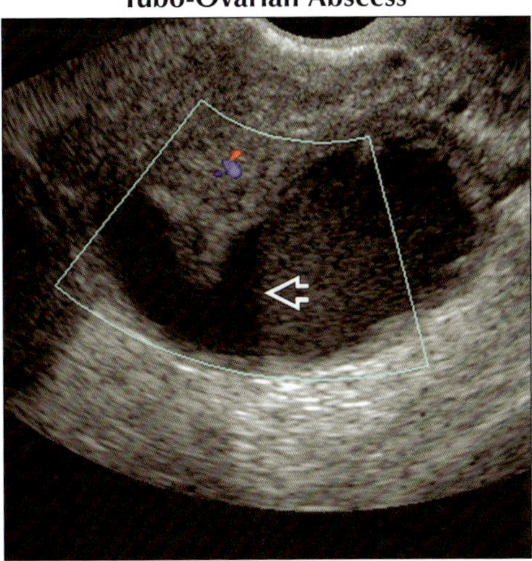

(Left) Oblique transvaginal ultrasound shows the oblong nature of a "cyst" folded on itself, typical of a hydrosalpinx. (Right) Oblique color Doppler ultrasound shows a dilated fallopian tube filled with debris. Note the layering of the debris within the tube.

Peritoneal Inclusion Cysts

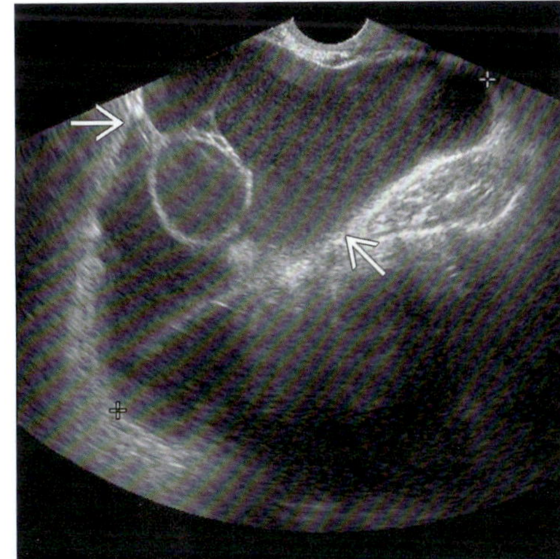

Appendicitis

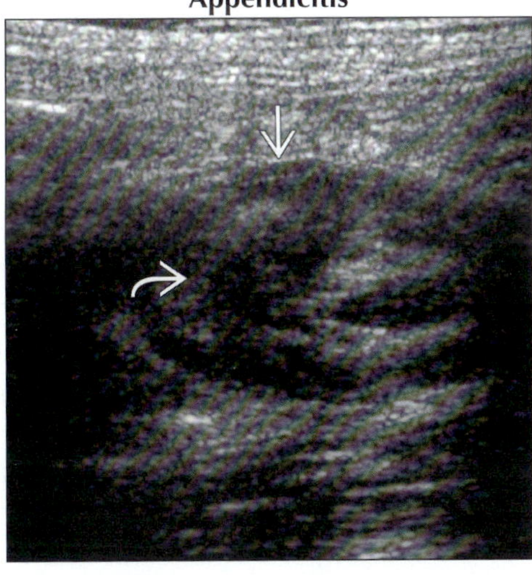

(Left) Longitudinal transvaginal ultrasound shows a septated fluid collection. Peritoneal inclusion cysts typically form around the ovaries but at times the ovaries are not visualized. (Right) Oblique transabdominal ultrasound in the right iliac fossa shows an enlarged and inflamed appendix. There is heterogeneity at the tip of the appendix, consistent with acute appendicitis with gangrenous changes at the tip.

Renal Ectopia (Pelvic Kidney)

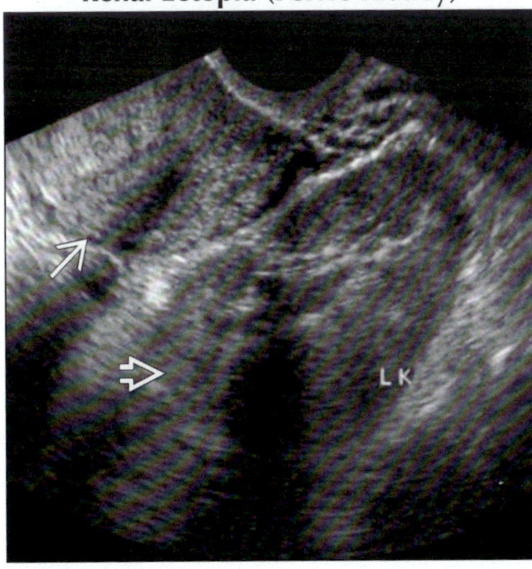

Heterotopic Pregnancy

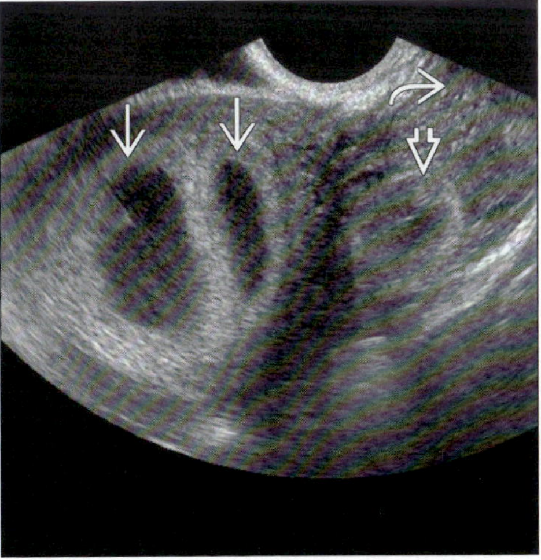

(Left) Oblique transvaginal ultrasound shows a left pelvic kidney (LK,) posterior to the uterus. (Right) Longitudinal transvaginal ultrasound shows 2 gestational sacs in the uterus with a thick dividing membrane, consistent with dichorionic diamniotic twins. In addition, there is an echogenic ring-like mass in the cul-de-sac with an adjacent blood clot.

DIFFERENTIAL DIAGNOSIS

Common
- Leiomyoma
- Adenomyosis
- Multiparous Patient
- Postpartum
  - Normal Postpartum
  - Endometritis

Less Common
- Cervical Stenosis
- Endometrial Cancer

Rare but Important
- Uterine Leiomyosarcoma
- Cervical Lesion
  - Cervical Leiomyoma
  - Cervical Cancer

ESSENTIAL INFORMATION

Key Differential Diagnosis Issues
- Enlarged uterus without focal mass
  - Diffuse adenomyosis
  - Multiparous patient
- Multiple masses
  - Round, well-defined masses
    - Intramural leiomyoma
  - Ovoid, ill-defined masses
    - Focal adenomyosis
- Fluid in endometrial cavity causing uterine enlargement
  - Cervical stenosis
- Ill-defined mass in uterine cavity
  - Endometrial cancer
- Lesion centered in cervix
  - Cervical leiomyoma
  - Cervical cancer

Helpful Clues for Common Diagnoses
- **Leiomyoma**
  - Focal, well-defined masses
  - May have pseudocapsule
  - Lobulated contour of uterus
- **Adenomyosis**
  - Asymmetric myometrial thickening
  - Cystic spaces in endometrium
  - Alternating bands of increased through transmission and shadowing
  - Uterus may be tender during examination

Helpful Clues for Less Common Diagnoses
- **Cervical Stenosis**
  - Patient with history of curettage or childbearing
  - Fluid in endometrial cavity
  - No lesion seen
  - Thin surrounding endometrium
- **Endometrial Cancer**
  - Patient typically presents with bleeding
  - Diffuse uterine enlargement
  - Ill-defined endometrium

Helpful Clues for Rare Diagnoses
- **Cervical Lesion**
  - Hypoechoic, ill-defined lesion suggests malignancy
  - Well-defined lesion could be leiomyoma

Leiomyoma

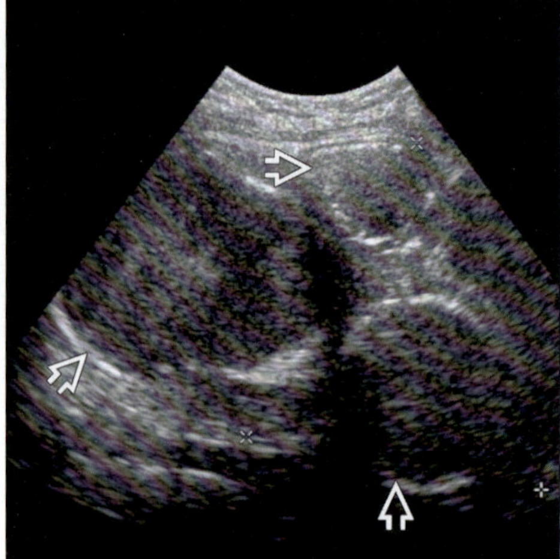

Longitudinal transabdominal ultrasound shows an enlarged uterus (over 20 cm in length) with multiple masses ➡ surrounded by calcific rims consistent with necrotic leiomyomas.

Adenomyosis

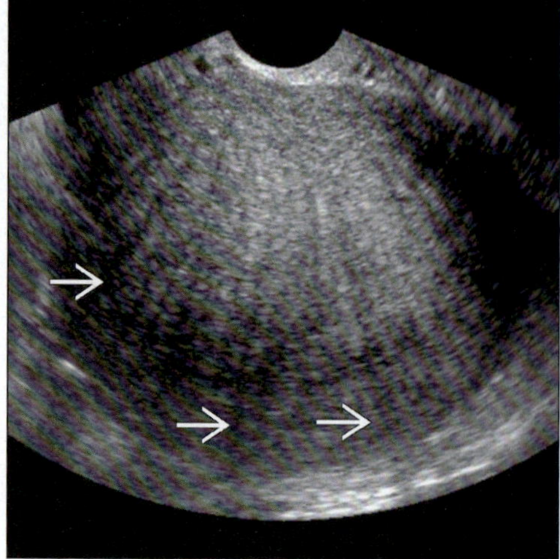

Transverse transvaginal ultrasound shows an enlarged, diffusely heterogeneous uterus measuring 10 x 10 x 10 cm with alternating bands of increased echogenicity and shadowing ➡.

ENLARGED UTERUS

Endometritis

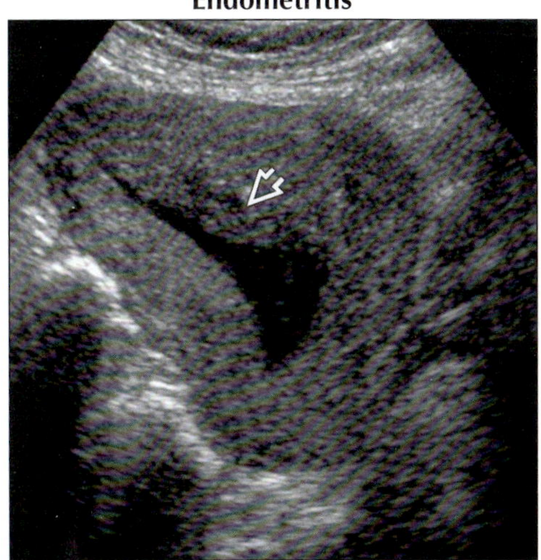

Cervical Stenosis

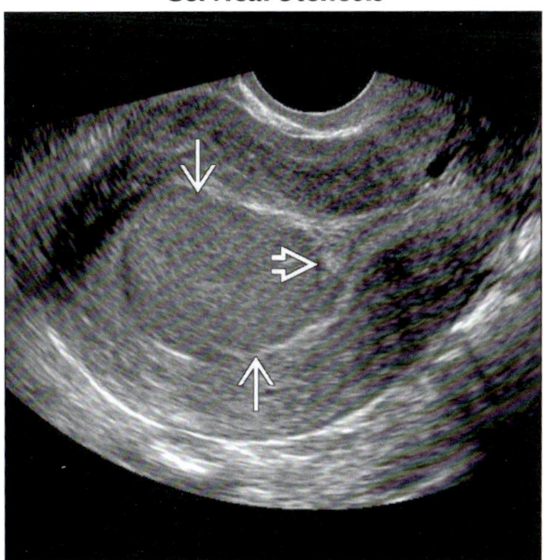

(Left) Longitudinal transabdominal ultrasound shows an enlarged uterus with endometrial fluid and a shaggy irregular appearance to the endometrium anteriorly ➡. (Right) Longitudinal transvaginal ultrasound in a woman after endometrial ablation shows that the endometrial cavity is filled with complex fluid ➡ with some echogenic debris ➡. The surrounding endometrium is thin.

Endometrial Cancer

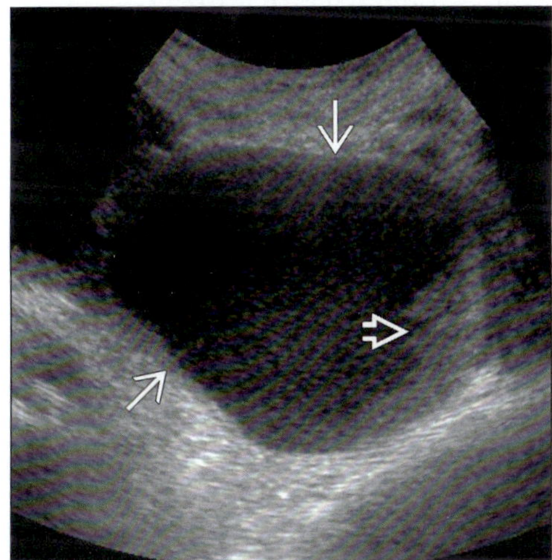

Uterine Leiomyosarcoma

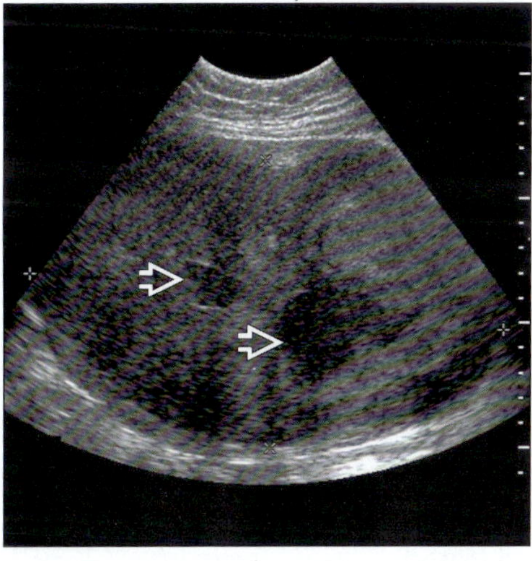

(Left) Oblique transabdominal ultrasound in 91-year-old woman shows an enlarged uterus ➡ distended with fluid and debris, consistent with blood products. A solid tissue mass ➡ is seen inferiorly. (Right) Longitudinal transabdominal ultrasound shows an enlarged uterus with a hypoechoic mass (calipers) with areas of necrosis ➡. The uterus had rapidly increased in size since a study 3 months before, raising the likelihood of malignancy.

Cervical Leiomyoma

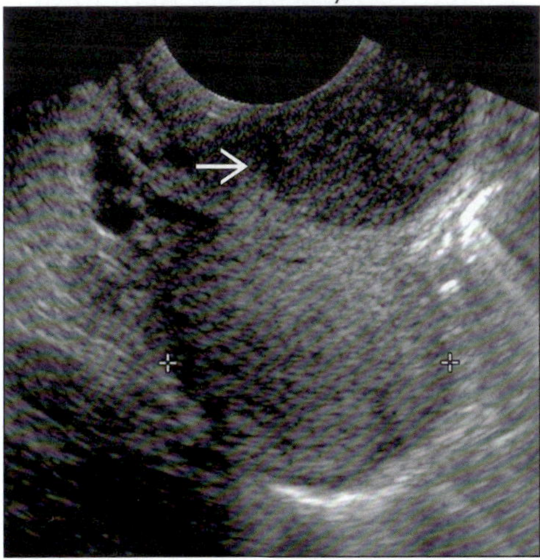

Cervical Cancer

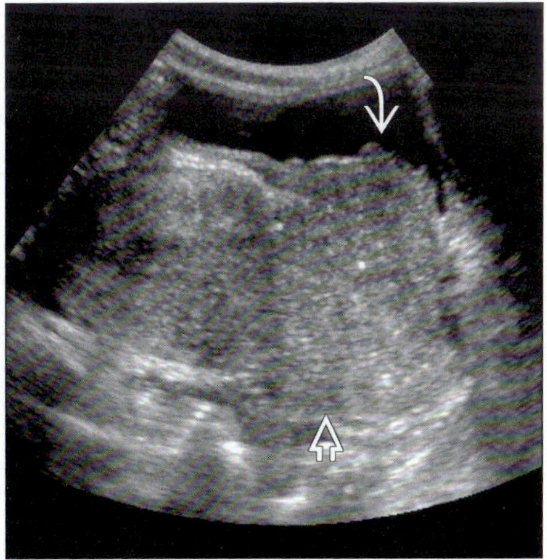

(Left) Transverse transvaginal ultrasound in a 55-year-old postmenopausal woman shows a well-defined hypoechoic mass ➡ in the cervix. Since the woman is postmenopausal, her uterus is relatively small (calipers), and therefore the cervical mass, although only 3.5 cm, is almost as large as the body of her uterus. (Right) Longitudinal transabdominal ultrasound shows a large, irregular, hypoechoic mass in the region of the cervix ➡. The mass invades the bladder ➡.

ABNORMAL UTERINE BLEEDING

DIFFERENTIAL DIAGNOSIS

Common
- Endometrial Polyps
- Endometrial Atrophy
- Leiomyoma
- Pregnancy and Complications
  - Normal Pregnancy
  - Subchorionic Hematoma
  - Tubal Ectopic Pregnancy
  - Hydatiform Mole

Less Common
- Adenomyosis
- C-Section Defect
- Endometrial Hyperplasia
- Endometrial Cancer
- Endocervical Polyp
- Cervical Cancer
- Endometritis
- Retained Products of Conception

Rare but Important
- Uterine Leiomyosarcoma
- Vulva Carcinoma
- Vaginal Carcinoma
- IUD Perforation
- Estrogen-Producing Tumor of Ovary
  - Granulosa Cell Tumor
  - Fibrothecoma, Ovary
- Ovarian Carcinoma
- Bleeding from GI or GU Tract

ESSENTIAL INFORMATION

Key Differential Diagnosis Issues
- Is patient premenopausal?
  - Pregnancy and complications
  - Endometrial polyps
  - Leiomyoma, submucosal
  - Endometrial hyperplasia
  - Malignancy (uterine, endometrial, cervical)
  - Nongynecologic sources of bleeding: Gastrointestinal or renal/bladder
- Is patient postmenopausal?
  - Bleeding due to hormone use
    - Hormones can affect endometrial thickness
  - Endometrial atrophy
  - Endometrial polyps
  - Endometrial cancer
  - Leiomyoma
  - Malignancy (uterine, endometrial, cervical)
  - Nongynecologic sources of bleeding: Gastrointestinal or urinary tract
- Is there focal thickening of endometrium?
  - Endometrial polyps: Most likely
  - Endometrial hyperplasia: Can be focal
  - Endometrial cancer, early stage
- Is endometrial-myometrial interface obscured?
  - Leiomyoma, submucosal
  - Endometrial cancer

Helpful Clues for Common Diagnoses
- **Endometrial Polyps**
  - Focal endometrial lesion
  - Echogenic
  - Smooth margins
  - ± vascular stalk
- **Endometrial Atrophy**
  - 75% of postmenopausal bleeding attributed to atrophy
  - Sonographic appearance of thin endometrium < 4 mm double layer thickness
- **Leiomyoma**
  - Shadowing
  - Iso- or hyperechoic
  - Submucosal leiomyomas most likely associated with bleeding
    - If > 50%, leiomyoma projects into endometrial cavity, this can be removed hysteroscopically
- **Pregnancy and Complications**
  - Positive urine/serum human chorionic gonadotropin
  - If intrauterine pregnancy
    - Normal pregnancy
    - Normal or abnormal intrauterine pregnancy with subchorionic hematoma
    - Miscarriage
    - Hydatidiform mole
  - If no intrauterine pregnancy visualized
    - Ectopic pregnancy
    - Normal pregnancy, too early to visualize
    - Miscarriage

Helpful Clues for Less Common Diagnoses
- **Adenomyosis**
  - Diffuse or asymmetric enlargement
  - ± tender uterus
  - ± small myometrial cysts
- **C-Section Defect**
  - Triangular collection anterior just above cervix

ABNORMAL UTERINE BLEEDING

- ○ Acts as reservoir for blood products, leading to intermenstrual bleeding
- **Endometrial Hyperplasia**
  - ○ Diffuse thickening most common but also can occur with focal thickening
  - ○ ± cystic spaces
- **Endometrial Cancer**
  - ○ Poor definition of endometrium
  - ○ Irregular, thickened, heterogeneous endometrium
  - ○ Loss of endometrial-myometrial interface

Other Essential Information

- Use transvaginal scanning for best evaluation of endometrium
  - ○ Sonohysterography helpful to distinguish if focal lesion present
  - ○ Diffuse thickening can be sampled with blind biopsy
  - ○ Focal mass best assessed with hysteroscopic biopsy
- In uterine duplication, anomalies must evaluate each endometrium separately
- Tamoxifen use leads to polyps, hyperplasia, and carcinoma, as well as reactivation of foci of adenomyosis
  - ○ Number of endometrial lesions related to cumulative dose
  - ○ Endometrial cancer in patients taking tamoxifen frequently arises in endometrial polyps
- Use endometrial thickness and appearance to triage postmenopausal patients with bleeding

- ○ Homogeneous endometrium: Measure combined thickness of anterior and posterior endometrium
- ○ < 4 mm likely atrophy, no need to biopsy
- ○ 4-8 mm, depends on hormone use
  - If taking continuous combined estrogen and progesterone, recommend biopsy
  - If taking sequential hormones, re-scan early or late in cycle to view endometrium at thinnest
- ○ > 8 mm, ↑ risk of neoplasm, recommend biopsy
- Any focal lesion needs biopsy

Alternative Differential Approaches

- Enlarged uterus
  - ○ Leiomyoma
  - ○ Adenomyosis
  - ○ Cervical stenosis with uterus distended with debris
  - ○ Endometrial carcinoma in advanced stage
- Solid or complex ovarian lesion in association with endometrial lesion
  - ○ Estrogenic effect from granulosa cell tumor leading to endometrial lesion
  - ○ Estrogen secretion from thecoma leading to endometrial lesion
  - ○ Concordant ovarian and endometrial carcinoma
  - ○ Endometrioid tumor
  - ○ Metastatic disease

Endometrial Polyps

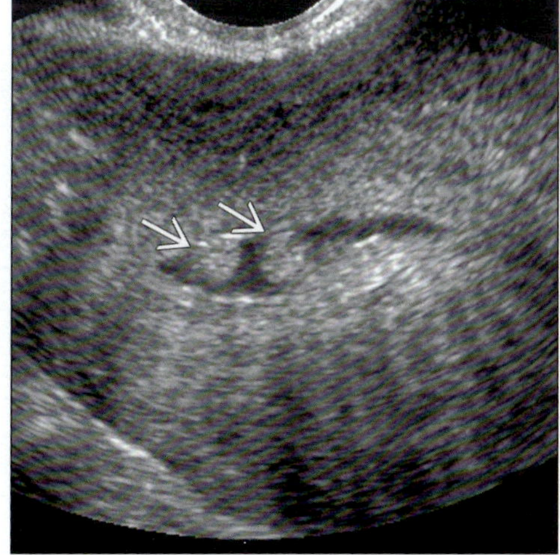

Transverse hysterosonogram shows multiple small echogenic masses ➔ arising from the endometrium.

Endometrial Polyps

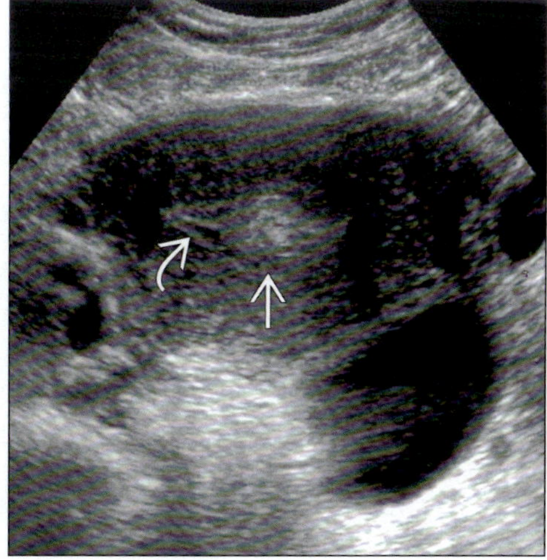

Transverse transabdominal ultrasound shows an echogenic mass ➔ in the endometrium. Note that the normal endometrial echo ➔ of the proliferative phase appearance is distorted by the endometrial lesion.

13

ABNORMAL UTERINE BLEEDING

(Left) Longitudinal transvaginal ultrasound shows a retroflexed uterus with a thin atrophic endometrium (calipers). (Right) Oblique transvaginal ultrasound shows a mass ➡ projecting into the endometrial cavity, with a small amount of endometrial fluid ➡. Note that more than 50% of the leiomyoma projects into the endometrial cavity. This will allow for hysteroscopic removal of the leiomyoma.

Endometrial Atrophy

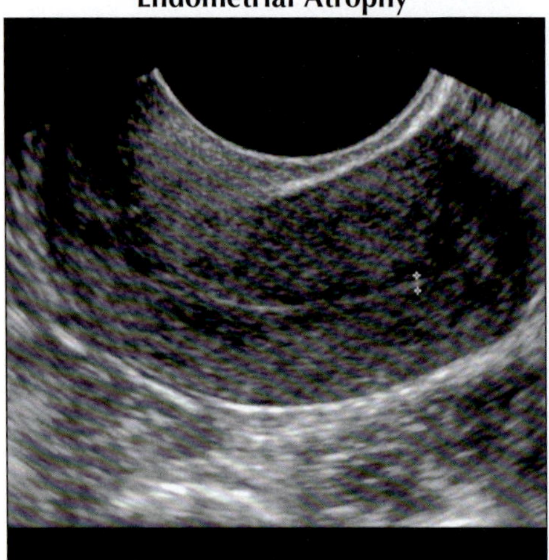

Leiomyoma

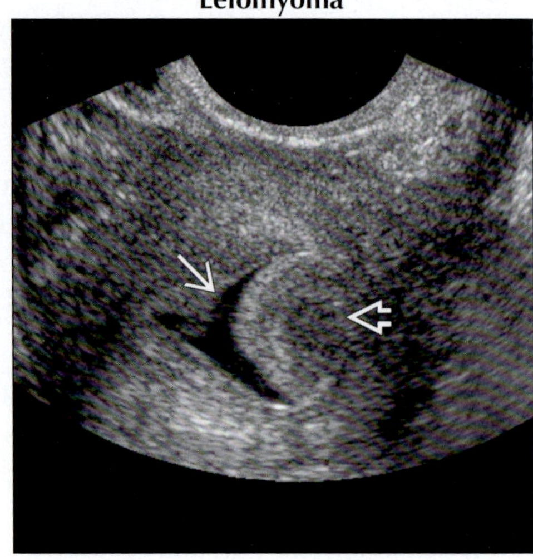

(Left) Longitudinal transabdominal ultrasound shows an enlarged heterogeneous uterus with multiple, solid, hypoechoic masses ➡ consistent with the leiomyomas. (Right) Oblique transabdominal ultrasound shows a marginal subchorionic hematoma ➡ in a patient 13 weeks pregnant with pain and bleeding.

Leiomyoma

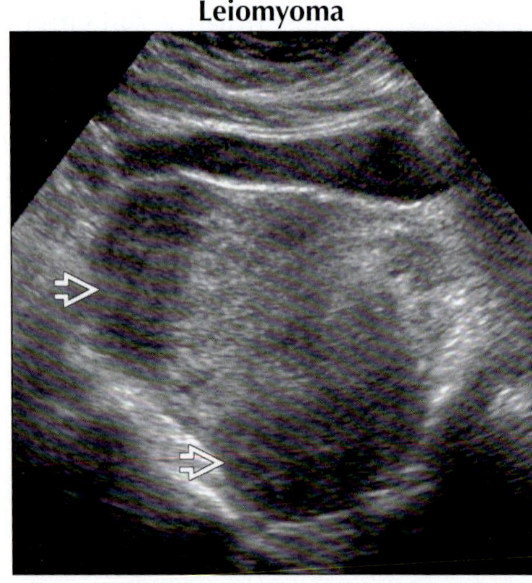

Subchorionic Hematoma

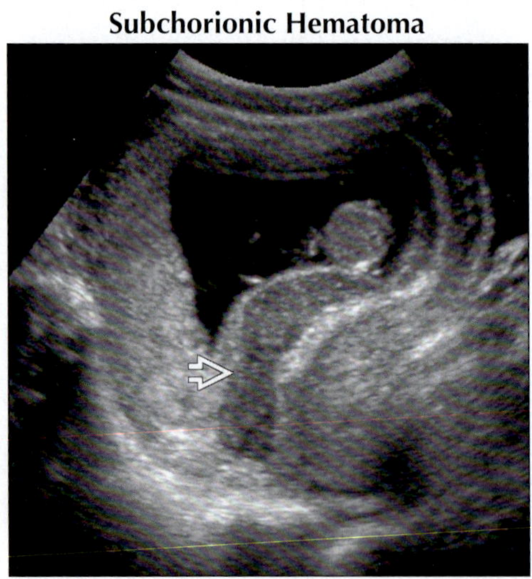

(Left) Longitudinal transabdominal ultrasound shows a complex fluid collection ➡ in the endometrial cavity in a woman with an ectopic pregnancy. This finding is consistent with a pseudosac. (Right) Transverse ultrasound shows a typical complete hydatidiform mole with the uterus filled by a complex cystic mass ➡. The fluid collection adjacent to the mass is hemorrhage ➡.

Tubal Ectopic Pregnancy

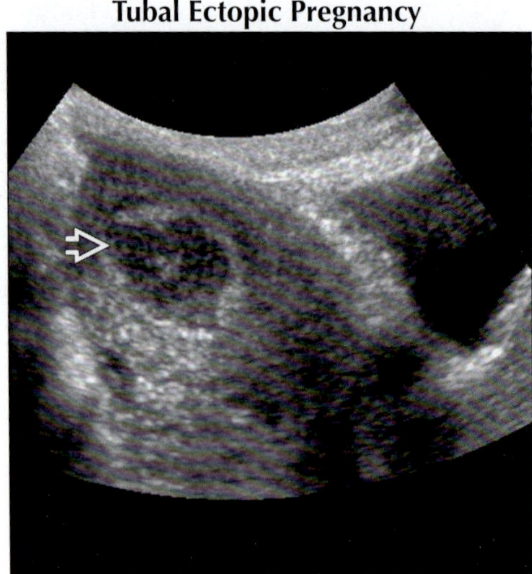

Hydatiform Mole

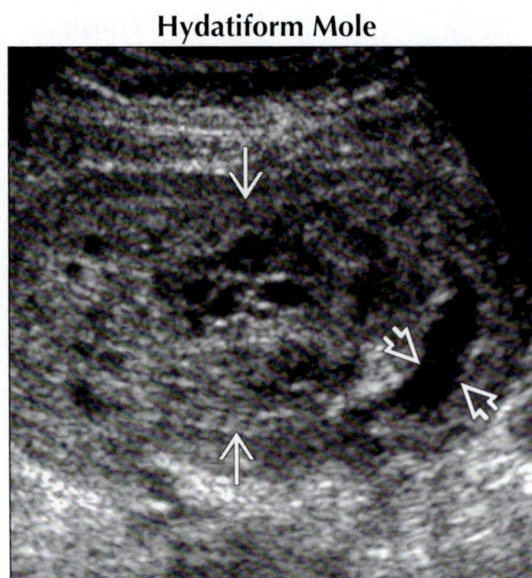

13

ABNORMAL UTERINE BLEEDING

C-Section Defect

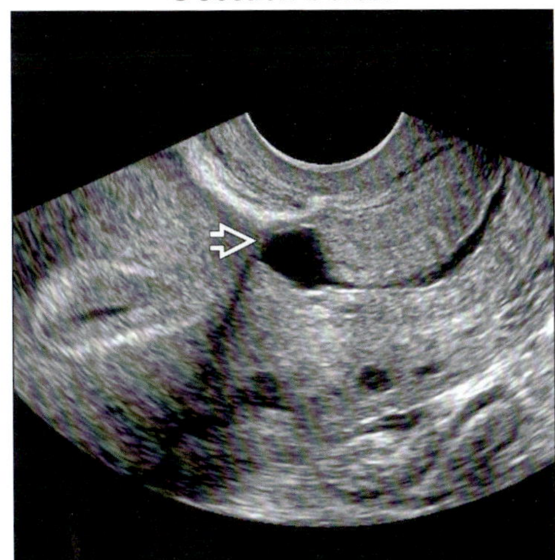

Endometrial Hyperplasia

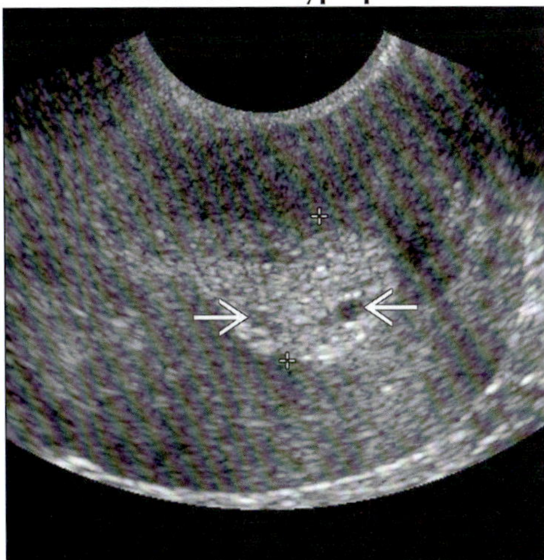

(Left) Longitudinal transvaginal ultrasound shows a fluid collection ➡ in the region of a prior cesarean section scar. This C-section defect can act as a reservoir for mid-cycle bleeding. (Right) Longitudinal transvaginal ultrasound in a patient with an ovarian granulosa cell tumor shows a thickened heterogeneous endometrium measuring 15 mm (calipers) with multiple cysts ➡.

Endometrial Cancer

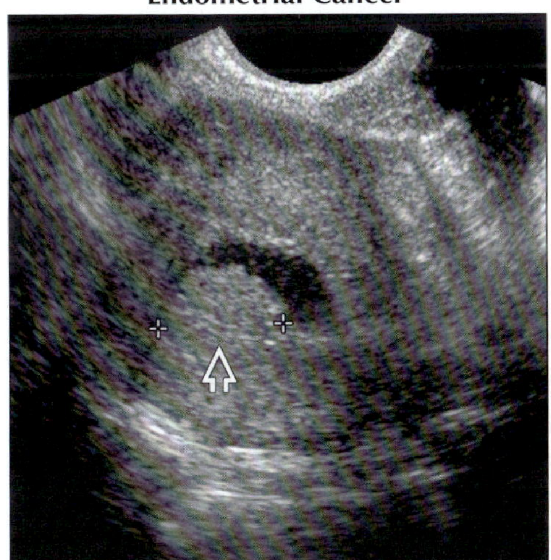

Endocervical Polyp

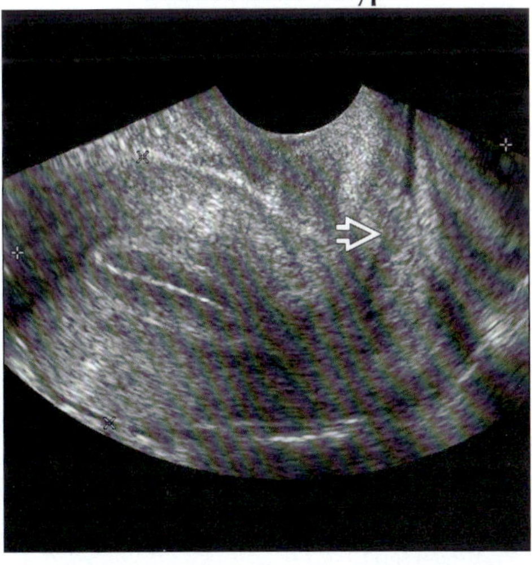

(Left) Transverse transvaginal ultrasound shows fluid in the endometrial cavity with a focal broad-based mass (calipers) in the posterior endometrium ➡. (Right) Longitudinal transvaginal ultrasound shows a well-defined, oblong, soft tissue echogenicity mass ➡ in the endocervical canal.

Cervical Cancer

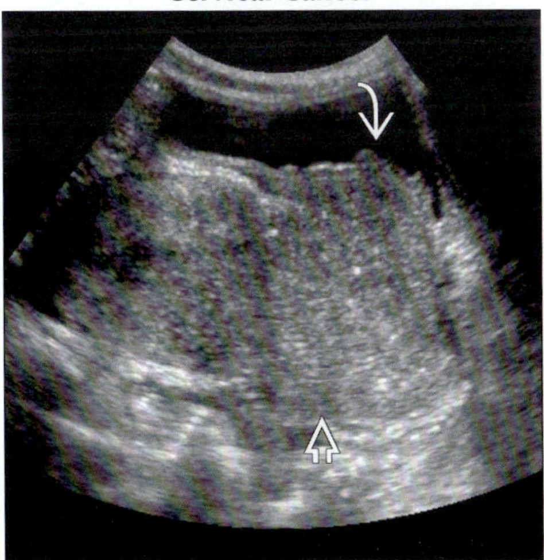

Bleeding from GI or GU Tract

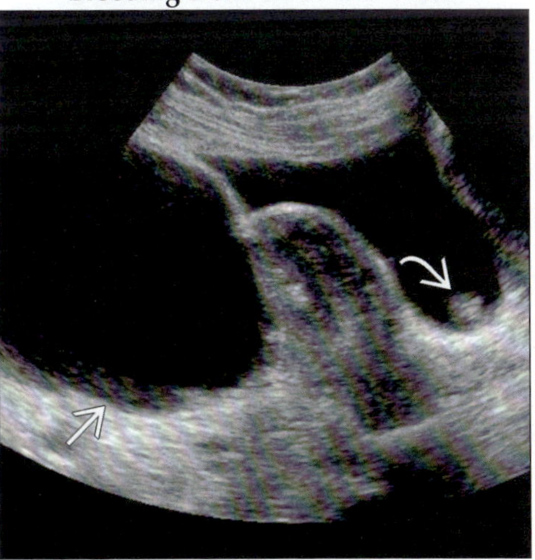

(Left) Longitudinal transabdominal ultrasound shows a large, irregular, hypoechoic mass in the region of the cervix ➡. The mass invades the bladder ➡. (Right) Longitudinal transabdominal ultrasound shows a 10 cm anechoic cyst ➡ and a solid mass ➡ in the bladder due to transitional cell carcinoma.

13

THICKENED ENDOMETRIUM

DIFFERENTIAL DIAGNOSIS

Common
- Menstrual-Related
  - Secretory Phase Endometrium
  - Pregnancy and Complications
- Mimic of Endometrial Thickening
  - Submucosal Leiomyoma
  - Intramural Leiomyoma
  - Hematometra
- Endometrial Polyps

Less Common
- Endometrial Hyperplasia
- Endometrial Cancer
- Tamoxifen-Induced Changes
- Retained Products of Conception

Rare but Important
- Endometritis
- Unopposed Estrogen Use
- Polycystic Ovary Syndrome
- Endometrial Stromal Sarcoma

ESSENTIAL INFORMATION

Key Differential Diagnosis Issues
- Is patient postpartum?
  - Endometritis
  - Retained products of conception
- Is thickening focal?
  - Endometrial polyps
  - Leiomyoma, submucosal
  - Endometrial cancer
  - Endometrial hyperplasia
  - Retained products of conception
- Does patient have abnormal bleeding?
  - Endometrial polyps
  - Leiomyoma, submucosal
  - Leiomyoma, intramural
  - Endometrial hyperplasia
  - Endometrial cancer
- Is endometrial-myometrial interface indistinct?
  - Endometrial cancer
  - Leiomyoma, submucosal

Helpful Clues for Common Diagnoses
- **Secretory Phase Endometrium**
  - In last 1/2 of menstrual cycle, endometrium can be thick, heterogeneous, and echogenic
  - Follow-up early in subsequent menstrual cycle will show thin endometrium
- **Pregnancy and Complications**
  - Positive urine/serum human chorionic gonadotropin
    - Normal early pregnancy
    - Miscarriage
    - Ectopic pregnancy
    - Hydatiform mole, complete mole
    - Hydatiform mole, partial mole
- **Submucosal Leiomyoma**
  - Submucosal lesions > 50% within endometrium
- **Intramural Leiomyoma**
  - Not true endometrial lesion but can cause appearance of endometrial thickening
  - Iso- or hypoechoic
  - Shadowing behind leiomyoma
- **Hematometra**
  - Look for underlying cause of obstruction
    - Uterine duplication anomaly
    - Leiomyoma
    - Endometrial cancer
    - Cervical cancer
    - If thin surrounding endometrium and no obstructing lesion, cervical stenosis is diagnosis of exclusion
- **Endometrial Polyps**
  - Focal endometrial lesion
  - Typically more echogenic than surrounding endometrium
  - May have cysts
  - Stalk with flow
  - May have broad base
  - Frequently multiple
  - Smooth margins
  - May have surrounding thin endometrium

Helpful Clues for Less Common Diagnoses
- **Endometrial Hyperplasia**
  - Peri- or postmenopausal woman
  - Association with polycystic ovarian syndrome
  - ± cystic spaces
  - Typically diffuse but may be focal
- **Endometrial Cancer**
  - Early stage
    - Appears as focal endometrial lesion
  - Later stage
    - Invades myometrium, leads to indistinct endometrial-myometrial interface

13

- Irregular thickened heterogeneous endometrium
- **Tamoxifen-Induced Changes**
  - ↑ incidence with ↑ dose and time of treatment
  - Reactivation of foci of adenomyosis
  - Due to estrogenic effect in endometrium, can lead to polyps, hyperplasia, and carcinoma
  - Endometrial cancer in patients taking tamoxifen is frequently in endometrial polyps
- **Retained Products of Conception**
  - Focal endometrial lesion
  - May have calcifications
  - May have blood flow, but lack of flow does not exclude diagnosis

Helpful Clues for Rare Diagnoses
- **Endometritis**
  - In postpartum patient, painful enlarged uterus
  - In nonpregnant patient, associated with pelvic inflammatory disease
  - Elevated white blood cell count
- **Unopposed Estrogen Use**
  - Estrogen use without progesterone ⇒ endometrial polyps, hyperplasia, and carcinoma
- **Polycystic Ovary Syndrome**
  - Enlarged ovaries with multiple, small, peripheral follicles
  - Central stroma echogenic
  - No dominant follicle

- Diffuse endometrial thickening due to prolonged proliferative phase or endometrial hyperplasia

Other Essential Information
- Use transvaginal scanning for best evaluation of endometrium
  - Sonohysterography helpful to distinguish if focal lesion present
  - Diffuse thickening can be sampled with blind biopsy
  - Focal mass best assessed with hysteroscopic biopsy
- In uterine duplication, anomalies must evaluate each endometrium separately

Alternative Differential Approaches
- Solid or complex ovarian lesion in association with endometrial lesion
  - Estrogenic effect from granulosa cell tumor ⇒ endometrial lesion
  - Estrogen secretion from thecoma ⇒ endometrial lesion
  - Concordant ovarian and endometrial carcinoma
  - Endometrioid tumor
  - Metastatic disease

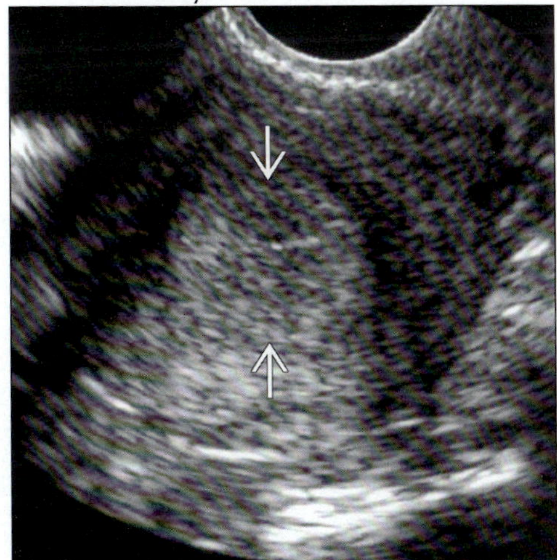

Secretory Phase Endometrium

Oblique transvaginal ultrasound shows a thick echogenic endometrium ➡ with through transmission in a woman in the secretory phase of a menstrual cycle.

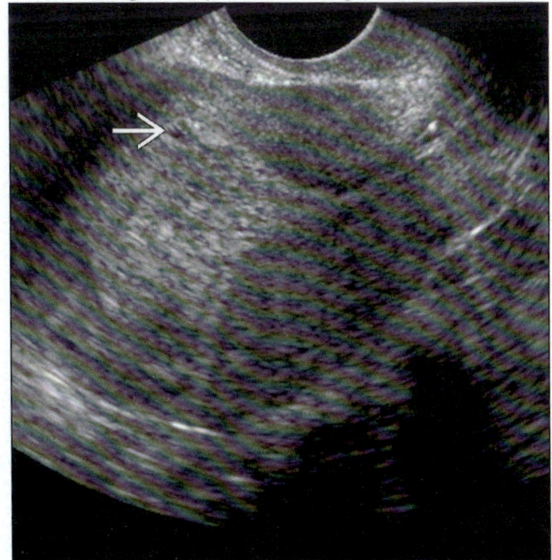

Pregnancy and Complications

Longitudinal transvaginal ultrasound in a woman with bleeding in the 1st trimester shows a heterogeneous endometrium with small cysts ➡. Follow-up showed a normal early pregnancy.

13

THICKENED ENDOMETRIUM

(Left) Longitudinal transvaginal ultrasound shows a hypoechoic mass ➡ projecting into the endometrial cavity with the appearance of a thick endometrium (calipers). (Right) Transverse transvaginal ultrasound in the same patient, but during the secretory phase, shows how the leiomyoma (➡, calipers) is now more apparent when surrounded by the echogenic endometrium.

Submucosal Leiomyoma

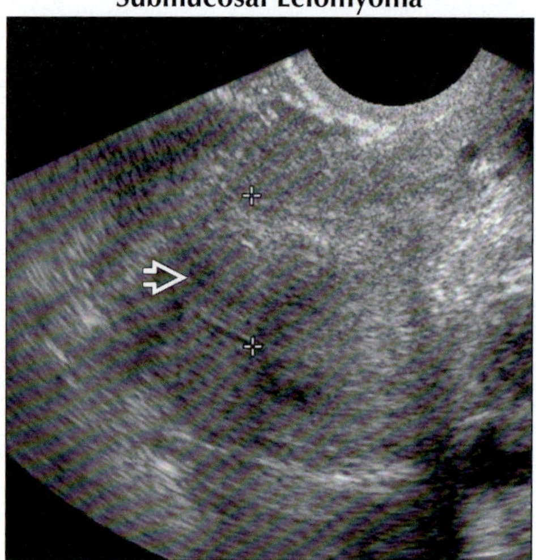

Submucosal Leiomyoma

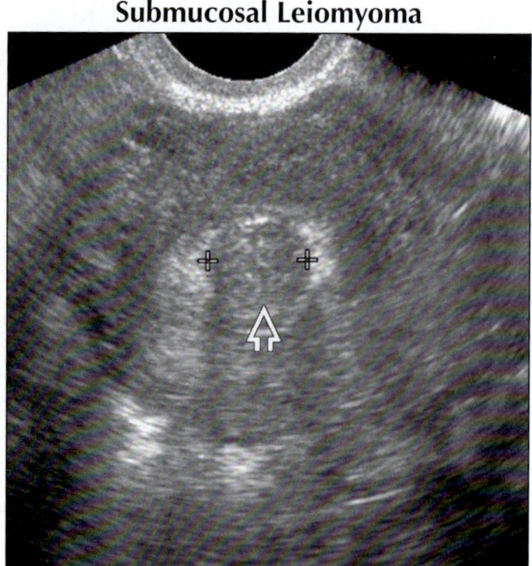

(Left) Transverse sonohysterogram shows 2 small echogenic masses ➡ surrounded by fluid. (Right) Longitudinal transvaginal ultrasound in an 89-year-old woman shows a thick heterogeneous endometrium (calipers). Pathology showed polyps.

Endometrial Polyps

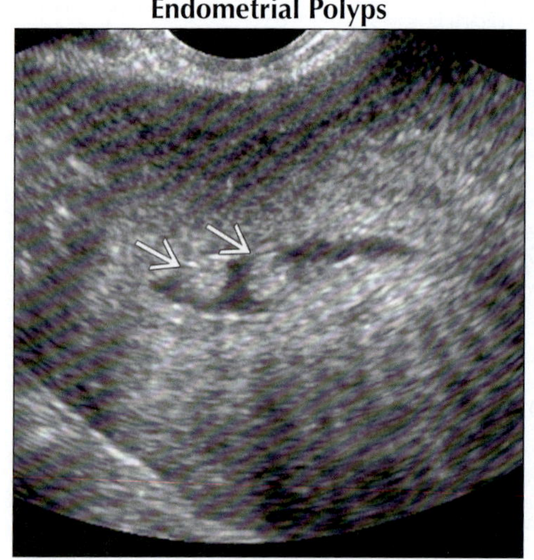

Endometrial Polyps

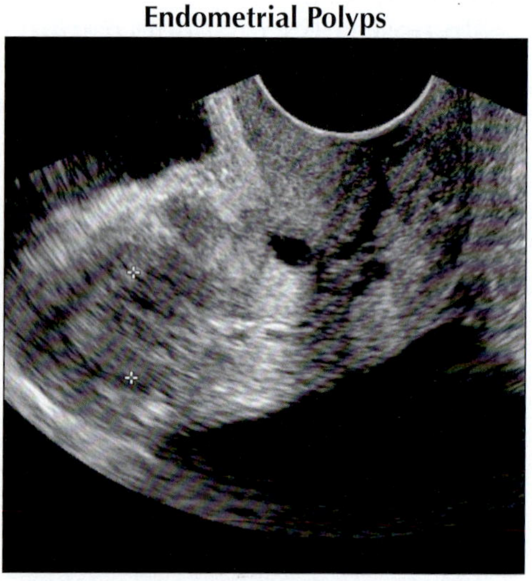

(Left) Longitudinal transvaginal ultrasound in a 47 year old with a granulosa cell tumor of the ovary shows a thickened endometrium measuring 15 mm (calipers) with multiple cysts. (Right) Longitudinal transvaginal ultrasound shows fluid in the endometrial cavity with a focal area of endometrial thickening ➡ in the fundal region.

Endometrial Hyperplasia

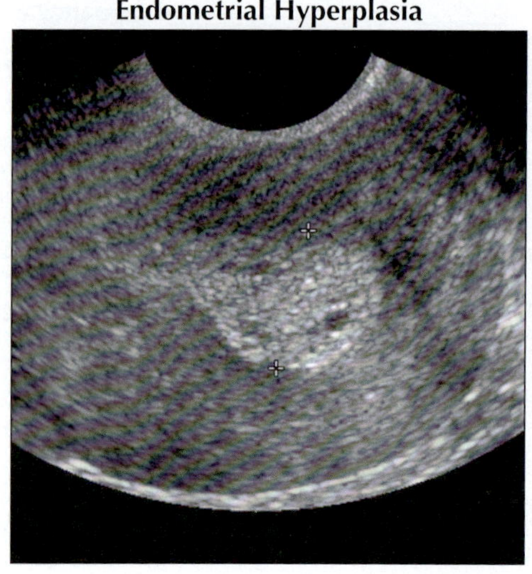

Endometrial Cancer

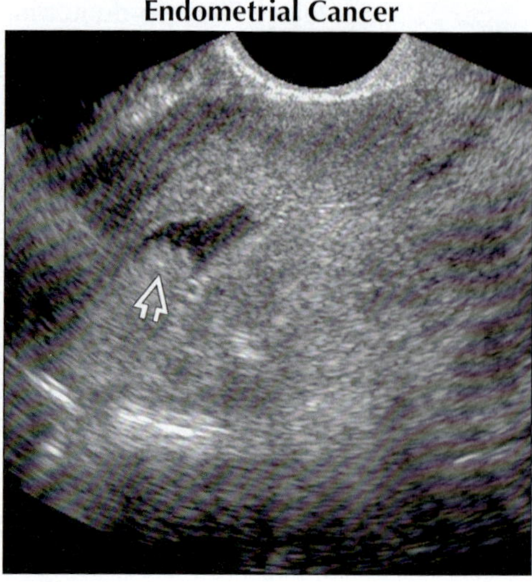

13

THICKENED ENDOMETRIUM

Tamoxifen-Induced Changes

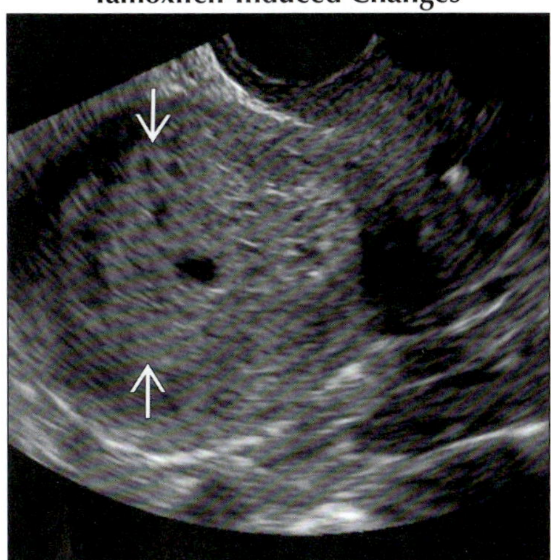

Tamoxifen-Induced Changes

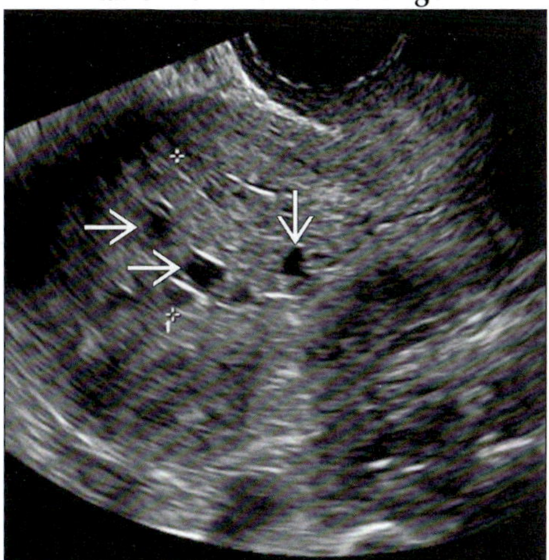

(Left) Longitudinal transvaginal ultrasound in a 76-year-old woman taking tamoxifen shows a thickened heterogeneous endometrium ➡ with multiple cysts. *(Right)* Another longitudinal image in the same patient shows more cysts ➡ within the thickened endometrium (calipers). This was endometrial carcinoma that arose within a polyp.

Retained Products of Conception

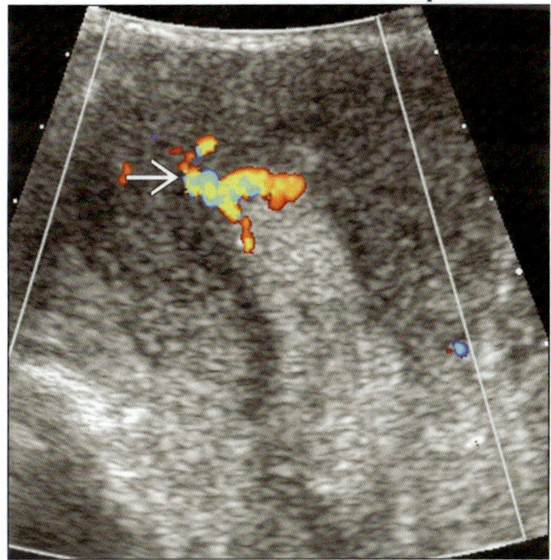

Retained Products of Conception

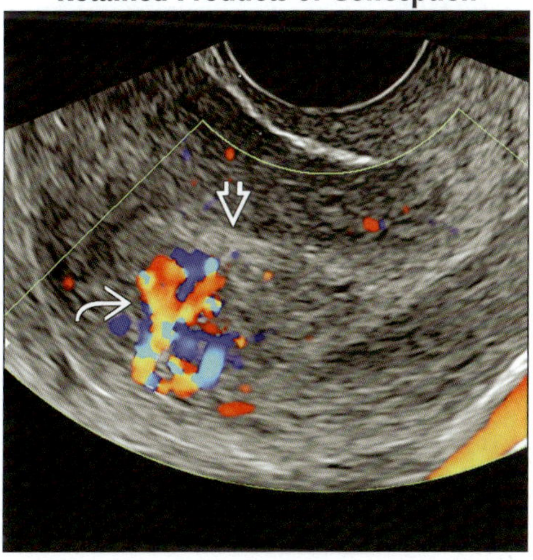

(Left) Longitudinal color Doppler ultrasound shows echogenic material in the endometrium in a patient 4 weeks post partum. Doppler interrogation reveals a large feeding vessel at the fundus ➡. Histology confirmed retained products of conception. *(Right)* Longitudinal color Doppler US shows a thickened heterogeneous endometrium ➡ with feeding vessels ➡ to the region of retained placental tissue. Histology showed partially necrotic decidua with hemorrhage.

Endometritis

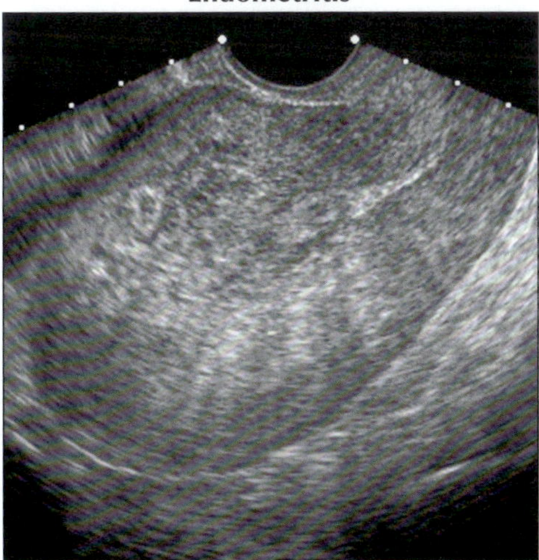

Polycystic Ovary Syndrome

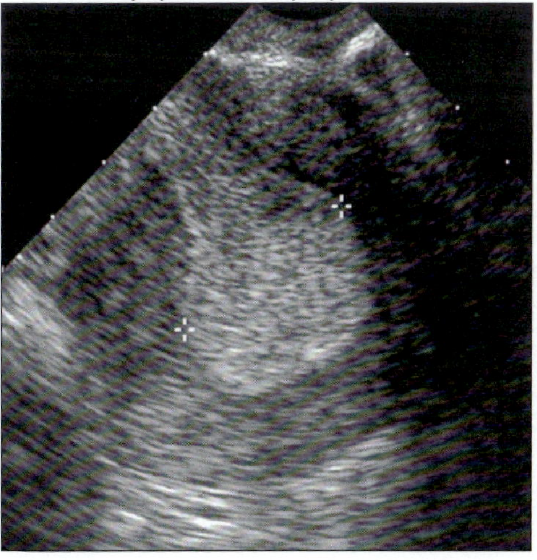

(Left) Longitudinal transvaginal ultrasound in a postpartum patient with a fever and elevated white blood cell count shows an ill-defined endometrium but no focal lesion to suggest retained products of conception. *(Right)* Longitudinal transvaginal ultrasound in a 24-year-old woman with oligomenorrhea and polycystic ovarian syndrome shows a thickened 23 mm endometrium (calipers) due to a prolonged proliferative phase.

13

ENDOMETRIAL FLUID

DIFFERENTIAL DIAGNOSIS

Common
- Normal Menstruation
- Pregnancy and Complications
- Cervical Stenosis
- Leiomyoma

Less Common
- Endometrial Polyps
- Endometrial Cancer
- Endometritis

Rare but Important
- Cervical Cancer
- Cervical Leiomyoma
- Müllerian Anomaly with Obstruction
- Imperforate Hymen

ESSENTIAL INFORMATION

Key Differential Diagnosis Issues
- Is patient pregnant?
  - Ectopic pregnancy
  - Normal or abnormal early intrauterine pregnancy
- Postmenopausal, no endometrial lesion seen
  - Cervical stenosis
- Endometrial lesion present
  - Endometrial polyps
  - Endometrial cancer
  - Leiomyoma, submucosal
- Obstructing lesion present
  - Leiomyoma
  - Endometrial cancer
  - Cervical cancer

Helpful Clues for Common Diagnoses
- **Pregnancy and Complications**
  - Positive urine/serum human chorionic gonadotropin
  - Intra- or extrauterine pregnancy visualized
- **Cervical Stenosis**
  - Typically asymptomatic, although may be painful if uterus enlarges
  - Thin surrounding endometrium

Helpful Clues for Less Common Diagnoses
- **Endometrial Polyps**
  - Focal endometrial lesion(s) as echogenic or more echogenic than surrounding endometrium
  - May have cysts
- **Endometrial Cancer**
  - Broad-based lesion surrounded by fluid
  - ± loss of endometrial/myometrial interface

Helpful Clues for Rare Diagnoses
- **Cervical Cancer**
  - Heterogeneous hypoechoic mass in cervix
  - Originates from endocervical canal; therefore mass centered in stroma unlikely to be cervical carcinoma
- **Cervical Leiomyoma**
  - Hypoechoic, well-defined mass
- **Imperforate Hymen**
  - Low vaginal obstruction with hematometrocolpos

Pregnancy and Complications

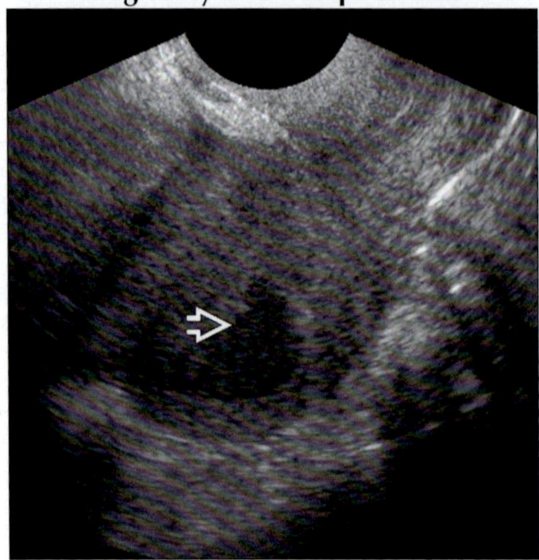

Longitudinal transvaginal US in a patient 5 wks pregnant shows a complex fluid collection ➤ centrally located in the endometrial cavity. This is consistent with a pseudosac in a patient with an ectopic pregnancy.

Cervical Stenosis

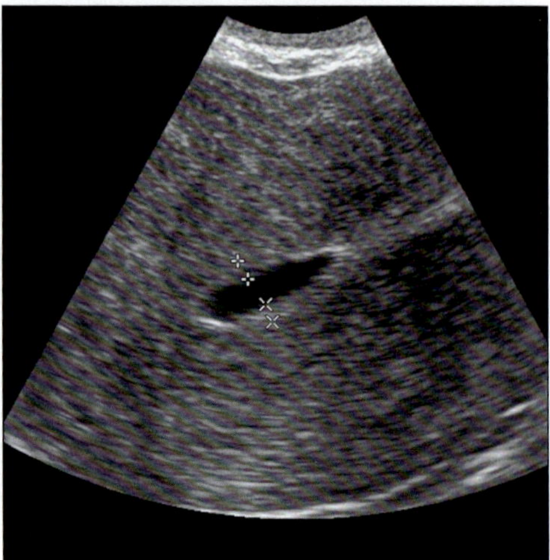

Longitudinal transvaginal ultrasound shows a small amount of fluid with a thin surrounding endometrium. Note that the endometrial thickness measurement (calipers) should be taken to exclude the fluid.

13

ENDOMETRIAL FLUID

Cervical Stenosis

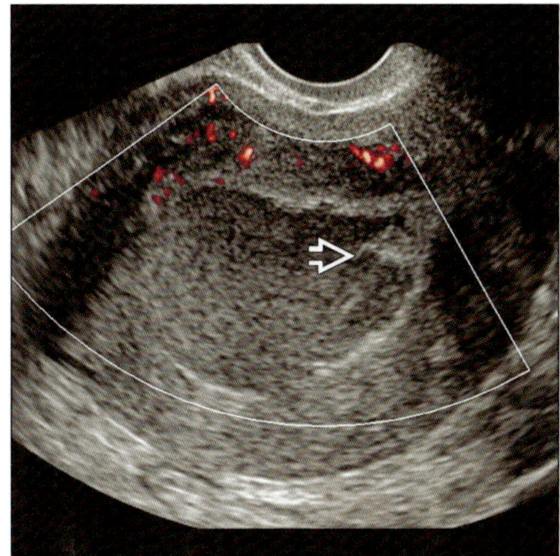

Leiomyoma

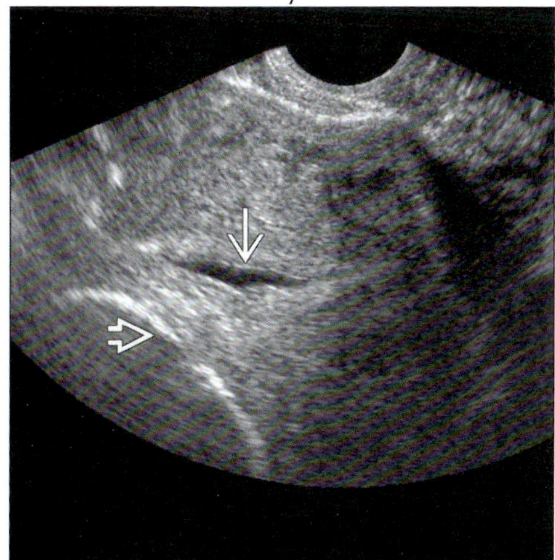

(Left) Longitudinal power Doppler US in a woman after endometrial ablation shows the endometrial cavity is filled with complex fluid with some echogenic debris ➡. The surrounding endometrium is thin. Power Doppler shows no flow to the endometrial contents. *(Right)* Longitudinal transvaginal ultrasound shows a portion of a calcified leiomyoma ➡ and a small amount of endometrial fluid ➡. The leiomyoma leading to partial obstruction is out of the plane of view.

Endometrial Polyps

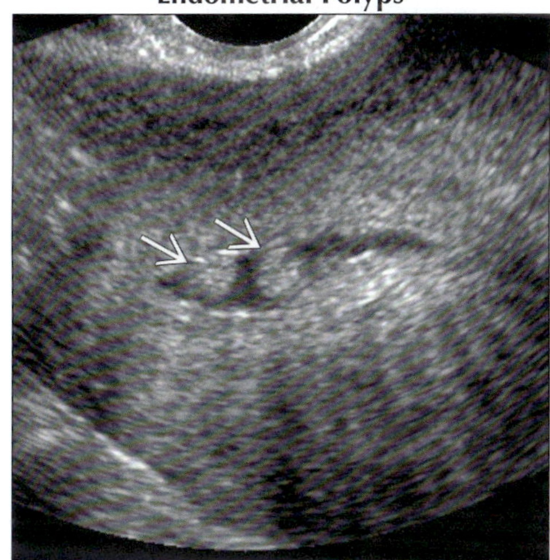

Endometrial Cancer

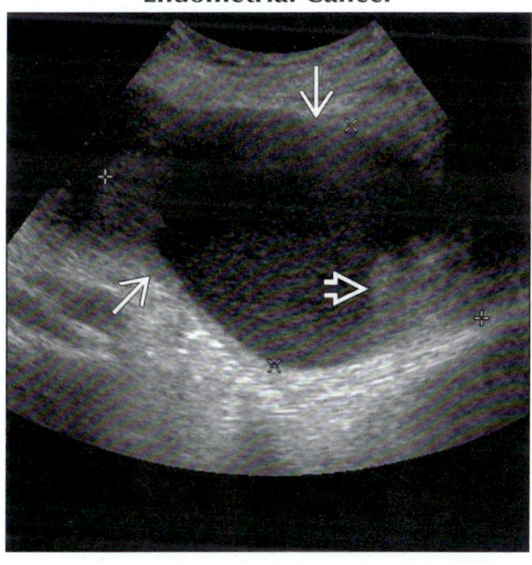

(Left) Transverse transvaginal ultrasound shows 2 small echogenic masses ➡ surrounded by fluid. *(Right)* Longitudinal transabdominal ultrasound shows the uterus ➡ distended with fluid and debris, consistent with blood products. An irregular, solid, soft tissue mass is seen inferiorly ➡.

Endometritis

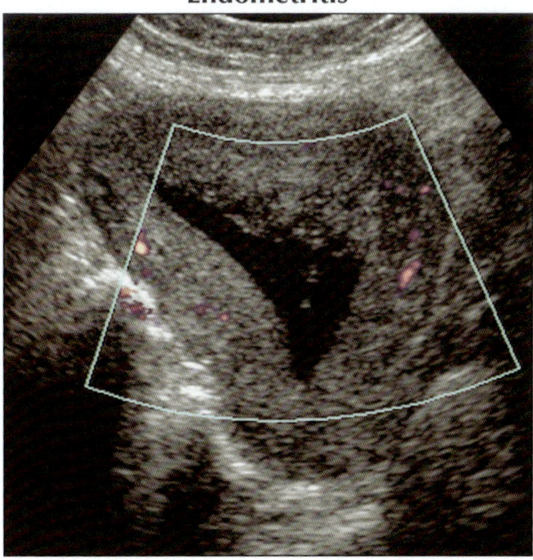

Cervical Cancer

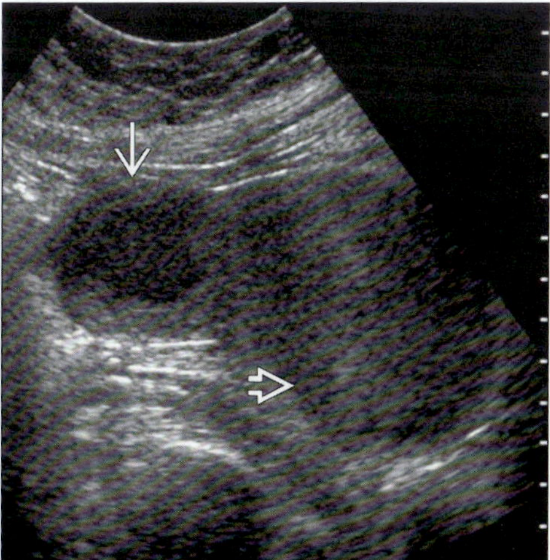

(Left) Longitudinal power Doppler ultrasound shows an enlarged uterus with endometrial fluid and debris and a shaggy irregular appearance to the endometrium anteriorly (without vascularity). *(Right)* Longitudinal transabdominal ultrasound shows a large mass ➡ that circumferentially encompasses the cervix. There is fluid within the endometrial cavity ➡ due to obstruction from a grade 2b cervical carcinoma.

13

PELVIC FLUID

DIFFERENTIAL DIAGNOSIS

Common
- Age-Related Physiologic Alterations
- Hemorrhagic Cysts, Rupture
- Ectopic Pregnancy, Rupture

Less Common
- Peritoneal Inclusion Cysts
- Abscess
  - Tubo-Ovarian Abscess
  - Pelvic Abscess due to Bowel Disease
    - Appendicitis
    - Other Bowel Related Abscess
- Ascites
- Endometriosis

Rare but Important
- Ovarian Cancer
- Ovarian Metastases
- Ovarian Hyperstimulation Syndrome

ESSENTIAL INFORMATION

Key Differential Diagnosis Issues
- Anechoic fluid
  - Small amount of anechoic fluid in asymptomatic woman likely physiologic
  - Large amount of anechoic fluid likely ascites
  - If signs of metastatic disease, check ovaries
- Fluid with debris in cul-de-sac
  - Blood: Patient may be hemodynamically unstable
    - Hemorrhagic cysts, rupture
    - Ectopic pregnancy, rupture
    - Endometriosis
  - Pus: Patient acutely ill with elevated white blood cell count and fever
    - Tubo-ovarian abscess
    - Appendicitis
    - Pelvic abscess due to other bowel disease
  - Cells: Metastatic disease
- Fluid with septations
  - Peritoneal inclusion cysts
  - Endometriosis

Helpful Clues for Common Diagnoses
- **Hemorrhagic Cysts, Rupture**
  - Hematocrit may initially be normal if patient has not had time to hemodilute after rehydration
  - Check for fluid by kidneys to demonstrate hemoperitoneum
- **Ectopic Pregnancy, Rupture**
  - Positive pregnancy test
  - May see tubal ring ± yolk sac and embryonic pole
  - Hematocrit may initially be normal if patient has not had time to hemodilute after rehydration

Helpful Clues for Less Common Diagnoses
- **Abscess**
  - Patient acutely tender in region of complex fluid collection
  - May see abnormal loop of bowel/appendix in region
  - May see dilated pus-filled tube in cases of tubo-ovarian abscess

Hemorrhagic Cysts, Rupture

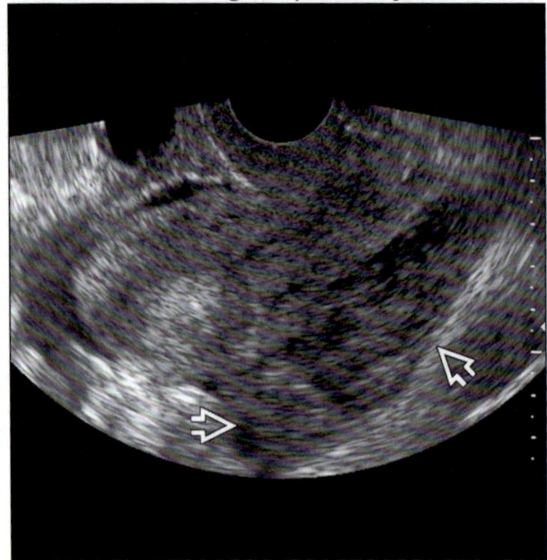

Longitudinal transvaginal ultrasound shows heterogeneous material posterior to the uterus, consistent with a blood clot ➡. The patient was not pregnant. This was a ruptured corpus luteum cyst.

Ectopic Pregnancy, Rupture

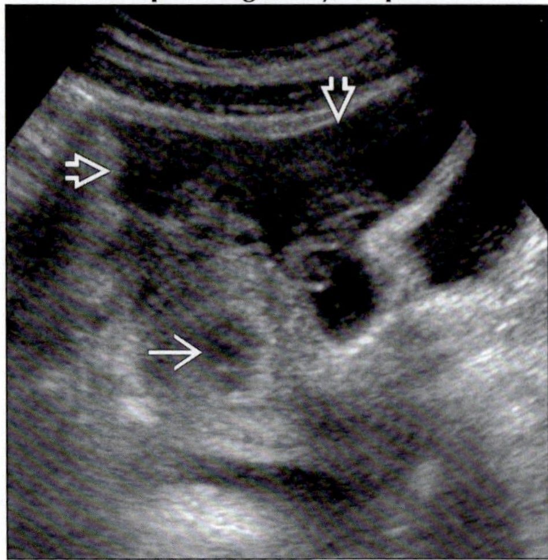

Longitudinal transabdominal ultrasound in a pregnant patient shows a large amount of complex fluid consistent with blood ➡ around the uterus. Note "pseudosac" of blood in the endometrial cavity ➡.

PELVIC FLUID

Peritoneal Inclusion Cysts

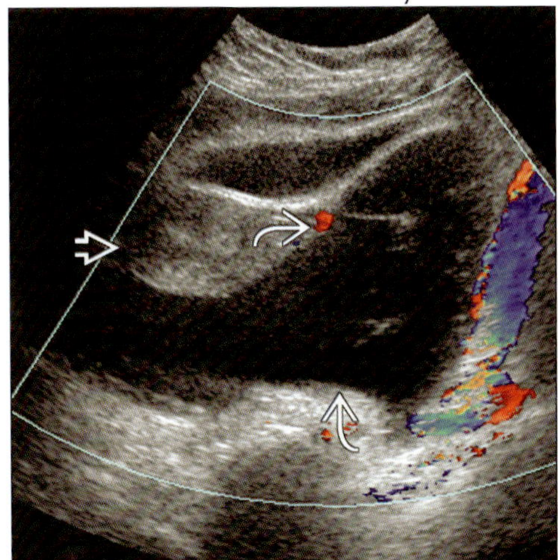

Peritoneal Inclusion Cysts

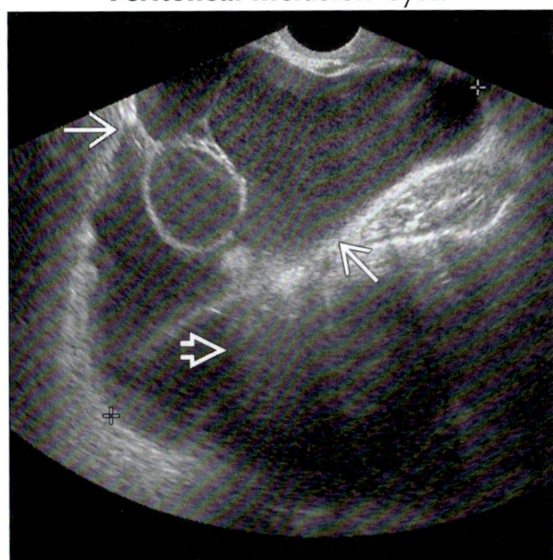

(Left) Transverse color Doppler ultrasound shows a septated fluid collection ➡ posterior to the uterus ➡. (Right) Longitudinal transvaginal ultrasound in the same patient shows a septated cyst ➡ with debris. This appearance is consistent with a peritoneal inclusion cyst. Note that the loops of bowel ➡ impress upon the cyst.

Tubo-Ovarian Abscess

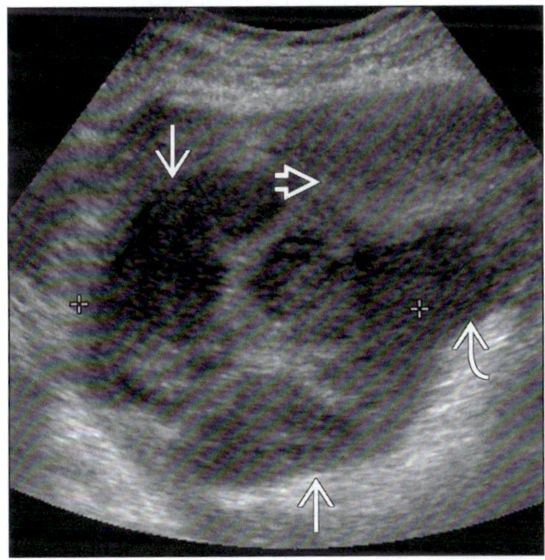

Ascites

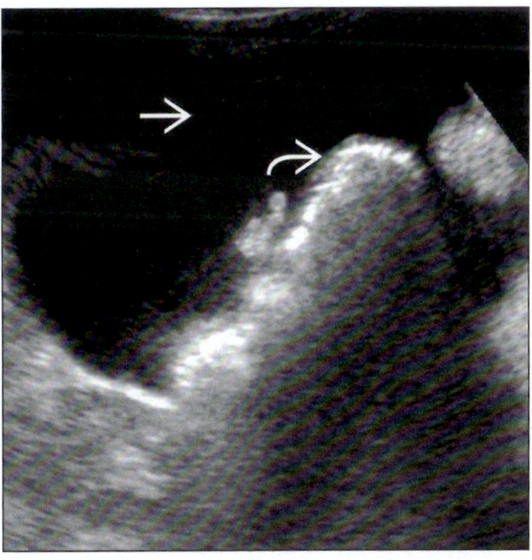

(Left) Transverse transabdominal ultrasound shows a large complex fluid collection ➡ posterior to the uterus ➡. There are low-level internal echoes within the fluid and thick septations. There is adjacent free fluid with debris ➡. (Right) Transverse transabdominal ultrasound shows anechoic ascites ➡ in the pelvis with floating bowel loops ➡.

Ovarian Hyperstimulation Syndrome

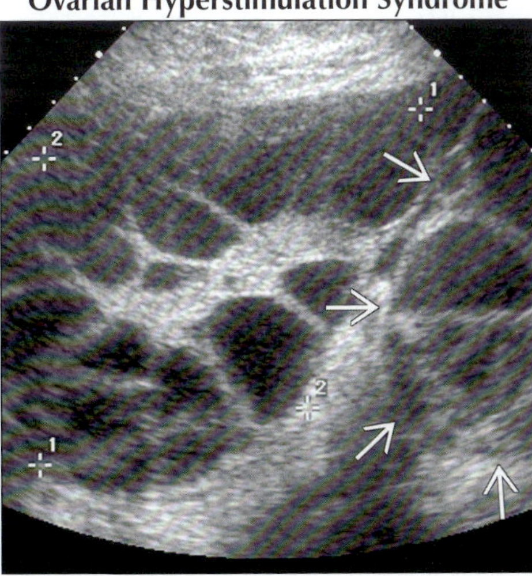

Ovarian Hyperstimulation Syndrome

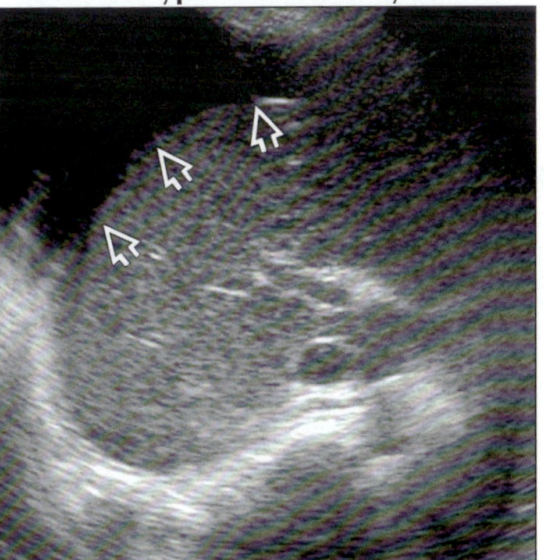

(Left) Transverse transabdominal ultrasound shows a typical case of markedly enlarged hyperstimulated ovaries (calipers, ➡). (Right) Transverse ultrasound in the same patient shows ascites ➡ extending into the upper abdomen.

PELVIC PAIN

DIFFERENTIAL DIAGNOSIS

Common
- Menstrual-Related Pain
- Cyst Development and Rupture
  - Corpus Luteal Cyst
  - Hemorrhagic Ovarian Cysts
- Pain Related to Pregnancy
  - Normal Pregnancy
  - Threatened Abortion
  - Ectopic Pregnancy
- Appendicitis

Less Common
- Endometriosis
- Adenomyosis
- Pelvic Inflammatory Disease
- Adnexal Torsion
- Leiomyoma Degeneration
- Pain Related to Pregnancy
  - Preterm Labor
  - Placental Abruption
  - Uterine Rupture
- Urinary Tract Causes of Pain
  - Urolithiasis
  - Cystitis
- Gastrointestinal Causes of Pain
  - Diverticular Disease
  - Crohn Disease

Rare but Important
- Ovarian Hyperstimulation Syndrome
- Cervical Stenosis with Distended Uterus

ESSENTIAL INFORMATION

Key Differential Diagnosis Issues
- Pain localized to area being scanned can determine etiology
  - Pain in uterus
    - If localized to leiomyoma, consider degeneration
    - If diffuse overenlarged uterus, consider adenomyosis
    - If obstructed uterus, consider cervical stenosis or other obstructing lesion
  - Pain over cyst due to size of cyst, hemorrhage in cyst, or rupture
    - Corpus luteal cyst
    - Hemorrhagic cysts, ovary
  - Pain in region of blood clot, but no cyst visualized
    - Ectopic pregnancy, rupture
    - Hemorrhagic cysts, ovary
  - Cervical motion tenderness due to pelvic inflammatory disease
    - Tubo-ovarian abscess
- Ill-defined mass in adnexa
  - Tubo-ovarian abscess
  - Ectopic pregnancy, rupture

Helpful Clues for Common Diagnoses
- **Menstrual-Related Pain**
  - May see normal pelvic US in women with pain due to normal cycle
    - Normal menstruation
    - Mittelschmerz (pain on ovulation)
    - Development of corpus luteal cyst and other hemorrhagic ovarian cysts
- **Cyst Development and Rupture**
  - Cysts can cause pain due to large size, hemorrhage, or rupture
  - Pain localized to region of cyst
  - Debris within cyst due to hemorrhage
    - Acute hemorrhage appears echogenic
    - Subacute hemorrhage has complex appearance with strands of internal density
    - Follow-up in 6 weeks with patient at different phase of menstrual cycle to ensure resolution of cyst
  - Free fluid with debris due to rupture
    - Check for fluid in upper abdomen to ensure no large amount of hemoperitoneum
- **Ectopic Pregnancy**
  - Pain localized to site of ectopic pregnancy
  - Bleeding
  - Adnexal mass present in 20% of cases
    - Ectopic ring more echogenic than wall of corpus luteum
    - Ectopic pregnancy typically in tube as opposed to corpus luteum location in ovary
  - Pseudosac of fluid centrally located in endometrial cavity
  - Rare forms of ectopic pregnancy in isthmic and interstitial tube, abdomen, cervix, and uterine scars
  - Visualization of intrauterine pregnancy ↓ risk of ectopic pregnancy except in patients who have been hyperstimulated
- **Appendicitis**
  - Graded compression in right lower quadrant

13

PELVIC PAIN

- Elongated tubular structure connects to cecum
- Noncompressible
- Rebound tenderness when ultrasound probe is lifted off
- Appendicolith suggestive of either ruptured appendix or impending rupture

Helpful Clues for Less Common Diagnoses

- **Endometriosis**
  - Functioning endometrial glands and stroma in ectopic site
  - Small implants not visualized with ultrasound
  - Endometrioma
    - "Chocolate" cyst with diffuse homogeneous low-level internal echoes
    - Thick wall
    - Layering debris
    - ± septations
    - Punctate calcifications in wall
- **Pelvic Inflammatory Disease**
  - Pain in both lower quadrants
  - Cervical motion tenderness
  - Elevated white blood cell count
  - ± rebound tenderness
  - ± metrorrhagia
  - Thickened heterogeneous endometrium with fluid ± gas
  - Dilated, thick-walled, hyperemic fallopian tube
- **Adnexal Torsion**
  - Pain localized to ovary

- Enlarged ovary with small peripheral cysts or mass 4-8 cm acting as lead point for torsion
- Blood flow may be normal or abnormal
  - Dual blood supply of ovary from ovarian artery and ovarian branch of uterine artery can preserve flow
  - Venous flow predictive of ovarian viability

- **Leiomyoma Degeneration**
  - Pain localized to leiomyoma
  - Cystic areas within leiomyoma indicate necrosis has already occurred
- **Urolithiasis**
  - Typically causes flank pain, but stone at ureterovesical junction can cause pelvic pain
  - Small stones at ureterovesical junction seen as echogenic foci with shadowing
  - ± dilated ureter above stone
  - ± absent ureteral jet on side of pain

Alternative Differential Approaches

- Is patient pregnant?
  - Ectopic pregnancy
  - Normal or abnormal intrauterine pregnancy
  - All other causes of pain can also occur in pregnant patients

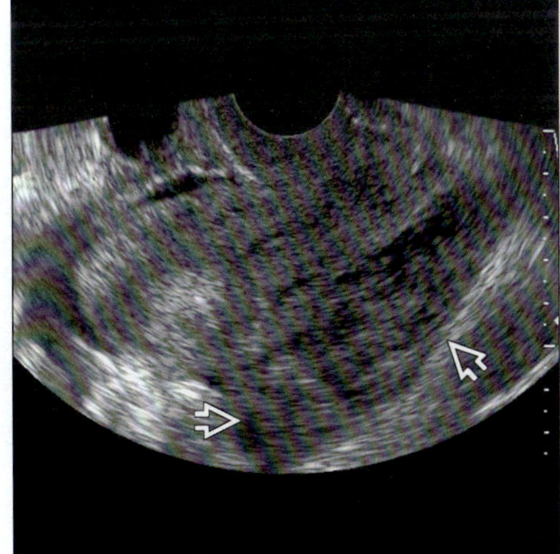

Cyst Development and Rupture

Longitudinal transvaginal US shows heterogeneous material ⊳ posterior to the uterus, consistent with a blood clot. The patient was not pregnant. This was a ruptured hemorrhagic corpus luteum cyst.

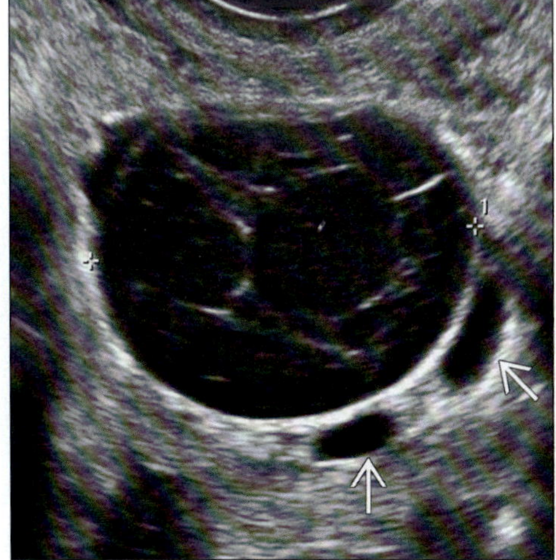

Corpus Luteal Cyst

Transverse transvaginal ultrasound shows a 4 cm right adnexal cyst (calipers) with a classic "cobweb" appearance of clot. Note the adjacent ovarian follicles ⊳.

(Left) Oblique transabdominal ultrasound shows a marginal subchorionic hematoma ⇨ in a patient 13 weeks pregnant with pelvic pain and bleeding. *(Right)* Transverse transvaginal ultrasound in a pregnant patient in her 1st trimester with left lower quadrant pain shows an echogenic ring-like mass ⇨ with a yolk sac ➡ adjacent to the ovary ➥.

Threatened Abortion

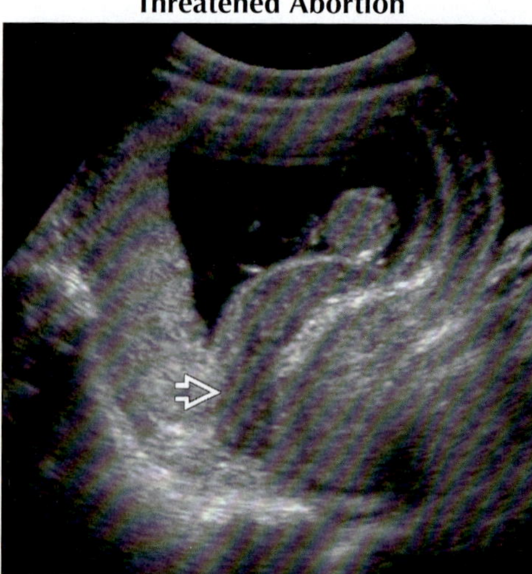

Ectopic Pregnancy

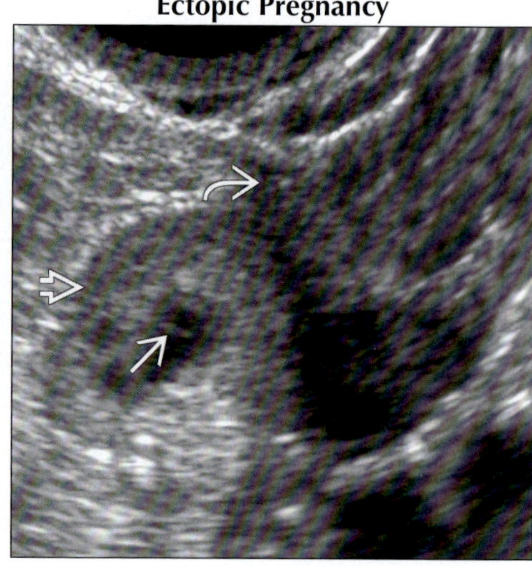

(Left) Transverse transabdominal ultrasound in a pregnant patient shows a large amount of complex fluid ⇨ consistent with blood around the uterus. The endometrial cavity has blood products ➡ within it, consistent with a pseudosac. *(Right)* Oblique transabdominal ultrasound shows a thickened and inflamed blind-ending tubular structure ➡ that was noncompressible and aperistaltic.

Ectopic Pregnancy

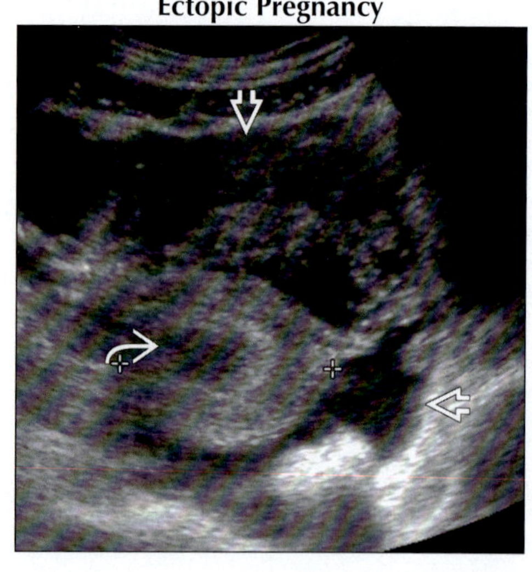

Appendicitis

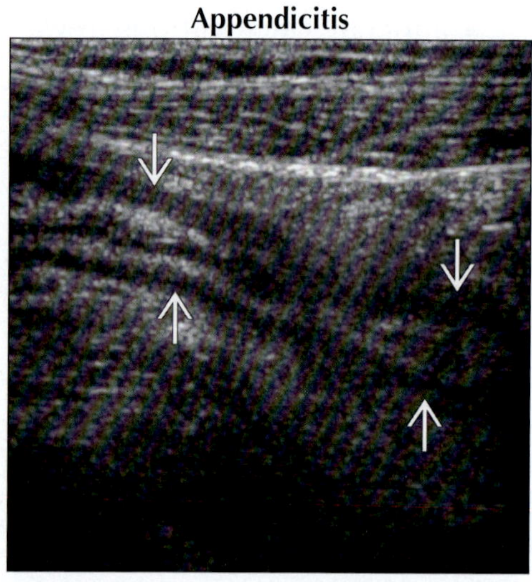

(Left) Transverse transvaginal ultrasound shows a cyst with diffuse homogeneous low-level internal echoes. Note a punctate echogenicity in the cyst ⇨ and a septation ➡. *(Right)* Transverse transvaginal ultrasound shows an enlarged heterogeneous uterus with alternating bands of increased through transmission and shadowing ➡.

Endometriosis

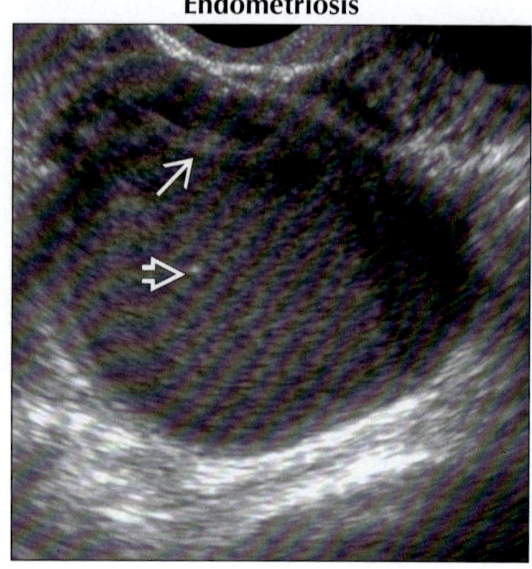

Adenomyosis

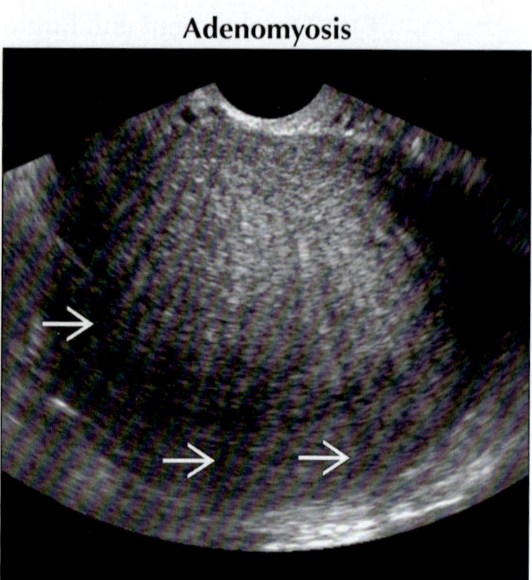

PELVIC PAIN

Pelvic Inflammatory Disease

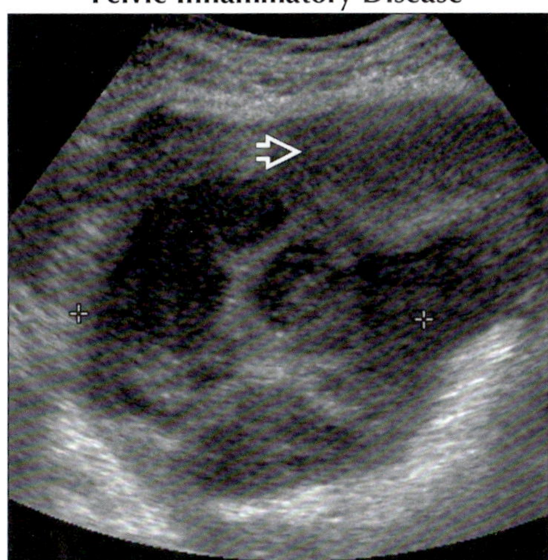

Adnexal Torsion

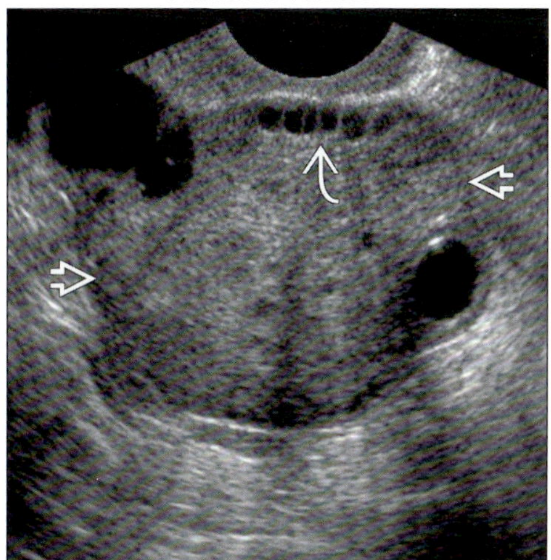

(Left) Transverse transabdominal US shows a large complex fluid collection (calipers) posterior to the uterus ➡. There are low-level internal echoes within the fluid and thick septations. This was a tubo-ovarian abscess complicating PID. *(Right)* Longitudinal transvaginal US in a pregnant patient with severe pelvic pain shows right ovarian enlargement ➡, measuring 6 cm. The ovary has a round appearance with peripherally located follicles ➡.

Leiomyoma Degeneration

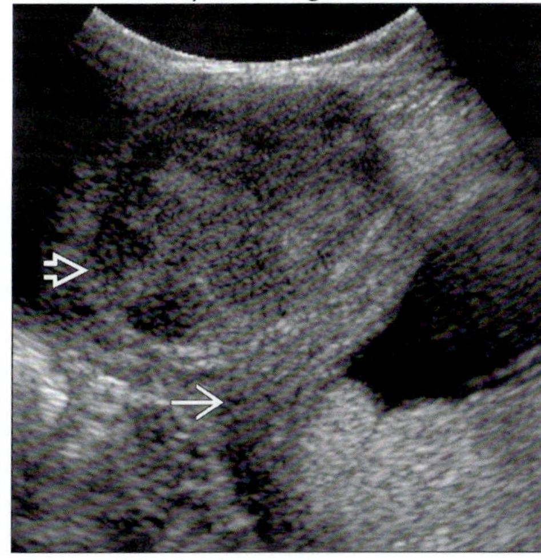

Urinary Tract Causes of Pain

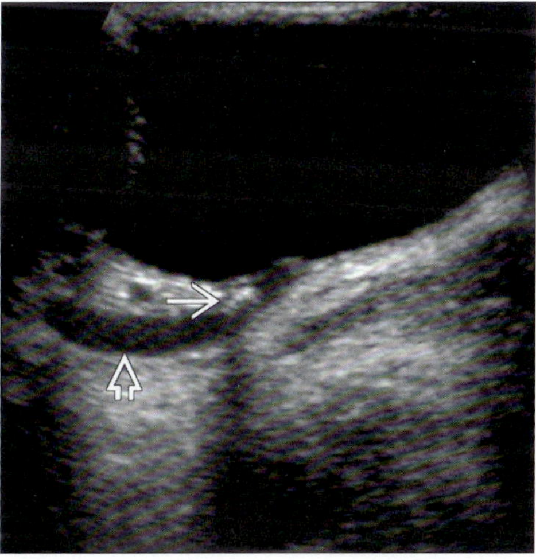

(Left) Oblique transabdominal ultrasound in a pregnant patient at 16 weeks gestation shows a heterogeneous solid mass ➡ exophytic from the gravid uterus ➡. *(Right)* Oblique transabdominal ultrasound shows a stone ➡ with shadowing just above the ureterovesical junction. Note the dilated ureter ➡ above the stone.

Crohn Disease

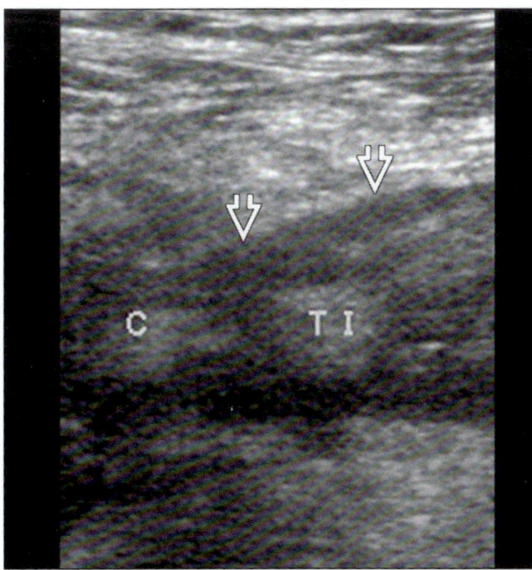

Ovarian Hyperstimulation Syndrome

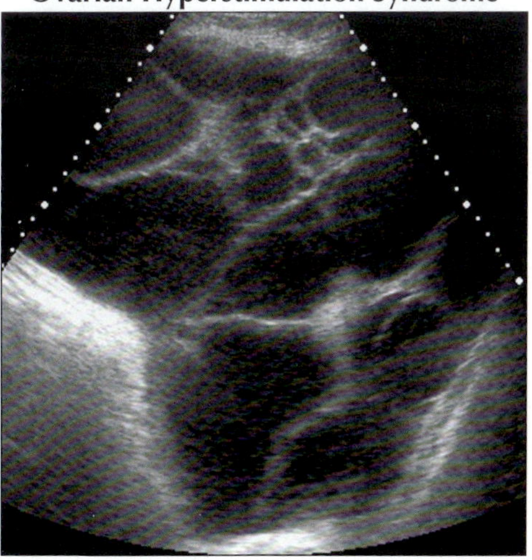

(Left) Oblique transabdominal ultrasound shows a thickened bowel wall ➡ in the terminal ileum in a pregnant patient with Crohn disease. Terminal ileum (TI), cecum (C). *(Right)* Transverse ultrasound in patient who underwent in vitro fertilization shows a typical presentation of hyperstimulation syndrome with a gigantic hyperstimulated ovary, measuring up to 31 cm.

13

SECTION 14
Vascular

Arteries

Veins

Vascular

DIFFERENTIAL DIAGNOSIS

Common
- Dilation/Aneurysm from Diseases of Aortic Wall
  - Atherosclerotic Aneurysm
  - Traumatic Aneurysm
  - Arterial Dissection
  - Infective Aneurysm
    - Mycotic Aneurysm
    - Syphilitic Aneurysm
  - Degenerative Aneurysm
    - Ehlers-Danlos Syndrome
    - Marfan Syndrome
    - Repetitive Aortic Injury and Repair Associated with Aging
  - Inflammatory Aneurysm
    - Vasculitis
    - Connective Tissue Disease
- Dilation from Increased Flow
  - Vascular Malformation
  - Arteriovenous Fistula
  - Aortic Regurgitation
- Dilation from Increased Pressure
  - Aortic Valve Stenosis
  - Systemic Hypertension
  - Post-Stenotic Dilation

ESSENTIAL INFORMATION

Key Differential Diagnosis Issues
- Artery considered aneurysmal when its diameter ≥ 1.5x normal diameter (outer wall to outer wall)
- In true aneurysms, composite layers of vessel are intact but stretched
- In false aneurysms, hole in arterial wall (through composite layers) allows escape of blood, which is subsequently confined by surrounding tissue

Helpful Clues for Common Diagnoses
- **Atherosclerotic Aneurysm**
  - Leading cause of aneurysms in thoracic (diameter > 5 cm) and abdominal aorta (diameter > 3 cm)
  - Location: Distal abdominal aorta most common
    - Iliac arteries > popliteal arteries > common femoral arteries > rest of abdominal aorta & descending thoracic aorta > carotid arteries & ascending aorta

- More commonly fusiform (80%) than saccular (20%)
  - Frequently contain calcified thrombus with irregular inner contour
- **Traumatic Aneurysm**
  - After trauma ~ 2-5% of patients with aortic disruption develop false aneurysm
  - Perfused false aneurysm may partially clot and organize with fibrous wall
    - Potentially evolves into saccular or fusiform aneurysm
    - Late enlargement and even rupture may occur
  - 90% of cases involve isthmus of aorta
- **Arterial Dissection**
  - Occurs when blood enters media through defect (entry site) in intima and dissects along length of artery
    - Intima may be stripped away in some parts and false lumen may be formed
    - May in turn cause increase in overall diameter of artery
  - Predisposing causes
    - Hypertension
    - Marfan syndrome
    - Ehlers-Danlos syndrome
    - Relapsing polychondritis
    - Valvular aortic stenosis
    - Trauma
    - Bicuspid aortic valves
    - Turner syndrome
    - Behçet syndrome
    - Coarctation
    - Aortitis
- **Mycotic Aneurysm**
  - Primary mycotic aneurysms that are not associated with demonstrable intravascular inflammatory processes are rare
  - Secondary mycotic aneurysms (nonsyphilitic) are more common
  - Predisposing factors to secondary aneurysms
    - IV drug abuse
    - Bacterial endocarditis
    - Immunocompromise (malignancy, chemotherapy, systemic steroids)
    - Autoimmune diseases
    - Diabetes
    - Atherosclerosis
    - Aortic trauma (accidental and iatrogenic causes)

14

ARTERIAL DILATION

- ○ Common organisms include *Staphylococcus aureus*, *Salmonella*; nonhemolytic *Streptococcus*, *Pneumococcus*, *Gonococcus*, and *Mycobacterium* (spread from contiguous lymph nodes)
- **Syphilitic Aneurysm**
  - ○ Predominantly affects ascending aorta and aortic arch
    - Less commonly involved: Proximal descending aorta > distal descending aorta > aortic sinuses
  - ○ Spectrum of disease
    - Uncomplicated syphilitic aortitis
    - Syphilitic aortic aneurysm
    - Syphilitic aortic vasculitis (leading to aortic regurgitation)
- **Degenerative Aneurysm**
  - ○ Equivalent to medial degeneration
  - ○ Most common cause of aneurysm in ascending aorta
  - ○ Can be seen in genetically inherited disorders such as
    - Marfan syndrome
    - Ehlers-Danlos syndrome
  - ○ Also can be seen in degenerative changes associated with aging
- **Inflammatory Aneurysm**
  - ○ Wide range of vasculitides and connective tissue diseases may cause inflammation of media and adventitia, resulting in arterial dilation
    - Takayasu arteritis
    - Giant cell arteritis
    - Relapsing polychondritis

- Rheumatoid arthritis
- Rheumatic fever
- Ankylosing spondylitis
- Ulcerative colitis
- Systemic lupus erythematosus
- Scleroderma
- Behçet disease
- Radiation
- **Dilation from Increased Flow**
  - ○ **Vascular Malformation**
    - Mainly occurs in high-flow arteriovenous vascular malformations where hypertrophy, dilation, and aneurysmal formation may occur in artery supplying malformation
  - ○ **Arteriovenous Fistula**
    - Whether traumatic, iatrogenic, or surgically created, increased shunting of blood through arteriovenous fistula may cause dilation of supplying artery
  - ○ **Aortic Regurgitation**
    - Results in abnormal volume increase, leading to dilation of ascending aorta
- **Dilation from Increased Pressure**
  - ○ Systemic hypertension causes diffuse increase in arterial luminal pressure
  - ○ Aortic valve stenosis and post-stenotic dilation cause increase in arterial luminal pressure and subsequent dilatation, distal to obstruction

Atherosclerotic Aneurysm

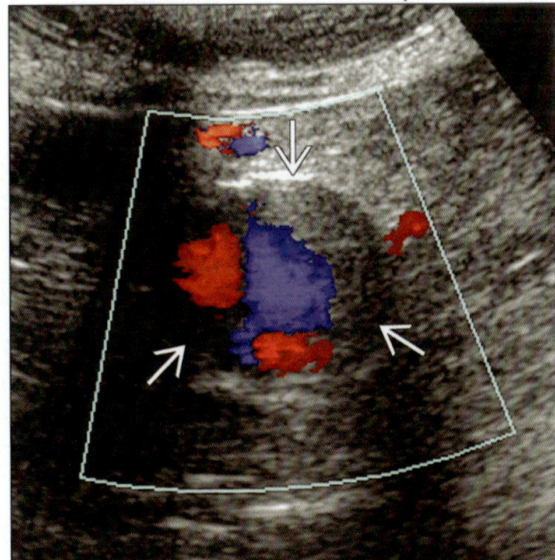

Transverse color Doppler ultrasound shows abdominal aneurysm with a circumferential mural thrombus ➡ in its lumen.

Atherosclerotic Aneurysm

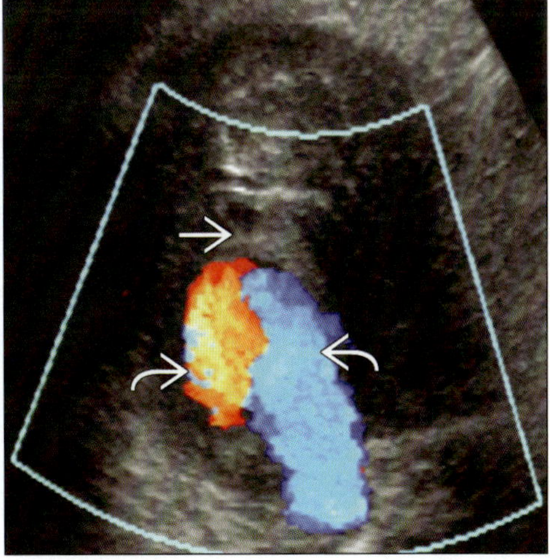

Transverse color Doppler ultrasound shows an abdominal aortic aneurysm (AAA) with mural thrombus in its anterior aspect ➡. Note that the outer diameter of the AAA is much wider than the lumen ➡.

ARTERIAL DILATION

(Left) Longitudinal color Doppler ultrasound shows an abdominal aortic aneurysm ➡ involving the bifurcation of the aorta ➡. Note that the left common iliac artery also appears aneurysmal ➡. *(Right)* Transverse transabdominal ultrasound in the same patient shows the left common iliac artery, demonstrating dilation of the artery ➡ with intramural thrombus ➡.

Atherosclerotic Aneurysm

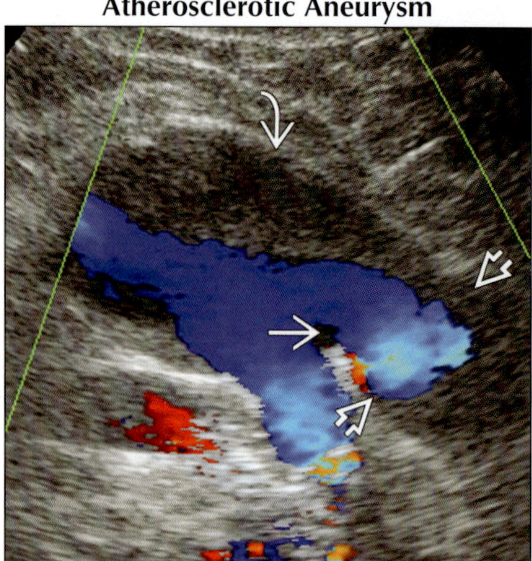

Atherosclerotic Aneurysm

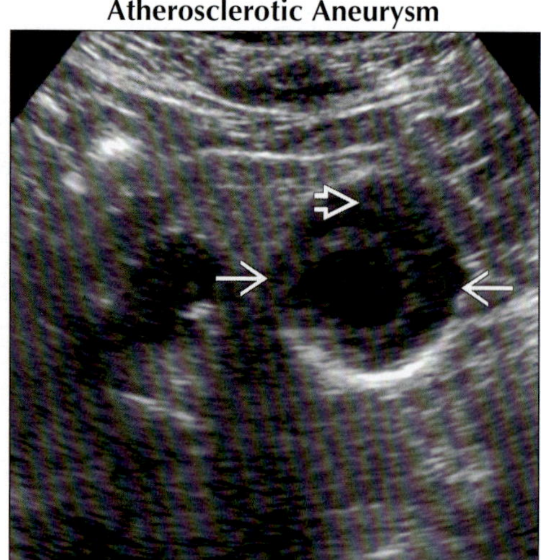

(Left) Transverse NECT shows an aneurysm ➡ in the infrarenal aorta. Note the low-attenuation collections ➡ in the aortic wall and in the left psoas muscle, which may represent pus. *(Right)* Transverse CECT shows the same infected aneurysm ➡. The low-attenuation collection in the aortic wall ➡ is better seen with contrast enhancement. Salmonella was subsequently identified in the blood culture of this patient.

Infective Aneurysm

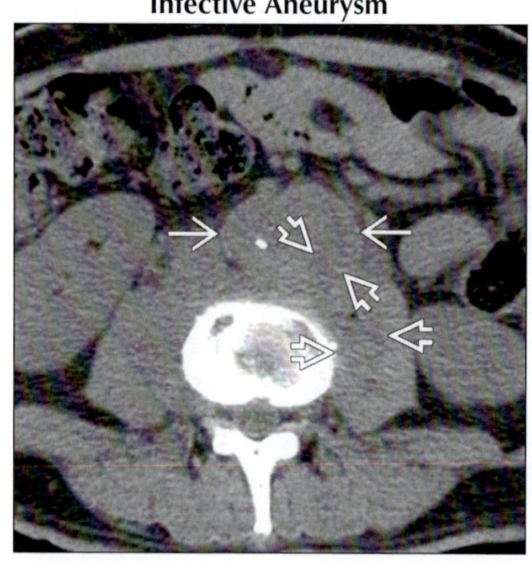

Infective Aneurysm

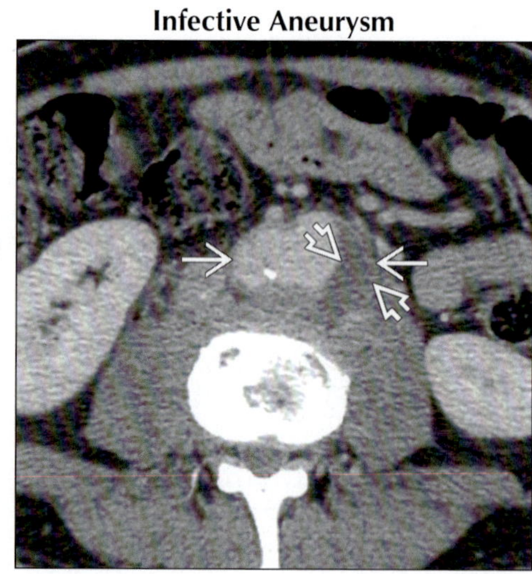

(Left) Oblique ultrasound shows a hypoechoic mycotic aneurysm ➡ in the buttock region of a patient with known infective endocarditis. *(Right)* Oblique color Doppler ultrasound in the same patient shows that the color signal fills the lumen of the mycotic aneurysm ➡. Note the thickening of the arterial wall ➡.

Mycotic Aneurysm

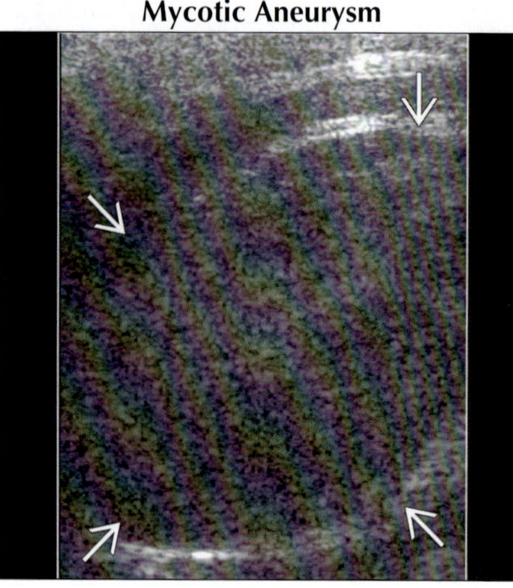

Mycotic Aneurysm

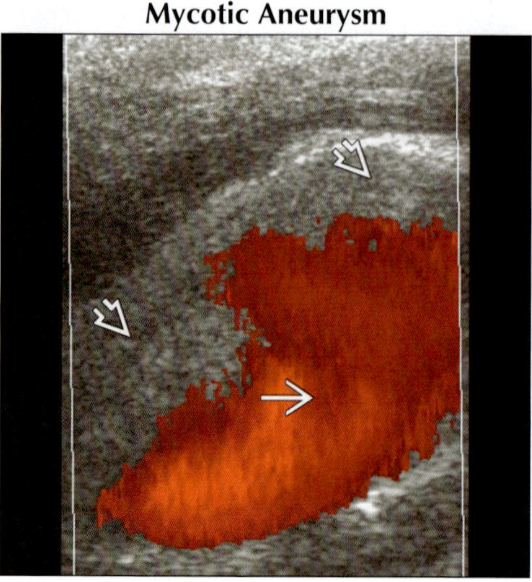

ARTERIAL DILATION

Mycotic Aneurysm

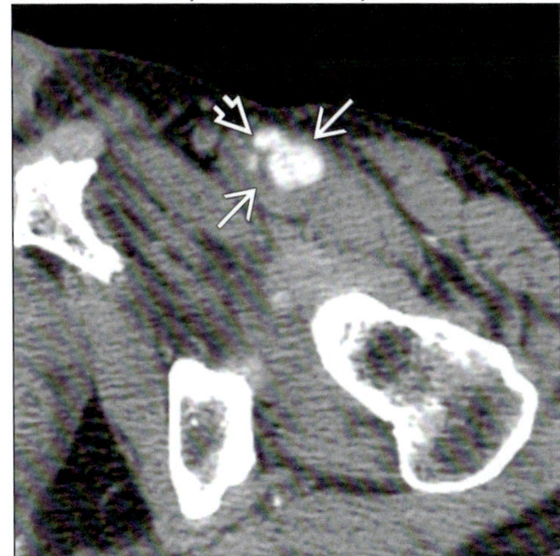

Mycotic Aneurysm

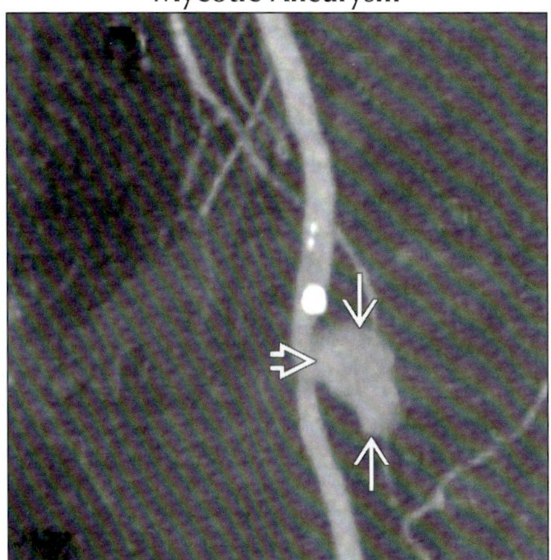

(Left) Transverse CECT shows a saccular mycotic aneurysm ➡ in the left common femoral artery ⮕ of a patient with known infective endocarditis. *(Right)* CTA maximal intensity projection shows the morphology of the same saccular mycotic aneurysm ➡. Note the neck of the aneurysm ⮕ arising from the lateral aspect of the artery.

Inflammatory Aneurysm

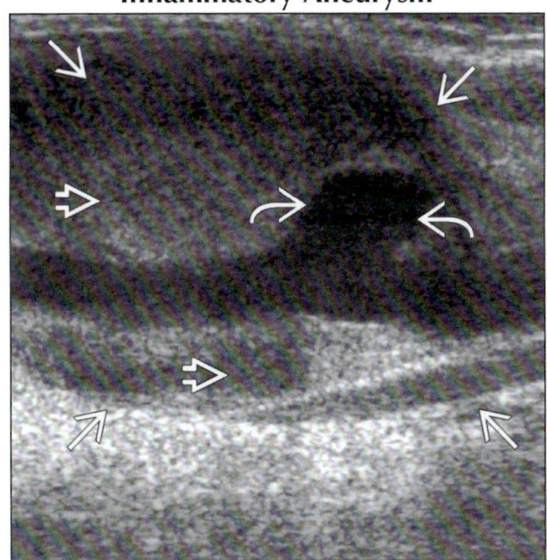

Inflammatory Aneurysm

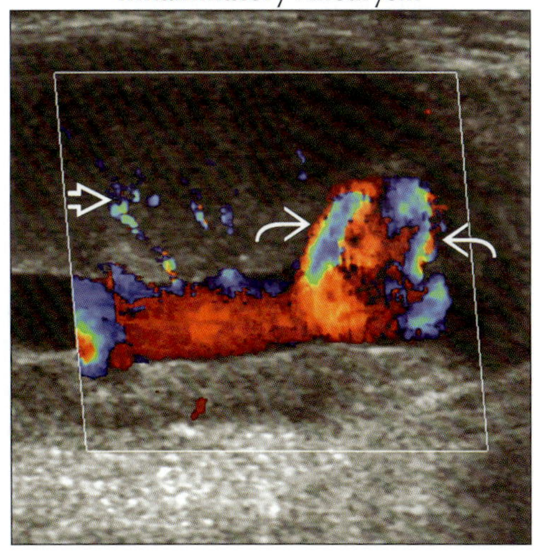

(Left) Oblique ultrasound shows an inflammatory aneurysm ➡ in the axillary artery of a patient with vasculitis. Note the marked thickening of the arterial wall ⮕ and the presence of a saccular aneurysm ➡ arising from the arterial lumen. *(Right)* Oblique color Doppler ultrasound in the same patient better shows the lumen of the saccular aneurysm ➡. Flashes of color signal are also seen in the arterial wall ⮕.

Vascular Malformation

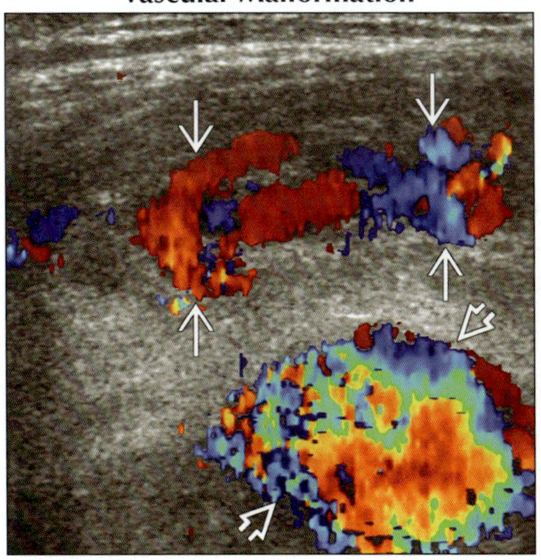

Post-Stenotic Dilation

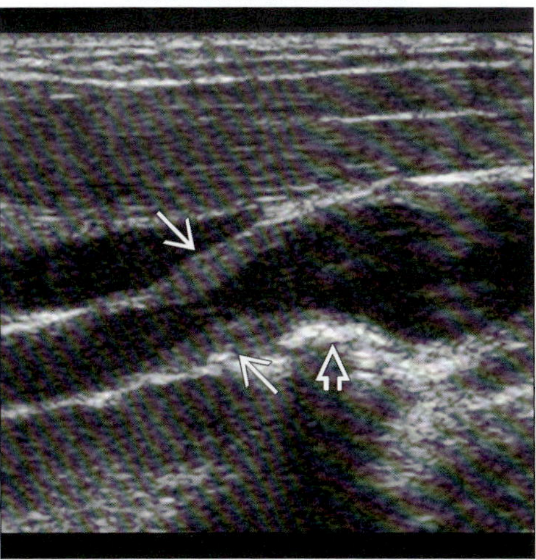

(Left) Oblique color Doppler ultrasound shows a superficial vascular malformation ➡, which is associated with aneurysmal dilation of the supplying artery ⮕. *(Right)* Longitudinal ultrasound shows internal carotid artery stenosis caused by fibrous plaque ➡ with foci of calcification ⮕.

DIFFERENTIAL DIAGNOSIS

Common
- Atherosclerosis
- Fibromuscular Dysplasia (FMD)

Less Common
- Neointimal Hyperplasia
- Arterial Dissection
- Arteritis
- Embolism
- Vasospasm
- Adventitial Cystic Disease
- Aneurysms
- Vessel Kinking

Rare but Important
- Extrinsic Compression by Tumor

ESSENTIAL INFORMATION

Key Differential Diagnosis Issues
- Clinical factors important in forming differential diagnosis
  - Age of patient
    - In older patients: Consider atherosclerosis, adventitial cystic disease, vessel kinking due to tortuous vessels, aneurysms
    - In younger patients: Consider FMD, arteritis, vasospasm
  - Predisposing factors to arterial disease
    - Smoking: Consider atherosclerosis, aneurysms, and possibility of embolism (e.g., embolization from aortic aneurysm)
    - Hypertension: Consider atherosclerosis, arterial dissection
    - Diabetes: Consider atherosclerosis
    - Atrial fibrillation: Consider embolism
    - Connective tissue disease: Consider arteritis
  - Previous endovascular intervention or surgical arterial anastomosis? or arterial stenosis close to known dialysis arteriovenous fistula?
    - Consider neointimal hyperplasia
- Imaging findings
  - Sonographic findings of stenosis
    - Increased stenotic zone velocity
    - Disturbed flow in post-stenotic zone
    - Proximal pulsatility changes
    - Distal pulsatility changes
  - Look for indirect findings in collateral vessels
    - Increased size, velocity, and volume flow
  - Document location
    - Near ostium or origin of artery: Consider atherosclerosis
    - In mid-portion of artery but sparing origin of artery: Consider FMD
    - Diffuse narrowing of entire artery: Consider atherosclerosis, arteritis, and vasospasm
  - Evaluate nature of wall thickening if present
    - Wall thickening and atheromatous plaques present: Consider atherosclerosis
    - Wall thickening present but atheromatous plaques not seen: Consider arteritis
    - Wall thickening absent: Consider vasospasm, vessel kinking, embolism
  - Look for dissection flap
    - If present, diagnostic of arterial dissection

Helpful Clues for Common Diagnoses
- **Atherosclerosis**
  - By far most common cause of arterial stenosis
  - Risk factors
    - Smoking
    - Diabetes mellitus
    - Hypertension
    - Hyperlipidemias
    - Obesity
    - Hypercoagulable states
- **Fibromuscular Dysplasia (FMD)**
  - Disorder of unknown etiology affecting medium-sized arteries
  - Women more commonly affected than men (M:F = 1:3)
  - Usually affects adults age 25-50
  - Familial association in 11% but not strictly genetic disorder
  - Overgrowth of smooth muscle cells and fibrous tissue within arterial wall
  - Not inflammatory or degenerative
  - Media is primarily involved in 85% of cases with intima and adventitia affected in remaining cases
  - Medial form gives classic "string of beads" appearance

14

- Caused by alternating areas of medial fibroplasia and focal aneurysmal dilation
  ○ Sonographically, FMD is seen as series of ridges in arterial wall
    - Most common locations: Renal arteries > internal carotid arteries
    - Internal carotid arteries may also present as long tubular stenosis or asymmetrical outpouching of artery

Helpful Clues for Less Common Diagnoses

- **Neointimal Hyperplasia**
  ○ Common cause of restenosis in artery following endovascular intervention, including angioplasty and stenting
  ○ Also common cause of stenosis in surgical bypass graft or at sites of arterial stenosis
  ○ Can also cause arterial stenosis around dialysis arteriovenous fistula
- **Arterial Dissection**
  ○ Entry of blood into wall of artery
    - Separates layers of wall & creates false lumen through which blood flows
    - False lumen may then cause narrowing of true lumen and compromise blood flow
- **Arteritis**
  ○ Large vessels
    - Takayasu arteritis, systemic giant cell arteritis, radiation-induced arteritis
  ○ Small vessels
    - Vasculitis of connective tissue disease, scleroderma, rheumatoid arthritis, SLE, Buerger disease

- **Embolism**
  ○ Acute onset
    - Cardiac source (atrial fibrillation or endocarditis)
    - Aortic source (thrombus in aneurysm)
- **Vasospasm**
  ○ Transient constriction of vessel
  ○ Seen with Raynaud phenomenon
    - Disorder characterized by episodic vasospasm and vasoconstriction of digital arteries
- **Adventitial Cystic Disease**
  ○ Cystic degeneration in wall of artery causes stenosis of arterial lumen
- **Aneurysms**
  ○ Popliteal artery aneurysms are often associated with stenosis or occlusion of popliteal artery
- **Vessel Kinking**
  ○ May give impression of stenosis

Helpful Clues for Rare Diagnoses

- **Extrinsic Compression by Tumor**
  ○ Any large mass may compress adjacent vessels
  ○ In neck, consider carotid body tumor
    - Highly vascular paraganglioma of low malignant potential, arising from carotid body
    - Tumor may encase external or internal carotid artery, causing stenosis or potentially complicating surgical excision

Atherosclerosis

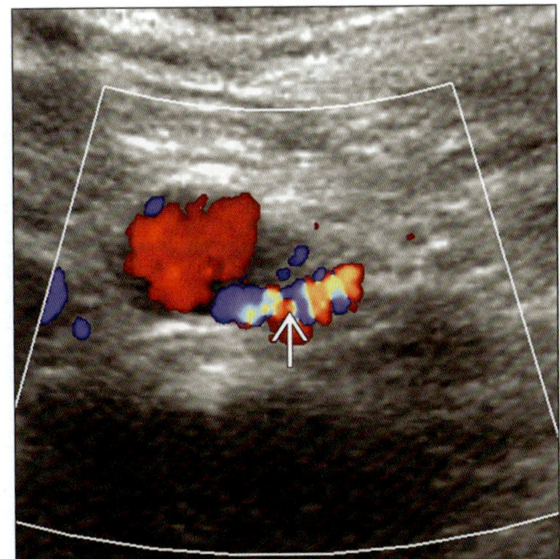

Transverse color Doppler ultrasound shows focal color "aliasing" ➡, *indicating turbulent flow at the ostium of the left renal artery. Stenosis at the renal ostium is most commonly due to atherosclerosis.*

Atherosclerosis

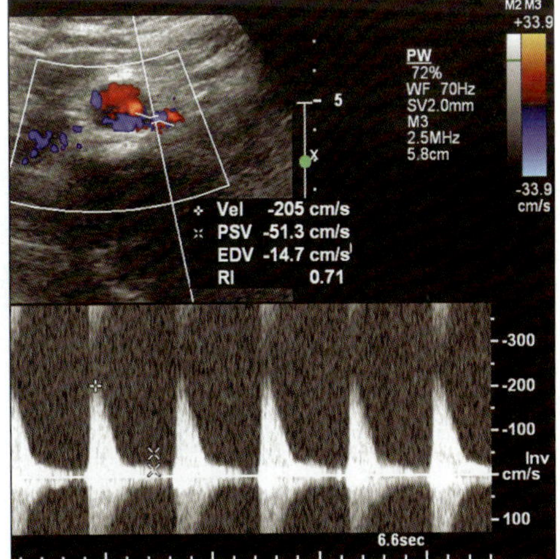

Transverse pulsed Doppler ultrasound in the same patient shows the peak velocity in the left renal artery ostium stenosis exceeds 200 cm/s with "wraparound" artifact also seen.

ARTERIAL STENOSIS

(Left) Longitudinal color Doppler ultrasound shows high-grade internal carotid artery stenosis. The arterial lumen is significantly narrowed with an "aliasing" flow artifact seen ➡ due to increased flow velocity. *(Right)* Longitudinal pulsed Doppler ultrasound shows the typical findings of stenosis. Both peak systolic velocity and end diastolic velocity are markedly increased, suggesting that the degree of stenosis exceeds 70%.

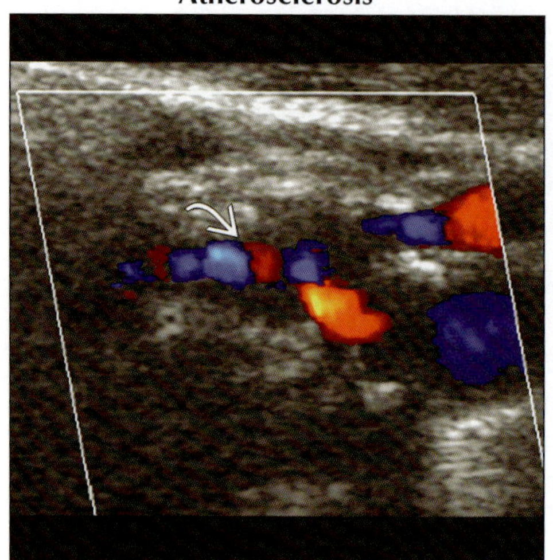

Atherosclerosis

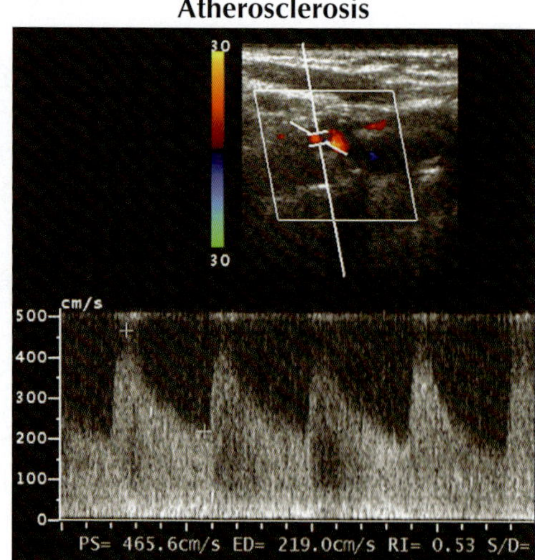

Atherosclerosis

(Left) Longitudinal power Doppler ultrasound shows a soft plaque ➡, which is typically hypoechoic, and is easily missed with grayscale imaging alone. Such a plaque has a high risk of embolization. *(Right)* Longitudinal ultrasound shows an irregular fibrous plaque ➡ in the common carotid artery causing tight stenosis. Such plaques are relatively stable and carry a low risk of cerebral embolism.

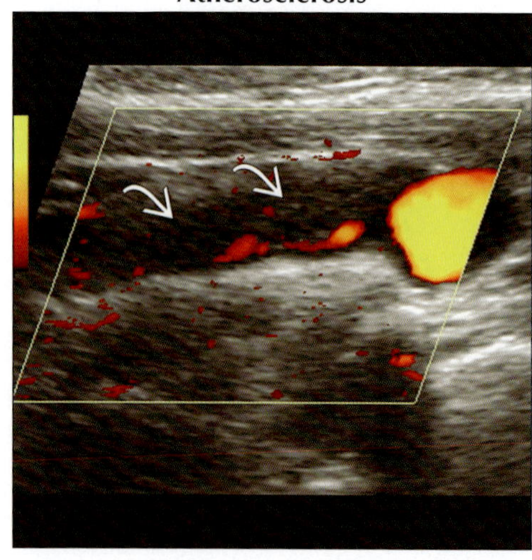

Atherosclerosis

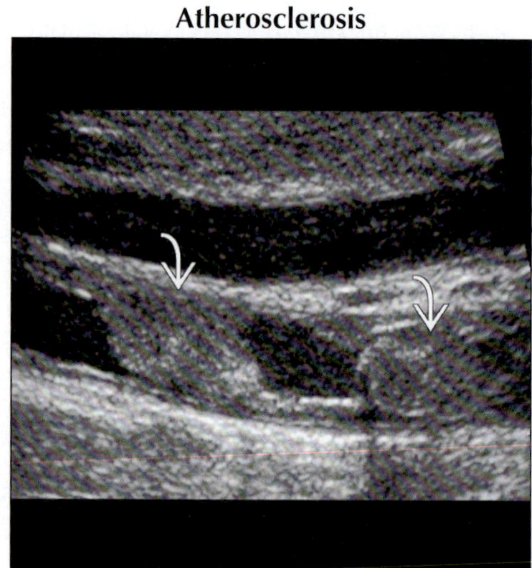

Atherosclerosis

(Left) Longitudinal ultrasound shows a calcified plaque ➡ characterized by posterior acoustic shadowing ➡. Such a plaque has a minimal risk of an embolic event. *(Right)* Longitudinal ultrasound shows a heterogeneous plaque with areas of calcification ➡ and hypoechogenicity ➡. Such a plaque has an increased risk of cerebral embolism.

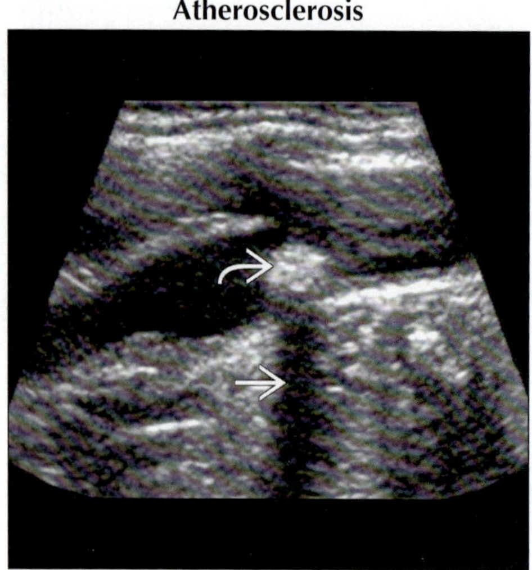

Atherosclerosis

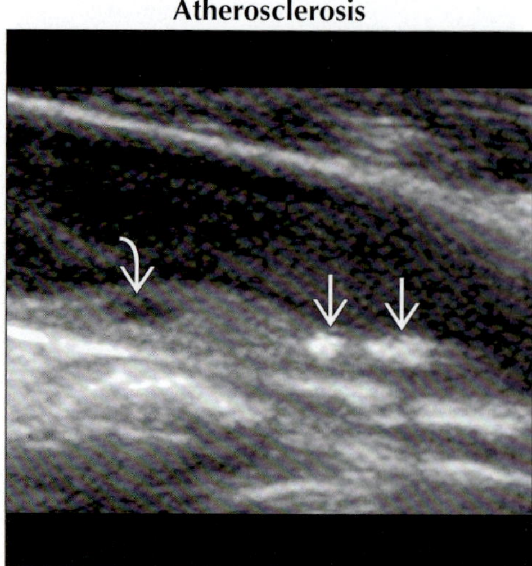

Atherosclerosis

14

Atherosclerosis

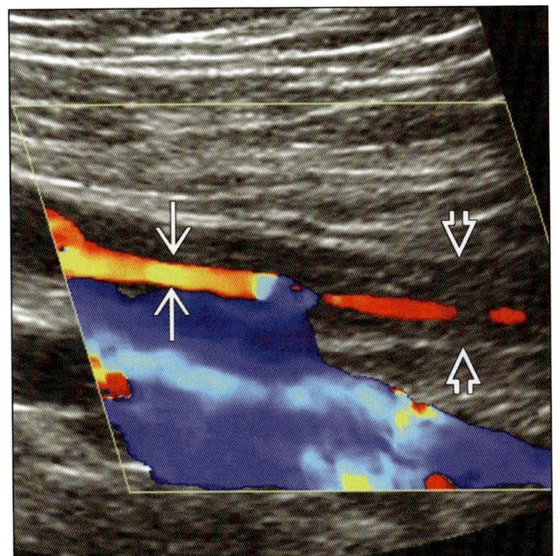

Atherosclerosis

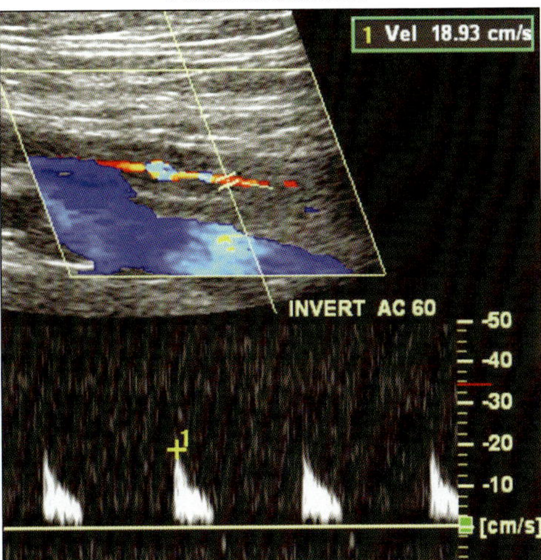

(Left) Longitudinal color Doppler ultrasound shows a long, stenotic, superficial, femoral artery segment with a trickle of flow. Note the lumen ➡, is considerably narrower than the diameter of the artery ➡. (Right) Longitudinal pulsed Doppler ultrasound shows monophasic, low-velocity flow in the same patient.

Fibromuscular Dysplasia (FMD)

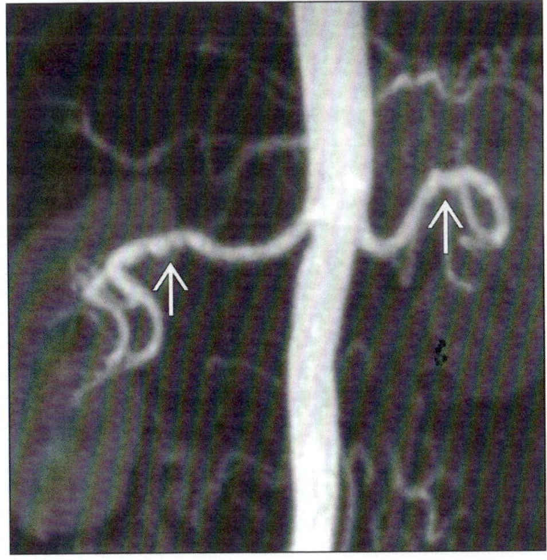

Neointimal Hyperplasia

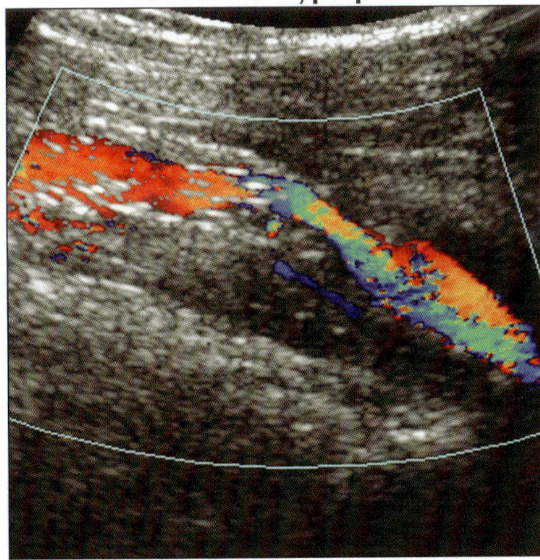

(Left) Coronal MRA shows the typical appearance of bilateral, mid-segment renal artery stenosis caused by fibromuscular dysplasia. Note the characteristic "string of beads" appearance ➡ in the renal arteries, bilaterally. (Right) Longitudinal color Doppler ultrasound shows turbulent flow within a previously placed popliteal artery stent, indicative of restenosis, likely due to neointimal hyperplasia.

Neointimal Hyperplasia

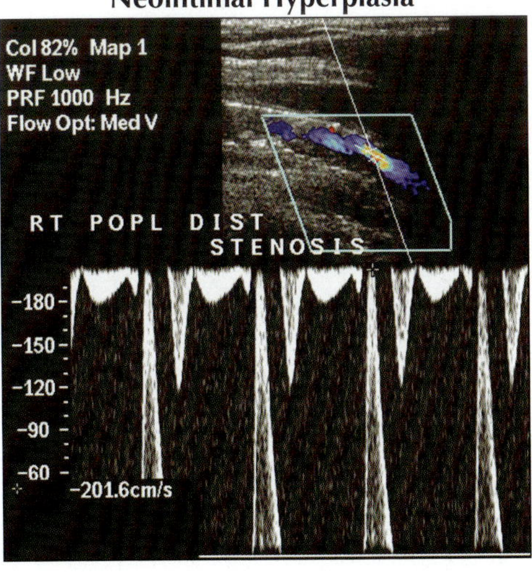

Neointimal Hyperplasia

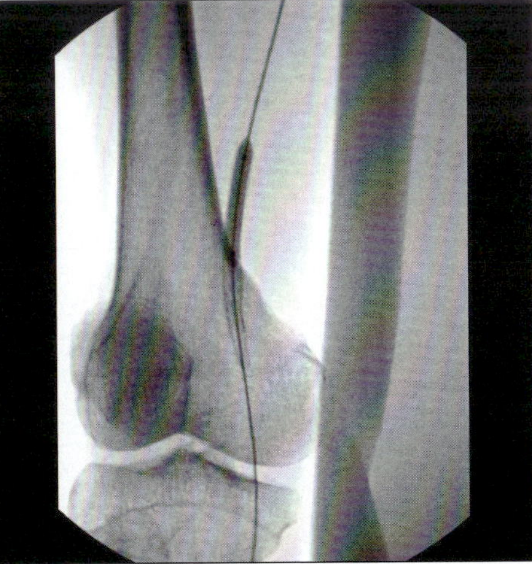

(Left) Longitudinal pulsed Doppler ultrasound in the same patient shows increased peak systolic velocity with a "wraparound" artifact, suggestive of turbulent flow and significant stenosis. (Right) DSA shows a balloon angioplasty of a new stent placed coaxially through the previously placed and stenosed stent, as seen on the 2 preceding ultrasound images.

ARTERIAL STENOSIS

Neointimal Hyperplasia

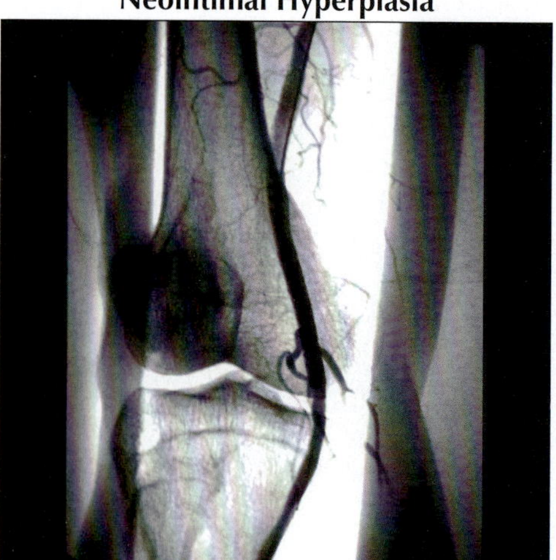

Neointimal Hyperplasia

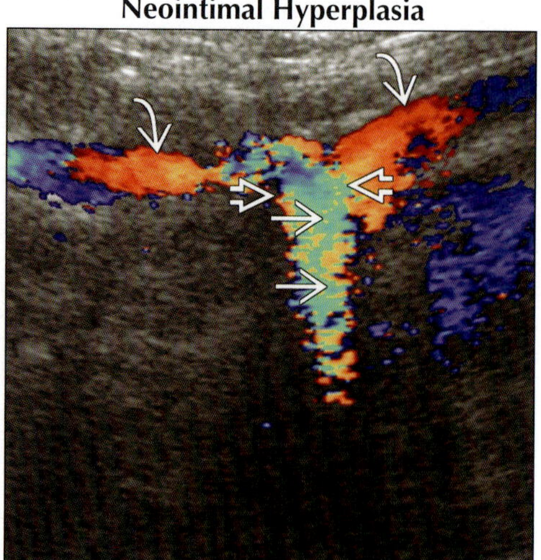

(Left) DSA performed after stenting and angioplasty shows no significant residual stenosis. *(Right)* Longitudinal color Doppler ultrasound shows focal color aliasing ➡ in a patient with transplant renal artery stenosis, close to the anastomotic site ➡ with the external iliac artery ➡. Transplant renal artery stenosis may be caused by neointimal hyperplasia, anastomotic technical problem, surgical injury, or rejection/scarring.

Neointimal Hyperplasia

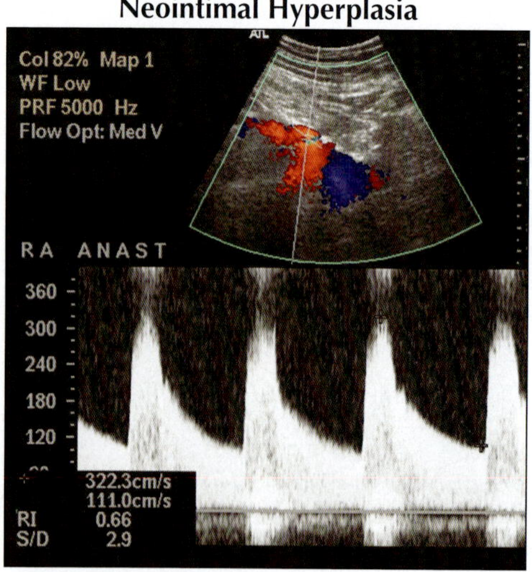

Neointimal Hyperplasia

(Left) Longitudinal pulsed Doppler ultrasound in the same patient shows peak systolic velocity of 322 cm/s, indicating stenosis in a transplanted renal artery. *(Right)* Longitudinal pulsed Doppler ultrasound shows a dampened "tardus parvus" waveform in the intrarenal arcuate artery. Note the sloped early systolic waveform ➡. This is an indirect method to demonstrate renal artery stenosis.

Arterial Dissection

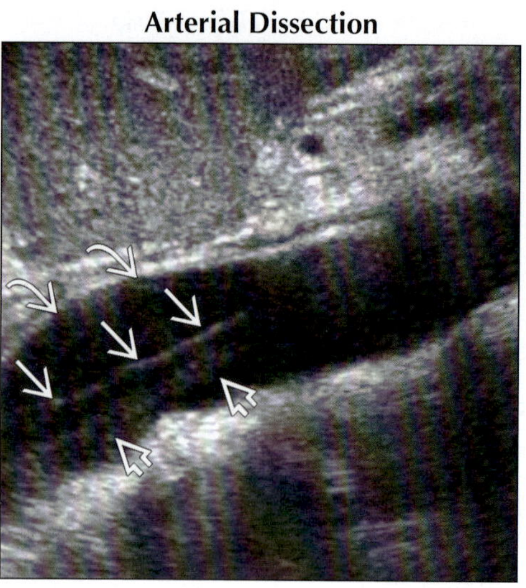

Arteritis

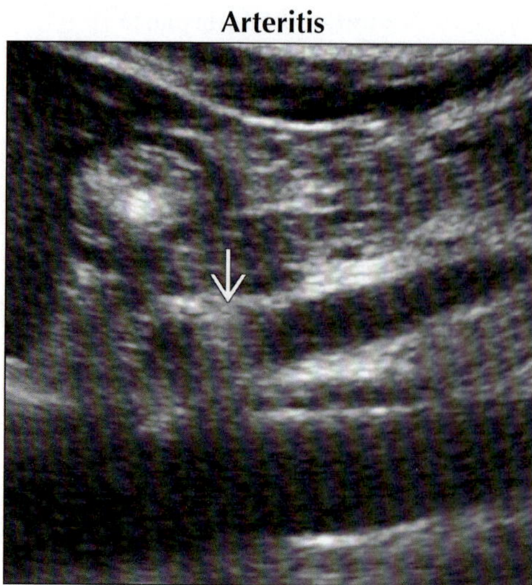

(Left) Longitudinal ultrasound shows arterial dissection within the abdominal aorta. Note the dissection flap ➡ and the false lumen ➡ that are causing significant narrowing of the true lumen ➡. *(Right)* Longitudinal ultrasound shows stenosis ➡ at the origin of the superior mesenteric artery in a patient with Takayasu arteritis. The disease typically affects the aorta, the aortic arch vessels, and the visceral and renal arteries.

ARTERIAL STENOSIS

Arteritis

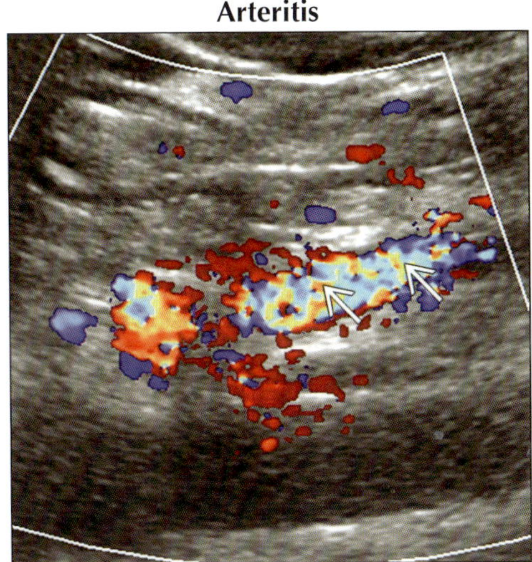

Arteritis

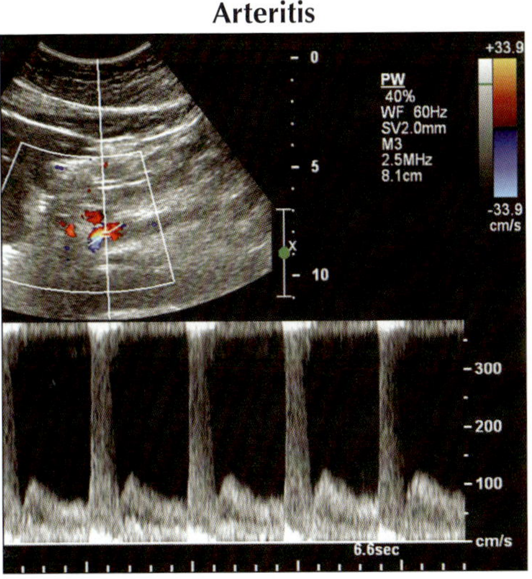

(Left) Longitudinal color Doppler ultrasound shows color "aliasing" ➡, indicative of significant stenosis, in the superior mesenteric artery of the same patient. *(Right)* Longitudinal pulsed Doppler ultrasound shows the peak systolic velocity in excess of 300 cm/s with aliasing at the origin of the superior mesenteric artery, again indicating significant stenosis in this patient.

Arteritis

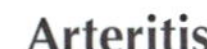
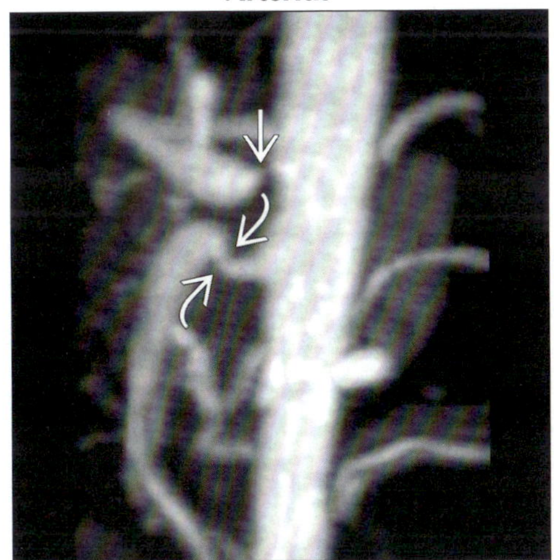

Adventitial Cystic Disease

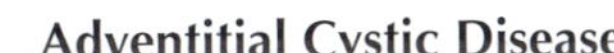
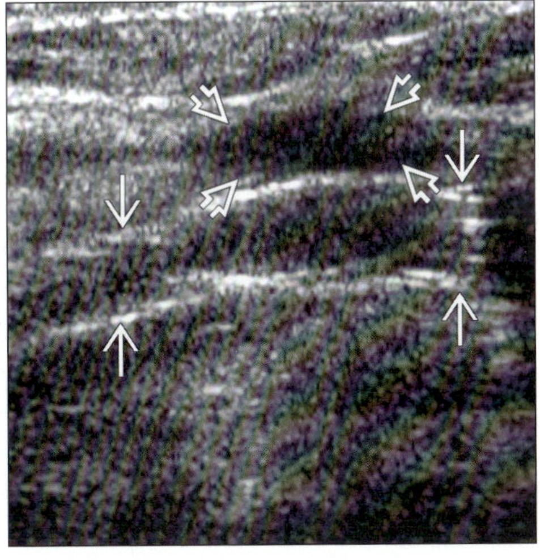

(Left) Sagittal MRA performed on the same patient shows significant stenoses at the origins of the celiac axis ➡ and the superior mesenteric artery ➡. *(Right)* Longitudinal ultrasound shows an echogenic stent ➡ in the lumen of a popliteal artery narrowed by adventitial cystic disease. The hypoechoic area ➡ indicates the area of cystic degeneration of the arterial wall.

Extrinsic Compression by Tumor

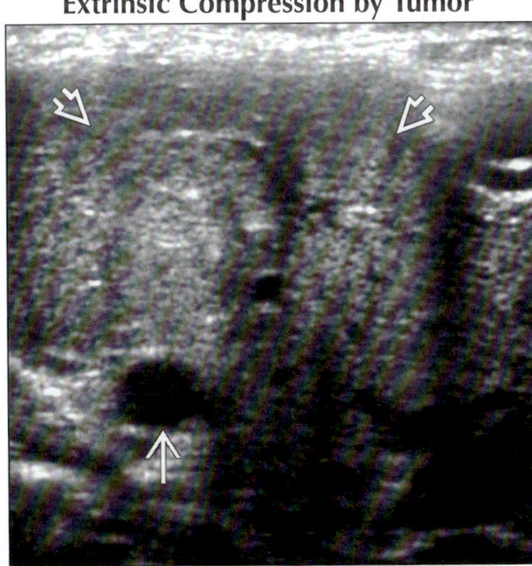

Extrinsic Compression by Tumor

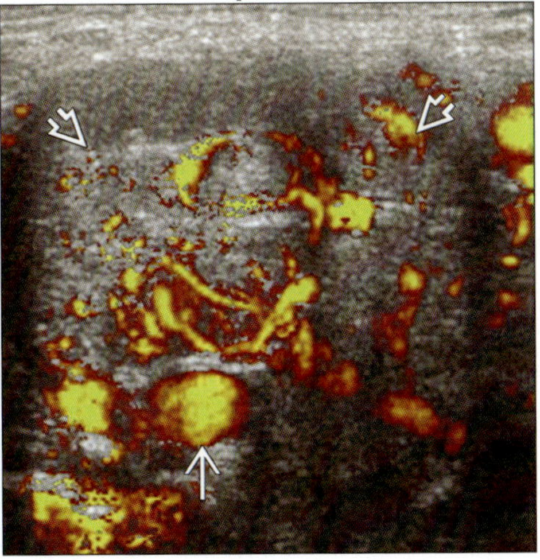

(Left) Transverse ultrasound shows a large, well-defined, noncalcified, homogeneous, carotid body paraganglioma ➡ in close relation to the carotid artery ➡. *(Right)* Transverse power Doppler ultrasound shows prominent vascularity in the tumor parenchyma, as well as the relationship between the carotid artery ➡ and the carotid body paraganglioma ➡.

INTRALUMINAL ARTERIAL MASS

DIFFERENTIAL DIAGNOSIS

Common
- Atherosclerotic Plaque
  - Fatty or "Soft" Plaque
  - Fibrous Plaque
  - Calcified Plaque
  - Ulcerated Plaque
  - Homogeneous Plaque
  - Heterogeneous Plaque
- Fibromuscular Dysplasia (FMD)
- Thrombus
- Iatrogenic Foreign Bodies
  - Endovascular Stents
  - Intraarterial Embolization Coils
  - Surgical Sutures

Less Common
- Neointimal Hyperplasia
- Embolism
- Arterial Dissection

ESSENTIAL INFORMATION

Key Differential Diagnosis Issues
- Differential diagnosis list for intraluminal arterial masses is relatively short
- Useful clinical factors to consider
  - In older patients: Atherosclerotic plaques and arterial dissection
  - In younger patients: Fibromuscular dysplasia
  - In acute presentation of arterial occlusion: Acute thrombosis, embolism, or arterial dissection
  - History of hypertension or trauma: Arterial dissection

Helpful Clues for Common Diagnoses
- **Atherosclerotic Plaque**
  - **Fatty or "Soft" Plaque**
    - Hypoechoic or slightly echogenic; ↑ risk of embolization
  - **Fibrous Plaque**
    - Mildly echogenic, stable; ↓ risk of embolization
  - **Calcified Plaque**
    - Highly echogenic with posterior acoustic shadowing; focal/diffuse, dystrophic, ↓ risk of embolization
  - **Ulcerated Plaque**
    - Focal crypt in plaque with sharp overhanging edges; ↑ risk of embolization
  - **Homogeneous Plaque**
    - Uniform medium-level echogenicity; ↓ risk of embolization
  - **Heterogeneous Plaque**
    - Focal or scattered areas of hypoechogenicity; ↑ risk of embolization
- **Fibromuscular Dysplasia (FMD)**
  - Medial is involved in 85% of cases, with intima and adventitia affected in remaining cases
  - Medial form gives classic "string of beads" appearance caused by alternating areas of medial fibroplasia and focal aneurysmal dilation
  - Sonographically, FMD is seen as series of ridges in arterial wall
    - Renal arteries > internal carotid arteries
  - In internal carotid arteries, may present as long tubular stenosis or asymmetrical outpouching of artery
- **Thrombus**
  - Acute thrombosis
    - May be related to emboli, endovascular stenting, or surgery (such as endarterectomy)
    - Vessel lumen is usually of normal caliber or slightly expanded, as opposed to luminal narrowing or obliteration in chronic thrombosis
    - Usually low echogenicity
    - Swirling sludge-like flow may be seen at interface between thrombosed and patent lumen
    - Spectral Doppler may show high impedance, hammer-like or "to and fro" configuration
  - Mural thrombus
    - Frequently seen within lumen of aneurysmal segments
    - Sonographically seen as hypoechoic material adherent to arterial wall
    - Color Doppler useful to depict flow in lumen
  - Chronic thrombosis
    - Lumen filled with echogenic material; absent flow on color and spectral Doppler
    - Smaller caliber

14

INTRALUMINAL ARTERIAL MASS

- **Iatrogenic Foreign Bodies**
  - **Endovascular Stents**
    - Used for treatment of arterial stenosis in common & internal carotid arteries, native & transplanted renal arteries, and arteries in upper & lower limbs
    - Covered stents increasingly used for treatment of aortic aneurysms and aortic dissection
    - Commonly made from stainless steel or nitinol
    - Metallic struts visible as echogenic linear structures on ultrasound
  - **Intraarterial Embolization Coils**
    - Used for treatment of arterial trauma in organs & peripheral arteries, arteriovenous fistulas, pseudoaneurysms, and gastrointestinal bleeding
    - Commonly made from stainless steel or platinum
    - Metal component is echogenic on ultrasound
  - **Surgical Sutures**
    - May be seen as echogenic material protruding into arterial lumen around arterial or graft anastomosis

Helpful Clues for Less Common Diagnoses
- **Neointimal Hyperplasia**
  - Major cause of in-stent restenosis, anastomotic site narrowing, central venous stenosis associated with hemodialysis arteriovenous fistulas
  - Seen on ultrasound as hypoechoic thickening of intimal layer
- **Embolism**
  - Cardiac source
    - Atrial thrombus in atrial fibrillation, septic emboli from infective endocarditis, or thrombus from ventricular aneurysm in myocardial infarction
  - Arterial source
    - Mural thrombus in aortic aneurysms, iliac aneurysms, or critical stenosis
  - Venous source
    - Possible if presence of right to left communication, such as patent foramen ovale, ASD, or VSD, with right to left shunt
  - Seen sonographically as abrupt occlusion with lack of collateralization in acute occlusion
- **Arterial Dissection**
  - Occurs when blood enters media through defect (entry site) in intima and dissects along length of artery
  - Intima may be stripped away in some parts, and new lumen (false lumen) may be formed
  - Blood may flow through both true and false lumens; compression of true lumen by false lumen may occur
  - Sonographic appearance typically shows presence of diagnostic dissection flap

Fatty or "Soft" Plaque

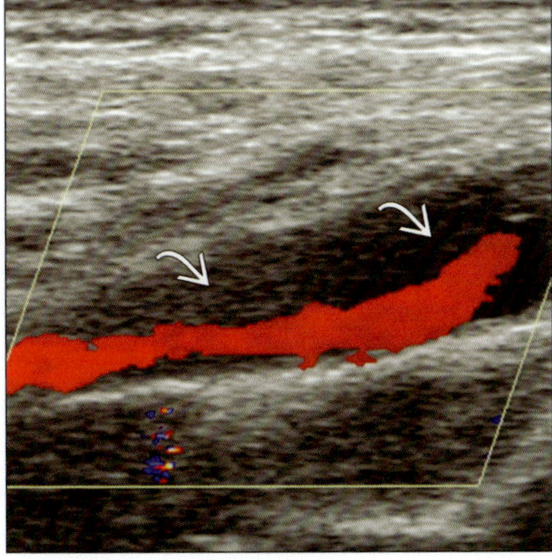

Longitudinal color Doppler ultrasound shows a soft plaque 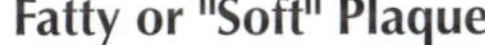, which is typically hypoechoic. Such plaque has a high risk of embolization and is easily missed with grayscale imaging alone.

Fibrous Plaque

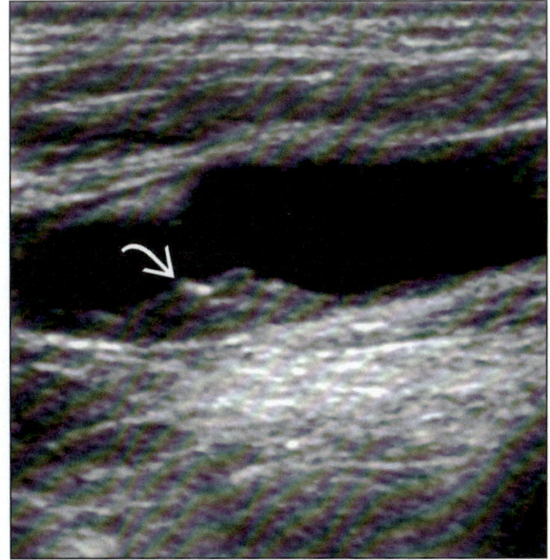

Longitudinal ultrasound shows an irregular fibrous plaque ➔ in the common carotid artery. Such plaque is relatively stable and carries a low risk of embolism.

INTRALUMINAL ARTERIAL MASS

Calcified Plaque

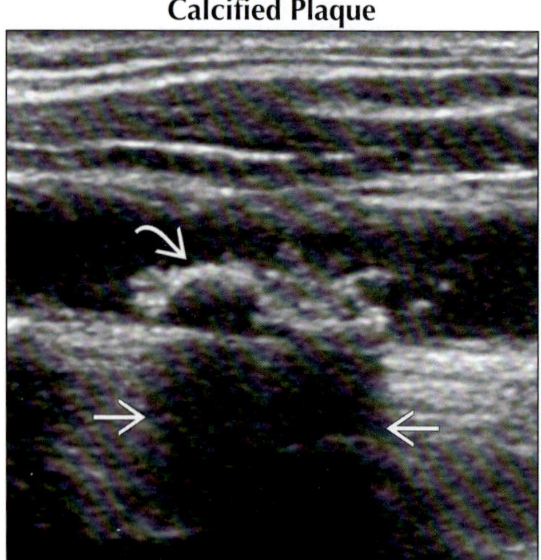

Ulcerated Plaque

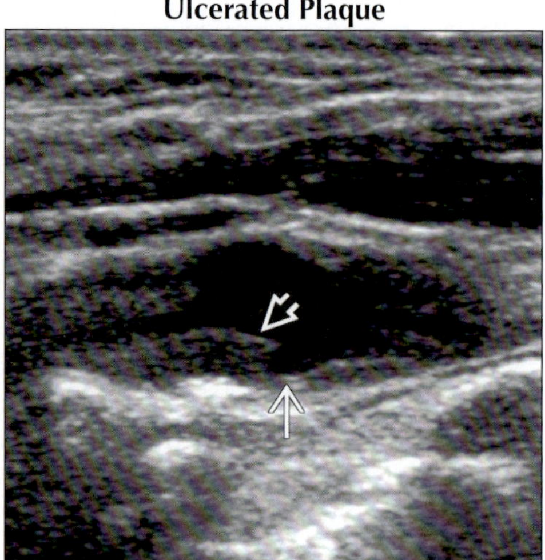

(Left) Longitudinal ultrasound shows a calcified plaque ➨ with posterior acoustic shadowing ➡. Such plaque carries minimal risk of embolization. (Right) Longitudinal ultrasound shows an ulcerated plaque with a typical focal crypt ➡, featuring sharp or overhanging edges ➨. Such a plaque carries an increased risk of embolization.

Homogeneous Plaque

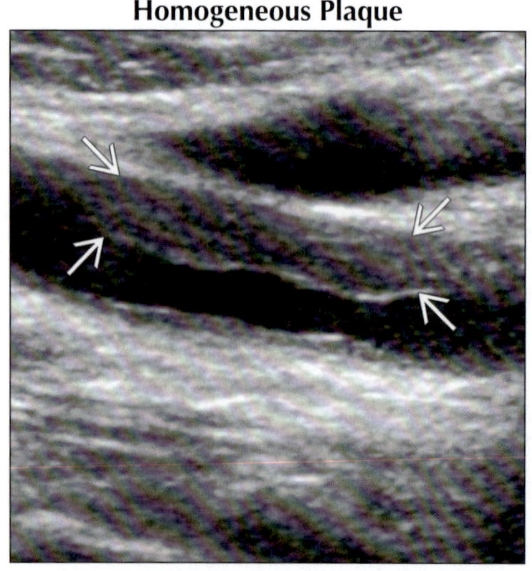

Heterogeneous Plaque

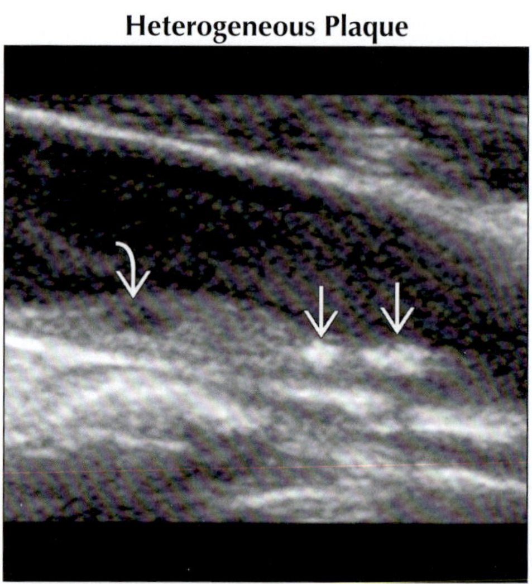

(Left) Longitudinal ultrasound shows a homogeneous plaque ➡ with a uniform medium level echotexture in the common carotid artery. Such a plaque has reduced risk of embolization. (Right) Longitudinal ultrasound shows a heterogeneous plaque with areas of calcification ➡ and hypoechogenicity ➡. Such plaque carries increased risk of embolism.

Fibromuscular Dysplasia (FMD)

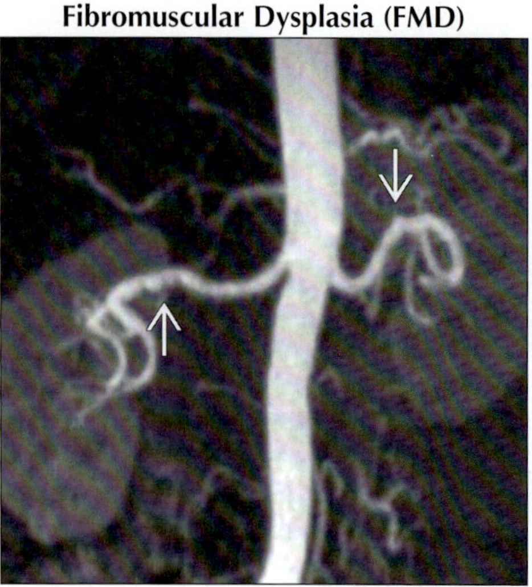

Thrombus

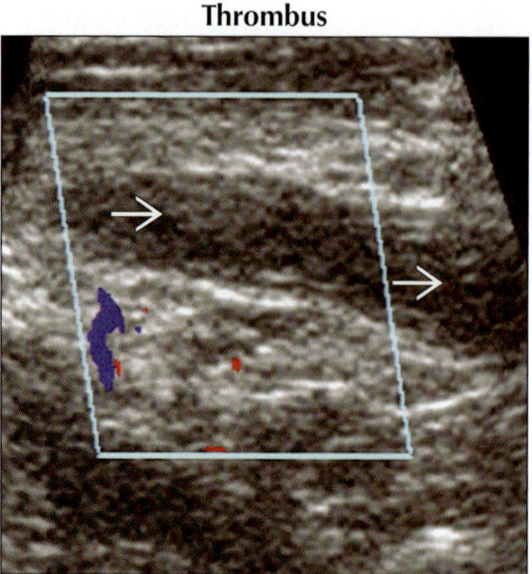

(Left) MRA shows the typical "string of beads" appearance ➡ of fibromuscular dysplasia of the renal arteries in its characteristic location at the mid-segment. (Right) Longitudinal color Doppler ultrasound shows total occlusion of the common carotid artery. Note the presence of a low echogenicity thrombus ➡ and the lack of color signal within the lumen of the artery.

INTRALUMINAL ARTERIAL MASS

Thrombus

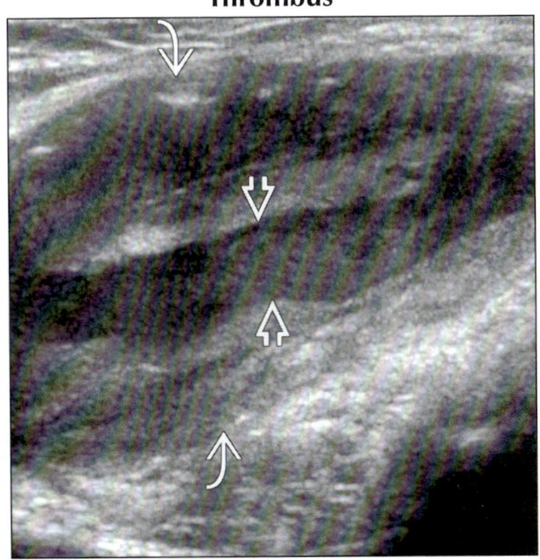

Thrombus

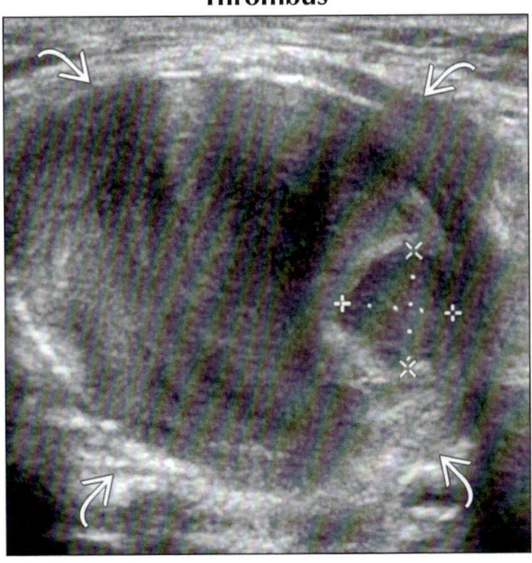

(Left) Longitudinal ultrasound shows a popliteal artery aneurysm containing a large amount of mural thrombus. Note that the luminal diameter ➡ is considerably less than the diameter of the aneurysm ➡. *(Right)* Transverse ultrasound in the same patient shows an eccentric arterial lumen marked by the calipers. Note the large amount of mural thrombus within the lumen of the popliteal artery aneurysm ➡.

Endovascular Stents

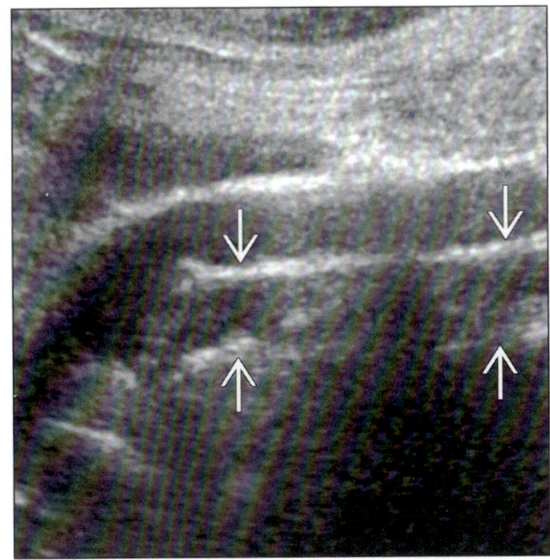

Endovascular Stents

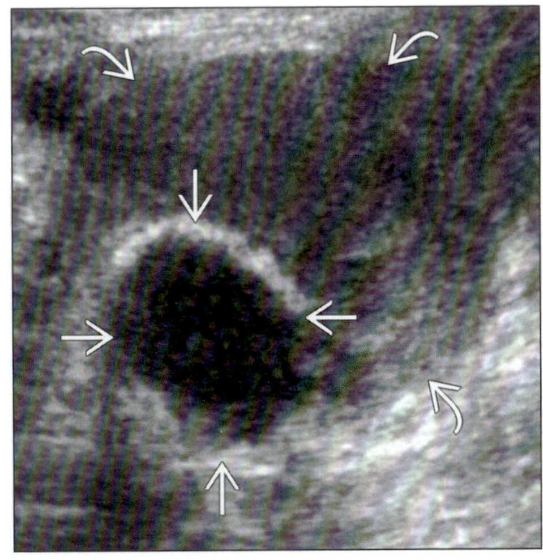

(Left) Longitudinal ultrasound shows an aortic stent graft lying within an aortic aneurysm. Note the 2 parallel echogenic lines ➡ correlating with the walls of the stent graft. *(Right)* Transverse ultrasound in the same patient shows the main body of the aortic stent graft. In transverse section, this portion of the stent graft appears as an echogenic ring ➡. Note the mural thrombus within the aneurysm ➡.

Endovascular Stents

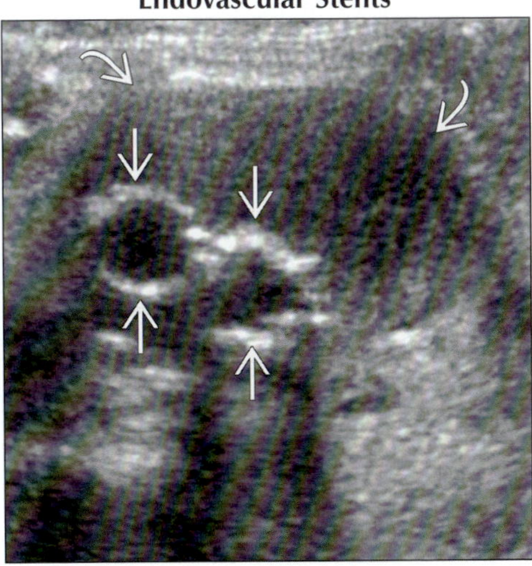

Endovascular Stents

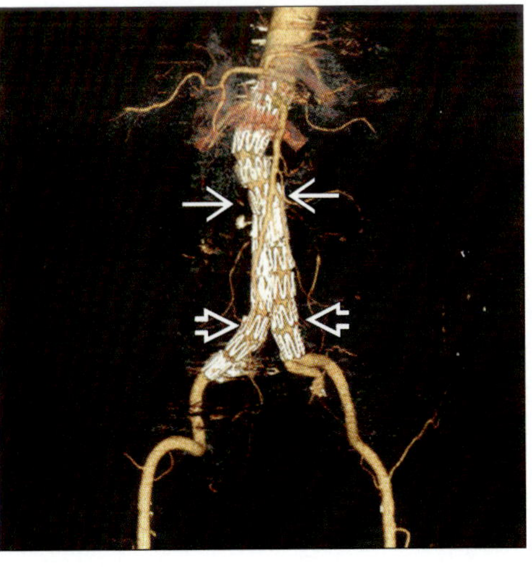

(Left) Transverse ultrasound through the proximal end of the limb extensions shows the same aortic stent graft. Note that the limb extensions appear as echogenic rings ➡ within the aortic aneurysm ➡. *(Right)* Corresponding CTA shows the volume-rendered image of the aortic stent graft. Note the configuration of the main body ➡ and the limb extensions ➡ of the aortic stent graft.

INTRALUMINAL ARTERIAL MASS
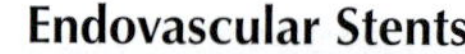

Endovascular Stents

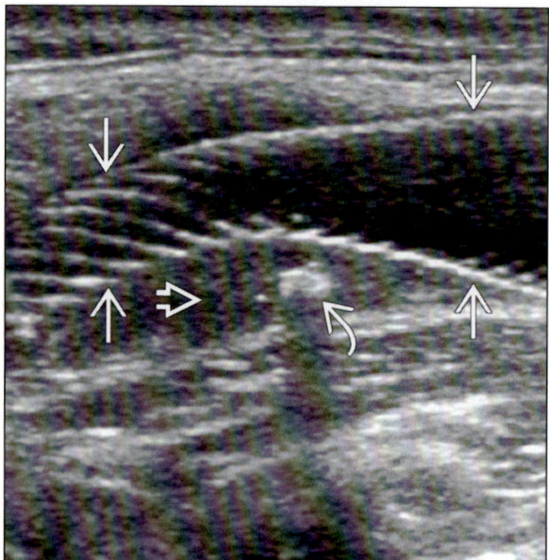

(Left) Longitudinal ultrasound shows a stent ➡ within the common carotid artery. Note the echogenic struts within the graft. Also note the underlying heterogeneous plaque ➡ with a focus of shadowing calcification ➡. (Right) Transverse ultrasound in the same patient shows the graft ➡, heterogeneous plaque ➡, and calcification ➡.

Endovascular Stents

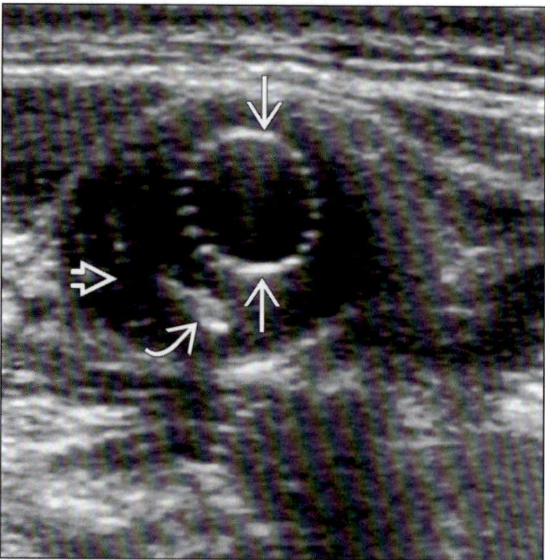

Endovascular Stents

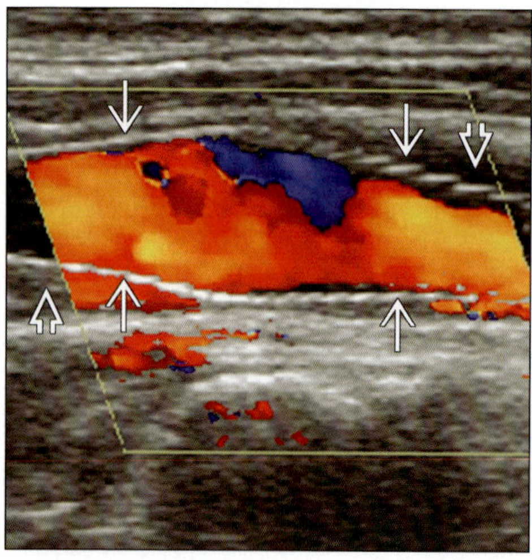

(Left) Longitudinal color Doppler ultrasound shows the widely patent lumen within a recently deployed carotid stent ➡ with no significant in-stent stenosis. Note the underlying fibrous plaque ➡. (Right) Longitudinal ultrasound shows the presence of 2 stents ➡ within the proximal internal carotid artery. The distal end ➡ of the inner 2nd stent is extended beyond the underlying plaque ➡.

Endovascular Stents

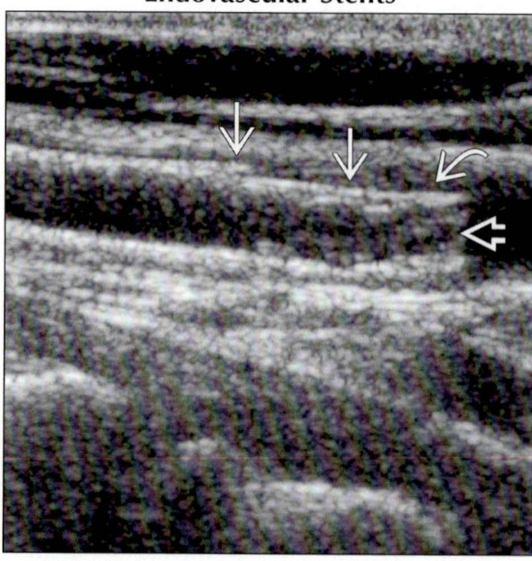

Intraarterial Embolization Coils

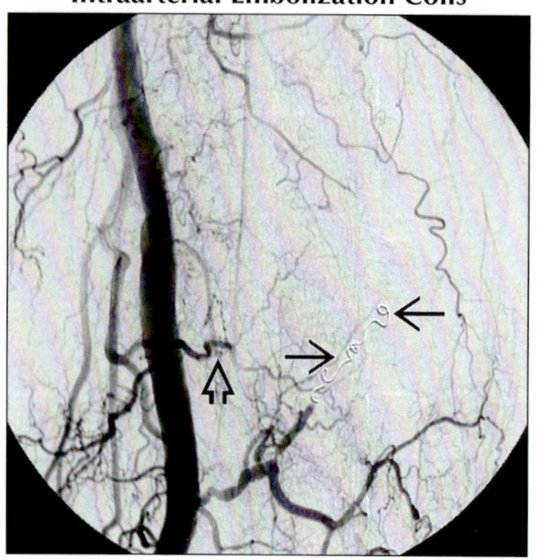

(Left) DSA following embolization of a pseudoaneurysm arising from the left lateral geniculate artery ➡ shows the intraarterial embolization coils ➡. Such coils appear echogenic on ultrasound. (Right) Oblique ultrasound shows surgical sutures around the anastomosis between the external iliac artery ➡ and transplanted renal artery ➡. The surgical sutures appear as small echogenic dots ➡.

Surgical Sutures

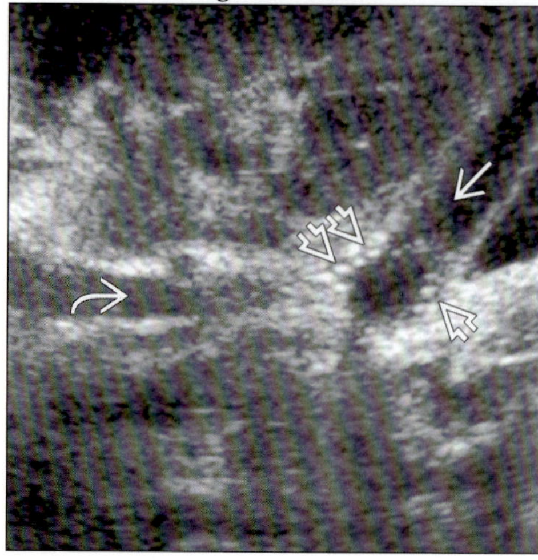

Neointimal Hyperplasia

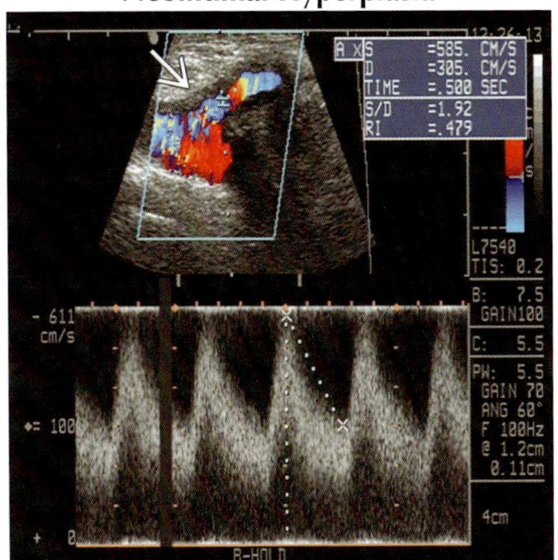

Neointimal Hyperplasia

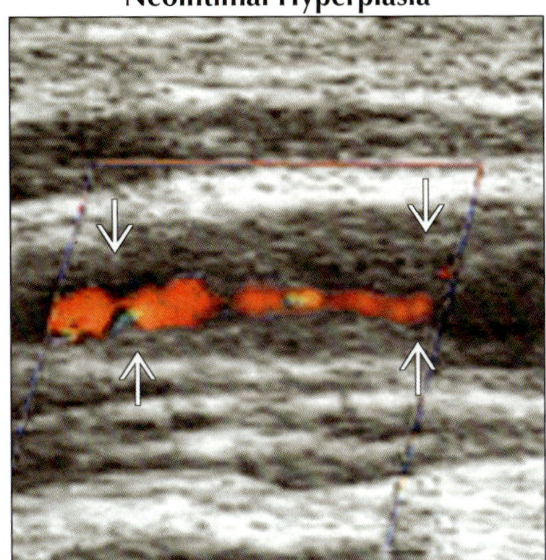

(Left) Longitudinal pulsed Doppler ultrasound shows an elevated peak systolic velocity at the stenotic proximal anastomotic site of a femoropopliteal bypass graft. This is usually caused by neointimal hyperplasia, which is seen as moderately echogenic wall thickening ➡. *(Right)* Longitudinal color Doppler ultrasound shows narrowing of the lumen within an in-situ carotid stent. Note the in-stent stenosis caused by medium echogenicity neointimal hyperplasia ➡.

Embolism

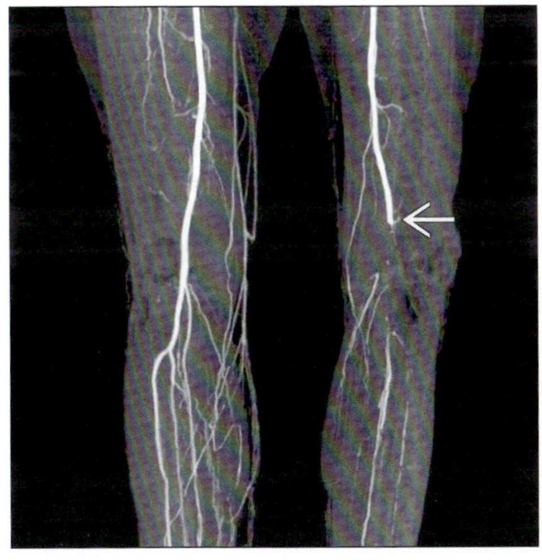

Arterial Dissection

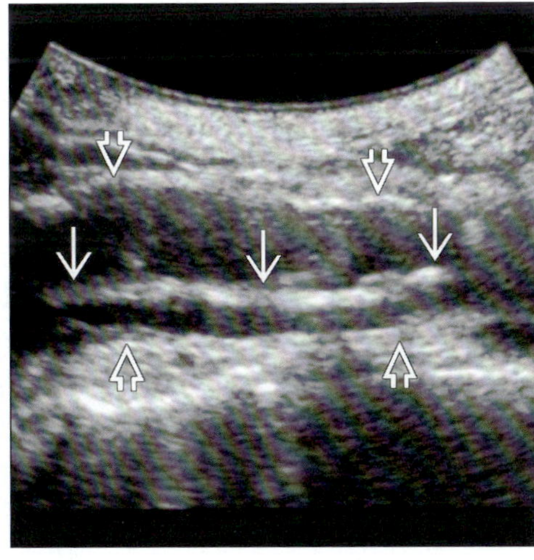

(Left) CTA shows the abrupt occlusion of the left popliteal artery ➡ with a paucity of adjacent collaterals, indicating embolism as a likely cause. Though ultrasound will show the occlusion, the images may not clearly define distal run-off and collaterals. *(Right)* Longitudinal transabdominal ultrasound shows a dissecting abdominal aortic aneurysm ➡. Note the echogenic intimal flap ➡, which is diagnostic of arterial dissection.

Arterial Dissection

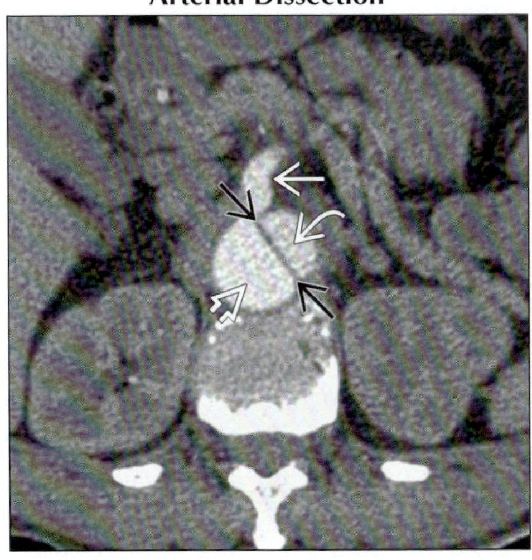

Arterial Dissection

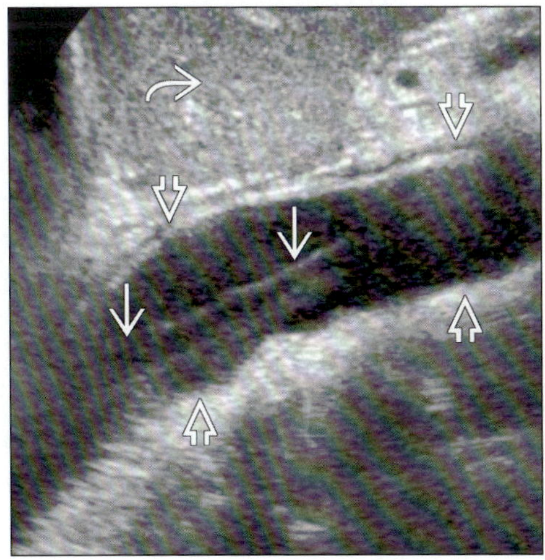

(Left) Transverse CECT shows a dissection flap ➡ at the level of the celiac axis ➡. Note the contrast enhancement within both the true lumen ➡ and the false lumen ➡, indicating patency in both. *(Right)* Longitudinal transabdominal ultrasound shows a dissection flap ➡ extending from the thoracic aorta into the abdominal aorta ➡ deep to the liver ➡. The majority of aortic dissections originate from the thoracic aorta.

PERIVASCULAR MASS

DIFFERENTIAL DIAGNOSIS

Common
- Vascular Origin
  - Hematoma
  - Pseudoaneurysm
  - Aneurysm
  - Normal Anatomical Variants
  - Vascular Malformation
    - Arteriovenous Malformation
    - Venous Malformation
    - Lymphatic Malformation
  - Hemangioma
- Lymphatic Origin
  - Reactive Node
  - Metastatic Node
  - Lymphoma
- Neural Origin
  - Peripheral Nerve Sheath Tumor
  - Carotid Body Paraganglioma
- Mass Arising from Adjacent Glandular Structure, Organs, or Tissues
  - Salivary and Thyroid Masses
  - Horseshoe Kidney
  - Hepatocellular Carcinoma
  - Gynecological Tumors
  - Soft Tissue Sarcomas
- Infective/Inflammatory Mass
  - Abscess
  - Granulomatous Deposit
  - Retroperitoneal Fibrosis

Less Common
- Embryological Remnants
  - 2nd Branchial Cleft Cyst
  - Thyroglossal Duct Cyst

ESSENTIAL INFORMATION

Key Differential Diagnosis Issues
- Perivascular masses present as common clinical problem with very wide differential diagnoses
- Key to accurate diagnosis lies in good understanding of anatomy around vascular structure in question
- Is mass of vascular origin? If so, is it high or low flow?
  - High-flow lesions
    - Arterial causes such as aneurysms, pseudoaneurysms, and arteriovenous malformations
  - Low-flow lesions
    - Venous causes, such as normal anatomical variants, venous malformation, or venous insufficiency
    - Lymphatic malformations, including lymphangiomas and lymphoceles
  - Color, power, and spectral Doppler ultrasound often useful for defining presence of vessels and flow characteristics within lesion
- If mass is not vascular in origin, then adjacent structures should be evaluated
  - Always consider nodal origin masses
    - Vessels in head and neck, chest, abdomen, and pelvis are invariably related to regional lymph nodes
  - If mass arises from/is adjacent to neurovascular bundles, consider neural origin masses
    - Mass may be directly linked to peripheral nerve as in peripheral nerve sheath tumors
  - Masses arising from adjacent organs (both anatomical variants and pathological masses) should be included in differential diagnosis
- After exhausting above possibilities, consider embryological remnants

Helpful Clues for Common Diagnoses
- **Vascular Origin**
  - **Hematoma**
    - No flow on Doppler
    - Echogenicity varies with age of blood products
  - **Pseudoaneurysm**
    - No true wall (may be surrounded by thrombus)
    - Connected to artery via neck
    - Color Doppler may have characteristic "yin-yang" sign with pulsed Doppler showing "to-and-fro" motion in neck
  - **Aneurysm**
    - Dilation of normal artery up to 1.5x its normal diameter
    - True outer arterial wall
    - May be saccular or fusiform in shape and contain mural thrombus
  - **Normal Anatomical Variants**
    - Multiple arteries (e.g., renal arteries), duplicated veins around arteries (e.g., double IVC, duplicated lower limb veins)

14

- ○ **Vascular Malformation**
  - ▪ Color, power, and spectral Doppler help to determine presence and type of flow to classify type of vascular malformation
  - ○ **Hemangioma**
  - ▪ Characterized by endothelial proliferation followed by involution
- **Lymphatic Origin**
  - ○ **Reactive Node**
    - ▪ Normal or mildly enlarged nodes with preserved echogenic hila
    - ▪ Hilar vascularity; low RI & PI on spectral Doppler
  - ○ **Metastatic Node**
    - ▪ Commonly round, hypoechoic, loss of hila, eccentric cortical hypertrophy
    - ▪ Large peripheral vessels; high RI and PI on spectral Doppler
    - ▪ Infiltration of adjacent fat or invasion of adjacent structures
  - ○ **Lymphoma**
    - ▪ Non-Hodgkin lymphoma nodes tend to show posterior acoustic enhancement and are commonly hypoechoic ("pseudocystic")
- **Neural Origin**
  - ○ **Peripheral Nerve Sheath Tumor**
    - ▪ Well-defined hypoechoic mass arising from peripheral nerves or in paraspinal position
    - ▪ Intratumoral vascularity
  - ○ **Carotid Body Paraganglioma**
    - ▪ Vascular mass splaying external carotid artery and internal carotid artery

- **Mass Arising from Adjacent Glandular Structures, Organs, or Tissues**
  - ○ Head and neck: Consider salivary glands and thyroid masses
  - ○ Abdomen and pelvis: Consider adjacent organs
  - ○ Extremity: Consider adjacent tissues such as fat, muscles, or bone
- **Infective/Inflammatory Mass**
  - ○ **Abscess**
    - ▪ May occur anywhere in body and may have variable internal appearance, thick walls ± adjacent hyperemia
  - ○ **Granulomatous Deposit**
    - ▪ May present as calcified echogenic shadowing masses in affected organs
  - ○ **Retroperitoneal Fibrosis**
    - ▪ Usually presents as hypoechoic, homogeneous masses in paraaortic region/perinephric space

Helpful Clues for Less Common Diagnoses
- **Embryological Remnants**
  - ○ **2nd Branchial Cleft Cyst**
    - ▪ Has characteristic location posterolateral to submandibular gland, lateral to carotid space, and anteromedial to sternocleidomastoid muscle
  - ○ **Thyroglossal Duct Cyst**
    - ▪ Midline cystic mass embedded in infrahyoid strap muscles ("claw" sign)

Hematoma

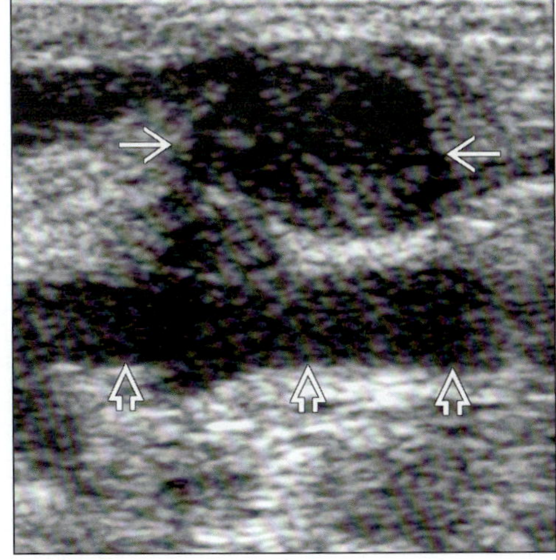

Longitudinal ultrasound shows a heterogeneous hematoma ➜ lying superficial to the common femoral artery ➔. This is a common complication after a femoral puncture for angiography.

Hematoma

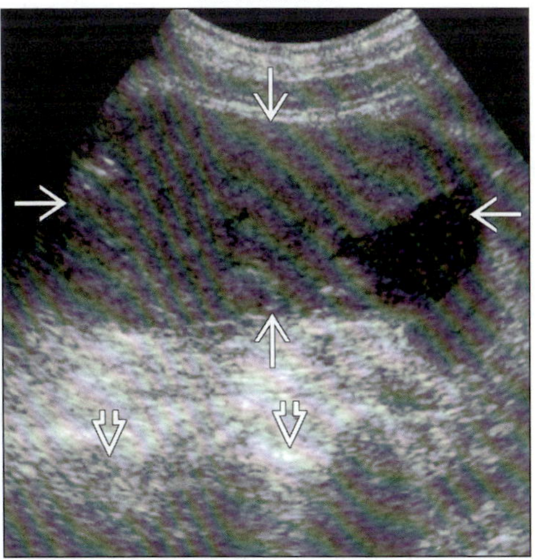

Oblique ultrasound shows a heterogeneous paraaortic hematoma ➜ with mixed echogenic and hypoechoic components adjacent to the spine ➔, following an aortic aneurysm rupture.

14

PERIVASCULAR MASS

(Left) Transverse ultrasound shows a pseudoaneurysm ➡ in the lateral aspect of the left knee in a patient after joint replacement surgery. (Right) Transverse color Doppler ultrasound shows the characteristic "yin-yang" sign ➡ within the same pseudoaneurysm. The different color signals within the pseudoaneurysm indicate swirling flow. Note the arterial flow in the adjacent source artery ➡.

Pseudoaneurysm
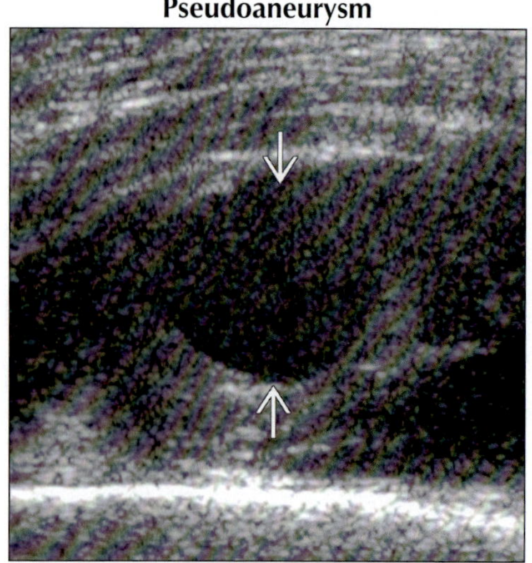

Pseudoaneurysm
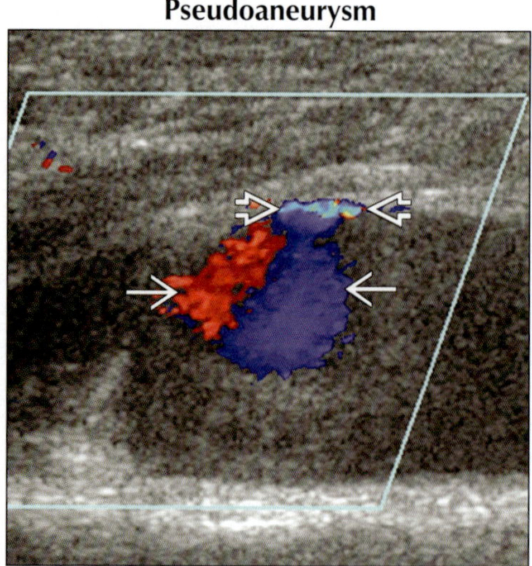

(Left) DSA in the same patient shows a pseudoaneurysm ➡ arising from a branch of the lateral geniculate artery. (Right) DSA shows the corresponding post-embolization image with coils ➡ occluding the arterial branch leading to the pseudoaneurysm.

Pseudoaneurysm
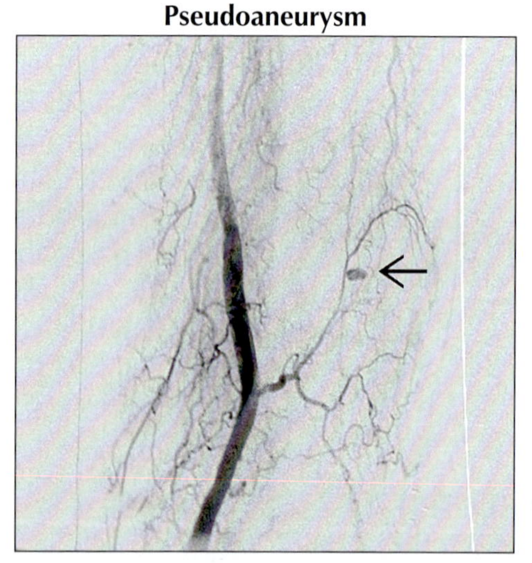

Pseudoaneurysm
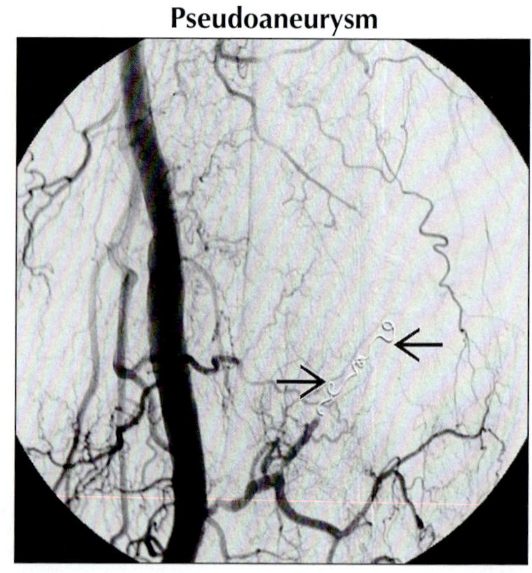

(Left) Transverse pulsed Doppler ultrasound shows characteristic "to-and-fro" flow in the neck ➡ of a pseudoaneurysm. (Right) Transverse transabdominal ultrasound shows a left inferior vena cava ➡, which is located to the left of the abdominal aorta ➡. Recognition of normal variants in vascular anatomy is important prior to a diagnosis of vascular perivascular masses.

Pseudoaneurysm
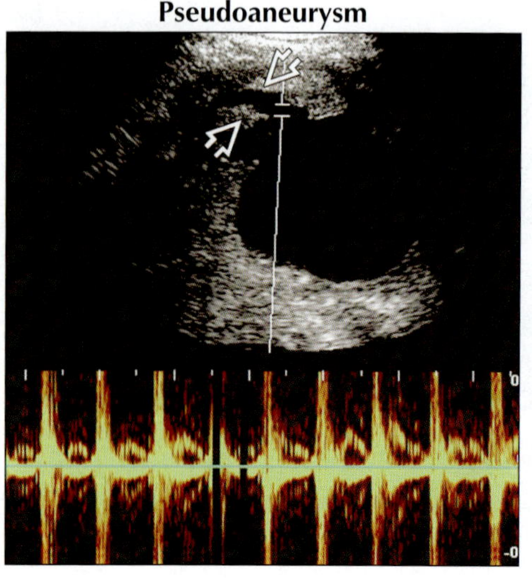

Normal Anatomical Variants
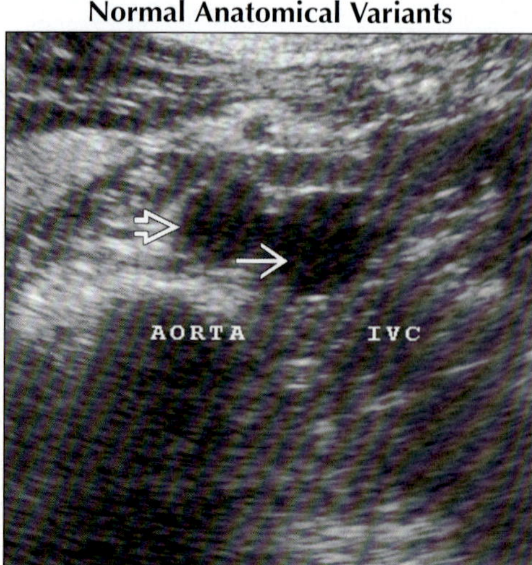

14

PERIVASCULAR MASS

Vascular Malformation

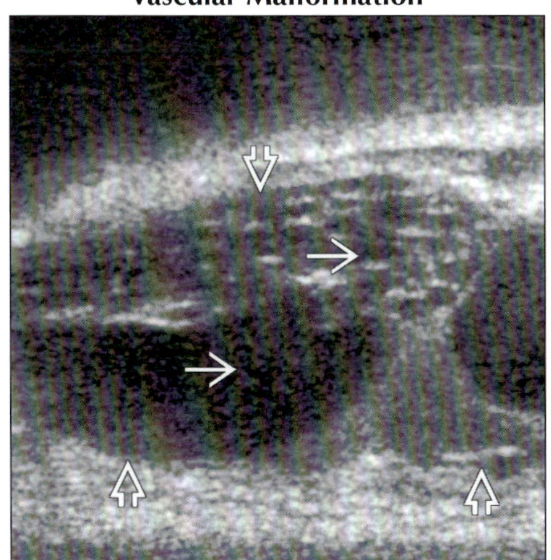

Vascular Malformation

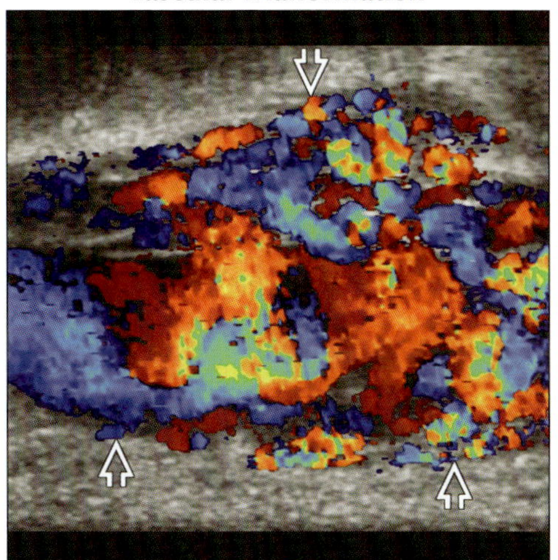

(Left) Longitudinal ultrasound of the forefoot shows a vascular malformation ⇒ with both large and small vascular spaces → adjacent to the metatarsal shaft. (Right) Correlative longitudinal color Doppler ultrasound shows flow throughout the vascular spaces in the malformation ⇒. Spectral Doppler confirmed arterial flow, indicative of high flow within an arteriovenous malformation.

Reactive Node

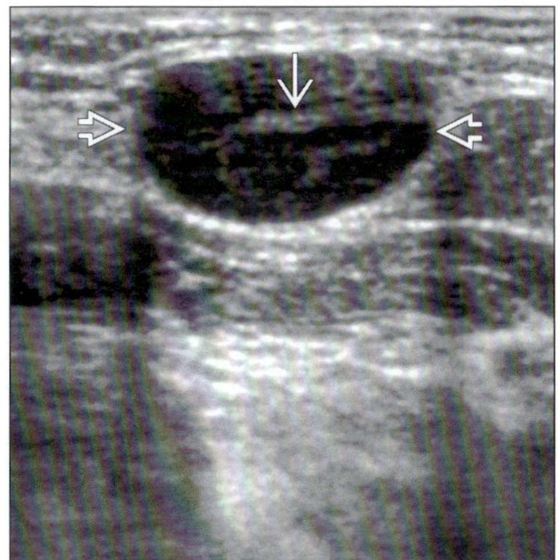

Reactive Node

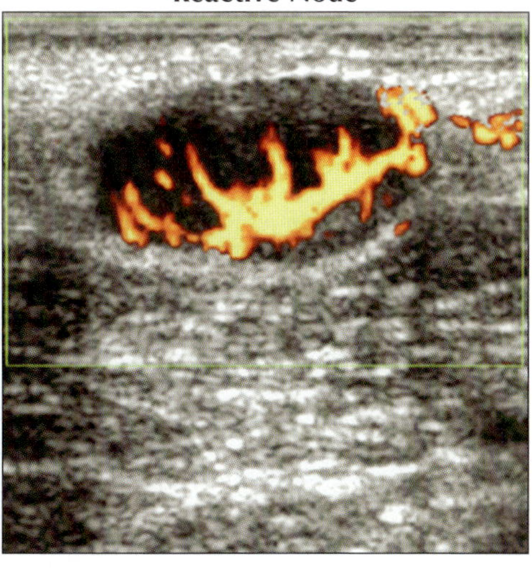

(Left) Transverse ultrasound shows a hypoechoic elliptical/oval node ⇒ with a linear echogenic hilus →. Note the lack of intranodal necrosis, calcification, or associated soft tissue edema. (Right) Transverse power Doppler ultrasound shows characteristic hilar vascularity within a reactive node. Note the absence of any peripheral vascularity.

Metastatic Node

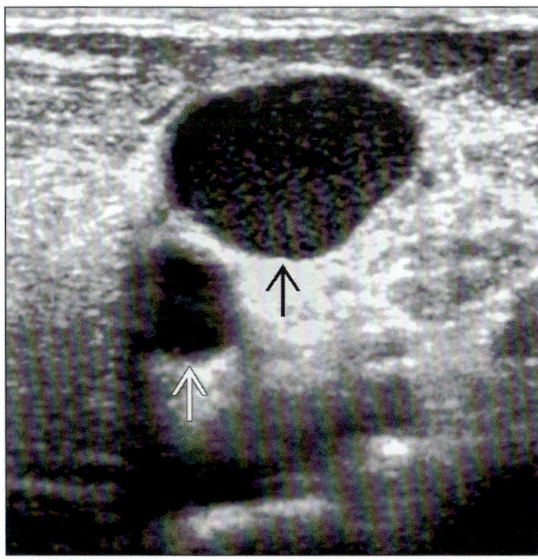

Metastatic Node

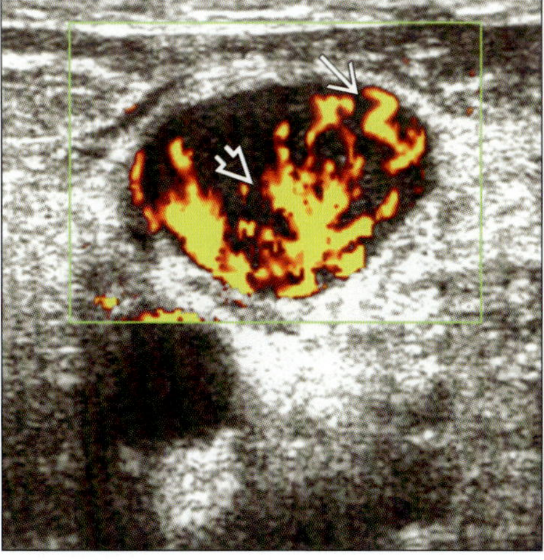

(Left) Transverse ultrasound shows a round, well-defined, hypoechoic node → with loss of the echogenic hilum in a patient with head and neck squamous cell carcinoma. This appearance is typical of a metastatic node adjacent to the carotid artery ⇒. (Right) Corresponding transverse power Doppler ultrasound shows abnormal peripheral vessels →, consistent with a metastatic node. Prominent hilar vessels ⇒ are seen as well.

14

PERIVASCULAR MASS

(Left) Transverse color Doppler ultrasound shows extensive lymphadenopathy ➡ around the celiac axis ➡ in a patient with lymphoma.
(Right) Longitudinal ultrasound shows a brachial plexus schwannoma ➡. Note its continuity with the brachial plexus trunk ➡.

Lymphoma

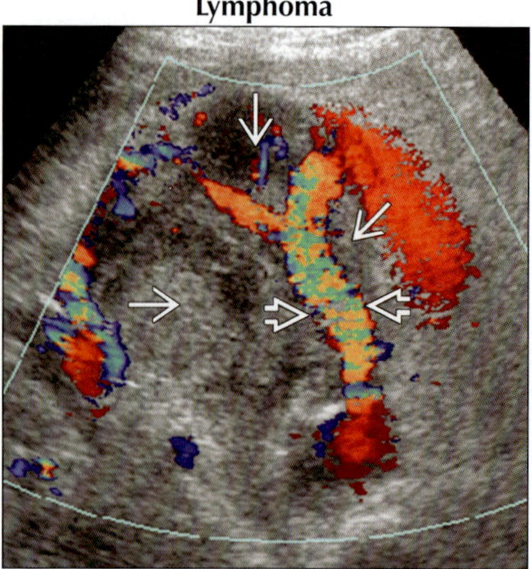

Peripheral Nerve Sheath Tumor

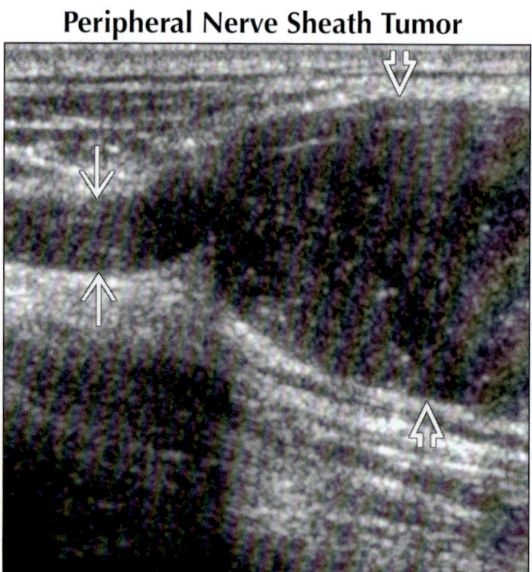

(Left) Transverse color Doppler US shows a solid, well-defined, hypoechoic mass ➡ insinuating between the internal and external carotid arteries ➡, typical of a carotid body paraganglioma. These are often very vascular on color Doppler. (Right) Transverse ultrasound shows a classic horseshoe kidney with an isthmus of renal tissue ➡ crossing the midline, anterior to the spine ➡, inferior vena cava, and aorta ➡.

Carotid Body Paraganglioma

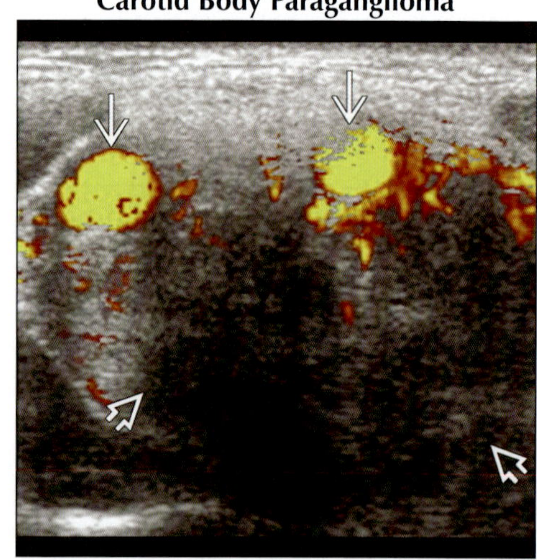

Horseshoe Kidney

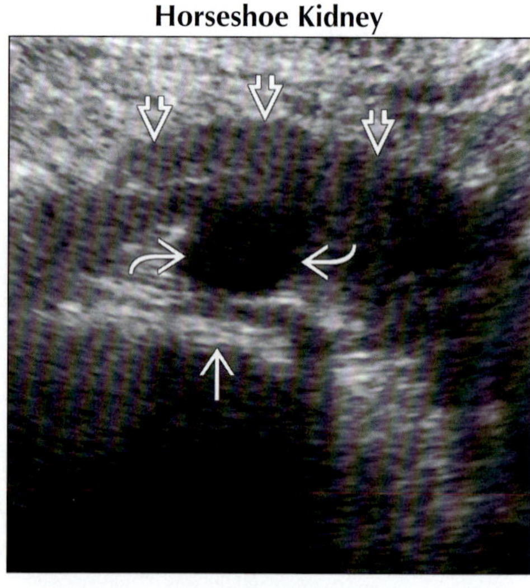

(Left) Tc-99m DMSA scan in the same patient shows symmetrical midline fusion to create a horseshoe kidney with its characteristic U-shape. (Right) Transverse transabdominal ultrasound shows a large, complex, cystic tumor ➡ compressing the inferior vena cava ➡.

Horseshoe Kidney

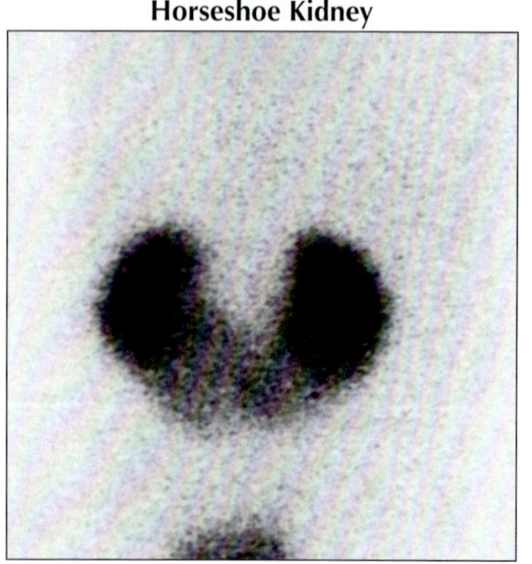

Gynecological Tumors

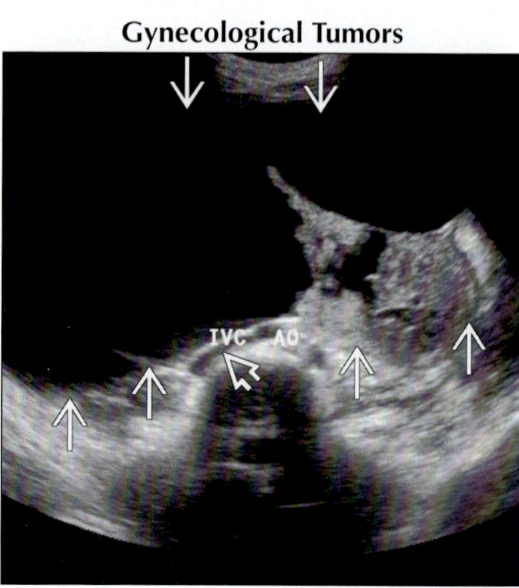

14

PERIVASCULAR MASS

Gynecological Tumors

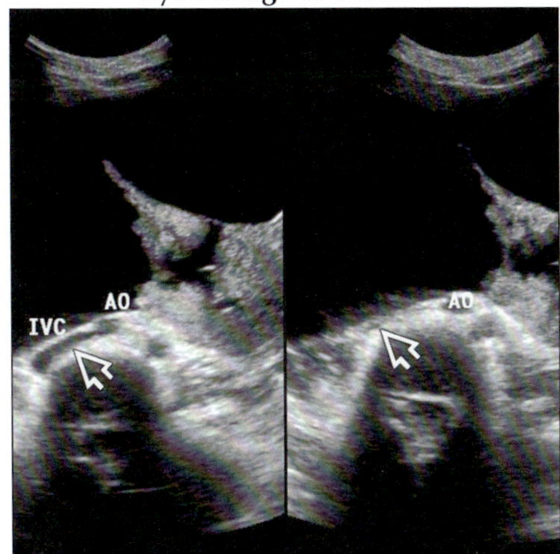

Soft Tissue Sarcomas

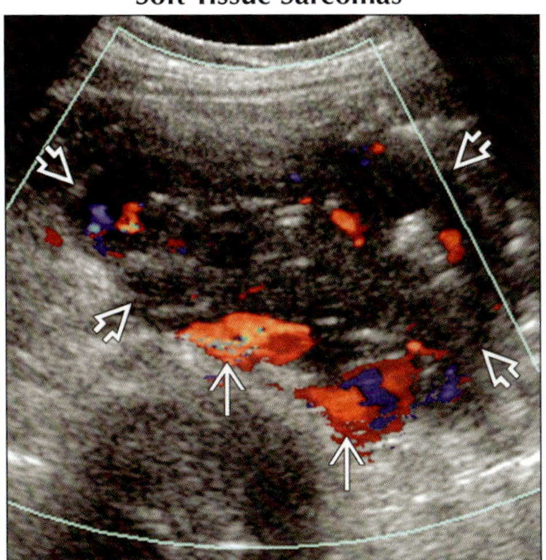

(Left) Composite image in the same patient, without (left) and with (right) compression, shows the IVC ➡ is compressible. This indicates that, despite its narrowing, the IVC is patent. *(Right)* Transverse color Doppler US shows a heterogeneous, predominantly hypoechoic sarcoma ➡ anterior to the common iliac arteries ➡. Note the presence of internal vascularity within the sarcoma.

Soft Tissue Sarcomas

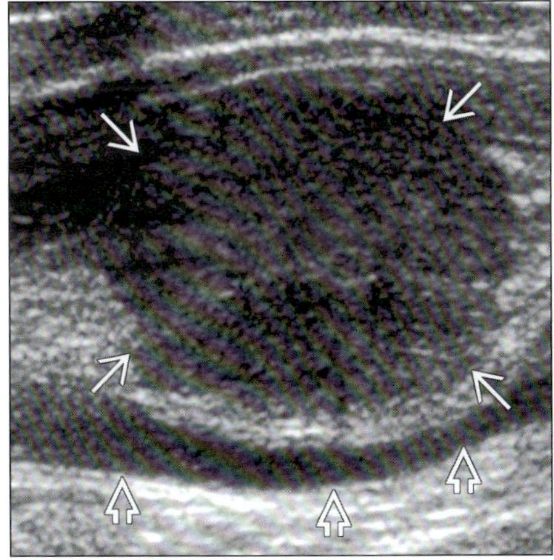

Retroperitoneal Fibrosis

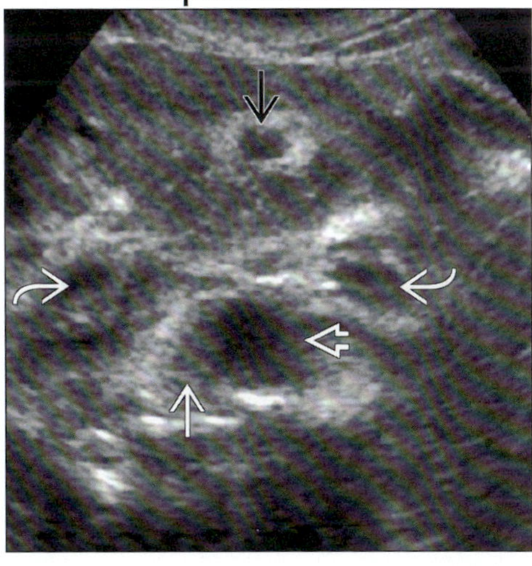

(Left) Longitudinal ultrasound shows a hypoechoic soft tissue tumor ➡ causing mild compression of the adjacent popliteal vein ➡. *(Right)* Transverse transabdominal ultrasound shows abnormal tissue ➡ encasing the abdominal aorta ➡ in a patient with retroperitoneal fibrosis diagnosed on CT. Note the similar abnormal tissue encasing the renal arteries ➡ and the superior mesenteric artery ➡.

2nd Branchial Cleft Cyst

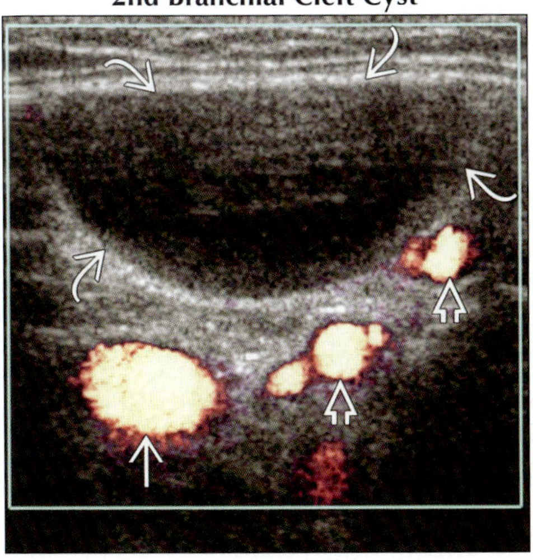

Thyroglossal Duct Cyst

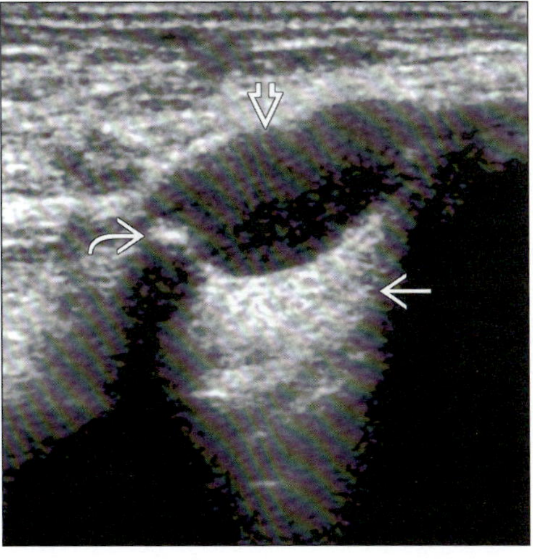

(Left) Transverse power Doppler ultrasound shows an avascular anechoic mass ➡ and confirms its relationship to the carotid arteries ➡ and the internal jugular vein ➡. *(Right)* Longitudinal ultrasound shows a well-defined anechoic, infrahyoid, thyroglossal duct cyst ➡ with thin walls and posterior acoustic enhancement ➡. Note the cyst's close relationship with the hyoid bone ➡, which is seen as an echogenic shadowing focus.

14

DIFFERENTIAL DIAGNOSIS

Common
- Intraluminal Venous Mass
  - Acute Thrombosis
  - Tumor Thrombus
- Obstruction to Outflow of Venous Blood
  - Extrinsic Compression by Perivascular Masses
  - Extrinsic Compression by Adjacent Vascular Structures
- Elevated Venous Pressure
  - Right Heart Failure
  - Tricuspid Regurgitation
  - Chronic Venous Insufficiency
- Increase in Inflow of Blood
  - Traumatic Arteriovenous Fistula
  - Iatrogenic Arteriovenous Fistula
  - Surgically Created Arteriovenous Fistula
- Vascular Malformation
  - Arteriovenous Malformation
  - Venous Malformation

ESSENTIAL INFORMATION

Key Differential Diagnosis Issues
- Is there obstructing lesion?
  - Is it caused by intravascular mass?
    - If yes, consider acute thrombosis or tumor thrombus
  - Is it caused by extrinsic mass?
    - If yes, consider mass lesions, such as tumors, abscesses, or hematoma arising from adjacent organs, glandular structures, or lymph nodes
  - Is it caused by adjacent arterial structure?
    - Consider anatomical variants and obstruction by normal arterial structures
- If there is no obstructive lesion, are there any causes for elevated venous pressure, increase in flow of blood, or vascular malformation?
- Color Doppler
  - Shows reverse direction of flow in venous reflux
  - Aliasing seen with turbulent arterial inflow
- Spectral Doppler
  - Useful to demonstrate duration of reflux
  - Arterial waveform in arteriovenous fistula and arteriovenous malformation
  - Venous flow in venous malformations

Helpful Clues for Common Diagnoses
- **Intraluminal Venous Mass**
  - **Acute Thrombosis**
    - Venous distension: Recently thrombosed veins are distended and substantially larger than accompanying artery
    - Low echogenicity thrombus: Acute thrombus may be virtually anechoic; flow may be seen within recanalized thrombus
    - Loss of compressibility: Thrombus is suspected if vein cannot be completely compressed
    - Free-floating thrombus: Recently formed clot may not adhere to vein wall (usually on side closer to heart)
    - Collateralization: Tortuous and braided veins, typically smaller than normal vein, may open up around site of venous obstruction
  - **Tumor Thrombus**
    - Color Doppler study useful in depicting vascularity within thrombus, which is key to diagnosis of tumor thrombus
    - Power Doppler is more sensitive to detection of slow intrathrombus flow
- **Extrinsic Compression by Perivascular Masses**
  - Vascular origin
    - Pseudoaneurysm/hematoma, aneurysm, normal anatomical variants, vascular malformation (arteriovenous malformation, venous malformation, lymphatic malformation), hemangioma
  - Lymph node origin
    - Reactive nodes, metastatic nodes, lymphoma
  - Neural origin
    - Peripheral nerve sheath tumor, carotid body paraganglioma
  - Mass arising from adjacent organs or tissue
    - Salivary and thyroid gland masses, horseshoe kidney, hepatocellular carcinoma, gynecological tumor, soft tissue tumor
  - Infective/inflammatory mass
    - Abscesses, granulomatous deposits, retroperitoneal fibrosis
  - Embryological remnants
    - 2nd branchial cleft cyst, thyroglossal duct cyst, duplication cyst

14

VENOUS DILATION

- **Extrinsic Compression by Adjacent Vascular Structures**
  - Anatomical variants
  - Compression of left renal vein by aorta in retroaortic left renal vein
  - Obstruction by normal arterial structures
  - Iliac vein obstruction (May-Thurner) syndrome
    - Compression of left common iliac vein by right common iliac artery
  - Left renal vein entrapment (nutcracker) syndrome
    - Obstruction of left renal vein by superior mesenteric artery
- **Elevated Venous Pressure**
  - **Right Heart Failure**
    - Causes: Cor pulmonale, ischemic heart disease, pulmonary stenosis, tricuspid regurgitation, endocarditis, atrial septal defect, ventricular septal defect, dilated cardiomyopathy, left heart failure
  - **Tricuspid Regurgitation**
    - Flow reversal during regurgitation may be seen in proximal veins, such as inferior vena cava and proximal hepatic veins
  - **Chronic Venous Insufficiency**
    - Caused by primary or secondary valvular incompetence; congenital valvular absence may also be seen
    - Duration of reflux > 0.5 seconds at any level is clinically significant
- **Increase in Inflow of Blood**
  - **Traumatic Arteriovenous Fistula**
    - Stab or penetrating injury, gunshot wounds
  - **Iatrogenic Arteriovenous Fistula**
    - Needle puncture from angiography; inadvertent damage to vessels during surgery, biopsy
  - **Surgically Created Arteriovenous Fistula**
    - Created for purpose of hemodialysis or bypass grafts
  - Characterized by single feeding artery and single draining vein
  - Duplex Doppler may demonstrate site of arteriovenous communication
    - Allows quantification and assessment of flow through AV fistula
- **Vascular Malformation**
  - **Arteriovenous Malformation**
    - Congenital abnormal communication between dilated tortuous arteries and veins, bypassing capillary bed
  - **Venous Malformation**
    - Poorly circumscribed vascular malformation consisting of irregular venous channels
    - Slow moving ("to-and- fro") blood flow may be better seen on grayscale
    - Phleboliths may be present

Acute Thrombosis

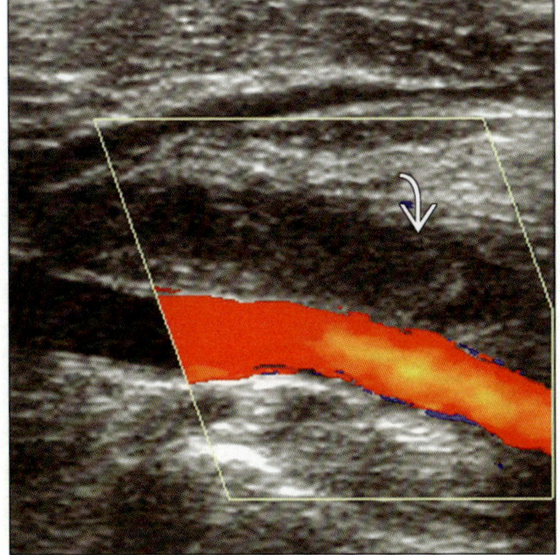

Longitudinal color Doppler ultrasound shows acute thrombosis of the popliteal vein ➔. Note that the thrombus is hypoechoic and that the popliteal vein is dilated and larger than the accompanying artery.

Tumor Thrombus

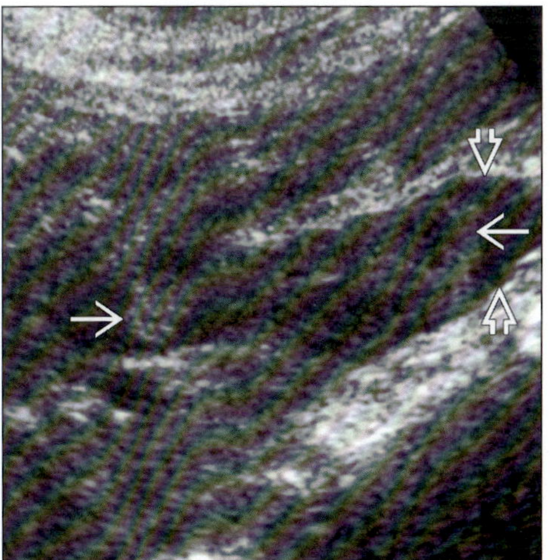

Transverse transabdominal ultrasound shows a tumor thrombus ➔ in a dilated right renal vein due to renal cell carcinoma. Note the extension of the tumor thrombus into the inferior vena cava ➔.

14

Extrinsic Compression by Adjacent Vascular Structures

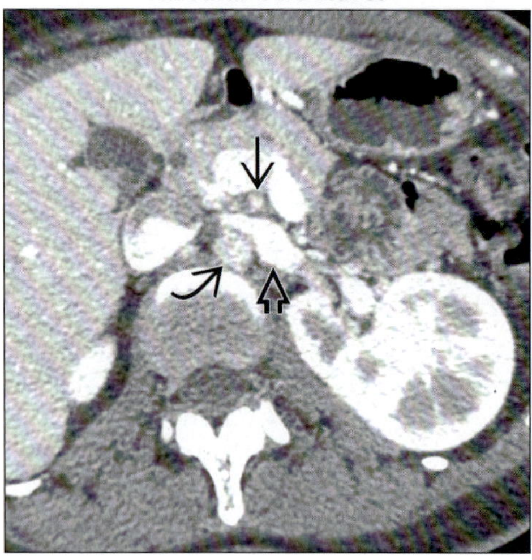

Extrinsic Compression by Adjacent Vascular Structures

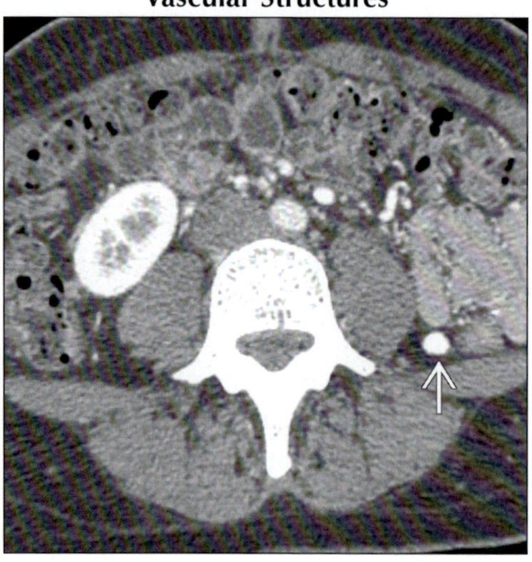

(Left) Axial CECT shows compression of the left renal vein ⇨ by the superior mesenteric artery ➡. Note the reduction in caliber of the left renal vein as it passes between the aorta ⇨ and the superior mesenteric artery in this patient with left renal vein compression syndrome. *(Right)* Axial CECT in the same patient shows reflux of contrast filling the dilated left ovarian vein ➡.

Extrinsic Compression by Adjacent Vascular Structures

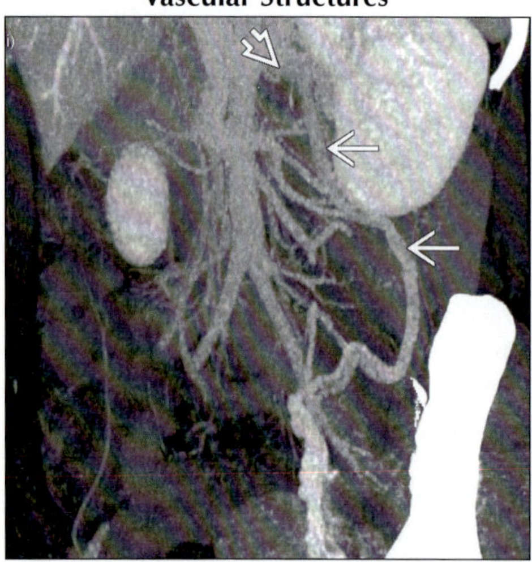

Extrinsic Compression by Adjacent Vascular Structures

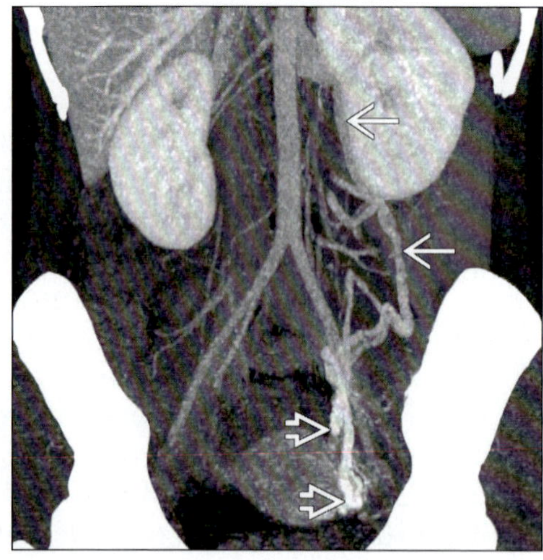

(Left) CTA 3D reconstruction in the same patient shows the left ovarian vein ➡ dilation from reverse flow via the left renal vein ➡. *(Right)* CTA 3D reconstruction in the same patient shows the inferior extent of the left ovarian vein reflux. Note the filling of the dilated left ovarian vein ➡ and the dilated veins around the uterine venous plexus ⇨.

Right Heart Failure

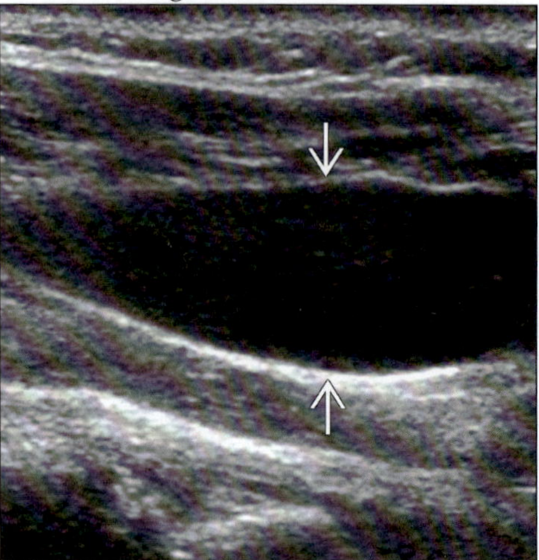

Right Heart Failure

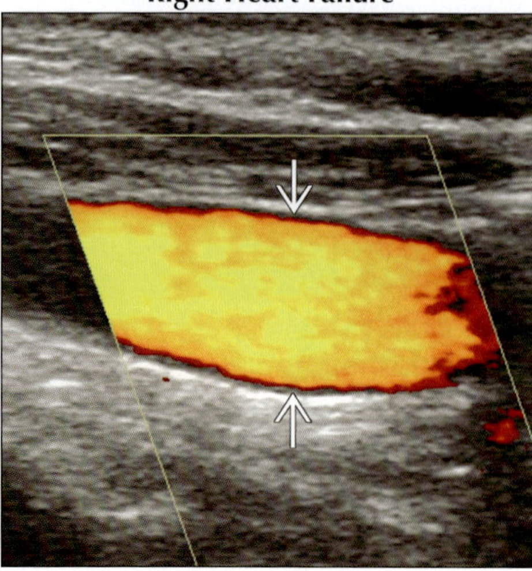

(Left) Longitudinal ultrasound shows an engorged internal jugular vein ➡ in a patient with right heart failure. *(Right)* Longitudinal power Doppler ultrasound in the same patient shows flow in the internal jugular vein ➡. Acutely thrombosed dilated veins may appear hypoechoic. Color and power Doppler studies are important to demonstrate patency in engorged veins.

VENOUS DILATION

Tricuspid Regurgitation

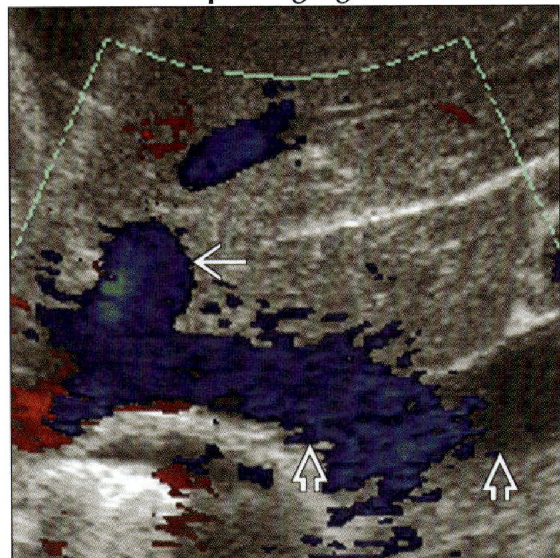

Tricuspid Regurgitation

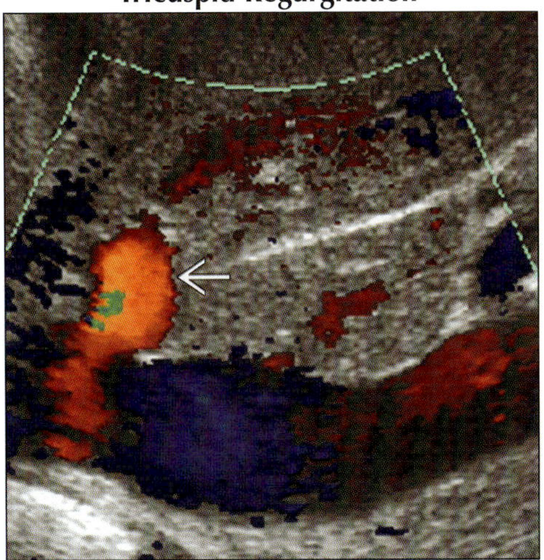

(Left) Longitudinal color Doppler ultrasound shows a dilated hepatic vein ➡ and inferior vena cava ⇉ in a patient with tricuspid regurgitation. (Right) Longitudinal color Doppler ultrasound in the same patient shows reversal of flow in the hepatic vein ➡, caused by tricuspid regurgitation.

Chronic Venous Insufficiency

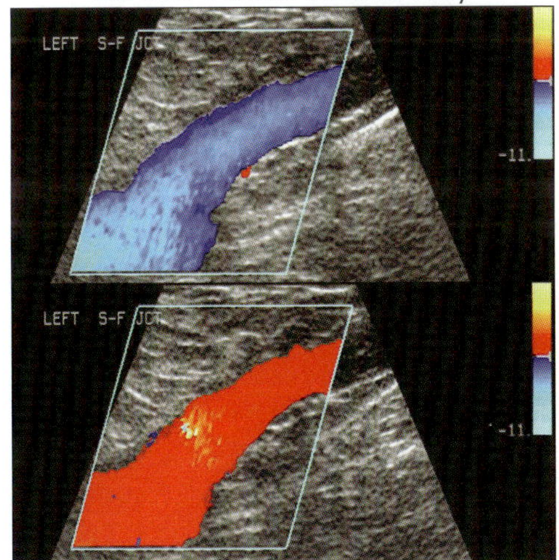

Chronic Venous Insufficiency

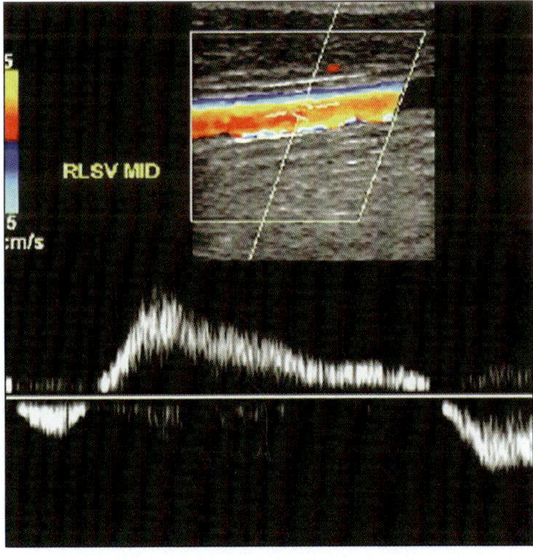

(Left) Longitudinal color Doppler ultrasound shows reflux at the saphenofemoral junction. Note the change in color from blue to red, indicating a reversal of flow at the saphenofemoral junction during a Valsalva maneuver. (Right) Longitudinal color Doppler ultrasound shows an incompetent long saphenous vein with significant reflux (more than 2.0 seconds) during Valsalva maneuver, findings consistent with valvular incompetence.

Chronic Venous Insufficiency

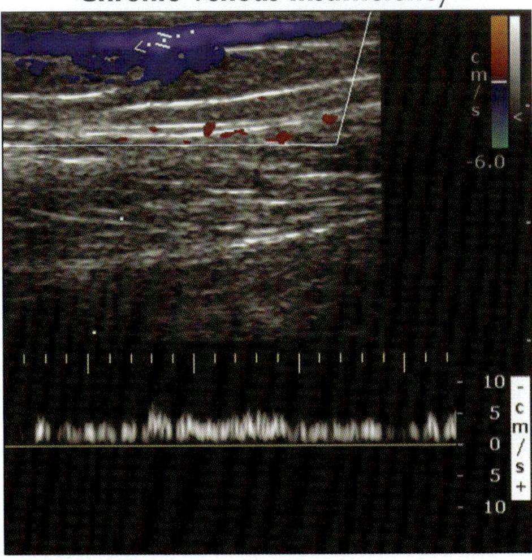

Chronic Venous Insufficiency

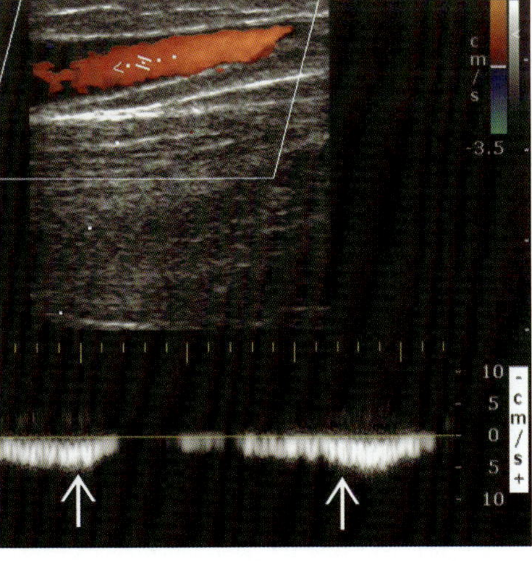

(Left) Longitudinal pulsed Doppler ultrasound shows venous flow with respiratory variations in a patient with congenital absence of valves in the long saphenous vein. This patient had varicose veins over the medial calf since childhood. (Right) Longitudinal pulsed Doppler ultrasound shows the corresponding spectral Doppler trace in the distal long saphenous vein during Valsalva maneuver. Note the reflux and flow reversal ➡.

VENOUS DILATION

Chronic Venous Insufficiency

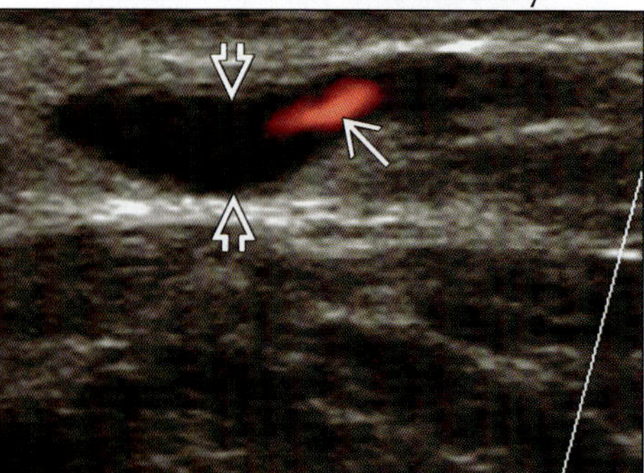

Chronic Venous Insufficiency

(Left) Oblique power Doppler ultrasound in the same patient shows slow flow → within a subcutaneous dilated varicose vein ⇒ over the medial aspect of the mid-calf. *(Right)* Oblique pulsed Doppler ultrasound shows venous flow with respiratory variations. Note the reversal of flow during inspiration → and forward flow during expiration ⇒ in the same small dilated varicose vein.

Chronic Venous Insufficiency

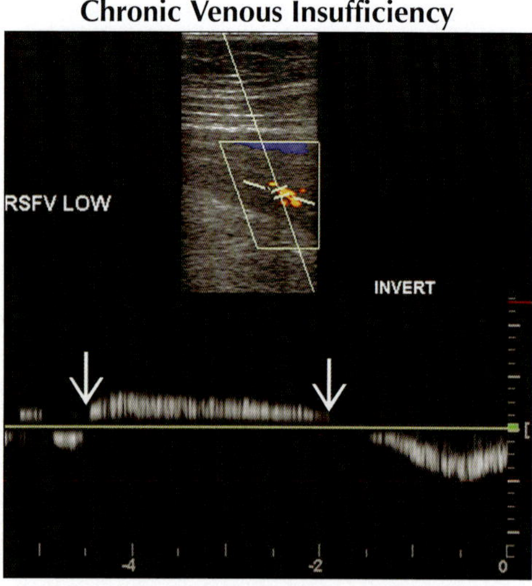

Chronic Venous Insufficiency

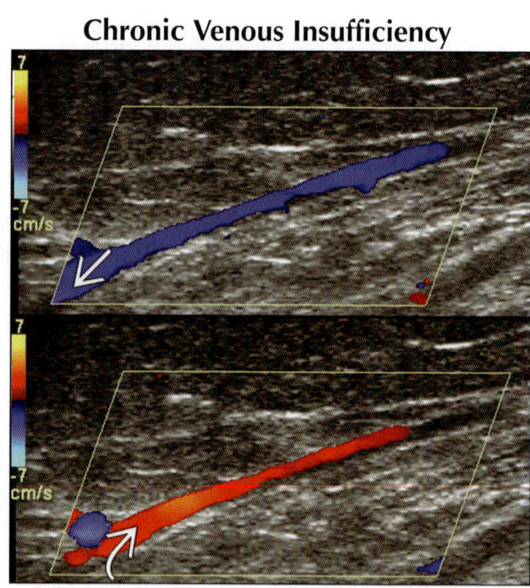

(Left) Longitudinal color Doppler ultrasound shows an incompetent, superficial femoral vein with significant reflux →. Abnormal reflux time is > 0.5 seconds, patient standing, and > 2.0 seconds, patient supine. *(Right)* Longitudinal color Doppler ultrasound shows an incompetent, dilated, short saphenous vein with antegrade flow → demonstrated during normal respiration (top). Flow reflux ⇒ is noted during Valsalva maneuver (bottom).

Traumatic Arteriovenous Fistula

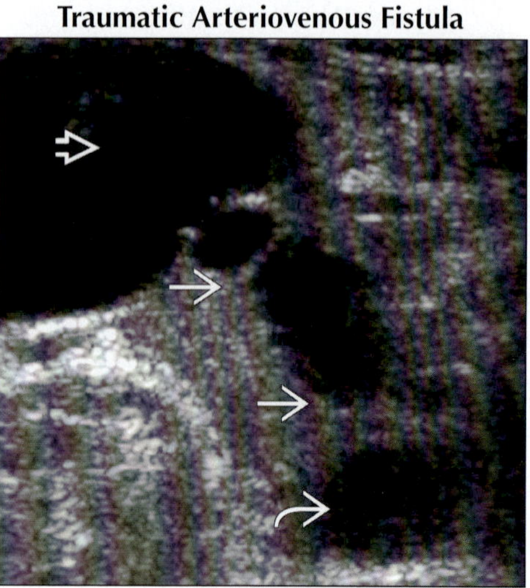

Traumatic Arteriovenous Fistula

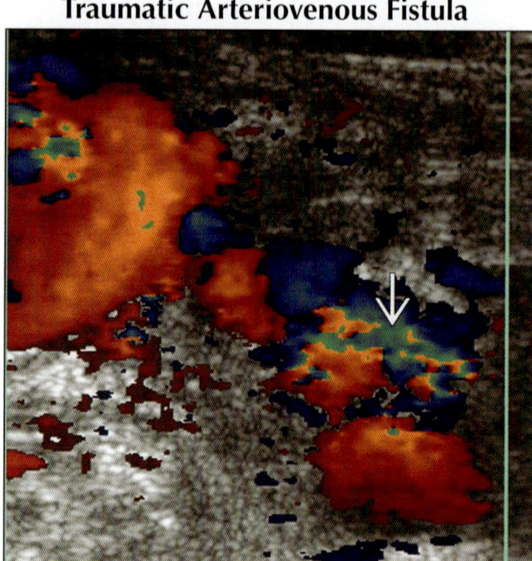

(Left) Transverse ultrasound shows an arteriovenous fistula → between the right internal jugular vein ⇒ and the right common carotid artery ⇒, resulting from a stab injury. Note the dilation of the internal jugular vein. *(Right)* Transverse color Doppler ultrasound of a corresponding image demonstrates turbulent flow through the arteriovenous fistula with an "aliasing" appearance →.

VENOUS DILATION

Surgically Created Arteriovenous Fistula

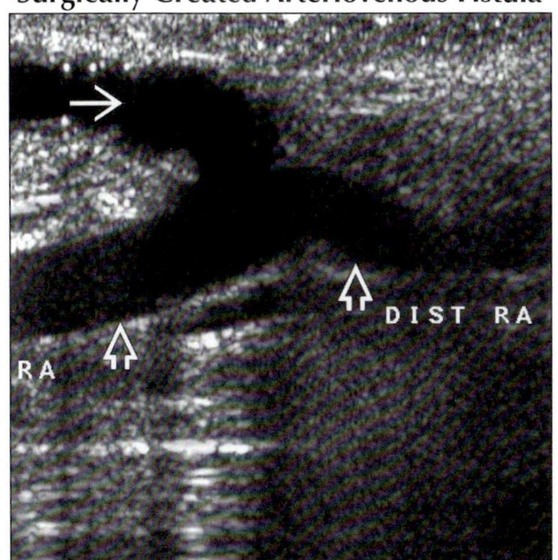

Surgically Created Arteriovenous Fistula

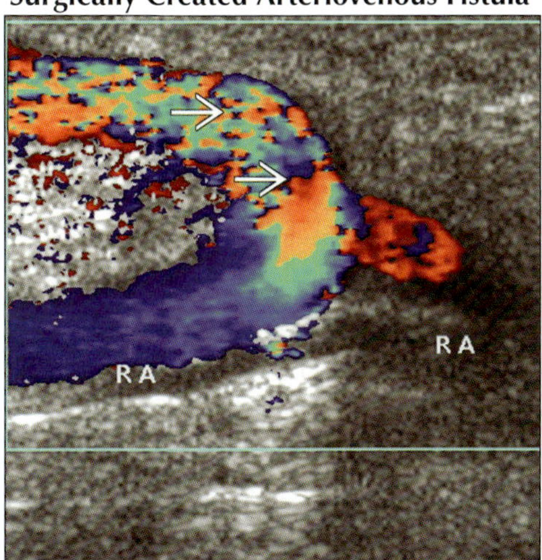

(Left) Oblique ultrasound shows an end-to-side radial artery hemodialysis fistula with a branch of the cephalic vein ➡ anastomosed onto the distal radial artery ➡. Note the dilation of the cephalic vein from increased flow. *(Right)* Oblique color Doppler ultrasound shows the same hemodialysis fistula. Note the "aliasing" artifact ➡, indicative of turbulent arterialized flow in the cephalic vein.

Arteriovenous Malformation

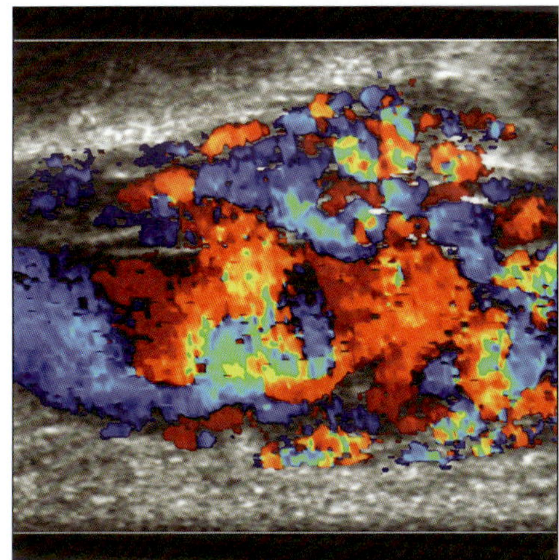

Arteriovenous Malformation

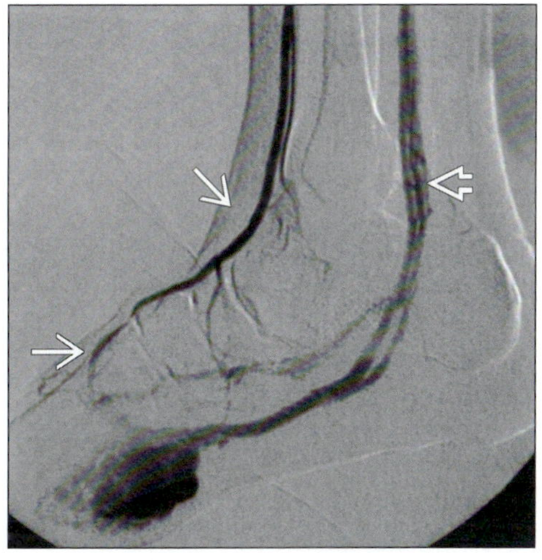

(Left) Longitudinal color Doppler ultrasound shows color signal present throughout a forefoot vascular malformation. Spectral analysis (not shown) revealed predominant arterial flow, indicative of a high-flow arteriovenous malformation. *(Right)* DSA shows the corresponding angiogram image of the same arteriovenous malformation. Note the feeding dorsalis pedis artery ➡ and dilation of the draining posterior tibial vein ➡.

Venous Malformation

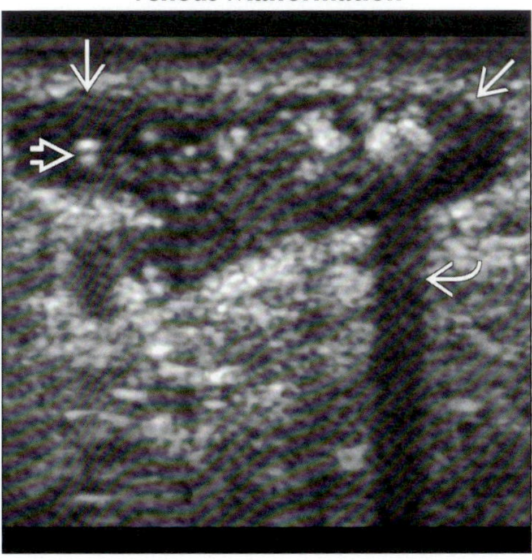

Venous Malformation

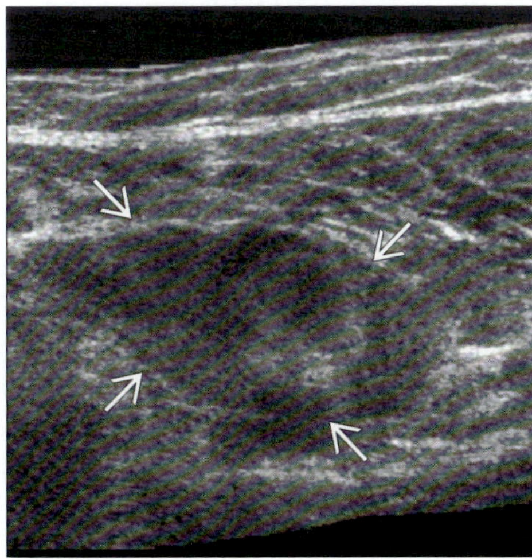

(Left) Transverse ultrasound shows a well-defined, subcutaneous venous malformation ➡ of the heel, with phleboliths indicated by echogenic foci with posterior acoustic shadowing ➡ and "comet tail" artifacts ➡. *(Right)* Longitudinal ultrasound with an extended field-of-view shows a large venous lake ➡ as part of a venous malformation within the gastrocnemius muscle. The echogenic contents represent slow-flowing blood.

14

INTRALUMINAL VENOUS MASS

DIFFERENTIAL DIAGNOSIS

Common
- Venous Thrombosis
  - Acute Thrombosis
  - Subacute Thrombosis
  - Chronic Thrombosis
- Tumor Thrombus
  - Renal Cell Carcinoma
  - Hepatocellular Carcinoma
  - Intravenous Leiomyomatosis
  - Leiomyosarcoma
- Foreign Bodies
  - Venous Catheter
  - Vena Cava Filter
  - Metallic Stent
  - Cardiac Pacing Wire
- Normal Structures
  - Valves
- Ultrasound Artifacts (Mimic)

Less Common
- Congenital Membranes

ESSENTIAL INFORMATION

Helpful Clues for Common Diagnoses
- **Acute Thrombosis**
  - Up to 14 days
  - Low echogenicity thrombus
    - May be virtually anechoic
    - Flow may be seen within recanalized thrombus
  - Recently thrombosed veins are distended and substantially larger than accompanying artery
  - Loss of compressibility
    - Thrombus is reliably excluded if vein can be completely compressed
  - Free-floating thrombus
    - Recently formed clot (usually on end closer to heart) may not adhere to vein wall
  - Collateralization begins to develop
    - Tortuous and braided collateral veins, usually smaller than normal vein
- **Subacute Thrombosis**
  - ~ 2 weeks to 6 months
  - Thrombus becomes more echogenic, variable appearance
  - Decreased thrombus and vein size
    - Retraction and lysis may reduce size of vein, which may even be normal
  - Adherence of thrombus
    - Free-floating thrombus becomes attached to vein wall
  - Vein may remain occluded, or luminal flow may be restored
  - Collateral venous channels continue to develop
- **Chronic Thrombosis**
  - ≥ 6 months
  - Post-thrombus scarring
    - Unlysed thrombus will be invaded by fibroblasts in process of being organized as fibrous tissue
    - Appear as echogenic plaque-like areas along vein and may occasionally calcify
    - Scarred veins are thick walled with reduced luminal diameter
  - Synechiae form from unlysed thrombus attached to 1 side of vein wall and gradually transform into fibrous band
  - Fibrous cord may form in veins, which fail to recanalize
    - Vein may be reduced to echogenic cord, which is much smaller than normal vein
  - Valve damage is frequently associated with venous thrombosis
    - Thickening of valve cusps and restricted cusp motion may lead to reflux and venous stasis
- **Tumor Thrombus**
  - Color Doppler study is useful for depicting flow in tumor, and vascularity is key to diagnosis of tumor thrombi
  - Power Doppler study is more sensitive to slow flow within tumor thrombi
  - Spectral Doppler may show pulsatile flow in tumor thrombi
  - When tumor thrombus is identified, look for tumor within adjacent organ
  - **Renal Cell Carcinoma**
    - Propensity to invade renal vein on side of tumor with tumor spreading to inferior vena cava (IVC) or right atrium
  - **Hepatocellular Carcinoma**
    - Propensity to invade hepatic veins and portal veins with spread of tumor to IVC or right atrium
    - Tumor may also arise from vein itself
  - **Intravenous Leiomyomatosis**

INTRALUMINAL VENOUS MASS

- Rare condition characterized by uterine leiomyomas with intravascular extension
- Convoluted, worm-like masses growing within veins
- Often extending into broad ligament, other pelvic veins, IVC, or even heart
  - **Leiomyosarcoma**
    - Leiomyosarcoma of IVC is most common venous intravascular tumor
    - M:F = 1:5, with preponderance in older women
    - Both intravascular and extravascular components may be present
    - Blood flow in IVC and hepatic veins may be absent, reversed, or turbulent
    - Collateral pathways bypassing IVC (e.g., via azygous/hemiazygous system) may be detected
- **Foreign Bodies**
  - Most common foreign bodies encountered in venous system are iatrogenic
  - Common categories of iatrogenic intravenous foreign bodies include
    - Intravenous catheters for venous access and hemodialysis
    - IVC filters for prevention of pulmonary embolism
    - Metallic stents for relieving venous obstruction; typically in large veins like superior vena cava or iliac veins
    - Pacing wires for cardiac pacing
  - Thrombi are not uncommonly seen around long-term iatrogenic intravenous foreign bodies

- **Normal Structures**
  - Valves are visible within veins
- **Ultrasound Artifacts (Mimic)**
  - Reverberation artifact
    - If 2 or more reflectors are in sound path, multiple reflections (i.e., reverberations) occur and may result in linear reverberation artifact

Helpful Clues for Less Common Diagnoses
- **Congenital Membranes**
  - Membranous obstruction may occur in IVC
  - May be developmental anomaly or result of organization of thrombus in hepatic portion of IVC
  - Occurs more frequently in Nepal, South Africa, Japan, India, China, and Korea
  - Occlusive lesion always occurs at approximately level of diaphragm
  - Commonly takes form of membrane but may be fibrotic occlusion of variable length
  - Ultrasound can identify site of obstruction in > 90% of cases in some reports

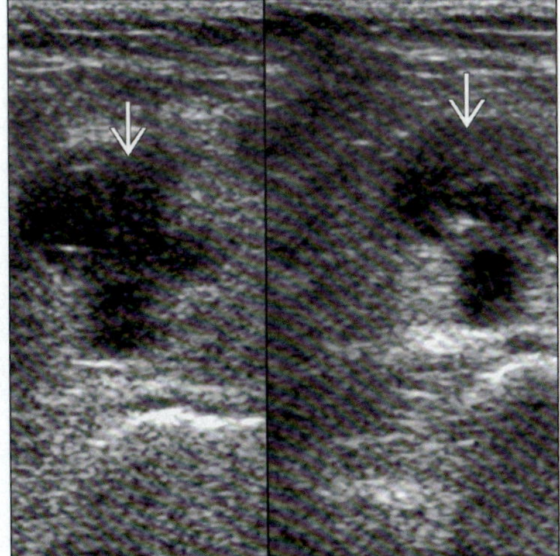

Acute Thrombosis

Transverse ultrasound without (left) and with (right) compression shows acute thrombosis of the popliteal vein. The vein is filled with hypoechoic thrombus ➡ and is noncompressible.

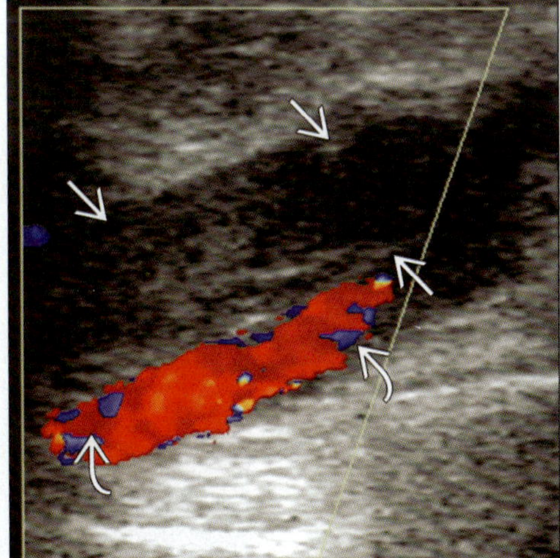

Acute Thrombosis

Longitudinal color Doppler ultrasound shows the corresponding distended, thrombosed popliteal vein ➡ with absent intravascular signal. The popliteal artery ➡ demonstrates normal color flow.

14

INTRALUMINAL VENOUS MASS

Acute Thrombosis

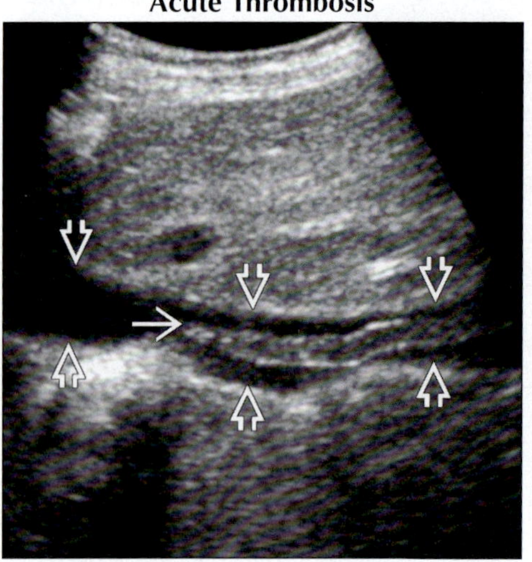

Acute Thrombosis

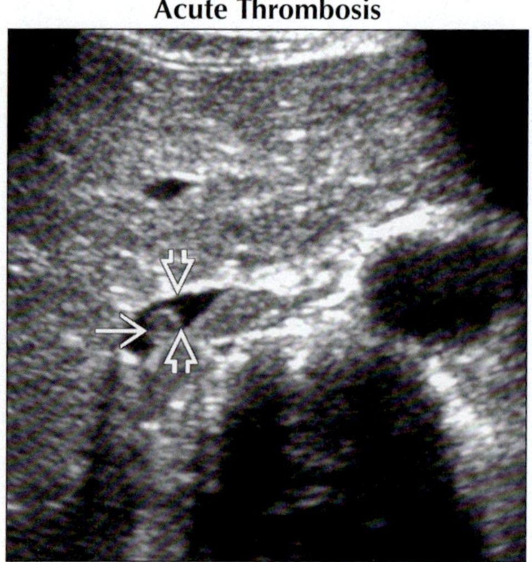

(Left) Longitudinal transabdominal ultrasound shows an echogenic "tongue" of thrombus ➡, extending from the iliac veins into the partially patent IVC ⮕. The free-floating nature of this "tongue" suggests the thrombus is relatively recently formed despite its increased echogenicity. Such a thrombus is prone to embolization. *(Right)* Transverse transabdominal ultrasound shows the corresponding "tongue" of thrombus ➡ within the IVC ⮕.

Subacute Thrombosis

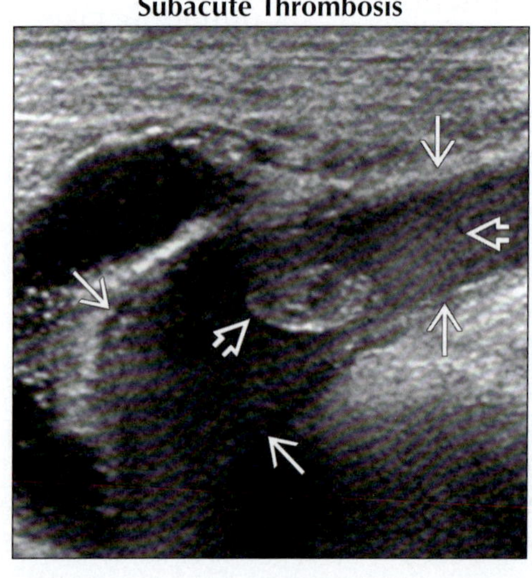

Subacute Thrombosis

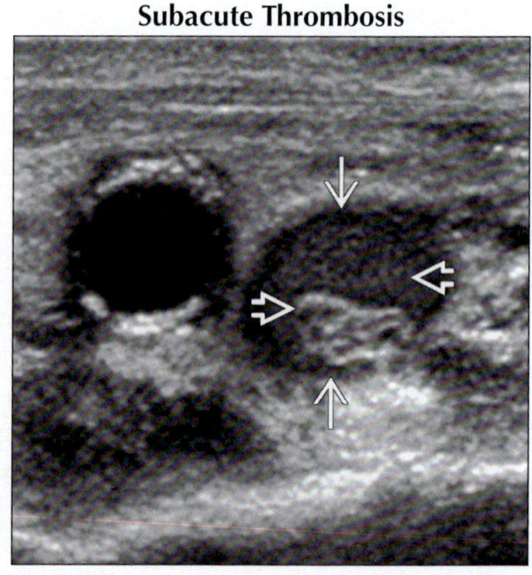

(Left) Longitudinal ultrasound shows the external iliac vein ➡ and a heterogeneously echogenic thrombus ⮕ within the normal-sized external iliac vein with no significant retraction. *(Right)* Transverse ultrasound shows subacute thrombosis of the external iliac vein ➡ in the same patient. Note that the vein is filled with heterogeneously echogenic thrombus ➡, but the vein remains normal-sized and is not significantly contracted.

Chronic Thrombosis

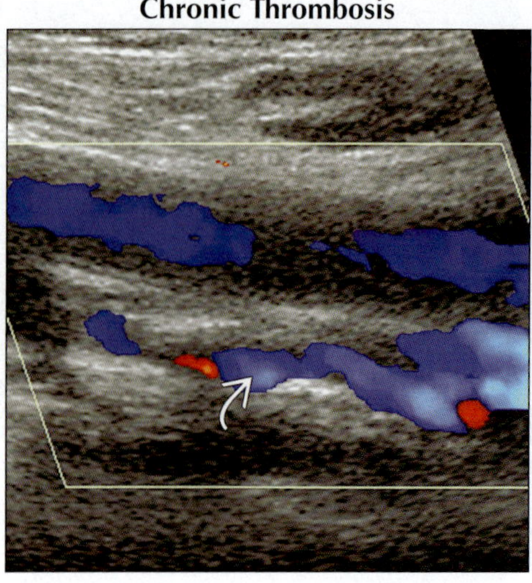

Chronic Thrombosis

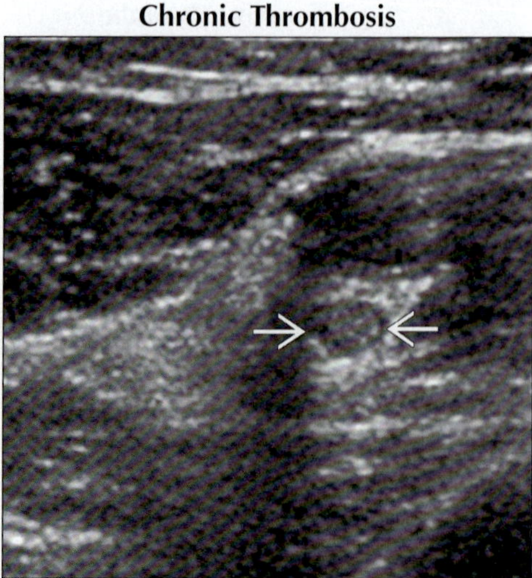

(Left) Longitudinal color Doppler ultrasound shows chronic thrombosis of the superficial femoral vein with partial recanalization of the thrombus ⮕. *(Right)* Transverse ultrasound shows chronic thrombosis of the superficial femoral vein. The thrombosed vein ➡ is contracted and filled with echogenic thrombus.

14

Tumor Thrombus

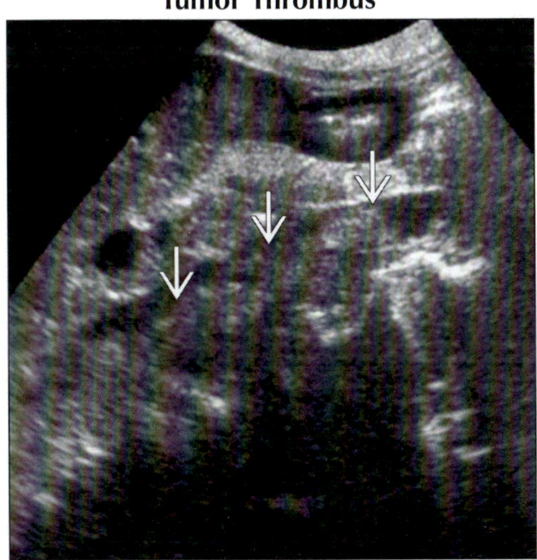

Tumor Thrombus

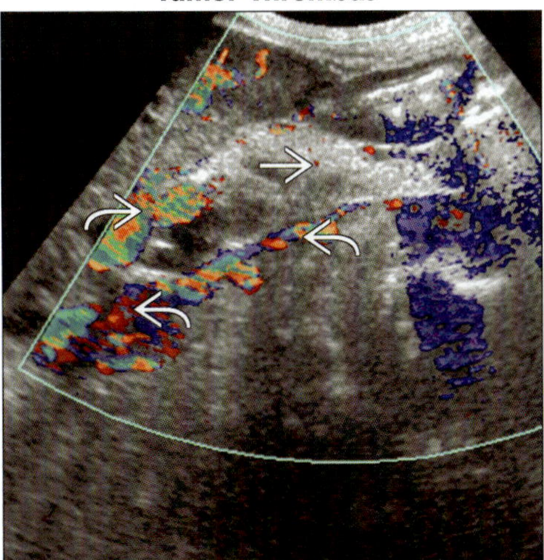

(Left) Longitudinal transabdominal ultrasound shows a partially occlusive tumor thrombus ➡ in a patient with a history of colonic carcinoma. *(Right)* Longitudinal color Doppler ultrasound shows color signal filling the residual lumen ➡ around the intraluminal venous mass in the same patient. Note the suggestion of color flow signal ➡ within the tumor thrombus.

Renal Cell Carcinoma

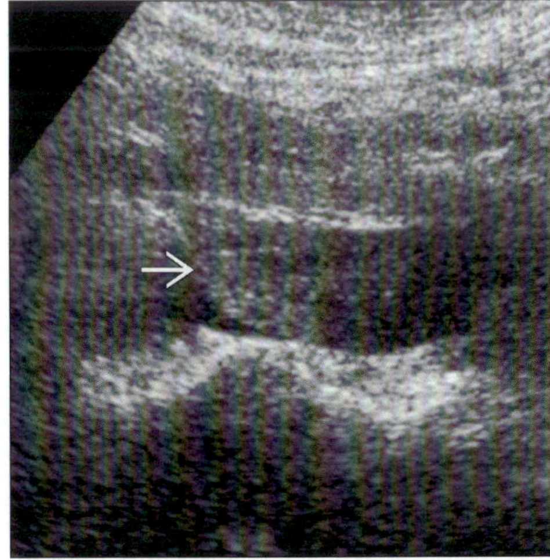

Renal Cell Carcinoma

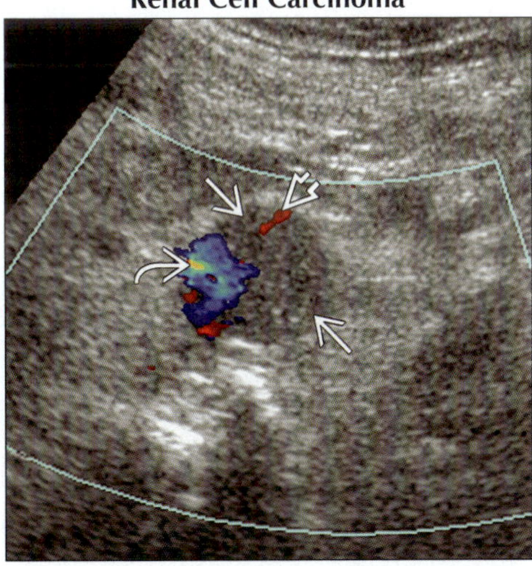

(Left) Longitudinal transabdominal ultrasound shows tumor thrombus ➡ in a patient with known renal cell carcinoma. *(Right)* Transverse color Doppler ultrasound in the same patient shows partial obstruction ➡ with incomplete color filling of the lumen ➡. Note the presence of color signal ➡ within the tumor thrombus.

Venous Catheter

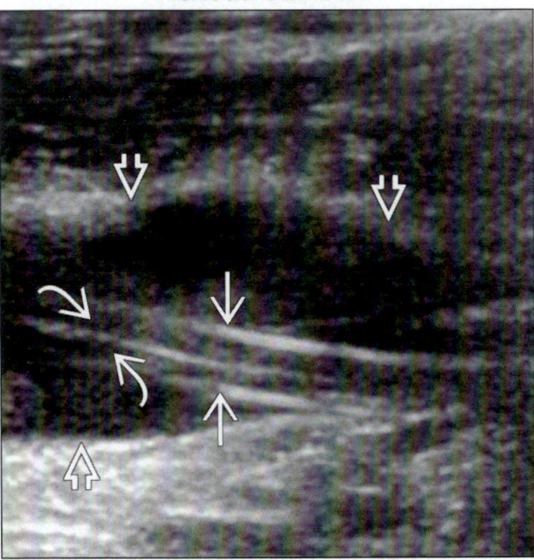

Venous Catheter

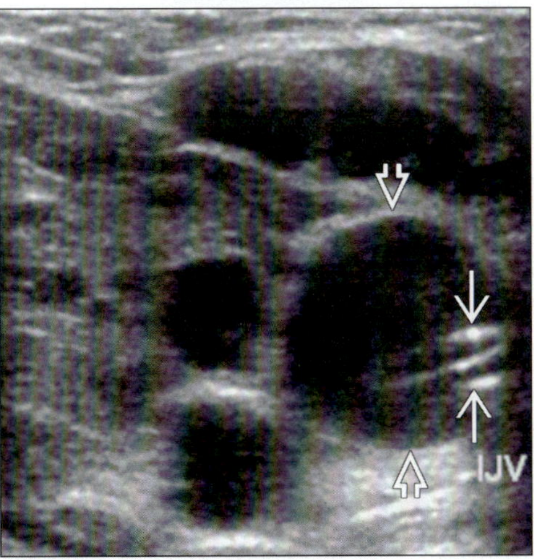

(Left) Longitudinal ultrasound shows a double lumen dialysis catheter ➡ within the internal jugular vein ➡. Note the 2 hypoechoic lumens ➡ within the catheter. *(Right)* Transverse ultrasound of the same dialysis catheter ➡ within the internal jugular vein (IJV) ➡.

INTRALUMINAL VENOUS MASS

(Left) Longitudinal transabdominal ultrasound shows suprarenal placement of an IVC filter ➡. Note that the echogenic IVC filter is placed below the hepatic venous confluence ⮞. This method of placement can be considered if thrombus extends above the renal veins. *(Right)* Transverse transabdominal ultrasound in the same patient shows the echogenic, suprarenal, IVC filter ➡.

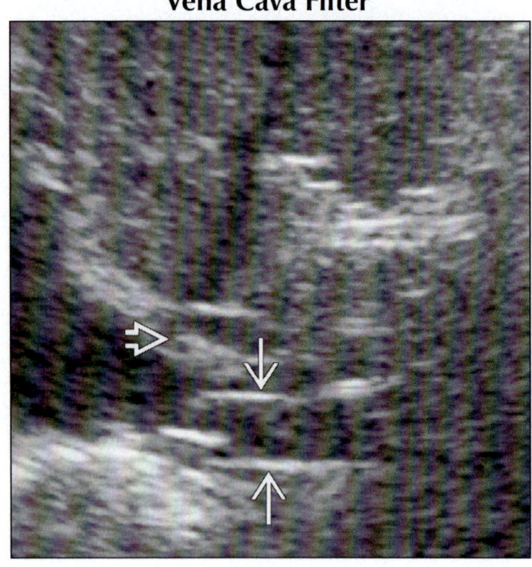

Vena Cava Filter

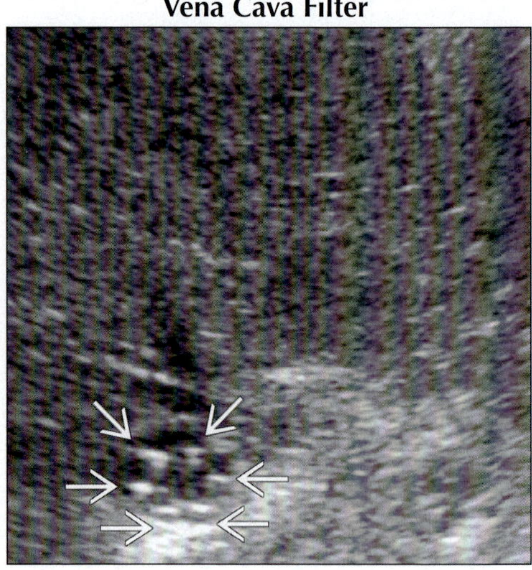

Vena Cava Filter

(Left) Longitudinal transabdominal ultrasound shows an echogenic filter ➡ within the infrarenal IVC. Note the echogenic material within the filter, suggestive of thrombus. *(Right)* Longitudinal color Doppler ultrasound in the same patient shows residual color flow through the partially thrombosed IVC lumen, likely related to the in-situ IVC filter.

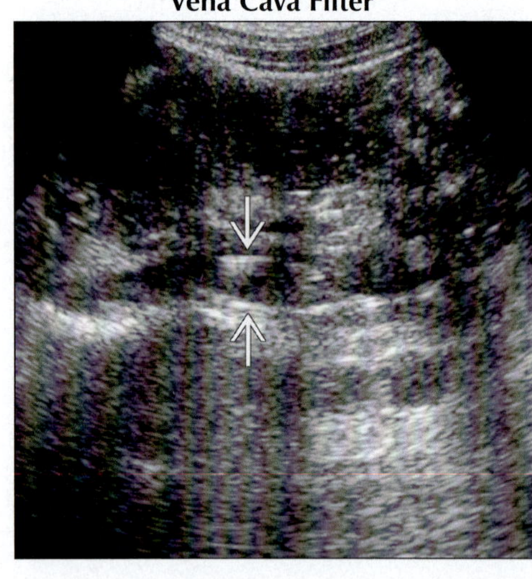

Vena Cava Filter

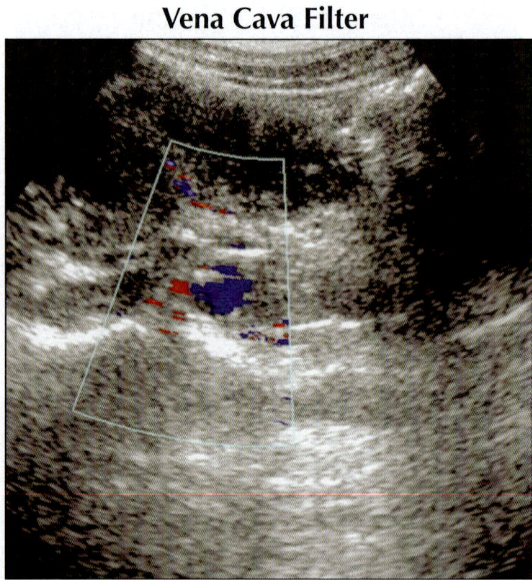

Vena Cava Filter

(Left) Nonsubtracted cavogram in the same patient shows a filling defect ⮞ within the filter ➡. *(Right)* Corresponding digital subtracted intraluminal cavogram better demonstrates the filling defect ⮞ (thrombus) within the intraluminal filter ➡.

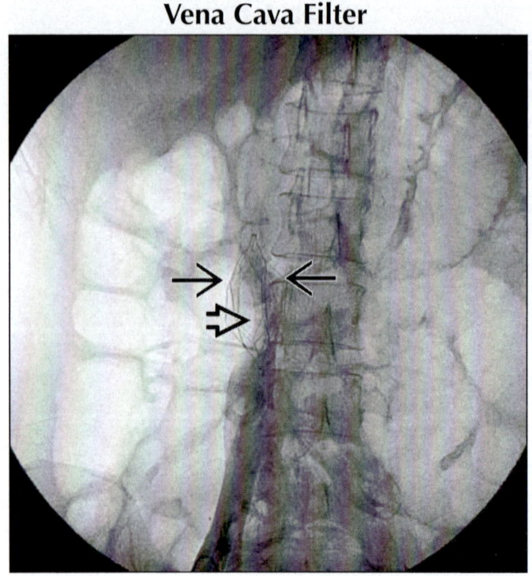

Vena Cava Filter

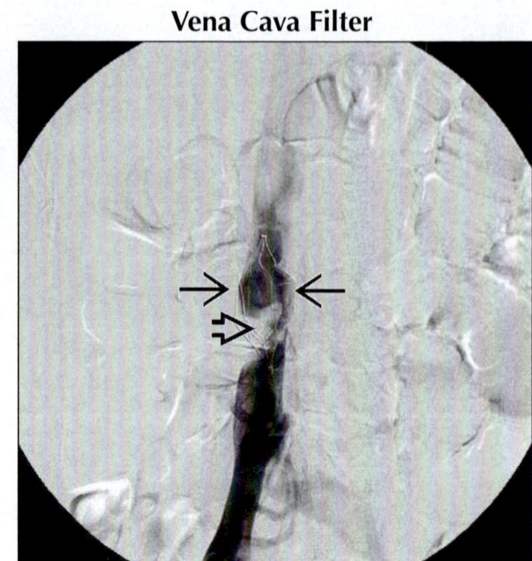

Vena Cava Filter

14

INTRALUMINAL VENOUS MASS

Valves

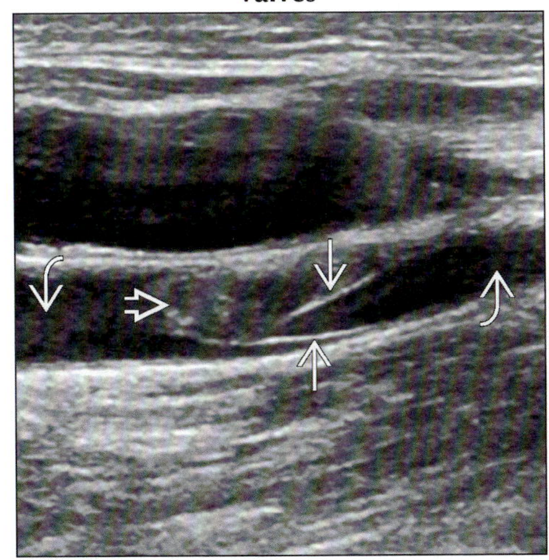

Valves

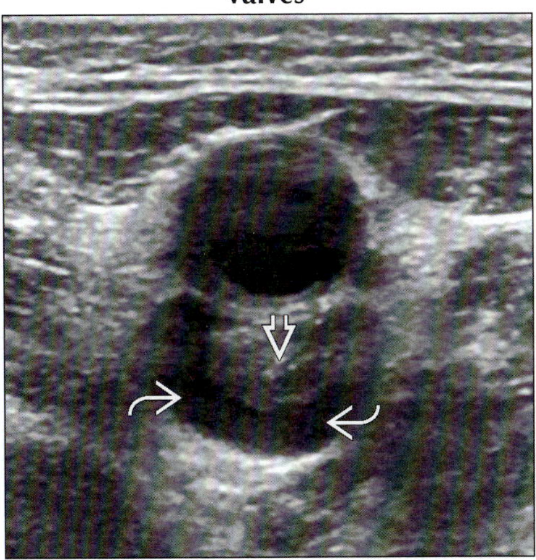

(Left) Longitudinal ultrasound shows the presence of an echogenic thrombus ➡ adherent to the echogenic valve ➡ within the superficial femoral vein ➡. (Right) Transverse ultrasound shows the echogenic thrombus ➡ adherent to a valve in the superficial femoral vein ➡ in the same patient. Note that the valve is not as visible on the transverse image.

Congenital Membranes

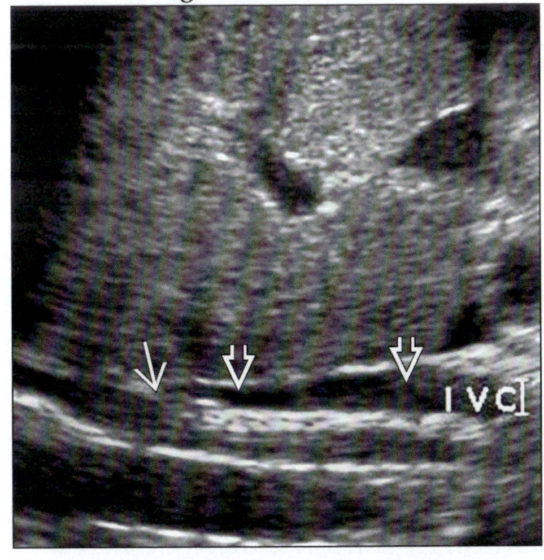

Congenital Membranes

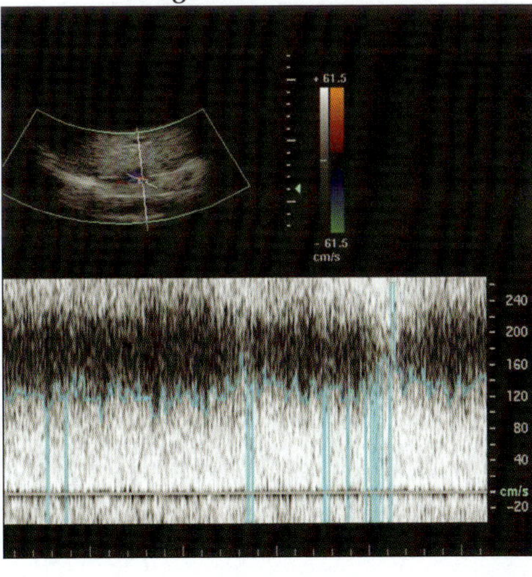

(Left) Oblique transabdominal ultrasound shows a partial membrane ➡ in the IVC that causes significant narrowing of the lumen ➡. (Right) Oblique pulsed Doppler ultrasound in the same patient shows turbulent flow at the luminal narrowing site caused by the partial membrane. Note the markedly increased peak velocity with a "wraparound" artifact, suggesting significant stenosis.

Ultrasound Artifacts (Mimic)

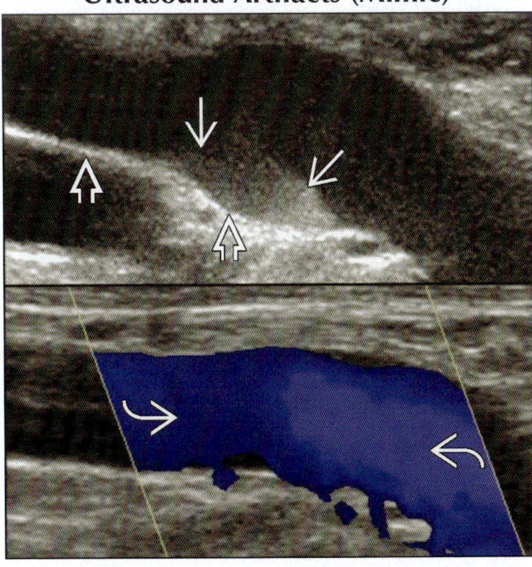

Metallic Stent

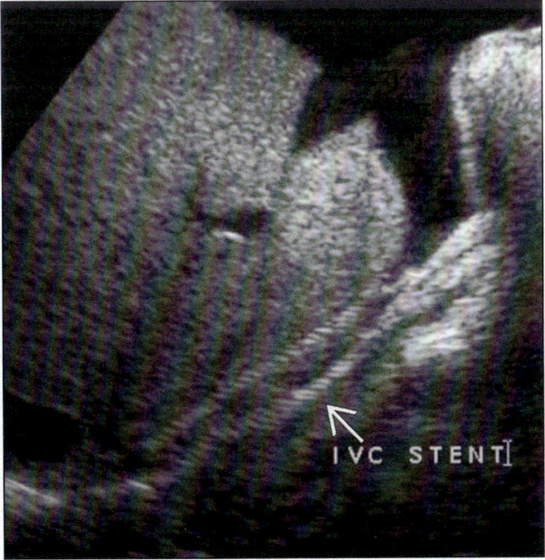

(Left) Longitudinal ultrasound shows apparent bright echoes ➡ within the vein ➡ resulting from a reverberation artifact (top). Note the complete filling of the lumen of the vein with color signal ➡, indicating complete luminal patency of the vein (bottom). (Right) Oblique ultrasound after treatment shows an echogenic IVC stent ➡ placed across the intrahepatic IVC.

14

VENOUS COMPRESSION/INFILTRATION

DIFFERENTIAL DIAGNOSIS

Common
- Vascular Origin Masses
  - Hematoma
  - Pseudoaneurysm
  - Aneurysm
  - Normal Anatomical Variants/Vascular Structures
- Tumor Thrombus
  - Intravenous Leiomyomatosis
  - Leiomyosarcoma
- Lymph Node Origin Masses
  - Metastatic Nodes
  - Lymphoma
- Neural Origin Masses
  - Peripheral Nerve Sheath Tumor
- Masses Arising from Adjacent Organs or Tissues
  - Salivary and Thyroid Masses
  - Hepatocellular Carcinoma
  - Hepatic Metastases
  - Renal Cell Carcinoma
  - Gynecological Tumor
  - Soft Tissue Sarcoma
- Infective/Inflammatory Masses
  - Abscesses

Less Common
- Embryological Remnants
  - 2nd Branchial Cleft Cyst
  - Duplication Cyst

ESSENTIAL INFORMATION

Key Differential Diagnosis Issues
- Accurate diagnosis depends on sound anatomical knowledge and understanding of structures adjacent to compressed vein
- When mass causes both compression and infiltration of venous structures, malignant tumors should be considered
- Grayscale ultrasound
  - Site of compression/infiltration may often be identifiable
  - Thrombus of different ages may be seen distal or proximal to site of narrowing from slow or disrupted flow
  - Tumor thrombus may be traced into tumor or organ of origin
  - Collateral veins may be seen around site of compression

- Pulsed Doppler
  - Normal flow
    - Proximal portion of inferior vena cava (IVC) and hepatic veins have pulsatile flow pattern due to changes in right atrial pressure during cardiac cycle
    - Distal portion of IVC shows respiratory variations
    - In medium to large veins, spontaneous and phasic flow (variations in flow velocity with respiration) are expected
  - Flow when compression is present proximally
    - Pulsatile flow in proximal IVC/hepatic veins may be dampened
    - Respiratory variations in flow in distal IVC, large, and medium-sized veins may be lost (resulting in continuous flow with no phasic variations)
  - Useful to confirm arterial masses, that are causing venous compression
    - Iliac vein compression syndrome
    - Left renal vein compression syndrome
    - Aneurysms
- Color Doppler/power Doppler
  - Useful to detect hypoechoic/anechoic acute thrombus proximal or distal to site of compression, which may be missed on grayscale US
  - Demonstrate recanalized lumen in thrombus, vascularity within tumor thrombus, and collateralization
  - Assess nature of any compressing mass

Helpful Clues for Common Diagnoses
- **Vascular Origin Masses**
  - All have potential to compress or involve adjacent veins
  - **Hematoma**
    - Echogenicity changes over time
    - No flow on Doppler imaging
  - **Pseudoaneurysm**
    - No true wall; (may be surrounded by thrombus)
    - Connected to artery via neck; may have characteristic "yin-yang" sign
  - **Aneurysm**
    - Dilation of normal artery up to 1.5x its normal diameter; genuine outer wall
    - May contain mural thrombus
    - May be saccular or fusiform in shape

14

VENOUS COMPRESSION/INFILTRATION

- ○ **Normal Anatomical Variants/Vascular Structures**
  - Compression of left renal vein by aorta in retroaortic left renal vein
  - Iliac vein obstruction (May-Thurner) syndrome: Compression of left common iliac vein by right common iliac artery
  - Left renal vein entrapment (nutcracker) syndrome: Obstruction of left renal vein by superior mesenteric artery
- **Tumor Thrombus**
  - ○ Tumor may invade from a primary neoplasm or arise from vein itself, causing infiltration and obstruction to venous flow
  - ○ Renal, hepatocellular and adrenal carcinoma most common abdominal primaries to show intravascular invasion
  - ○ **Intravenous Leiomyomatosis**
    - Rare condition characterized by leiomyomas with growth of smooth muscle cells into venous vasculature
    - Presents as convoluted, worm-like masses growing within veins
    - Often extend into broad ligament, other pelvic veins, IVC, or even heart
  - ○ **Leiomyosarcoma**
    - Most common intravascular tumor, preponderance in old women (M:F = 1:5)
    - Both intravascular and extravascular components may be present
    - Blood flow in IVC and hepatic veins may be absent, reversed, or turbulent
- **Lymph Node Origin Masses**
  - ○ **Metastatic Nodes**
    - Commonly round, may be hypoechoic, loss of fatty hila, eccentric cortical hypertrophy and
    - Large peripheral vessels
    - Infiltration of adjacent fat or invasion of adjacent structures
  - ○ **Lymphoma**
    - Loss of hila and round shape, non-Hodgkin lymphoma nodes
    - Commonly hypoechoic, ± reticulated
    - Tend to show posterior acoustic enhancement ("pseudocystic")
- **Neural Origin Masses**
  - ○ **Peripheral Nerve Sheath Tumor**
    - Well-defined hypoechoic masses arising from nerve
    - Located along peripheral nerves or in paraspinal position
- **Masses Arising from Adjacent Organs or Tissues**
  - ○ Head and neck
    - Consider salivary glands and thyroid masses
  - ○ Abdomen and pelvis
    - Any mass can potentially compress adjacent veins
    - Renal, adrenal and hepatocellular carcinoma may also have intravascular invasion
  - ○ Extremity
    - Consider masses arising from adjacent tissue; such as fat, muscles, or bone

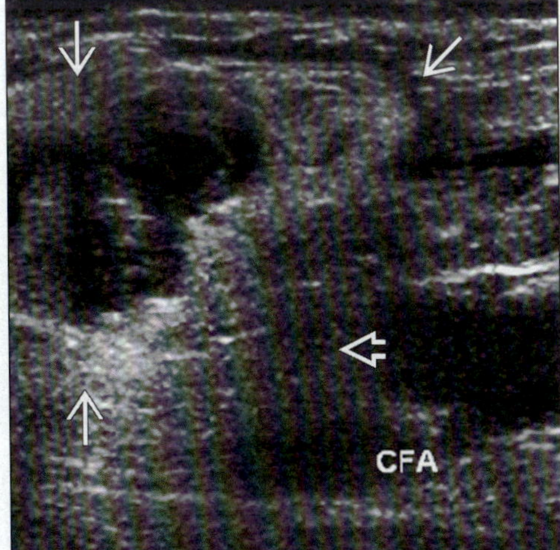

Hematoma

Oblique ultrasound shows a heterogeneous hematoma ➡ overlying the common femoral artery (CFA) after femoral artery puncture during angiography. Note the compression of the adjacent common femoral vein ⇨.

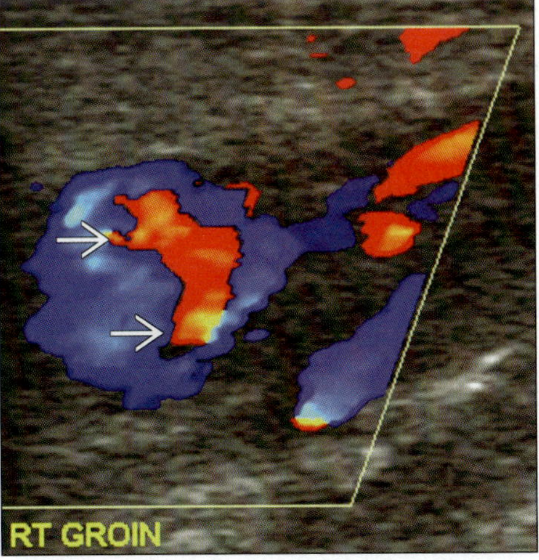

Pseudoaneurysm

Oblique color Doppler ultrasound shows a pseudoaneurysm arising from the right common femoral artery after femoral puncture during angiography. Note the "yin-yang" sign ➡ caused by swirling flow.

14

VENOUS COMPRESSION/INFILTRATION

(Left) Transverse color Doppler US shows infiltration of the IVC by tumor thrombus → in a child with an invasive presacral germ cell tumor. Note the vascularity within the tumor thrombus → and the patent adjacent abdominal aorta →. (Right) Longitudinal pulsed Doppler US in the same patient shows an arterial waveform within the tumor thrombus →. This distinguishes tumor thrombus from recanalization of an ordinary thrombus.

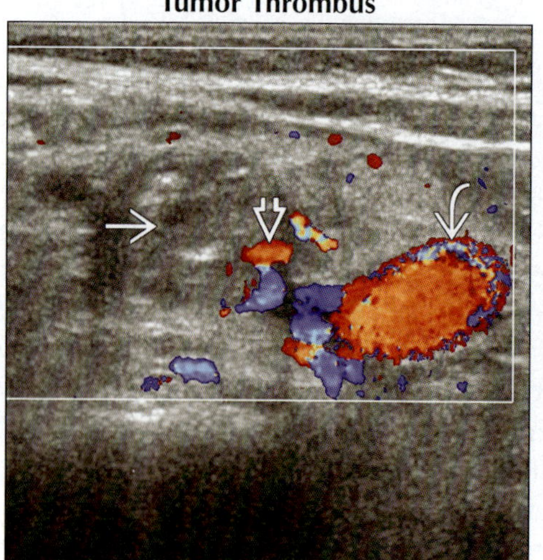

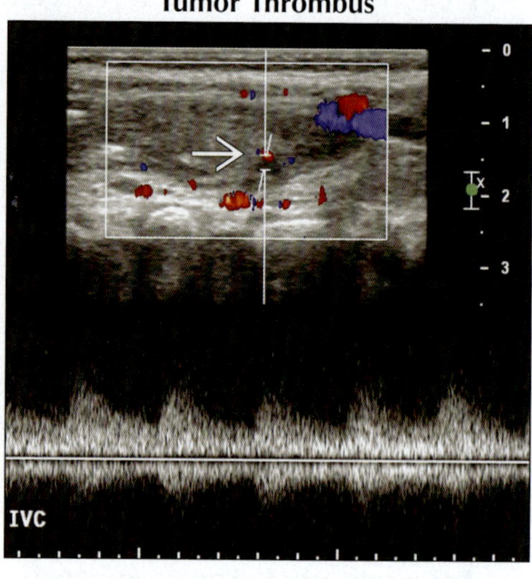

(Left) Transverse color Doppler ultrasound in the same patient shows the tumor thrombus also infiltrating the left common iliac vein →. Note the color flow within the tumor thrombus → and the patency of the adjacent common iliac arteries →. (Right) Transverse pulsed Doppler ultrasound shows vascularity within the same tumor thrombus →. The presence of vascularity is key to the diagnosis of a tumor thrombus.

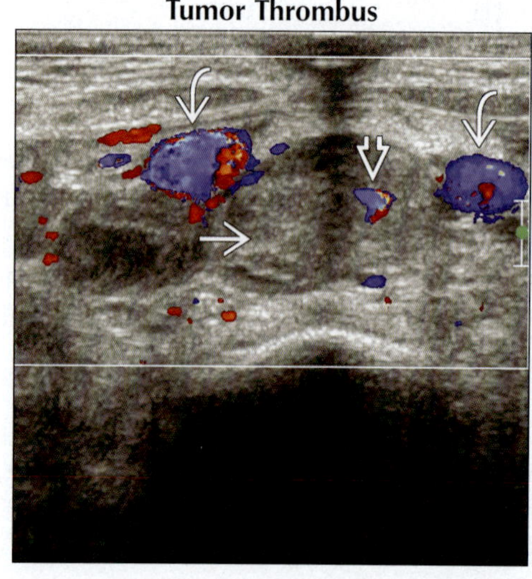

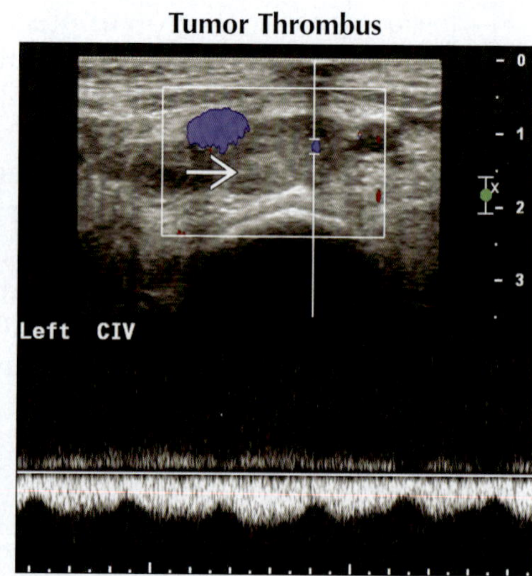

(Left) Oblique color Doppler ultrasound shows patency in the left external iliac vein →, distal to the IVC and common iliac vein infiltrated by tumor thrombi. (Right) Oblique pulsed Doppler ultrasound in the same patient shows continuous flow in the left external iliac vein →, with abolishment of normal respiratory phasic variation, indicating obstruction proximally in the common iliac vein and IVC.

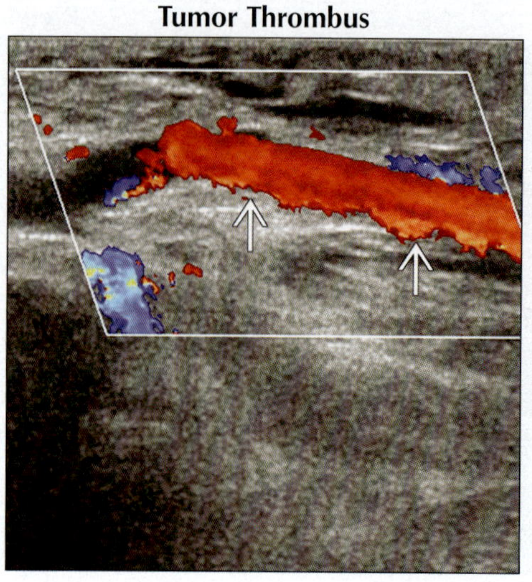

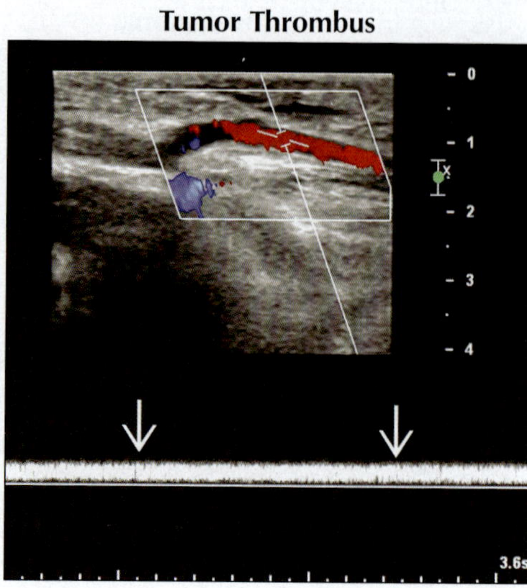

14

VENOUS COMPRESSION/INFILTRATION

Metastatic Nodes

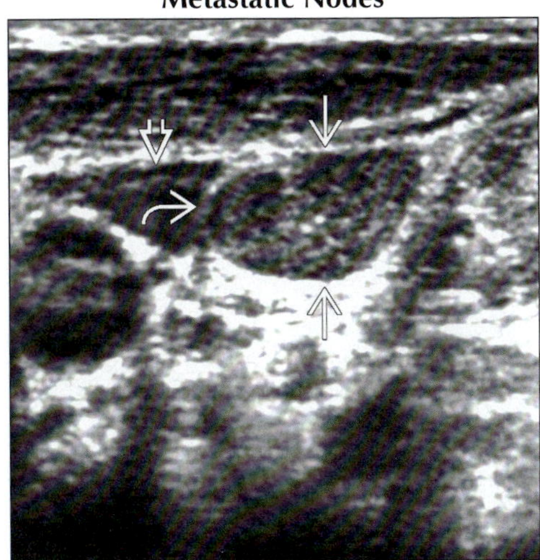

Metastatic Nodes

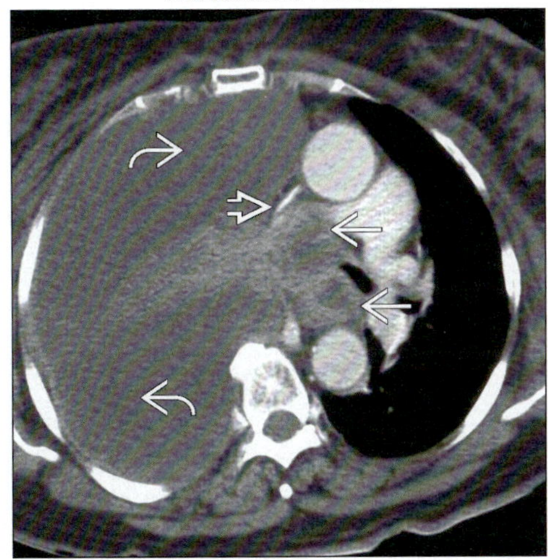

(Left) Transverse ultrasound shows a metastatic lymph node ➡ with loss of its normal echogenic hilus, which causes mild compression ➡ of the adjacent left internal jugular vein ➡. (Right) Axial CECT shows necrotic mediastinal nodes ➡ compressing the superior vena cava ➡ in a patient with metastatic lung carcinoma and a large right pleural effusion ➡. The superior vena cava is not easily imaged with ultrasound.

Lymphoma

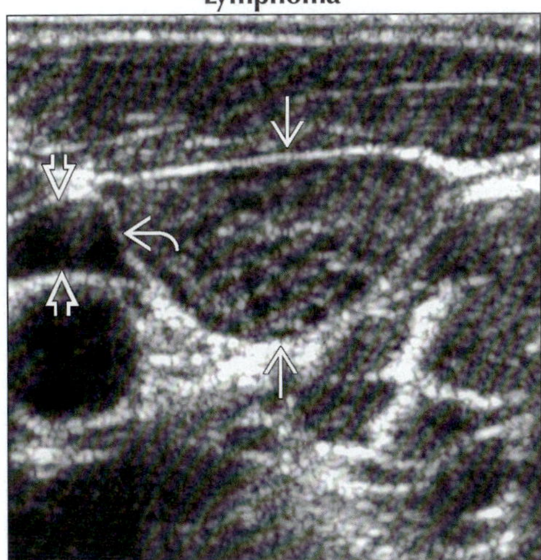

Peripheral Nerve Sheath Tumor

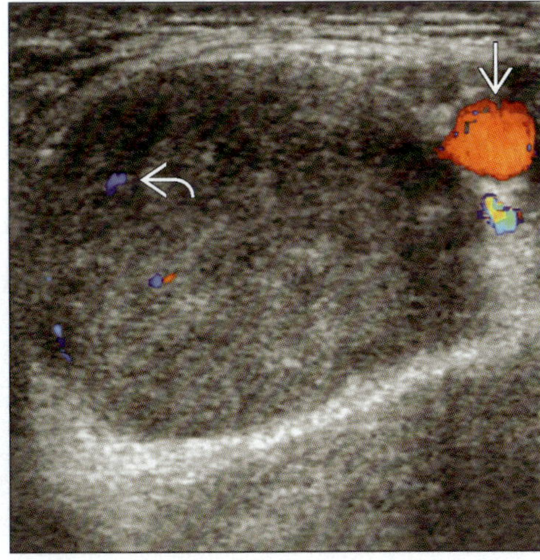

(Left) Transverse ultrasound shows a reticulated, intranodal echopattern that is typical of non-Hodgkin lymphoma ➡. Note the mild compression ➡ of the adjacent internal jugular vein ➡. (Right) Transverse color Doppler ultrasound of the axilla shows a peripheral nerve sheath tumor of the median nerve with minimal vascularity ➡. Note the proximity of the adjacent vascular bundle ➡ and the potential for venous compression.

Hepatocellular Carcinoma

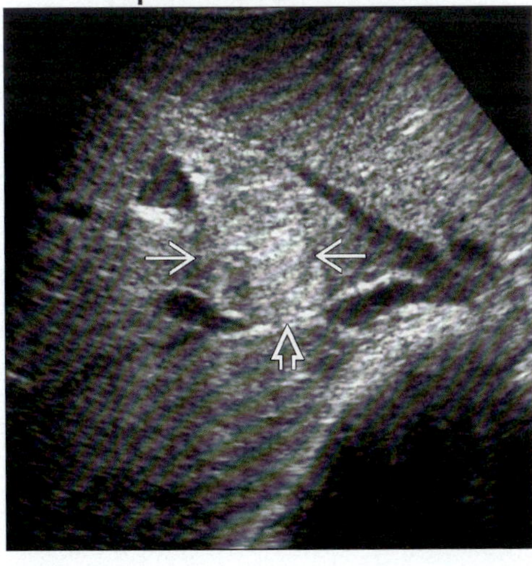

Hepatocellular Carcinoma

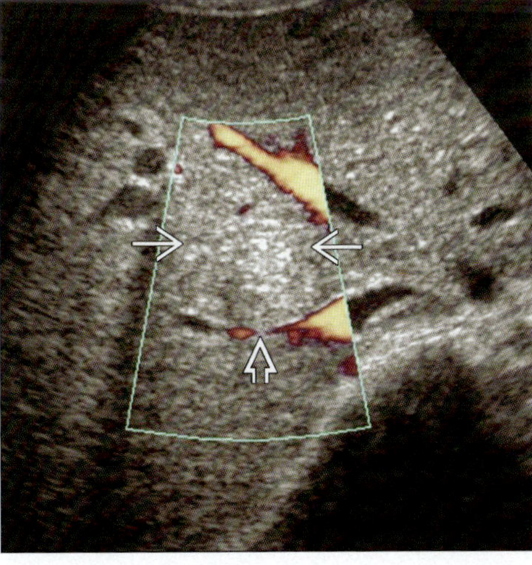

(Left) Transverse transabdominal ultrasound shows a small, mildly hyperechoic hepatocellular carcinoma ➡ causing obliteration of the hepatic vein lumen ➡. (Right) Transverse power Doppler ultrasound shows the same hepatocellular carcinoma ➡ with no color flow in the hepatic vein ➡ due to compression/infiltration. Hepatic veins are less commonly involved than portal veins by hepatocellular carcinoma.

14

VENOUS COMPRESSION/INFILTRATION

(Left) *Transverse transabdominal ultrasound shows numerous hyperechoic liver metastases* ➡ *with distortion and compression of the right portal vein* ➡. **(Right)** *Transverse transabdominal ultrasound shows multiple target lesions* ➡ *in the liver representing multiple hepatic metastases from lung carcinoma. Note the mass effect on the hepatic vein* ➡ *caused by 1 of the metastases.*

Hepatic Metastases

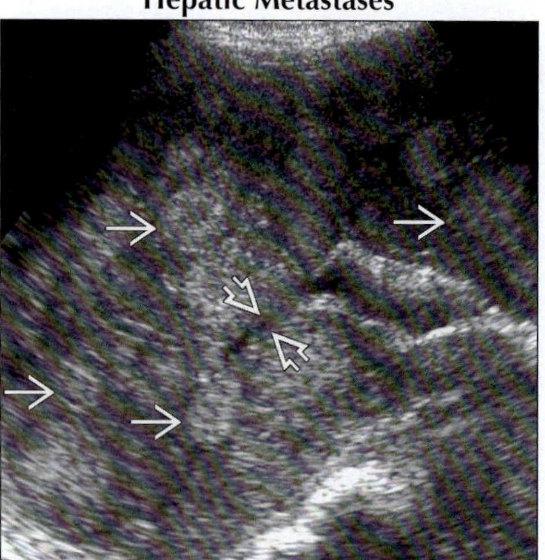

Hepatic Metastases

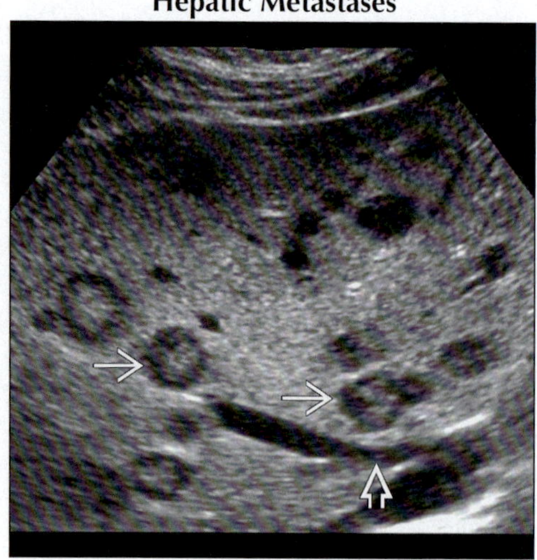

(Left) *Longitudinal transabdominal ultrasound shows a heterogeneous metastatic deposit* ➡ *causing compression of the inferior vena cava* ➡. **(Right)** *Longitudinal color Doppler ultrasound shows the patency of the IVC despite compression by the metastasis* ➡. *Note the slightly turbulent flow through the narrowed portion of the IVC as illustrated by "aliasing" of the color signal* ➡.

Hepatic Metastases

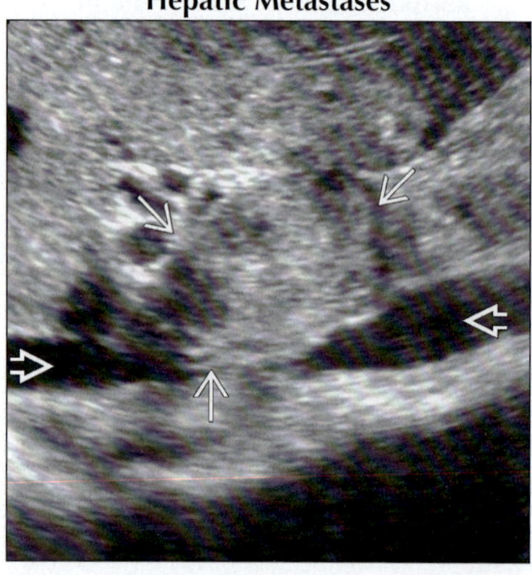

Hepatic Metastases

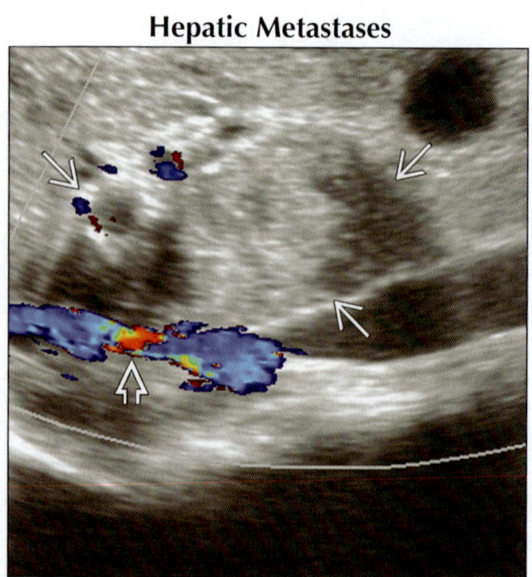

(Left) *Transverse transabdominal ultrasound shows tumor thrombus* ➡ *infiltrating the lumen of the right renal vein in a patient with renal cell carcinoma, a tumor with a propensity to invade venous structures. Renal vein invasion should always be looked for in patients with renal cell carcinoma.* **(Right)** *Transverse transabdominal ultrasound shows tumor thrombus* ➡ *infiltrating the lumen of the IVC in the same patient.*

Renal Cell Carcinoma

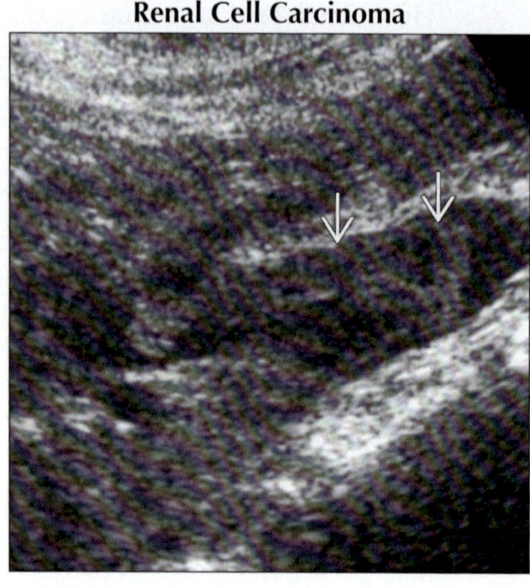

Renal Cell Carcinoma

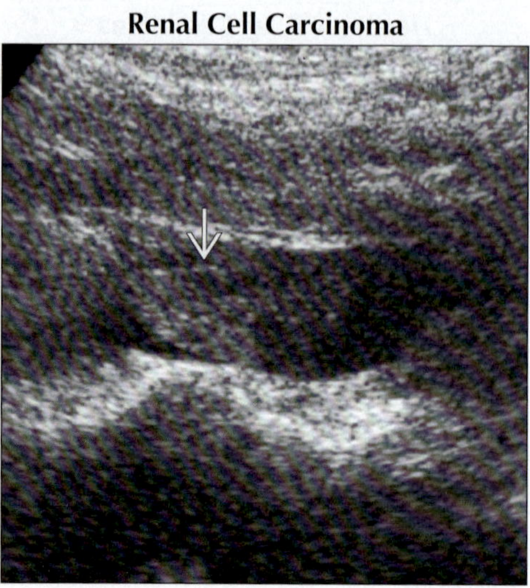

VENOUS COMPRESSION/INFILTRATION

Gynecological Tumor

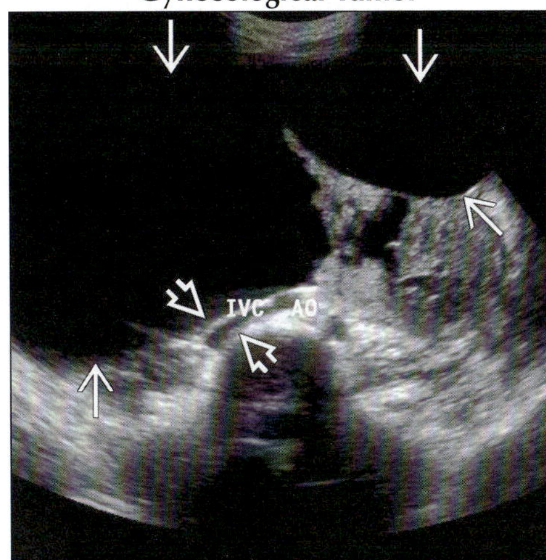

Gynecological Tumor

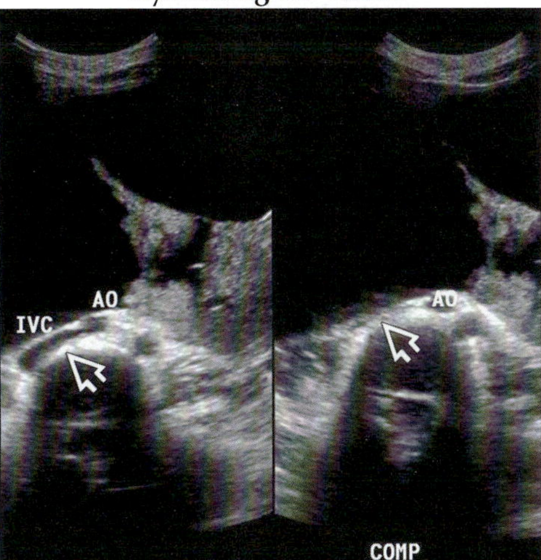

(Left) Transverse transabdominal ultrasound shows a large, complex, cystic tumor ➡ arising from the pelvis and compressing the IVC ➡. *(Right)* Composite image in the same patient, without (left) and with (right) compression, shows the IVC ➡ is compressible. This indicates that, despite its narrowing, the IVC is patent.

Infective/Inflammatory Masses

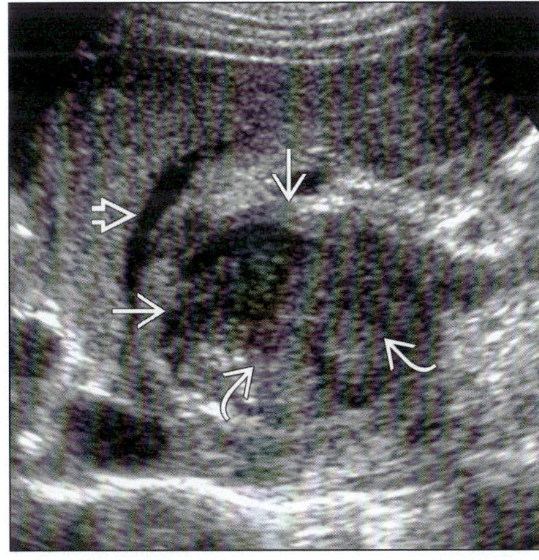

Infective/Inflammatory Masses

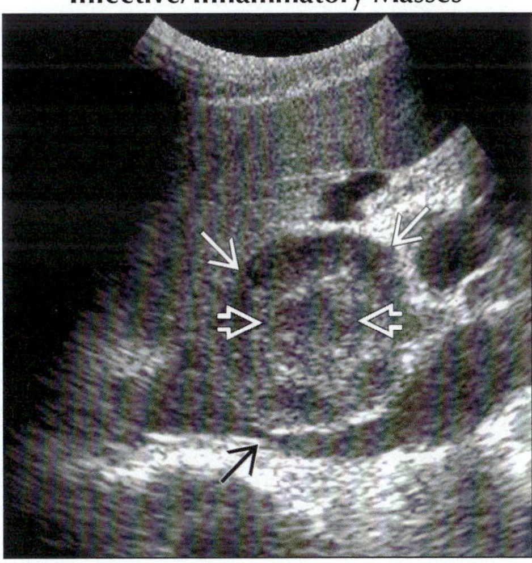

(Left) Transverse transabdominal ultrasound shows a pyogenic liver abscess with a thick and irregular wall ➡, heterogeneous internal echoes ➡, and mass effect on the adjacent hepatic vein ➡. *(Right)* Oblique transabdominal ultrasound shows an amebic abscess ➡ that is hypoechoic with low-level internal echoes ➡. Note the compression of the inferior vena cava ➡ by the protruding abscess.

2nd Branchial Cleft Cyst

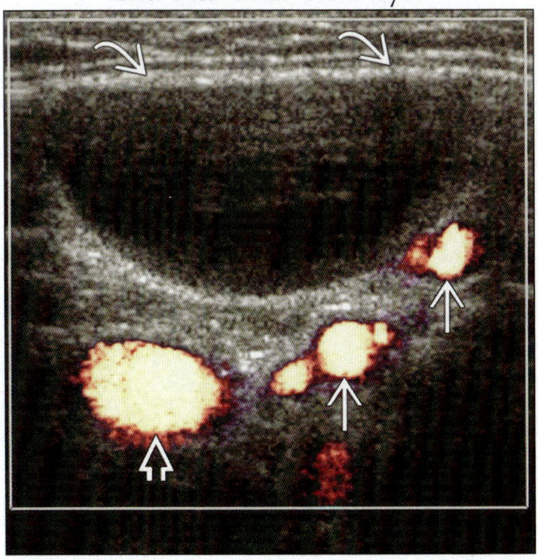

2nd Branchial Cleft Cyst

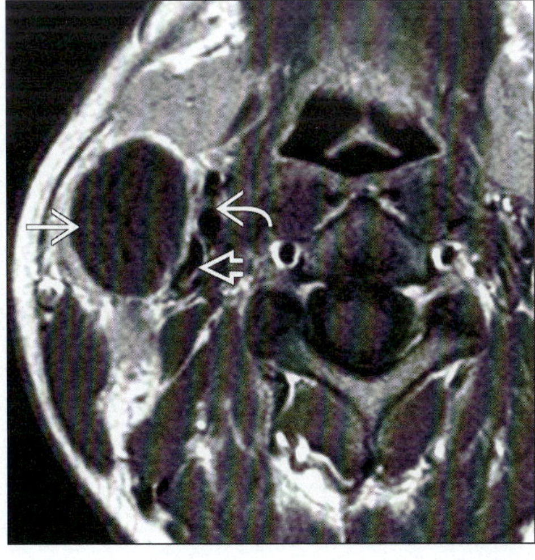

(Left) Transverse power Doppler ultrasound shows an anechoic 2nd branchial cleft cyst ➡ in its characteristic location lateral to the carotid sheath. Note its relationship to the carotid arteries ➡ and the internal jugular vein ➡. *(Right)* Axial T1 C+ MR shows a typical 2nd branchial cleft cyst ➡ with no central enhancement. The cyst is lateral to the carotid bifurcation ➡ and compresses the right internal jugular vein ➡.

SECTION 15
Musculoskeletal

HYPOECHOIC SUBCUTANEOUS MASS

DIFFERENTIAL DIAGNOSIS

Common
- Ganglion Cyst
- Nerve Sheath Tumor
- Lipoma

Less Common
- Epidermoid Cyst
- Vascular Anomaly
- Lymphangioma
- Foreign Body Granuloma
- Hidradenoma
- Pilomatrixoma
- Metastatic Nodule
- Sarcoma
- Lymph Node
- Fat Necrosis
- Rheumatoid Nodule

ESSENTIAL INFORMATION

Key Differential Diagnosis Issues
- Ensure lesion is confined to subcutaneous tissues
  - Important implications for diagnosis and treatment
- Use minimal transducer pressure to avoid distorting lesion
  - Copious gel will allow stand-off effect if mass is producing cutaneous nodule
- Compressibility readily assessed for subcutaneous masses

Helpful Clues for Common Diagnoses
- **Ganglion Cyst**
  - Wrist and hand most common sites of clinical presentation, particularly dorsal aspect
    - Scapholunate joint, radiocarpal joint, scapho-trapezio-trapezoid joint, ulnocarpal joint
    - Metacarpophalangeal joint just proximal to A1 pulley
  - Foot next most common site
    - Subtalar joint, talonavicular joint, navicular-cuneiform joint, intercuneiform joint
  - Ganglia arising from large joints, such as shoulder, hip, and knee, will not be subcutaneous in location
  - Well-defined hypoechoic mass with stalk extending to or pointing toward joint
    - Often irregular in outline
    - ± loculations
    - ± "comet tail" artifacts
    - Not compressible
    - No hyperemia, though color Doppler will allow detection of arteries alongside ganglion cyst
    - Often not possible to trace neck to joint
    - May no longer communicate with joint
    - Ganglia that occur close to A1 pulley have no visible communication with flexor tendon sheath or metacarpophalangeal joint
- **Nerve Sheath Tumor**
  - Well-defined hypoechoic mass
  - Occasionally heterogeneous
    - Heterogenicity due to areas of myxoid tissue, hemorrhage, fibrosis, or calcification
  - Fusiform-shaped along course of nerve
    - Entering or exiting nerve seen in majority of cases
    - If nerve sheath tumor arises from small peripheral nerves, entering/exiting nerves may not be seen
  - Posterior acoustic enhancement is common
    - ± edge shadowing artifact at margin of tumor
- Vascular pattern on color Doppler imaging varied
  - Usually moderately vascular, but some have minimal demonstrable vascularity
- Ultrasound features usually typical enough to make diagnosis without need for biopsy
  - Cannot distinguish between schwannoma and neurofibroma based on ultrasound appearances
- **Lipoma**
  - Well-defined usually hypoechoic, though occasionally hyperechoic tumor
    - Fusiform-shaped → rounded, aligned parallel to skin
    - Multiple, fine, internal striations parallel to skin
    - Compressible
    - Absent or minimal vascularity

Helpful Clues for Less Common Diagnoses
- **Epidermoid Cyst**
  - 3 potential causes

HYPOECHOIC SUBCUTANEOUS MASS

- From sequestration of epidermal rests during embryonic life
- From occlusion of pilosebaceous unit
- From traumatic implantation of epithelial elements
  - ○ Hypoechoic masses with multiple echoes
    - Echoes due to aggregates of keratin debris
- **Vascular Anomaly**
  - ○ Hemangioma
    - Childhood tumor (does not persist into adulthood)
    - Natural progression: Proliferation → stabilization → involution
  - ○ Vascular malformation
    - Venous, capillary, arteriovenous, or mixed
    - Grow proportional to patient growth ± more rapid growth precipitated by puberty, pregnancy, trauma
  - ○ Variable ultrasound appearances
    - Usually irregular though may be rounded
    - Hypoechoic most common but may be hyperechoic depending on degree of fibrous or fatty stroma & calcification
    - Moderately vascular, though some may have minimal or high vascularity
    - ± phleboliths
    - ± venous lakes
- **Lymphangioma**
  - ○ Congenital lesions that develop from sequestered lymphatic channels
  - ○ 4 different ultrasound appearances
    - Cystic with thin septae
    - Cystic with thick septae
    - Cystic with solid areas
    - Mainly solid with scattered cystic areas
  - ○ Solid areas result from clumps of thin lymphatic channels too small to resolve
- Majority are ovoid or spherical, typically 1-5 cm
  - ○ Minority are lobulated or tubular
    - Lobulation due to localized rupture of cyst
  - ○ Posterior acoustic enhancement
  - ○ Color Doppler signal typically absent
    - Vascularity may be evident in areas of granulation tissue due to recent cyst rupture
- **Foreign Body Granuloma**
  - ○ Variable thickness rim of hyperemic granulation tissue forms around foreign bodies
    - Makes echogenic foreign bodies more conspicuous
- **Hidradenoma**
  - ○ Tumor of sweat glands
  - ○ Hypoechoic heterogeneous nodule of low vascularity ± cystic areas
- **Pilomatrixoma**
  - ○ Benign skin neoplasms with differentiation toward hair matrix seen mainly in children
  - ○ Oval-shaped, well-defined, partially calcified lesion with acoustic shadowing
    - Some lesions may be almost completely calcified
  - ○ ± peripheral hypoechoic halo ± peripheral vascularity

Ganglion Cyst

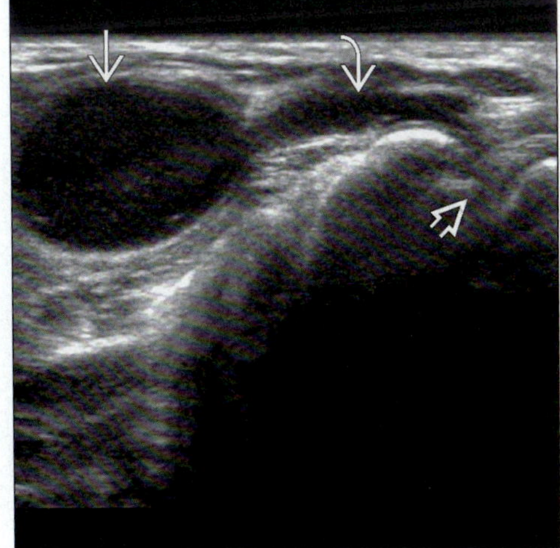

Oblique ultrasound shows a well-defined ganglion cyst ⇨ extending into the thenar muscle with a clearly defined subcutaneous stalk ⇨ arising from scaphotrapezium articulation ⇨.

Nerve Sheath Tumor

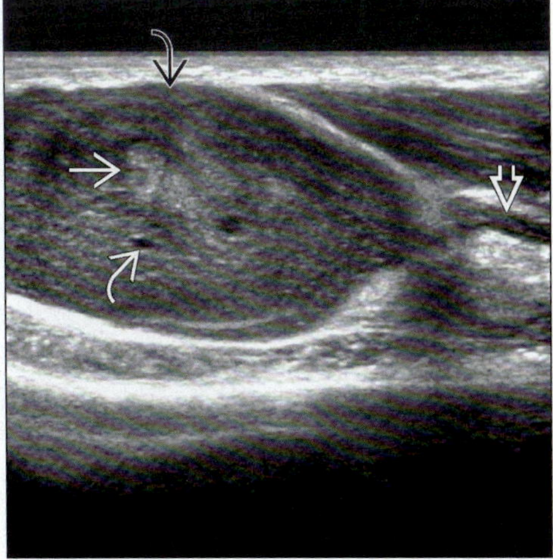

Longitudinal US shows a fusiform-shaped nerve sheath tumor ⇨ of median nerve ⇨ in the distal forearm. Hyperechoic areas ⇨ may present hemorrhage, while hypoechoic areas ⇨ represent myxoid matrix.

HYPOECHOIC SUBCUTANEOUS MASS

Lipoma

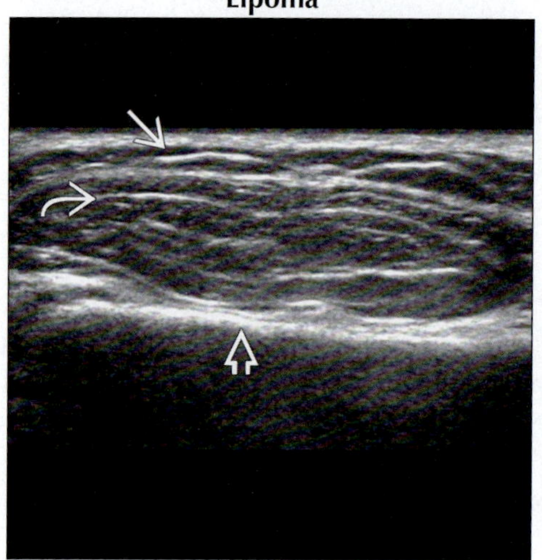

Epidermoid Cyst

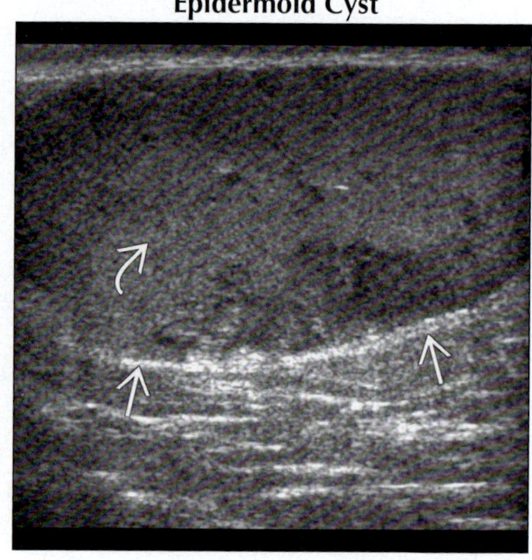

(Left) Transverse US shows a well-defined subcutaneous lipoma ➡ posterior to the acromion ➡. The tumor has characteristic fine internal echogenic lines ➡. A distinct margin must be confirmed before a lipoma is diagnosed. *(Right)* Transverse US shows a well-defined subcutaneous mass ➡, consistent with an epidermoid cyst. A nearly uniform finely speckled pattern ➡ throughout the mass is characteristic. Gravitational layering of contents may be seen.

Vascular Anomaly

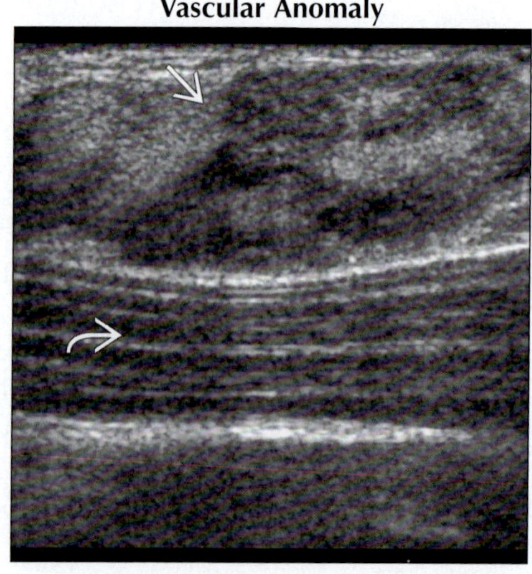

Vascular Anomaly

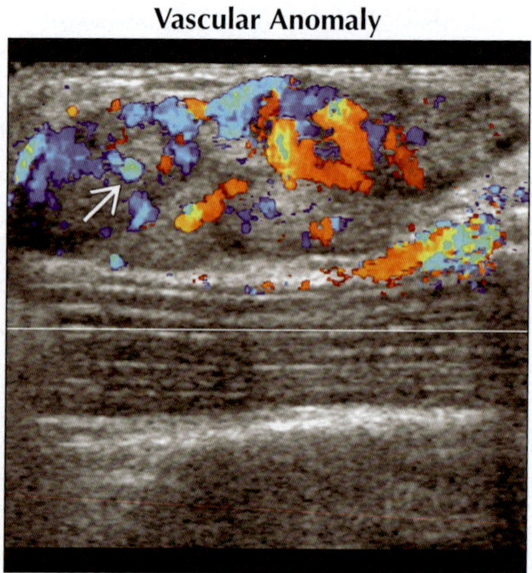

(Left) Transverse ultrasound shows a heterogeneous, largely hypoechoic, well-defined mass ➡ in the subcutaneous tissues of the upper chest wall in a 12-year-old patient. The pectoralis major muscle ➡ lies deep to the mass. *(Right)* Correlative transverse color Doppler US shows marked hypervascularity ➡ of the mass. Note how color Doppler imaging shows high vascularity, even though very few discernible vessel-like structures were evident on grayscale imaging.

Foreign Body Granuloma

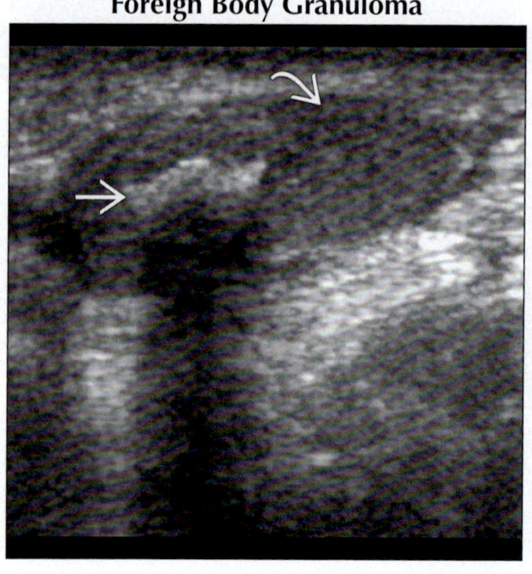

Hidradenoma

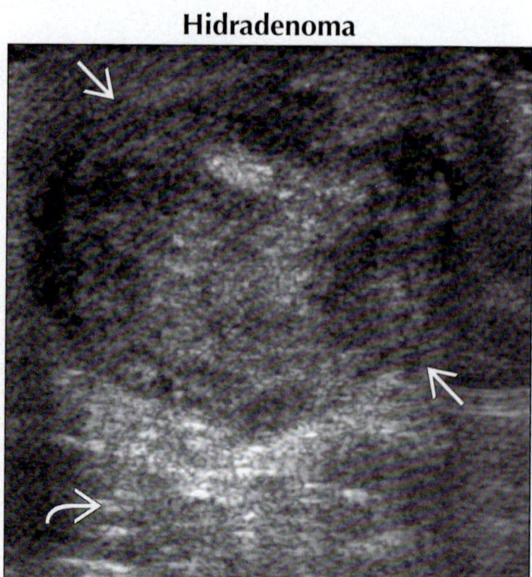

(Left) Longitudinal US shows a foreign body granuloma of the forearm. A hyperechoic region ➡ from a retained glass fragment is surrounded by a hypoechoic region ➡ of granulation tissue. The amount of granulation tissue loosely reflects reactivity and the duration of a retained foreign body. *(Right)* Transverse ultrasound shows a heterogeneous, well-marginated tumor ➡ with posterior acoustic enhancement ➡. No discernible cystic areas are seen.

15

HYPOECHOIC SUBCUTANEOUS MASS

Pilomatrixoma

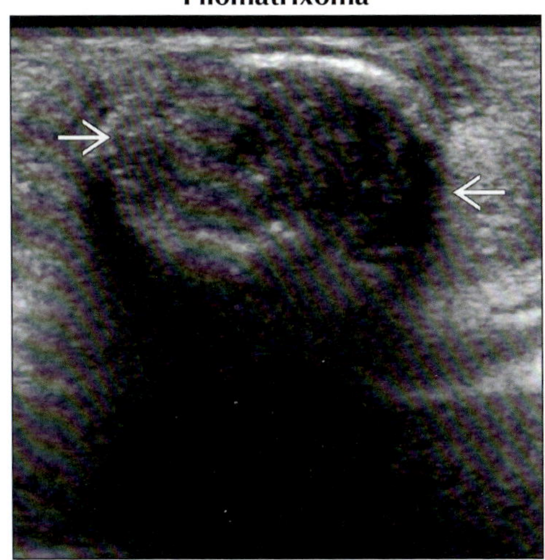

Metastatic Nodule

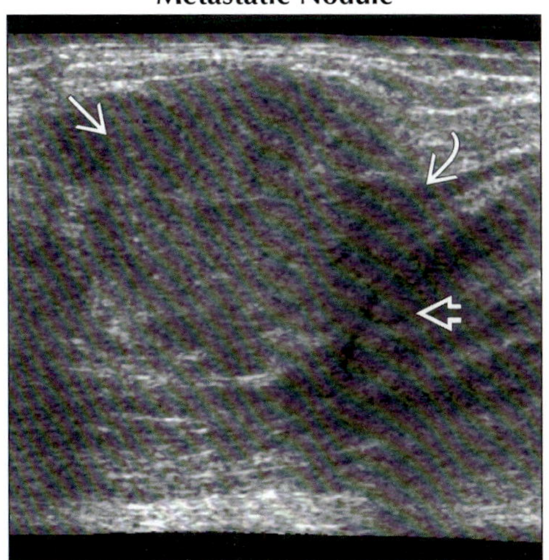

(Left) Transverse US shows a partially calcified mass ➡ with posterior acoustic shadowing, consistent with pilomatrixoma. A calcified granuloma does not have the same degree of internal heterogeneity. (Right) Longitudinal US shows a hypoechoic mass ➡ in the subcutaneous tissues of the anterior chest wall in a patient with cervical carcinoma. The mass invades the investing fascia ➡. The underlying muscle is distorted ➡. Biopsy showed metastatic cervical cancer.

Sarcoma

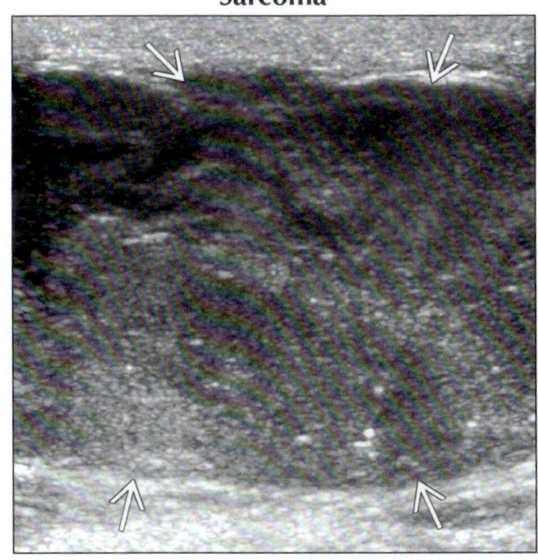

Lymph Node

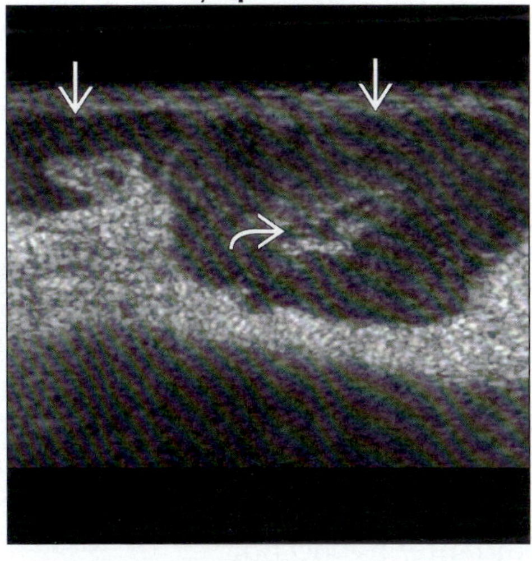

(Left) Longitudinal ultrasound shows a large mass ➡ entirely contained within subcutaneous layer. The mass was hypervascular on color Doppler (not shown). Biopsy specimen revealed malignant fibrous histiocytoma. Although uncommon, soft tissue sarcomas can arise within subcutaneous tissues. (Right) Transverse ultrasound shows 2 reactive-type nodes ➡ in the groin. In the larger node, fatty hilum ➡ is nearly effaced by hypertrophied cortex.

Fat Necrosis

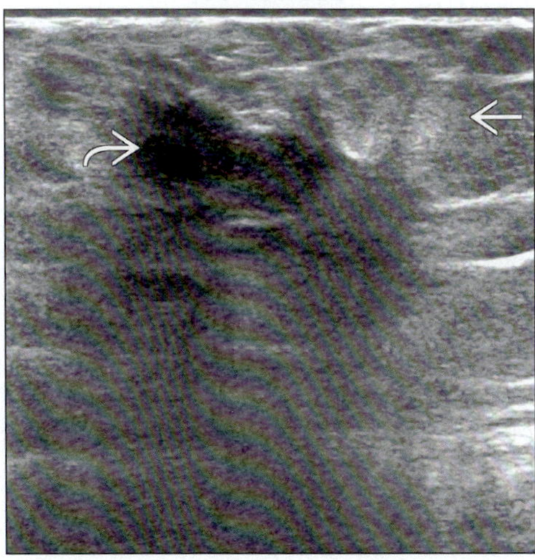

Rheumatoid Nodule

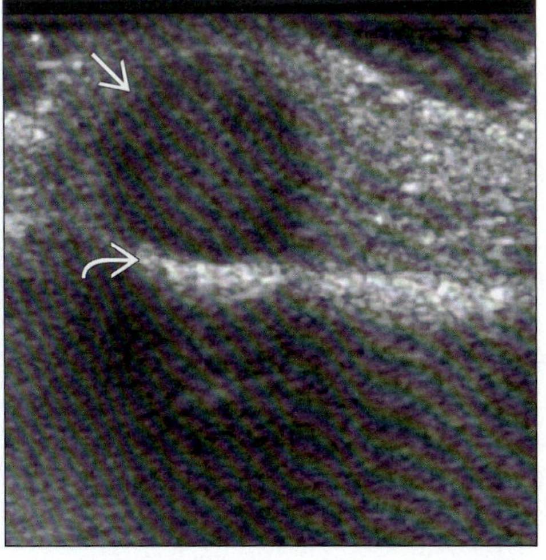

(Left) Oblique US shows findings consistent with fat necrosis with early liquefaction. The disruption & swelling of subcutaneous fat ➡ with increased echogenicity reflects edema, and an irregular focal hypoechoic area ➡ represents fluid. (Right) Oblique US shows a round, hypoechoic finger nodule ➡ in a patient with rheumatoid arthritis. Characteristic posterior acoustic enhancement is present ➡. No discernible cystic area or liquefaction is seen.

15

HYPERECHOIC SUBCUTANEOUS MASS

DIFFERENTIAL DIAGNOSIS

Common
- Lipoma

Less Common
- Cellulitis
- Panniculitis
- Fat Necrosis
- Granuloma and Fibroma
- Hematoma
- Venous Vascular Malformation
- Gouty Tophus
- Abscess
- Normal Lymph Node

ESSENTIAL INFORMATION

Key Differential Diagnosis Issues
- Use light transducer pressure
  - Otherwise subcutaneous fat will be compressed and subcutaneous lesions made less conspicuous
- Subcutaneous fat may vary from hyperechoic to hypoechoic depending on location
- In some regions, particularly gluteal region, subcutaneous fat looks similar to muscle
  - Take care in defining correct layer as this has important diagnostic and surgical implications

Helpful Clues for Common Diagnoses
- **Lipoma**
  - Variable echogenicity from predominantly hyperechoic → predominantly hypoechoic
  - Characteristic feature of lipoma is well-marginated, compressible, fusiform-shaped mass
    - Multiple, thin, echogenic lines parallel to skin surface
    - Usually no detectable vascularity on color Doppler
    - Large lipomas may have 1-2 small, detectable vessels
    - Vascularized lipoma → consider angiolipoma
    - Echogenicity comparable to surrounding fat
  - Lipohypertrophy = localized area of subcutaneous fat accumulation
    - Increase in size of fat lobules and depth of subcutaneous fat

- Usually affects middle-aged women
- Lack of distinct border or margin allows distinction of lipohypertrophy from lipoma
- Similar echogenicity to adjacent fat, so normally hypoechoic as opposed to lipomas, which are usually hyperechoic

Helpful Clues for Less Common Diagnoses
- **Cellulitis**
  - Infective inflammation of subcutaneous fat
    - Characterized by edema & hyperemia
  - Group A *Streptococcus* and *Staphylococcus aureus* organisms usually responsible
  - Certain condition predispose to more severe cellulitis
    - Immunodeficiency, diabetes, steroid treatment
    - Peripheral circulatory impairment and lymphedema
  - Subcutaneous fat → more echogenic when edematous
  - Subcutaneous edema = nonspecific finding seen with many conditions
    - Heart failure, venous insufficiency, immobility, and dependency
  - Cellulitis should have combination of edema and hyperemia
    - Thickened interlobular septa
    - ± periseptal fluid or fluid above investing fascia
  - Phlegmon = localized, intense inflammation of subcutaneous fat prior to development of abscess
- **Panniculitis**
  - Focal inflammation of subcutaneous fat
  - Often idiopathic
  - Also associated with pancreatitis, autoimmune disease, tuberculosis infection
  - Variant known as subcutaneous, panniculitis-like T-cell lymphoma
    - Multiple nodules
  - Ill-defined hyperechoic subcutaneous nodules (2-5 cm wide) with hyperemia
    - No necrosis or atrophy
    - Ultrasound-guided biopsy should be considered to establish underlying cause
- **Fat Necrosis**
  - Swelling of subcutaneous fat in early stages

HYPERECHOIC SUBCUTANEOUS MASS

- Hyperechoic edematous fat with loss of normal echogenic striation
  - Subcutaneous fat becomes more hypoechoic with increasing chronicity
    - ± liquefaction with discrete irregular hypoechoic areas
    - ± calcification
    - ± fat atrophy in later stages
    - Usually investing fascia and muscle unaffected
- **Granuloma and Fibroma**
  - Common in gluteal region
    - Frequently follow subcutaneous injection
  - May also occur elsewhere without any recognizable cause
  - Usually hypoechoic though occasionally hyperechoic
    - Often calcified
- **Hematoma**
  - Echogenic in acute stages
  - ± circular echogenic layering due to sequential deposition of layers of hemorrhage
  - ± moving echoes on real-time imaging
  - ± linear layering due to separation of cellular and serous components
  - ± liquefaction after several days to weeks
  - ± calcification as late feature
- **Venous Vascular Malformation**
  - Hemangioma
    - Childhood tumor: Endothelial proliferation followed by involution
  - Vascular malformation
    - Error of vascular morphogenesis

- No endothelial proliferation or involution
    - Capillary, venous, arteriovenous, or mixed
  - Variable ultrasound appearances
    - Well- or ill-defined
    - Mixed echogenicity depending on relative stromal, fatty, or vascular components
    - Variable vascularity from no detectable flow → very hypervascular
    - Moderately compressible
    - ± phleboliths
    - ± venous lakes
- **Gouty Tophus**
  - Soft or hard tophi depending on concentration of crystals deposited
    - Soft tophi → echogenic with mild to moderate posterior acoustic shadowing
    - Hard tophi → echogenic with strong posterior acoustic shadowing
- **Abscess**
  - May be echogenic due to aggregates of inflammatory debris
  - Surrounding edema and hyperemia
  - ± moving echoes on real-time imaging
- **Normal Lymph Node**
  - May appear largely echogenic if large central fatty hilum and thin hypoechoic cortex
    - Particularly in subcutaneous lymph nodes medial aspect proximal thigh

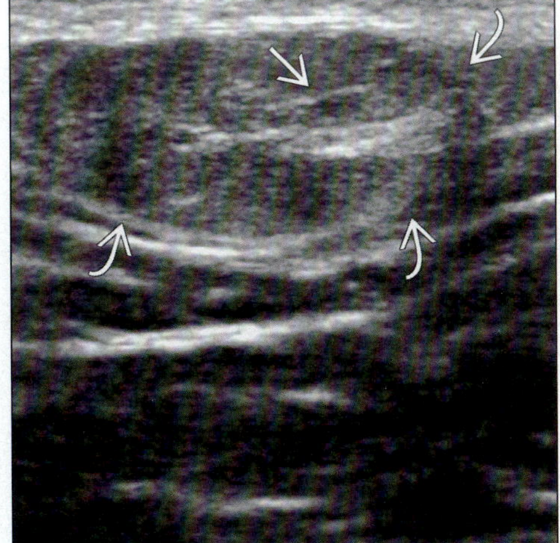

Lipoma

Transverse ultrasound shows a lipoma ➡ *of subcutaneous fat as a well-defined echogenic mass with fine linear internal striations* ➡. *Acoustic enhancement is comparable to that of the surrounding fat.*

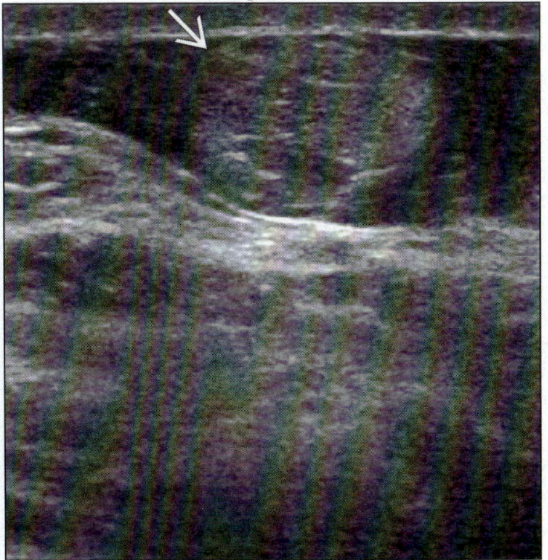

Lipoma

Transverse ultrasound shows a small well-defined echogenic lipoma ➡ *in a patient with multiple subcutaneous lipomas. In such patients, many (up to 100) small lipomas of varying size may be present.*

HYPERECHOIC SUBCUTANEOUS MASS

(Left) Transverse ultrasound of the ankle in a patient with venous insufficiency shows swelling and edema of the subcutaneous ➡ and deeper tissues. This is a nonspecific finding. The tibialis posterior tendon ➡ and posterior tibial artery ➡ are shown. (Right) Transverse color Doppler ultrasound of the same area shows marked hyperemia ➡ of the subcutaneous and deep fat, consistent with cellulitis. Edema of noninflammatory origin is not hyperemic.

Cellulitis

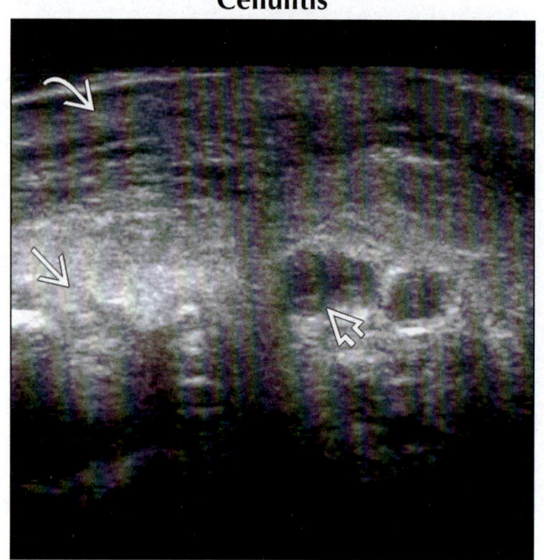

Cellulitis

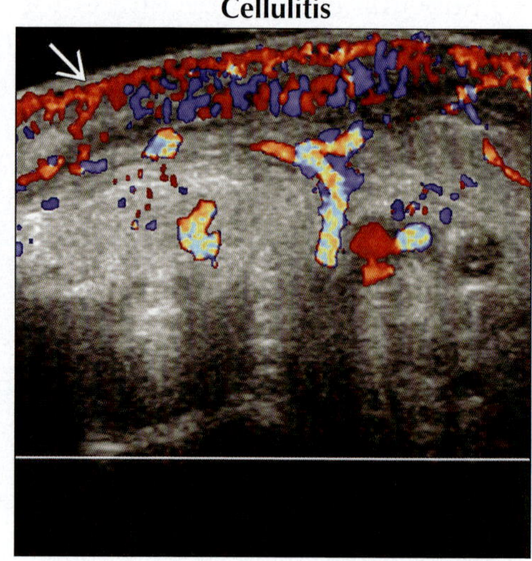

(Left) Transverse ultrasound of the lateral aspect of the leg shows a nodular area of edema ➡ confined to the subcutaneous tissues. The nodule arose insidiously about 2 weeks earlier. No discrete mass lesion is present. (Right) Correlative transverse color Doppler US of the same area shows mild hyperemia ➡ of subcutaneous fat edema, consistent with nodular subcutaneous panniculitis. A similar smaller area of panniculitis is present on the contralateral leg.

Panniculitis

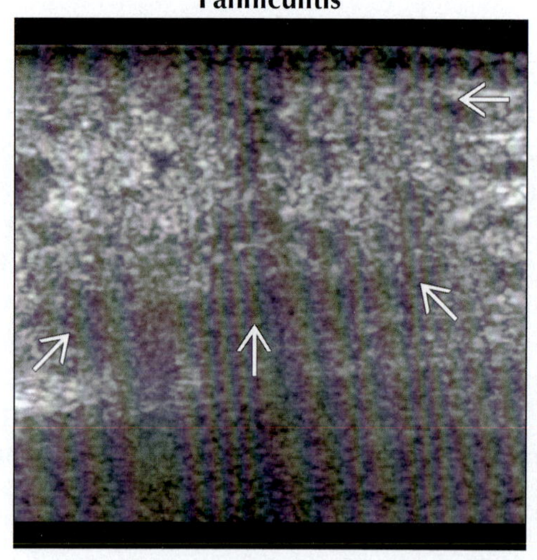

Panniculitis

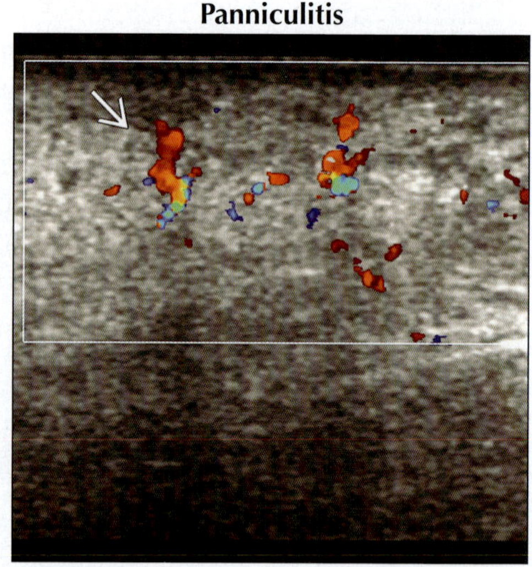

(Left) Transverse ultrasound shows a localized ill-defined area of increased echogenicity ➡ of subcutaneous fat with mild swelling, edema, and loss of normal striations following recent trauma, appearances that are consistent with a fat injury. (Right) Transverse US of the anterior abdominal wall shows a well-defined, mildly hyperechoic nodule ➡ at the surgical scar (not shown). Faint suture material ➡ is present, giving the appearance of a suture granuloma.

Fat Necrosis

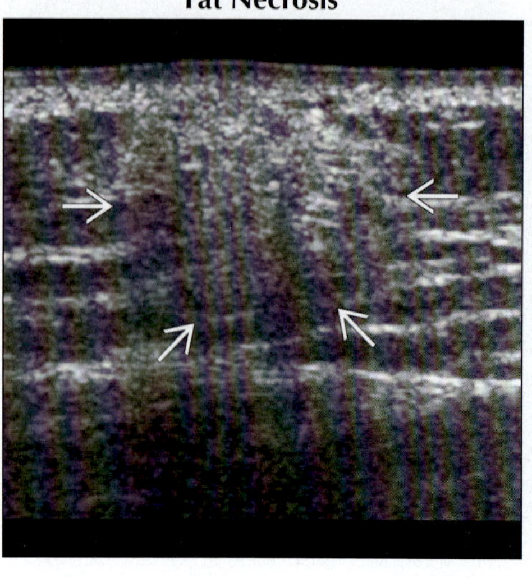

Granuloma and Fibroma

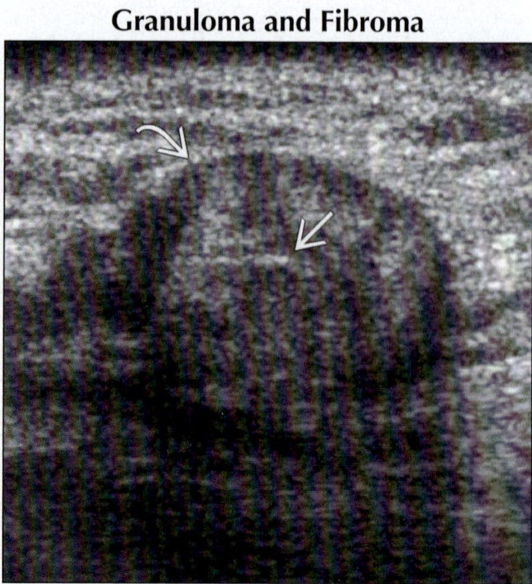

HYPERECHOIC SUBCUTANEOUS MASS

Hematoma

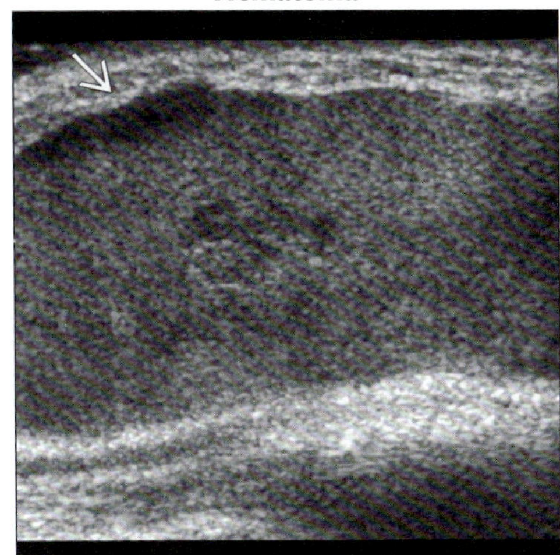

Gouty Tophus

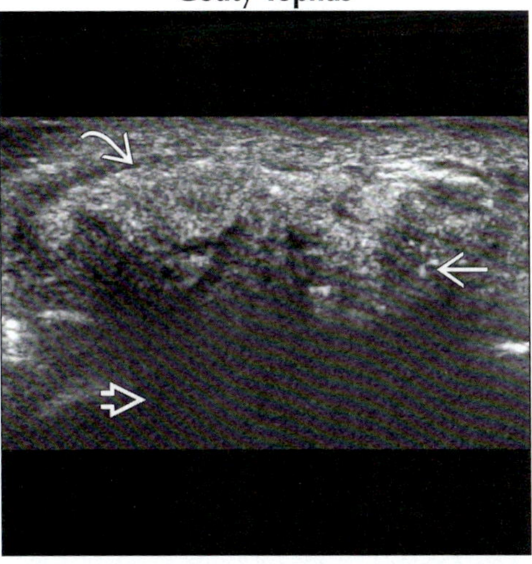

(Left) Transverse US shows a large post-traumatic hematoma ➡ in the subcutaneous tissues of the lower chest wall. No associated vascular malformation or rib fracture was present. It resolved over the ensuing 6 months. *(Right)* Longitudinal US shows an echogenic gouty tophus ➡ in subcutaneous tissues overlying the 3rd metatarsophalangeal joint. There are "comet tail" artifacts ➡ present with posterior acoustic shadowing ➡.

Venous Vascular Malformation

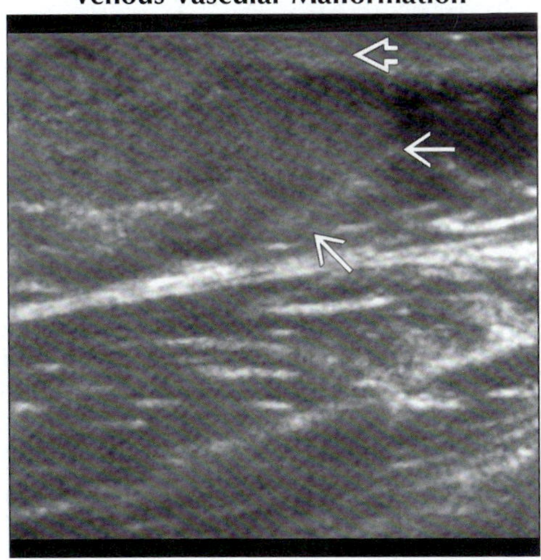

Venous Vascular Malformation

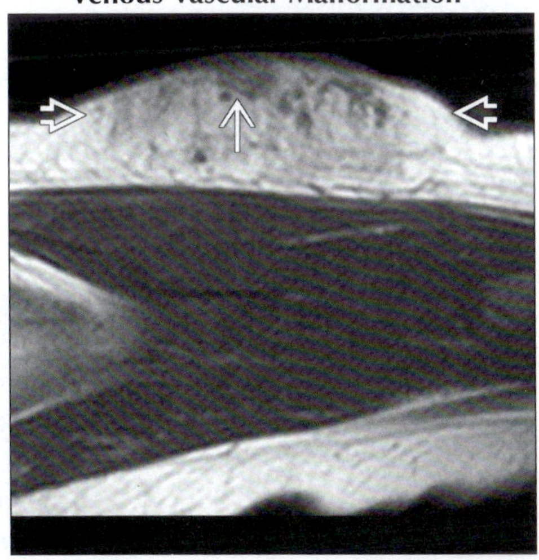

(Left) Transverse US of the thigh in a young child shows a large hyperechoic mass ➡ in subcutaneous tissues extending into the dermis ➡. Color Doppler imaging (not shown) revealed mild internal vascularity. *(Right)* Sagittal T1WI MR of the same lesion shows a lipomatous subcutaneous mass ➡ with some vascular & nonlipomatous elements. A tuft of hair was present on the skin over the more solid component ➡. These features are consistent with an angiolipoma.

Abscess

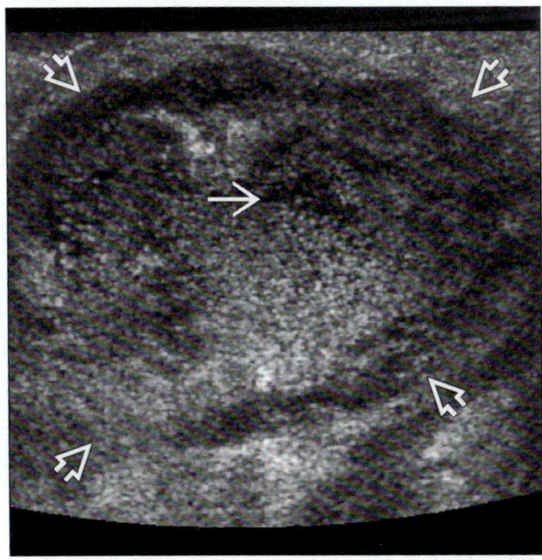

Normal Lymph Node

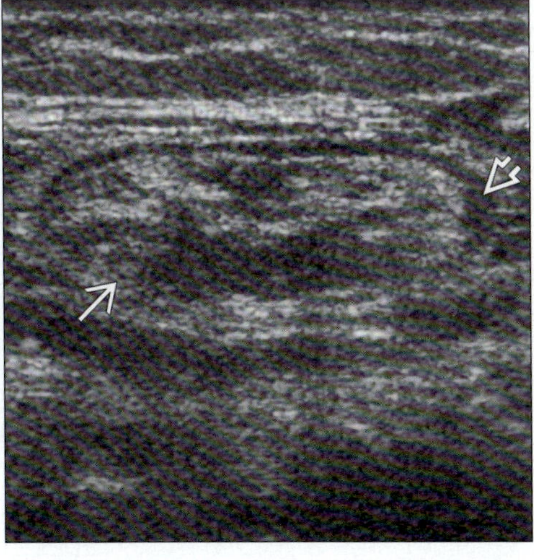

(Left) Longitudinal ultrasound in an intravenous drug user shows a large hyperechoic abscess ➡ within the subcutaneous fat of proximal thigh. There are small areas of more distinct liquefaction ➡ present. Purulent fluid was aspirated. *(Right)* Longitudinal US shows a large, fatty lymph node ➡ in the medial aspect of the proximal thigh. This node, located near the long saphenous vein, is a common finding. Thin hypoechoic cortex ➡ thickens in a reactive node.

15

DIFFERENTIAL DIAGNOSIS

Common
- Plantar Fasciitis
- Plantar Fibromatosis

Less Common
- Plantar Fascial Tear
- Investing Fascial Tear
- Nodular Fasciitis
- Necrotizing Fasciitis
- Vascular Malformation Involving Fascia
- Eosinophilic Fasciitis

ESSENTIAL INFORMATION

Key Differential Diagnosis Issues
- Plantar fascia seen as thin, laminated, echogenic aponeurosis stretching between calcaneus and forefoot
- Investing fascia seen as thin, laminated, echogenic tissue enveloping muscles of appendicular skeleton and trunk
- Fascial lesions tend to be site-specific
- For most lesions, ultrasound is as accurate as MR or CT
- Fascial insertional lesions may be 1st manifestation of inflammatory enthesopathy

Helpful Clues for Common Diagnoses
- **Plantar Fasciitis**
  - Probably caused by repetitive microtrauma ± microvascular injury
  - Common in runners
    - Other risk factors include faulty shoes, high-arched feet, short Achilles tendon, obesity, and prolonged weightbearing
  - Affects plantar fascial attachment to medial aspect of calcaneus
    - Bilateral in 1/3 patients
  - Manifested as thickening of plantar fascia at calcaneal insertion
  - > 4.3 mm thickness considered abnormal
    - Hypoechogenicity and thickening of plantar fascia over short segment (~ 10 mm) at calcaneal insertion
    - ± loss of echogenic laminar pattern of plantar fascia
    - ± perifascial edema
    - 4.3 mm = guideline; no absolute measure as normal & abnormal range exists

- Measurements taken at leading edge of calcaneus
- The greater plantar fascial thickening, the more likely diagnosis of plantar fasciitis
- Subclinical fascitis may be present on opposite side, so be careful about using contralateral side as normal reference
  - ± plantar calcaneal spur
    - Echogenic bony spur about 1-3 mm long at deep surface of plantar fascia
  - Hyperemia, calcification, or macroscopic fascial tears not feature of plantar fasciitis
  - Associated calcaneal edema &/or inflammation at plantar fascial insertional area not visible with ultrasound
    - Best seen with MR
    - However, not known to be useful prognostic indicator
  - Temporary symptom relief provided by steroid ± local anesthetic injection
    - Using ultrasound guidance
    - 23-g needle to edge of plantar fascia medially
    - Do not inject directly into plantar fascia; inject to perifascial area
- **Plantar Fibromatosis**
  - Focal nodular fibroblastic proliferation of plantar fascia away from calcaneal insertion
    - No specific risk factors identified
  - Most commonly affects medial aspect of plantar fascia in mid-foot region
    - Often multiple
    - Bilateral in 1/3 of patients
  - Discrete fusiform-shaded nodule expanding plantar fascia
    - Either hypoechoic (75%) or isoechoic (25%) to plantar fascia
  - Posterior acoustic enhancement (20%)
  - Internal vascularity (10%)
  - Does not extend beyond plantar fascia
    - If present, consider aggressive plantar fibromatosis

Helpful Clues for Less Common Diagnoses
- **Plantar Fascial Tear**
  - May be acute or chronic
    - Localized and does not extend across width of plantar fascia
  - Acute tears are usually precipitated by specific traumatic event

- May be precipitated by steroid injection for plantar fasciitis
  - More common on medial side
  - Involve proximal 1/3 and middle 1/3 of plantar fascia equally
    - Involvement of forefoot region rare
  - Acute tears characterized by focal disruption, perifascial edema, and inflammation
  - Chronic tears characterized by focal disruption, tendon thickening, perifascial fibrosis, and hyperemia
- **Investing Fascial Tear**
  - Investing fascia envelopes muscles of appendicular skeleton and trunk
  - Either complete focal defect in fascia or linear intrasubstance fascial tear
  - Focal defect may result in muscle hernia
    - Accentuated by muscle contraction
    - Often occurs spontaneously in athletic muscular individuals
  - Linear tear follows specific injury to affected region
- **Nodular Fasciitis**
  - Benign proliferation of fibroblasts and myofibroblasts of investing fascia
    - Lesions are generally small and solitary
    - Most commonly involves upper limb
    - Patient may have history of preceding trauma, though usually no traumatic history and no known cause
- **Necrotizing Fasciitis**
  - Advancing soft tissue infection characterized by widespread fascial necrosis
  - May occur after trauma or surgery
  - Either monomicrobial or polymicrobial infection can cause necrotizing fasciitis
    - Group A β-hemolytic *Streptococcus* is a common organism
  - Thickened disrupted fascia with perifascial fluid
  - Severe subcutaneous and muscle edema
  - ± muscle necrosis
  - ± gas locules due to gas-forming organisms
- **Vascular Malformation/Tumors Involving Fascia**
  - Vascular malformations may arise within or involve fascia
  - Appearances akin to similar tumors arising beyond fascia
- **Eosinophilic Fasciitis**
  - Disorder characterized by peripheral eosinophilia and fasciitis
    - Investing fascia and intermuscular fascia of forearm and calf most commonly affected
  - Thickening and hyperemia of muscle fascia on ultrasound
  - Diagnostic MR appearances
    - Isolated fascial thickening, edema, and inflammation in affected areas
    - Little or no myositis

Plantar Fasciitis

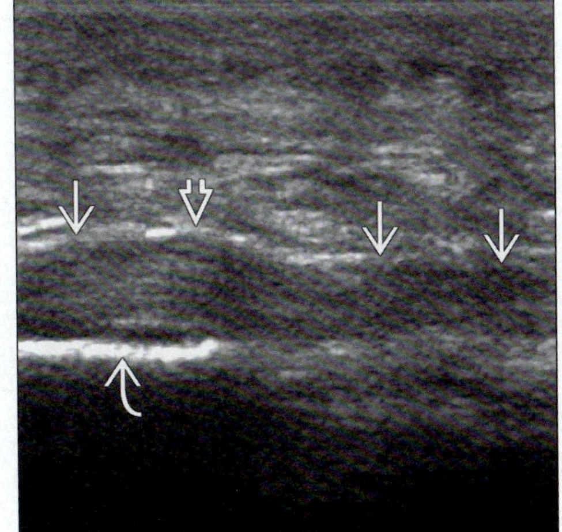

Longitudinal US of the plantar fascia ➡ shows mild thickening (4.8 mm) ➡ at medial calcaneal attachment ➡. Plantar fascial thickness > 4.3 mm is considered abnormal, though this is a guide, not absolute standard.

Plantar Fasciitis

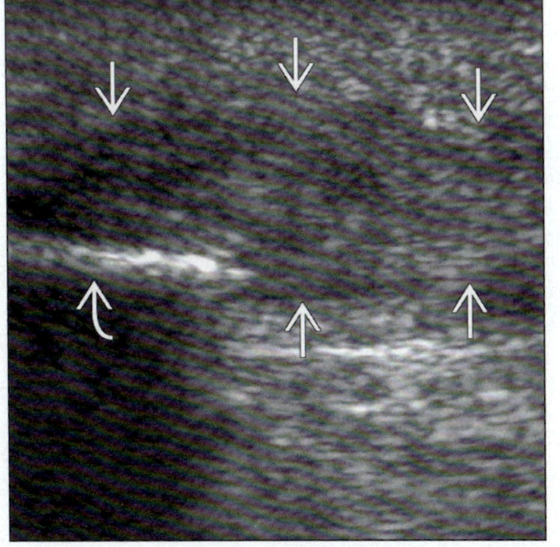

Longitudinal ultrasound shows markedly thickened (10.7 mm) plantar fascia ➡ at the medial calcaneal attachment ➡. This indicates disease chronicity and the likelihood of recurrent symptoms.

FASCIAL LESION

(Left) Longitudinal ultrasound shows hypoechoic concentric fusiform thickening ➡ of the plantar fascia ➡ in the mid-foot, away from the calcaneal attachment. (Right) Longitudinal ultrasound shows an eccentric, discrete, hypoechoic fusiform thickening ➡ on the more superficial aspect of the plantar fascia ➡ in the mid-foot removed from the calcaneal attachment.

Plantar Fibromatosis

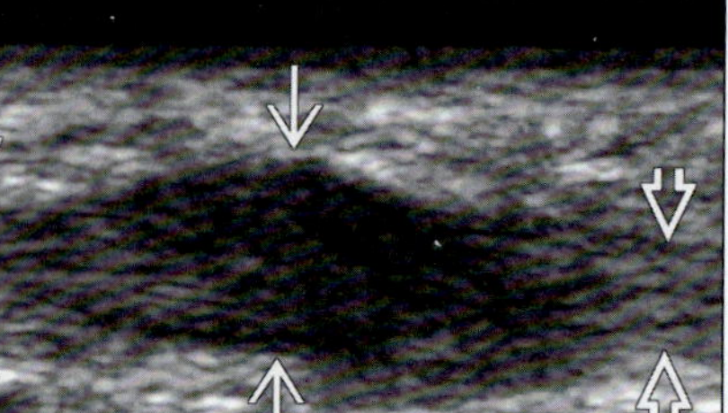

Plantar Fibromatosis

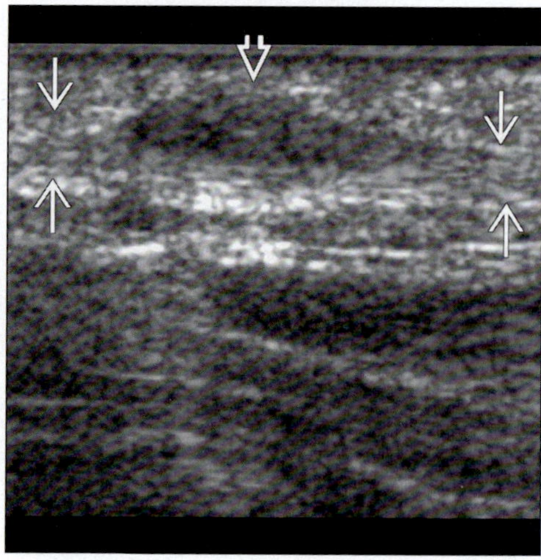

(Left) Sagittal T1WI MR shows fusiform thickening ➡ of the plantar fascia in the mid-foot away from the calcaneal attachment ➡. (Right) Longitudinal ultrasound shows a small, fibrotic-type mass ➡ involving superficial layers of the thickened investing fascia ➡ of the arm in a young patient with no history of trauma. The underlying muscle ➡ is normal. The mass completely resolved on follow-up at 9 months.

Plantar Fibromatosis

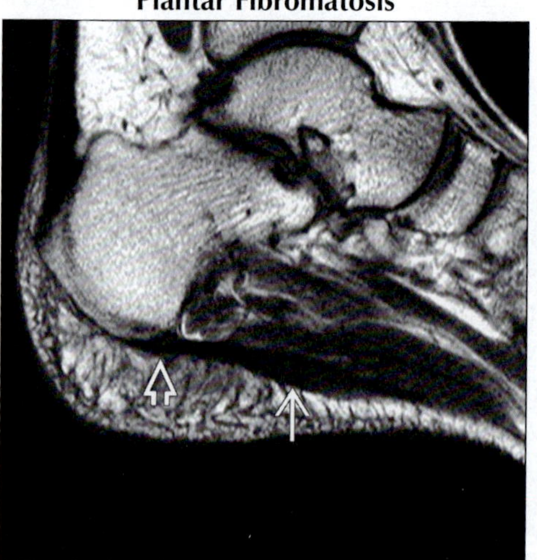

Nodular Fasciitis

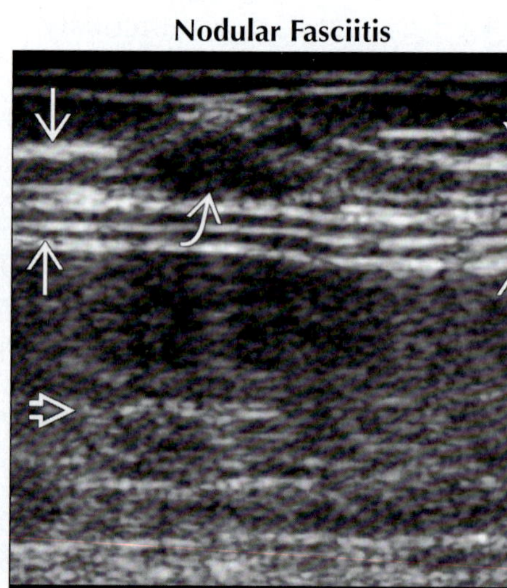

(Left) Longitudinal ultrasound shows a tear ➡ in the plantar fascia ➡ immediately distal to the calcaneal ➡ insertion. There is fluid just deep to this tear ➡. (Right) Sagittal T1WI MR in the same patient shows a localized tear ➡ in the plantar fascia just distal to the calcaneal attachment. There is fluid ➡ deep and superficial to this tear.

Plantar Fascial Tear

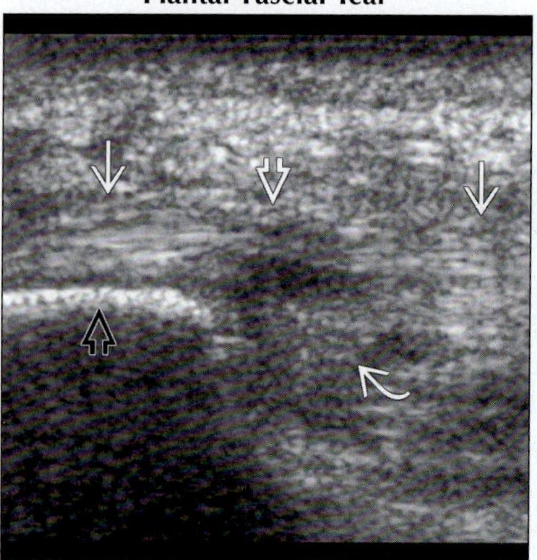

Plantar Fascial Tear

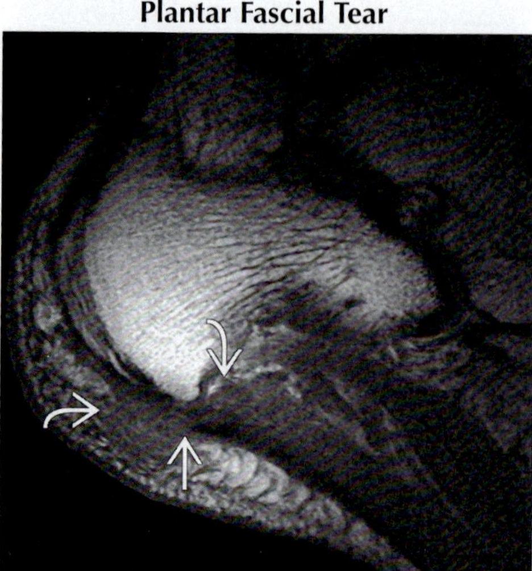

15

FASCIAL LESION

Investing Fascial Tear

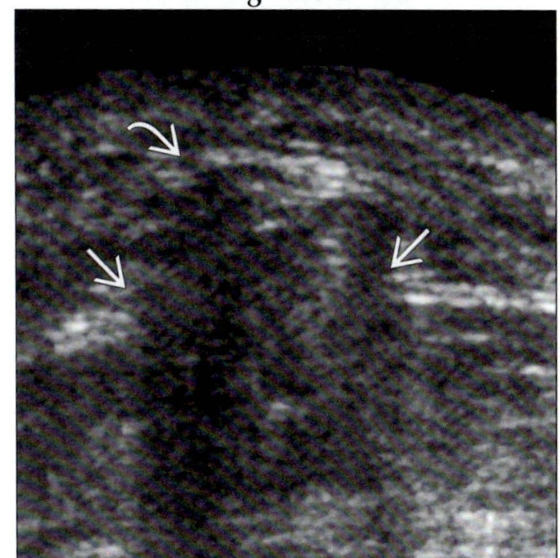

Investing Fascial Tear

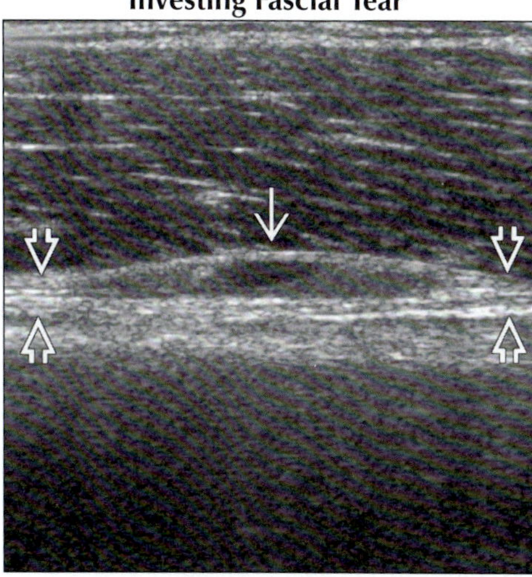

(Left) Transverse ultrasound shows herniation ➘ of the peroneal muscle into the subcutaneous tissues though a defect ➔ in the investing fascia. This patient had point tenderness at this location aggravated by exercise. *(Right)* Longitudinal ultrasound shows an elongated tear ➔ within the substance of vastus medialis fascia ➘ of the thigh. This tear occurred during a fall while the patient was playing basketball.

Necrotizing Fasciitis

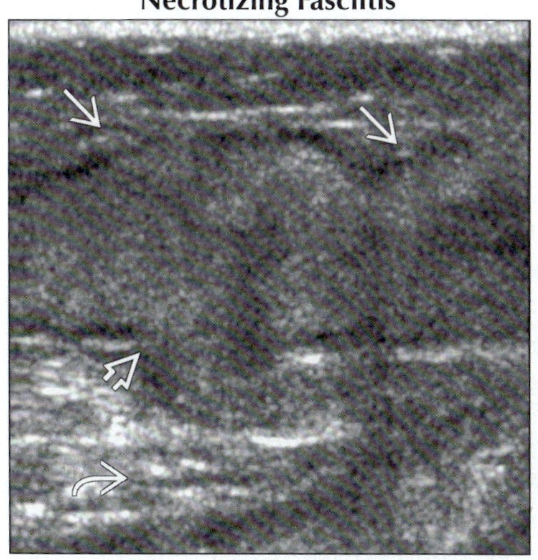

Vascular Malformation Involving Fascia

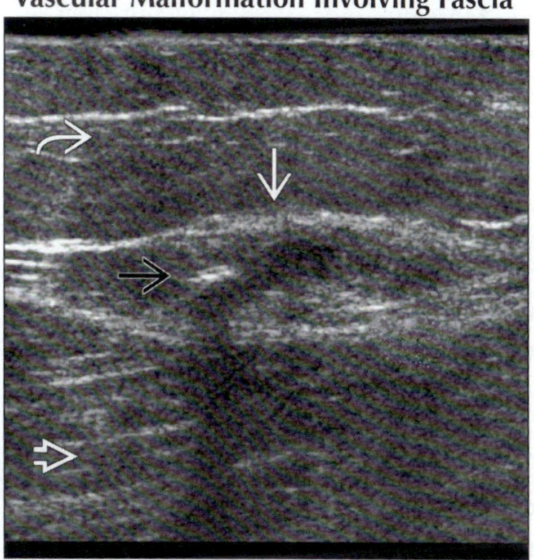

(Left) Longitudinal US of the thigh shows a lobulated abscess ➔ extending through the investing fascia ➘ into the vastus lateralis muscle ➔. Surgery confirmed necrotizing fasciitis. *(Right)* Transverse ultrasound of the thigh shows expansion of investing fascia by a hypoechoic mass ➔ with a phlebolith ➔. Minimal internal vascularity was present. Histology revealed a venous vascular malformation. Subcutaneous fat ➘ and muscle ➘ were not involved.

Eosinophilic Fasciitis

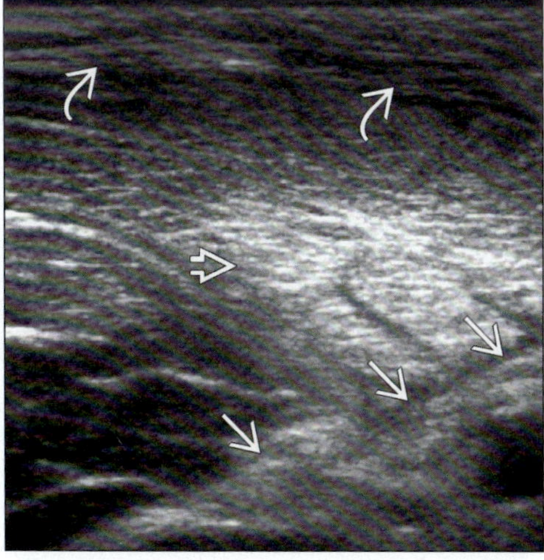

Eosinophilic Fasciitis

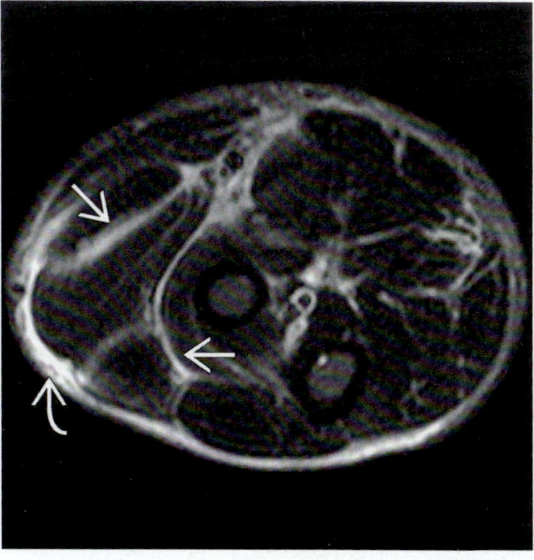

(Left) Transverse ultrasound of the forearm shows thickening of the investing fascia ➘ and intermuscular fascia ➘ in a patient with eosinophilia. Muscle edema is also present ➘. *(Right)* Transverse T2WI MR with fat suppression in the same patient shows edema and thickening of the investing fascia ➘ and intermuscular fascia ➘.

HYPOECHOIC MUSCLE MASS

DIFFERENTIAL DIAGNOSIS

Common
- Hematoma
- Muscle Tear
- Nerve Sheath Tumor

Less Common
- Soft Tissue Sarcoma
- Myxoma
- Desmoid Tumor
- Abscess
- Diabetic Muscle Infarction
- Granuloma
- Metastases

Rare but Important
- Parasitic Infection

ESSENTIAL INFORMATION

Key Differential Diagnosis Issues
- History important when differentiating hematoma from sarcoma or infection

Helpful Clues for Common Diagnoses
- **Hematoma**
  - Due to trauma, anticoagulation, or vascular malformation
  - Anterior thigh common location, because it is susceptible to compression injury against femoral shaft and muscle contraction injury
  - Initially hyperechoic or isoechoic
    - Becomes more hypoechoic with ↑ liquefaction after several days to weeks
    - ± layering or whorled pattern due to sequential episodes of bleeding
  - Minor hemorrhage may not be apparent on ultrasound, as ill-defined hyperechoic areas of blood blend with hyperechoic muscle
    - No disturbance of muscle architecture with minor bleeding
    - MR more sensitive than ultrasound at detection of tumor hemorrhage
- **Muscle Tear**
  - Discontinuity ± retraction of muscle fibers within muscle bulk or at myofascial junction
    - Myofascial junction most common site of tear
  - ± tear filled with hematoma or fluid

- ± surrounding muscle and subcutaneous edema
  - Do not confuse with muscle contusion
    - Contusion shows no fiber discontinuity
    - May cross muscle fascial boundaries
    - Ill-defined hyperechogenicity of muscle due to edema ± blood
    - Hyperemia during reparative stage
- **Nerve Sheath Tumor**
  - Arises along course of peripheral nerve
  - Well-defined, fusiform-shaped, hypoechoic mass
    - Anechoic areas due to myxoid accumulation (very common)
    - ± additional areas of hyperechogenicity due to hemorrhage, calcification, or fibrosis
  - Posterior acoustic enhancement
  - Thickened entering or exiting nerve (very common)
    - Entering or exiting nerve may not be visible if tumor arises from small peripheral nerve
  - Mild to moderate hyperemia on color Doppler imaging
    - Very occasionally, minimal demonstrable vascularity
  - Cannot differentiate between schwannoma and neurofibroma based on ultrasound findings alone

Helpful Clues for Less Common Diagnoses
- **Soft Tissue Sarcoma**
  - Usually seen as large, well-defined, hypoechoic mass within muscle layer
    - Moderately to highly vascular
    - Occasionally hypovascular or even avascular on color Doppler imaging (due to tumor infiltration of vessels)
    - Any large (> 5 cm), solid, nonfatty, soft tissue tumor should be considered sarcoma unless proven otherwise by biopsy
    - Biopsy not very helpful in differentiating well-differentiated liposarcoma from lipoma
    - Better to decide likelihood of malignancy by clinical and MR criteria, full tumor histology analysis
- **Myxoma**

- ○ Composed of a few spindle-shaped cells within mucoid material supported by loose collagen framework
  - ■ Derived from modified fibroblasts producing ↑ proteoglycan
- ○ Hypoechoic, cystic-type, intramuscular mass ± "comet tail" artifacts
  - ■ Peripheral rim of increased echogenicity ("bright rim" sign), corresponding to perilesional muscle edema
  - ■ Triangular hyperechoic area adjacent to mass ("bright cap" sign), corresponding to muscle atrophy
  - ■ Main differential diagnosis is myxoid liposarcoma
- **Desmoid Tumor**
  - ○ Also known as fibromatosis
  - ○ Locally aggressive overgrowth of fibrous tissue with well-defined or infiltrative border
    - ■ Typically absent or minimal vascularity on color Doppler imaging
- **Abscess**
  - ○ More frequent in immunosuppressed patients
  - ○ Many variable appearances
  - ○ From solid-type hyperechoic mass to necrotic-type hypoechoic mass to well-defined hypoechoic area similar to intramuscular tear
    - ■ + surrounding edema and hyperemia
    - ■ ± intralesional gas locules
- **Diabetic Muscle Infarction**
  - ○ Occurs in diabetics with established vasculopathy
  - ○ Ill-defined hypoechoic area → better defined after 1 week
    - ■ Muscle architecture remains vaguely detectable within hypoechoic area
    - ■ No necrosis
    - ■ No detectable vascularity at onset → mild to moderate hyperemia after/around 1 week
- **Granuloma**
  - ○ Much more common in subcutaneous tissues, especially gluteal region
  - ○ Usually following injection
    - ■ Occasionally following trauma or foreign body implantation
  - ○ Majority have calcified rim
- **Metastases**
  - ○ Usually seen only in setting of widely disseminated disease
  - ○ Most common tumor = adenocarcinoma lung
  - ○ Similar in appearance to soft tissue sarcoma though generally smaller

Helpful Clues for Rare Diagnoses

- **Parasitic Infection**
  - ○ Cysticercosis = most common parasitic infection of soft tissue
  - ○ Well-defined, small, hypoechoic mass with eccentric echogenic nidus representing scolex
    - ■ Diagnosis can be confirmed by therapeutic response

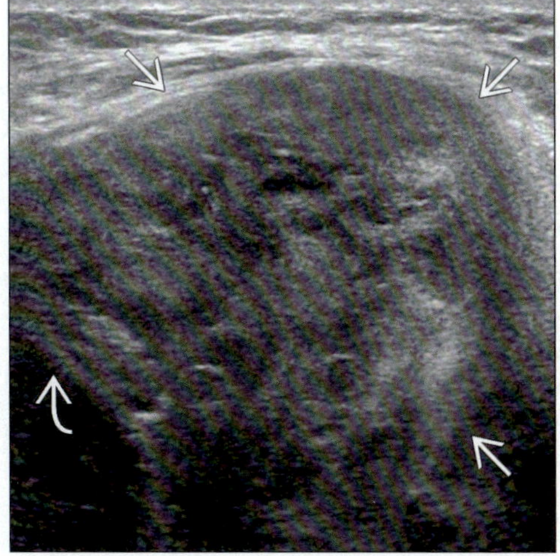

Hematoma

Transverse ultrasound of the thigh in a patient with cerebral palsy shows a large, well-defined hematoma ➡ with a whorled echopattern in the adductor compartment, alongside the femoral shaft ➡.

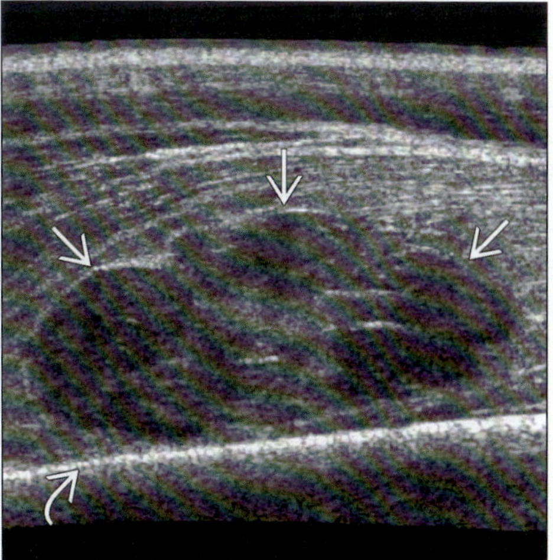

Hematoma

Oblique ultrasound of the thigh shows a well-defined hematoma ➡ within the vastus intermedius muscle adjacent to the femoral shaft ➡ 2 weeks after a blunt football injury.

HYPOECHOIC MUSCLE MASS

(Left) Longitudinal ultrasound of the calf shows a localized tear ➡ at the distal myofascial junction of the medial belly of the gastrocnemius ➡ with muscle stripped off the fascia. This is the most common location of calf muscle tears. The soleus muscle lies deep to region of tear ➡. *(Right)* Longitudinal ultrasound shows a large hematoma ➡ at the site of a myofascial tear of the medial belly of the gastrocnemius muscle ➡ following a sprain injury sustained 1 day earlier.

Muscle Tear

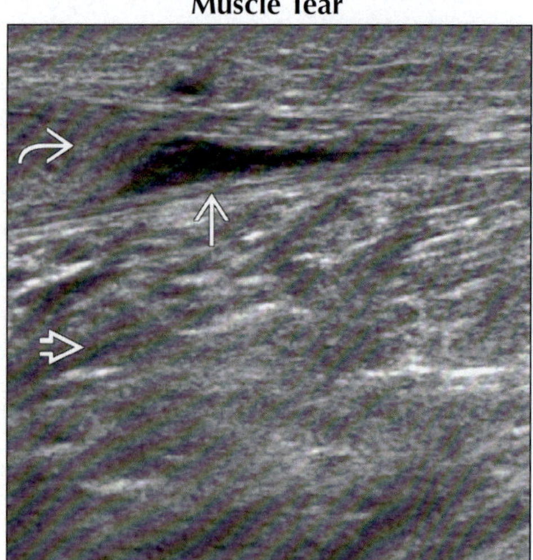

Muscle Tear

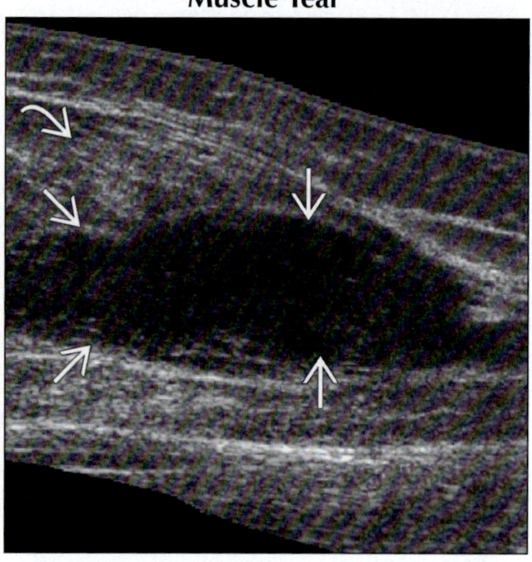

(Left) Transverse ultrasound shows a large, well-defined, soft tissue sarcoma ➡ (alveolar soft portion of sarcoma) bulging out between the tibia ➡ and fibula ➡. *(Right)* Transverse ultrasound shows an intramuscular myxoma ➡ located in the superficial aspect of the soleus muscle ➡. The tumor is largely hypoechoic with small internal echogenic speckles ➡.

Soft Tissue Sarcoma

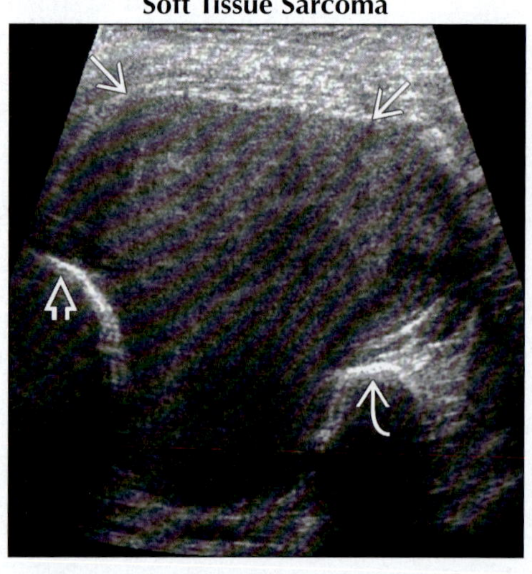

Myxoma

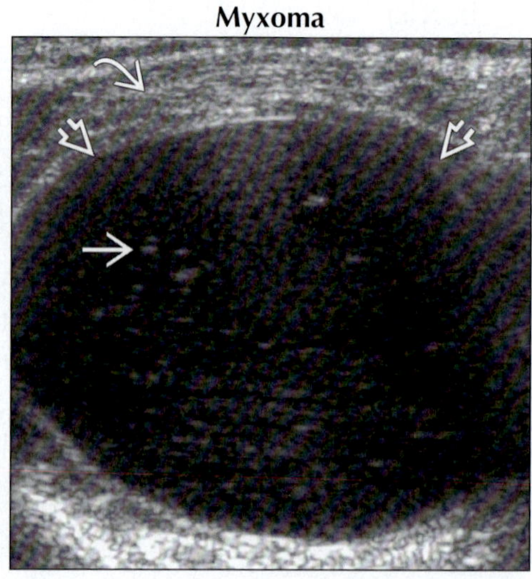

(Left) Transverse US shows a well-defined myxoma ➡ within the vastus intermedius muscle of the thigh anterior to the femur ➡. The tumor has a less myxomatous component & is more solid-looking than the myxoma in the previous image. Histology confirmed myxoma. *(Right)* Transverse US shows a well-defined, heterogeneous mass ➡ near the coracoid process ➡. There was no detectable vascularity on color Doppler imaging. Biopsy confirmed desmoid tumor.

Myxoma

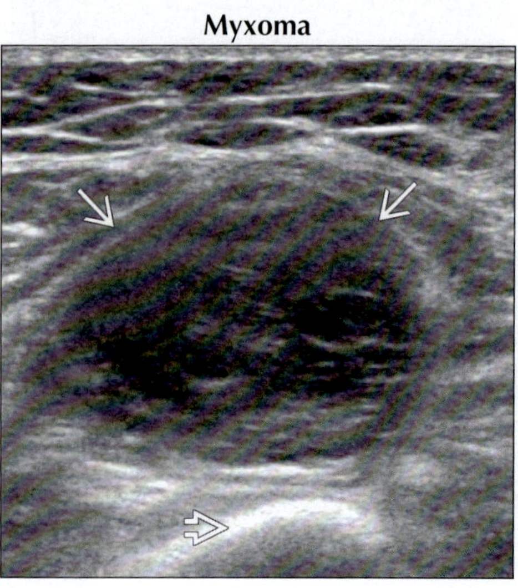

Desmoid Tumor

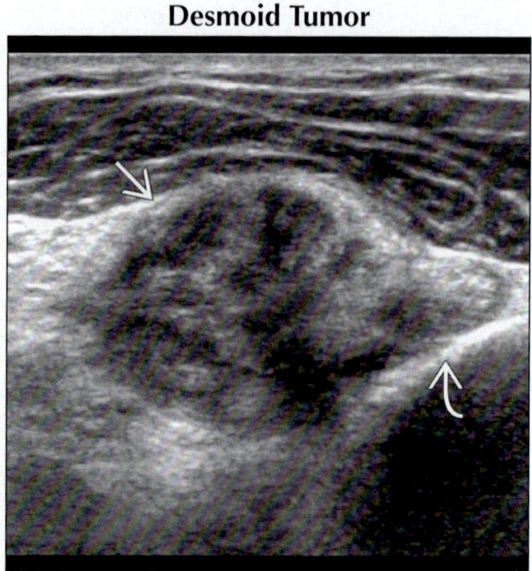

15

HYPOECHOIC MUSCLE MASS

Desmoid Tumor

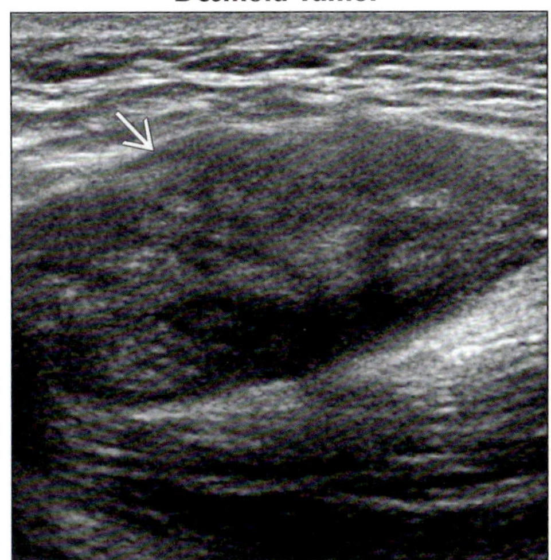

Abscess

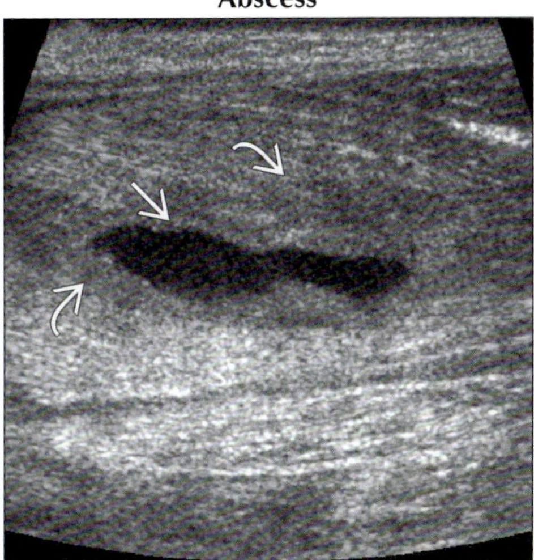

(Left) Oblique US in a patient with a confirmed buttock desmoid tumor shows a well-defined, ovoid, hypoechoic mass ➡ just deep to investing fascia. No detectable vascularity on color Doppler imaging was seen. (Right) Longitudinal US of the calf shows a well-defined hypoechoic area ➡ with surrounding echogenic edema ➡ within the gastrocnemius muscle. The appearance is similar to a muscle tear, though the patient was septic. Aspiration yielded purulent fluid.

Abscess

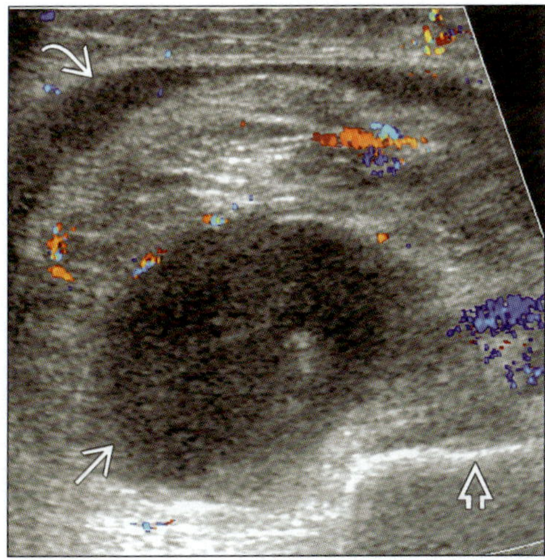

Diabetic Muscle Infarction

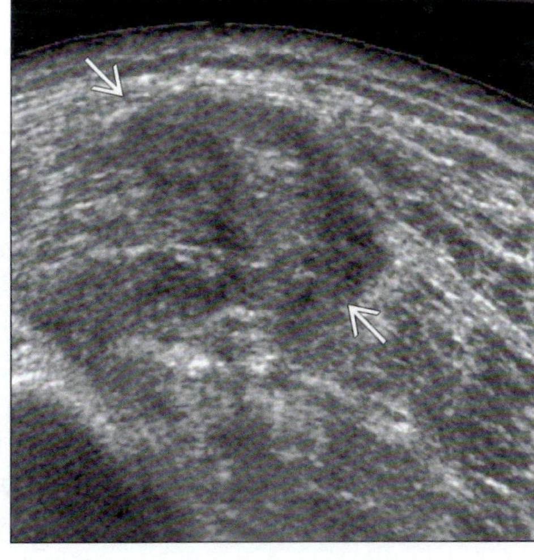

(Left) Transverse color Doppler US in a patient with SLE shows a large abscess cavity ➡ within the brachialis muscle anterior to the humeral shaft ➡. There is perimuscular fluid exudate ➡ with mild hyperemia. (Right) Transverse US in a diabetic following aortic aneurysm repair shows marked swelling of the flexor hallucis muscle with a more central hypoechoic area ➡. Mild hyperemia was present. Clinical progression was compatible with diabetic muscle infarction.

Metastases

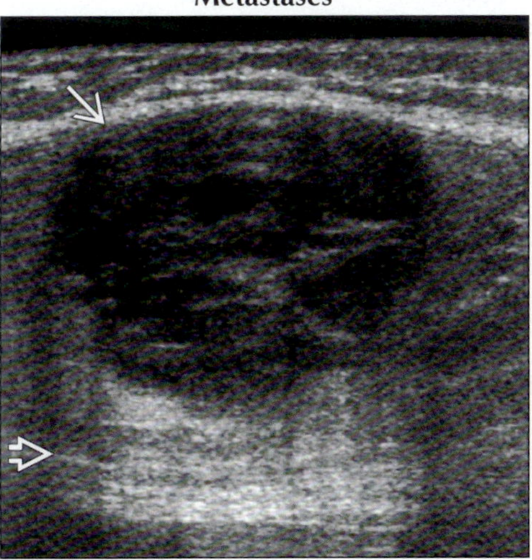

Parasitic Infection

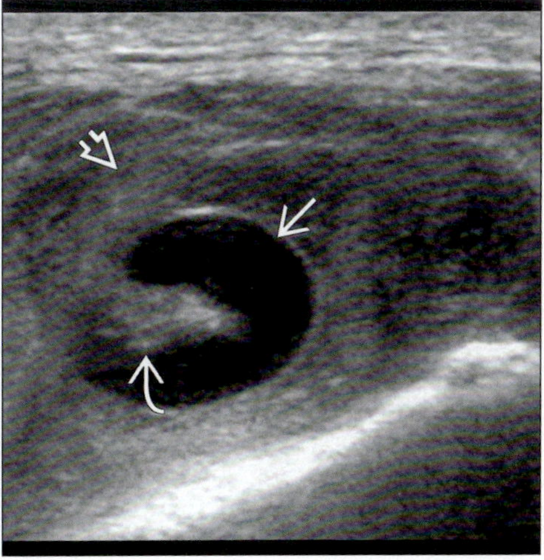

(Left) Longitudinal US in a patient with metastatic malignant thymoma shows a large, partially cystic, hypoechoic mass ➡ in the hamstring muscles. Note the posterior acoustic enhancement ➡. Biopsy confirmed metastasis. (Right) Transverse US shows a cysticercosis infestation as a small, hypoechoic, intramuscular mass ➡ with an eccentric echogenic nidus ➡ representing the scolex. There is surrounding muscle edema ➡. (Courtesy V. Hardas, MD.)

15

DIFFERENTIAL DIAGNOSIS

Common
- Intermuscular Lipoma
- Intramuscular Lipoma
- Muscle Edema
- Vascular Malformation
- Hematoma

Less Common
- Foreign Body
- Rhabdomyolysis
- Myositis
- Peripheral Nerve Sheath Tumor
- Soft Tissue Sarcoma

ESSENTIAL INFORMATION

Key Differential Diagnosis Issues
- Often need low frequency transducer to visualize full depth of muscle
- Muscle echogenicity varies according to orientation of fiber, transducer, and relative amount of lean or fatty tissue
  - Leaner muscle → more hypoechoic
  - More fatty muscle ("fatty atrophy") → more hyperechoic
- Scanning along muscle length in transverse plane indicates whether mass is present or delineates its boundaries
- Dynamic scanning not as helpful for muscle as it is for tendons, nerves, and joints
  - Muscle may be hyperechoic when edematous
  - MR more sensitive than ultrasound at depicting muscle edema

Helpful Clues for Common Diagnoses
- **Intermuscular Lipoma**
  - Located deep to investing fascia
  - May be classified as subfascial, intermuscular, intramuscular, or submuscular in location
    - Subfascial: Between investing fascia and muscle
    - Intermuscular: Between muscles is most common location
    - Intramuscular: Within muscle
    - Submuscular: Beneath muscle (i.e., juxtacortical); least common location
  - Ultrasound appearances of deep lipomas similar to subcutaneous lipomas but more variable
    - Usually larger than subcutaneous lipomas at presentation
    - Less compressible
    - Occasional vessels detected as opposed to subcutaneous lipoma, which are nearly always avascular
  - Discrete noninfiltrative mass with well-defined convex margins
  - Fusiform or oblong in shape with long axis parallel to skin
  - Echogenic stroma may be hypoechoic (infrequent)
  - Fine linear echogenic striations running parallel to long axis of tumor
  - ± acoustic enhancement, as ultrasound transmission in fat > muscle
  - No vascularity in or around lipoma on color Doppler imaging
    - Occasionally, several vessels traversing lipoma may be visible
  - Consider malignancy if following features are present
    - Large mass
    - Thick (> 2 mm) septations
    - Nodular areas of nonlipomatous tissue
    - Cyst-like or necrotic areas within tumor
    - Majority of tumor is nonlipomatous
  - 4 distinct histological types of liposarcoma
    - Well-differentiated liposarcoma
    - Myxoid liposarcoma
    - Pleomorphic liposarcoma
    - Dedifferentiated liposarcoma
- **Vascular Malformation**
  - 4 types depending on predominant vascular feature
    - Capillary, venous vascular malformation (VVM), arteriovenous, mixed
  - Hemangioma
    - Vascular tumor of childhood: Progressive → regressive stages
  - Vascular malformation
    - Vascular dysmorphogenesis
    - Enlarges in line with skeletal development
    - Changes shape in adulthood due to thrombosis and revascularization
  - Ultrasound extremely helpful in establishing diagnosis, assessing flow, and relative amount of stroma vs. vascular component

15

HYPERECHOIC MUSCLE MASS

- ▪ MR better at assessing extent and multiplicity
- • **Hematoma**
  - ○ Intramuscular hematoma may occur due to trauma, anticoagulation, or vascular malformation
    - ▪ Anterior thigh common, because it is prone to muscle contusion injury
  - ○ Acute hematoma usually isoechoic or hyperechoic to muscle
    - ▪ ± layering due to repeated hemorrhage
    - ▪ Becomes more hypoechoic with increasing liquefaction after several days
  - ○ Minor hemorrhage may be overlooked on ultrasound, as ill-defined hyperechoic areas blend with muscle
    - ▪ MR more sensitive than ultrasound at detecting mild muscle injury

Helpful Clues for Less Common Diagnoses

- • **Foreign Body**
  - ○ Lodges in subcutaneous tissues much more commonly than muscle
  - ○ Nearly all foreign bodies echogenic
  - ○ ± reverberation artifacts or acoustic shadowing
  - ○ Bamboo or noncompact wood difficult to see, because they absorb fluid and have similar echogenicity to soft tissue
    - ▪ Always repeat ultrasound after 1-3 days if foreign body not detected initially
  - ○ Missed foreign bodies often develop hypoechoic rim

- ▪ Composed of hyperemic granulation and fibrous tissue
- ▪ Makes foreign body more conspicuous
- • **Rhabdomyolysis**
  - ○ Necrosis of skeletal muscle
    - ▪ Contents of injured muscle cells leak into circulation
    - ▪ If severe → electrolyte imbalance, acidosis, coagulopathy, hypovolemia, and acute renal failure
  - ○ Many causes, including trauma, strenuous muscle exercise, and prolonged muscle compression
  - ○ Diffusely echogenic muscle or muscles
- • **Myositis**
  - ○ Ill-defined increase in muscle echogenicity and swelling of muscle, decreased definition of muscle architecture ± focal hyperemia
    - ▪ Inflammatory myositis often symmetrical
  - ○ MR more sensitive than ultrasound at detecting myositis
- • **Peripheral Nerve Sheath Tumor**
  - ○ Usually hypoechoic
    - ▪ Similar appearance to subcutaneous nerve sheath tumor
    - ▪ Areas of hyperechogenicity usual imply internal hemorrhage
- • **Soft Tissue Sarcoma**
  - ○ Occur most frequently in muscle layer
    - ▪ Mostly hypoechoic
    - ▪ Occasionally hyperechoic due to fat, fibrosis, or hemorrhage

Intramuscular Lipoma

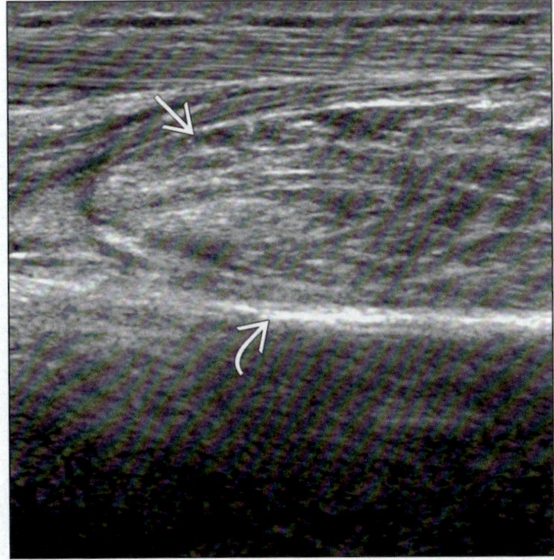

Longitudinal ultrasound shows an intramuscular lipoma ➡ on surface of fibula ➡ within the peroneal brevis muscle. The tumor is slightly more heterogeneous than a subcutaneous lipoma, though otherwise very similar.

Intramuscular Lipoma

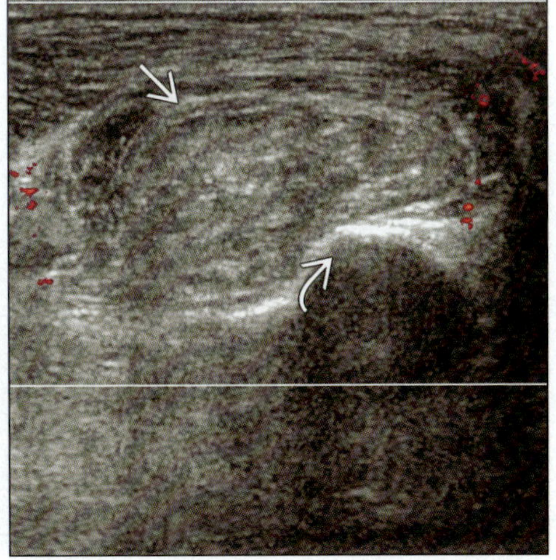

Correlative transverse color Doppler ultrasound of the same tumor demonstrates that there is no intrinsic tumor vascularity within the well-defined, intramuscular lipoma ➡ (fibula ➡).

15

HYPERECHOIC MUSCLE MASS

Muscle Edema

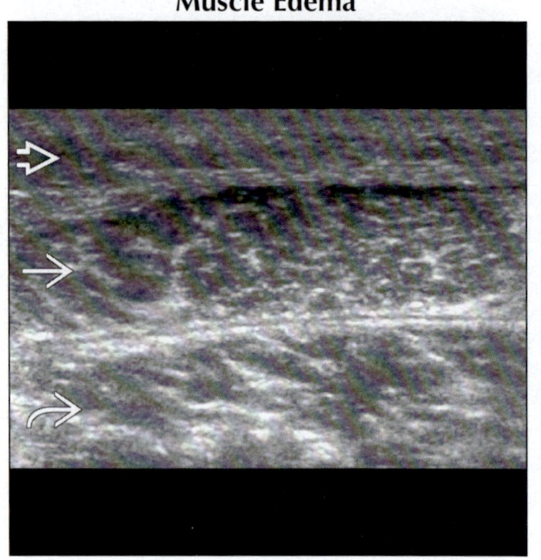

Muscle Edema

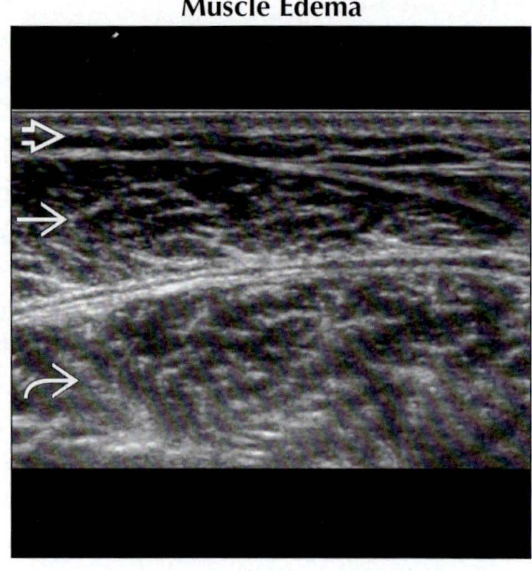

(Left) Longitudinal ultrasound shows moderate edema of the subcutaneous tissues ⇨ as well as the gastrocnemius ➡ and soleus muscles ➡ of the calf. Edematous muscle is diffusely hyperechoic with the preservation of muscle architecture. (Right) Transverse ultrasound shows a normal contralateral limb for comparison. The normal hypoechogenicity and appearance of gastrocnemius ➡ and soleus ➡ muscles, as well as subcutaneous fat ⇨, can be appreciated.

Vascular Malformation

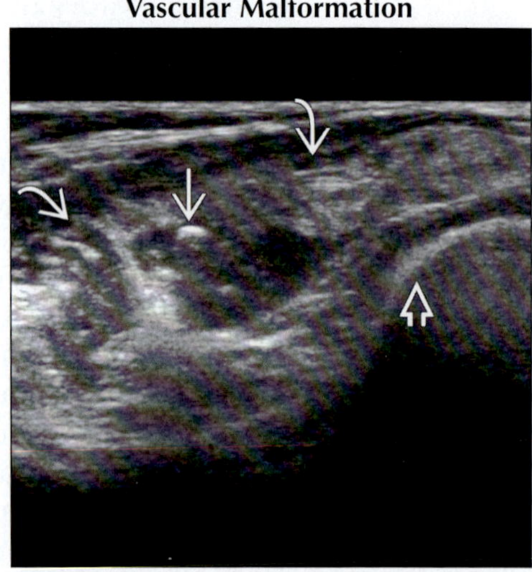

Vascular Malformation

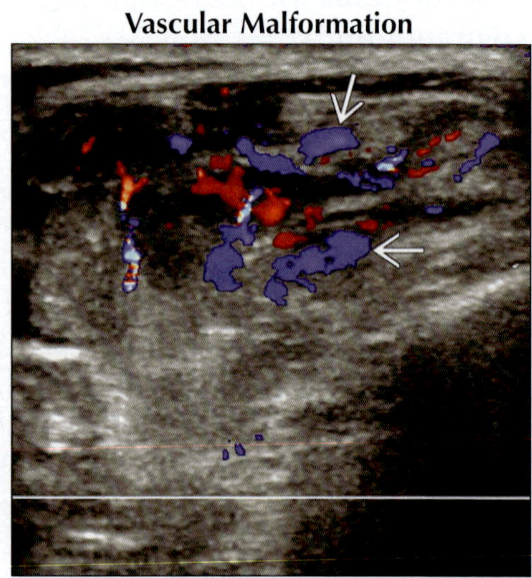

(Left) Transverse ultrasound shows a moderate-sized, hyperechoic vascular malformation ➡ within the distal part of the triceps alongside the olecranon ⇨. Vascular malformation is comprised mainly of large vessels. A single phlebolith ➡ present. (Right) Correlative transverse color Doppler ultrasound in the same patient shows slow-flowing vascular channels ➡ occupying most of the lesion, findings consistent with venous vascular malformation.

Vascular Malformation

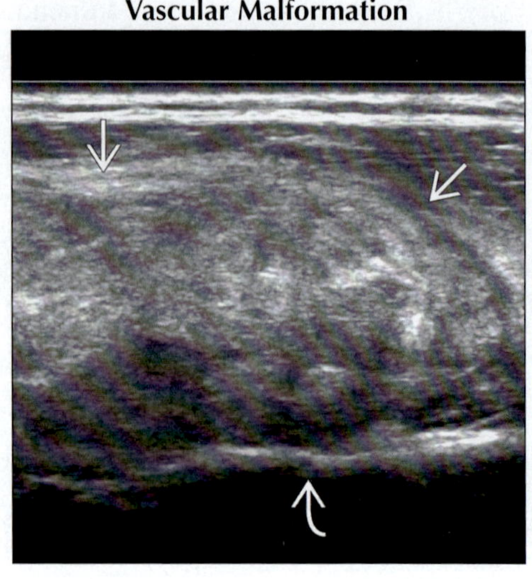

Vascular Malformation

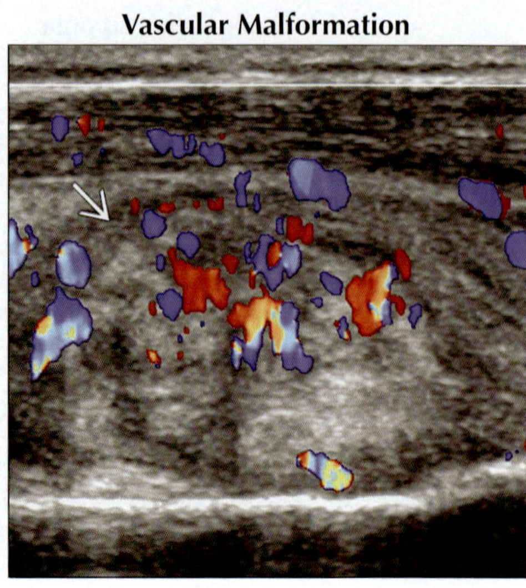

(Left) Longitudinal US shows a large, hyperechoic, soft tissue mass ➡ present in the flexor muscle on the surface of the radius ➡. No vascular channels are evident. (Right) Correlative transverse color Doppler US in the same patient shows a moderately hypervascular, hyperechoic mass ➡ in the flexor compartment. Appearances would favor either a soft tissue sarcoma or a vascular malformation. Ultrasound guided-biopsy revealed a venous vascular malformation.

15

HYPERECHOIC MUSCLE MASS

Vascular Malformation

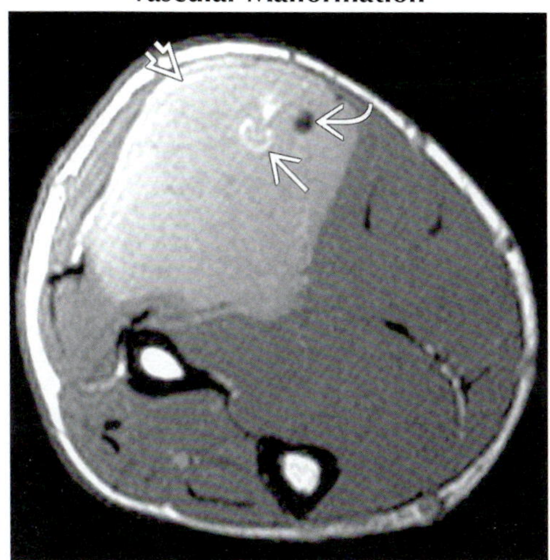

Hematoma

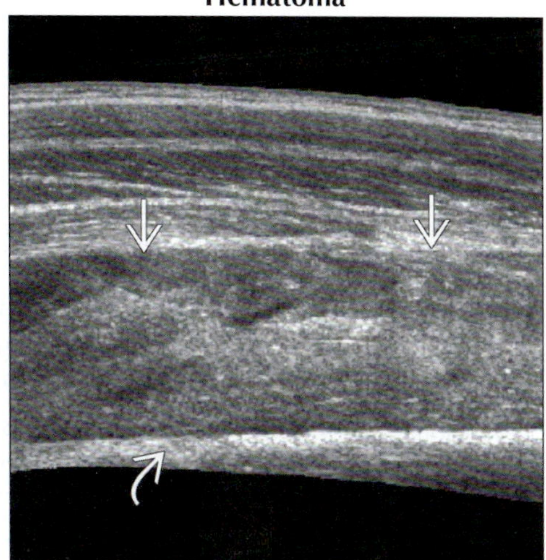

(Left) Axial T1WI MR in the same patient shows a large T1 hyperintense tumor within the flexor compartment of the forearm ➡. The radial artery is encased ➡. A small amount of intratumoral hemorrhage is present ➡. US-guided biopsy confirmed a venous vascular malformation. *(Right)* Longitudinal ultrasound shows a large intramuscular hematoma ➡ on the surface of the femoral shaft ➡ within the vastus intermedius muscle.

Foreign Body

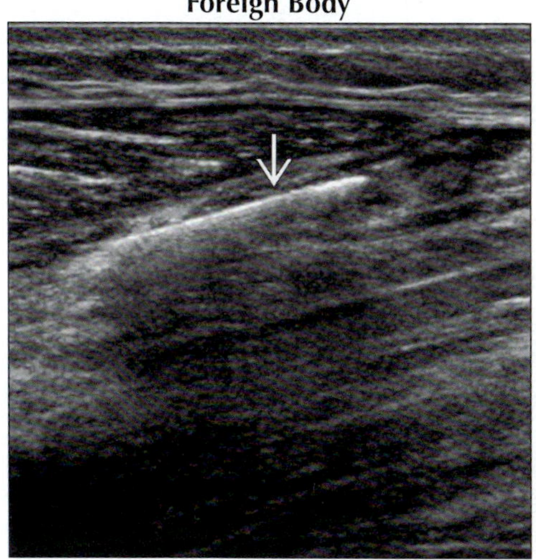

Peripheral Nerve Sheath Tumor

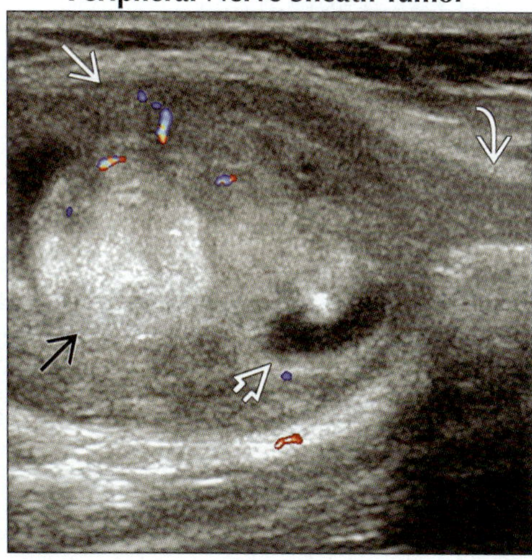

(Left) Longitudinal US shows a retained needle ➡ in the calf muscle, which had been present for many years. In an US-guided removal with forceps, the needle was found to be firmly adherent to the adjacent muscle and had to be pried off. *(Right)* Longitudinal color Doppler US shows a mildly vascular, hyperechoic nerve sheath tumor ➡ of the median nerve ➡. There are myxoid ➡ as well as hyperechoic areas ➡, the later usually indicating hemorrhage.

Rhabdomyolysis

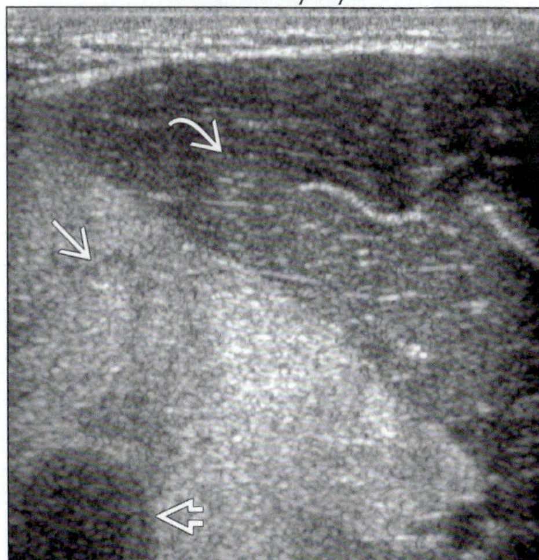

Rhabdomyolysis

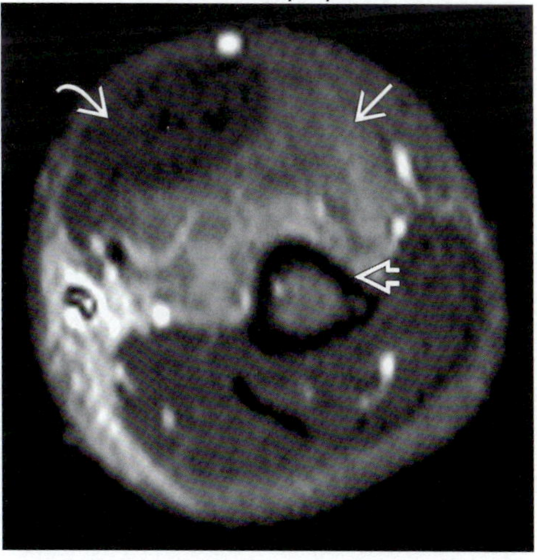

(Left) Transverse US shows a hyperechoic brachialis muscle ➡ following unaccustomed exertion on a rowing machine, indicative of delayed-onset muscle soreness with rhabdomyolysis. Biceps brachii muscle ➡ is normal. Note the humeral shaft ➡. *(Right)* Correlative axial T2WI MR with fat suppression in the same location shows the edematous brachialis muscle ➡ with a normal biceps brachii muscle ➡. Note the humeral shaft ➡.

CALCIFIED SOFT TISSUE MASS

DIFFERENTIAL DIAGNOSIS

Common
- Venous Vascular Malformation
- Granuloma
- Gout or Pseudogout
- Fat Necrosis

Less Common
- Panniculitis
- Pilomatrixoma
- Sarcoma
- Soft Tissue Metastases
- Nerve Sheath Tumor
- Fibroma
- Soft Tissue Chondroma
- Hematoma
- Calcifying Aponeurotic Fibroma
- Myositis Ossificans

ESSENTIAL INFORMATION

Key Differential Diagnosis Issues
- Visibility of lesion on ultrasound very dependent on level of calcification
  - Heavy peripheral calcification → only superficial margin visible
  - Light peripheral calcification → much of lesion visible
  - Mild matrix mineralization → most or all of lesion visible
- Align transducer obliquely to obtain views not obscured by calcification
- Review of radiographs ± computed tomography very helpful for analyzing type of calcification

Helpful Clues for Common Diagnoses
- **Venous Vascular Malformation**
  - Calcified phleboliths common but not invariable feature
    - More common with slow-flowing vascular malformations
    - Represent calcified thrombi
  - Small to medium-sized phleboliths, depending on size of vein
    - Echogenic with acoustic shadowing
    - Ultrasound more sensitive than radiographs for detection
- **Granuloma**
  - Commonly located in subcutaneous tissues of buttock and frequently multiple

- Often have history of previous subcutaneous injection at site
  - Variable rim calcification → posterior acoustic shadowing
  - Rounded hypoechoic mass
    - → width gives indication of depth; posterior margin may not be visualized due to dense posterior acoustic shadowing
  - Typically little or no hyperemia on Doppler
  - ± indentation of adjacent investing fascia or muscle when large
- **Gout or Pseudogout**
  - Located around joints, ligament, and fascial insertions
    - Tophi more common with gout
    - Pseudogout → hydroxyapatite deposition
  - Soft tophi or deposits contain little mineralized component
    - "Comet tail" artifacts secondary to crystal aggregates
  - Hard tophi or deposits often heavily mineralized
    - Dense posterior acoustic shadowing limit ultrasound assessment
- **Fat Necrosis**
  - Subcutaneous fat is prone to trauma, particularly on
    - Anterolateral aspect of thigh, lateral aspect arm, and gluteal region
  - Blunt subcutaneous trauma → injury and necrosis of fat cells
    - → focal swelling and edema of subcutaneous tissues
    - → reparative change with mild localized hyperemia on color Doppler imaging
    - → encapsulated fat necrosis ± heterotopic ossification ± fibrosis
  - More severe forms of fat necrosis tend to undergo calcification and ossification

Helpful Clues for Less Common Diagnoses
- **Panniculitis**
  - Calcification or ossification occurs following panniculitis (panniculitis ossificans)
    - Difficult to distinguish from fat necrosis
- **Pilomatrixoma**
  - Benign skin neoplasm with differentiation toward hair matrix

15

- Round, well-defined, hypoechoic mass with partially calcified rim and posterior acoustic shadowing
  - Some lesions may be completely calcified
  - ± peripheral hypoechoic halo ± mild peripheral hyperemia on color Doppler
- **Sarcoma**
  - Both benign and malignant soft tissue tumors may calcify
    - Chondroid mineralization → "ring and arc" type
    - Osteoid mineralization → cloud-like or hazy or akin to mature bone
  - Calcification may be intrinsic part of tumor or may represent residual bone in tumor extending from bone
  - Synovial sarcoma most common malignant soft tissue tumor to calcify
    - About 50% show foci of calcification
  - Other sarcomas that contain foci of calcification include
    - Liposarcoma, malignant fibrous histiocytoma, extraskeletal osteosarcoma, leiomyosarcoma, and alveolar soft part sarcoma
- **Soft Tissue Metastases**
  - Soft tissue metastases that contain foci of calcification usually arise from
    - Adenocarcinoma of colon, stomach, or pancreas
    - Medullary carcinoma of thyroid and ovarian carcinoma
- **Nerve Sheath Tumor**
  - Similar to nerve sheath tumors elsewhere
    - Calcification uncommon
- **Fibroma**
  - Subcutaneous fibrous nodules, which may calcify or ossify
  - Not locally aggressive
- **Soft Tissue Chondroma**
  - Often quite heavily calcified at periphery, limiting visibility
    - Well-defined hypoechoic rim of cartilage visible beyond echogenic calcified front
    - Mild or absent hyperemia on color Doppler
- **Hematoma**
  - Rarely can show peripheral calcification
- **Calcifying Aponeurotic Fibroma**
  - a.k.a. juvenile aponeurotic fibroma
  - Locally aggressive fibroblastic tumor of children and young adults, usually located in hands and feet
    - Occur next to dense fibrous connective tissue (fascia or periosteum)
    - May erode bone
  - Nodular or ill-defined infiltrating mass with fine stippled calcification
    - About 50% recur after resection
- **Myositis Ossificans**
  - 2 types, depending on trauma history
  - Soft tissue trauma ⇒ known as myositis ossificans circumscripta
  - No soft tissue trauma ⇒ atraumatic myositis ossificans
    - May be due to nondocumented trauma, repeated minor injury, ischemia, or inflammation

Venous Vascular Malformation

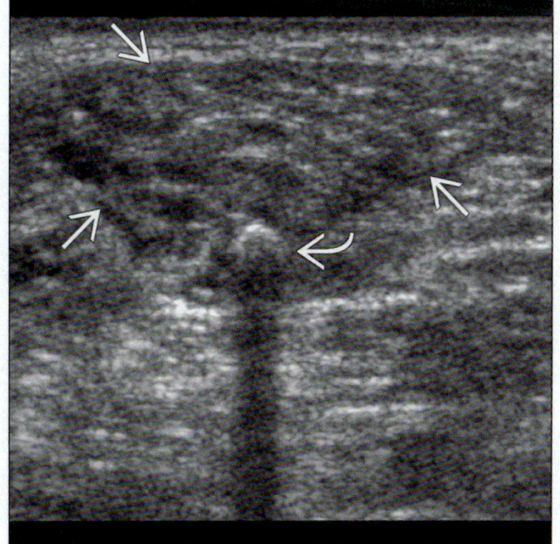

Transverse ultrasound of the volar aspect forearm shows a venous vascular malformation ➡ with a single phlebolith ➡. Color and pulsed Doppler imaging (not shown) demonstrated mild vascularity with slow flow.

Venous Vascular Malformation

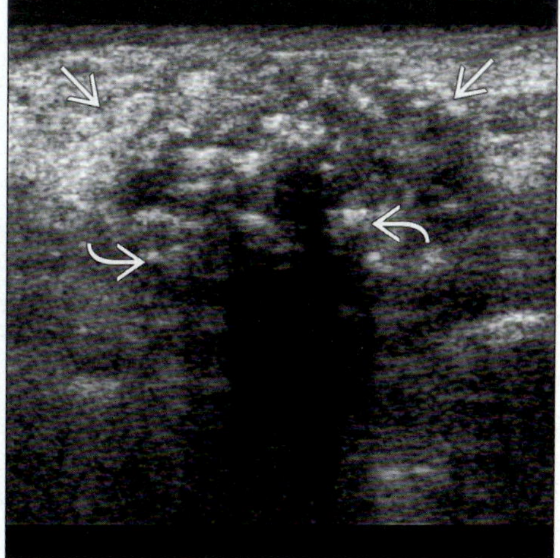

Transverse ultrasound of the foot shows a venous vascular malformation ➡ in the abductor hallucis muscle containing numerous phleboliths ➡. Doppler ultrasound revealed mild vascularity with slow flow.

(Left) Transverse ultrasound shows a heavily calcified granuloma ➡ within the subcutaneous tissues of the gluteal region. Although dense acoustic shadowing prevents visualization of the deep margin of the granuloma, the muscle and investing fascia ➡ is not displaced. (Right) Longitudinal ultrasound in a patient with chronic gout shows a hard tophus of the forefoot. Dense acoustic shadowing ➡ impedes visibility of all but the outer margin ➡.

Granuloma

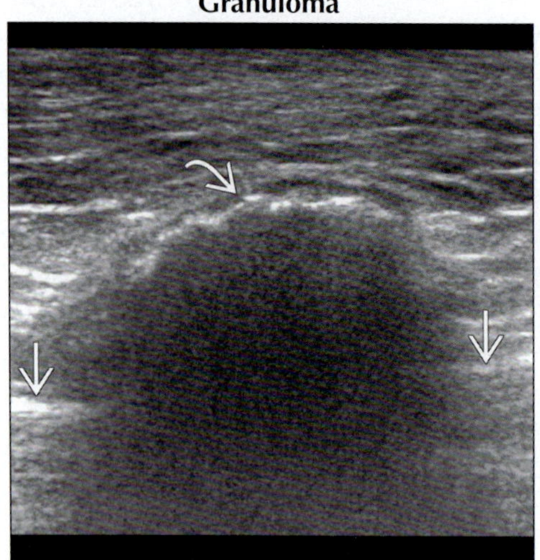

Gout or Pseudogout

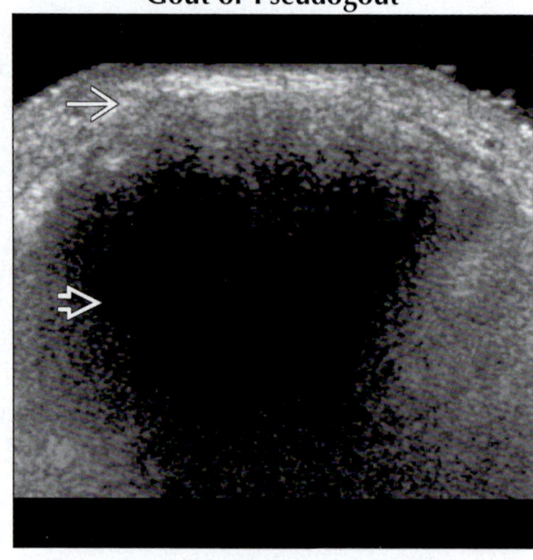

(Left) Longitudinal US of the forefoot shows an echogenic mass ➡ near the 3rd metatarsophalangeal joint with many small echogenic foci ➡ and shadowing ➡ due to crystal aggregation in a soft tophus. Biopsy revealed pyrophosphate crystals with focal chondroid proliferation. (Right) Transverse US of a buttock shows a well-defined, subcutaneous, hypoechoic mass ➡ due to fat necrosis. There is prominent calcification ➡ with dense acoustic shadowing ➡.

Gout or Pseudogout

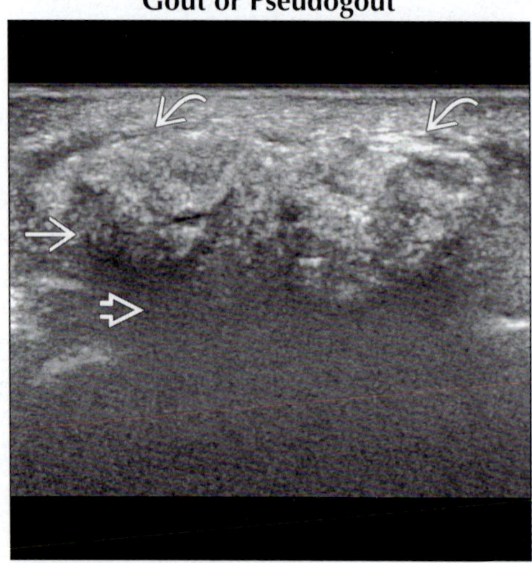

Fat Necrosis

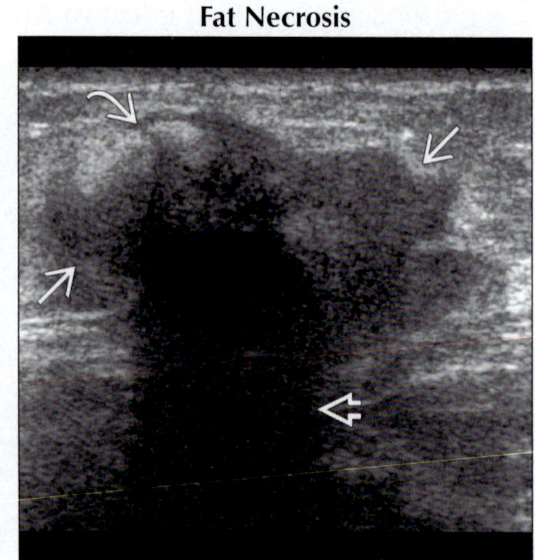

(Left) Transverse US in a patient with a tender leg nodule and no history of trauma shows a heavily calcified subcutaneous nodule ➡ anterior to the tibia. Other nodules appeared similar (not shown). Histology was compatible with panniculitis ossificans. (Right) Transverse US shows a well-defined, hypoechoic, subcutaneous nodule ➡ with peripheral calcification ➡ and dense acoustic shadowing ➡. Histology confirmed pilomatrixoma.

Panniculitis

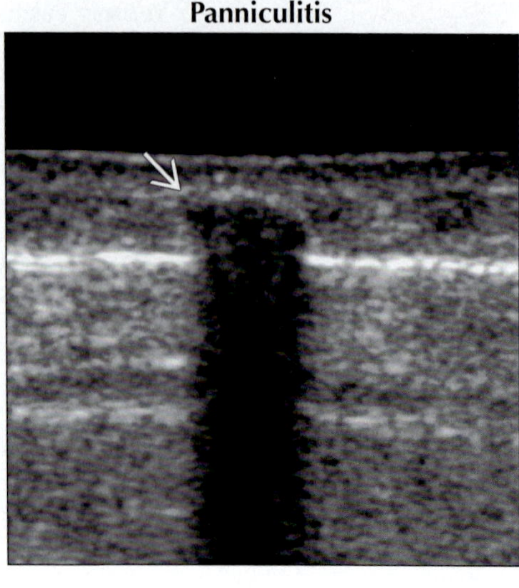

Pilomatrixoma

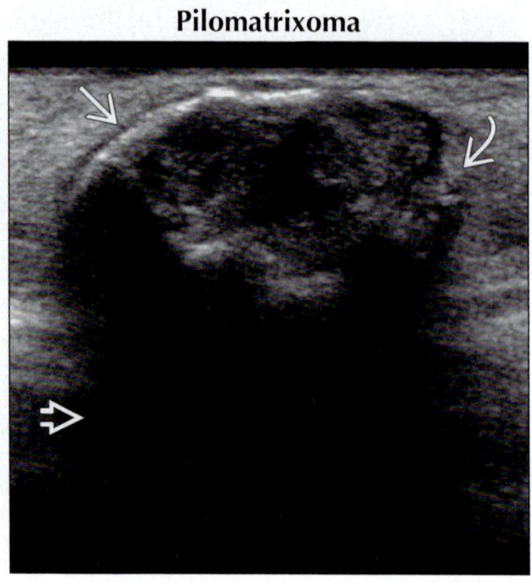

15

CALCIFIED SOFT TISSUE MASS

Pilomatrixoma

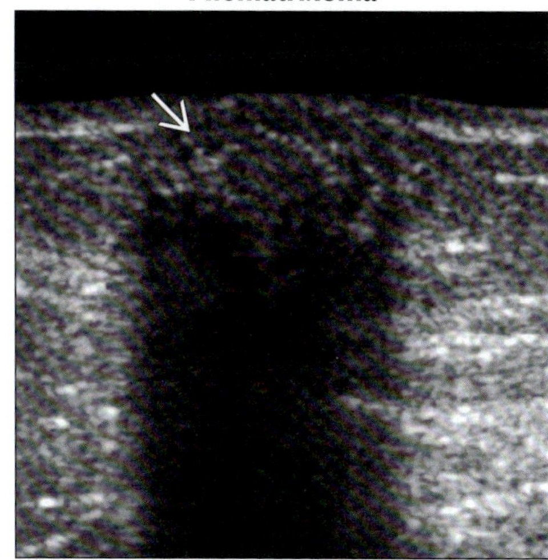

Pilomatrixoma

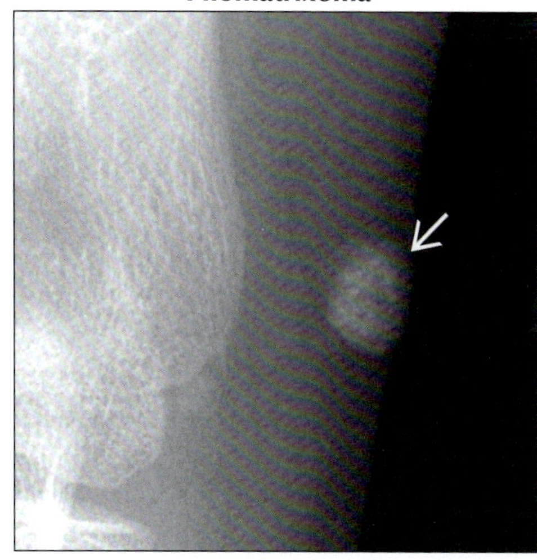

(Left) Longitudinal ultrasound of an elbow nodule present for many years shows a mass ➡ with speckled calcification within the subcutaneous tissues. Most of the mass is visible, except for the deep margin. (Right) Radiograph at the same location shows a heavily calcified nodule ➡ within the subcutaneous tissues. Calcification is best characterized by radiography. Histology revealed pilomatrixoma.

Sarcoma

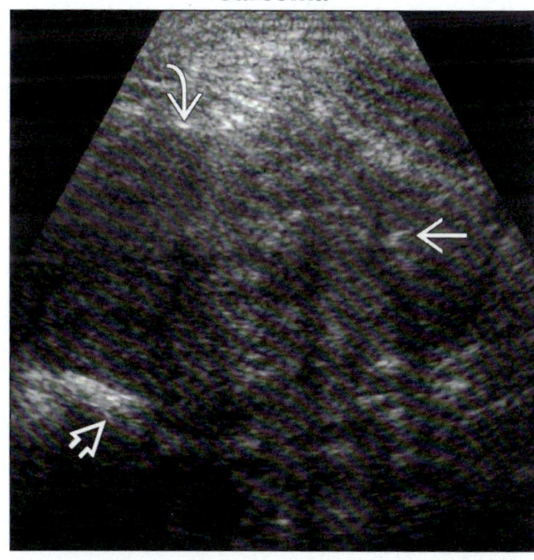

Soft Tissue Metastases

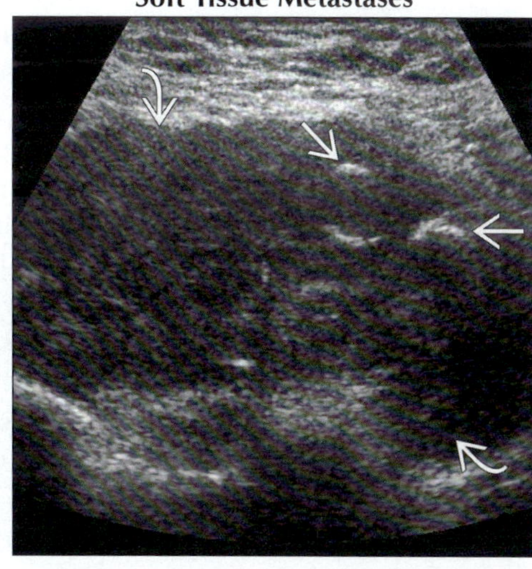

(Left) Transverse ultrasound shows a large hypoechoic mass ➡ with foci of calcification ➡ adjacent to the scapula ➡. Percutaneous biopsy and histology revealed a leiomyosarcoma. (Right) Transverse ultrasound of the axilla in a patient with carcinoma of the colon resected 4 years ago shows a large hypoechoic mass ➡ with foci of calcification ➡, consistent with a metastatic deposit. This was confirmed by fine-needle aspiration.

Nerve Sheath Tumor

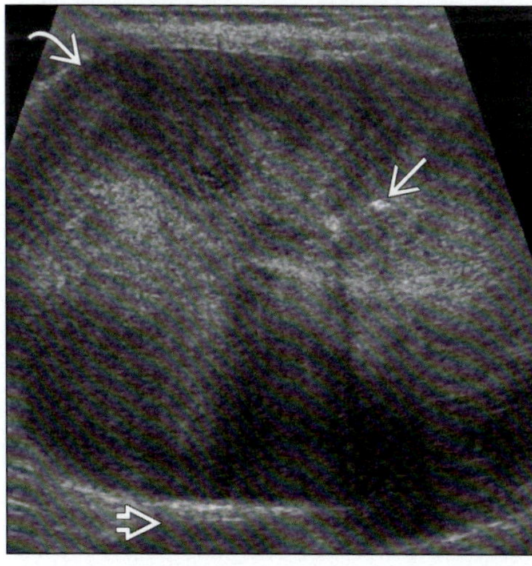

Soft Tissue Chondroma

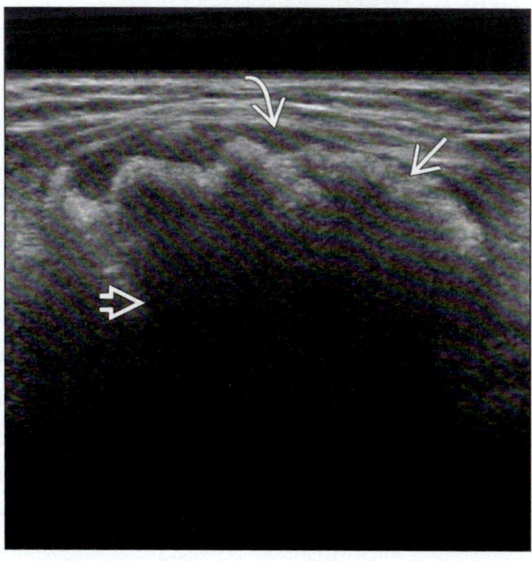

(Left) Longitudinal ultrasound in a patient with a mass in the lateral aspect of the leg, slowly growing for 10 years, shows a large nerve sheath tumor ➡ of the peroneal nerve with small foci of calcification ➡. Note the fibula ➡. (Right) Transverse ultrasound of the thenar eminence shows a densely calcified mass ➡ with a thin, hypoechoic chondroid rim ➡. Dense acoustic shadowing ➡ limits the evaluation of the central and deeper aspects of the mass.

15

HYPERVASCULAR SOFT TISSUE MASS

DIFFERENTIAL DIAGNOSIS

Common
- Vascular Anomaly
- Nerve Sheath Tumor
- Soft Tissue Sarcoma

Less Common
- Glomus Tumor
- Granulation Tissue
- Giant Cell Tumor of Tendon Sheath
- Inflammatory Mass
- Peri-articular Giant Cell Tumor
- Pigmented Villonodular Synovitis
- Fibroma
- Focal Myositis
- Diabetic Muscle Infarction
- Metastases

ESSENTIAL INFORMATION

Key Differential Diagnosis Issues
- Vascularity can be assessed on grayscale, color Doppler, and power Doppler imaging
  - Color Doppler provides information about flow direction but is not as sensitive as power Doppler in detection of flow
    - Power Doppler does not assess flow direction
  - Additional spectral analysis usually not helpful or necessary
- Apply minimal transducer pressure to avoid obliterating vascularity
- Note whether vascularity pattern is predominantly central or peripheral, organized, chaotic, or mixed pattern
- Color Doppler not quite as sensitive to hyperemia as contrast enhancement on MR or CT
  - Contrast enhancement on MR or CT also dependent on features such as permeability or interstitial flow

Helpful Clues for Common Diagnoses
- **Vascular Anomaly**
  - For all vascular malformations assess
    - Size and location of lesion
    - Predominant vascular structure (arterial or venous)
    - Relative amount of vascular vs. stromal tissue
    - Presence of phleboliths or recognizable areas of thrombosis
  - Lesion characteristics and flow best assessed with ultrasound
    - Lesion extent (of large and ill-defined lesions) and multiplicity best assessed with MR imaging
  - 2 main types of vascular anomaly vary in regards to age of onset and clinical course
  - Hemangioma
    - Present at birth and grows during childhood
    - Involutes spontaneously after childhood
    - Proliferation → stabilization → involution
  - Vascular malformation
    - Grow proportional to patient growth
    - More rapid growth of vascular malformation precipitated by puberty, pregnancy, trauma
    - 3 main types of vascular malformation with considerable overlap: Capillary, venous, and arteriovenous
- **Nerve Sheath Tumor**
  - Hypoechoic, typically fusiform-shaped
  - ± anechoic areas due to myxoid deposition
    - ± hyperechoic areas due to hemorrhage, calcification, or fibrosis
  - Posterior acoustic enhancement
  - Variable vascularity, which diminishes with transducer pressure
    - Mostly moderate to highly vascular
    - Rarely no detectable vascularity
- **Soft Tissue Sarcoma**
  - Usually hypervascular
    - Cannot predict aggressiveness of lesion based on degree or pattern of vascularity
  - Occasionally hypo-/avascular
    - Particularly fibrosarcoma or liposarcoma
  - Alveolar soft part sarcoma may mimic vascular malformation on imaging

Helpful Clues for Less Common Diagnoses
- **Glomus Tumor**
  - Most common location: Distal extremities, especially subungual areas
    - Hypoechoic, hypervascular nodule between nail and cortex of distal phalanx
  - Arises from glomus body, which is arteriovenous shunt in dermis that contributes to temperature regulation
  - Glomus tumors also arise in extracutaneous locations, which do not normally contain glomus cells

15

HYPERVASCULAR SOFT TISSUE MASS

- ▪ May arise from perivascular cells that can differentiate into glomus cells
- ▪ Small, well-defined, hypoechoic, hypervascular masses
- **Granulation Tissue**
  - ○ Hypoechoic irregular tissue
  - ○ Within scar tissue or around foreign body
- **Giant Cell Tumor of Tendon Sheath**
  - ○ Mostly eccentrically located to tendon growing along length of tendon sheath
  - ○ Moderately → highly vascular
  - ○ Hypoechoic, peritendinous in location
- **Pigmented Villonodular Synovitis**
  - ○ a.k.a. benign proliferative synovial disorder
  - ○ 2 forms, diffuse or focal
    - ▪ Diffuse: Affects entire synovial lining of joint
    - ▪ Focal: Less common = focal nodular synovitis
  - ○ Thickened synovium with villous & nodular proliferation
  - ○ Locally aggressive, involves paraarticular soft tissues and subchondral bone
- **Fibroma**
  - ○ Localized tumorous collection of collagen, + sparse number of fibroblasts
    - ▪ Nuchal fibromas in midline nape of neck
    - ▪ Tendon sheath fibromas of hands and feet
- **Focal Myositis**
  - ○ Ill-defined area of muscle is hyper-/hypoechoic with hyperemia
    - ▪ Underlying muscle architecture visible

- ○ Manifestation of generalized inflammatory arthropathy such as Behçet disease
- ○ MR more sensitive than ultrasound for diagnosis
- **Diabetic Muscle Infarction**
  - ○ Hypovascular stage → hypervascular stage after about 10 days
    - ▪ Ill-defined hypoechoic area evolves into better-defined hypoechoic area
    - ▪ Underlying muscle architecture remains visible to some degree
    - ▪ Painful area without palpable mass evolves into less painful area with harder small mass
    - ▪ Biopsy not necessarily required
    - ▪ Longstanding diabetes with established vasculopathy, including retinopathy and nephropathy
- **Metastases**
  - ○ Manifestation of end-stage metastatic disease
  - ○ Ultrasound appearances similar to soft tissue sarcoma, though metastases seem to present at smaller size than sarcomas
    - ▪ Average size of muscle metastases larger than sarcomas
  - ○ Adenocarcinoma of lung is most common primary
  - ○ Most common site: Lower limb muscles
    - ▪ Biopsy necessary for diagnosis

Vascular Anomaly

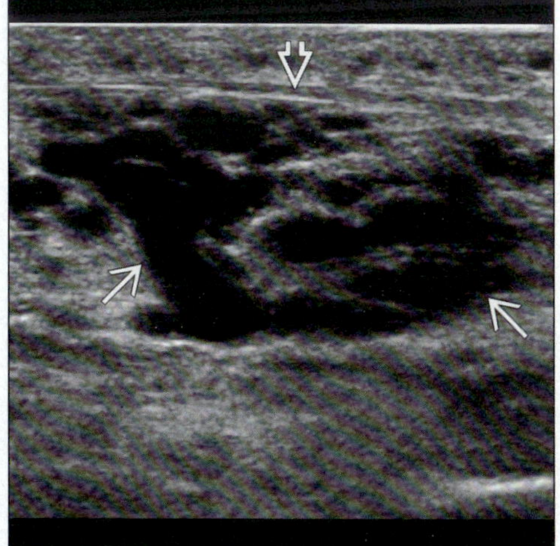

Longitudinal ultrasound of plantar aspect of the foot, in a patient with 10 years of foot swelling, shows multiple, large, dilated, vascular channels ➡ with a small stromal component deep to the plantar fascia ➡.

Vascular Anomaly

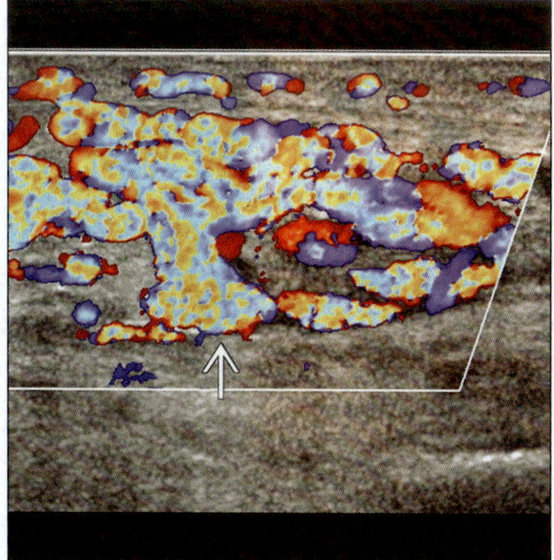

Longitudinal color Doppler ultrasound in the same lesion shows high flow (with arterial pattern on pulsed Doppler) within the vascular channels ➡, consistent with an arteriovenous malformation.

HYPERVASCULAR SOFT TISSUE MASS

(Left) Longitudinal ultrasound of the distal forearm shows a nerve sheath tumor of the median nerve. Characteristic myxoid ⮕ and echogenic areas ⮕, as well as posterior acoustic enhancement ⮕, are present. **(Right)** Longitudinal power Doppler ultrasound at the same site shows moderate hyperemia of the tumor. This is very typical of nerve sheath tumors. However, this type of tumor may show little or no vascularity.

Nerve Sheath Tumor

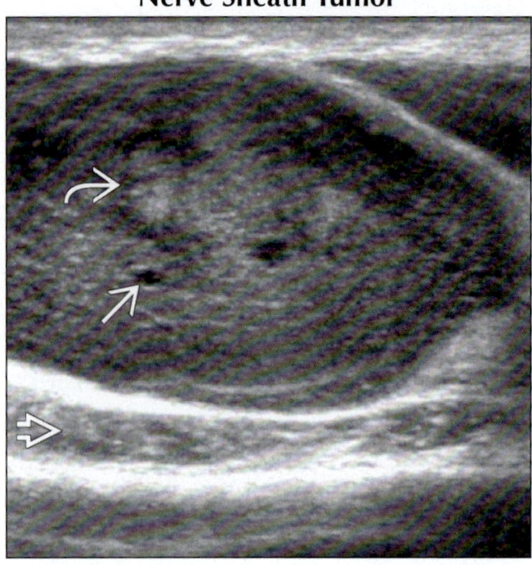

Nerve Sheath Tumor

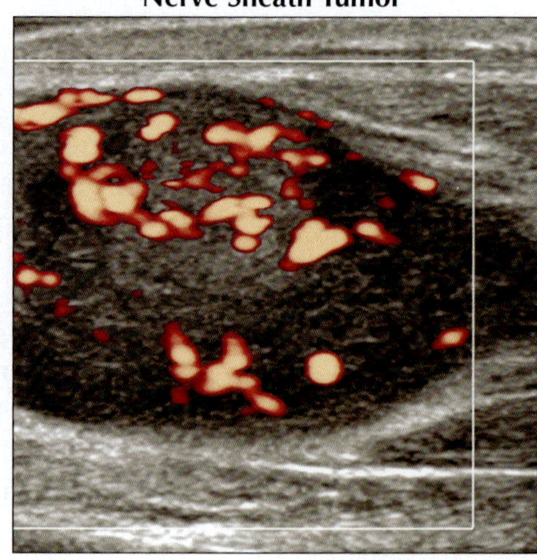

(Left) Transverse US in a patient with a slowly growing mass for 10 years shows the more superficial aspect of a large solid mass ⮕ between the flexor muscles of the forearm. Biopsy confirmed myxoid malignant fibrous histiocytoma. **(Right)** Transverse color Doppler US of the same area shows that the tumor is hypervascular ⮕ with evenly spaced intratumoral vessels. Neither this nor any other vascular pattern is predictive of tumor aggressiveness.

Soft Tissue Sarcoma

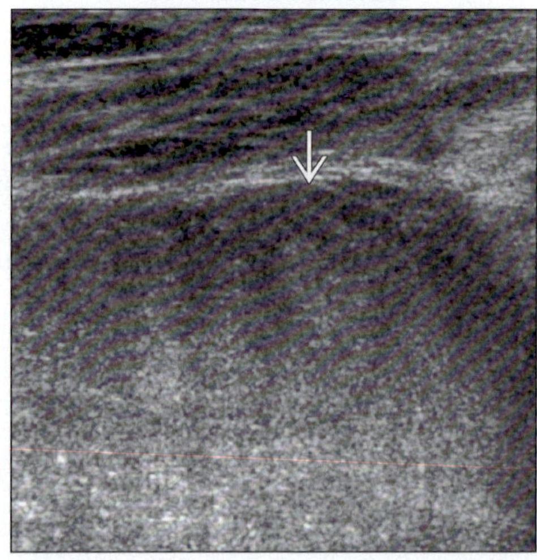

Soft Tissue Sarcoma

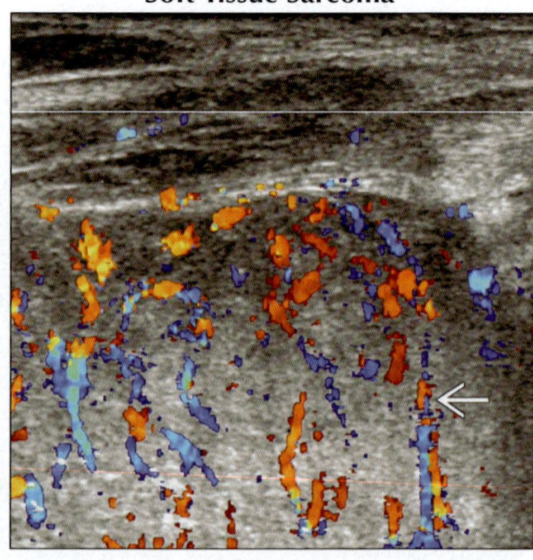

(Left) Longitudinal ultrasound of the nailbed of a thumb shows a rounded, mildly hypoechoic tumor ⮕ deep to the nail ⮕. Mild scalloping of the underlying cortex ⮕ is present with no intraosseous extension. There is also prominent posterior acoustic enhancement ⮕. **(Right)** Longitudinal color Doppler ultrasound of the same lesion shows it to be hypervascular ⮕, consistent with subungual glomus tumor. This was confirmed by histology.

Glomus Tumor

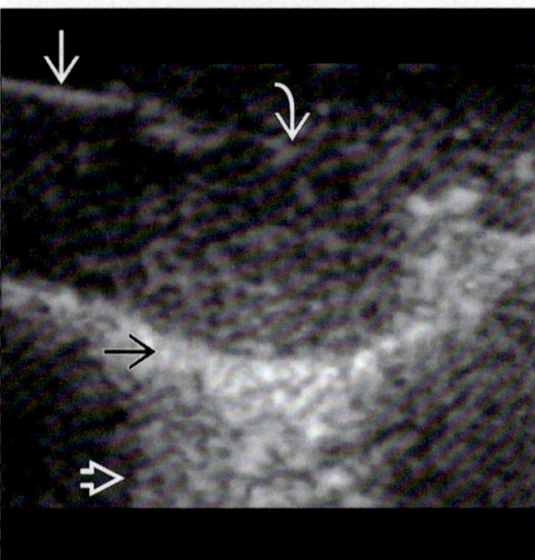

Glomus Tumor

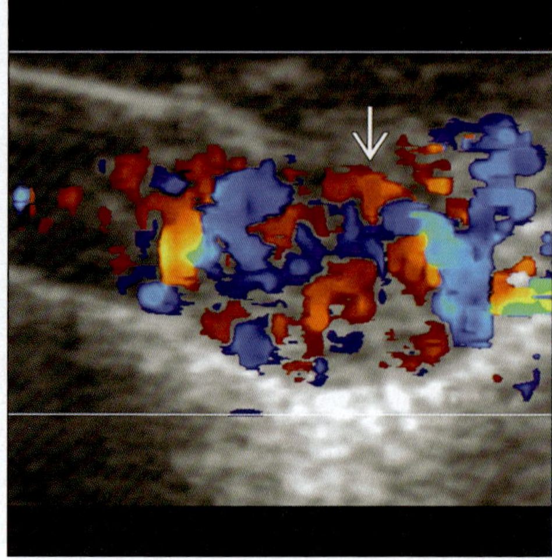

15

HYPERVASCULAR SOFT TISSUE MASS

Granulation Tissue

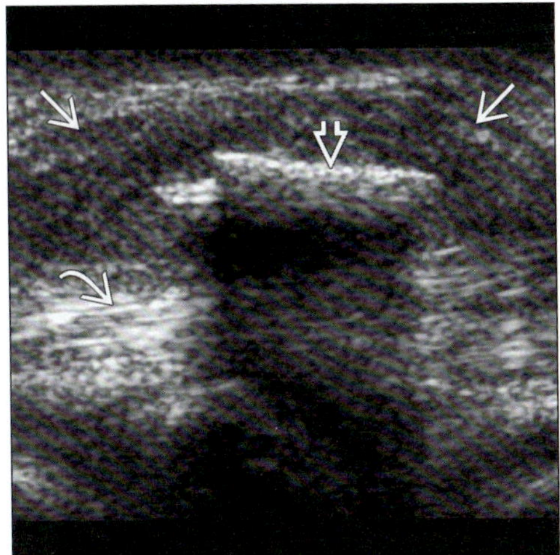

Granulation Tissue

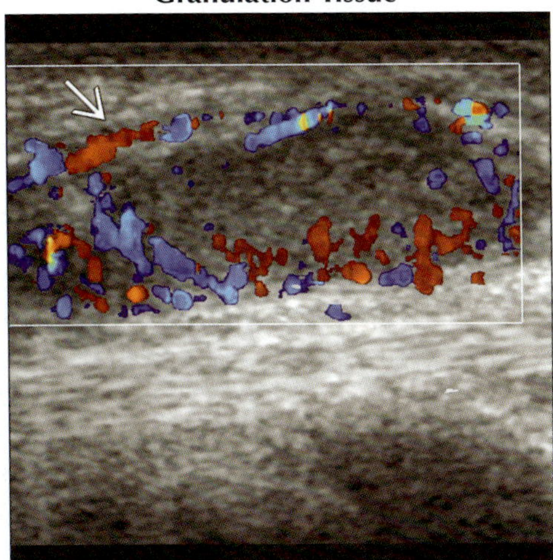

(Left) Longitudinal US of the palm shows a wood fragment ⊡ in the subcutaneous tissues superficial to the flexor tendons ⊡. A thick rind of hypoechoic granulation tissue ⊡ is seen. Although the foreign body was in the palm, the entry site was proximal to the wrist crease. (Right) Longitudinal color Doppler US of the palm medial to the previous image shows typical peripheral hyperemia ⊡ of granulation tissue surrounding the wooden fragment.

Giant Cell Tumor of Tendon Sheath

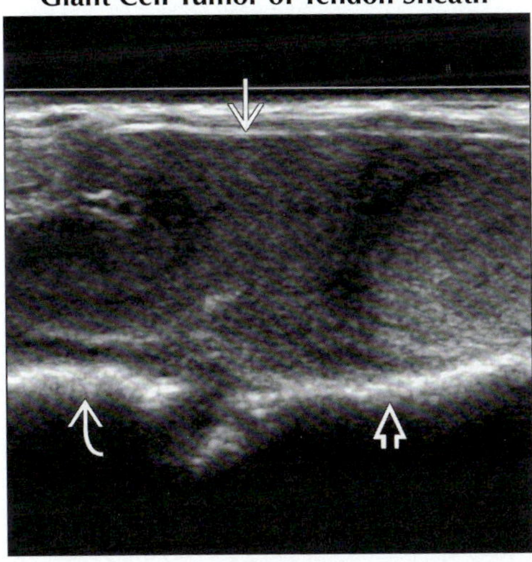

Giant Cell Tumor of Tendon Sheath

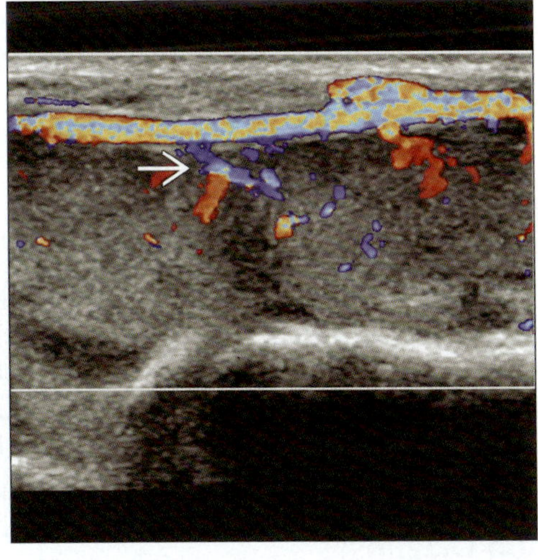

(Left) Longitudinal ultrasound of the dorsum of the foot shows an elongated hypoechoic mass ⊡, extending along the dorsum of the mid-foot, in contact with the underlying navicular ⊡ and cuneiform ⊡ bones. (Right) Longitudinal color Doppler ultrasound in the same patient at a more distal location shows moderate vascular ingrowth ⊡ from the artery lying on the dorsal surface of the tumor. Biopsy confirmed a giant cell tumor of the tendon sheath.

Fibroma

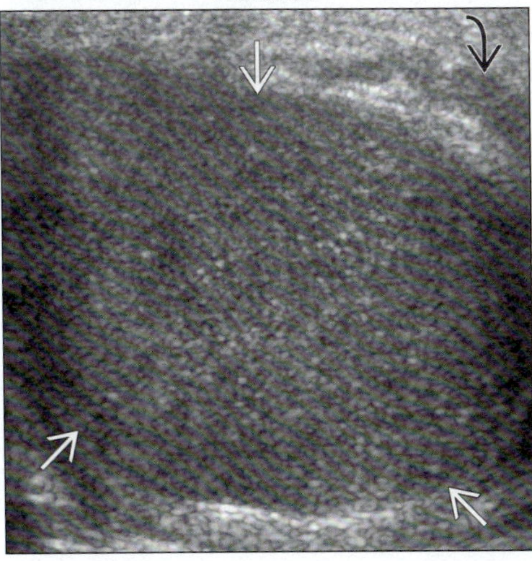

Fibroma

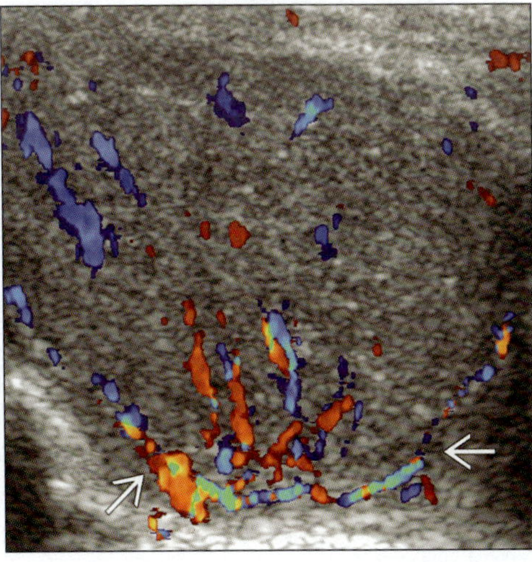

(Left) Transverse ultrasound of a neck mass present for more than 20 years shows a well-defined, hypoechoic mass ⊡ deep to the paravertebral musculature ⊡. (Right) Transverse color Doppler ultrasound of the same lesion shows well-organized vascularity ⊡ radiating from the deep margin of the tumor. Histology confirmed a fibroma.

15

DIFFERENTIAL DIAGNOSIS

Common
- Tenosynovitis
- Ganglion Cyst
- Giant Cell Tumor of Tendon Sheath
- Nerve Sheath Tumor
- Annular Pulley Thickening

Less Common
- Bursitis
- Gouty Tophus
- Fibrosis

ESSENTIAL INFORMATION

Key Differential Diagnosis Issues
- Note whether affected tendon has tendon sheath
  - Only some tendons, notably those around wrist and ankle, have tendon sheaths
  - Some tendons, such as patellar and Achilles tendons, have incomplete tendon sheaths known as paratenon
  - Occurrence of tenosynovitis and giant cell tumor of tendon sheath is dependent on presence of tendon sheath or paratenon
- Relationship of mass to tendon ± tendon sheath is important
  - Dynamic assessment by tendon movement is helpful in this respect
- Color Doppler allows differentiation of hypoechoic synovial proliferation from hypoechoic tendon fluid

Helpful Clues for Common Diagnoses
- **Tenosynovitis**
  - Acute exudative tenosynovitis
    - Usually due to acute infection
    - Echogenic fluid accumulation within tendon sheath
    - Echogenic speckles are due to aggregation of purulent debris
    - Hyperemia around, rather than within, tendon sheath
    - Tendon sheath may rupture with spread of infection into peritendinous tissues
    - Tendon usually only mildly thickened ± indistinct margins
    - Ultrasound-guided aspiration helpful to confirm infection and isolate organism
  - Acute nonexudative tenosynovitis
    - Due to inflammation or infection
    - Synovial proliferation predominates over tendon sheath effusion
    - Hyperemia around, more than within, sheath
    - Fluid aspiration often unfruitful
  - Chronic active tenosynovitis
    - Due to inflammation or infection
    - Hyperemia within, rather than around, sheath
  - Chronic inactive tenosynovitis
    - Mild thickening of tendon sheath with clear tendon sheath effusion
    - ± stenosing tenosynovitis with entrapped, noncompressible fluid
- **Ganglion Cyst**
  - Anechoic, cystic-like structure closely related to joint
    - Noncompressible
    - Filled with gelatinous-type material of variable consistency
    - Common sites are wrists, base of fingers, and tarsus
  - May be irregular in outline
  - Usually points toward or closely related to particular joint
    - Try to identify joint of origin since this has treatment implications
    - Usually neck or stalk cannot be actually followed into joint
  - ± "comet tail" artifacts
  - ± leakage/rupture
- **Giant Cell Tumor of Tendon Sheath**
  - Composed of multinucleated cells and fibroblast-like cells that may have hemosiderin deposits
    - Pathologically, giant cell tumors of tendon sheath are identical to pigmented villonodular synovitis
  - Common in hand, wrist, and feet
    - May also occur around elbow or knee or anywhere tendon sheaths exist
  - All giant cell tumors contact tendon to some degree
    - Most often tendon sheath is only partially encased with complete encasement being less common
    - Tendon movement is not affected since tumor expands on outer margin of tendon sheath
  - Hypoechoic tumor, which may be irregular, fusiform, or rounded in outline

15

PERITENDINOUS MASS

- Tends to extend along long axis of tendon sheath
- Posterior acoustic enhancement, cystic areas, or calcification are not seen
  - Usually moderately vascular; infrequently may have no demonstrable flow on color Doppler imaging
  - ± bone erosions
  - May be multifocal
- **Nerve Sheath Tumor**
  - Often occur in proximity to tendons particularly at wrist and ankle
  - Arise along course of peripheral nerve
  - Fusiform-shaped, hypoechoic with posterior acoustic enhancement and moderate vascularity
    - ± thickening of entering or exiting parent nerve (very common)
    - ± areas of myxoid accumulation (very common)
    - ± areas of hemorrhage of calcification (much less common)
    - If tumors arise from small peripheral nerves, entering or exiting nerve may not be visible
    - Cannot differentiate between schwannoma and neurofibroma based on ultrasound appearance alone
- **Annular Pulley Thickening**
  - Pulleys are series of fibrous slings that maintain close proximity between flexor tendons and fingers during finger flexion

- Pulley thickening usually affects A1 pulley, which is located at metacarpophalangeal joint level
    - Leads to restriction of flexor tendon movement known as "trigger finger"
  - Normal pulley seen as thin hypoechoic band looping over tendon from bony attachment
    - Normally ~ 0.5 mm thick at area most distant from bone
  - In "trigger finger," A1 pulley thickens to 1-2 mm
    - ± hyperemia of pulley
    - ± tendinosis or tenosynovitis of flexor tendons
  - Dynamic imaging allows depiction of flexor tendon movement restriction
    - Superficialis tendon movement restricted more than profundus tendon

Helpful Clues for Less Common Diagnoses
- **Bursitis**
  - Bursa usually located alongside tendons
    - Variably distended with echogenic fluid
- **Gouty Tophus**
  - Deposition in proximity of tendon is common
    - Soft or hard tophi depending on level of crystal deposition
    - Crystal aggregates → "comet tail" artifacts
- **Fibrosis**
  - Peritendinous fibrosis is normal following injury or surgery

Tenosynovitis

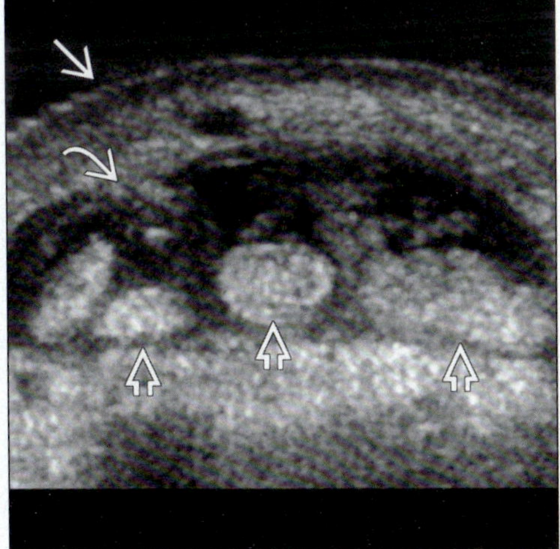

Transverse US shows acute on chronic tenosynovitis of extensor digitorum tendons with dorsal soft tissue swelling ➡, distended tendon sheath with synovial proliferation ➤, and edematous extensor tendons ➤.

Ganglion Cyst

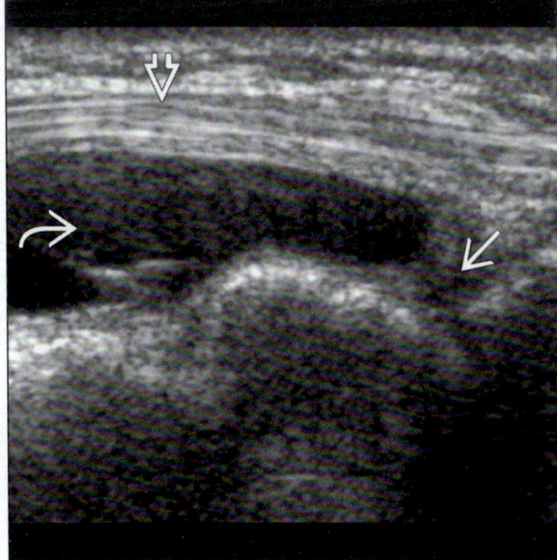

Longitudinal ultrasound shows an anechoic ganglion cyst ➡ on the dorsum of the wrist, which seems to be arising from the radiolunate articulation ➡. Normal extensor tendons ➤ overlie the ganglion.

15

(Left) Longitudinal ultrasound shows a large hypoechoic mass ➡ deep to the extensor hallucis longus tendon ➡ of the foot. Note the mass does not envelop the tendon. There is a broad erosion ➡ on the dorsal surface of the medial cuneiform. *(Right)* Longitudinal US shows the proximal end ➡ of the same tumor. Note the acute angle of the tumor with the tendon ➡. Giant cell tumors of the tendon sheath tend to grow along the axis of the tendon.

Giant Cell Tumor of Tendon Sheath

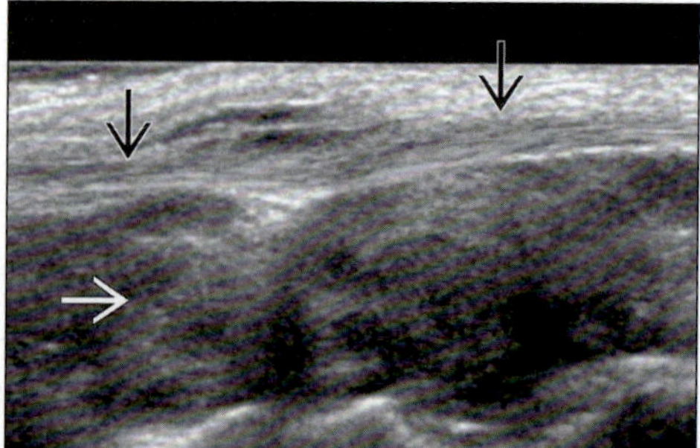

Giant Cell Tumor of Tendon Sheath

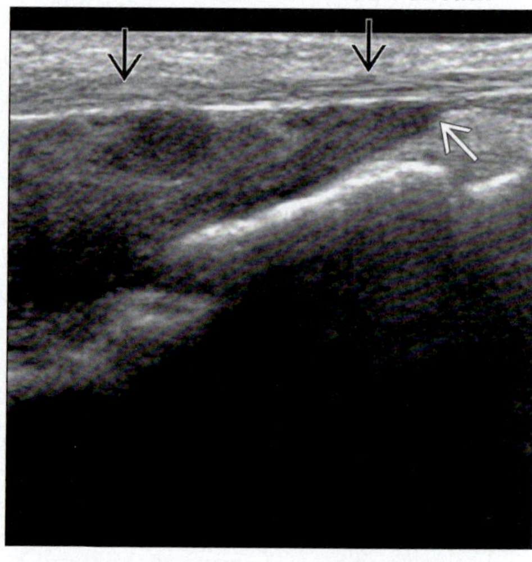

(Left) Transverse US shows a globular, hypoechoic tumor ➡ along the flexor pollicis longus tendon ➡. Note that the tumor contacts only a small area of the tendon sheath. Complete encasement of tendon sheath by a giant cell tumor is relatively uncommon compared to partial contact. *(Right)* Correlative transverse color Doppler US shows marked hyperemia ➡ in and around a giant cell tumor of the tendon sheath. Most giant cell tumors show moderate to high vascularity.

Giant Cell Tumor of Tendon Sheath

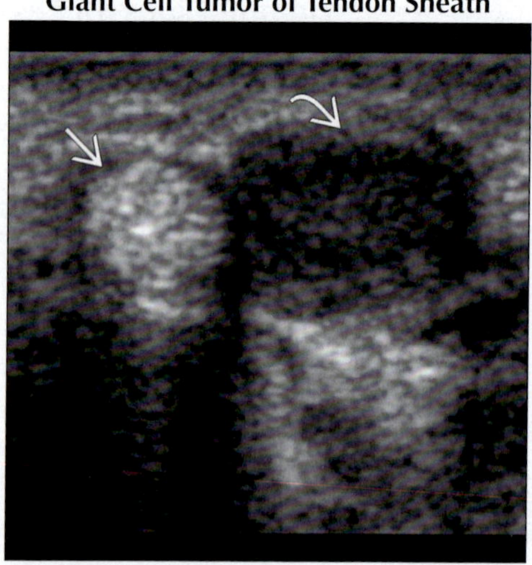

Giant Cell Tumor of Tendon Sheath

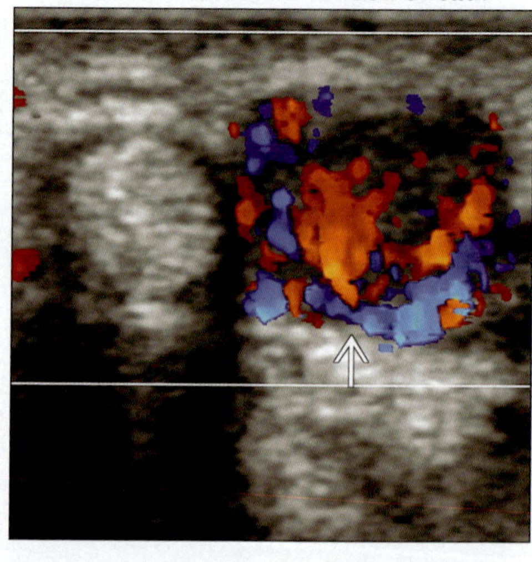

(Left) Longitudinal ultrasound shows 2 discrete, hypoechoic nodules ➡ alongside the flexor digitorum tendon ➡ in a patient with recurrence of a giant cell tumor of the tendon sheath. Usually there is only a single tumor focus. *(Right)* Longitudinal ultrasound shows thickening of the A1 pulley ➡ overlying the flexor tendons ➡ and metacarpophalangeal joint ➡ of the middle finger in a patient with "trigger finger."

Giant Cell Tumor of Tendon Sheath

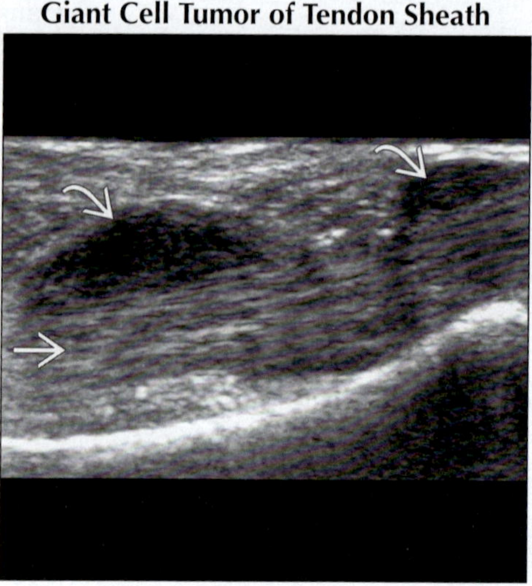

Annular Pulley Thickening

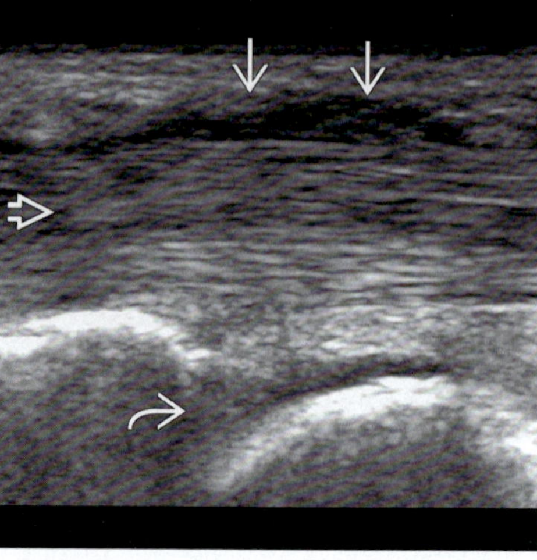

15

PERITENDINOUS MASS

Annular Pulley Thickening

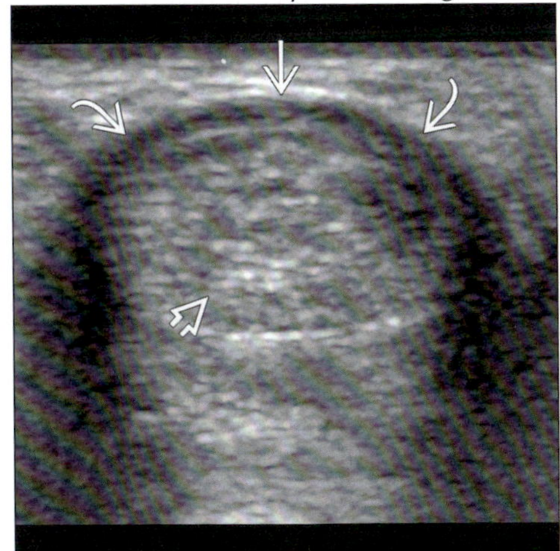

Annular Pulley Thickening

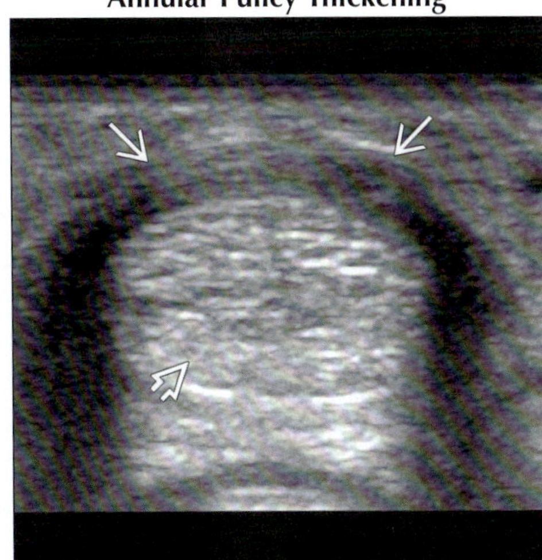

(Left) Transverse ultrasound shows a normal A1 pulley ➡ of the middle finger surrounding the flexor tendons ➡. The thickness of the pulley is best measured at its top ➡ because it always widens toward its basal attachments. Normal pulley thickness is 0.3-0.5 mm. *(Right)* Transverse ultrasound shows a thickened A1 pulley ➡ overlying the flexor tendons ➡ of the middle finger in a patient with "trigger finger." Pulley thickness measured 1.2 mm.

Bursitis

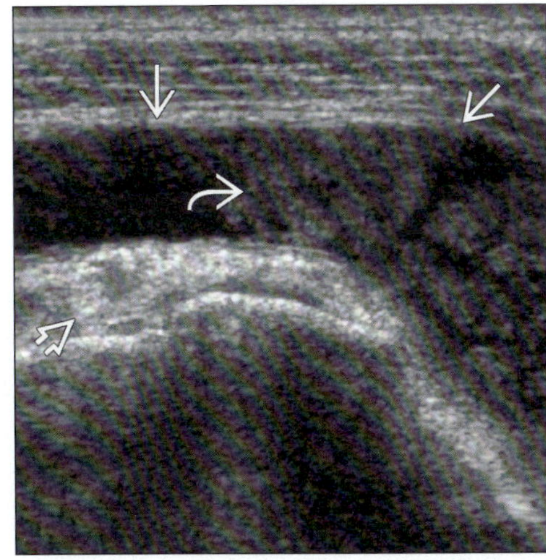

Bursitis

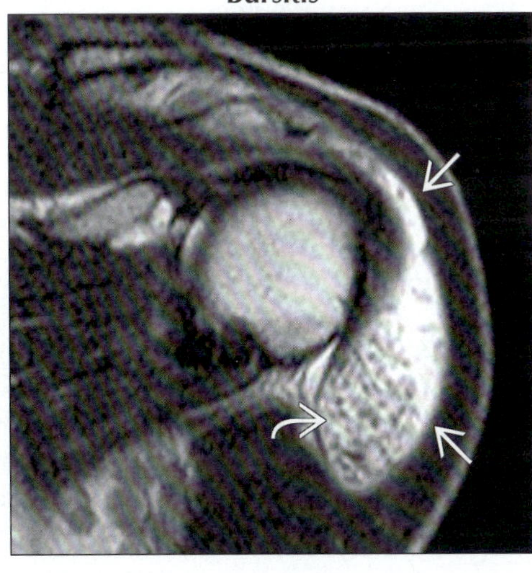

(Left) Transverse ultrasound shows a distended subacromial-subdeltoid bursa ➡ overlying the supraspinatus tendon ➡. The bursa contains several mobile, echogenic nodules ➡ consistent with rice bodies, which represent fibrin aggregates. *(Right)* Correlative longitudinal T2WI MR shows a distended subacromial-subdeltoid bursa ➡ with many small hypointense nodules ➡, consistent with rice bodies.

Gouty Tophus

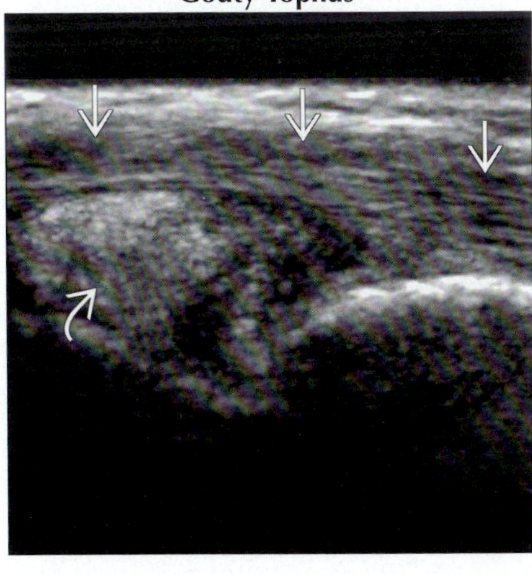

Gouty Tophus

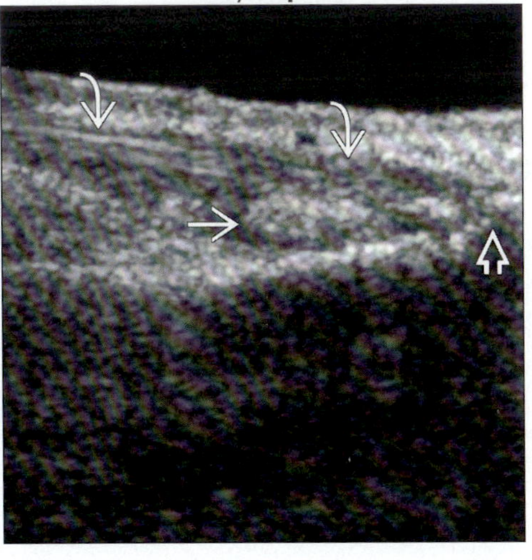

(Left) Longitudinal shows echogenic soft tophus ➡ at the dorsal aspect of the wrist deep to the extensor tendons ➡. Soft tophi contain relatively few crystals and little posterior acoustic shadowing. Gouty tophi are commonly found in peritendinous locations. *(Right)* Longitudinal ultrasound shows a small, echogenic, soft gouty tophus ➡ just deep to the extensor hallucis longus tendon ➡ at the tendon insertion ➡ into the distal phalanx.

TENDON HYPOECHOGENICITY

DIFFERENTIAL DIAGNOSIS

Common
- Anisotropy
- Tendon Tear
- Tendinosis

Less Common
- Xanthoma

ESSENTIAL INFORMATION

Key Differential Diagnosis Issues
- Have clear idea of normal appearances of tendon and insertion before commenting on abnormality
- Changing position of limb can optimize tendon visibility
  - Particularly important in evaluating shoulder
- Always confirm abnormality on orthogonal view
- Dynamic assessment to view tendon movement is useful
- Color Doppler useful to assess tendon vascularity and distinguish between tears and vascular channels
  - Stretching tendon may compress vascularity
  - Also assess when tendon is relaxed
  - Normal tendons show no internal vascularity on color Doppler imaging
- Some tendons more susceptible to angiogenesis than others
  - Achilles, posterior tibialis, patellar, and common extensor tendon origin prone to vascular ingrowth with disease
  - Rotator cuff tendons less frequently show vascular ingrowth

Helpful Clues for Common Diagnoses
- **Anisotropy**
  - Reflectivity of normal tendon, nerve, and muscle is dependent on angle
  - Tendon best seen when incident beam is perpendicular to tendon
  - Any alteration from perpendicular irrespective of direction can lead to loss of reflectivity = anisotropy
    - Tendinosis and tears also lead to loss of echogenicity, so ensure that ultrasound beam is maintained at right angles to tendon

- **Tendon Tear**
  - Ultrasound accurate at detecting macroscopic tendon tears
  - May occur at insertion (avulsive-type), at tendon surface, or within tendon substance (intrasubstance)
  - Tears usually on background of tendinosis
    - Uncommon to see tears in normal healthy tendons
  - Tears tend to happen at specific sites for each tendon
    - Supraspinatus most commonly torn tendon (avulsive-type tear anterior fibers)
    - Achilles tendon tears occur at junction of proximal and middle 1/3 of tendon
    - Common extensor tendon origin → intrasubstance or deep avulsive-type tears
    - Biceps tendon, peroneal and posterior tibialis tendons → longitudinal tears within bicipital groove and just distal to malleoli
  - Tendon discontinuity with hypoechoic area
    - Retraction gap may be filled with echogenic blood, making tear less conspicuous
    - ± tendon indentation and contour deformity
    - ± peritendinous or bursal fluid
  - Peritendinitis
    - Edema and hyperemia of peritendinous tissues
    - Important feature to note as it will respond to antiinflammatory medication
- **Tendinosis**
  - Failed wound healing cascade after microtear sustained during specific injury or repetitive microtrauma due to overuse
  - Pathologically represents degenerative process of tendons
    - Hypercellularity and irregular vascular ingrowth
    - Collagen fiber disorganization and thinning
    - ↑ interfibrillar glycosaminoglycan deposition
    - Inflammatory cell infiltrate not feature of tendinosis
  - Tendons more prone to tendinosis in upper limb

15

TENDON HYPOECHOGENICITY

- Supraspinatus, infraspinatus, subscapularis, and long head of biceps
- Common tendon extensor origin, extensor carpi ulnaris, abductor pollicis longus, and extensor pollicis brevis
  - Tendons more prone to tendinosis in lower limb
    - Hamstrings at ischial tuberosity attachment; gluteus minimus and medius at greater trochanteric insertion
    - Quadriceps, patellar, Achilles tendon, and posterior tibialis
  - Seen on ultrasound as tendon thickening, hypoechogenicity, loss of normal fibrillar pattern ± focal hyperemia
    - ± cortical irregularity ± hyperostosis at insertional area
    - ± intrinsic tendon calcification
    - ± variable degree of peritendinitis
  - May be focal or diffuse
  - Tendon thickening
    - Tendon cross-sectional area larger than expected (compare with asymptomatic side if normal in appearance)
  - Loss of normal fibrillar pattern and hypoechogenicity
    - Due to proteoglycan matrix deposition between tendon fibrils
  - Hyperemia
    - Vessels not present within normal tendons
    - Level of hyperemia is proportional to level of tendinosis disease activity
    - May be related to disease progression or repair; reduction in hyperemia correlates with ↓ of symptoms
    - Subjectively graded as mild, moderate, or severe
    - For Achilles tendon, mild is ≤ 2 vessel ingrowth, moderate is 3-4 vessel ingrowth, & severe is ≥ 5 vessel ingrowth

Helpful Clues for Less Common Diagnoses
- **Xanthoma**
  - Tendon xanthomas are manifestation of familial hyperlipidemia
  - Appear as fusiform enlargement of tendon ± discrete or confluent hypoechoic areas
    - Xanthomas composed of lipid-filled foamy histiocytes, extracellular cholesterol, and giant cells
  - Most commonly occur in Achilles tendon, though patellar tendon and extensor tendons of hands and feet may also be affected
  - May regress with lipid-lowering treatment
  - May be difficult to distinguish from tendinosis
    - Lack of pain, atypical distribution in affected tendon, and less hyperemia on color Doppler imaging may be helpful distinguishing features

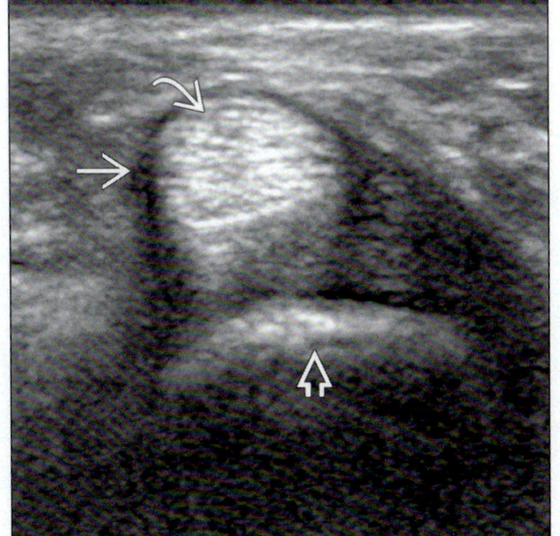

Anisotropy

Transverse ultrasound of the middle finger shows normal echogenicity of flexor tendons ⇗ at the level of the A1 pulley ⇗ and metacarpal head ⇒.

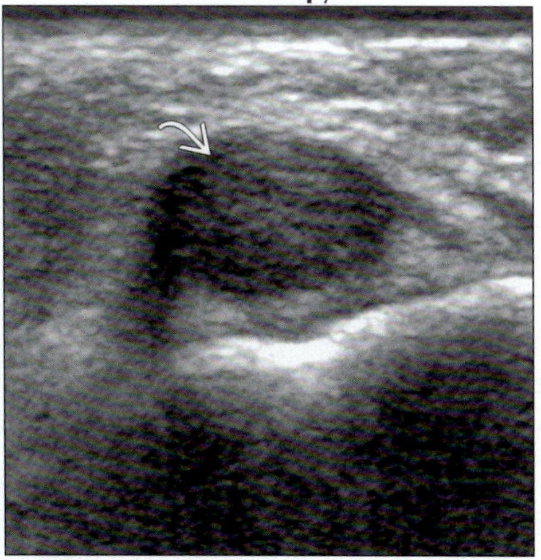

Anisotropy

Transverse ultrasound at the same level shows that tendon echogenicity ⇗ changes from hyperechoic to hypoechoic when the transducer is not aligned at a right angle to the tendon.

TENDON HYPOECHOGENICITY

Tendon Tear

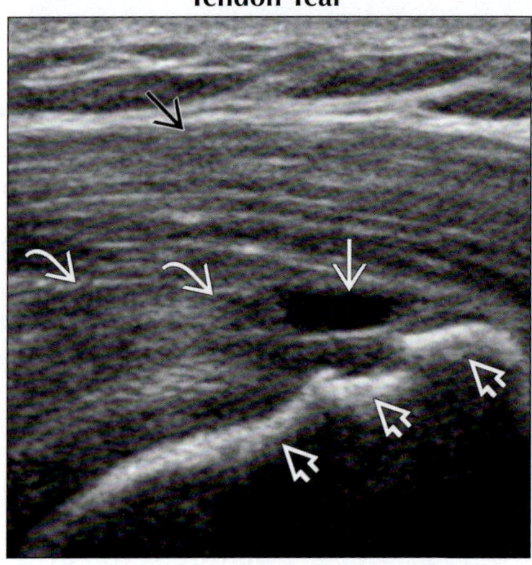

Tendon Tear

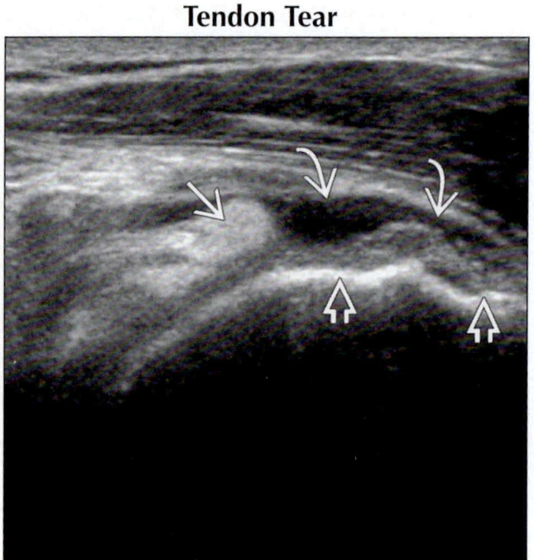

(Left) Longitudinal US of the supraspinatus tendon ➔ shows a medium-sized partial thickness bursal-surface tear ➔ at the lateral end of greater tuberosity ➔, a common site of a tear. Note overlying deltoid muscle ➔. *(Right)* Longitudinal US shows a large avulsive-type tear from the greater tuberosity ➔ of the retracted supraspinatus tendon ➔. Only some short fibers remain attached to greater tuberosity. Note fluid in subacromial-subdeltoid bursa ➔.

Tendon Tear

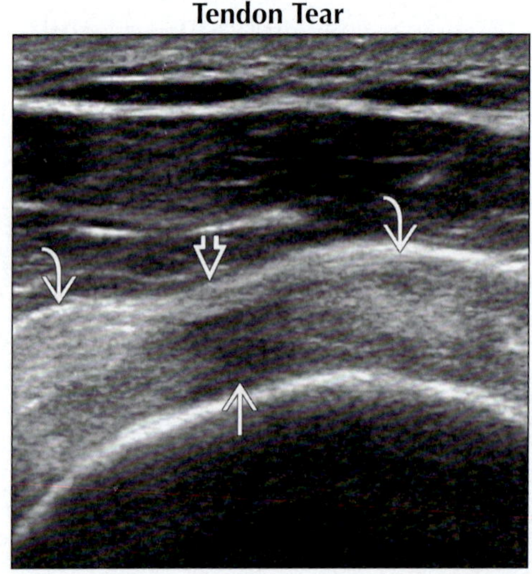

Tendon Tear

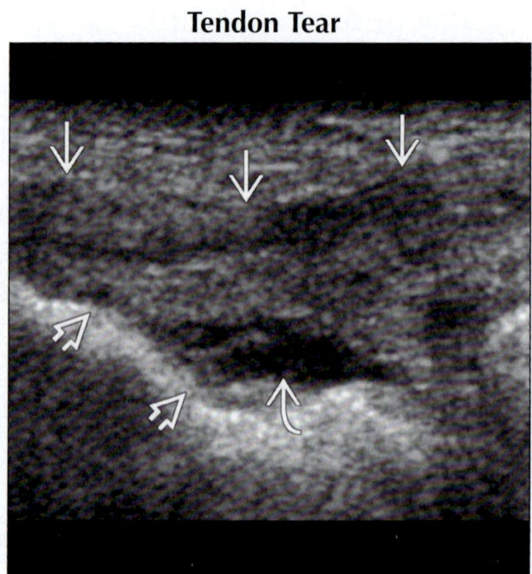

(Left) Transverse ultrasound shows a full-thickness tear ➔ of the supraspinatus tendon ➔ proximal to the greater tuberosity with flattening of the bursal contour ➔. *(Right)* Longitudinal ultrasound shows a large avulsive-type tear ➔ of the deep common extensor tendon ➔ from its attachment to the lateral humeral condyle ➔.

Tendon Tear

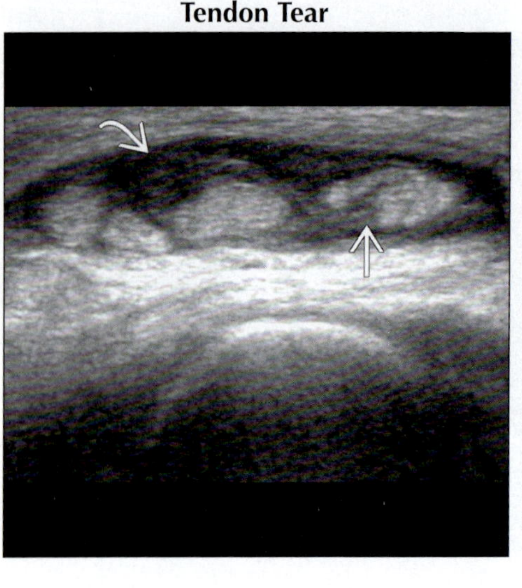

Tendinosis

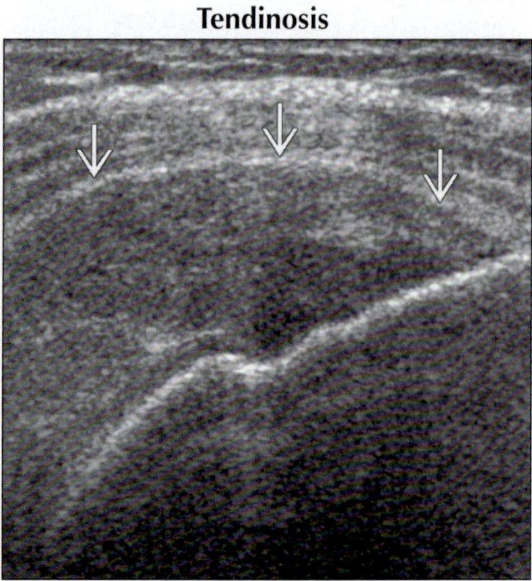

(Left) Transverse ultrasound shows a partial thickness longitudinal tear ➔ of the extensor tendon of the ring finger and background tenosynovitis with distension and synovial proliferation ➔ of the tendon sheath. Minimal hyperemia was present on color Doppler (not shown). *(Right)* Transverse ultrasound shows severe tendinosis of the supraspinatus tendon ➔. The tendon is thickened with complete loss of its normal fibrillar pattern.

15

TENDON HYPOECHOGENICITY

Tendinosis

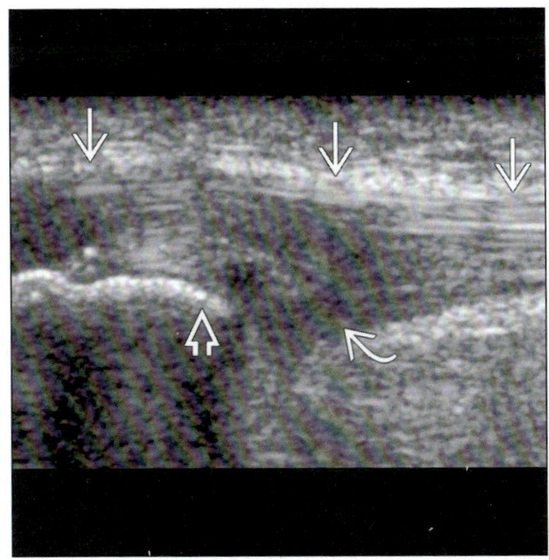

Tendinosis

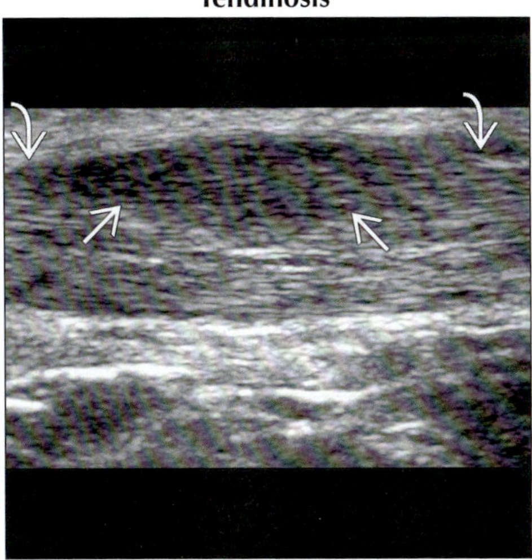

(Left) Longitudinal US of the patellar tendon ➡ shows severe tendinosis with focal hypoechogenicity ➘ due to proteoglycan accumulation, mainly affecting the tendon undersurface near the lower pole of the patella ⮞. *(Right)* Longitudinal US of the Achilles tendon ➘ shows a focal area of hypoechogenicity and swelling ➡ due to moderately severe tendinosis in the mid-portion of the Achilles tendon. Mild focal hyperemia was present (not shown).

Tendinosis

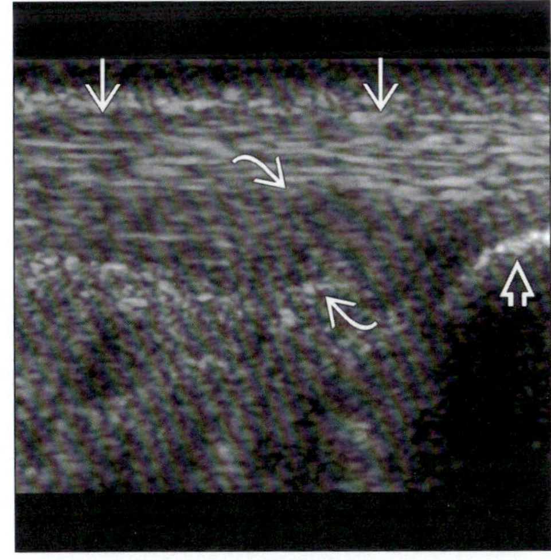

Tendinosis

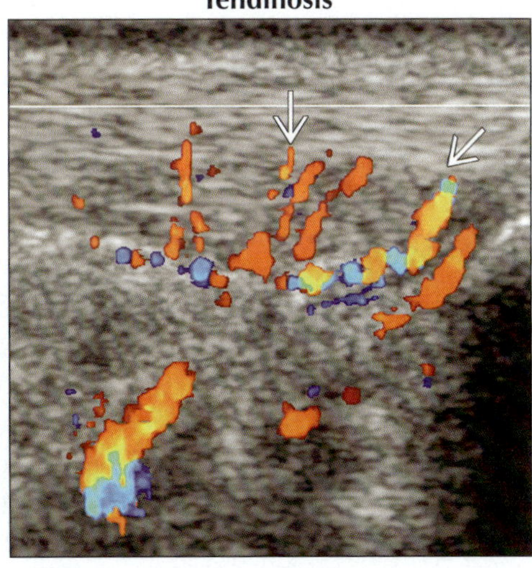

(Left) Longitudinal ultrasound of the Achilles tendon ➡ shows moderately severe insertional tendinosis with hypoechogenicity ➘ on the undersurface of the tendon at the upper border of the calcaneum ⮞. *(Right)* Longitudinal color Doppler ultrasound at the same location shows moderate hyperemia ➡ of the Achilles tendon entering from the deep surface of the tendon. This is consistent with active disease.

Xanthoma

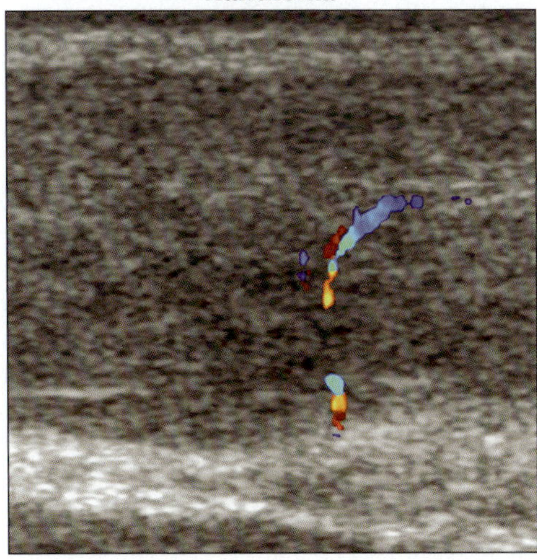

Xanthoma

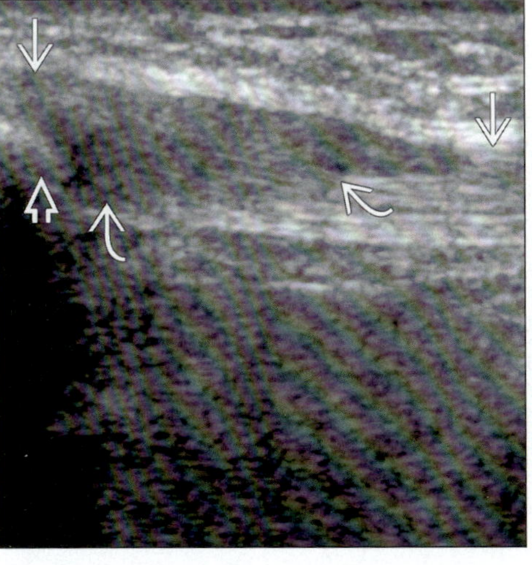

(Left) Longitudinal ultrasound of the Achilles tendon shows diffuse swelling, hypoechogenicity, loss of normal fibrillar pattern, and mild hyperemia of the tendon in this patient with hyperlipidemia. *(Right)* Longitudinal ultrasound of the patellar tendon ➘ in a patient with hyperlipidemia shows a focal hypoechoic area ➘ at the inferior pole of the patella ⮞ due to deposition of cholesterol-rich lipids within the tendon. Any part of the tendon may be affected.

DIFFERENTIAL DIAGNOSIS

Common
- Calcific Tendinitis
- Calcification within Tendinosis
- Gouty Tenosynovitis

Less Common
- Tendon Tear
- Accessory Ossicles
- Suture Material within Tendon

ESSENTIAL INFORMATION

Key Differential Diagnosis Issues
- Normal tendons are echogenic with distinct fibrillar pattern
- Areas of tendon hyperechogenicity are usually due to crystal deposition within tendon substance
  - Alternatively gas, blood, or suture
- US more sensitive than radiograph or MR at detecting crystal deposition within tendons
- Large areas of crystal deposition within tendon may limit assessment of adjacent tears

Helpful Clues for Common Diagnoses
- **Calcific Tendinitis**
  - Due to deposition of hydroxyapatite crystal within tendon substance
  - Leads to severe pain and restriction of movement
    - Can affect any joint or tendon
  - Some tendons more commonly affected than others
  - Tendons around shoulder are most commonly affected
    - Supraspinatus tendon
    - Infraspinatus tendon
    - Subscapularis tendon
  - Focal hyperechoic area of varying size and shape
    - Arch-shaped (most common)
    - Punctuate or fragmented
    - Nodular
    - Cystic type (uncommon)
  - ± shadowing depending on size
  - ± tendinosis
  - ± tendon tear
  - ± bursitis
  - ± intraarticular hydroxyapatite crystal deposition
  - ± peri-calcific color flow on Doppler imaging
    - Grade 0 = no flow
    - Grade 1 = weak spot of color flow signal
    - Grade 2 = few linear color flow signals
    - Grade 3 = many linear color flow signals
  - Color Doppler may be able to distinguish between formative and resorptive phases of calcific tendinitis
    - If no peri-calcific color flow visible → formative phase → aspiration may be indicated
    - If peri-calcific color flow visible → resorptive phase → conservative treatment may be indicated, better clinical outcome
  - Several tendons may be affected simultaneously
  - Contralateral side also frequently affected, even though asymptomatic
    - Any joint may be affected but mostly shoulder
  - Treatment includes analgesia and local heat
  - ± ultrasound-guided needling ± aspiration or surgery
  - ± ultrasound-guided steroid or long-acting local anesthetic
- **Calcification within Tendinosis**
  - Usually only found within Achilles tendon and to lesser extent posterior tibialis and patellar tendons
    - Site-specificity allows easy differentiation from calcific tendinitis, which mainly affects rotator cuff tendons
  - Affects tendons close to insertional area
    - Posterosuperior aspect calcaneus of Achilles tendon
    - Medial inferior navicular bone and adjacent bones for posterior tibialis tendon
  - Background tendinosis
  - Discrete areas of calcification within tendon from few mm to few cm
    - Strong propensity to ossify
    - Not possible to aspirate, unlike calcific tendinitis
  - Strong posterior acoustic shadowing
  - Usually associated with reactive changes at insertional area
    - Cortical irregularity

15

- Cortical surface fragmentation
- Cortical hyperostosis and spur formation
  - ○ May occur in asymptomatic subjects with no other US features of tendinosis
- **Gouty Tenosynovitis**
  - ○ Crystal deposition within tendon substance
  - ○ Most crystal deposition tends to be around tendons, ligaments, and joints
    - Intratendinous deposition is more feature of chronic gouty arthropathy
    - Rare feature of hydroxyapatite crystal deposition
  - ○ Focal tendon thickening
    - Loss of normal fibrillar pattern
  - ○ Intratendinous crystal aggregates seen as "comet tail" artifacts within tendon
    - ± posterior acoustic shadowing depending on level of crystal deposition
    - ± mild peritendinous or intratendinous hyperemia
  - ○ Usually associated with other features of gout
    - Gouty arthropathy
    - Soft or hard extraarticular gouty tophi
  - ○ Normally affects tendons of wrist/hand or ankle/foot
    - Uncommon in larger tendons

Helpful Clues for Less Common Diagnoses
- **Tendon Tear**
  - ○ Often associated with hemorrhage
    - Acute hemorrhage may be echogenic on ultrasound

- Makes tear less readily visible on ultrasound
  - ○ Look for associated secondary signs of tear
    - Flattening or indentation of tendon surface
    - Loss of continuity of tendon fibrillar pattern
    - Widening of gap on dynamic movement
    - ± compression of hematoma in gap on dynamic scanning
  - ○ Chronic tears may also be filled with echogenic fat, particularly in Achilles tendon
- **Accessory Ossicles**
  - ○ Most common accessory ossicles within tendon are accessory navicular bone (within posterior tibialis tendon) and os peroneum (within peroneus longus)
  - ○ May be confused with dystrophic ossification
    - Accessory ossicle has smooth convex superficial border, while dystrophic ossification is more irregular
  - ○ Fractures or displacement of os peroneum can be clue to peroneus longus tear
- **Suture Material within Tendon**
  - ○ Often nonabsorbable and thus may be visible many years after tendon repair
    - Easily recognized as tubular echogenic material within tendon substance

Calcific Tendinitis

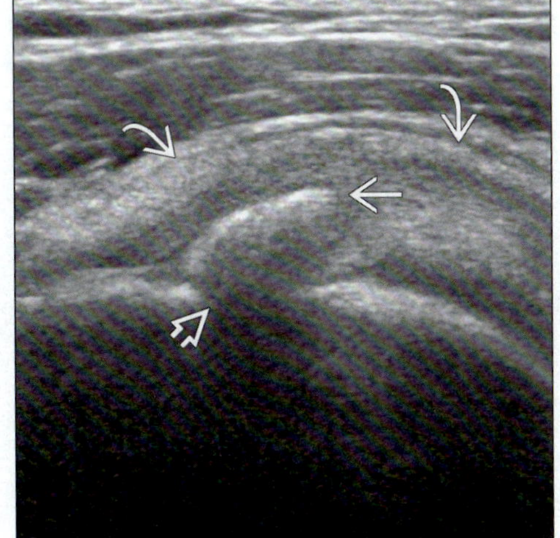

Longitudinal ultrasound shows an area of calcific tendinitis ➡ within the supraspinatus tendon ➡ at its insertion. Posterior acoustic shadowing limits visibility of the insertional area ➡.

Calcific Tendinitis

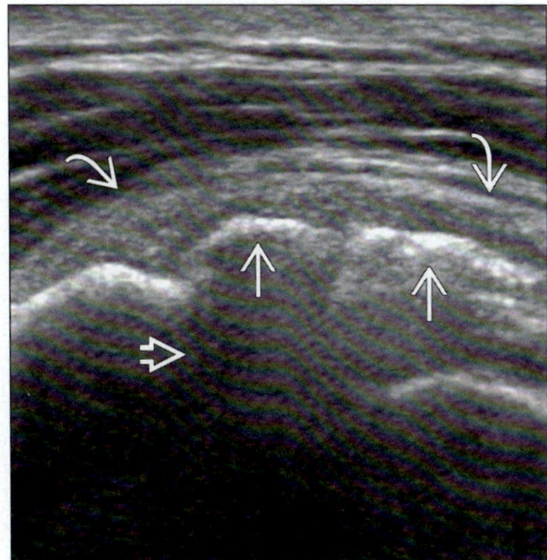

Longitudinal ultrasound shows a large area of calcific tendinitis ➡ close to the insertion site of the supraspinatus tendon ➡. Posterior acoustic shadowing gives the impression of a humeral cortical defect ➡.

TENDON HYPERECHOGENICITY

(Left) Longitudinal ultrasound shows a focal area of calcific tendinitis ➡ within the infraspinatus tendon ➡, close to the insertion. A surrounding hypoechogenic rim ➡ is present. *(Right)* Transverse ultrasound shows nonconfluent calcific tendinitis ➡ within the subscapularis tendon ➡ close to the insertion site. There is moderate distension of the overlying subacromial-subdeltoid bursa ➡.

Calcific Tendinitis

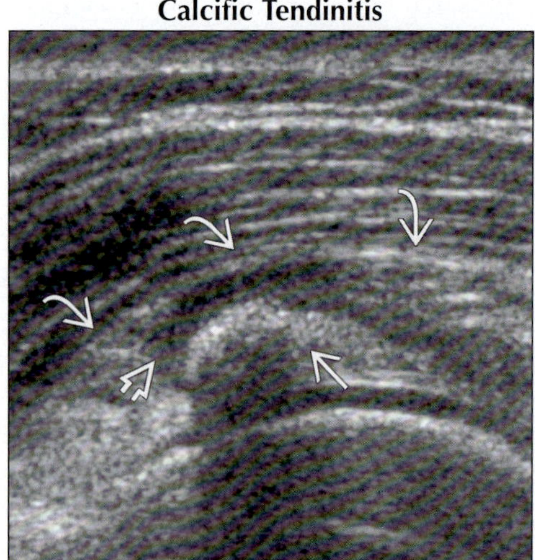

Calcific Tendinitis

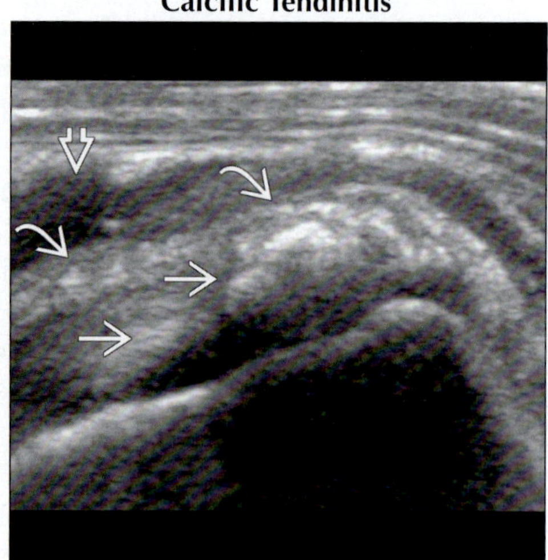

(Left) Longitudinal US shows localized calcific tendinitis ➡ involving the coracobrachialis tendon ➡ at the attachment to coracoid process of the scapula ➡. The patient had localized pain and tenderness in this area. *(Right)* Longitudinal US shows a focal area of hypoechoic tendinosis, associated with early calcification exhibiting "comet tail" artifacts ➡ at the common extensor tendon origin ➡ from the lateral humeral condyle ➡.

Calcific Tendinitis

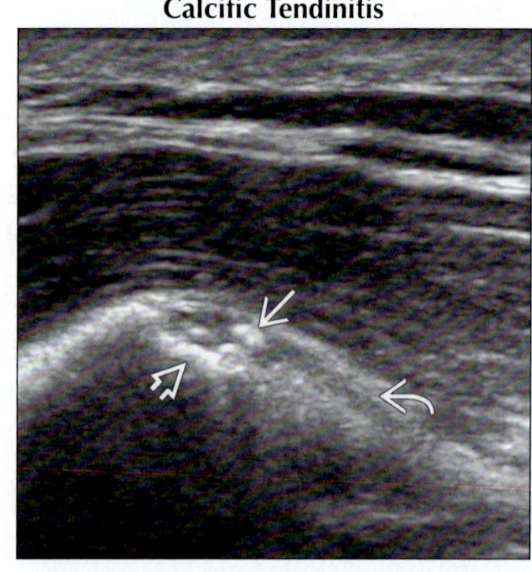

Calcification within Tendinosis

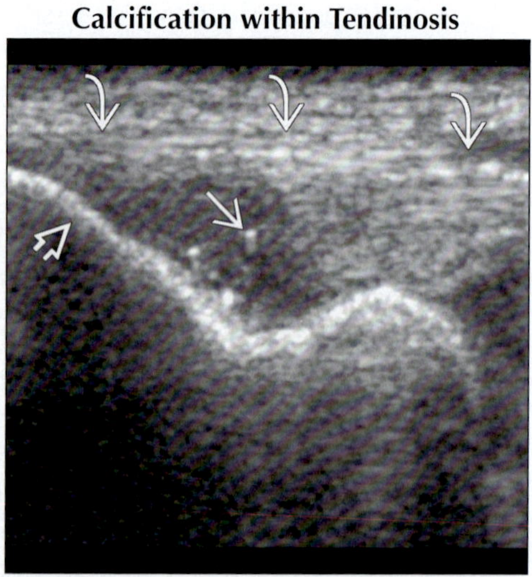

(Left) Longitudinal US shows focal insertional tendinosis of the posterior tibialis tendon ➡. It was hyperemic on color Doppler and has internal dystrophic calcification ➡ (navicular bone ➡). *(Right)* Longitudinal US shows a focal area of dystrophic calcification ➡ within the middle 1/3 of the Achilles tendon ➡. Tendon calcification associated with tendinosis is often asymptomatic, while calcific tendinitis can be very painful.

Calcification within Tendinosis

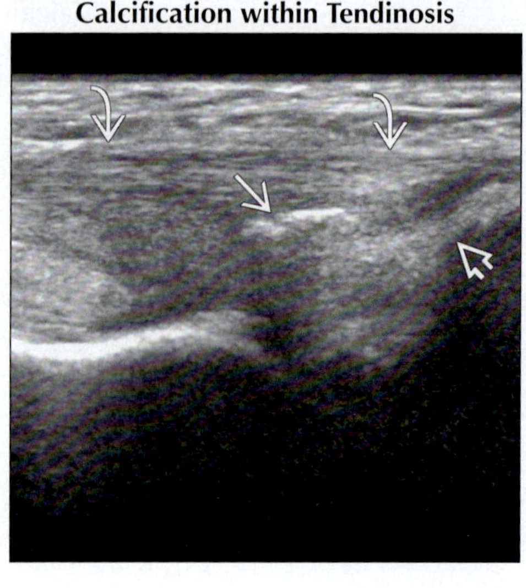

Calcification within Tendinosis

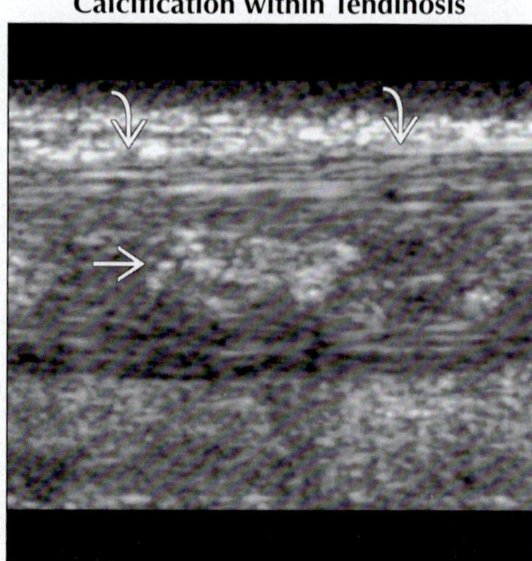

15

TENDON HYPERECHOGENICITY

Gouty Tenosynovitis

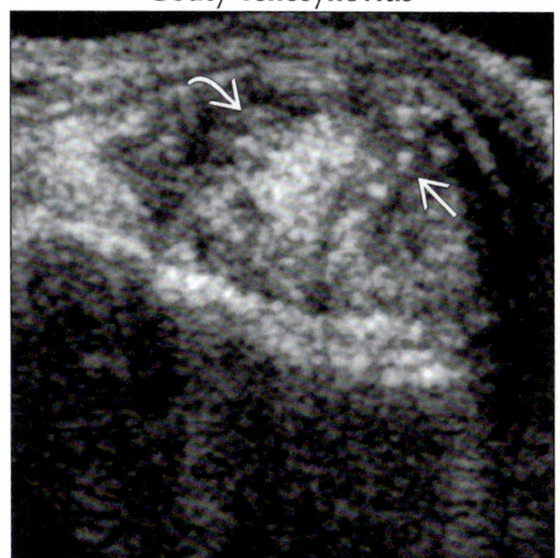

Gouty Tenosynovitis

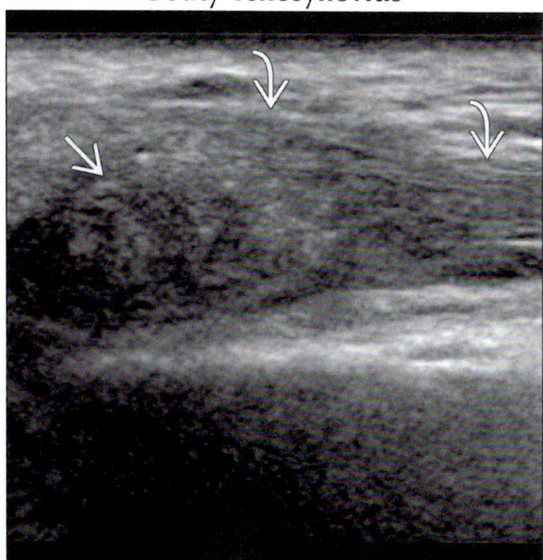

(Left) Transverse US shows an enlarged, hyperechoic extensor carpi ulnaris tendon ➡ containing several small "comet tail" artifacts ➡, consistent with intratendinous crystal deposition. This patient had chronic tophaceous gout. *(Right)* Longitudinal US shows echogenic gouty tophus ➡ expanding the extensor tendon ➡ on the dorsum of the hand. There are several small "comet tail" artifacts representing crystal aggregation within the tophus.

Tendon Tear

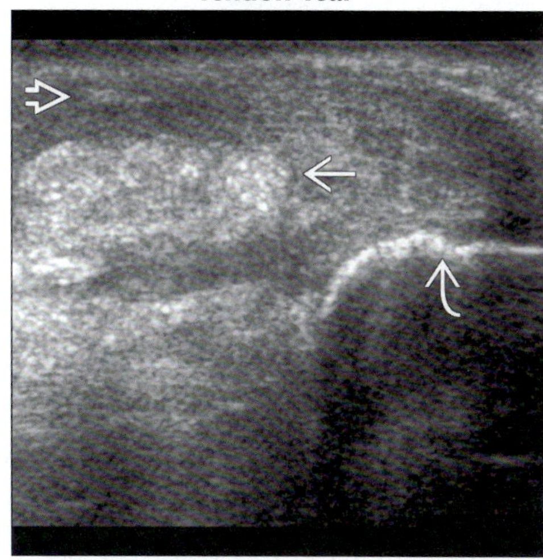

Tendon Tear

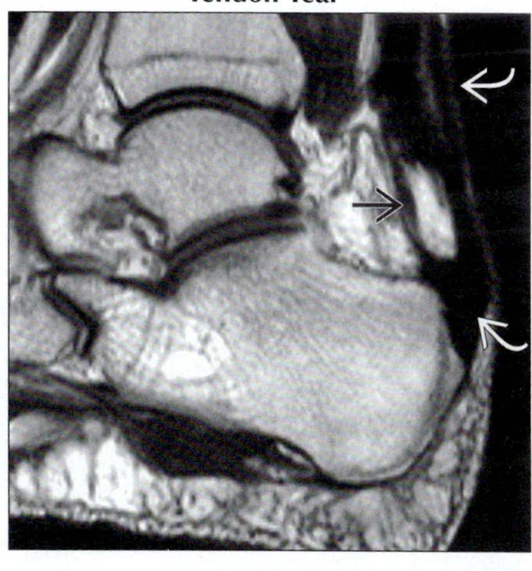

(Left) Longitudinal US shows a thickened distal Achilles tendon ➡ just proximal to the calcaneus ➡. There is a large tear on the deep surface of the tendon, which is filled with echogenic fat ➡. Note lack of both strong reflective echoes & acoustic shadowing, often seen with calcification. *(Right)* Sagittal T2WI MR in the same patient shows a thickened Achilles tendon ➡ with hyperintense tissue ➡ in the defect at the deep margin of the tendon, consistent with a fat-filled, chronic tendon tear.

Tendon Tear

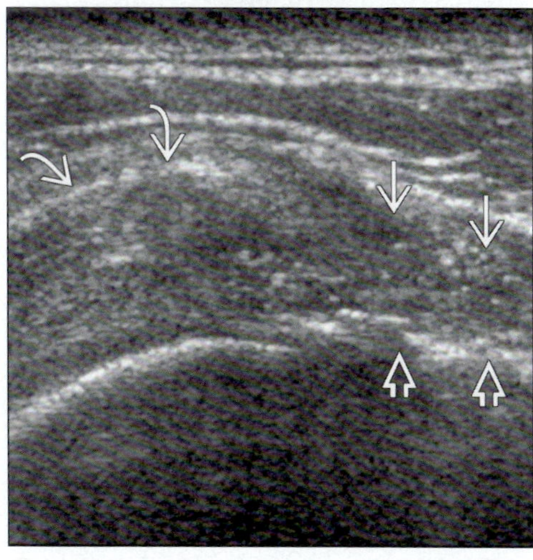

Accessory Ossicles

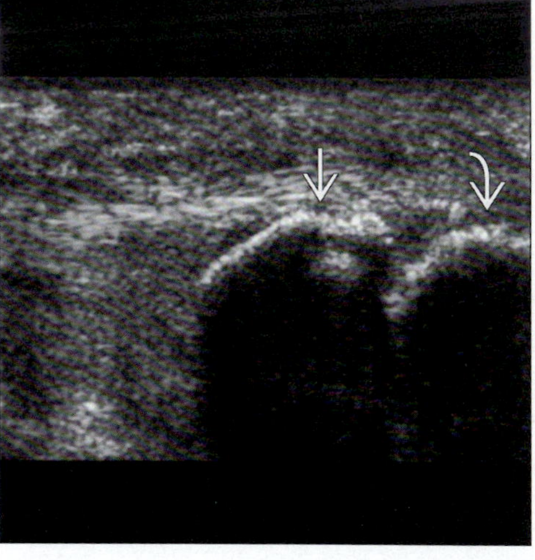

(Left) Longitudinal US shows a complete tear of the supraspinatus tendon ➡, which is retracted from the greater tuberosity ➡. The retraction gap is filled with echogenic blood ➡, making the tendon tear less visible. *(Right)* Longitudinal ultrasound shows a large accessory navicular bone ➡ with a rounded superior border in close proximity to the medial pole of the navicular bone ➡.

TENDON SWELLING

DIFFERENTIAL DIAGNOSIS

Common
- Tendinosis

Less Common
- Acute Nonexudative Tenosynovitis
- Acute Exudative Tenosynovitis
- Chronic Active Tenosynovitis
- Chronic Inactive Tenosynovitis
- Gout and Pseudogout
- Xanthomatosis

ESSENTIAL INFORMATION

Key Differential Diagnosis Issues
- Need to determine whether primary pathology affects tendon or tendon sheath
- Distinction between tendinosis and tenosynovitis has important therapeutic and prognostic implications
  - Tendinosis = tendon disease with secondary involvement of peritendinous structures
    - Tenosynovitis = disease of tendon sheath with secondary involvement of tendon
  - Tendinosis results from microtears, proteoglycan deposition, and collagen disorganization
    - Tenosynovitis results from tendon sheath inflammation due to bacteria, crystals, inflammatory mediators, or repetitive movement
  - Tendinosis = not primary inflammatory disease
    - Tenosynovitis = primary inflammatory disease
  - Tendinosis effects any tendon
    - Tenosynovitis only affects tendons with tendon sheath
  - Tendinosis often affects only segment of tendon
    - Tenosynovitis usually affects all of tendon contained by tendon sheath
  - Tendinosis often subclinical
    - Tenosynovitis rarely subclinical
  - Tendinosis frequently predisposes to tendon tear or rupture
    - Tenosynovitis infrequently predisposes to tendon tear or rupture
  - Tendinosis treated primarily by rest and is likely to recur

- Tenosynovitis treated primarily by antibiotics and not likely to recur
- Note that mild tendon and tendon sheath swelling occurs in presence of cellulitis or edema as feature of generalized soft tissue swelling
  - Do not misdiagnose as tenosynovitis

Helpful Clues for Common Diagnoses
- **Tendinosis**
  - Very common, especially in rotator cuff tendons and long head of biceps tendon
  - Supraspinatus > infraspinatus > subscapularis > teres minor
  - Long head of biceps near top of bicipital groove
  - Progressive tendon thickening from mild → severe
  - Progressive loss of normal fibrillar pattern
  - Increasing tendon hypoechogenicity
  - Tendon hyperemia
    - More common in some tendons than others
    - Uncommon around shoulder, hip, and posterior aspect of knee
    - Common around elbow, wrist, anterior aspect of knee, and ankle/foot
  - ± tendon tear
    - Intrasubstance, avulsive-type, or full-thickness tears
  - ± tendon sheath effusion or peritendinous bursal distension
  - ± peritendinitis with inflammation of soft tissues around tendon
    - Important to note as it will respond to antiinflammatory treatment
  - ± reactive changes at bony insertional area
    - Hyperostotic or resorptive changes
  - ± dystrophic calcification within tendon

Helpful Clues for Less Common Diagnoses
- **Acute Nonexudative Tenosynovitis**
  - Due to inflammation or infection
  - Synovial proliferation within tendon sheath > tendon sheath fluid
  - Hyperemia predominates around, rather than within, tendon sheath
  - Commonly affects common flexor tendon sheath (ulnar bursa) of hand
    - Ulnar bursa extends from just proximal → just distal to carpal tunnel
    - Communicates with 1 of digital flexor tendon sheaths in ~ 10% normal subjects

15

- Communicates with radial bursa in ~ 5% of normal subjects
- Ulnar bursal infection may also spread → space of Parona
- Space of Parona = potential space superficial to pronator quadratus muscle, which extends to mid-forearm

- **Acute Exudative Tenosynovitis**
  - Due to acute infection
  - Fluid accumulation within sheath with little or no synovial proliferation
  - Speckled echogenic fluid
    - Speckles due to aggregates of purulent material
  - Mild tendon swelling
    - ± indistinct tendon margins if infection established and severe
  - Hyperemia around, rather than within, tendon sheath
  - Infection may spread → surrounding tissues
  - Ultrasound-guided aspiration helpful to identify infective organism
- **Chronic Active Tenosynovitis**
  - Due to inflammation or infection
  - Synovium is visibly hypervascular on color Doppler imaging; in acute tenosynovitis, synovium is NOT visibly hypervascular
- **Chronic Inactive Tenosynovitis**
  - Tendon sheath thickening with fluid or synovial proliferation, though little or no hypervascularity

- In stenosing tenosynovitis, tendon sheath markedly distended focally and noncompressible
- Some expected overlap exists among various categories of tenosynovitis
- **Gout and Pseudogout**
  - Tophi within tendons seen commonly in chronic crystal deposition disease
  - Range from soft tophi → hard tophi
    - Soft tophi → scattered crystal aggregates with "comet tail" artifacts
    - Hard tophi → only superficial margin seen due to dense posterior acoustic shadowing
- **Xanthomatosis**
  - Feature of familial hyperlipidemia
  - Accumulation of foamy histiocytes, cholesterol, and giant cells
  - Achilles tendon > patellar tendon > extensor tendons of hands and feet
  - Focal or more generalized tendon swelling, increased tendon hypoechogenicity, and mild hypervascularity
  - Difficult to distinguish from tendinosis
    - Known hyperlipidemia, lack of pain, ↓ hyperemia, and atypical location in affected tendon may be helpful distinguishing features
  - Xanthomas may regress with lipid-lowering treatment

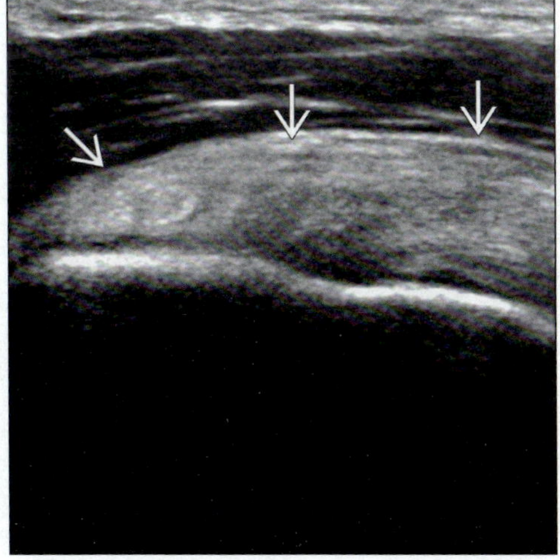

Tendinosis

Transverse ultrasound along the long axis of the supraspinatus tendon ➡ shows mild tendinosis as evidenced by mild tendon thickening and a decrease in the normal fibrillar pattern of the tendon.

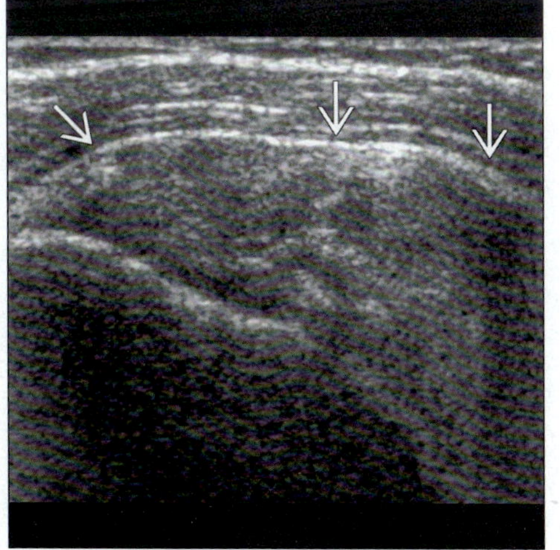

Tendinosis

Transverse ultrasound of the long axis of the supraspinatus tendon ➡ shows severe tendinosis with marked tendon thickening, severe hypoechogenicity, and loss of normal fibrillar pattern.

TENDON SWELLING

(Left) Transverse US shows marked thickening of the extensor pollicis brevis ➜ & abductor pollicis ➡ tendons, consistent with de Quervain tenosynovitis. Although termed tenosynovitis, histologically this is tendinosis. The extensor retinaculum ➡ is mildly thickened. *(Right)* Oblique US shows severe tendinosis of the posterior tibialis tendon with small longitudinal tears ➜, sheath thickening ➡, and moderate peritendinitis. Retinaculum ➥ is mildly thickened.

Tendinosis

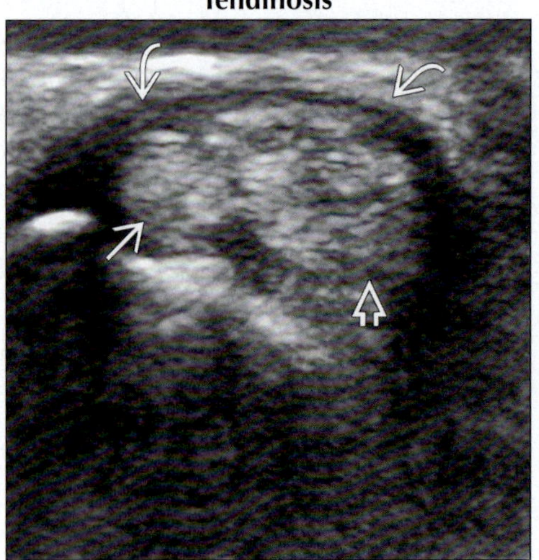

Tendinosis

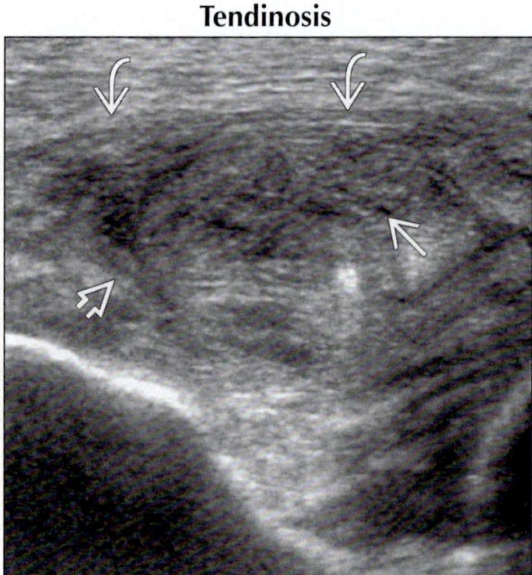

(Left) Transverse ultrasound proximal to carpal tunnel shows swelling of the flexor digitorum tendons and synovial proliferation within the tendon sheath ➡. Fluid accumulation in the space of Parona ➥, overlying the pronator quadratus muscle ➡, is also present. *(Right)* Transverse ultrasound of the mid-palm in the same patient shows swelling of the flexor digitorum tendon sheath ➜ with synovial proliferation and tendon ➥ swelling.

Acute Nonexudative Tenosynovitis

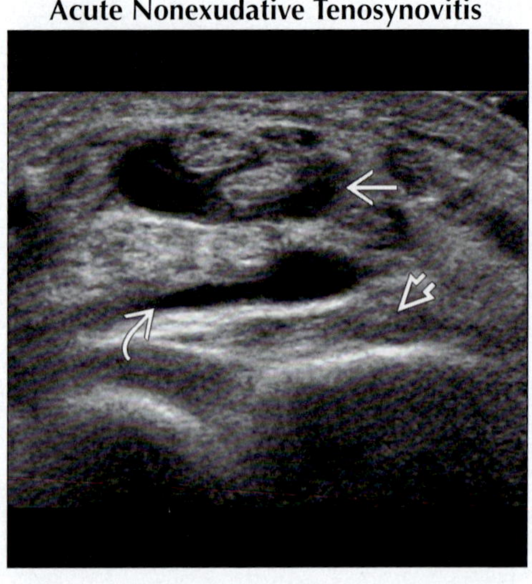

Acute Nonexudative Tenosynovitis

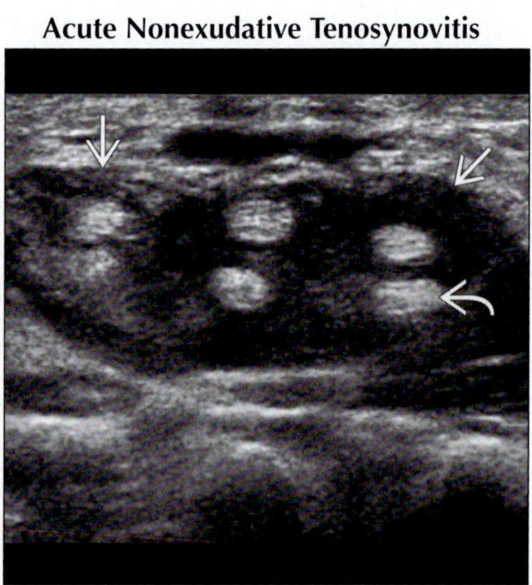

(Left) Transverse ultrasound of a finger shows moderate swelling of the flexor digitorum tendons ➜ and rupture of the tendon sheath, with leakage of inflammatory content ➥ into the swollen peritendinous soft tissues. *(Right)* Transverse color Doppler ultrasound in the same location shows moderate peritendinous hypervascularity ➜.

Acute Nonexudative Tenosynovitis

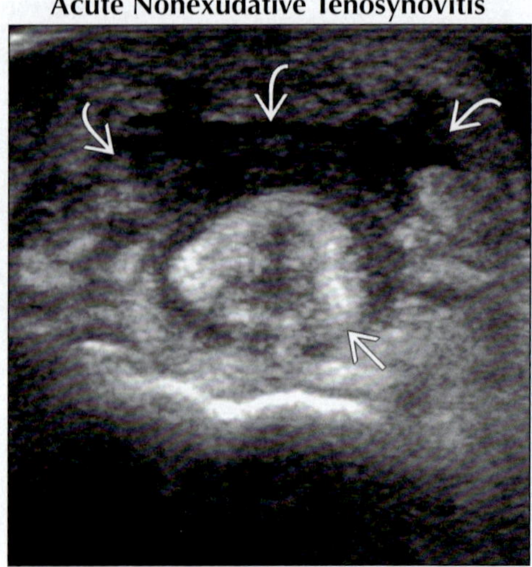

Acute Nonexudative Tenosynovitis

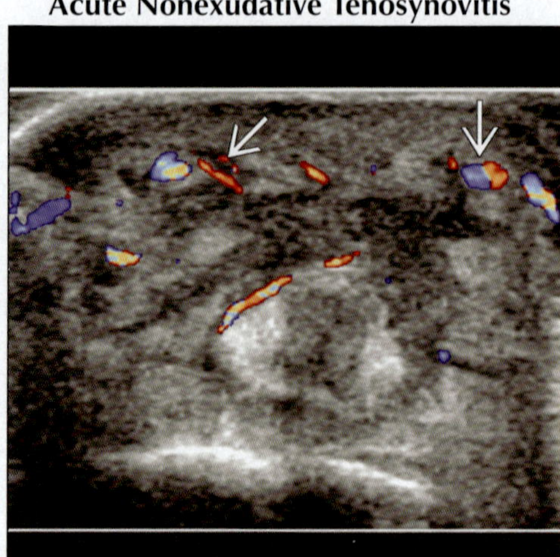

TENDON SWELLING

Acute Exudative Tenosynovitis

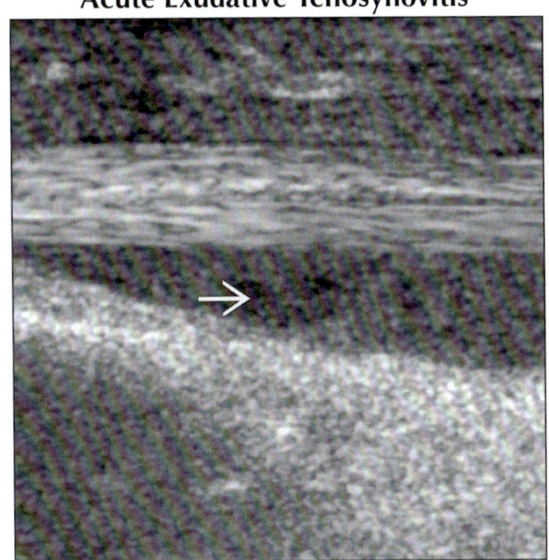

Acute Exudative Tenosynovitis

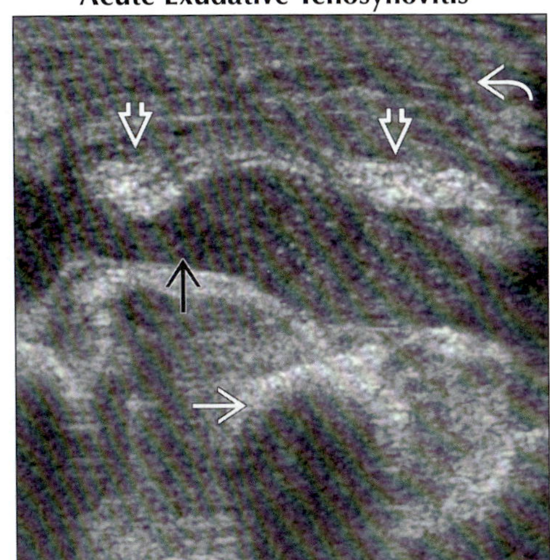

(Left) Longitudinal US on the dorsum of the hand shows a mildly thickened extensor digitorum tendon of the middle finger with an echogenic tendon sheath effusion ➡. Aspirate yielded pus, which grew coagulase negative Staphylococci. (Right) Transverse US dorsum of the wrist shows echogenic fluid ➡ deep to the mildly thickened extensor digitorum tendons ➡ with severe subcutaneous edema ➡. Note the 3rd metacarpal bone ➡.

Chronic Active Tenosynovitis

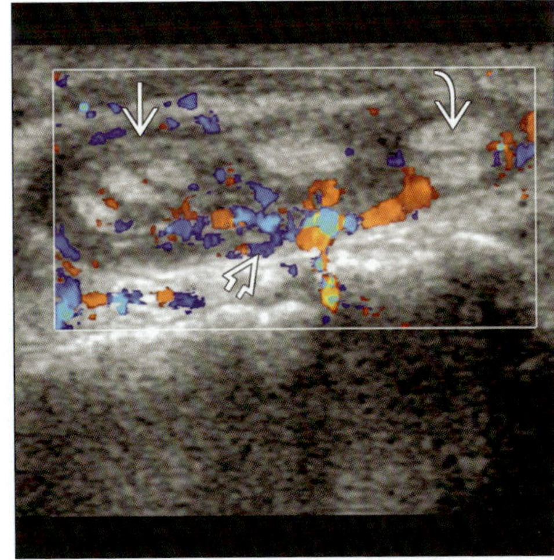

Chronic Inactive Tenosynovitis

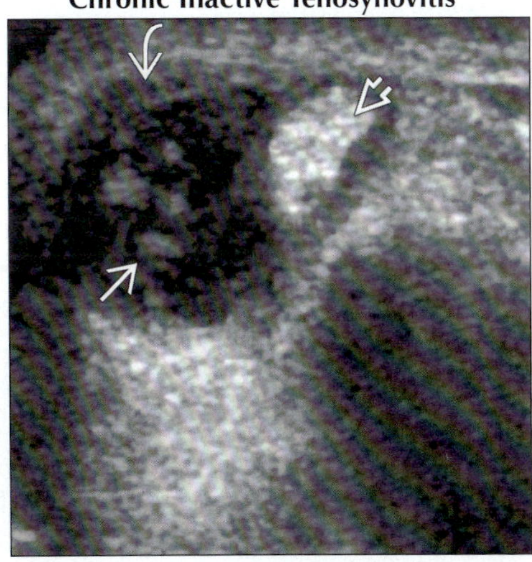

(Left) Transverse color Doppler US of the dorsum of the wrist shows mild extensor digitorum tendon thickening ➡ and moderate synovial proliferation ➡ with synovial hypervascularity ➡. (Right) Transverse US of the wrist shows a markedly distended tendon sheath ➡ of the extensor carpi ulnaris tendon ➡, containing some fibrinous aggregates ➡, appearances that are consistent with stenosing tenosynovitis, a form of chronic tenosynovitis.

Gout and Pseudogout

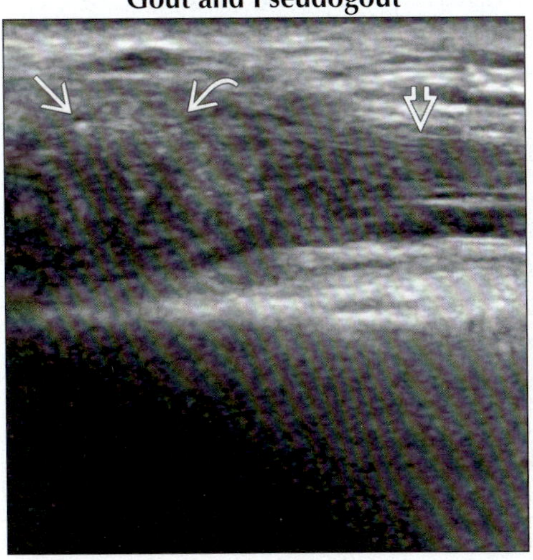

Xanthomatosis

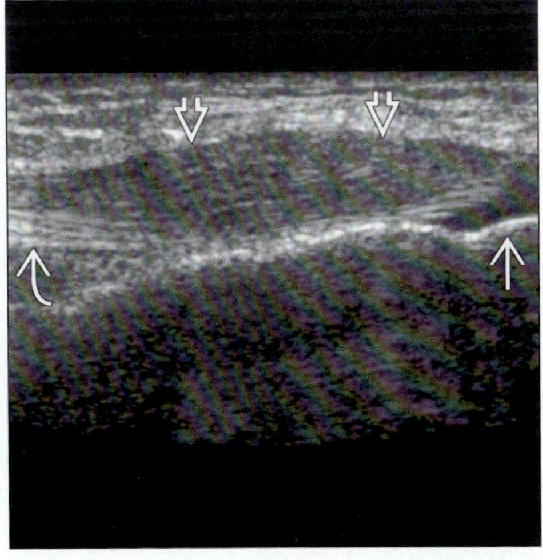

(Left) Longitudinal ultrasound of the distal forearm shows a soft tophus ➡ containing a few small echogenic foci ➡ with "comet tail" artifacts within the flexor digitorum profundus tendon ➡. (Right) Longitudinal ultrasound of the knee in a patient with hyperlipidemia shows a hypoechoic nodule ➡ within the superficial aspect of the patellar tendon ➡ close to the tibial insertion ➡, consistent with xanthoma.

SWOLLEN NERVE

DIFFERENTIAL DIAGNOSIS

Common
- Nerve Compression
- Nerve Sheath Tumor

Less Common
- Nerve Injury
- Fibrolipomatous Hamartoma
- Metastases
- Acromegaly
- Charcot-Marie-Tooth Disease
- Leprosy

ESSENTIAL INFORMATION

Key Differential Diagnosis Issues
- Familiarity with appearances and course of main peripheral nerves is essential to identifying nerve injuries
- Nerves show honeycomb-like pattern on transverse imaging
  - Roundish, hypoechoic fascicles within hyperechoic background of epineurium
- When assessing nerve compression, important to measure cross-sectional area (CSA) of nerve at specific locations
  - Continuous boundary tracing of nerve provides more correct area measurement than best-fitting ellipse method
  - Contralateral side is unreliable internal reference since contralateral, subclinical, compressive neuropathy is common

Helpful Clues for Common Diagnoses
- **Nerve Compression**
  - Most commonly within fibroosseous tunnels
    - Less commonly within muscular or fascial tunnels
  - Fibroosseous tunnels in upper limb
    - Carpal tunnel ↔ median nerve
    - Cubital and Guyon tunnels ↔ ulnar nerve
  - Fibroosseous tunnels in lower limb
    - Fibular neck ↔ common peroneal nerve
    - Tarsal tunnel ↔ tibial nerve
    - Intermetatarsal spaces ↔ interdigital nerves
  - Swelling of nerve proximal to or at site of compression is overriding sign of nerve compression
    - No swelling → no compression
  - Carpal tunnel syndrome
    - Measure CSA of median nerve at 4 sites
    - Proximal border pronator quadratus, proximal to tunnel inlet, at tunnel inlet and tunnel outlet
    - Maximum CSA ≥ 12 mm² → diagnostic of carpal tunnel syndrome
    - Maximum CSA = 9-12 mm² → borderline
    - Maximum CSA ≤ 9 mm² → normal
    - Or, if largest carpal tunnel CSA minus proximal pronator quadratus CSA > 2 mm² → diagnostic of carpal tunnel syndrome
  - Cubital tunnel syndrome
  - Swelling of ulnar nerve CSA posterior to medial epicondyle
    - ≥ 2.5x ulnar nerve CSA mid-arm or mid-forearm → diagnostic of cubital tunnel syndrome
    - ≤ 1.5x ulnar nerve CSA mid-arm or mid-forearm → normal
- **Nerve Sheath Tumor**
  - Tumor of peripheral nerve
    - Schwannoma: Tumor of Schwann cells lining axons
    - Neurofibroma: Tumor of connective tissue between axons
  - Hypoechoic, fusiform-shaped tumor of nerve
  - Thickening of entering or exiting nerve
    - Tumors arising from small nerves may not have visible thickening of parent nerve
  - Anechoic areas
    - Due to myxoid or fluid accumulation
    - Some schwannomas may be predominantly anechoic and cyst-like ("ancient schwannoma")
  - Posterior acoustic enhancement
  - Moderately hyperemic on Doppler
  - ± hyperechoic areas
    - Due to hemorrhage or calcification
  - Malignant peripheral nerve sheath tumor more likely if
    - Patient has neurofibromatosis type 1
    - Tumor is large (> 5 cm) ± ill-defined ± heterogeneous ± rapidly growing
  - FDG PET has quite high (~ 80-90%) sensitivity and specificity for diagnosing malignant peripheral nerve sheath tumor associated with neurofibromatosis

15

Helpful Clues for Less Common Diagnoses

- **Fibrolipomatous Hamartoma**
  - Benign, fibrofatty malformations of peripheral nerves
  - Most cases present before 30 years of age
    - 1/3 associated with finger enlargement or macrodactyly (macrodystrophia lipomatosa)
  - Majority involve median nerve
    - Less frequently affects ulnar nerve, radial nerve, brachial plexus, or plantar nerves
  - Soft, slow-growing, fusiform swelling of nerve
    - ± increasing pain, tenderness, and diminished sensation
    - ± symptoms of compression neuropathy such as carpal tunnel syndrome
- **Metastases**
  - Usually involve brachial plexus
    - Hypoechoic, irregular, hypervascular mass infiltrating brachial plexus
    - May need aspiration for cytology to differentiate from radiotherapy-induced perineural fibrosis
- **Acromegaly**
  - Peripheral nerves ~ 2x as large in acromegalic patients as normal subjects
  - Degree of nerve enlargement related to clinical control, duration, and insulin-like growth factor 1 level
- **Charcot-Marie-Tooth Disease**
  - Heterogeneous group of inherited peripheral nervous system disorders
    - Most common types are autosomal dominant types 1A, 2, and X-linked type
  - Onset usually before 30 years of age
    - Progressive peripheral weakness, ↓ tendon reflexes, peroneal muscle atrophy, pes cavus, and mild sensory loss
  - Ultrasound can show median nerve hypertrophy
    - Can allow differentiation of Charcot-Marie-Tooth type 1A from other types
    - Useful screening tool for next of kin who may need genetic assessment
- **Leprosy**
  - Chronic granulomatous disease due to *Mycobacterium leprae*
  - Affects peripheral nerves, upper respiratory tract mucosa, and skin
  - Wide spectrum of ultrasound abnormalities depending on disease duration, activity ± compression
    - Early disease affects intradermal nerves → no visible ultrasound abnormality
    - Active disease → swelling of endoneural space, thickening of individual fascicles, and endoneural hyperemia
    - Longstanding inactive disease → nerves less swollen than active disease with overall ↑ echogenicity and ↓ visibility of fascicles

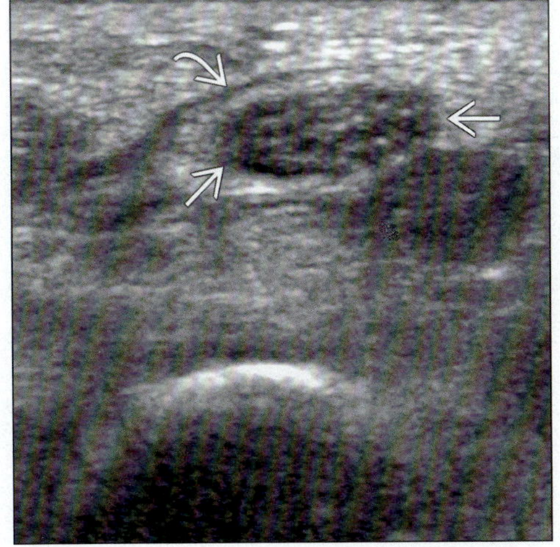

Nerve Compression

Transverse ultrasound immediately proximal to the carpal tunnel in a patient with carpal tunnel syndrome shows a swollen median nerve ➡ (14 mm²). Overlying the nerve is the thin antebrachial fascia ➡.

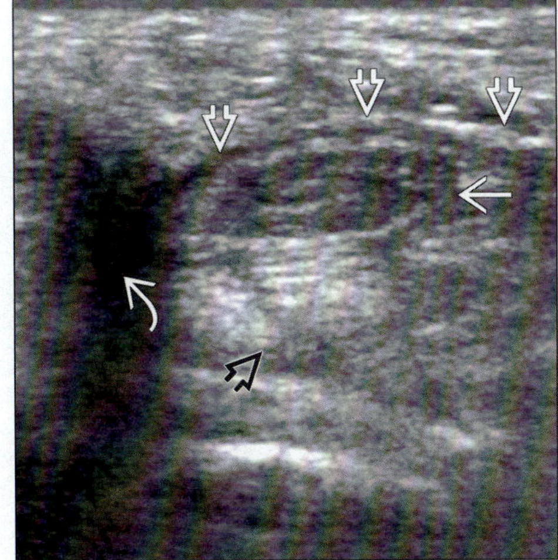

Nerve Compression

Transverse ultrasound at tunnel inlet in the same patient shows a swollen median nerve ➡ (15 mm²) with overlying thick flexor retinaculum ➡. Note flexor tendons ▷ and scaphoid retinacular attachment ➡.

15

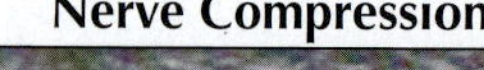

SWOLLEN NERVE

Nerve Compression

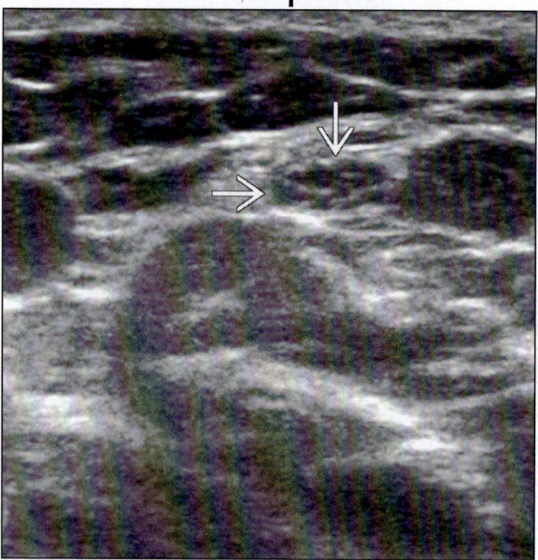

Nerve Compression

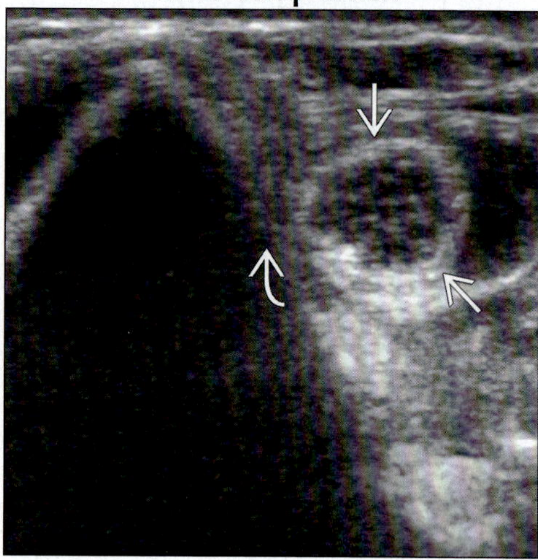

(Left) Transverse ultrasound of the ulnar nerve in the distal arm in a patient with cubital tunnel syndrome shows a normal caliber (7 mm²) ulnar nerve ➡. *(Right)* Transverse ultrasound posterior to the median humeral epicondyle ➡ in the same patient shows a thickened ulnar nerve ➡ (14 mm²) in the cubital tunnel, consistent with cubital tunnel syndrome.

Nerve Sheath Tumor

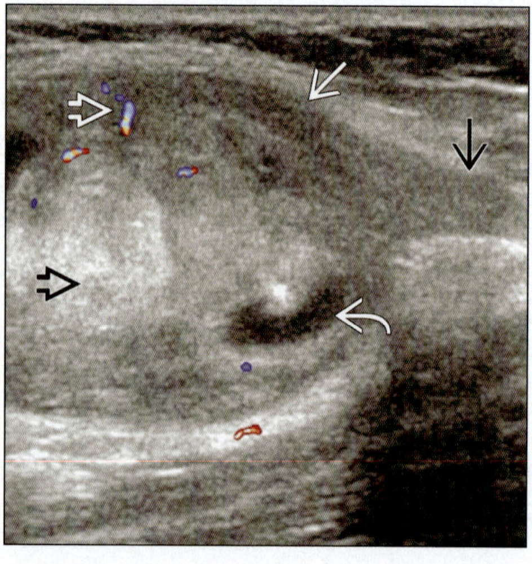

Nerve Sheath Tumor

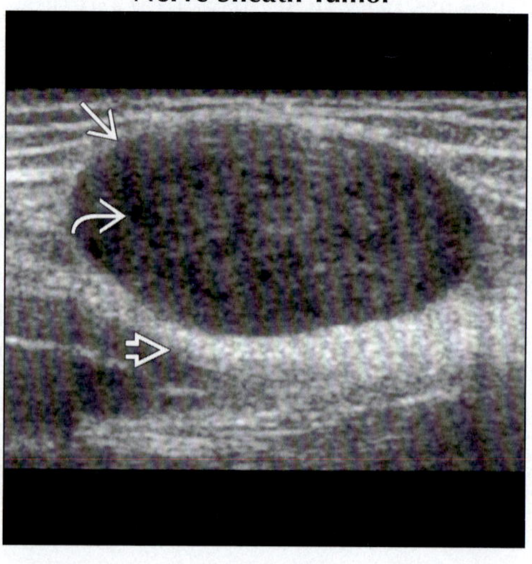

(Left) Longitudinal color Doppler US of the arm shows a nerve sheath tumor ➡ of the median nerve with mild vascularity ➡, myxoid components ➡, hyperechoic areas ➡, and thickening of the median nerve ➡ proximally. *(Right)* Oblique US of the thigh shows a subcutaneous mass ➡. No entering or exiting nerve is visible. Nevertheless, size, shape, anechoic areas within hypoechoic tumor ➡, and posterior acoustic enhancement ➡ are typical of a nerve sheath tumor.

Nerve Sheath Tumor

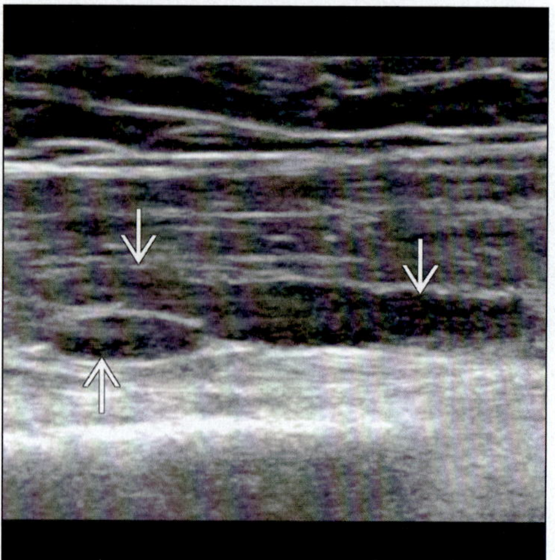

Nerve Injury

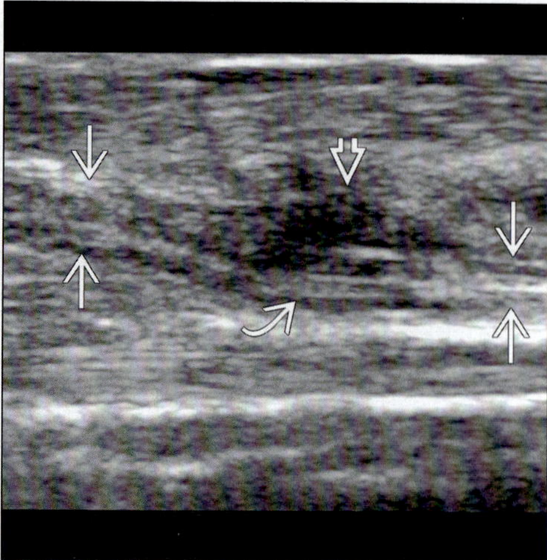

(Left) Longitudinal ultrasound of the arm shows an elongated, branching, hypoechoic mass ➡, consistent with a plexiform nerve sheath tumor. This was separate from the musculocutaneous and other nerves. *(Right)* Longitudinal ultrasound of the forearm shows injury ➡ to the median nerve ➡ from a dog bite. The deeper fascicles ➡ of the median nerve are intact. Appearances are consistent with an incomplete nerve injury.

15

SWOLLEN NERVE

Fibrolipomatous Hamartoma

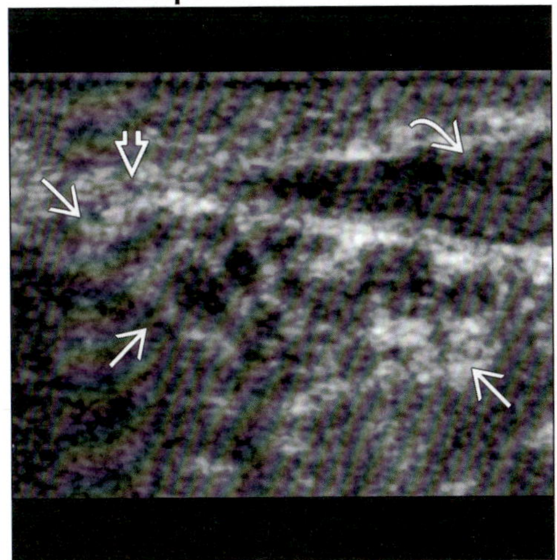

Fibrolipomatous Hamartoma

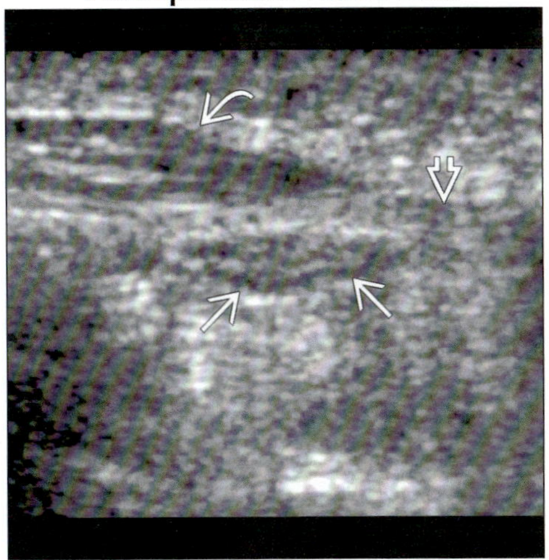

(Left) Transverse ultrasound of a carpal tunnel inlet in the middle finger of a patient with macrodactyly shows a severely thickened median nerve (56 mm²) ➡ with thickened nerve fascicles. Note the hypothenar eminence ➡ and flexor retinaculum ➡. (Right) Transverse ultrasound of the contralateral palm in the same patient shows a normal caliber median nerve (8 mm²) ➡. Note the hypothenar eminence ➡ and flexor retinaculum ➡.

Fibrolipomatous Hamartoma

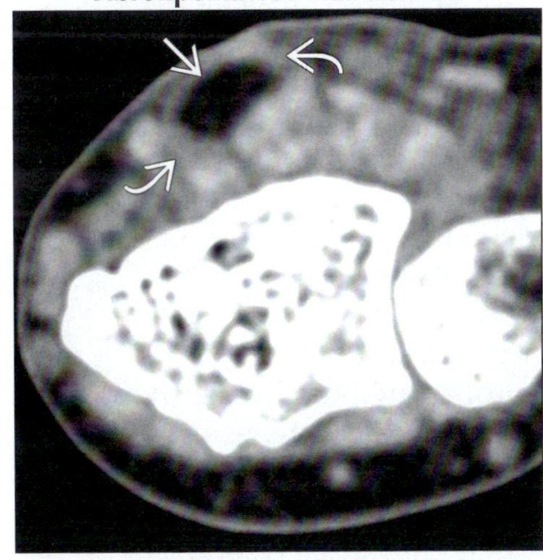

Fibrolipomatous Hamartoma

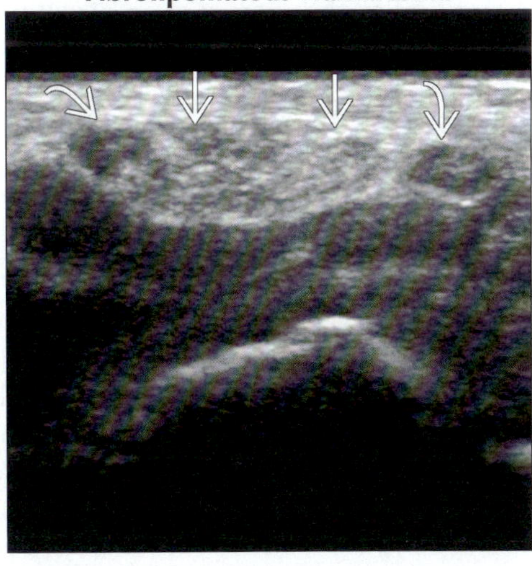

(Left) Transverse CECT just proximal to the carpal tunnel, in a patient with volar wrist swelling for 1 year, shows a lipoma ➡ located between the widely separated components of the bifid medial nerve ➡. (Right) Transverse ultrasound of the wrist shows a lipoma ➡ located between 2 components ➡ of the bifid median nerve.

Metastases

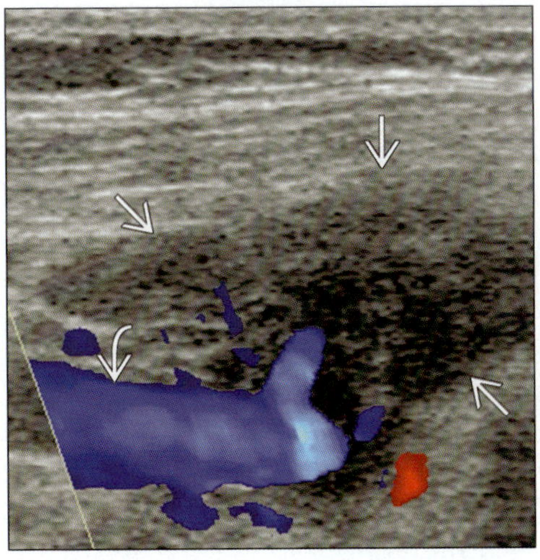

Leprosy

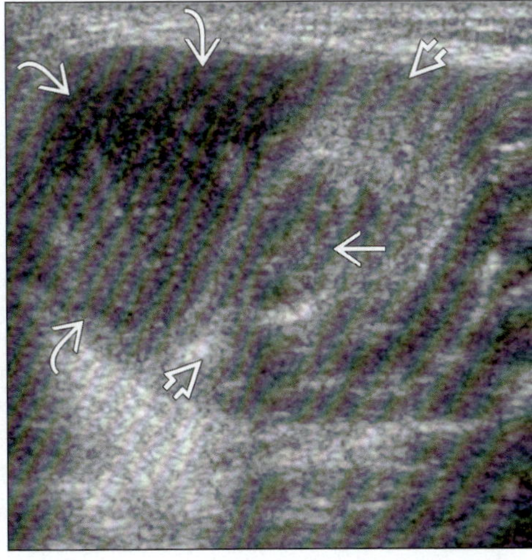

(Left) Transverse color Doppler US of the infraclavicular region shows a large, irregular, hypoechoic mass ➡ infiltrating the brachial plexus (subclavian vein ➡). This proved to be metastatic breast cancer. (Right) Transverse US proximal to the elbow shows a thickened ulnar nerve ➡ with marked surrounding edema, echogenic granulation tissue ➡, and abscess ➡. Perineural abscess is an uncommon feature of leprosy. (Courtesy S.J. Lodge, MD.)

DIFFERENTIAL DIAGNOSIS

Common
- Ganglion Cyst
- Bursal Distension

Less Common
- Seroma
- Vascular Malformation
- Abscess
- Fat Necrosis
- Hematoma
- Parameniscal Cyst
- Myxoma
- Schwannoma
- Sarcoma
- Lymph Node
- Aneurysm
- Pseudoaneurysm

ESSENTIAL INFORMATION

Key Differential Diagnosis Issues
- All cystic-type masses should be evaluated with color Doppler imaging
  - May reveal internal vascularity in lesion initially considered to be entirely cystic
  - May reveal previously unrecognized vascular structures alongside cystic-type mass
- Adjust gain setting to maximize visualization of internal contents
  - Cystic-type mass is not necessarily anechoic
  - Many cystic lesions contain hyperechoic fluid or echogenic foci

Helpful Clues for Common Diagnoses
- **Ganglion Cyst**
  - Most common cystic-type mass
  - Filled with gelatinous material of variable viscosity
  - Occurs alongside joints
  - Synovial fluid squeezed out from joint through capsular defect
  - Communication with joint not always apparent
  - Usually can see cyst point toward nearby joint
  - Increase in extent through process of cyst enlargement → rupture → consolidation
    - Some ganglion cysts can be extensive, serpiginous, multiloculated, and quite removed from joint of origin
    - May extend into muscle and simulate myxoma
- **Bursal Distension**
  - Synovial or adventitial bursae
  - Baker cyst = distended semimembranous, gastrocnemius bursa

Helpful Clues for Less Common Diagnoses
- **Seroma**
  - Only occurs following tissue disruption due to surgery or trauma
  - Does not occur spontaneously
  - Fluid collection usually deep to investing fascia
    - ± septations
- **Vascular Malformation**
  - Proliferative
    - Hemangioma: Proliferation → stabilization → involution
    - Kaposiform hemangioendothelioma, Kaposi sarcoma, and angiosarcoma
  - Static
    - Arterial, venous, capillary, lymphatic, or mixed depending on predominant vascular pattern
    - Best assessed with color and pulsed Doppler ultrasound
    - Do not proliferate but change shape due to thrombosis, hemorrhage, or infection
    - Microvascular component looks like supporting stroma on imaging, because microvessels cannot be resolved
  - Each type of vascular malformation may also
    - Be focal or diffuse
    - Possess ectatic vessels
    - Have variable microvascular component
- **Abscess**
  - Usually in immunosuppressed or at-risk patient
  - Majority are hypoechoic; some are hyperechoic if contents are viscous
    - Look for moving echoes within lesion on real-time imaging
    - Surrounding edema or inflammation
    - Peripheral hyperemia
- **Fat Necrosis**
  - Fat trauma → fat inflammation → fat necrosis → liquefaction

- Visible liquefaction occurs with large areas of fat necrosis
  - ± calcification due to combination of fatty acids combining with calcium to form calcium soap
- **Hematoma**
  - All hematomas start to visibly liquefy after about 1 week
    - Some → margination with complete liquefaction
    - Others → gradually reduce in size without margination and liquefaction
    - ± calcification (uncommon)
- **Parameniscal Cyst**
  - Fluid squeezed from peripheral part of meniscus
  - Normally associated with meniscal tear
    - Nearly always horizontal tear
- **Myxoma**
  - Occur in muscle
  - Well-defined, roundish masses ± surrounding muscle compression or atrophy
    - Variable amount of thick myxoid material
- **Schwannoma**
  - Majority of peripheral schwannomas contain small amount (≤ 10%) of myxoid or cystic components
    - Minority contain larger (> 30%) myxoid or cystic components

- Cystic competent may be due to necrosis, hemorrhage, or fluid accumulation due to altered tumor barrier
  - Cystic schwannoma tends to be larger and more compressive with shorter duration of neurological symptoms
- **Sarcoma**
  - Will appear cystic if it has fluid, hemorrhagic, necrotic, or myxoid component
    - Tumors with myxoid component include myxoid liposarcoma, malignant peripheral nerve sheath tumor, and malignant fibrous histiocytoma
- **Lymph Node**
  - Appendicular cystic nodes most commonly due to tumor necrosis or tuberculosis
- **Aneurysm**
  - Popliteal aneurysm most common appendicular aneurysm
    - Associated with increase in age, male gender, and atherosclerosis
    - ~ 50% bilateral
  - Most other appendicular aneurysms associated with vasculopathy, such as polyarthritis nodosa or arterial malformation
- **Pseudoaneurysm**
  - Associated with trauma, vascular surgery, or impingement from pedunculated osteochondroma
  - Characteristic "to-and-fro" spectral pattern at narrow aneurysm neck

Ganglion Cyst

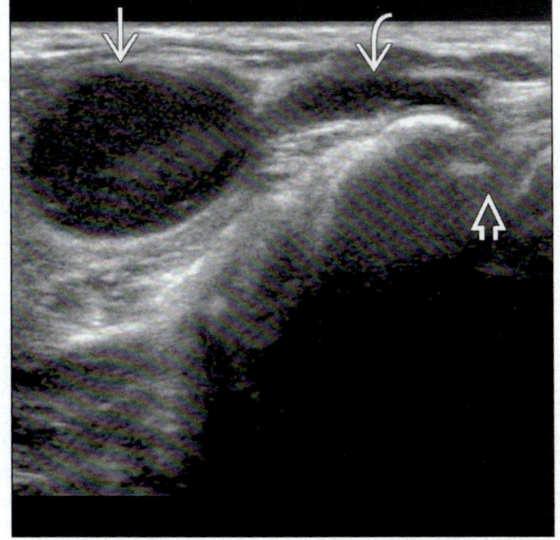

Oblique US of the thenar eminence shows a unilocular, thin-walled ganglion cyst ➡ between opponens and adductor muscles. There is a tail ➡ extending proximally to scapho-trapezium articulation ➡.

Ganglion Cyst

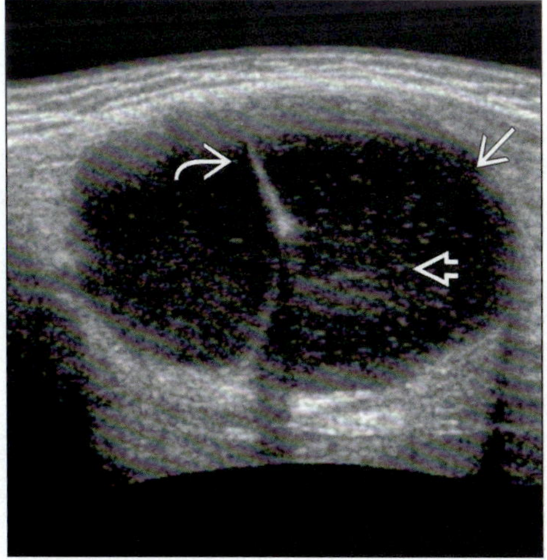

Longitudinal ultrasound of proximal leg shows a large, septated ➡, thin-walled cyst ➡ with fine echoes ➡ within tibialis anterior muscle. Other images revealed a small tail extending to the proximal tibiofibular joint.

EXTREMITY CYSTIC MASS

(Left) Longitudinal ultrasound of the buttock region shows a large, septated, cystic mass ➡ overlying the hamstring tendon ➡ at the attachment to the ischial tuberosity ➡, consistent with distended ischial tuberosity bursa. The patient had fallen 1 month earlier. *(Right)* Longitudinal US of the proximal thigh 1 month following a hip replacement shows a large cystic collection ➡ located just deep to the investing fascia ➡. Aspiration confirmed seroma.

Bursal Distension

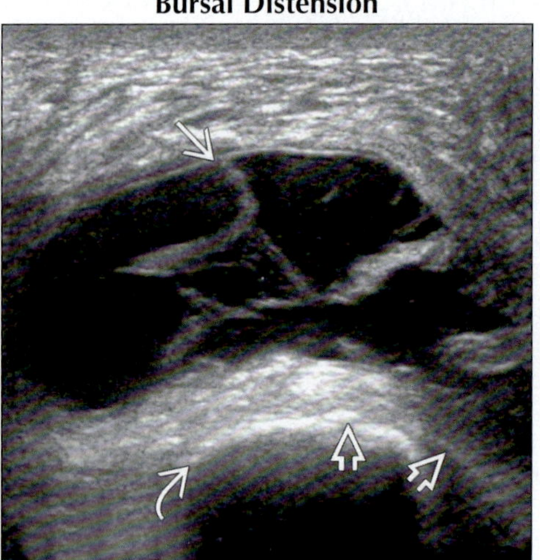

Seroma

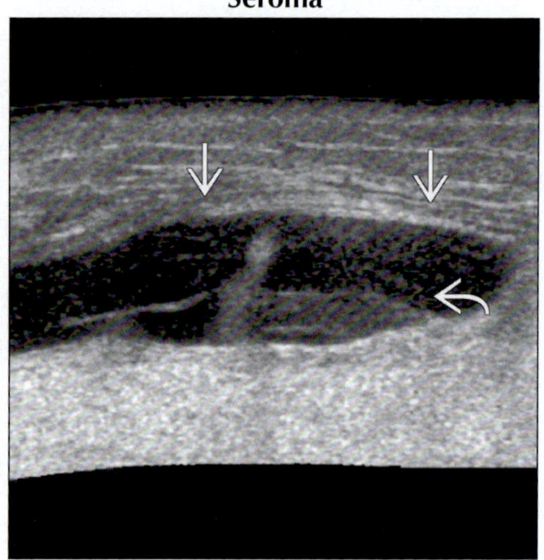

(Left) Longitudinal ultrasound of the leg in an adult shows a well-defined, subcutaneous, cystic mass ➡ with minimal marginal vascularity detected during real-time scanning, consistent with a slow-flow vascular malformation and dilated vascular channels. *(Right)* Transverse ultrasound of an intravenous drug user shows an irregular abscess cavity ➡ within the gluteus maximus muscle. Percutaneous needle ➡ aspiration for culture is being undertaken.

Vascular Malformation

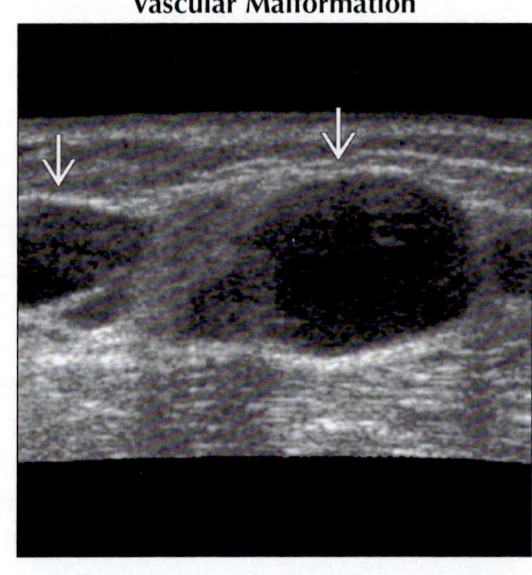

Abscess

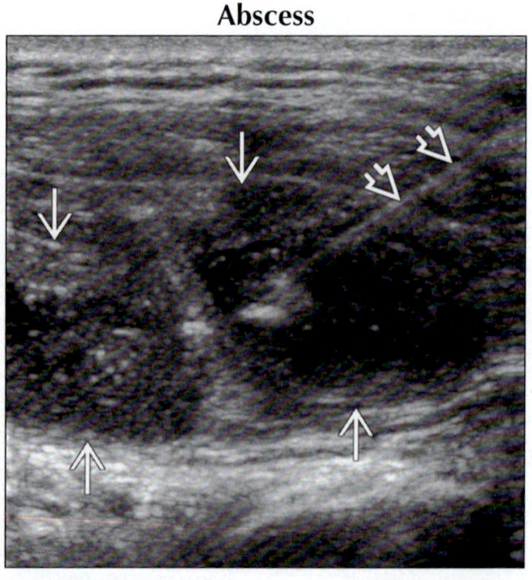

(Left) Transverse ultrasound in a patient 3 years following revision of a hip prosthesis shows a large, subcutaneous, cystic mass ➡ with internal fronds ➡ in the proximal aspect of the thigh. Aspiration grew Candida parapsilosis. *(Right)* Longitudinal US of the buttock 1 month following blunt trauma to this area shows a well-defined, largely cystic mass ➡ with early calcification ➡ within the subcutaneous tissues, findings consistent with liquefied fat necrosis.

Abscess

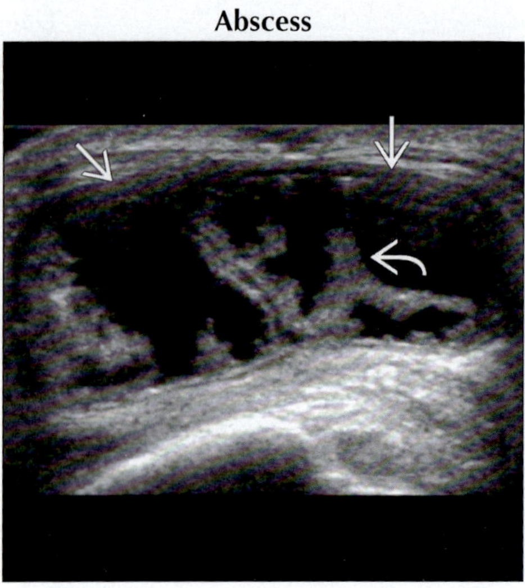

Fat Necrosis

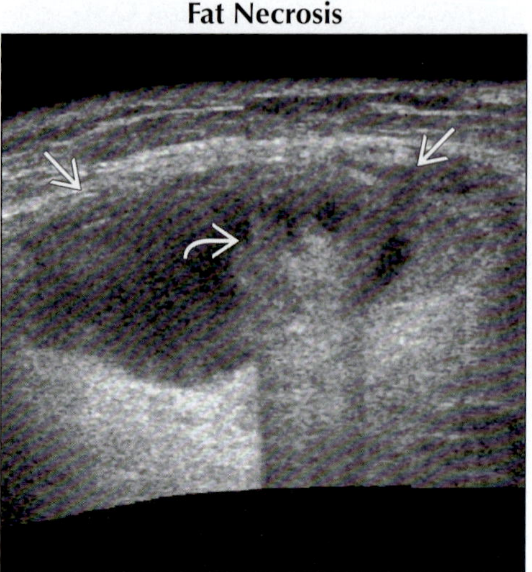

EXTREMITY CYSTIC MASS

Hematoma

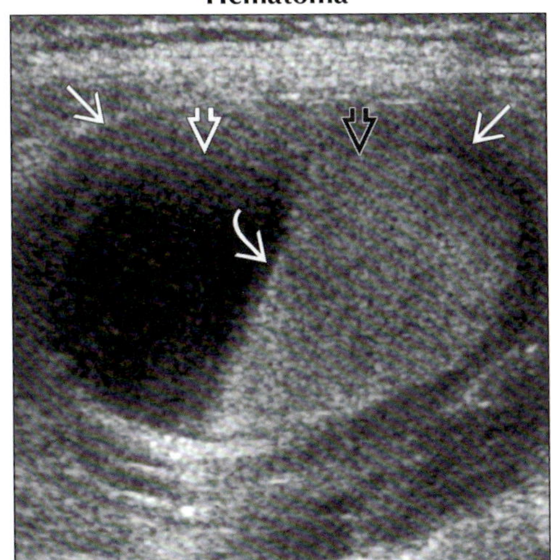

Myxoma

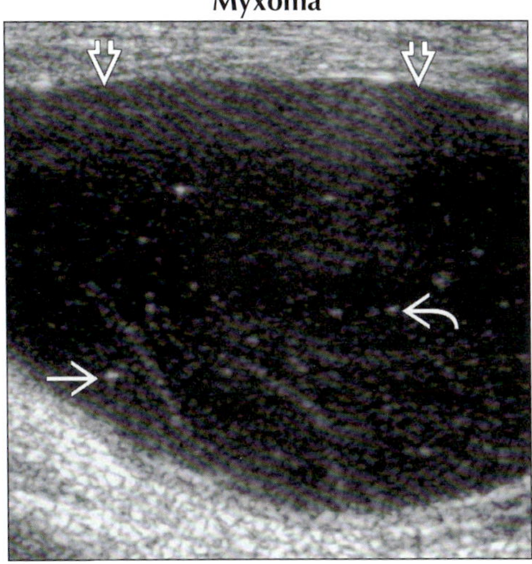

(Left) Transverse ultrasound of the scapular region 1 month following trauma shows a large, well-defined liquefied hematoma ➡ with serous ➡ and cellular ➡ components and an intervening fluid level ➡. *(Right)* Transverse ultrasound shows a well-defined myxoid tumor ➡ within the soleus muscle. Many small, fine, internal echoes ➡ are present, some with "comet tail" artifacts ➡. These may be seen in myxoma or ganglia.

Sarcoma

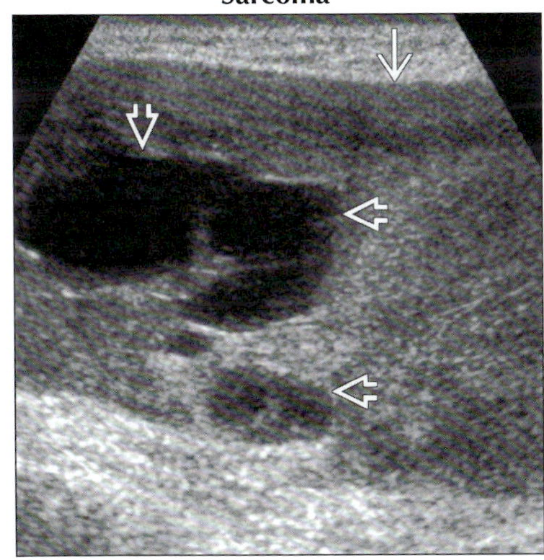

Sarcoma

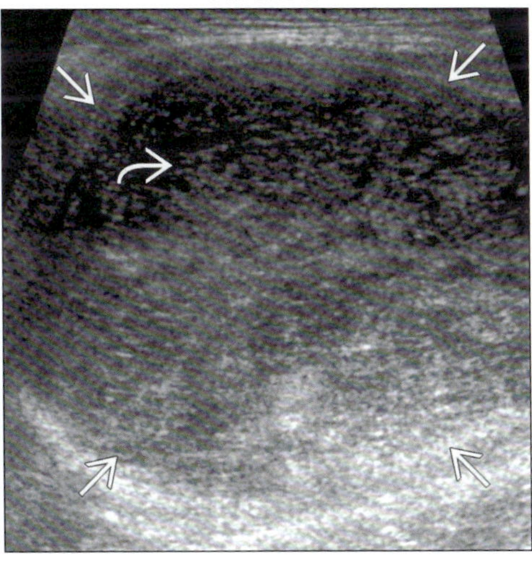

(Left) Longitudinal US shows a section of a large subcutaneous mass ➡ in the shoulder region. There are large cystic or myxoid areas ➡ present. Biopsy specimen confirmed malignant fibrous histiocytoma. *(Right)* Longitudinal US of the thigh shows an intramuscular mass ➡ with large amounts of myxoid-type tissue demonstrating fine internal echoes ➡. Most of the mass showed little or no vascularity with a single clump of vessels on the proximal border.

Sarcoma

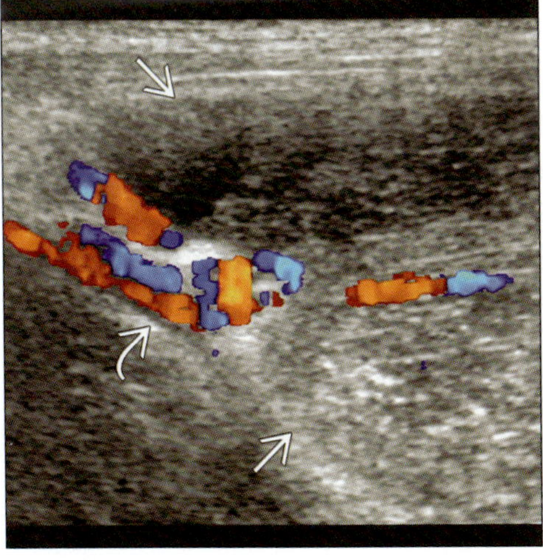

Lymph Node

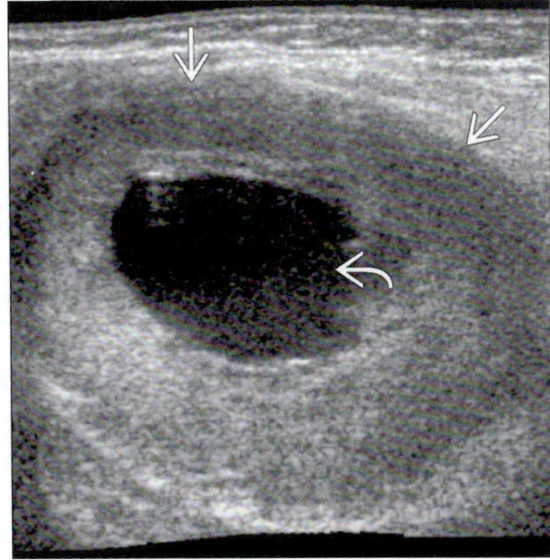

(Left) Longitudinal color Doppler ultrasound of the same patient shows a clump of vessels ➡ at the proximal border of the tumor ➡ extending into the tumor matrix. Biopsy specimen confirmed myxoid liposarcoma. *(Right)* Transverse ultrasound of the groin region shows a large, malignant, inguinal node ➡ with a central cystic area ➡ from primary alveolar soft part sarcoma of the thigh.

15

DIFFERENTIAL DIAGNOSIS

Common
- Ganglion Cyst
- Baker Cyst
- Parameniscal Cyst
- Bursal Distension

ESSENTIAL INFORMATION

Key Differential Diagnosis Issues
- Establishing whether mass is intra- or extracapsular is key to diagnosis and therapeutic approach
  - If extracapsular, does mass communicate with joint?

Helpful Clues for Common Diagnoses
- Ganglion Cyst
  - Mucinous fluid contained within pseudocapsule
    - Not lined by synovial tissue
  - Most common in hands and feet
    - 80% of soft tissue masses of hands & feet
    - Dorsal wrist ganglia are more commonly symptomatic, though volar wrist ganglia are overall more common
    - Most volar wrist ganglia are asymptomatic
  - Typical locations reflect weakness in joint capsule
    - Dorsal radiocarpal joint
    - Dorsal scapholunate joint
    - Scapho-trapezio-capitate joint
  - Near A1 pulley on middle, index, and ring fingers
    - Does not appear to communicate with metacarpophalangeal joint or flexor tendon sheath
  - Anechoic, well-defined, rounded or irregular mass alongside joint
    - ± "comet tail" artifacts
    - Infrequently hyperechoic, possibly due to hemorrhage
  - Typically has neck pointing toward particular joint
    - Usually neck cannot be traced to joint because it is too small
    - Important to identify potential joint of origin as it has therapeutic implications
  - About 1/2 recur after percutaneous aspiration
    - Hyaluronidase may facilitate aspiration by making contents less viscous
- Baker Cyst
  - Semimembranous-gastrocnemius bursa, which communicates with joint
    - Slit-like opening in capsule close to root of posterior horn medial meniscus
  - Classic "talk-bubble" configuration on transverse ultrasound with beak pointing between semimembranous tendon and medial head gastrocnemius muscle
    - Frequently bilateral
  - Has synovial membrane; therefore affected by synovial inflammatory or neoplastic disorders involving knee joint
    - Calcified bodies may also occur in Baker cyst
  - ± hemorrhage
  - ± leakage or rupture
  - Usually spreads distally over medial belly gastrocnemius
    - Less commonly spreads proximally along semimembranous muscle
    - Uncommonly spreads into semimembranous or gastrocnemius muscle
- Parameniscal Cyst
  - Cystic mass extending from peripheral aspect of meniscus
  - Usually associated with horizontal meniscal tear
  - Occasionally no meniscal tear present
    - Meniscal tear may have healed
    - Cyst may be arising from mucoid meniscal matrix in absence of tear
    - Cyst may be arising via tear in meniscocapsular ligaments
  - Percutaneous cyst aspiration helpful particularly in those cases without any apparent meniscal tear
- Bursal Distension
  - 2 types of bursae
  - Synovial bursae: Synovial-lined bursa, which occurs at defined anatomical locations
    - May become inflamed in systemic synovitis and in conditions affecting synovium, such as synovial osteochondromatosis

PARA-ARTICULAR CYSTIC MASS

- ○ Adventitial bursae: Non-synovial-lined bursae acquired due to friction between opposing structures
- ○ Some paraarticular bursa more affected than others
- ○ Subacromial-subdeltoid bursa
  - Fixed attachments to free edge of coracoacromial ligament & to greater tuberosity distal to attachment of supraspinatus and infraspinatus
  - Coracoid & proximal humeral recesses
  - Richly innervated
  - Most, if not all, pain from rotator cuff injury comes from subacromial-subdeltoid bursa
  - Hence, pain is poorly localized
  - If present, look closely for associated rotator cuff tear
  - If markedly thickened bursa with hyperemia, consider inflammatory arthropathy (e.g., systemic lupus erythematous) or infection
- ○ Olecranon bursa
  - Synovial bursa located between olecranon process and skin
  - Composed of synovium and extrasynovial fat
  - Common site of gouty bursitis
  - Commonly inflamed but uncommonly infected
- ○ Iliopsoas bursa
  - Synovial bursa located anterior to hip between iliopsoas tendon and hip capsule
  - Communicates with hip joint in 15% of patients
  - Consider iliopsoas infection, particularly tuberculous
- ○ Semimembranous bursa
  - Synovial bursa between anterior arm of semimembranous tendon complex and medial collateral ligament
  - Semimembranous tendon complex inserts to posteromedial corner of tibia
  - Located medial to Baker cyst and proximal to pes anserinus bursa
  - Distended bursa has "J"-shaped appearance
- ○ Pes anserinus bursa
  - Pes anserinus = conjoint tendons of sartorius, gracilis, and semitendinous
  - Insert into anteromedial aspect of proximal tibia ~ 5 cm distal to joint line
  - Bursa located between pes anserinus and medial collateral ligament
- ○ Pre-patellar, superficial, & deep infra-patellar bursae
  - Prepatellar bursa located between patella and skin
  - Superficial infrapatellar bursa located between tibial tuberosity and skin
  - Deep infrapatellar bursa located between distal portion of patellar tendon and tibia, beneath Hoffa fat pad
  - ≤ 3 mm distension of deep infrapatellar bursa common finding and considered normal

Ganglion Cyst

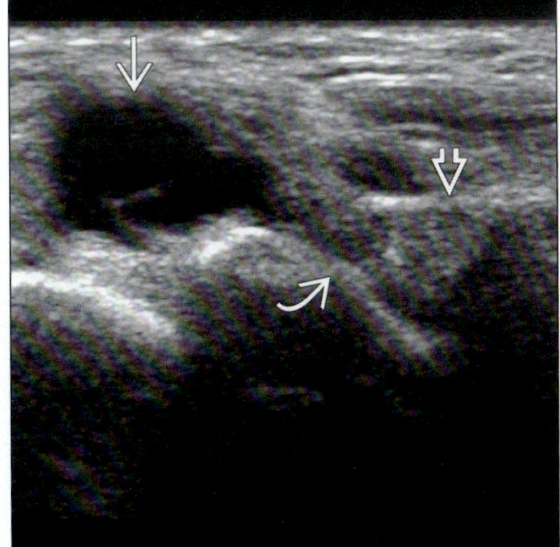

Longitudinal ultrasound dorsum of the wrist shows a small septated ganglion ➡, which points toward and seems to arise from articulation between the radius ➡ and lunate ➡.

Ganglion Cyst

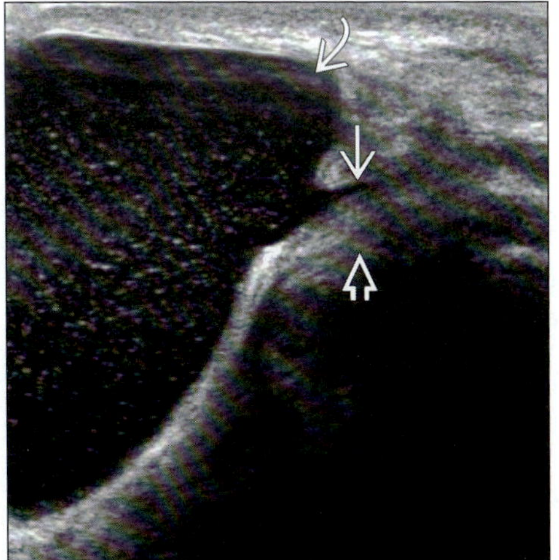

Transverse US of an ankle in a patient with acute swelling following trauma shows an acute ganglion cyst ➡ containing small echogenic speckles lying alongside the tibia ➡ and pointing ➡ toward the ankle joint.

15

PARA-ARTICULAR CYSTIC MASS

Ganglion Cyst

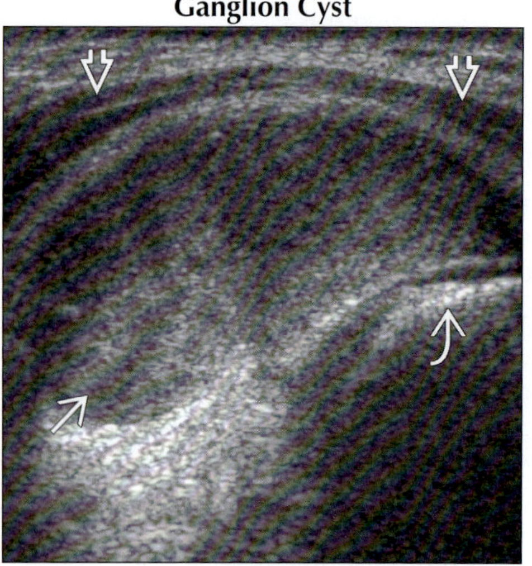

Baker Cyst

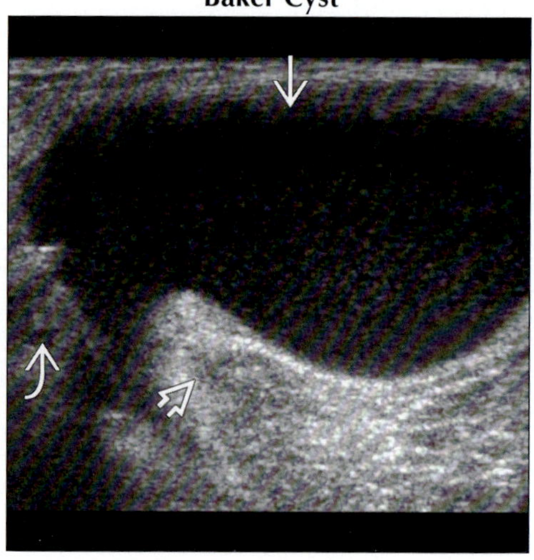

(Left) Transverse US of knee region shows a hyperechoic paraarticular ganglion ➡ alongside the medial femoral condyle ➡ & deep to the sartorius tendon ➡, communicating with joint (not shown). Ganglia may be echogenic due to the internal hemorrhage. *(Right)* Transverse US of popliteal fossa shows the typical "talk-bubble" configuration of a Baker cyst ➡ with the beak pointing between the semimembranous tendon ➡ and the medial head of the gastrocnemius muscle ➡.

Baker Cyst

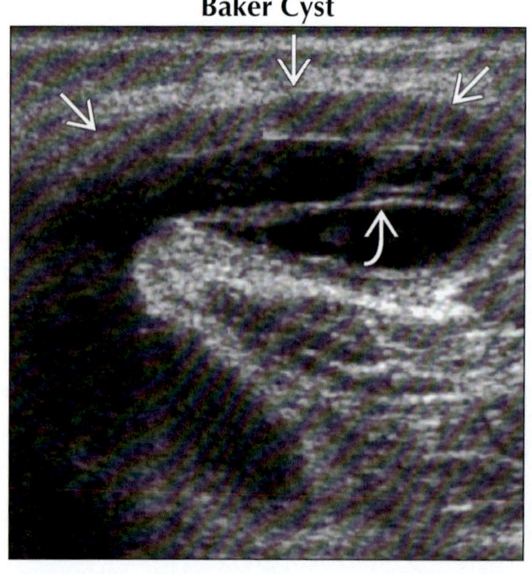

Baker Cyst

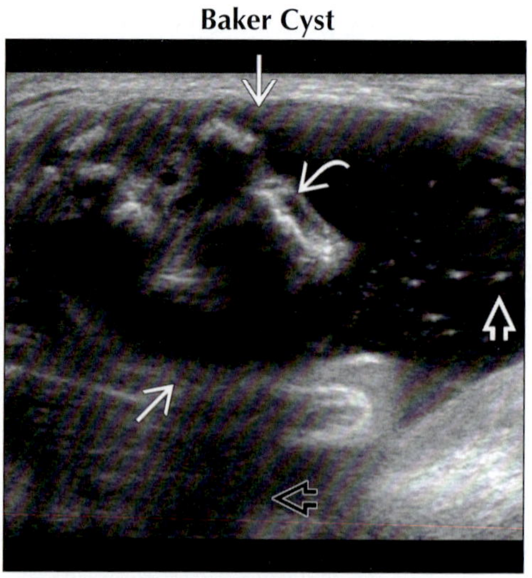

(Left) Transverse ultrasound shows a small, thick-walled Baker cyst ➡ containing several septations ➡. These findings are often seen with synovial inflammation of the knee. *(Right)* Transverse ultrasound shows a large, complicated Baker cyst with synovial thickening ➡, calcification ➡ with acoustic shadowing ➡, and echogenic speckles with "comet tail" artifacts ➡.

Parameniscal Cyst

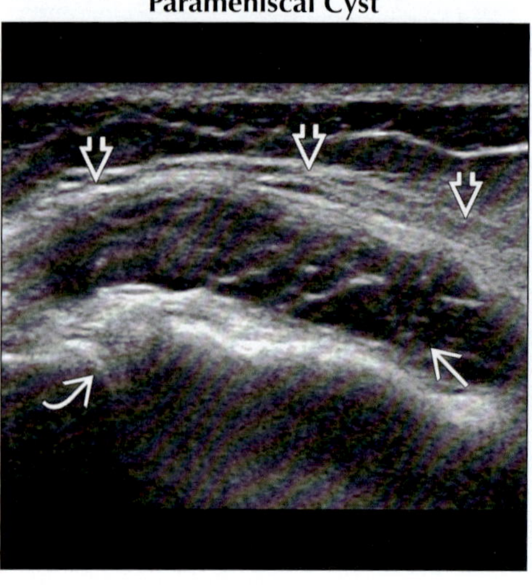

Parameniscal Cyst

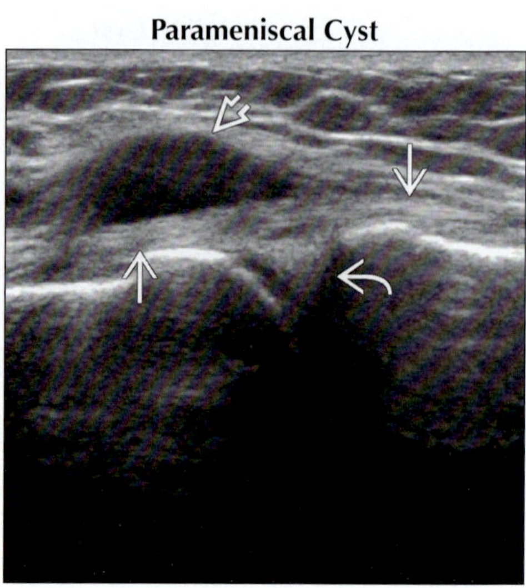

(Left) Longitudinal US of medial aspect of knee shows a parameniscal cyst ➡ lying deep to the medial collateral ligament ➡ and pointing toward the periphery of the medial meniscus ➡. *(Right)* Longitudinal US of knee shows a small parameniscal cyst ➡ located superficial to the medial collateral ligament ➡. This extracapsular part communicated more posteriorly with the intracapsular component alongside medial meniscus ➡.

15

PARA-ARTICULAR CYSTIC MASS

Bursal Distension

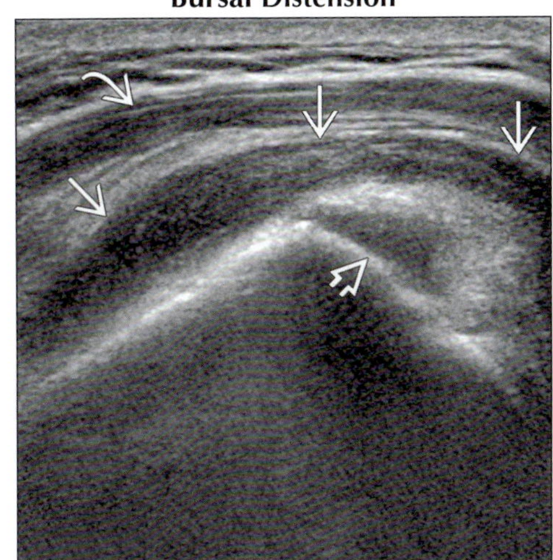

Bursal Distension

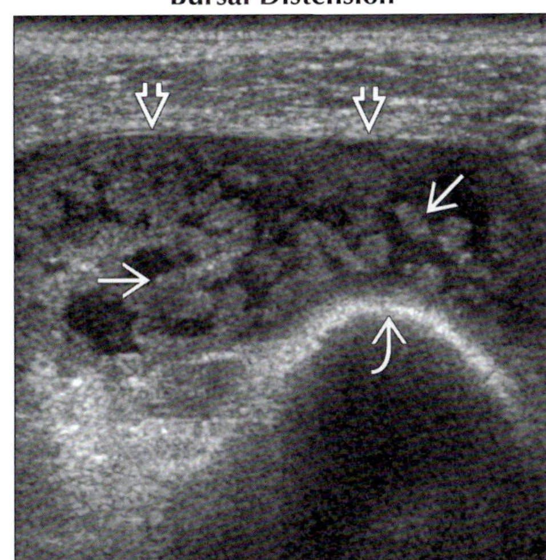

(Left) Longitudinal US shows a distended subacromial-subdeltoid bursa ➡ containing echogenic fluid. No tendon tear was present. The hypoechoic area ➡ within the supraspinatus tendon at insertion was artifactual. Note the deltoid muscle ➡. (Right) Transverse US of the shoulder in a patient with rheumatoid arthritis shows a subacromial-subdeltoid bursa ➡ distended with multiple rice bodies ➡. Note the humeral shaft ➡.

Bursal Distension

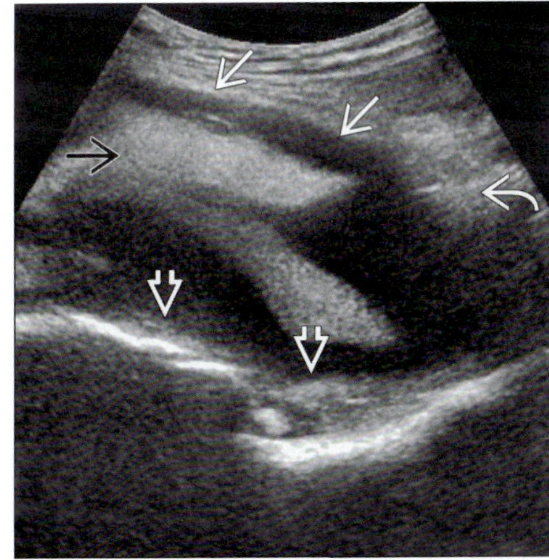

Bursal Distension

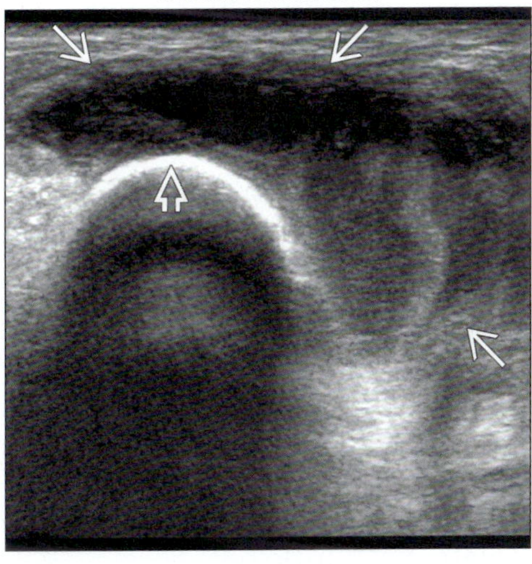

(Left) Longitudinal ultrasound shows a distended iliopsoas bursa ➡ anterior to a nondistended hip capsule ➡. The iliopsoas tendon ➡ is displaced anteriorly. The bursa contains blood clot ➡ and fluid. Aspirate grew Staphylococcus aureus. (Right) Transverse ultrasound of the posterior elbow shows a thick-walled, mildly distended, olecranon bursa ➡ overlying the olecranon process of the ulna ➡.

Bursal Distension

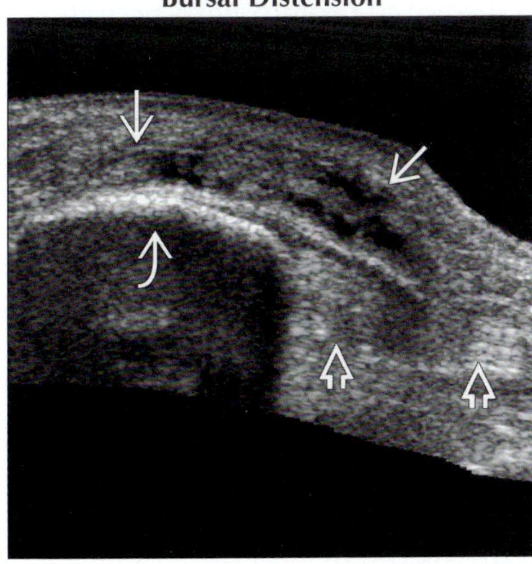

Bursal Distension

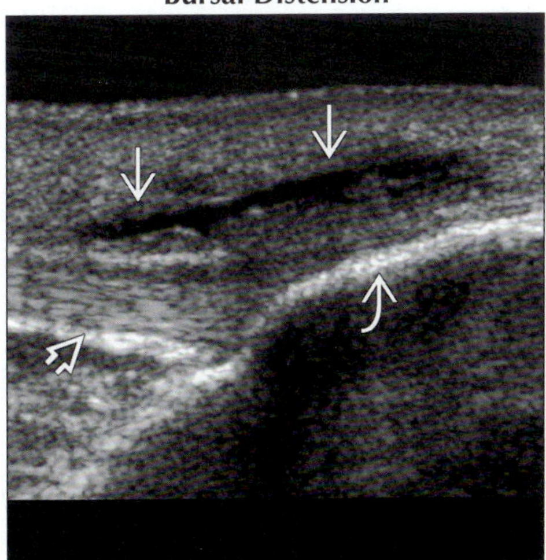

(Left) Longitudinal ultrasound shows a mildly distended prepatellar bursa ➡ with thickened irregular walls and a small amount of internal debris, overlying the patella ➡ and proximal patellar tendon ➡. (Right) Longitudinal ultrasound shows a mildly distended superficial, infrapatellar bursa ➡ overlying the tibial tuberosity ➡ and distal patellar tendon ➡.

15

DIFFERENTIAL DIAGNOSIS

Common
- Inflammatory Synovial Mass
- Tophi of Gout or Pseudogout

Less Common
- Pigmented Villonodular Synovitis
  - Focal Nodular Synovitis
- Synovial Sarcoma
- Amyloid
- Synovial Hemangioma
- Synovial Osteochondromatosis
- Lipoma Arborescens

ESSENTIAL INFORMATION

Key Differential Diagnosis Issues
- Deciding tissue of origin and whether intra- or extraarticular is often key to diagnosis
- For simple diarthrodial joints (acromioclavicular, small joints, hands, and feet), distinction between intra- and extraarticular origin is straightforward
- For more complex larger joints, distinction between intra- & extraarticular origin is less straightforward

Helpful Clues for Common Diagnoses
- **Inflammatory Synovial Mass**
  - Synovial proliferation with chronic inflammation or infection
    - Echogenic or hypoechoic synovial proliferation
    - With chronic infection, synovial proliferation predominates with little or no synovial fluid
  - Mild to moderate hyperemia typical
    - Severe hyperemia → pigmented villonodular synovitis more likely
  - Impossible to distinguish between tuberculous and pyogenic infection based on imaging alone
    - Phemister radiographic triad of severe periarticular osteopenia, marginal erosions, and progressive ↓ in joint space, not specific for tuberculosis
  - Ultrasound-guided synovial biopsy to identify infection and causative organism
- **Tophi of Gout or Pseudogout**
  - Commonly deposited around joints in chronic tophaceous gout
    - Particularly joints of hands, feet, and knee
  - Tophi more common in gout
    - Pseudogout → hydroxyapetite deposition
  - Periarticular location
    - Soft → hard tophi
    - ± synovial or intrameniscal deposition

Helpful Clues for Less Common Diagnoses
- **Pigmented Villonodular Synovitis**
  - Benign proliferative synovial disorder
    - Affects synovium of joint, bursa, or tendon sheath
  - Knee > hip > ankle > shoulder
  - Joint involvement may be diffuse or focal
    - Although histologically identical, focal disease behaves differently from diffuse disease
  - **Focal Nodular Synovitis**
    - Localized to 1 area of synovium
    - Contains less hemosiderin
    - Does not have frond-like projections
    - Becomes more pedunculated rather than more extensive with growth
- **Synovial Sarcoma**
  - Named because of similar appearance to synovial tissue at light microscopy
  - However, does not arise from synovium
  - Arises from primitive mesenchymal cells in extraarticular soft tissues
    - < 5% of synovial sarcomas arise from within joint
  - Calcification in up to 50%
    - ± myxoid areas, cystic areas, or hemorrhage
- **Amyloid**
  - Amyloid → abnormal accumulation of unrelated insoluble protein with tissues
  - Examples: β_2 microglobulin, immunoglobulin light chains, and serum amyloid A protein
    - Chronic hemodialysis → increased β_2 microglobulin
    - Myeloma → increased monoclonal immunoglobulin light chain fragments
    - Chronic inflammatory condition → ↑ acute phase protein serum amyloid A
    - May also be idiopathic occurring de novo with no recognizable associated systemic disease
  - Especially affects shoulder, hip, knee, and wrist; usually bilateral

15

ARTICULAR MASS

- Shoulder → thickening of rotator cuff, bursa, and long head of biceps; periarticular hypoechoic nodules ± bony erosions
- **Synovial Hemangioma**
  - Strictly speaking, most are not hemangiomas
    - Hemangioma = vascular tumor of childhood with proliferative, stable, and involutionary phases
  - Most synovial hemangiomas are synovial vascular malformations
    - Arteriovenous, venous, capillary, lymphatic, or mixed depending on flow and dominant vessel type
  - More common to see vascular malformation involving synovium than vascular malformation confined to synovium
  - Similar to vascular malformations elsewhere; synovial vascular malformations seem to have predominant vascular or stromal component
    - Vascular component largely composed of many small vessels too small to resolve on ultrasound
  - ± phleboliths (common)
  - ± ectatic vessels
  - ± venous lakes
  - Present in children and young adults → joint pain, swelling, and repeated hemarthroses
- **Synovial Osteochondromatosis**
  - Proliferation and metaplastic transformation of synovium
  - Affects any synovium and can occur in any synovium-lined joint, bursa, or tendon
    - Monoarticular
    - Joints most commonly affected are knee > elbow > hip > shoulder
  - Active synovial proliferation and cartilaginous metaplasia → inactive phase
    - Intrasynovial cartilage nodules → detach to lie free in joint and ossify
    - Nodules may consist of cartilage, cartilage/bone mixture, or mature bone with marrow fat
  - Variable-sized joint effusion
  - ± erosion of adjacent cartilage and bone
    - Especially in less distensible joints (hip)
  - ± secondary degenerative change
- **Lipoma Arborescens**
  - Proliferation of subsynovial fat → villous-like synovial swelling and proliferation
    - Probably secondary to inflammatory or traumatic stimuli
  - Usually presents around 50 years of age
    - Monoarticular with predilection for suprapatellar recess of knee
  - Hyperechoic, frond-like, synovial mass that bends and waves during joint movement on real-time scanning
  - MR appearance more specific with hypertrophied, subsynovial fatty tissue

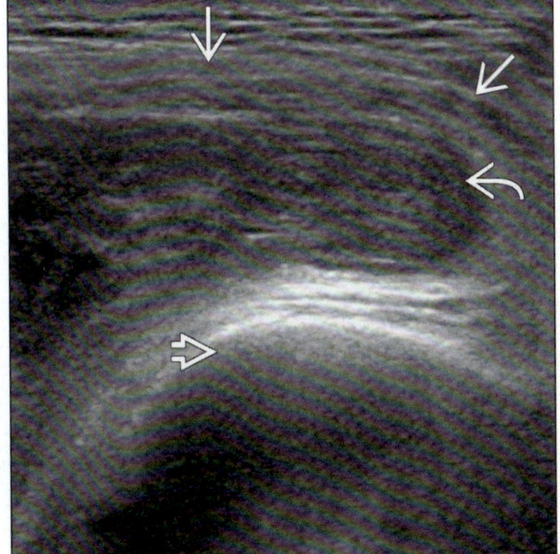

Inflammatory Synovial Mass

Transverse ultrasound shows lateral recess of knee with thickened synovium ⊅ and capsule ⊟ with no effusion. Mild hyperemia was present. Biopsy revealed tuberculous infection. Note the femoral condyle ⊟.

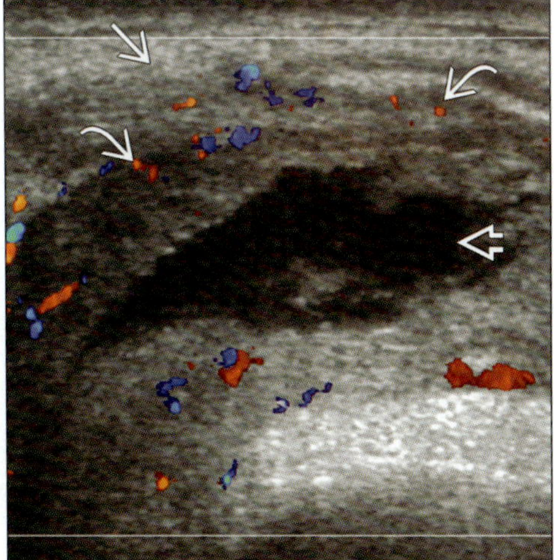

Inflammatory Synovial Mass

Transverse color Doppler US of the lateral recess of the knee shows a severely thickened capsule ⊟, hyperemic synovium ⊅, and joint effusion ⊟. Synovial biopsy showed a tuberculous infection.

ARTICULAR MASS

(Left) Longitudinal ultrasound shows a large heterogeneous mass ➡ with small cystic areas ➡ posterior to the distal femur ⮡, initially considered a soft tissue tumor. Mild hyperemia was present. Biopsy specimen grew Haemophilus influenzae. (Right) Sagittal T1 C+ MR in the same patient shows an enhancing mass ➡ with synovial enhancement throughout the knee ➡ and periarticular inflammation ⮡. The mass resolved with treatment.

Inflammatory Synovial Mass

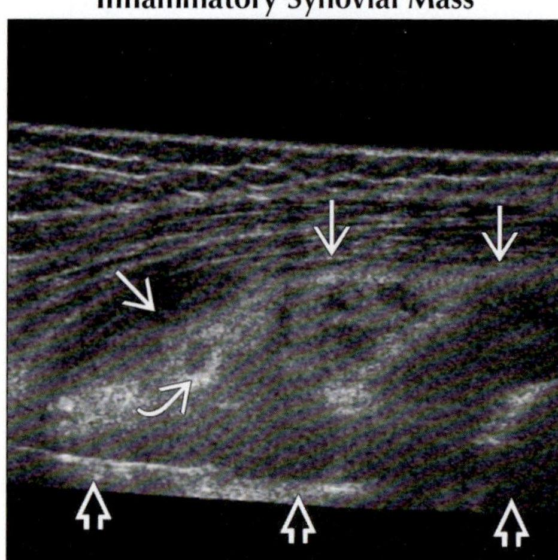

Inflammatory Synovial Mass

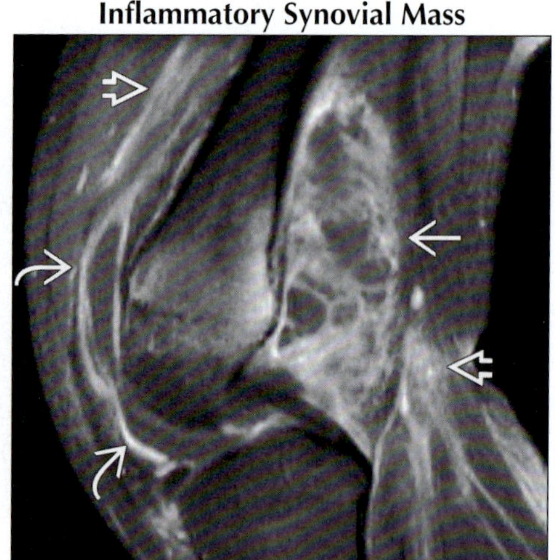

(Left) Longitudinal ultrasound of the medial hindfoot shows a large hypoechoic mass ➡ centered on talocalcaneal articulation ⮡. Biopsy confirmed pigmented villonodular synovitis (PVNS). (Right) Longitudinal power Doppler ultrasound in the same patient shows the mass ➡ is highly vascular. This level of hyperemia favors pigmented villonodular synovitis, though not all PVNS is so vascular.

Pigmented Villonodular Synovitis

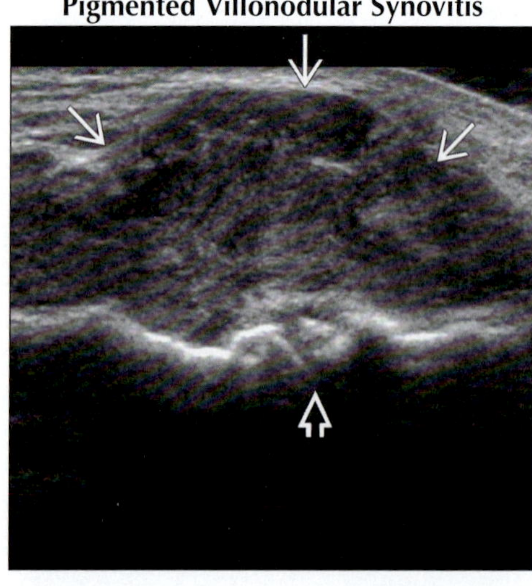

Pigmented Villonodular Synovitis

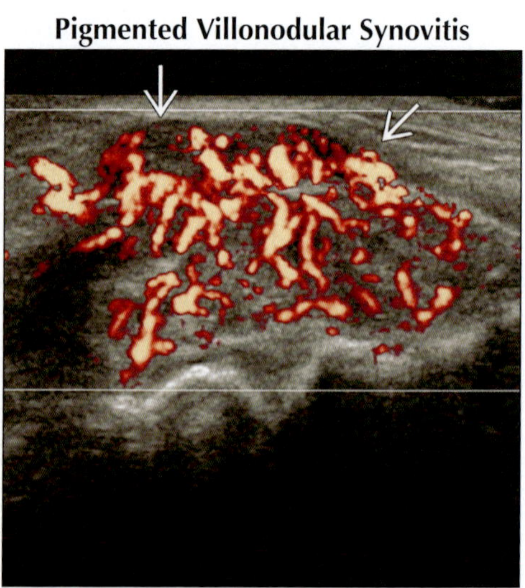

(Left) Longitudinal US shows a large mass ➡ arising from the lateral aspect of the subtalar joint ⮡. This tumor is hyperechoic ➡ in parts due to an intratumoral hemorrhage. The mass was moderately hyperemic (not shown). (Right) Transverse US shows a hypoechoic mass ➡ arising from the ankle and overlying the articular cartilage of the talar dome ⮡. The mass was moderately hyperemic. Biopsy specimen showed pigmented villonodular synovitis.

Pigmented Villonodular Synovitis

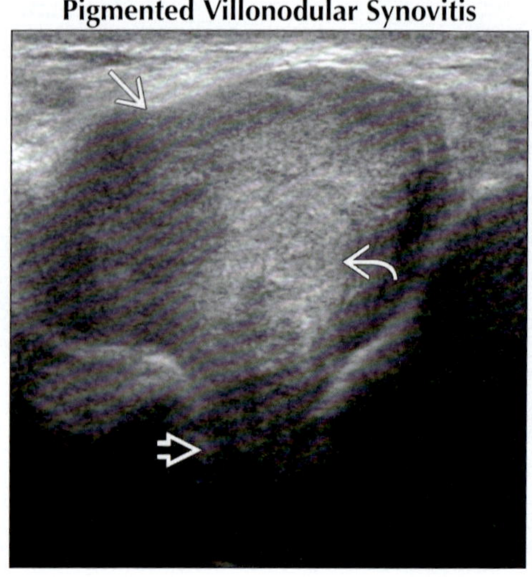

Pigmented Villonodular Synovitis

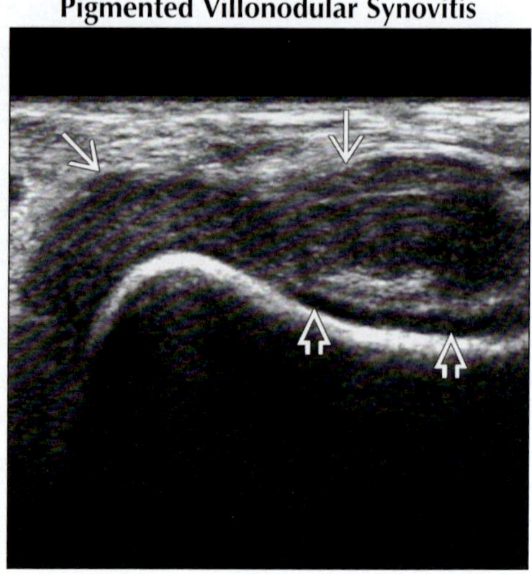

15

ARTICULAR MASS

Focal Nodular Synovitis

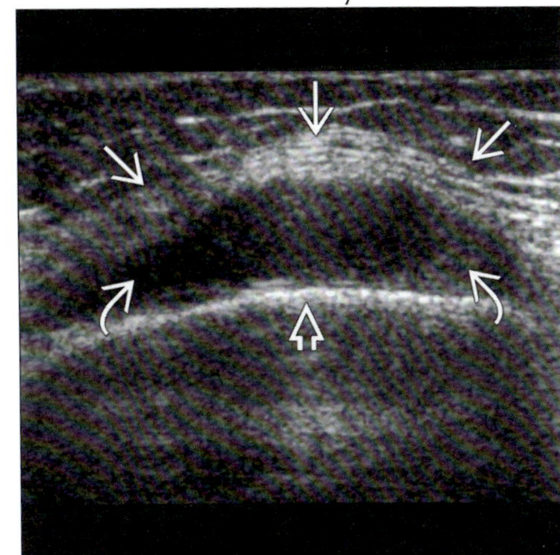

Focal Nodular Synovitis

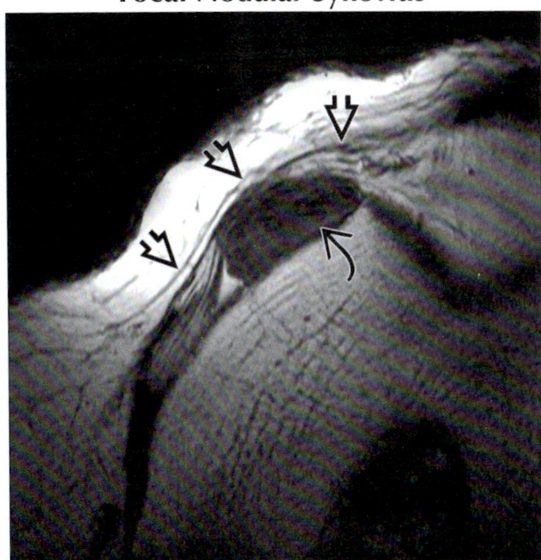

(Left) Transverse ultrasound of the knee shows a fusiform hypoechoic mass ➡ between the retinaculum ➡ and femoral cortex ➡. The mass was mildly hyperemic on color Doppler. The appearance suggests focal nodular synovitis. (Right) Axial T2WI MR shows a focal, heterogeneous, slightly low signal intensity mass ➡ between the retinaculum ➡ and femoral cortex, consistent with focal nodular synovitis.

Synovial Sarcoma

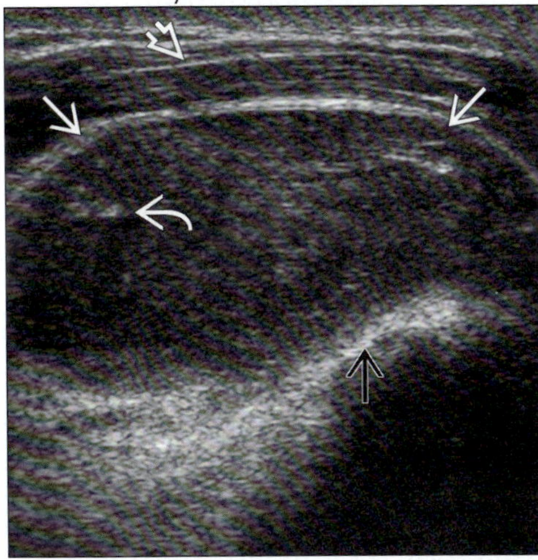

Synovial Sarcoma

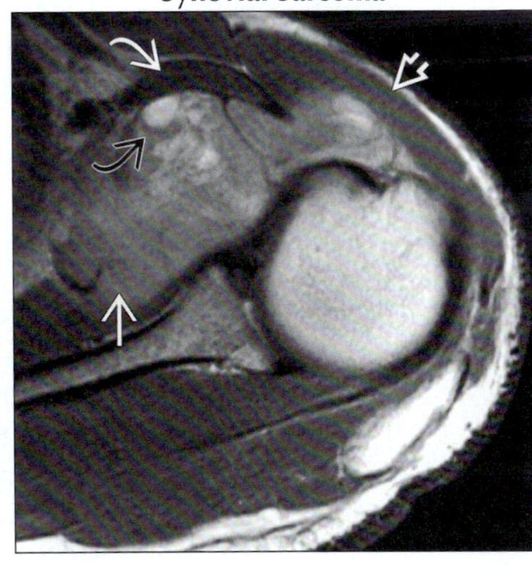

(Left) Transverse ultrasound shows a large hypoechoic mass ➡ with small echogenic areas ➡, which may represent hemorrhage, deep to the deltoid muscle ➡. Note the humerus ➡. (Right) Axial T2WI MR of the shoulder in the same patient shows a mildly hyperintense mass ➡ with small cyst-like areas ➡, deep to the pectoralis ➡ and deltoid ➡ muscles. Biopsy specimen confirmed synovial sarcoma.

Amyloid

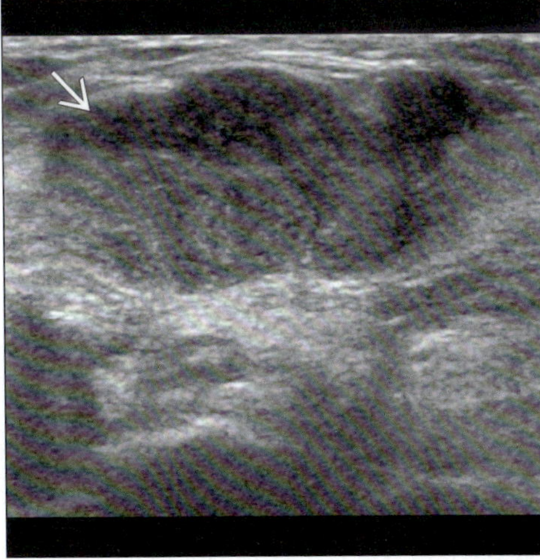

Synovial Hemangioma

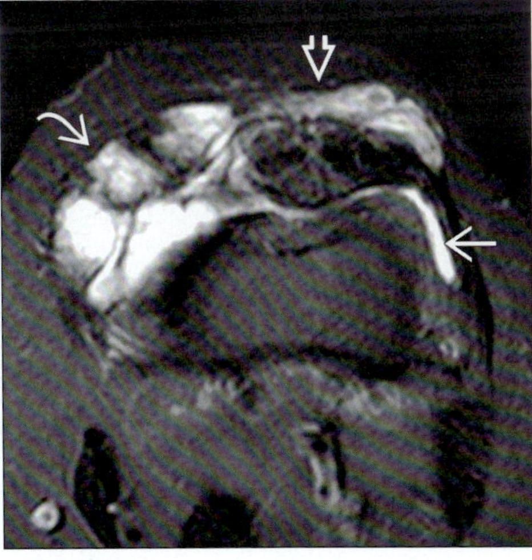

(Left) Transverse ultrasound shows a well-defined, hypoechoic, lobulated, peritendinous mass ➡ in the medial side of the ankle in a patient on hemodialysis. Biopsy specimen revealed amyloid. (Right) Axial T2WI MR with fat suppression shows a venous vascular malformation ➡ of the knee, particularly involving the medial retinaculum and extending to the prepatellar region ➡. There is a small joint effusion ➡.

JOINT EFFUSION

DIFFERENTIAL DIAGNOSIS

Common
- Osteoarthritis

Less Common
- Inflammatory Arthropathy
- Crystal Arthropathy
- Septic Arthritis
- Hemarthrosis
- Lipohemarthrosis

ESSENTIAL INFORMATION

Key Differential Diagnosis Issues
- Characterization of underlying arthropathy relies on disease pattern rather than single ultrasound characteristic
  - Speed of onset, joints affected, severity of disease, age of patient, associated features, radiographic and ultrasound appearances
  - Oligoarticular or polyarticular → inflammatory or degenerative arthropathy
- Ultrasound helpful in assessing disease activity and characterization
- Amount and echogenicity of fluid are useful to note but lack specificity
  - Amount and appearance of joint fluid in osteoarthritis, inflammatory arthropathy, repeated hemarthrosis, and septic arthritis may appear very similar
    - Distinguish among these by noting concurrent ultrasound features, history, and clinical presentation
- If joint fluid is hyperechoic → keep joint still for several minutes
  - Facilitates sedimentation of contents, which may help diagnosis
  - If 2-layered, more likely hemorrhagic
    - Infective fluid does not sediment readily
  - If 3-layered, diagnostic of lipohemarthrosis
  - Ultrasound-guided fluid aspiration often necessary and very helpful
    - Specimen for crystals → send fresh as saline or alcohol will dissolve crystals

Helpful Clues for Common Diagnoses
- **Osteoarthritis**
  - Especially knees, hips, fingers, carpometacarpal joint thumb
    - Characterized by joint space narrowing, cartilage thinning, and marginal osteophytosis on US

  - Variable increase in joint fluid
  - Variable degree of reactive-type inflammatory synovial proliferation
  - ± variable periarticular inflammation
    - Inflammatory component important to note because this can respond to antiinflammatory medication
  - ± particulate debris
  - ± subluxation

Helpful Clues for Less Common Diagnoses
- **Inflammatory Arthropathy**
  - Affects any synovial-lined joint
    - Often bilateral and symmetrical
  - Most common finding: Diffusely thickened hyperechoic or hypoechoic synovium
    - Frond-like or nodular synovial proliferation
  - Effusion may be anechoic or hyperechoic
  - ± speckles due to precipitated fibrin or inflammatory debris
  - ± marginal erosions
    - Well-defined, small, periarticular defects
    - Coalesce to form larger erosions & more generalized marginal irregularity of joint
    - Ultrasound more sensitive than radiography and MR at detecting small joint periarticular erosions
    - Ultrasound less sensitive than contrast-enhanced MR
  - Color Doppler helpful for estimating level of disease activity and distinguishing synovium from joint fluid
    - Hyperemia more readily apparent in small joints (e.g., hand, wrist, elbow) than large joints (e.g., shoulder, hip)
    - Active pannus ⇒ increased color flow
    - Hyperemia graded semiquantitatively as high, intermediate, or low/absent vascularity
    - Quantitative analysis of hyperemia is feasible, though semiquantitative analysis adequate for clinical use
  - Other signs include joint space narrowing, subluxation, deformity, and ankylosis
  - Coexistent soft tissue features include tenosynovitis, bursitis, and entrapment neuropathy
- **Crystal Arthropathy**
  - Always consider in any acute arthritis
  - Effusion anechoic or hyperechoic

15

JOINT EFFUSION

- ○ Gout ⇒ urate crystal deposition
  - ▪ 1st metatarsophalangeal joint is 1st affected joint in 50% → later becomes polyarticular
  - ▪ Best diagnostic clue: Identification of echogenic foci with "comet tail" artifacts within and around joint
  - ▪ ± "'urate sand" (fine punctuate echoes) or "sandstorm" (larger echogenic aggregates) appearance
  - ▪ ± urate deposition in articular cartilage surface → thin echogenic band
  - ▪ Soft tophi (no acoustic shadowing) → hard tophi (dense acoustic shadowing)
- ○ Pseudogout ⇒ calcium pyrophosphate deposition
  - ▪ Knee, wrist, scaphotrapezium articulation
  - ▪ More often associated with osteoarthritis
  - ▪ Crystal deposition in mid-zone of articular cartilage → more prolific cartilage loss
  - ▪ ± meniscal chondrocalcinosis
  - ▪ Paraarticular tophi less common in pseudogout
- **Septic Arthritis**
  - ○ Usually hematogenous spread
    - ▪ ↑ In immunosuppressed, diabetics, and patients with rheumatoid arthritis
  - ○ Joint effusion: Cardinal sign of septic arthritis
  - ○ For most joints, no effusion ⇒ no septic arthritis
  - ○ 2 exceptions to rule

- ▪ For nondistensible diarthrodial joints such as acromioclavicular joint, effusion is minimal
- ▪ If joint capsule not intact following rupture or recent surgery, no effusion
- ○ Echogenic due to aggregates of inflammatory debris
- ○ Ultrasound-guided fluid aspiration for Gram stain, culture, & cytology helpful
- **Hemarthrosis**
  - ○ History of trauma or coagulopathy
    - ▪ ± associated fracture
  - ○ Hyperechoic fluid initially ± layering → hypoechoic later
  - ○ Repeated hemarthroses
    - ▪ Variable synovial thickening
    - ▪ Common and severe in patients with hemophilia with repeated hemorrhage
    - ▪ ± bone overgrowth and secondary osteoarthritis-type picture
    - ▪ ± progressive joint disorganization
- **Lipohemarthrosis**
  - ○ Leakage of marrow fat into joint cavity
    - ▪ Presence of lipohemarthrosis implies fracture communicating with joint
  - ○ 3 layers that become evident are
    - ▪ Fat layer: Least dependent layer
    - ▪ Serum layer: Middle layer
    - ▪ Cellular layer: Most dependent layer

Osteoarthritis

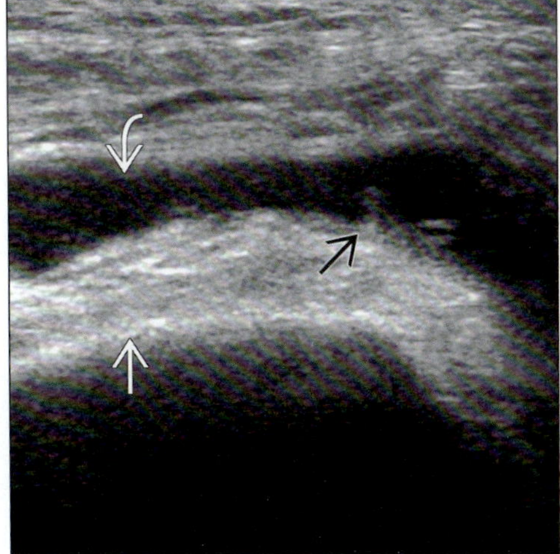

Transverse ultrasound of the knee shows a mildly distended medial patellar recess ➡ with mild synovial proliferation (very uncommon) and fronds ➡. Note the femoral condyle ➡.

Osteoarthritis

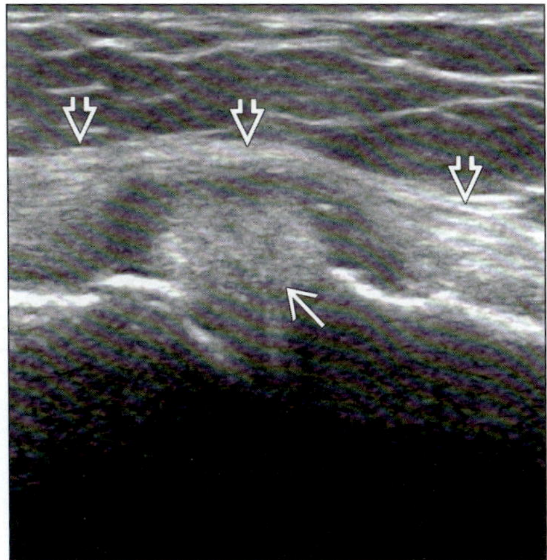

Longitudinal ultrasound of the medial joint line shows moderate extrusion of the medial meniscus ➡ with joint space narrowing, features of osteoarthritis. The medial collateral ligament ➡ is displaced.

JOINT EFFUSION

(Left) Transverse ultrasound shows marked synovial proliferation ➡ distending the medial recess of the knee in a patient with rheumatoid arthritis. This is not specific for inflammatory arthropathy and may be seen with infection or repeated hemarthrosis. Very little fluid ➡ is present. *(Right)* Longitudinal ultrasound of the medial aspect of the knee shows periarticular erosion ➡ of the proximal tibia in a patient with known enthesopathy.

Inflammatory Arthropathy

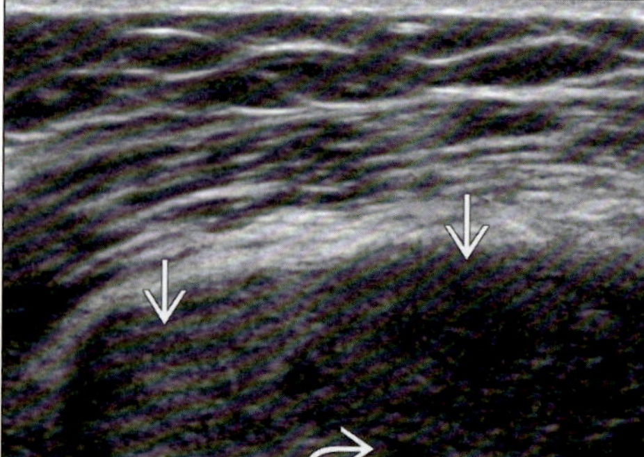

Inflammatory Arthropathy

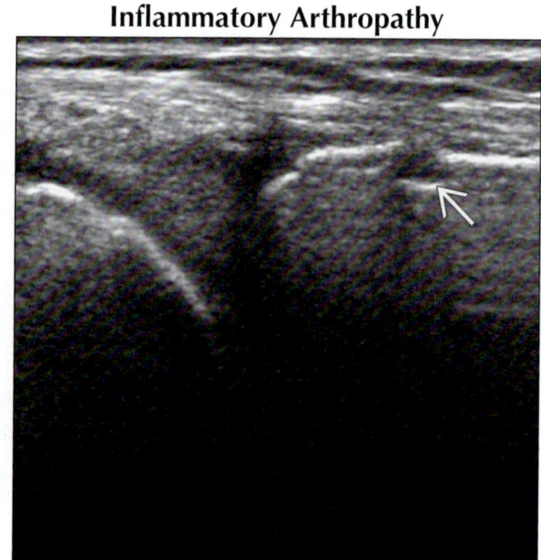

(Left) Longitudinal US in a patient with juvenile arthropathy shows a distended ankle joint ➡ with mildly echogenic fluid. The aspiration was sterile. Note the articular cartilage of the talar dome ➡, tibia ➡, & anterior tibial artery ➡. *(Right)* Longitudinal US shows an echogenic band ➡ in the articular cartilage along the posterior femoral condyle ➡, indicative of calcium pyrophosphate deposition. Other images showed meniscal chondrocalcinosis.

Inflammatory Arthropathy

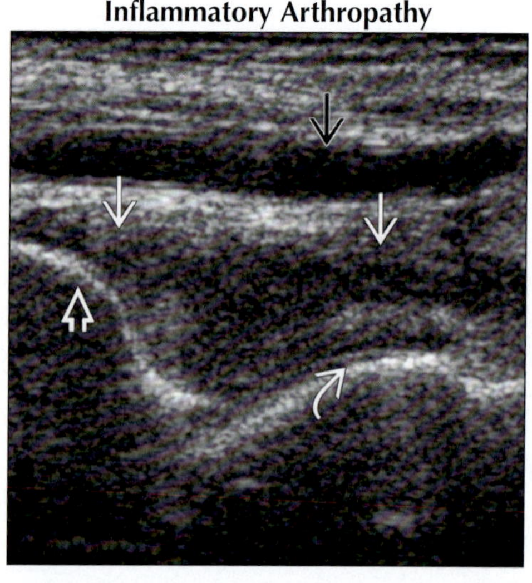

Crystal Arthropathy

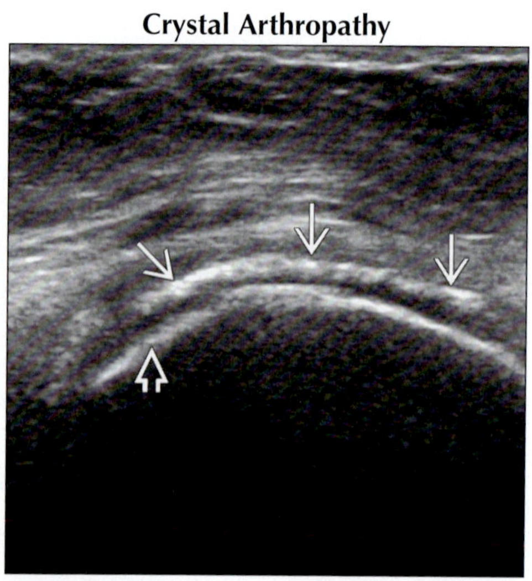

(Left) Longitudinal US shows marked distension ➡ of the 3rd metatarsophalangeal joint ➡ in a patient with chronic gout. The joint fluid is echogenic with small "comet tail" artifacts ➡ & larger crystal aggregates with acoustic shadowing ➡. *(Right)* Transverse US shows the posterior aspect of the glenohumeral joint ➡ distended by synovial proliferation and echogenic fluid due to chronic septic arthritis. Note humeral head ➡, glenoid ➡, and posterior labrum ➡.

Crystal Arthropathy

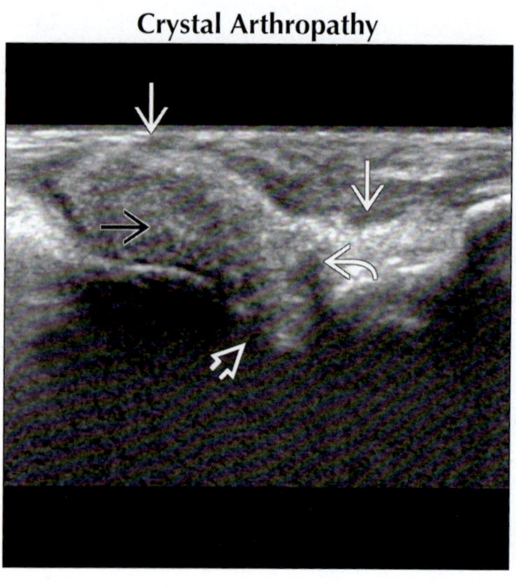

Septic Arthritis

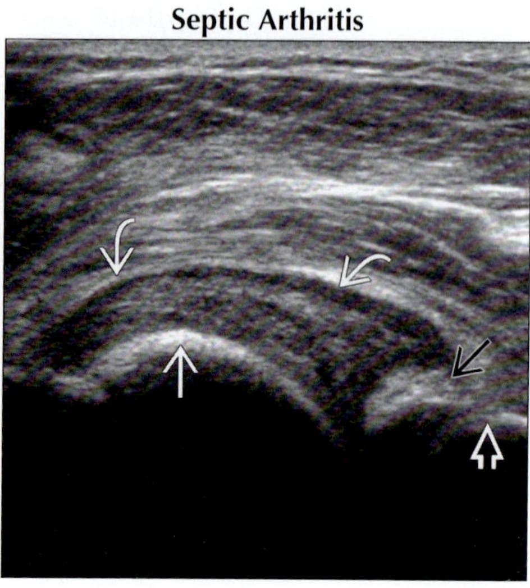

15

JOINT EFFUSION

Septic Arthritis

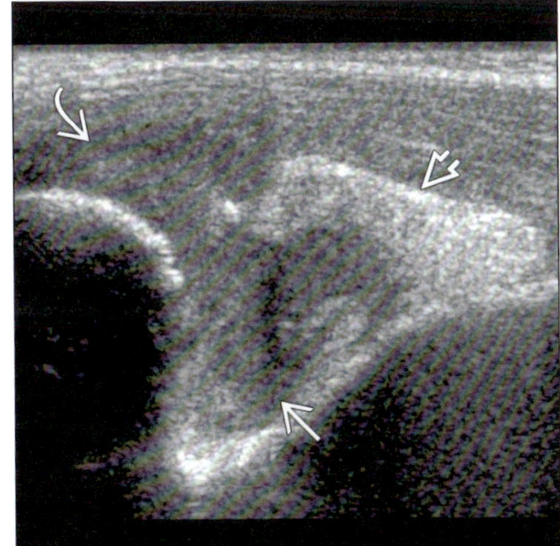

Septic Arthritis

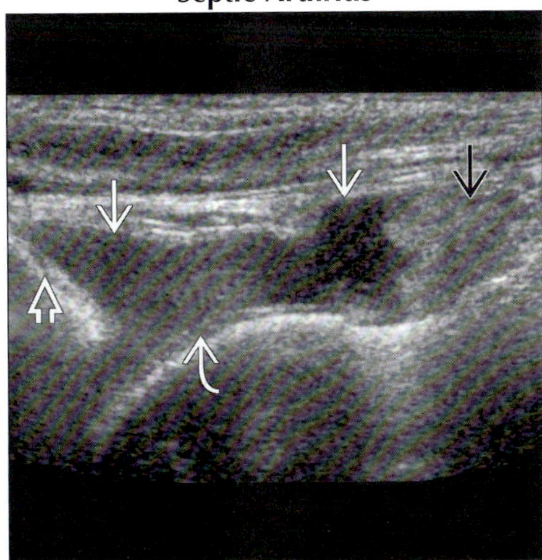

(Left) Longitudinal US of the posterior elbow shows echogenic fluid filling the olecranon recess ➡ with rupture of the posterior elbow capsule ➡ and leakage of contents ➡ deep to the triceps musculotendinous junction. *(Right)* Longitudinal US shows hypoechoic fluid distending the ankle joint ➡, displacing periarticular fat ➡. Aspiration yielded pus, which grew *Staphylococcus aureus*. Note articular cartilage of the talar dome ➡ & distal tibia ➡.

Hemarthrosis

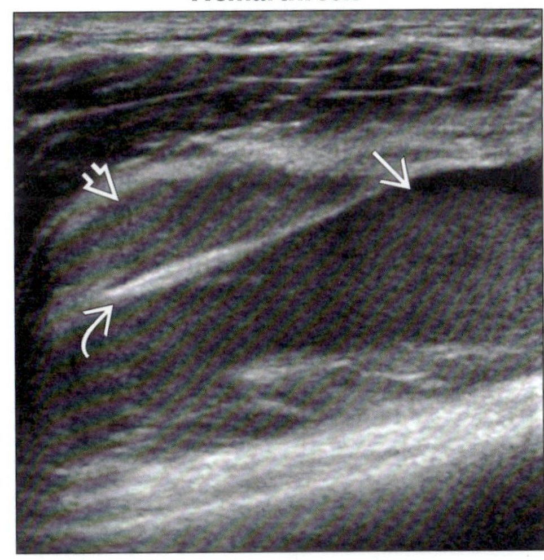

Hemarthrosis

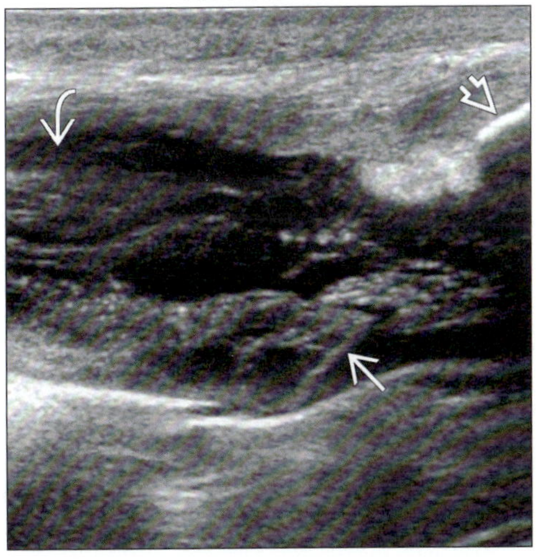

(Left) Longitudinal US shows echogenic fluid distending the suprapatellar recess ➡ due to acute hemarthrosis. Early separation with layering ➡ of cellular & serous components is present. A synovial plica ➡ is visible. *(Right)* Longitudinal US shows the chronic sequelae of hemarthrosis in a hemophiliac patient. There is a combination of synovial proliferation ➡ & septae ➡, with anechoic fluid moderately distending the suprapatellar recess. Note the patella ➡.

Lipohemarthrosis

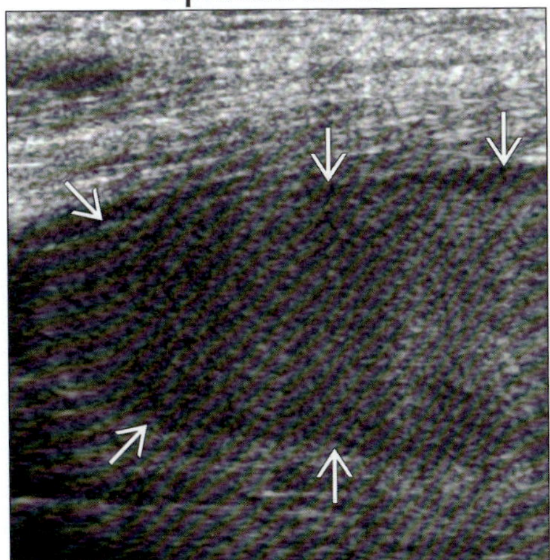

Lipohemarthrosis

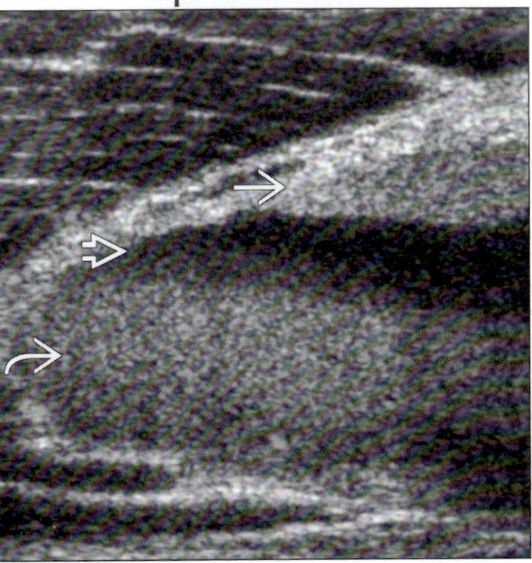

(Left) Longitudinal ultrasound of the knee in a patient with a tibial plateau fracture shows marked distention of the suprapatellar recess ➡ with echogenic fluid. *(Right)* Longitudinal ultrasound at the same location, after keeping the joint still for 15 minutes, shows separation of the fluid contents into fatty ➡, serous ➡, and cellular ➡ components.

BONE SURFACE LESION

DIFFERENTIAL DIAGNOSIS

Common
- Osteochondroma
- Other Benign Bone Tumor
- Malignant Bone Tumor

Less Common
- Metastases
- Acute Osteomyelitis
- Chronic Osteomyelitis
- Soft Tissue Masses

ESSENTIAL INFORMATION

Key Differential Diagnosis Issues
- Check radiographs or other imaging before commenting on bone lesions
- Ultrasound cannot assess intramedullary extent or surrounding bone quality
- Beware of normal bone irregularity at sites of muscle insertion and previous surgery
- Heavy calcification or ossification alongside bone may appear as attached to bone on ultrasound
- Only portion of bony lesion visible with ultrasound
  - Angulation of transducer can help with fuller evaluation
  - MR or CT often required for complete evaluation
- Determining etiology of surface bone lesions often helped by clinical features
  - Age of patient
  - Location of lesion
  - Duration and type of symptoms
- Ultrasound-guided biopsy of bone tumor possible if extraosseous mass present
- Ultrasound-guided biopsy of intramedullary component of bone tumor or infection is possible via cortical breach if present

Helpful Clues for Common Diagnoses
- **Osteochondroma**
  - Most common bone tumor
  - Metaphyseal or metadiaphyseal in location
    - Points away from joint
  - Majority are solitary
    - If multiple and metaphyseal dysplasia ⇒ multiple hereditary exostoses (diaphyseal aclasis)
  - Variable thickness in hypoechoic cartilage cap
  - Most osteochondromas are asymptomatic
  - Symptoms can be due to several causes
  - Reactive myositis secondary to friction between osteochondroma and adjacent muscle
    - Degree of myositis best evaluated on MR
  - Reactive bursitis
    - Friction between osteochondroma and muscle or tendon can produce intervening bursa
  - Pseudoaneurysm
    - Most common vascular complication
    - Arterial rupture → lumen contained by hematoma
    - Characteristic "to-and-fro" pattern on spectral analysis of narrow neck
  - Bleeding
    - From vascular injury, hemorrhagic bursitis, or myositis
  - Neurological sequelae
    - Depending on location, may be due to compressive neuropathy, radiculopathy, or myelopathy
    - Snapping nerve → reactive neuritis
  - Fracture
    - Affects pedunculated osteochondroma
  - Malignant transformation more common with
    - Diaphyseal aclasis (likelihood ≈ 1%)
    - Increase in age
    - Osteochondromas located in axial skeleton
- **Other Benign Bone Tumor**
  - Most intramedullary benign tumors remain intramedullary
    - May expand bone cortex or fracture → bone surface irregularity
  - Giant cell tumor of bone → not infrequently has extraosseous soft tissue component
    - Hypervascular ± hemorrhagic cystic areas
  - Common benign juxtacortical tumors
    - Chondroma
    - Fibroma
    - Lipoma
    - Schwannoma
- **Malignant Bone Tumor**
  - Osteosarcoma = most common malignant bone lesion of children
  - Arises most frequently at metaphyseal ends of long bones

15

- ▪ Areas of most rapid growth in childhood
- ○ Hypoechoic, broad-based, tumoral outgrowth from bone
- ○ Spiculated seams of tumoral osteoid deposition
- ○ Moderately hyperemic
- ○ Ultrasound-guided biopsy undertaken if significant extraosseous component
  - ▪ Intramedullary bone biopsy performed if cortical breach is present

Helpful Clues for Less Common Diagnoses
- **Metastases**
  - ○ Can be detected by ultrasound if periosteal margin of cortex is affected
    - ▪ Medullary or endosteal metastases not seen by US if periosteal cortical margin intact
  - ○ May arise from any primary site (lung most common)
  - ○ More common in diaphyseal location
  - ○ Compromise bone strength as cortical bone is particularly relevant for diaphyseal bone strength
- **Acute Osteomyelitis**
  - ○ Most frequently involves metaphyses of long bones in children
  - ○ Fine lamellar periosteal reaction
  - ○ Anechoic fluid accumulation alongside cortex
  - ○ Subperiosteal accumulation of fluid
  - ○ Subperiosteal abscess
  - ○ Color Doppler imaging → hyperemia within & around inflamed periosteum

- ○ ± concurrent joint involvement
  - ▪ Sympathetic effusion common
  - ▪ Infective arthritis can be excluded by aspiration
- ○ Ultrasound-guided aspiration of subperiosteal fluid or abscess for Gram stain and culture can be performed
- ○ MR best at assessing acute osteomyelitis
  - ▪ Acute osteomyelitis not excluded by ultrasound
- **Chronic Osteomyelitis**
  - ○ Most frequently involves diaphysis of long bones in young → middle-aged adults
  - ○ Coarse or fine periosteal reaction depending on level of activity
    - ▪ ± cortical defect (cloaca)
    - ▪ ± sequestrum within extraosseous tissues
    - ▪ ± juxtacortical inflammation or abscess
    - ▪ ± sinus tract extending towards skin
  - ○ MR best at assessing activity and extent of chronic osteomyelitis
    - ▪ US cannot evaluate intramedullary disease
    - ▪ US very helpful if metal implants in situ, which limit assessment by CT/MR
- **Soft Tissues Masses**
  - ○ Commonly lies against bone
    - ▪ i.e., juxtacortical
  - ○ Juxtacortical is descriptive term only
    - ▪ Difficult to distinguish between tumor arising from bone surface vs. tumor arising in soft tissues abutting bone

Osteochondroma

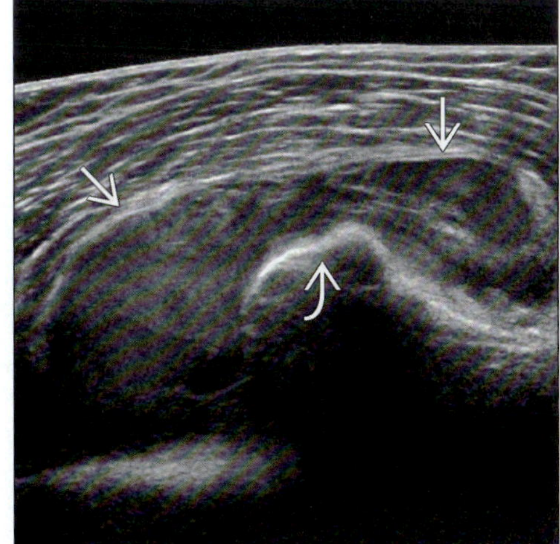

Longitudinal ultrasound of the thigh in a patient with acute swelling shows a femoral osteochondroma ⇨ surrounded by a large hematoma ⇨ due to vascular injury. No pseudoaneurysm was present.

Osteochondroma

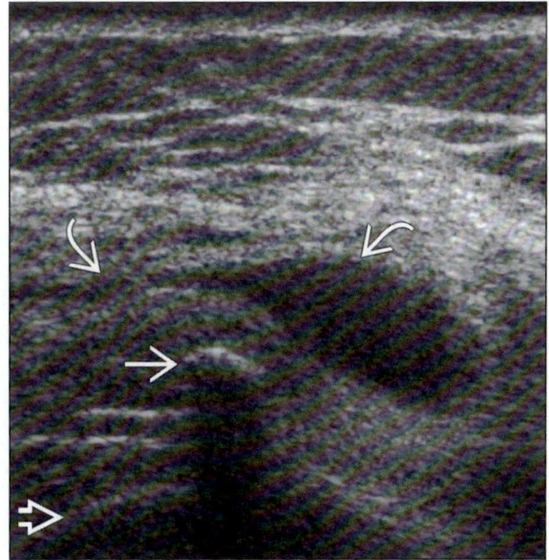

Transverse ultrasound in a patient with distal thigh pain shows a pedunculated osteochondroma ⇨ arising from the femur ⇨. The overlying bursa is distended with fluid ⇨ from a reactive bursitis.

BONE SURFACE LESION

(Left) Lateral radiograph in a patient with diaphyseal aclasis and recent onset thigh swelling shows a large soft tissue mass ⇒ proximal to a distal femoral osteochondroma ➡. *(Right)* Correlative oblique ultrasound of the same lesion shows a large, anechoic, fluid-filled mass ➡. There is a thin echogenic band of thrombus ➡ in the periphery.

Osteochondroma

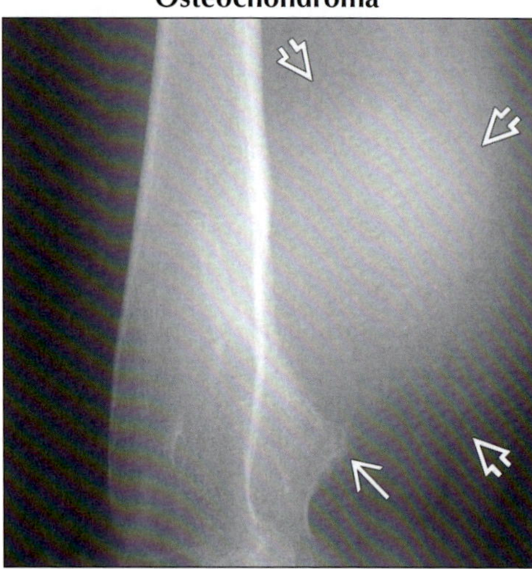

Osteochondroma

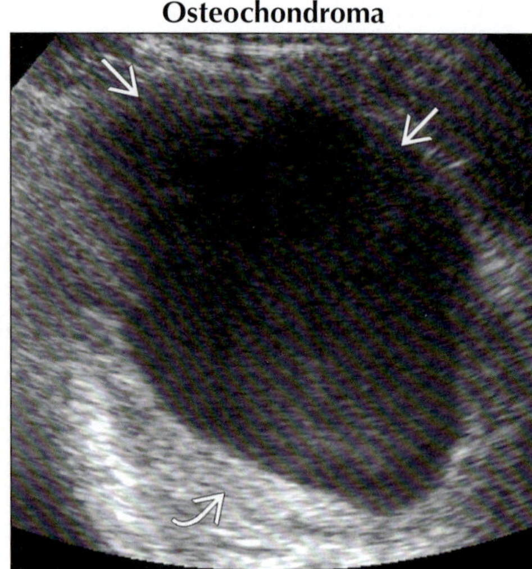

(Left) Corresponding oblique ultrasound shows pulsatile bi-directional flow within the lumen ➡. The superficial femoral artery ➡ lies adjacent to this large pulsatile mass. *(Right)* Pulsed Doppler ultrasound shows characteristic "to-and-fro" flow within the thin neck between the superficial femoral artery and the pulsatile mass. This is a pseudoaneurysm secondary to a vascular injury from the protruding osteochondroma.

Osteochondroma

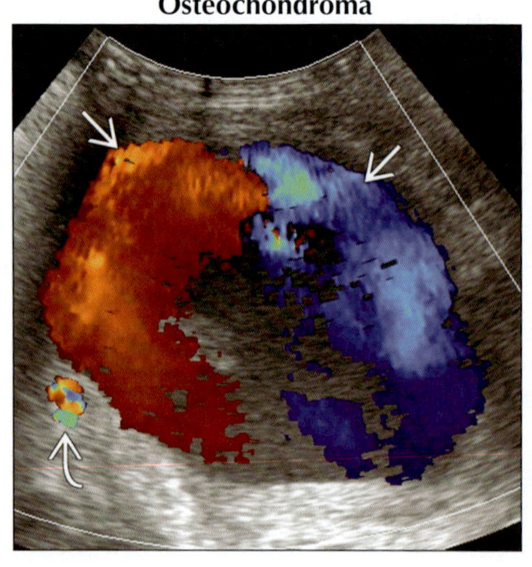

Osteochondroma

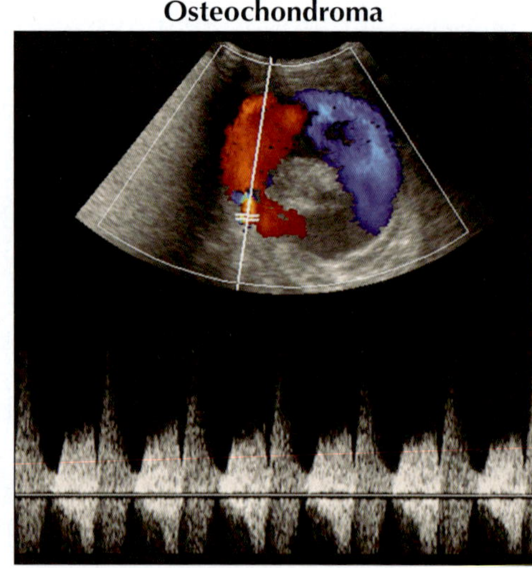

(Left) Transverse US of the leg shows a juxtacortical mass ➡ arising from a cortical defect ➡ on the anteromedial aspect of the tibia ➡ in a patient with a schwannoma extending from a nutrient foramen (which transmits intraosseous vessels and nerves). *(Right)* Longitudinal US shows a large, mainly extraosseous mass ➡ with osteolysis of the proximal fibula ➡, representing a largely extraosseous fibular osteosarcoma. Note the tibia ➡.

Other Benign Bone Tumor

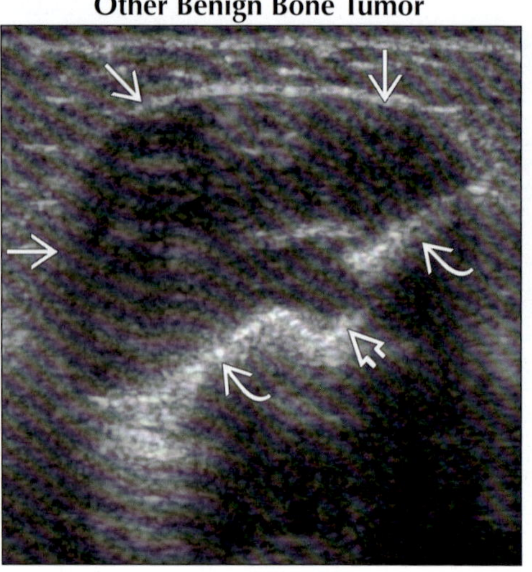

Malignant Bone Tumor

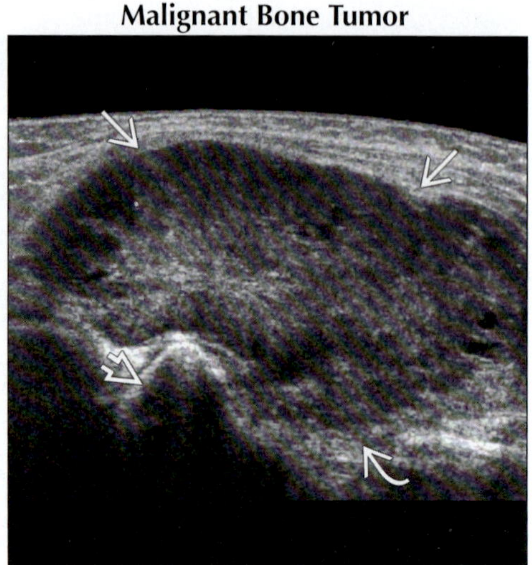

BONE SURFACE LESION

Malignant Bone Tumor

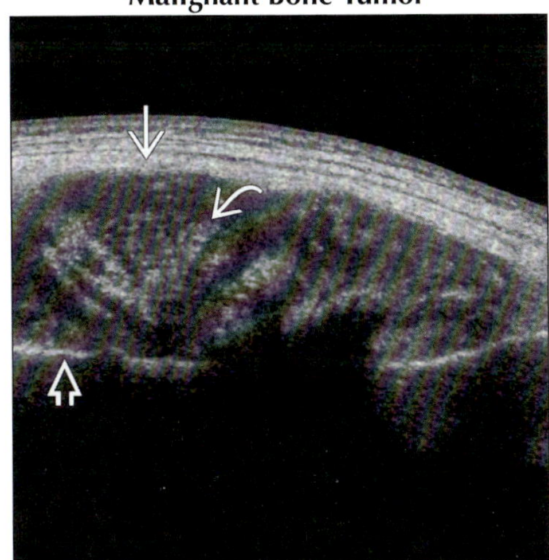

Malignant Bone Tumor

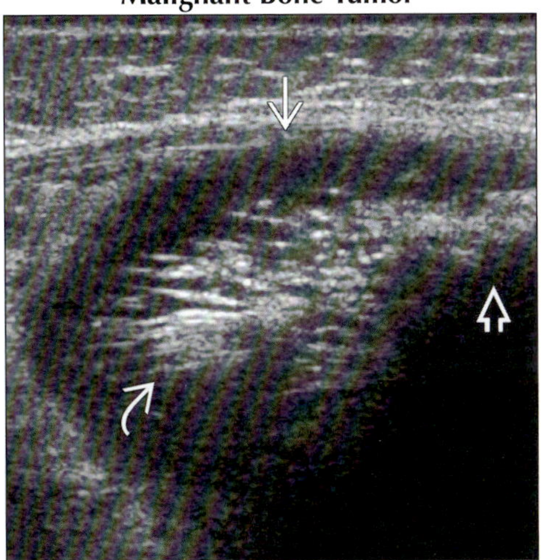

(Left) Longitudinal US shows a large hypoechoic osteosarcoma ➡ arising from the distal femur ➡. Note the spiculated echogenic seams ➡ of mineralized osteoid within the tumor matrix. *(Right)* Transverse US shows a large hypoechoic tumor ➡ arising from the distal ulna ➡ with many echogenic seams ➡ within the tumor matrix. Although appearances are compatible with osteosarcoma, the final diagnosis was Ewing sarcoma.

Acute Osteomyelitis

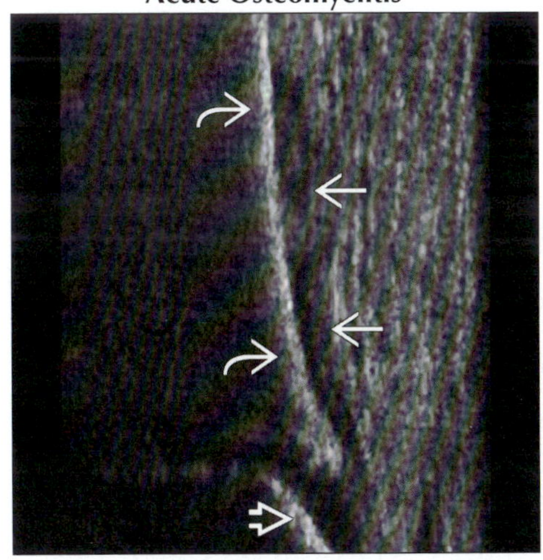

Acute Osteomyelitis

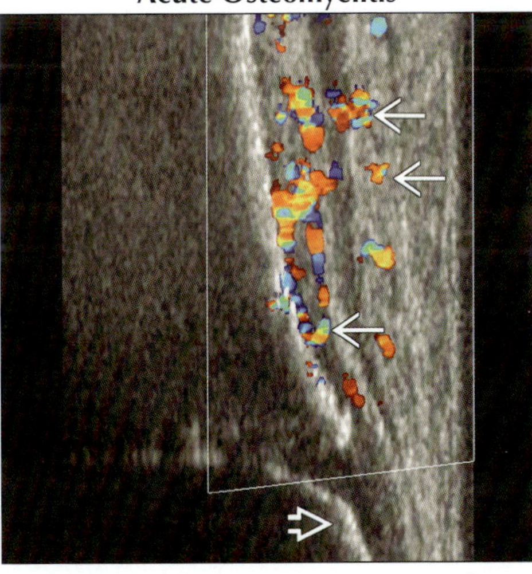

(Left) Longitudinal ultrasound in a child with leg pain and a fever shows periosteal thickening ➡ along the medial aspect of the distal tibial metaphysis ➡. The epiphysis ➡ is not affected. *(Right)* Correlative longitudinal color Doppler US at the same location shows marked hyperemia ➡ of the inflamed thickened periosteum and juxtacortical soft tissues. The epiphysis ➡ is spared. Subsequent MR confirmed acute osteomyelitis.

Acute Osteomyelitis

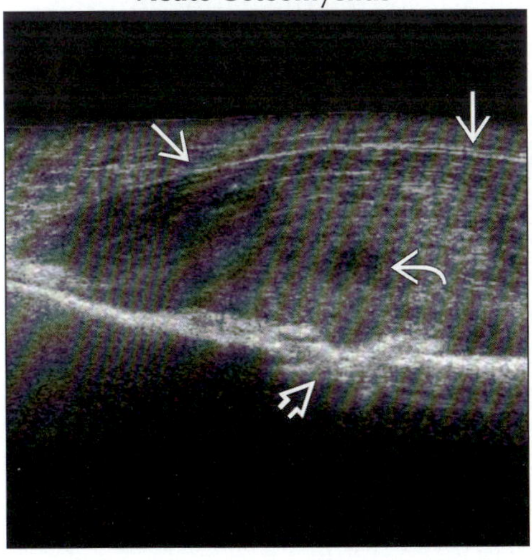

Chronic Osteomyelitis

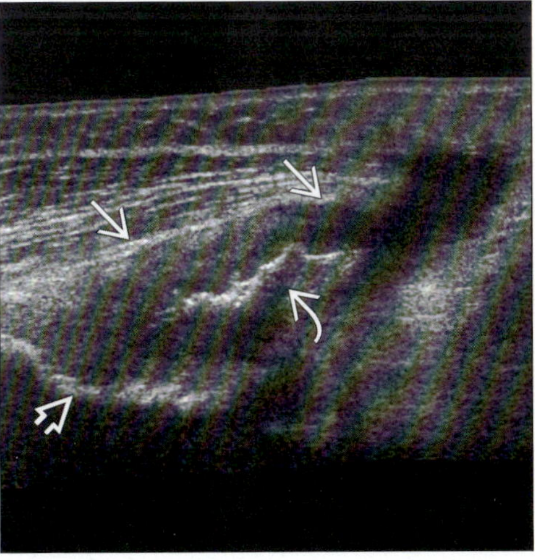

(Left) Transverse ultrasound in a patient with arm pain and a fever shows a large juxtacortical inflammatory mass ➡ with focal disruption of the underlying cortex ➡. An aspirate of the small cystic area ➡ grew Staphylococcus aureus. *(Right)* Longitudinal US of the thigh shows a sequestrum ➡ within a sinus tract ➡ extending from the femoral cortex ➡ to the investing fascia. Sequestra are detached dead bone fragments harboring bacteria.

15

CHEST WALL LESION

DIFFERENTIAL DIAGNOSIS

Common
- Acute Rib Fracture
- Healing Rib Fracture
- Rib Metastases

Less Common
- Muscle Metastases
- Hematoma
- Gynecomastia
- Carcinoma, Male Breast
- Lipoma
- Prominent Xiphoid Process
- Elastofibroma Dorsi

ESSENTIAL INFORMATION

Key Differential Diagnosis Issues
- Ultrasound is very useful for chest wall lesions as structures are superficial & readily visible on high-resolution ultrasound
  - Retroscapular region only area not accessible
- For rib fractures, examine around painful area only
- Ask patient to place finger over most painful area
  - Caveat: US less helpful in unconscious, uncooperative patients or young children
- No need to examine all ribs

Helpful Clues for Common Diagnoses
- **Acute Rib Fracture**
  - History of trauma
  - Localized tenderness
  - Sharp break in superficial bone cortex
    - ± displacement or angulation
    - ± adjacent soft tissue swelling or hypoechoic hematoma
    - Wide break in cortex or cortical irregularity suggests pathological fracture
  - Rib fractures usually occur in vertical line
    - Check adjacent ribs along rib fracture
  - Ultrasound will detect 10x more rib fractures than radiograph
    - Also able to accurately detect fractures of costal cartilage or costochondral junction
  - Ultrasound more accurate than radiograph at detecting pneumothorax
    - Loss of normal "to-and-fro" respiratory motion at pleural surface on real-time scans

- No movement at echogenic pleural surface
- **Healing Rib Fracture**
  - Fracture margin less sharp and more rounded
  - ± slight widening of fracture gap
  - ± bridging callus
    - Unossified hypoechoic mass ± localized hyperemia
    - Progressive ossification of callus with ↑ echogenicity & ↑ acoustic shadowing
    - After approximately 2 months, only cortical bump without visible fracture line will remain
    - Cortical contour will take from months to years to remodel to normal
- **Rib Metastases**
  - Common site of osseous metastases
  - Lung, kidney, hepatocellular carcinoma, and bowel are all common primary sites
  - Usually multiple
    - Randomly located, as opposed to linear location of rib fractures
  - Can be detected only if cortex is disrupted
    - Metastases usually originate in medullary canal prior to infiltrating cortices
    - Therefore, US has low sensitivity for detecting rib metastases
  - Bone destruction
    - Irregular thinning or loss of echogenic superficial cortex of rib
    - ± soft tissue mass at site of bony destruction

Helpful Clues for Less Common Diagnoses
- **Muscle Metastases**
  - Feature of advanced stage malignancy
  - Muscle metastases relatively uncommon, possibly due to
    - Destruction of tumor cells due to muscle motion
    - Muscle pH inhospitable to tumor cells
    - Muscle prevents build up of tumor-produced lactic acid that induces tumor neovascularity in other tissues
  - Varied primary tumors (melanoma, pancreatic, kidney, colon, lungs, stomach, ovary, hepatocellular carcinoma, etc.) → muscle metastases
  - Soft tissue mass
    - ± hyperemia
    - ± surrounding edema

15

- ■ ± central necrosis (uncommon)
- **Hematoma**
  - ○ Due to trauma, anticoagulation, strenuous, prolonged coughing, vascular malformation
  - ○ Often within pectoralis or intercostal muscles
  - ○ Mildly echogenic mass
    - ■ ± layering or liquefaction
    - ■ ± marginal hyperemia
- **Gynecomastia**
  - ○ Growth of glandular tissue in male breast
  - ○ Pseudogynecomastia = ↑ fat in male breast
  - ○ Most cases are idiopathic
  - ○ Identifiable causes include
    - ■ Congenital anorchia, Klinefelter syndrome
    - ■ Hermaphroditism, adrenal carcinoma
    - ■ Liver disorders, drugs (spirolactone, cimetidine, estrogen derivatives)
  - ○ Glandular proliferation → more diffuse fibrotic proliferation
    - ■ Glandular hyperplasia occurs in retroareolar region and is hypoechoic
    - ■ Branches out in triangular fashion beyond retroareolar region
  - ○ As glandular hyperplasia becomes more diffuse, fibrosis develops
    - ■ Leads to increase in echogenicity of proliferating tissues
- **Carcinoma, Male Breast**
  - ○ Multilobulated cystic pattern more common than mixed cystic-solid pattern

- ○ Ill-defined margin more common than well-defined margin
- ○ Mildly hypervascular, mainly peripheral
- **Lipoma**
  - ○ Similar appearances to lipoma elsewhere
  - ○ Hypoechoic, well-defined, soft tissue mass with fine echogenic striations
- **Prominent Xiphoid Process**
  - ○ Cartilaginous lower end of sternum, which normally points slightly forward
  - ○ If large, or if pectus excavatum, may be felt as palpable mass
- **Elastofibroma Dorsi**
  - ○ Uncommon; benign, slow-growing, connective tissue tumor
    - ■ Subscapular area in elderly women = most frequent occurrence
    - ■ ↑ in persons who perform manual labor involving shoulder girdle
    - ■ Tumor composed of abnormal elastic fibers
    - ■ Generally regarded as fibroblastic reactive process or pseudotumor
  - ○ Large, well-circumscribed tumor
  - ○ US appearances typically comprise arrays of linear echogenic strands within less echogenic background
  - ○ Occasionally US pattern similar to surrounding muscle with neither clear demarcation or specific vascular pattern seen
    - ■ Can be occasionally difficult to distinguish from surrounding muscle

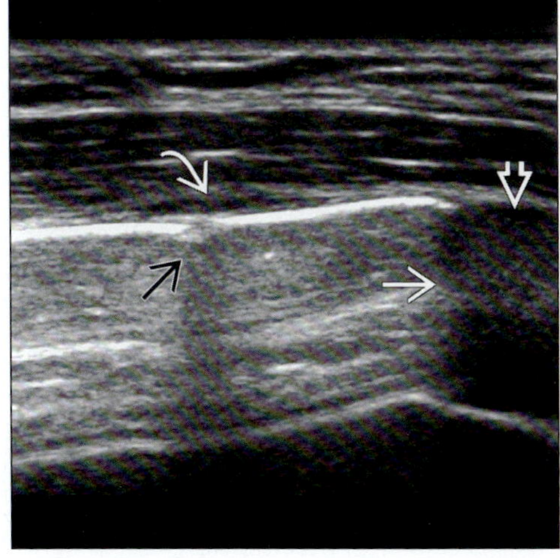

Acute Rib Fracture

Longitudinal ultrasound of a rib shows an undisplaced fracture ➡ of the anterior cortex of the rib with a small adjacent hematoma ➡. Hypoechoic costal cartilage ➡ and costochondral junction ➡ are shown.

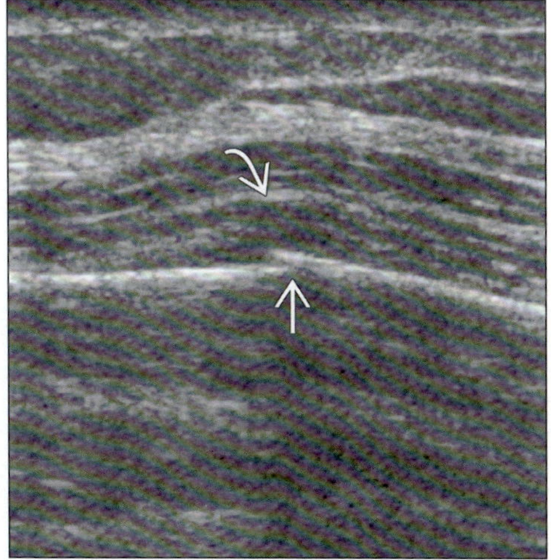

Acute Rib Fracture

Longitudinal ultrasound of a rib shows an undisplaced angulated fracture ➡ with adjacent soft tissue swelling ➡.

CHEST WALL LESION

Healing Rib Fracture

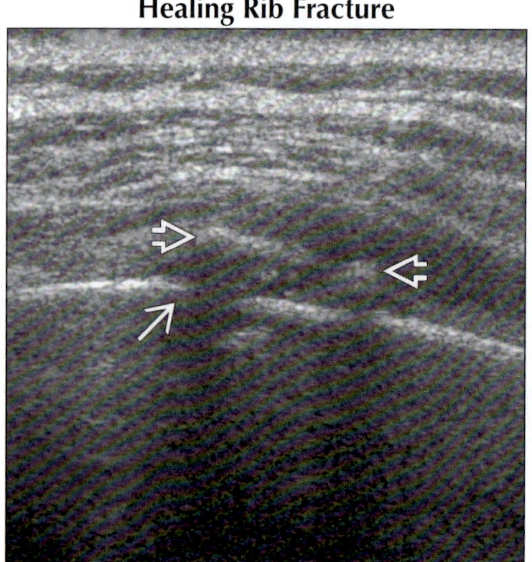

Rib Metastases

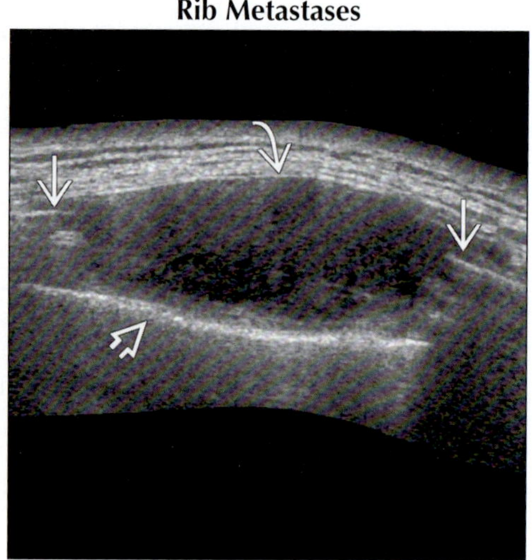

(Left) Longitudinal ultrasound shows a healing rib fracture with widened, rounded fracture margins ➡. Note the ossification ➡ within the callus. *(Right)* Longitudinal ultrasound shows a large, hypoechoic, metastatic deposit ➡ destroying the cortex of the rib ➡ and providing an acoustic window to view the underlying pleura ➡.

Muscle Metastases

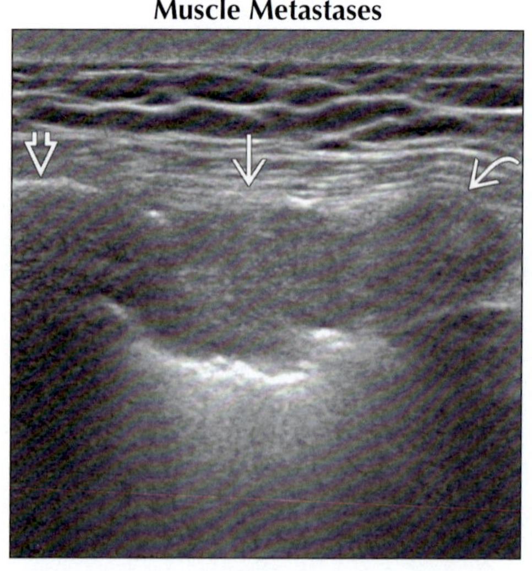

Hematoma

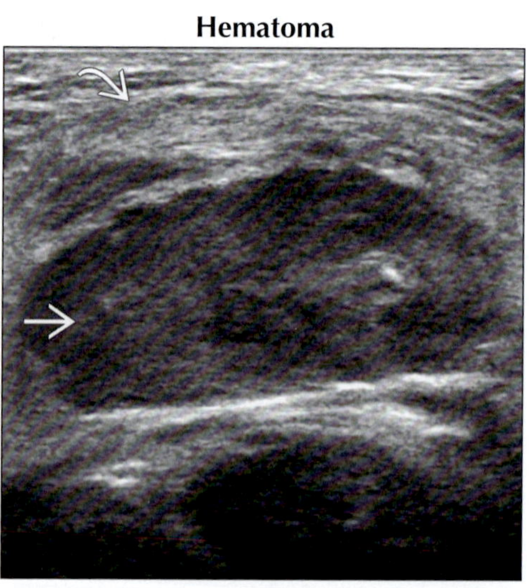

(Left) Transverse ultrasound of the upper chest wall shows a medium-sized hypoechoic mass ➡ with posterior enhancement at the interspace between the 2nd costal cartilage ➡ and 3rd rib ➡. While the mass indents and seems to invade the parietal pleura, the visceral pleura was seen moving freely on real-time imaging. *(Right)* Transverse ultrasound of the upper anterior chest wall shows a large hypoechoic hematoma ➡ deep to the pectoralis muscle ➡.

Hematoma

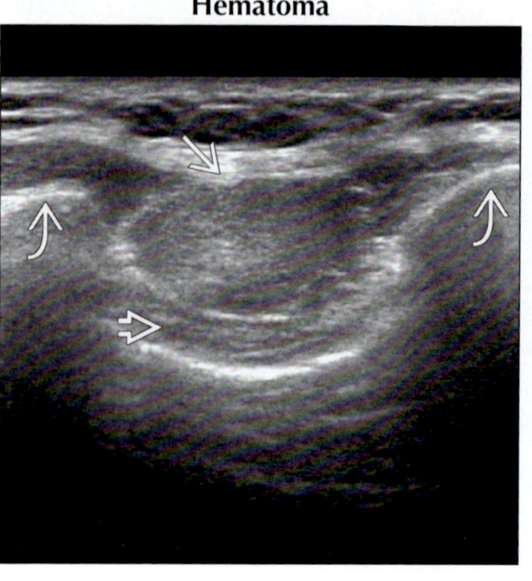

Hematoma

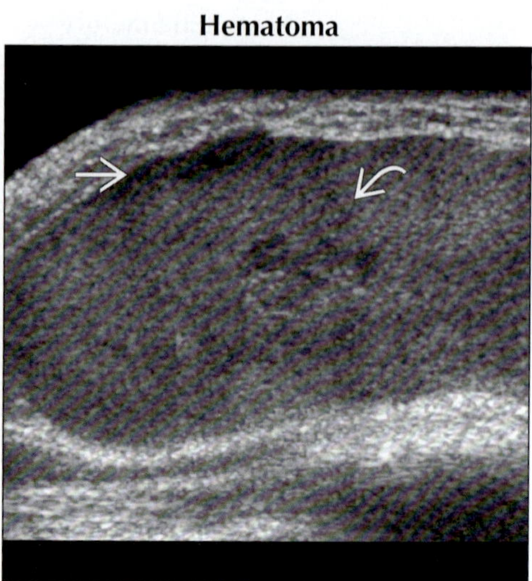

(Left) Transverse ultrasound following recent chest trauma shows a slightly hypoechoic, well-defined hematoma ➡ between the ribs ➡. No rib fracture was present. Intercostal muscle is displaced deep to the hematoma ➡. *(Right)* Transverse ultrasound of the lower anterior chest wall in a young boy shows a large, well-defined, hypoechoic hematoma. There is some early separation of cellular & serous elements superficially ➡, with hypoechoic debris centrally ➡.

15

CHEST WALL LESION

Gynecomastia

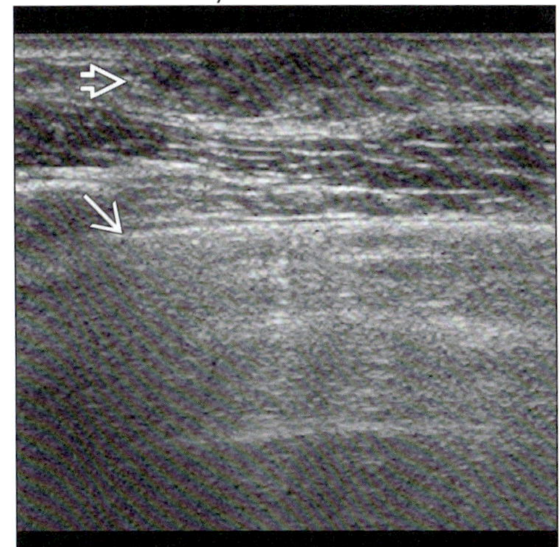

Gynecomastia

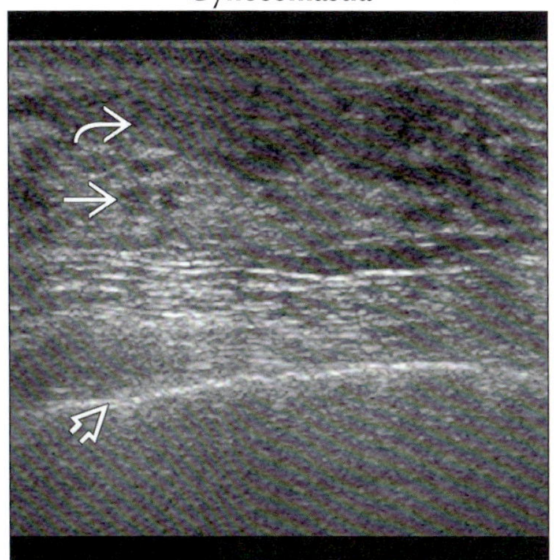

(Left) Transverse ultrasound of the normal side in a male patient with unilateral gynecomastia shows a normal areola and subareolar region ➡. *The underlying pleura is visible* ➡. *(Right) Transverse ultrasound of the contralateral breast in the same patient shows gynecomastia with subareolar hypoechoic glandular tissue* ➡ *and underlying hyperechoic fibrotic and fatty tissue* ➡. *The underlying pleura is again visible* ➡.

Carcinoma, Male Breast

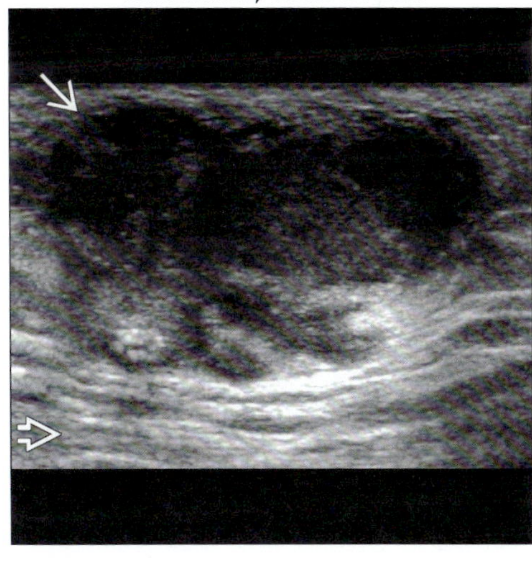

Prominent Xiphoid Process

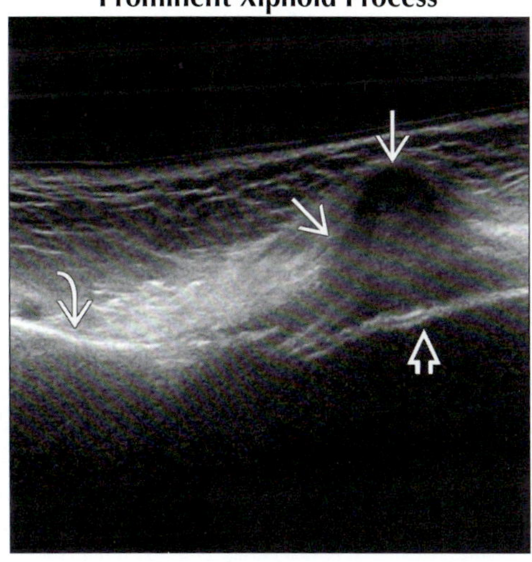

(Left) Transverse ultrasound shows a heterogeneous, mixed solid & cystic mass ➡ *with distinct margins, associated with edema & architectural distortion of the surrounding tissue. There is mild posterior acoustic enhancement* ➡. *Excision confirmed ductal carcinoma. (Right) Longitudinal ultrasound in an elderly male patient with an "epigastric" mass shows a prominent hypoechoic xiphoid process* ➡ *at the lower end of the sternum* ➡, *overlying the peritoneum* ➡.

Elastofibroma Dorsi

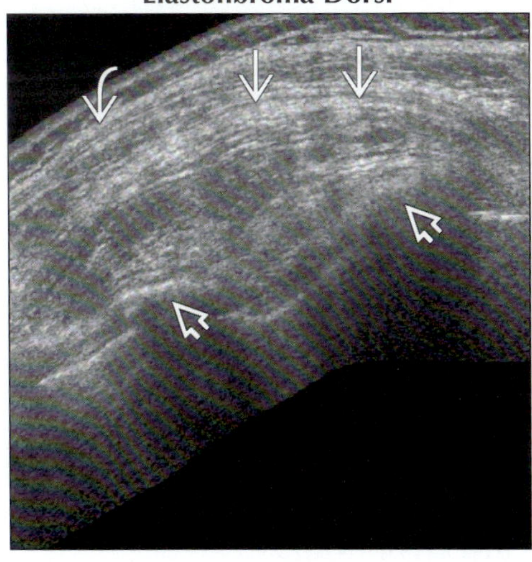

Elastofibroma Dorsi

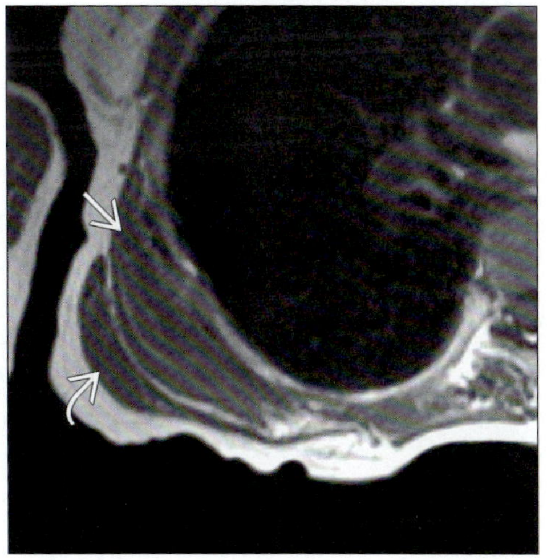

(Left) Oblique ultrasound of the infrascapular region in an elderly woman shows a mixed echogenic mass ➡ *lying between the ribs* ➡ *and a moderately atrophic latissimus dorsi muscle* ➡. *The mass shows layers of linear echogenic strands on a hypoechoic background. The biopsy confirmed elastofibroma. (Right) Axial T1WI MR of a comparable area shows a crescent-shaped mass* ➡ *deep to the latissimus dorsi* ➡ *comprised of isointense and hyperintense strands.*

15

DIFFERENTIAL DIAGNOSIS

Common
- Inguinal Hernia
- Ventral Hernia
- Incisional Hernia
- Diastasis Recti

Less Common
- Rectus Sheath Hematoma
- Endometrioma
- Muscle Tear
- Undescended Testis
- Umbilical Hernia
- Lumbar Hernia
- Subcutaneous Lipoma
- Nerve Sheath Tumor
- Desmoid Tumor
- Muscle Metastases
- Granuloma

ESSENTIAL INFORMATION

Key Differential Diagnosis Issues
- Pay close attention to deep margin of any anterior abdominal wall mass, because hernias may masquerade as abdominal wall masses
  - Defect may be small relative to size of mass and potentially overlooked
  - May be fixed and not reducible
  - May look like hypoechoic subcutaneous nodule or lipomatous mass
  - Check for peristalsis, vascularity, and perform Valsalva maneuver
    - Valsalva for groin hernia often better with patient standing upright
  - If deep border of mass not seen, reassess with either CT or MR

Helpful Clues for Common Diagnoses
- **Inguinal Hernia**
  - Most groin hernias more common in males
  - Indirect inguinal hernias 5x more common than direct inguinal hernias
  - Indirect hernia passes into deep inguinal ring, along inguinal canal, and out of deep inguinal ring
    - Elongated oblique course
    - In males, follows course of spermatic cord → scrotum
    - In females, follows course of round ligament → labia majora
    - Indirect hernia passes lateral to inferior epigastric vessels
  - Direct hernia passes through floor of inguinal canal
    - Broad and dome-shaped
    - Appears as small bulge in groin
    - Passes medial to inferior epigastric vessels
  - Ultrasound to accurately identify presence, type, and contents of groin hernias
    - Contents include fluid, omentum, and bowel
    - Omentum is echogenic due to omental fat and has no peristalsis
    - Bowel has visible bowel wall (± "target" echopattern) filled with fluid or bowel contents ± peristalsis
  - Hernia may be irreducible, obstructed, or strangulated
    - Irreducible: No change in hernia size with decrease in intraabdominal pressure or increase with cough or Valsalva
    - Obstructed: Associated with signs of intestinal obstruction ± reduced peristalsis
    - Strangulated: Swollen bowel wall with absence of vascularity within bowel wall or mesentery
- **Ventral Hernia**
  - Protrusion of extraperitoneal fat through defect in linea alba
    - Point where vessels perforate fascia
    - Usually occurs in young to middle-aged patients
  - Narrow defect in linea alba
    - Fatty contents can strangulate and infarct
  - Small hernia containing either echo-poor or echogenic fat in epigastric region
    - Often no change with Valsalva since neck of hernia is tight
- **Incisional Hernia**
  - Can occur after any abdominal operation
    - Presents months to years after surgery
- **Diastasis Recti**
  - Results from widened linea alba
  - Ultrasound to exclude presence of true ventral hernia

Helpful Clues for Less Common Diagnoses
- **Rectus Sheath Hematoma**

- Due to bleeding within rectus sheath from injury to superior or inferior epigastric arteries or direct tear of rectus muscle
- Inferior epigastric artery arises from external iliac artery
  - Ascends between rectus abdominis muscle and posterior rectus sheath
  - Prone to injury during strong muscle contractions
- Superior epigastric artery originates from external thoracic artery
  - Descends between rectus abdominis muscle and posterior rectus sheath
- **Endometrioma**
  - Palpable mass often near cesarean section scar or pelvic surgical scar
  - Pain ± cyclical pain occurring with menses
  - Solid, mainly hypoechoic, heterogeneous nodule
  - Infiltrating margins
  - Peripheral hyperechoic ring
  - Mild internal vascularity
  - Anechoic cystic areas uncommon
- **Muscle Tear**
  - Often affects oblique muscles in lower abdominal quadrants
    - Well-localized mechanical pain
    - Affects athletes and patients with chronic cough
- **Undescended Testis**
  - Ultrasound will locate undescended testis in nearly 90% of patients with cryptorchidism
    - Almost 90% of undescended testes will be located in inguinal canal
    - Remainder located in abdomen and pelvis
- **Umbilical Hernia**
  - Occurs in newborns
    - Large neck and therefore unlikely to strangulate
- **Lumbar Hernia**
  - Occurs through defect in posterolateral abdominal wall
  - Either spontaneous, postsurgical, or post-traumatic in origin
  - Herniation of retroperitoneal fat ± colon or small bowel
- **Subcutaneous Lipoma**
  - Fusiform mass with thin, parallel, echogenic internal striations
- **Nerve Sheath Tumor**
  - Fusiform, hyperemic, hypodense mass ± myxoid areas ± internal hemorrhage
- **Desmoid Tumor**
  - Benign fibrous tumor also known as fibromatosis with predilection for anterior abdominal wall
    - Hypoechoic tumor often with irregular margin
- **Granuloma**
  - May arise from retained suture or at apex of sinus tract
  - Hypoechoic mass ± suture material ± mild to moderate vascularity

Inguinal Hernia

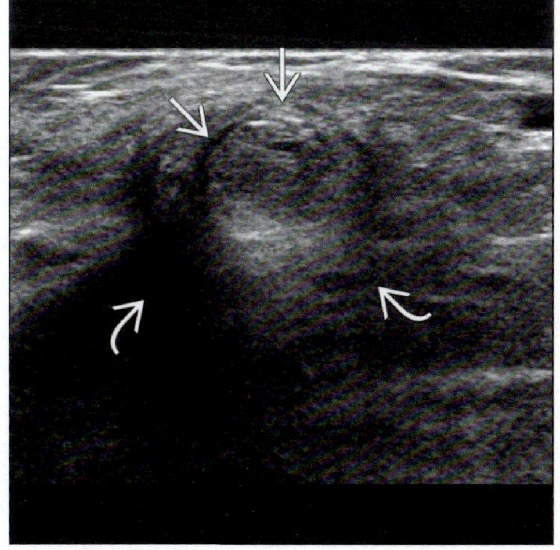

Transverse ultrasound shows indirect inguinal hernia ➡ containing fat & bowel extending along inguinal canal after emerging through deep inguinal ring ➡. Inferior epigastric vessels (not shown) lie medial to hernia neck.

Inguinal Hernia

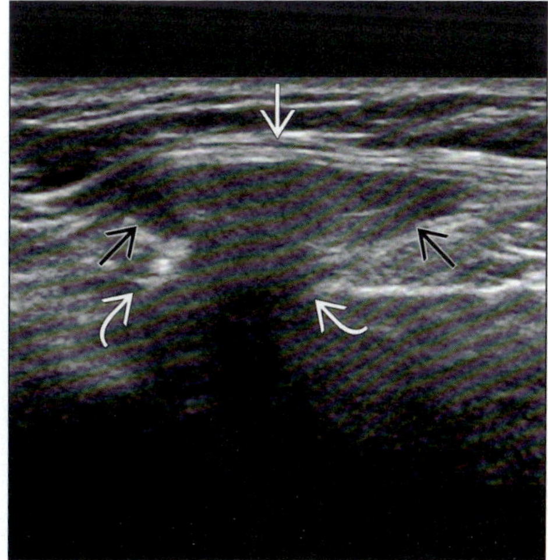

Transverse ultrasound shows a fat-containing direct inguinal hernia ➡ protruding through a defect in floor of inguinal canal ➡ medial to inferior epigastric vessels and lying deep to external aponeurosis ➡.

ABDOMINAL WALL MASS

Ventral Hernia

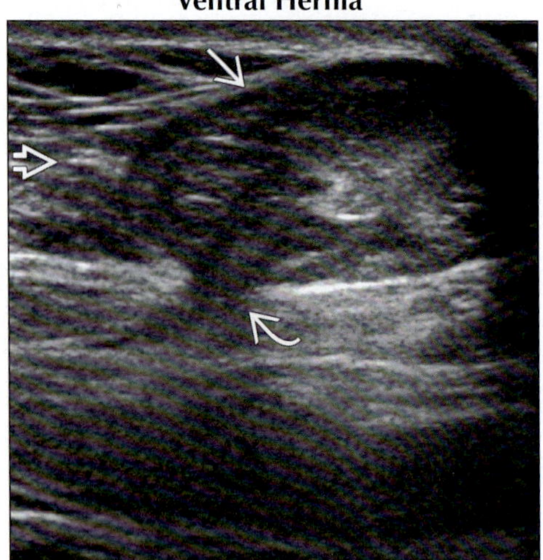

Incisional Hernia

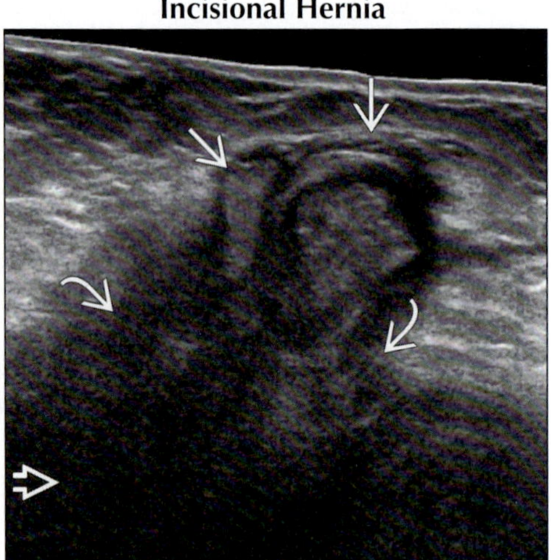

(Left) Longitudinal ultrasound shows a large ventral hernia ➡ at the linea alba protruding into the subcutaneous fat ⇨. The defect ➡ in the midline linea alba is narrow, making this hernia prone to strangulation. The hernia contains fat but no bowel. *(Right)* Transverse ultrasound shows loops of small bowel ➡ protruding from the peritoneal cavity ⇨ into the subcutaneous fat through a wide incisional fascial defect ➡ in the lower abdomen.

Diastasis Recti

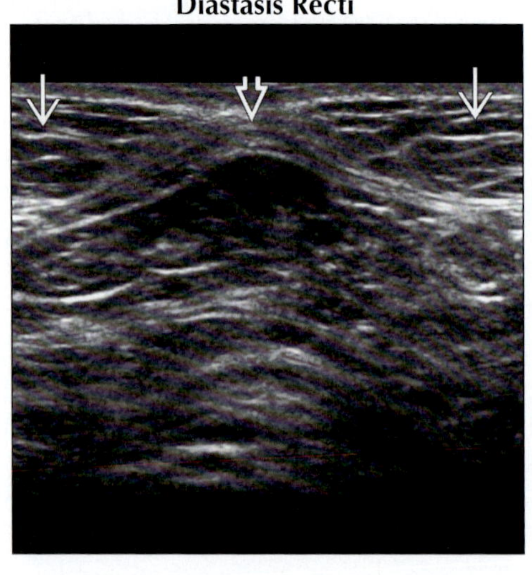

Rectus Sheath Hematoma

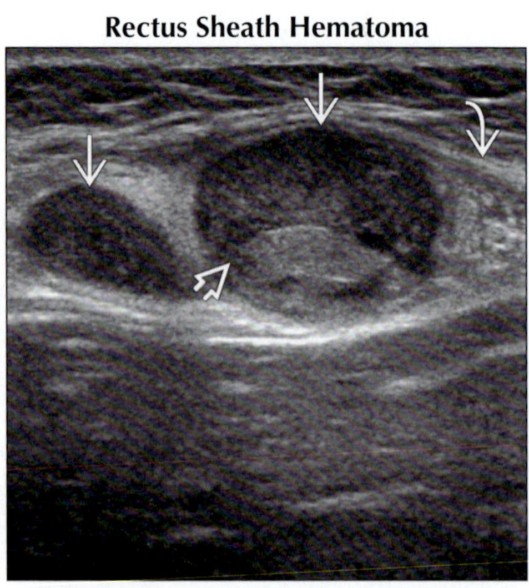

(Left) Transverse ultrasound shows a widened linea alba ⇨ connecting the rectus abdominus muscles ➡. The widened linea alba is bulging upwards in midline, simulating a hernia. No fascial defect or hernia is present. *(Right)* Transverse ultrasound shows 2 large traumatic hematomas ➡ within an edematous rectus abdominal muscle ➡. Note the typical layering debris ⇨. The hematomas are contained by the rectus sheath. There is no liquefaction present.

Endometrioma

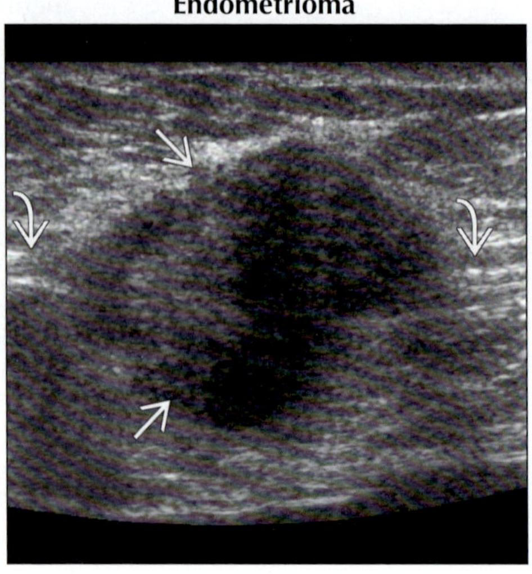

Muscle Tear

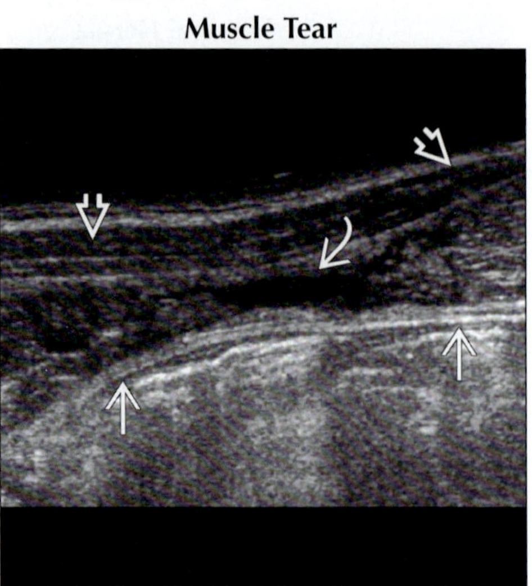

(Left) Transverse US shows a heterogeneous, hypoechoic mass ➡ straddling the oblique musculature ➡ of the lower abdominal wall. Endometriomas may have more spiculated edges. Excision confirmed an endometrioma. An alternative diagnosis was a desmoid tumor. *(Right)* Transverse US shows a tear ➡ of the internal oblique muscle of the lower abdomen. The external oblique muscle ⇨ and transversus fascia ➡ are intact.

ABDOMINAL WALL MASS

Undescended Testis

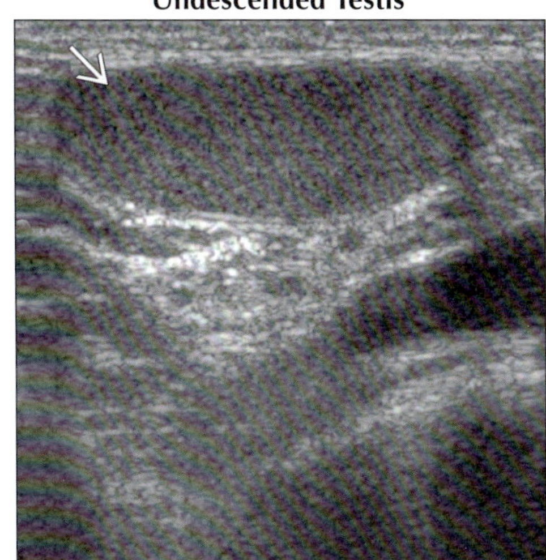

Umbilical Hernia

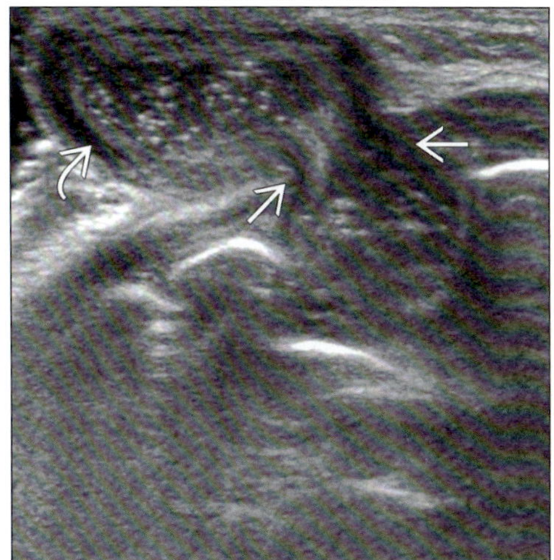

(Left) Transverse ultrasound shows an oval-shaped, hypoechoic testis ➡ within the inguinal canal in a patient with cryptorchidism. Most undescended testes are located in the inguinal canal. (Right) Transverse ultrasound shows bowel ➡ protruding though the umbilicus in this newborn with an umbilical hernia. Note that the neck of this type of hernia is wide ➡, allowing the hernia to be readily reduced and not prone to strangulation.

Lumbar Hernia

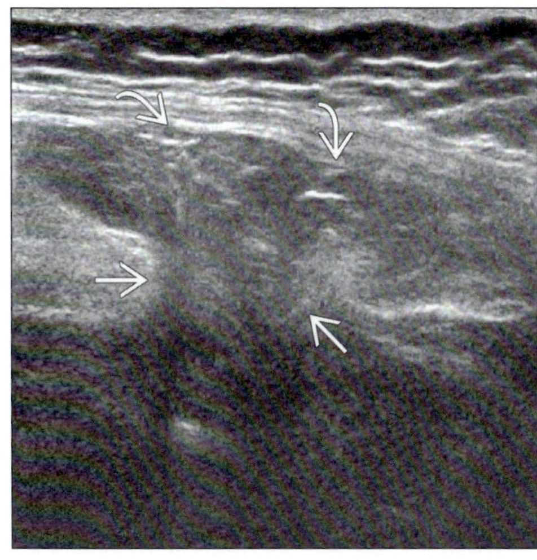

Lumbar Hernia

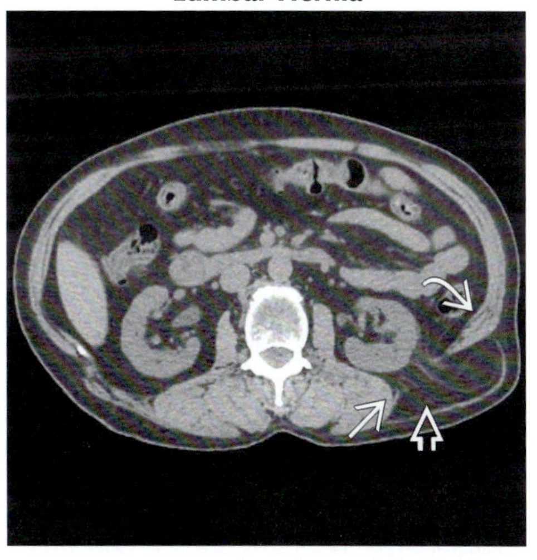

(Left) Oblique ultrasound shows a wide defect ➡ in the fascia of the posterior abdominal wall with herniation of retroperitoneal fat ➡ through this defect. (Right) Axial NECT in the same patient shows a large fascial defect posterior to the left kidney. The defect is bounded by the erector spinae muscle medially ➡ and retracted quadratus lumborum muscle laterally ➡. Retroperitoneal fat ➡ has herniated through this defect.

Subcutaneous Lipoma

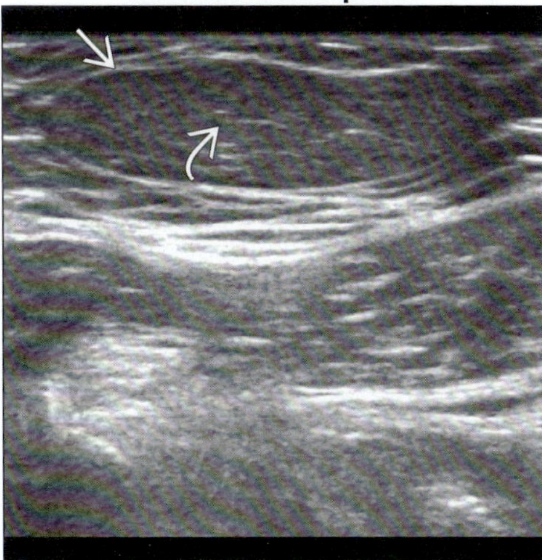

Granuloma

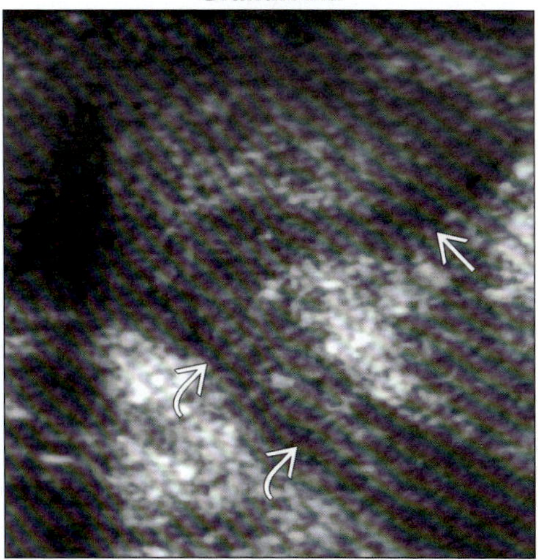

(Left) Transverse ultrasound shows a well-defined, hypoechoic mass ➡ in the subcutaneous fat of the anterior abdominal wall with fine, linear, internal striations ➡, typical of a lipoma. (Right) Transverse ultrasound shows a granuloma of the anterior abdominal wall ➡ in this patient with Crohn disease. There is a sinus tract ➡ extending down into the peritoneal cavity.

SECTION 16
Breast

DIFFERENTIAL DIAGNOSIS

Common
- Fibroadenoma
- Fibrosis
- Infiltrating Ductal Carcinoma
- Papilloma
- Lipoma

Less Common
- Infiltrating Lobular Carcinoma
- Phyllodes Tumor
- Medullary Carcinoma
- Fibroadenolipoma (Hamartoma)

Rare but Important
- Lactating Adenoma
- Pseudoangiomatous Stromal Hyperplasia (PASH)

ESSENTIAL INFORMATION

Key Differential Diagnosis Issues
- Breast ultrasound must be performed with high-frequency transducer (10-15 MHz)
- Scan planes: Radial and anti-radial, not longitudinal and transverse
  - Radial: Radiates from nipple, like spokes of wheel
  - Anti-radial: 90° orthogonal to radial
- Considerable overlap in ultrasound features of solid breast masses
  - Biopsy required for definitive diagnosis
- Clinical history and mammographic correlation important to distinguish among solid breast masses
  - Most solid masses warrant referral to specialist for appropriate treatment and follow-up

Helpful Clues for Common Diagnoses
- **Fibroadenoma**
  - Most common solid breast mass in women < 35 years, peak age 20-30 years
  - Typical US appearance in younger women
    - Circumscribed iso- to hypoechoic oval or gently lobulated mass
    - Homogeneous internal echoes
    - Variable posterior acoustic enhancement
  - Natural history is to involute and calcify
    - Coarse shadowing Ca++ on US
    - "Popcorn" Ca++ on mammogram
- **Fibrosis**

  - Maybe indistinguishable from malignancy and merits biopsy
  - Often associated with fibrocystic change
  - Varied US appearances include
    - Heterogeneous, hyperechoic, or hypoechoic mass
    - Non-mass-like irregular area of mixed echogenicity
    - Posterior acoustic shadowing
    - May be associated with cysts or microcysts in fibrocystic breast
  - Common cause of mammographic asymmetry or palpable mass
- **Infiltrating Ductal Carcinoma**
  - Irregular hypoechoic mass with posterior acoustic shadowing
  - Taller than wide
  - May have echogenic halo
  - Less often, circumscribed mass on US
  - Mammography
    - Spiculated irregular mass, ± architectural distortion
- **Papilloma**
  - Most present with bloody nipple discharge
  - Usually periareolar
  - Oval or round solid mass within dilated duct
  - Solid hypoechoic mass, with circumscribed or irregular margins
  - May be difficult to distinguish papilloma from debris in dilated ducts
  - Vascular flow within stalk excludes debris as cause of intraductal mass
- **Lipoma**
  - Palpable, soft, painless, mobile
    - Ovoid circumscribed mass, iso- or slightly hyperechoic to adjacent fat
    - Often corresponds to definitively benign, fat-containing lesion on mammography

Helpful Clues for Less Common Diagnoses
- **Infiltrating Lobular Carcinoma**
  - Presents as "thickening," often vaguely tender
  - Irregular ill-defined mass with dense posterior acoustic shadowing
  - May be solid, poorly circumscribed mass
  - US more sensitive at depicting lobular cancer than mammography
  - Mammography: Spiculated mass, architectural distortion, new focal asymmetry

- Both modalities may underestimate size/extent of tumor
- **Phyllodes Tumor**
  - Rapidly growing soft palpable mass
  - Clinically similar to medullary cancer but older age group (median age 45-49 years)
  - Indistinguishable from fibroadenoma on US
    - Circumscribed, hypoechoic, lobular mass
    - Variable posterior enhancement
    - Occasional peripheral cystic spaces, slit-like fluid-filled spaces, or septations
- **Medullary Carcinoma**
  - 10% of cancers in women < 35 years
  - Rapidly growing, soft, palpable mass
    - Clinically similar to phyllodes
  - Posterior acoustic enhancement
  - ± echogenic wall
  - ± septations and internal cystic spaces
  - Markedly hypoechoic, circumscribed, lobular mass
- **Fibroadenolipoma (Hamartoma)**
  - Circumscribed heterogeneous mass within pseudocapsule of compressed breast parenchyma
  - Contains hypoechoic areas of fat and hyperechoic glandular tissue
  - Correlates with oval circumscribed fat-containing mass with "breast within breast" appearance on mammogram

Helpful Clues for Rare Diagnoses
- **Lactating Adenoma**

- Palpable mass in pregnant or lactating woman
- Indistinguishable from FA clinically, as both may enlarge in pregnancy
- Indistinguishable from FA on US
  - Circumscribed, oval or gently lobulated, hypoechoic mass
  - Posterior acoustic enhancement
  - Echogenic septations
- Core needle biopsy often needed to distinguish from other pathology
- **Pseudoangiomatous Stromal Hyperplasia (PASH)**
  - Nonspecific, similar to FA on US, biopsy needed to confirm diagnosis
  - Well-circumscribed, oval or lobular, hypoechoic mass
  - Posterior enhancement, minimal vascularity

SELECTED REFERENCES

1. Mercado CL et al: Papillary lesions of the breast at percutaneous core-needle biopsy. Radiology. 238(3):801-8, 2006
2. Shetty MK et al: Sonographic findings in focal fibrocystic changes of the breast. Ultrasound Q. 18(1):35-40, 2002
3. Kirkpatrick UJ et al: Imaging appearances of pseudoangiomatous hyperplasia of mammary stroma. Clin Radiol. 55(7):576-8, 2000
4. Sickles EA: The subtle and atypical mammographic features of invasive lobular carcinoma. Radiology. 178(1):25-6, 1991

Fibroadenoma

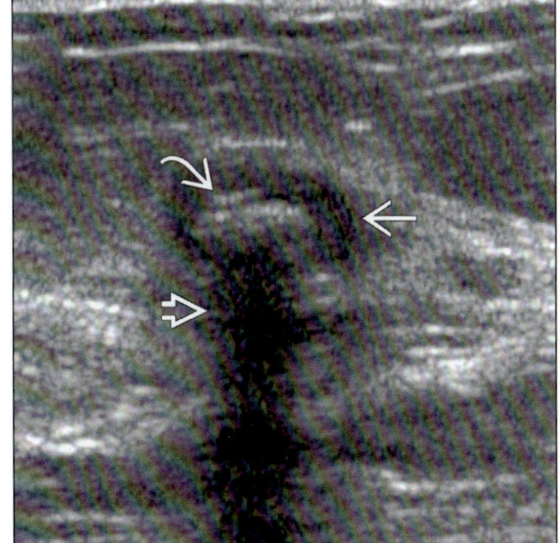

Radial ultrasound shows an oval, circumscribed, hypoechoic mass ➡ with coarse echogenic calcification ➡ causing posterior acoustic shadowing ➡, typical of an involuting FA.

Fibroadenoma

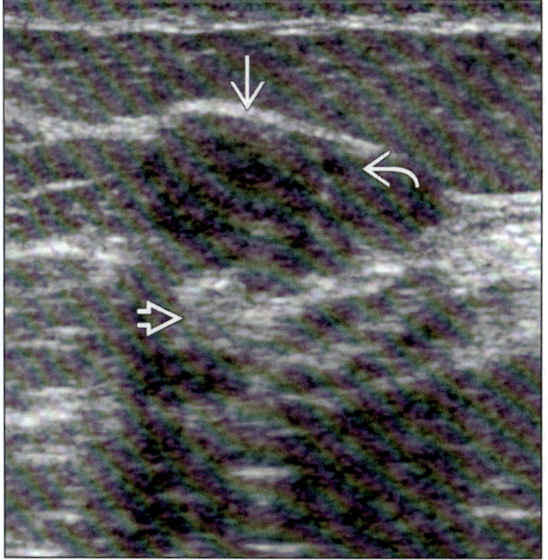

Radial ultrasound shows a fibroadenoma with lobular margins ➡ isoechoic to fat, with posterior acoustic enhancement ➡. Small cystic spaces ➡ may also be seen in phyllodes tumors.

SOLID BREAST MASS

(Left) CC mammogram of a palpable mass shows asymmetric tissue ➡ with interspersed fat in the upper outer right breast. The presence of fat in the lesion suggests benignity. *(Right)* Radial ultrasound in the same patient shows an ovoid mass ➡ containing interspersed hypoechoic fat ➡ typical of benign breast tissue. Because the mass was newly discovered, biopsy was performed and fibrosis was confirmed.

Fibrosis

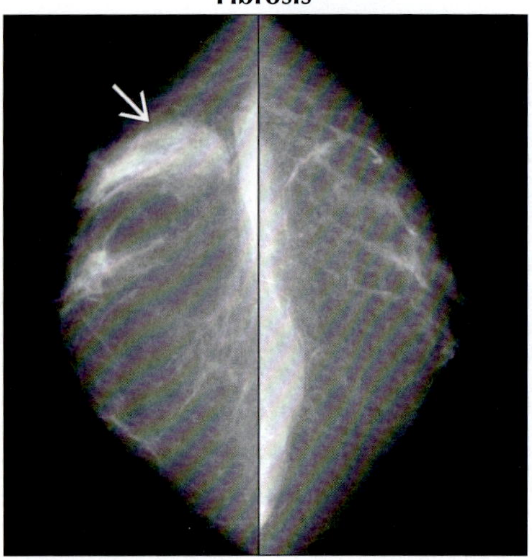

Fibrosis

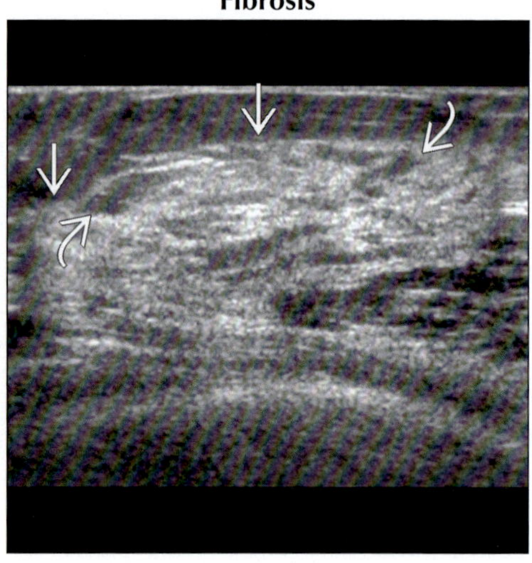

(Left) Radial ultrasound shows a small, spiculated, hypoechoic mass ➡ with posterior acoustic shadowing ➡. Pathology on ultrasound-guided core biopsy showed grade II infiltrating ductal carcinoma. *(Right)* CC mammogram spot compression of the same patient shows a mass ➡ with spiculated margins ➡, highly suspicious for malignancy.

Infiltrating Ductal Carcinoma

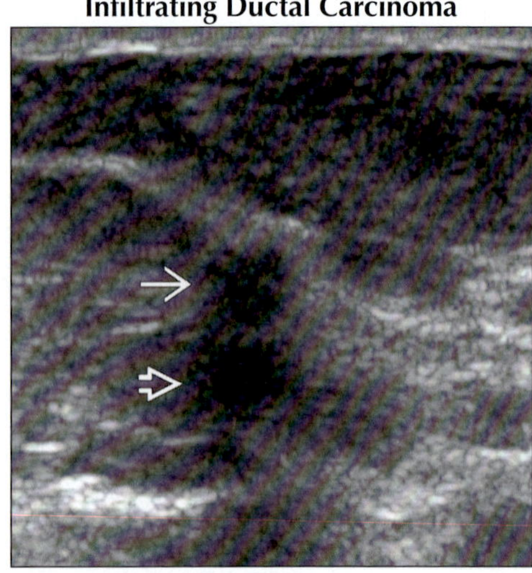

Infiltrating Ductal Carcinoma

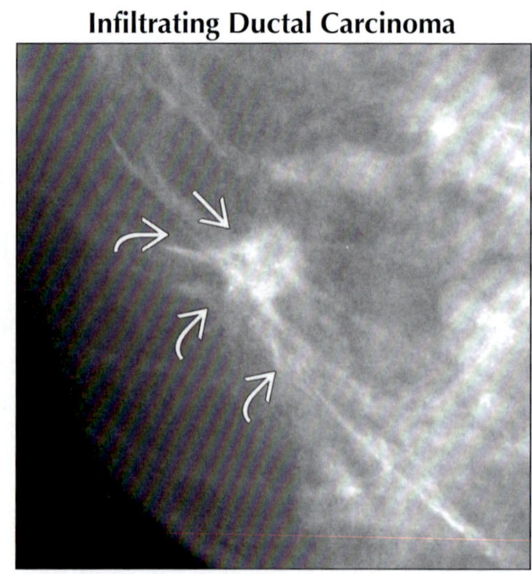

(Left) Radial ultrasound shows an irregular hypoechoic mass ➡ with posterior acoustic shadowing ➡ and an echogenic halo ➡, findings typical of infiltrating ductal carcinoma. *(Right)* Radial ultrasound shows a hypoechoic, irregular, cystic ➡ and solid thick-walled mass ➡ with posterior acoustic enhancement ➡, shown to be infiltrating ductal carcinoma with central necrosis on core biopsy.

Infiltrating Ductal Carcinoma

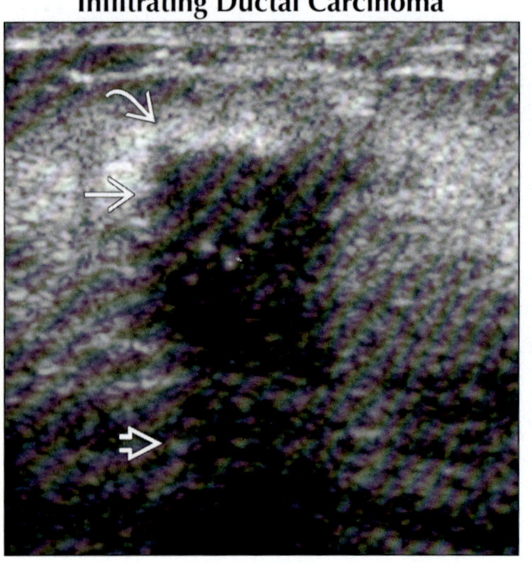

Infiltrating Ductal Carcinoma

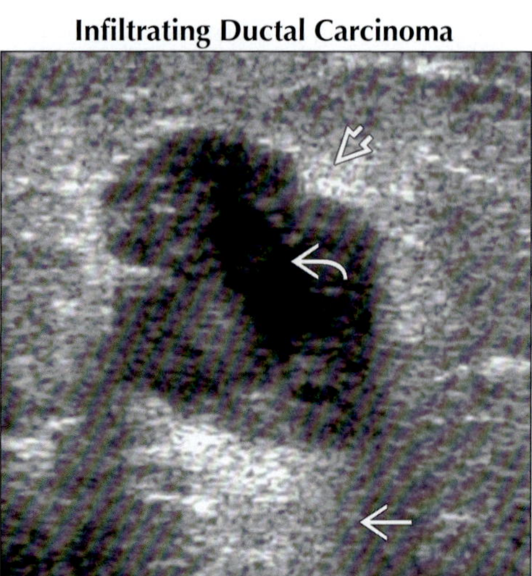

16

SOLID BREAST MASS

Papilloma

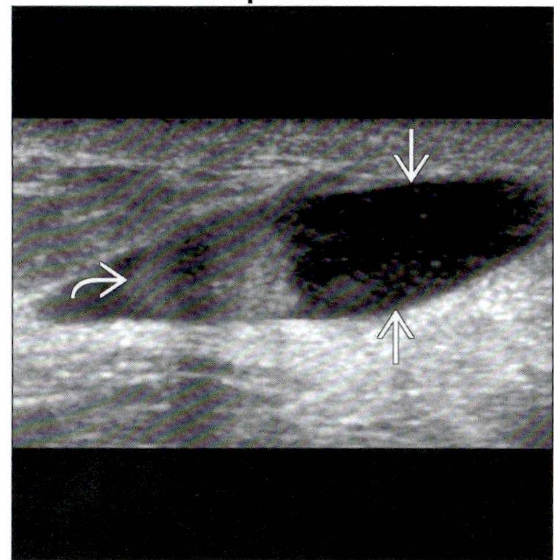

Papilloma

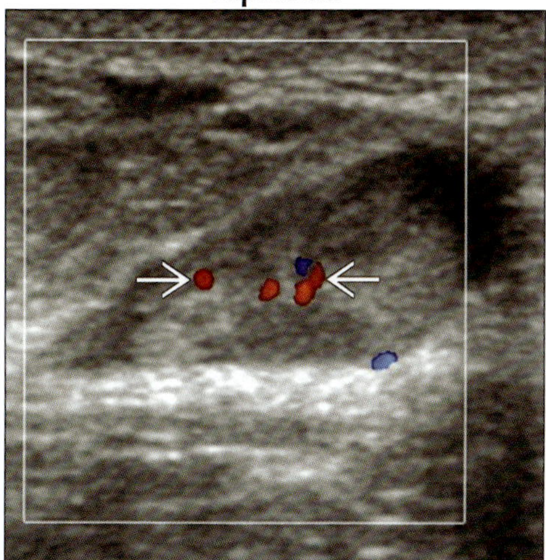

(Left) Radial ultrasound shows an intraductal mass ➡ in a large dilated duct ➡ near the nipple, typical for an intraductal papilloma, confirmed at excision. *(Right)* Radial color Doppler ultrasound of the same lesion shows internal vascularity ➡, typical of the vascular stalk often seen in papillomas. Nonmobile solid intracystic masses such as this warrant biopsy.

Papilloma

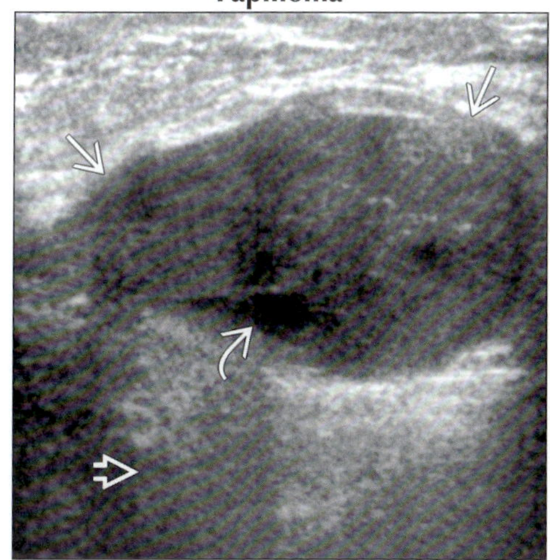

Papilloma

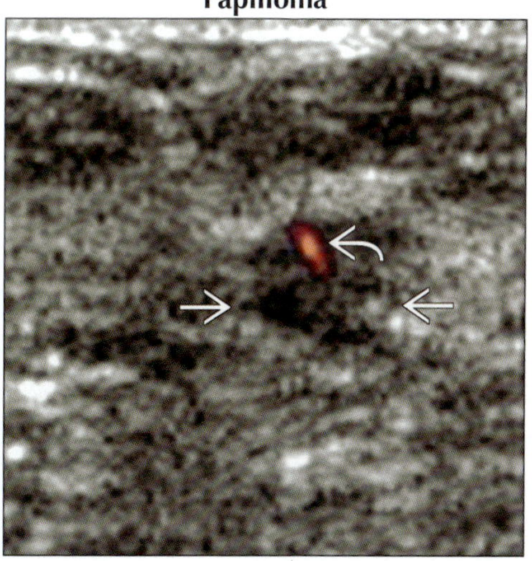

(Left) Anti-radial ultrasound of a biopsy-proven papilloma shows a large, hypoechoic, circumscribed mass ➡ with posterior acoustic enhancement ➡. Small cystic spaces ➡ in this patient are an atypical finding in a papilloma and can be seen in both fibroadenoma and phyllodes tumors, as well as malignant lesions. *(Right)* Radial power Doppler ultrasound shows flow in a vascular stalk ➡ in an irregular hypoechoic mass ➡, typical for papilloma.

Lipoma

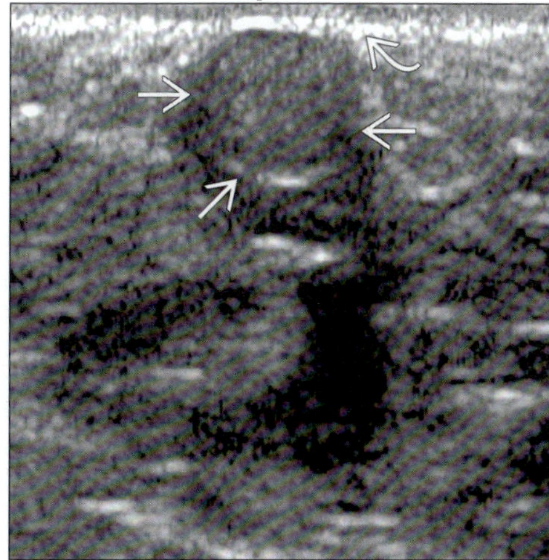

Lipoma

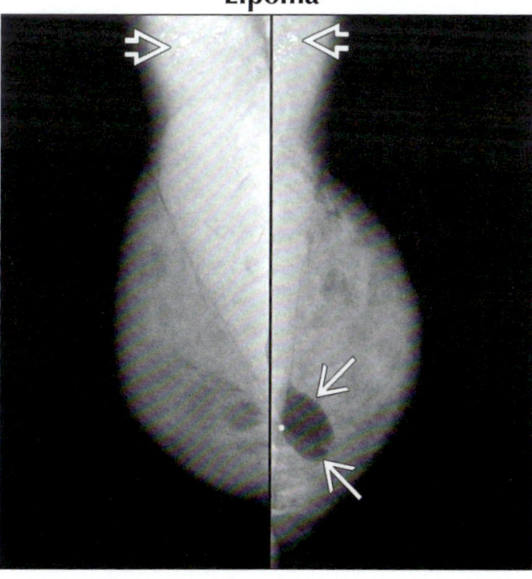

(Left) Anti-radial ultrasound of a superficial, mobile, palpable mass shows an oval circumscribed mass ➡ slightly hyperechoic to adjacent fat and just deep to the skin ➡ with no blood flow, typical findings for a lipoma. *(Right)* MLO mammogram shows a lobulated, fatty, palpable mass ➡ at the 6:00 o'clock position in the left breast, compatible with a lipoma. Incidentally noted are deodorant artifacts ➡ in both axillae.

Infiltrating Lobular Carcinoma

Infiltrating Lobular Carcinoma

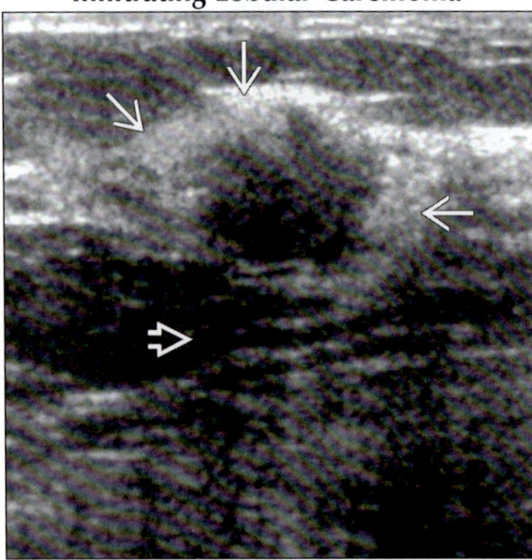

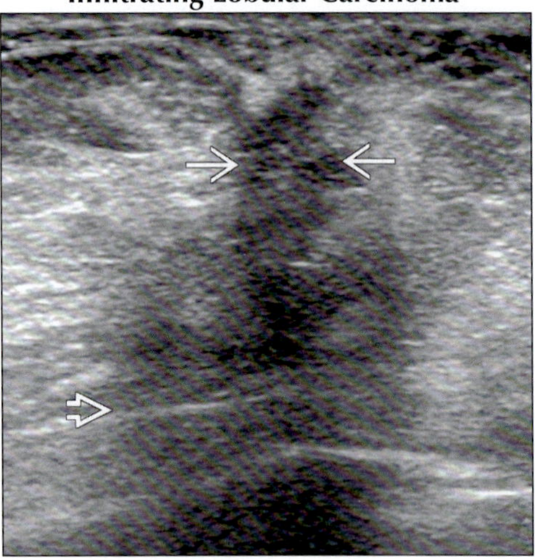

(Left) Anti-radial ultrasound shows an irregular, angular, hypoechoic mass with a surrounding echogenic halo ➡ and mild posterior acoustic shadowing ➡. This lesion corresponded to an ill-defined mass on mammogram. *(Right)* Anti-radial ultrasound shows an ill-defined, hypoechoic mass ➡ with extensive posterior acoustic shadowing ➡. Biopsy specimen proved this to be infiltrating lobular carcinoma.

Phyllodes Tumor

Phyllodes Tumor

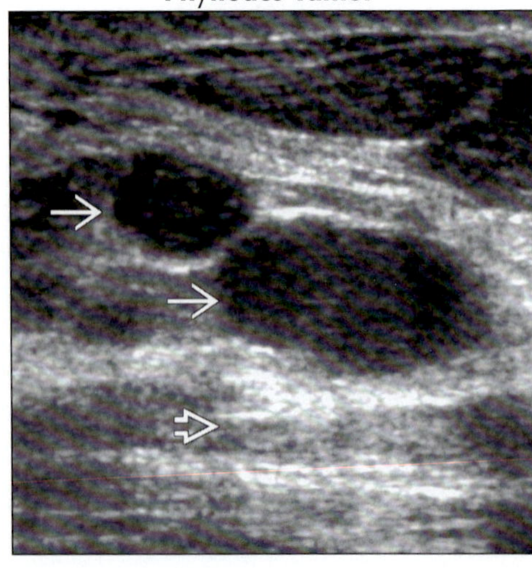

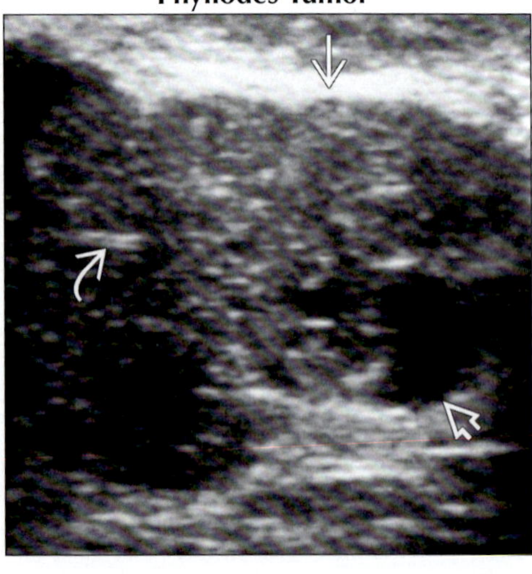

(Left) Radial ultrasound shows circumscribed, hypoechoic, oval masses ➡ with mild posterior acoustic enhancement ➡. These US features are nonspecific and overlap with FA. Because the solid masses were new, they were suspicious. Biopsy specimen confirmed phyllodes tumors. *(Right)* Anti-radial ultrasound shows typical US features of a phyllodes tumor: A lobular hypoechoic mass ➡ with eccentric cystic spaces ➡ and septations ➡.

Medullary Carcinoma

Medullary Carcinoma

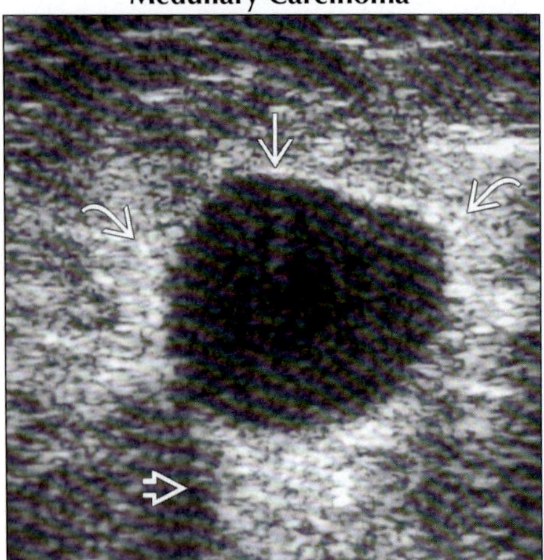

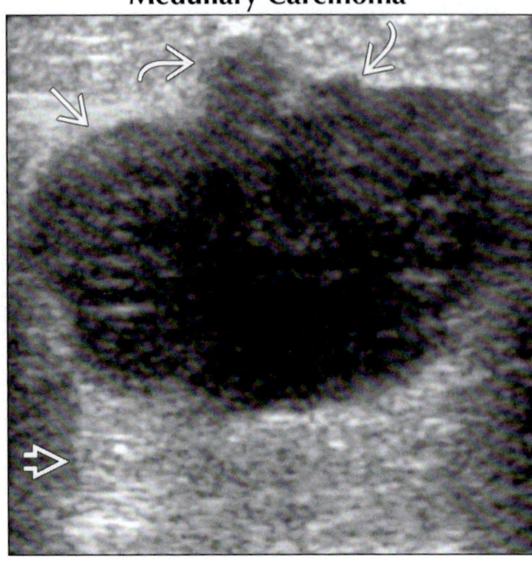

(Left) Radial ultrasound of a rapidly growing palpable mass shows a markedly hypoechoic mass ➡ with posterior acoustic enhancement ➡ and an echogenic halo ➡. *(Right)* Anti-radial ultrasound shows a very hypoechoic mass ➡ with microlobulated margins ➡ and posterior acoustic enhancement ➡. These features are nonspecific but suspicious, and they are typical for medullary carcinoma.

16

SOLID BREAST MASS

Fibroadenolipoma (Hamartoma)

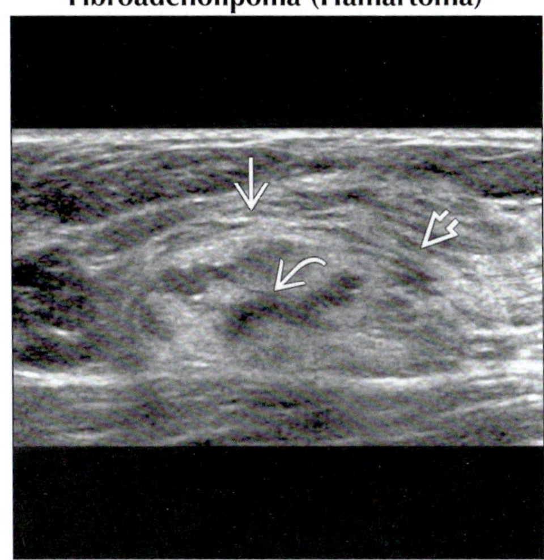

Fibroadenolipoma (Hamartoma)

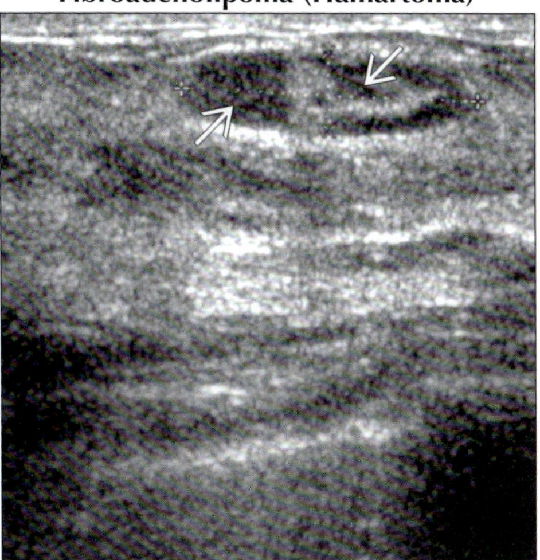

(Left) Anti-radial ultrasound shows a circumscribed ovoid mass ➡ containing areas of hypoechoic fat ➡, with an echogenic pseudocapsule of compressed tissue ➡ and no posterior acoustic enhancement or shadowing, typical fibroadenolipoma findings. This corresponded to a circumscribed fat-containing lesion on mammography. (Right) Anti-radial ultrasound shows a circumscribed ovoid mass with hypoechoic fat ➡, typical of a fibroadenolipoma.

Lactating Adenoma

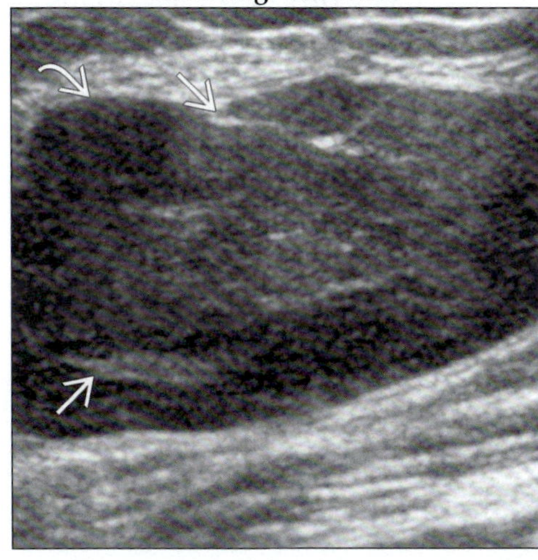

Lactating Adenoma

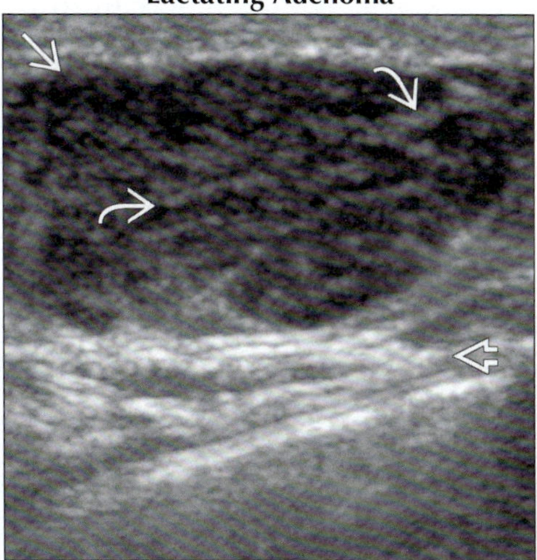

(Left) Anti-radial ultrasound shows a gently lobulated hypoechoic mass ➡ with echogenic septations ➡ and posterior acoustic enhancement, typical for lactating adenoma. (Right) Radial ultrasound of a palpable mass in a pregnant woman shows a hypoechoic solid mass ➡ with echogenic internal septations ➡ and posterior acoustic enhancement ➡. Biopsy showed a lactating adenoma.

Pseudoangiomatous Stromal Hyperplasia (PASH)

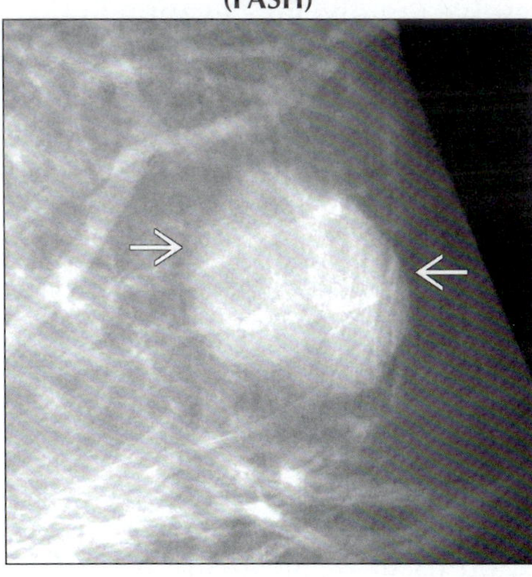

Pseudoangiomatous Stromal Hyperplasia (PASH)

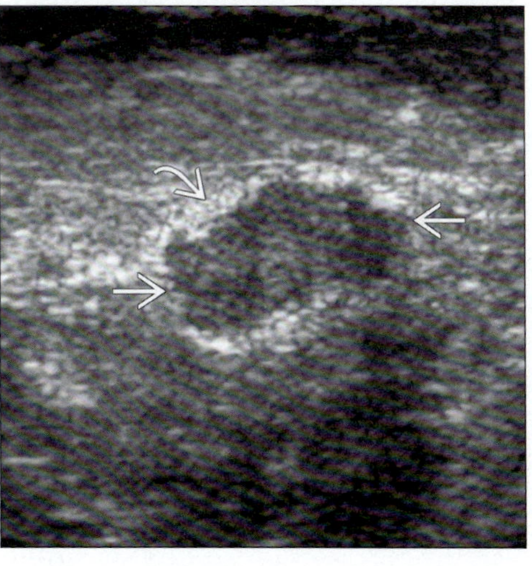

(Left) MLO mammogram shows a mostly circumscribed mass ➡, which warrants further evaluation with ultrasound. (Right) Anti-radial ultrasound in the same patient shows a microlobulated isoechoic mass ➡ with an echogenic halo ➡, suspicious features for any solid mass. Biopsy specimen showed fibrosis and pseudoangiomatous stromal hyperplasia.

16

DIFFERENTIAL DIAGNOSIS

Common
- Simple Cyst
- Complicated Cyst
- Clustered Microcysts

Less Common
- Abscess
- Hematoma
- Post-Treatment Changes

Rare but Important
- Complex Cystic Mass
- Galactocele
- Epidermal Inclusion Cyst

ESSENTIAL INFORMATION

Key Differential Diagnosis Issues
- Cystic definition of mass hinges on its ultrasound features
  - Cannot differentiate mass as cystic or solid on mammogram
  - US necessary part of evaluation and diagnosis of all potentially cystic breast lesions
- Breast US must be performed with high-frequency transducer (10-15 MHz)
- Scan planes: Radial and anti-radial, not longitudinal and transverse
  - Radial = radiates from nipple, like spokes of wheel
  - Anti-radial = 90° orthogonal to radial
- History of recent breast biopsy, surgery, or trauma → think hematoma, seroma, or fat necrosis
- Vascularity within intracystic nodule mandates biopsy to exclude carcinoma
- Mobile, avascular, solid component = debris
  - Excludes malignant nodule/mass

Helpful Clues for Common Diagnoses
- **Simple Cyst**
  - Most common mass in female breast
  - Often multiple and bilateral, waxing/waning on subsequent mammograms
  - Must meet following criteria on ultrasound
    - Well-circumscribed mass
    - Anechoic
    - Thin imperceptible wall
    - Posterior acoustic enhancement
  - Most often in women 35-50 years
- **Complicated Cyst**
  - Meets all US criteria of simple cyst and contains internal echoes
  - May contain mobile debris or fluid-debris level
  - May contain milk of calcium; correlate with mammogram
  - Follow-up in 6 months for stability or resolution
- **Clustered Microcysts**
  - Microlobulated cluster of tiny anechoic cystic foci, thin septae, no solid component
    - US clearly demonstrates internal structure of anechoic microcysts → benign finding
    - Too small to resolve with US → cannot exclude solid component, must biopsy

Helpful Clues for Less Common Diagnoses
- **Abscess**
  - Usually high clinical index of suspicion, often starts as mastitis: Pain, erythema, fever, ± ↑ white blood cell count
    - Thick-walled, complex, cystic/solid mass
    - Mastitis may start as solid mass on US and develop into abscess
    - Surrounding ↑ echogenicity due to edema
    - May have floating/mobile debris or air within cavity
    - Surrounding ↑ vascularity on color Doppler
- **Hematoma**
  - Check for history of trauma, surgery, or biopsy
  - Should resolve rapidly, may eventually evolve into fat necrosis
    - Initially may be anechoic collection
    - Can evolve into thick-walled, complex, cystic mass with debris, avascular nodules, and septations
    - May look similar to complicated cyst: Oval mass with low-level echoes
    - Internal flow raises suspicion for hemorrhagic tumor
- **Post-Treatment Changes**
  - Seroma
    - Anechoic, simple fluid collection at lumpectomy site, ± nodules of granulation tissue or fibrin strands

CYSTIC BREAST MASS

- • Thin walled, unlike hematoma, which often can be thick walled
- ○ Fat necrosis may develop around hematoma in lumpectomy cavity
  - • Cystic or solid on ultrasound; wide range of sonographic appearances, from anechoic cyst to complex cystic mass
  - • May have fat-fluid level and resemble galactocele
  - • Correlate with history of surgery, biopsy, trauma, and mammogram: Rim calcifications in fat-containing mass reassuring for fat necrosis

Helpful Clues for Rare Diagnoses
- • **Complex Cystic Mass**
  - ○ Has 1 or more of following US features
    - • Thick, indistinct wall > 0.5 mm
    - • Thick septations > 0.5 mm
    - • Nonmobile intracystic mass or solid component; reposition patient to exclude mobile debris mimicking mass
    - • Vascularity in solid component on color Doppler
    - • Extension of solid component into adjacent ducts
  - ○ Presence of 1 or more of above features mandates biopsy
  - ○ Bloody fluid on cyst aspiration raises concern for intracystic neoplasm
- • **Galactocele**
  - ○ Fat-fluid level in circumscribed mass; posterior enhancement; ± septations and solid debris

- ○ Associated with pregnancy and lactation; correlate with history
- ○ Milky fluid on aspiration confirms diagnosis
- • **Epidermal Inclusion Cyst**
  - ○ Hypoechoic, superficial, circumscribed mass in skin
  - ○ Use gel stand-off pad to show hypoechoic track to skin → confirms diagnosis
    - • Track to skin is dilated hair follicle
  - ○ Indistinguishable from sebaceous cyst on imaging; both are benign, and management is same
  - ○ Palpable, painless, usually located in axilla or inframammary fold

SELECTED REFERENCES

1. Berg WA: Sonographically depicted breast clustered microcysts: is follow-up appropriate? AJR Am J Roentgenol. 185(4):952-9, 2005
2. Versluijs-Ossewaarde FN et al: Subareolar breast abscesses: characteristics and results of surgical treatment. Breast J. 11(3):179-82, 2005
3. Berg WA et al: Cystic lesions of the breast: sonographic-pathologic correlation. Radiology. 227(1):183-91, 2003
4. Mendelson EB et al: Toward a standardized breast ultrasound lexicon, BI-RADS: ultrasound. Semin Roentgenol. 36(3):217-25, 2001
5. Venta LA et al: Management of complex breast cysts. AJR Am J Roentgenol. 173(5):1331-6, 1999

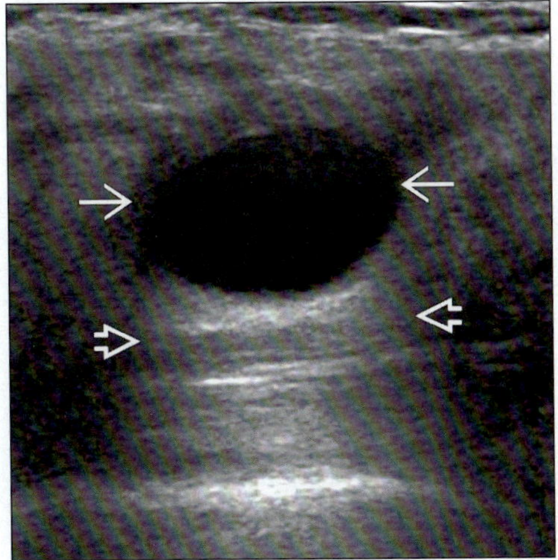

Simple Cyst

Anti-radial spatial compounding ultrasound shows a well-circumscribed anechoic mass ➡ with posterior acoustic enhancement ➡, typical of a simple cyst.

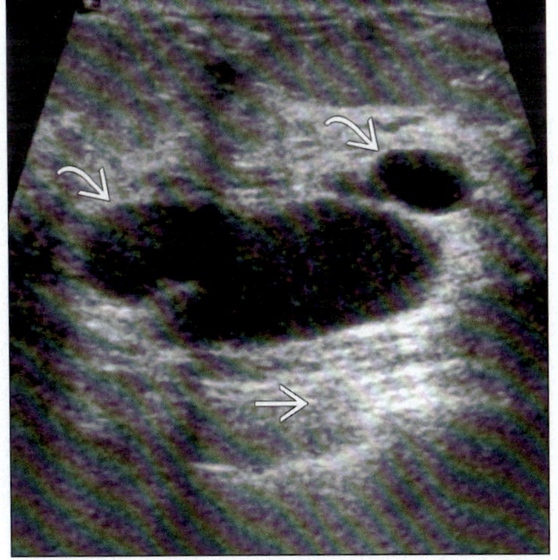

Simple Cyst

Anti-radial ultrasound demonstrates a bilobed, anechoic, thin-walled mass ➡ with posterior acoustic enhancement ➡, typical of a group of simple cysts.

CYSTIC BREAST MASS

Complicated Cyst

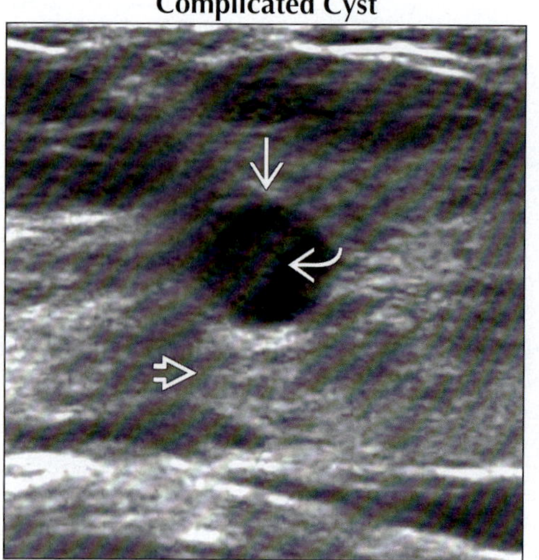

Complicated Cyst

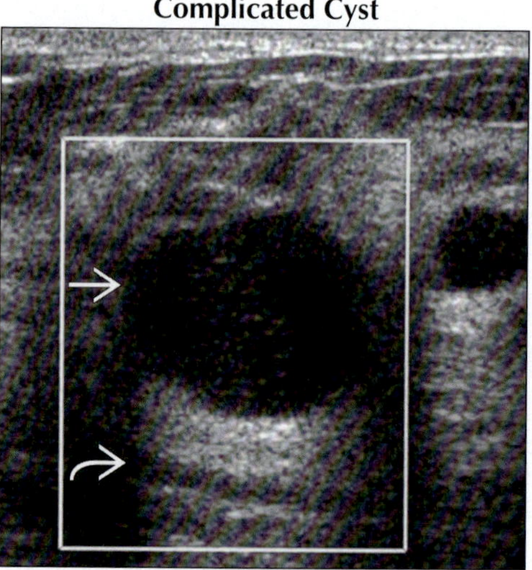

(Left) Radial spatial compounding ultrasound shows a circumscribed, oval, hypoechoic mass ➡ with posterior enhancement ➡ and a fluid-debris level ➡, compatible with a benign complicated cyst. *(Right)* Anti-radial power Doppler ultrasound shows an avascular, well-circumscribed, oval mass ➡ with homogeneous low-level internal echoes and posterior acoustic enhancement ➡, compatible with a benign complicated cyst.

Complicated Cyst

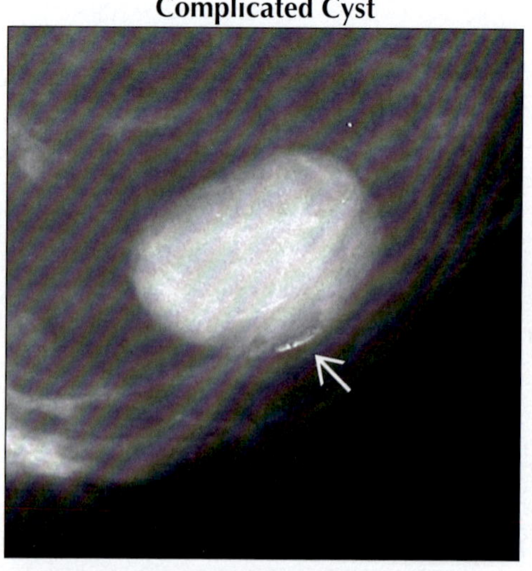

Complicated Cyst

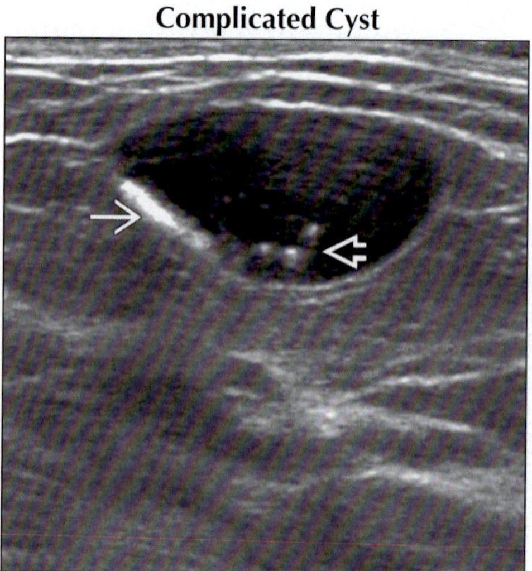

(Left) MLO mammogram shows milk of calcium calcifications ➡ layering dependently within a well-circumscribed mass. *(Right)* Radial ultrasound in the same patient shows an anechoic cyst with layering echogenic calcifications ➡ and floating punctate calcifications ➡. Because of the milk of calcium, this lesion qualifies as a complicated cyst.

Clustered Microcysts

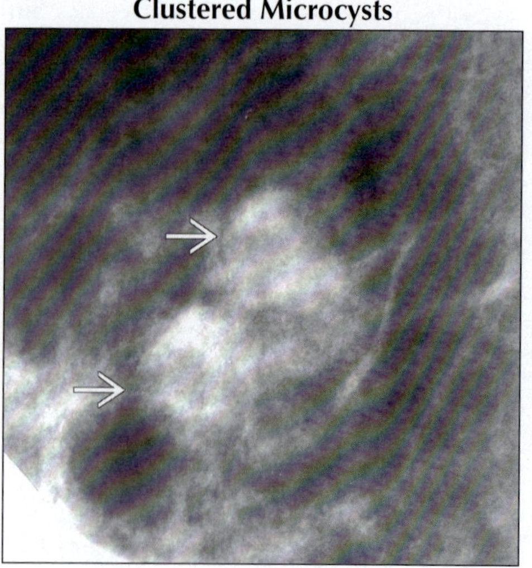

Clustered Microcysts

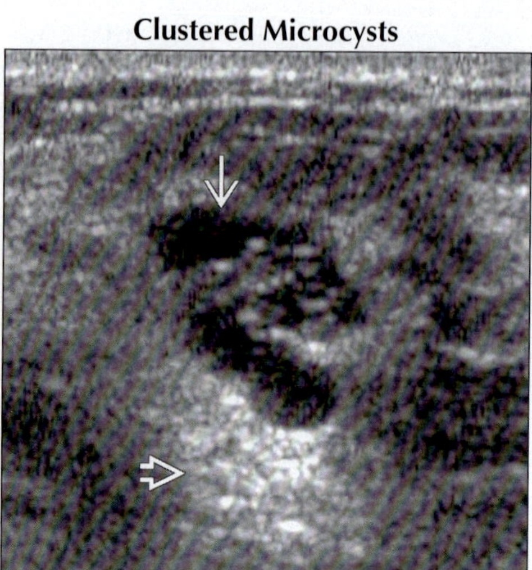

(Left) MLO mammogram spot compression shows 2 masses ➡ that cannot be characterized as cystic or solid. *(Right)* Radial ultrasound in the same patient shows the more superior mass with the typical ultrasound features of clustered microcysts ➡: A lobulated cluster of tiny anechoic foci with thin septae and posterior enhancement ➡.

CYSTIC BREAST MASS

Abscess

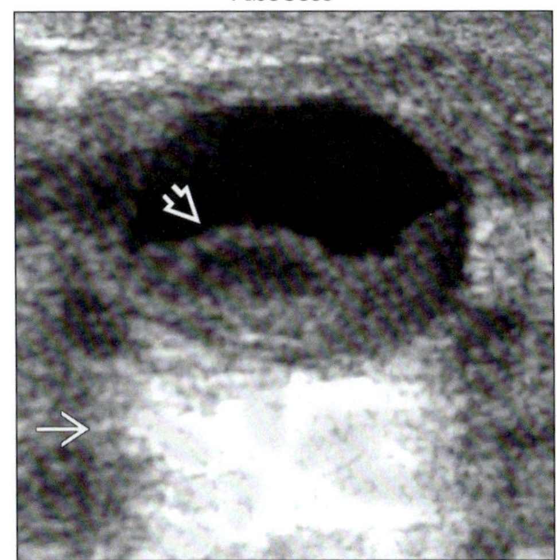

Abscess

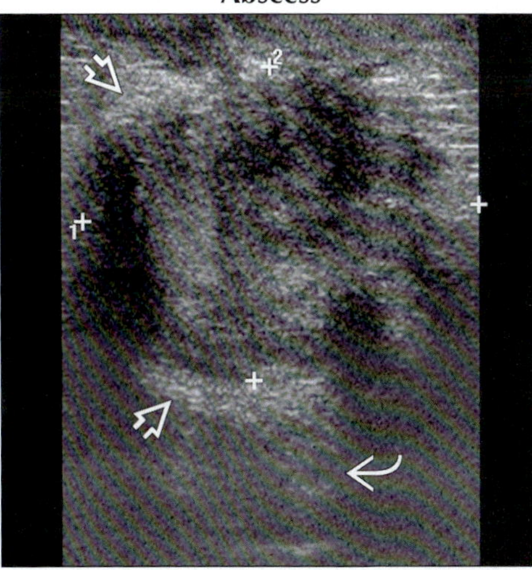

(Left) Radial US shows a complex thick-walled cystic mass with posterior enhancement ➡ and mobile debris ➡, typical features of an abscess. (Right) Anti-radial US in a patient with mastitis shows a developing abscess presenting as an irregular, mixed-echogenicity, solid, and cystic mass (calipers) with thick echogenic margins ➡ and posterior enhancement ➡. There is increased echogenicity in the surrounding tissue from edema.

Hematoma

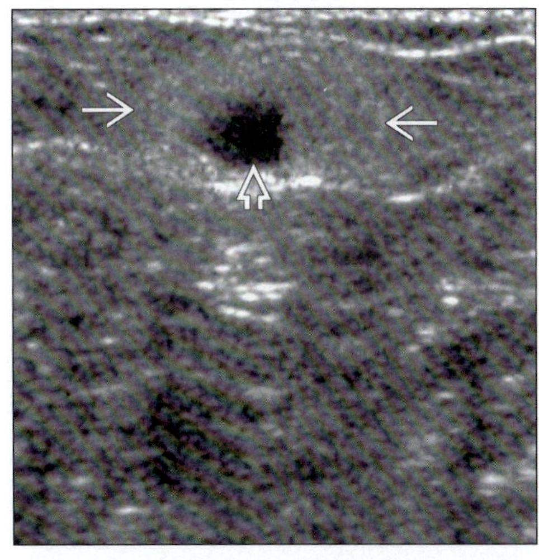

Hematoma

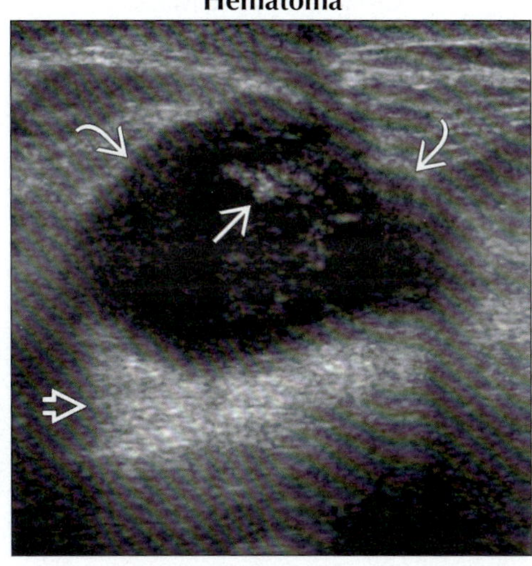

(Left) Radial ultrasound of a palpable mass following trauma to the breast shows a superficial hyperechoic mass ➡ with a central cystic area ➡, findings consistent with a hematoma. This lesion resolved on a 6 week follow-up ultrasound. (Right) Radial ultrasound following a recent lumpectomy shows the typical features of a hematoma including a thick-walled cystic mass ➡ with internal debris ➡ and posterior enhancement ➡ in the lumpectomy bed.

Post-Treatment Changes

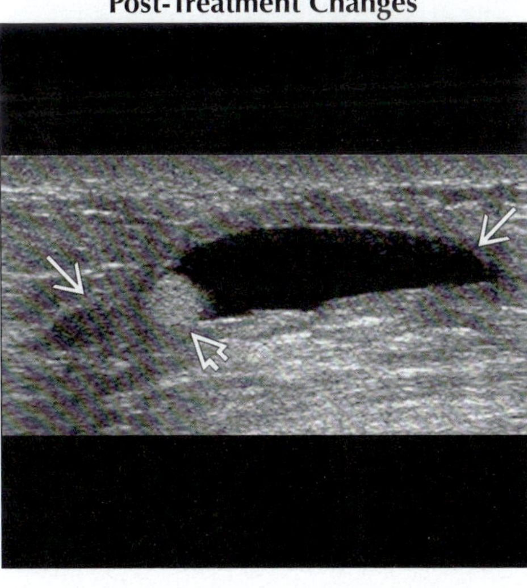

Post-Treatment Changes

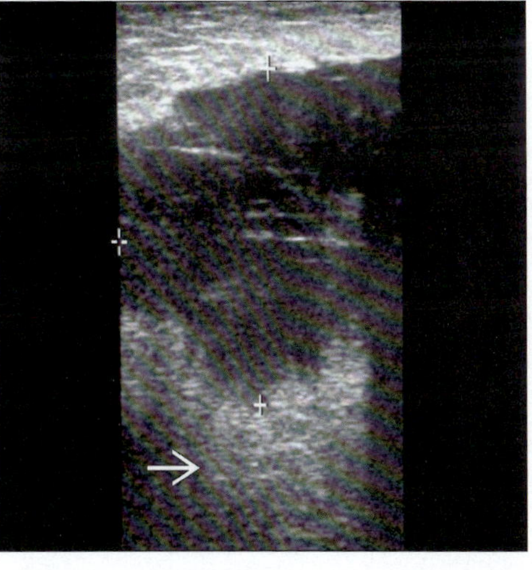

(Left) Radial ultrasound shows an anechoic, thick-walled, oval mass ➡ typical of a postsurgical seroma. The avascular echogenic nodule ➡ in the mass is granulation tissue. Seromas are seen months to weeks after lumpectomy. (Right) Radial ultrasound over a lumpectomy site shows an avascular hypoechoic collection with irregular margins (calipers) and posterior enhancement ➡, findings typical of a postoperative seroma/hematoma.

CYSTIC BREAST MASS

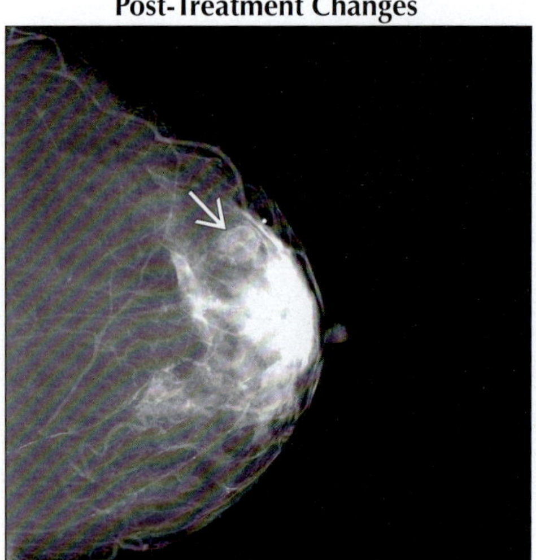

Post-Treatment Changes

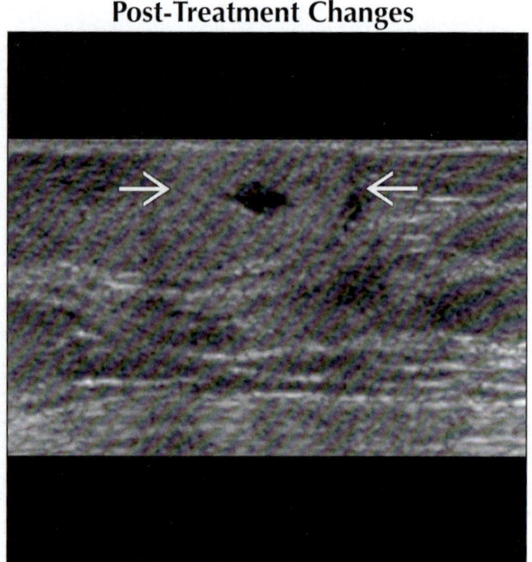

Post-Treatment Changes

(Left) CC mammography of the left breast shows a round well-circumscribed mass in the upper outer quadrant ➡ containing lucent central fat. This mammographic appearance is diagnostic of fat necrosis. *(Right)* Anti-radial ultrasound of the mammographic mass in the same patient shows an oval, well-circumscribed, primarily hyperechoic mass ➡, consistent with fat necrosis. The ultrasound appearance of fat necrosis may vary; the mammogram is diagnostic.

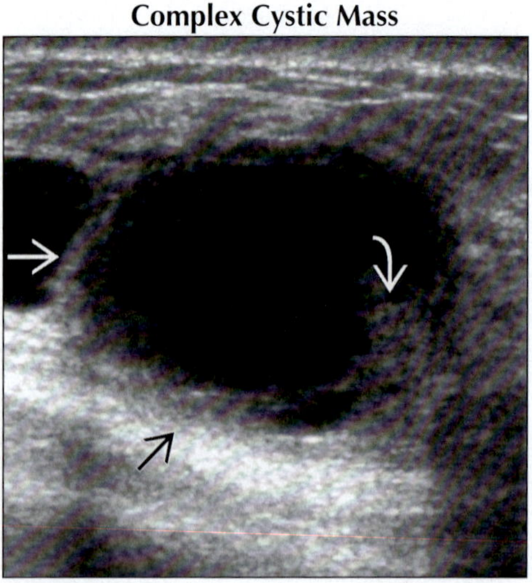

Complex Cystic Mass

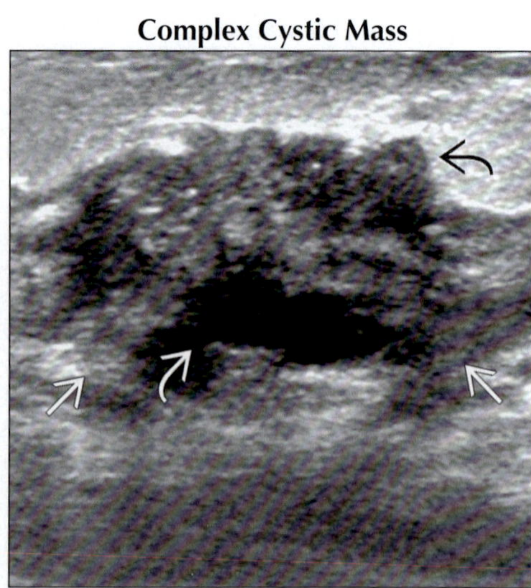

Complex Cystic Mass

(Left) Anti-radial ultrasound shows a cystic and solid mass with a thick wall ➡, thick septation ➡, and an apparent intracystic mass ➡. This complex cystic mass qualifies as BI-RADS-4 and warrants aspiration or biopsy. Pathology showed a ruptured cyst with chronic inflammation. *(Right)* Radial ultrasound of a palpable mass shows a hypoechoic cystic ➡ and solid mass ➡ with irregular margins ➡. Biopsy demonstrated DCIS.

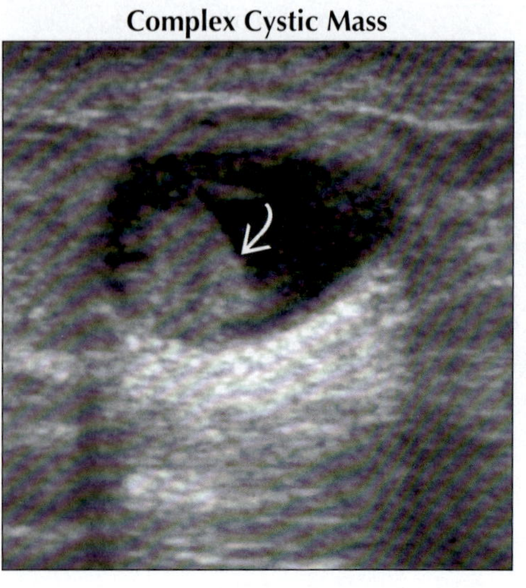

Complex Cystic Mass

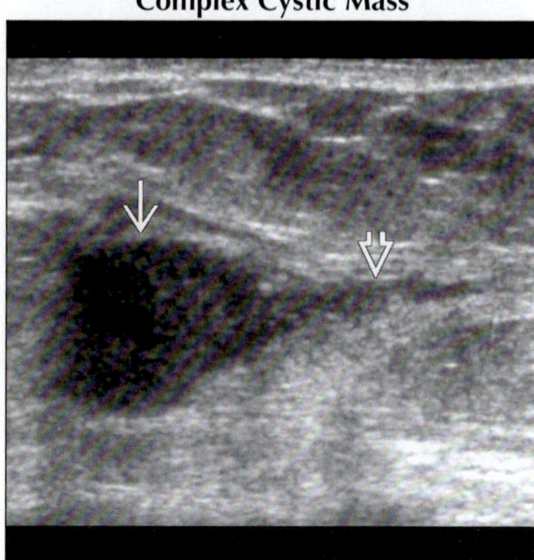

Complex Cystic Mass

(Left) Anti-radial ultrasound shows an irregular, nonmobile, solid, intracystic mass ➡. Internal vascularity was identified in the solid component, making this a BI-RADS-4 lesion, and biopsy was performed. Pathology showed intraductal papilloma. *(Right)* Radial ultrasound shows an irregular, complex, cystic and solid mass ➡ with extension into an adjacent duct ➡. This proved to be grade III invasive ductal carcinoma on biopsy.

16

CYSTIC BREAST MASS

Galactocele

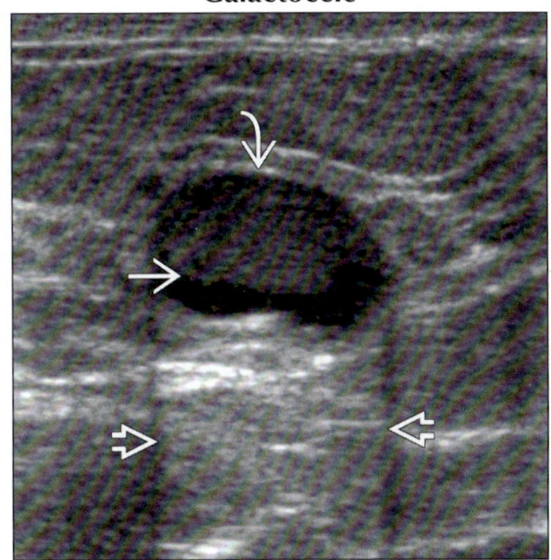

Galactocele

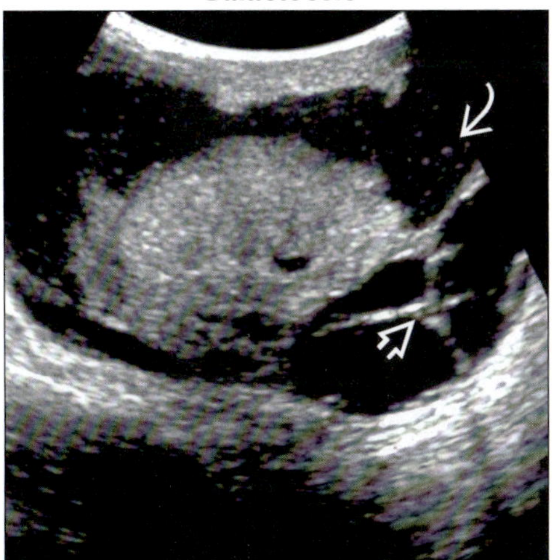

(Left) Radial ultrasound shows an oval, well-circumscribed, cystic mass ➤ with a fluid-debris level ➤ and posterior enhancement ➤. Aspiration yielded milk confirming the diagnosis of a galactocele. (Right) Radial ultrasound in a pregnant woman shows a 12 cm mixed cystic-solid mass with loculated fluid, septations ➤, and mobile solid debris ➤. Aspiration yielded breast milk, thereby confirming the diagnosis of a galactocele.

Epidermal Inclusion Cyst

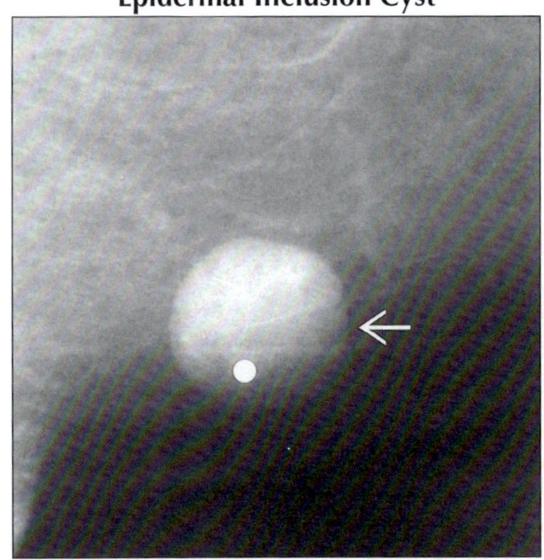

Epidermal Inclusion Cyst

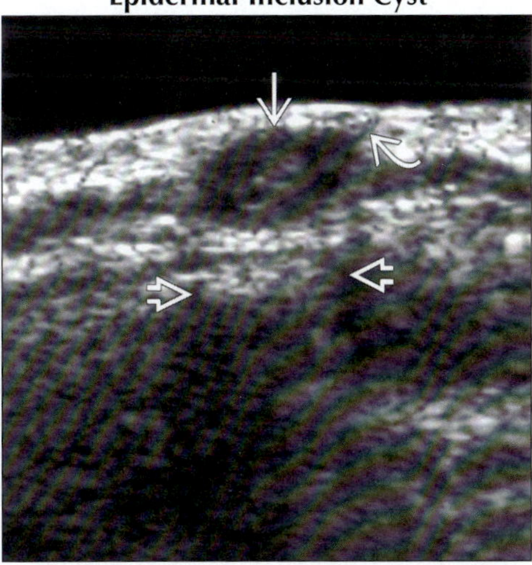

(Left) Lateral mammogram spot compression shows a well-circumscribed palpable mass ➤ in the inframammary fold marked by a BB. (Right) Radial US shows a well-circumscribed hypoechoic mass ➤ with posterior acoustic enhancement ➤ entirely within the skin. The tiny track of the blocked hair follicle ➤ is well seen with the gel standoff pad. These features are compatible with either a benign epidermal inclusion cyst or sebaceous cyst.

Epidermal Inclusion Cyst

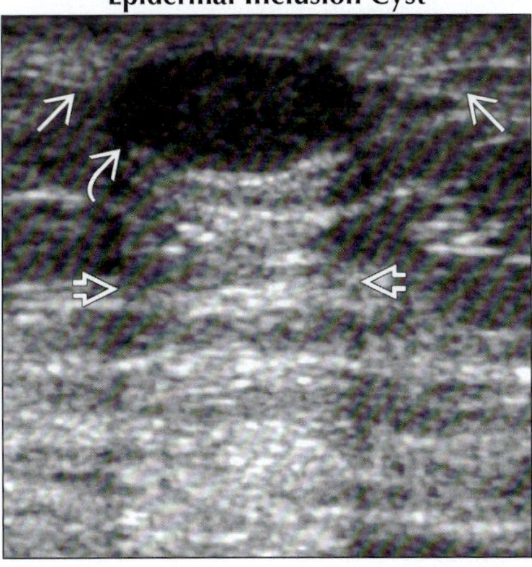

Epidermal Inclusion Cyst

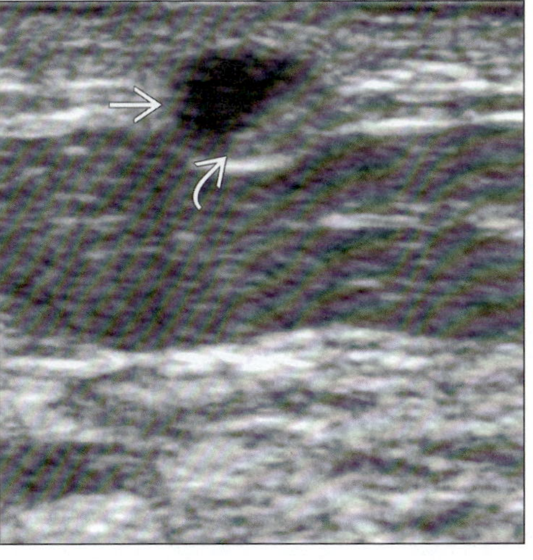

(Left) Radial ultrasound shows a circumscribed hypoechoic mass ➤ within the skin ➤ with posterior enhancement ➤, typical of an epidermal inclusion cyst. (Right) Anti-radial ultrasound shows a circumscribed oval mass ➤ found within the skin containing mobile, dependently layering material ➤, consistent with an epidermal inclusion cyst. These lesions often appear more solid than cystic, as in the previous examples.

16

INDEX

INDEX

INDEX

INDEX

INDEX

INDEX

INDEX

INDEX

INDEX

INDEX

INDEX

INDEX

INDEX

INDEX

INDEX

INDEX

INDEX

INDEX

INDEX

INDEX

INDEX

INDEX